CLINICAL
PHARMACOLOGY

'And I will use regimens for the benefit of the ill in accordance with my ability and my judgement.'
Hippocrates' Oath

'They used to have a more equitable contract in (ancient) Egypt: for the first three days, the doctor took on the patient at the patient's risk and peril: when the three days were up, the risks and perils were the doctor's. But doctors are lucky: the sun shines on their successes and the earth hides their failures.'
Michael de Montaigne 1533–92

'Nature is not only odder than we think, but it is odder than we can think.'
J B S Haldane 1893–1964

'Morals do not forbid making experiments on one's neighbour or on one's self … among the experiments that may be tried on man, those that can only harm are forbidden, those that are innocent are permissible, and those that may do good are obligatory.' 'Men who have excessive faith in their theories or ideas are not only ill prepared for making discoveries; they make very poor observations … they can see in [their] results only a confirmation of their theory … This is what made us say that we must never make experiments to confirm our ideas, but simply to control them.'

'Medicine is destined to get away from empiricism little by little; like all other sciences, it will get away by the scientific method.'

'Considered in itself, the experimental method is nothing but reasoning by whose help we methodically submit our ideas to experience – the experience of facts.'
Claude Bernard 1865

'I do not want two diseases – one nature-made, one doctor-made.'
Napoleon Bonaparte 1820

'The ingenuity of man has ever been fond of exerting itself to varied forms and combinations of medicines.'
William Withering 1785

'All things are poisons and there is nothing that is harmless, the dose alone decides that something is no poison.'
Paracelsus 1493–1541

Commissioning Editor: Timothy Horne
Development Editor: Janice Urquhart
Senior Project Manager: Andrew Palfreyman
Production Assistant: Camilla Cudjoe
Design Direction: Erik Bigland
Illustrations Manager: Gillian Richards
Illustrator: David Gardner

TENTH EDITION CLINICAL PHARMACOLOGY

Peter N. Bennett MD FRCP DPMSA
Formerly Reader in Clinical Pharmacology, University of Bath, and Consultant Physician,
Royal United Hospital, Bath, UK

Morris J. Brown MA MSc MD FRCP FAHA FMedSci
Professor of Clinical Pharmacology, University of Cambridge; Consultant, Physician,
Addenbrooke's Hospital, Cambridge, and Director of Clinical Studies,
Gonville and Caius College, Cambridge, UK

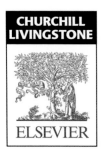

CHURCHILL
LIVINGSTONE

ELSEVIER

EDINBURGH LONDON NEWYORK OXFORD PHILADELPHIA ST LOUIS SYDNEY TORONTO 2008

CHURCHILL LIVINGSTONE
ELSEVIER

An imprint of Elsevier Limited

First edition 1960
Second edition 1962
Third edition 1966
Fourth edition 1973
Fifth edition 1980
Sixth edition 1987
Seventh edition 1992
Eighth edition 1997
Ninth edition 2003
Previous editions translated into
Italian, Chinese, Spanish, Serbo-Croat,
Russian, Malasian, Japanese

ISBN 9780443102448
IE ISBN 9780443102455

British Library Cataloguing in Publication Data
A catalogue record for this book is available from the British Library

Library of Congress Cataloging in Publication Data
A catalog record for this book is available from the Library of Congress

Note

Knowledge and best practice in this field are constantly changing. As new research and experience broaden our knowledge, changes in practice, treatment and drug therapy may become necessary or appropriate. Readers are advised to check the most current information provided (i) on procedures featured or (ii) by the manufacturer of each product to be administered, to verify the recommended dose or formula, the method and duration of administration, and contraindications. It is the responsibility of the practitioner, relying on their own experience and knowledge of the patient, to make diagnoses, to determine dosages and the best treatment for each individual patient, and to take all appropriate safety precautions. To the fullest extent of the law, neither the Publisher nor the Editors/Authors assume any liability for any injury and/or damage to persons or property arising out or related to any use of the material contained in this book.
The Publisher

The publisher's policy is to use **paper manufactured from sustainable forests**

Printed in Spain

Preface

For your own satisfaction and for mine, please read this preface![1]

A preface should tell the prospective reader about the subject of a book, its purpose, and its plan. This book is about the scientific basis and practice of drug therapy. It addresses medical students and doctors in particular, but also anyone concerned with evidence-based drug therapy and prescribing.

The scope and rate of drug innovation increase. Doctors now face a professional lifetime of handling drugs that are new to themselves – drugs that do new things as well as drugs that do old things better; and drugs that were familiar during medical training become redundant.

We write not only for readers who, like us, have a special interest in pharmacology. We try to make pharmacology understandable for those whose primary interests lie elsewhere but who recognise that they need some knowledge of pharmacology if they are to meet their moral and legal 'duty of care' to their patients. We are aware too, of medical curricular pressures that would reduce the time devoted to teaching clinical pharmacology and therapeutics, and such diminution is surely a misguided policy for a subject that is so integral to the successful practice of medicine. Thus, we try to tell readers what they need to know without burdening them with irrelevant information, and we try to make the subject interesting. We are very serious, but seriousness does not always demand wearying solemnity.

All who prescribe drugs would be wise to keep in mind the changing and ever more exacting expectations of patients and of society in general. Doctors who prescribe casually or ignorantly now face not only increasing criticism but also civil (or even criminal) legal charges. The ability to handle new developments depends, now more than ever, on comprehension of the principles of pharmacology. These principles are not difficult to grasp and are not so many as to defeat even the busiest doctors who take upon themselves the responsibility of introducing manufactured medicines into the bodies of their patients.

The principles of pharmacology and drug therapy appear in Chapters 1–8 and their application appears in the subsequent specialist chapters, which are offered as a reasonably brief solution to the problem of combining practical clinical utility with an account of the principles on which clinical practice rests.

The quantity of practical technical detail to include is a matter of judgement. In general, where therapeutic practices are complex, potentially dangerous, and commonly updated, e.g. anaphylactic shock, we provide more detail, together with websites for the latest advice; we give less or even no detail on therapy that specialists undertake, e.g. anticancer drugs. Nevertheless, especially with modern drugs that are unfamiliar, the prescriber should consult formularies, approved guidelines, or the manufacturer's current literature.

Use of the book. Francis Bacon[2] wrote that 'Some books are to be tasted, others to be swallowed, and some few to be chewed and digested.' Perhaps elements of each activity can apply to parts of our text. Students are, or should be, concerned to understand and to develop a rational, critical attitude to drug therapy and they should therefore chiefly concern themselves with how drugs act and interact in disease and with how evidence of therapeutic effect is obtained and evaluated.

To this end, they should read selectively and should not impede themselves by attempts to memorise lists of alternative drugs and doses and minor differences between them, which should never be required of them in examinations. Thus, we do not encumber the text with exhaustive lists of preparations, which properly belong in a formulary, although it is hoped that enough have been mentioned to cover much routine prescribing, and many drugs have been included solely for identification.

---

[1] St Francis of Sales: Preface to *Introduction to the devout life* (1609).

[2] Francis Bacon (1561–1626) *Essays* (1625) 'Of studies'. A philosopher and scientist, Bacon introduced the idea of the experimental or inductive method of reasoning for understanding nature.

The role and status of a textbook. A useful guide to drug use must offer clear conclusions and advice. If it is to be of reasonable size, it may often omit alternative acceptable courses of action. What it recommends should rest on sound evidence, where this exists, and on an assessment of the opinions of the experienced where it does not.

Increasingly, guidelines produced by specialist societies and national bodies have influenced the selection of drugs. We provide or refer to these as representing a consensus of best practice in particular situations. Similarly, we assume that the reader possesses a formulary, local or national, that will provide guidance on the availability, including doses, of a broad range of drugs. Yet the practice of medicinal therapeutics by properly educated and conscientious doctors working in settings complicated by intercurrent disease, metabolic differences or personality, involves challenges beyond the rigid adherence to published recommendations. The role of a textbook is to provide the satisfaction of understanding the basis for a recommended course of action and to achieve an optimal result by informed selection and use of drugs.

The guide to further reading at the end of each chapter comprises references to original papers, review articles, and web sources from a range of English language journals, mostly general but some more specialised. Our intent is to enable the reader to gain access to the original literature, to informed opinion, and to provide interest and sometimes amusement. We urge readers to select a title that looks interesting and to read the article. We do not attempt to document all of the statements we make, which would be impossible in a book of this size.

Bath, Cambridge P.N.B., M.J.B.
2007

Contributors

It is not possible for two individuals to cover the whole field of drug therapy from their own knowledge and experience. As with the previous edition, we invited selected experts to review chapters in their specialty. They were given free rein to add, delete or amend existing text as they deemed appropriate. We consider that the chapters have benefited greatly from the proficiency of these individuals and are deeply indebted for their contributions. They are:

Nigel S Baber BSc FRCP FRCPEd FFPM DipClinPharmacol
Head of Renewals, Reclassification and Patient Safety, Medicines Control Agency, London, UK and Visiting Professor, Queen Mary and Westfield College, University of London, London, UK

Chapter 3. *Discovery and development of drugs*
Chapter 4. *Evaluation of drugs in humans*
Chapter 5. *Official regulation of medicines*
Chapter 6. *Classification and naming of drugs*

Mark Farrington MA MB BChir FRCPath
Consultant Microbiologist, Addenbrooke's Hospital, Cambridge, UK

Chapter 11. *Chemotherapy of infections*
Chapter 12. *Antibacterial drugs*
Chapter 13. *Chemotherapy of bacterial infections*
Chapter 14. *Viral, fungal, protozoal and helminthic infections*

Frances Hall MA BM BCh MRCP DPhil
Consultant Rheumatologist, Department of Clinical Medicine, University of Cambridge, Cambridge, UK

Chapter 15. *Drugs for inflammation and rheumatological disease*

Thomas Ha MD FRACP
Consultant Dermatologist, Addenbrooke's Hospital, Cambridge, UK

Chapter 16. *Drugs and the skin*

Michael C Lee MB BS FRCA
Specialist Registrar in Anaesthesia, Addenbrooke's Hospital, Cambridge, UK

Mark Abrahams MB ChB DA FRCA
Consultant in Anaesthesia and Pain Management, Addenbrooke's Hospital, Cambridge, UK

Chapter 17. *Pain and analgesics*

Jerry Nolan FRCA
Consultant in Anaesthesia and Intensive Care, Royal United Hospital, Bath, UK

Chapter 18. *Anaesthesia and neuromuscular block*

Simon J C Davies MA(Oxon) MBBS(Lond) MRCPsych
Clinical Research Fellow, University of Bristol, Bristol, UK

Sue Wilson PhD
Research Fellow, University of Bristol, Bristol, UK

David J Nutt MB BChir MA DM FRCP FRCPsych FMedSci
Professor of Psychopharmacology, Head of the Department of Clinical Medicine, Dean of Clinical Medicine and Dentistry, University of Bristol, Bristol, UK

Chapter 19. *Psychotropic drugs*

Pankaj Sharma MD PhD
Consultant Neurologist & Senior Lecturer, Hammersmith Hospitals & Imperial College

Chapter 20. *Epilepsy, parkinsonism and allied conditions*

Kevin M O'Shaughnessy MA BM BCh DPhil FRCP
University Lecturer in Clinical Pharmacology and Honorary Consultant Physician, Addenbrooke's Hospital, Cambridge, UK

Chapter 21. *Cholinergic and antimuscarinic (anticholinergic) mechanisms and drugs*
Chapter 22. *Adrenergic mechanisms and drugs*
Chapter 23. *Arterial hypertension, angina pectoris, myocardial infarction*
Chapter 25. *Hyperlipidaemias*
Chapter 26. *Kidney and genitourinary tract*
Chapter 27. *Respiratory system*

Andrew Grace PhD FRCP FACC
Consultant Cardiologist, Papworth Hospital, Cambridge, UK
Chapter 24.   Cardiac arrhythmia and failure

Trevor Baglin MA MB PhD FRCP FRCPath
Consultant Haematologist, Addenbrooke's Hospital, Cambridge, UK
Chapter 28.   Drugs and haemostasis

Charles R J Singer BSc MB ChB FRCP FRCPath
Consultant Haematologist, Royal United Hospital, Bath, UK
Chapter 29.   Cellular disorders and anaemias

Pippa G Corrie PhD, FRCP
Consultant and Associate Lecturer in Medical Oncology, Addenbrooke's Hospital and University of Cambridge, Cambridge, UK

Charles R J Singer BSc MB ChB FRCP FRCPath
Consultant Haematologist, Royal United Hospital, Bath, UK
Chapter 30.   Neoplastic disease and immunosuppression

Michael Davis MD FRCP
Consultant Gastroenterologist, Royal United Hospital, Bath, UK
Chapter 31.   Oesophagus, stomach and duodenum
Chapter 32.   Intestines
Chapter 33.   Liver, biliary tract, pancreas

Diana C Brown MD MSc FRCP
Consultant Endocrinologist, Cromwell Hospital, London, UK
Chapter 34.   Adrenal corticosteroids, antagonists, corticotropin
Chapter 35.   Diabetes mellitus, insulin, oral antidiabetes agents, obesity
Chapter 36.   Thyroid hormones, antithyroid drugs

Diana C Brown MD MSc FRCP
Consultant Endocrinologist, Cromwell Hospital, London, UK

Gerard S Conway MB BS MD FRCP
Consultant Endocrinologist, University College Hospital, London, UK
Chapter 37.   Hypothalamic, pituitary and sex hormones

Diana C Brown MD MSc FRCP
Consultant Endocrinologist, Cromwell Hospital, London, UK

Chrysothemis C M Brown BA MB BS
House Officer, Royal Free Hospital, London, UK
Chapter 38.   Vitamins, calcium, bone

Acknowledgements

Aditionally, we express our gratitude to others who have, with such good grace, given us their time and energy to supply valuable facts and opinions for this and previous editions; they principally include: Dr E S K Assem, Dr N B Bennett, Dr Noeleen Foley, Dr Sheila Gore, Professor J Guillebaud, Dr P Jackson, Professor D H Jenkinson, Dr H Ludlam, Professor P J Maddison, Dr P T Macgee, Dr N J McHugh, Dr N J Mineur, the late Professor Sir William Paton, Professor B N C Prichard, Dr J P D Reckless, Dr Catriona Reid, Dr Andrew Souter, Professor P L Weissberg.

Drug doses were reviewed by Joy Craine MRPS and references by Anderley Askham librarian. Other acknowledgements appear in the appropriate places.

Much of any merit this book may have is due to the generosity of those named above as well as others too numerous to mention who have put their knowledge and practical experience of the use of drugs at our disposal. We hope that this collective acknowledgement will be acceptable. Errors are our own. We are grateful to readers who alert us to errors and make other suggestions for future editions.

In addition, we thank the authors and publishers who generously granted permission to quote directly from their writings. If we have omitted any due acknowledgement, we will make such amends as soon as we can.

P.N.B.
M.J.B.

Contents

Preface v
Contributors vii
Acknowledgements ix

SECTION 1: GENERAL
1 Clinical pharmacology 3
2 Topics in drug therapy 5
3 Discovery and development of drugs 32
4 Evaluation of drugs in humans 41
5 Official regulation of medicines 61
6 Classification and naming of drugs 69

SECTION 2: FROM PHARMACOLOGY TO TOXICOLOGY
7 General pharmacology 75
8 Unwanted effects and adverse drug reactions 115
9 Poisoning, overdose, antidotes 129
10 Drug abuse 142

SECTION 3: INFECTION AND INFLAMMATION
11 Chemotherapy of infections 175
12 Antibacterial drugs 188
13 Chemotherapy of bacterial infections 208
14 Viral, fungal, protozoal and helminthic infections 225
15 Drugs for inflammation and rheumatological disease 250
16 Drugs and the skin 274

SECTION 4: NERVOUS SYSTEM
17 Pain and analgesics 293
18 Anaesthesia and neuromuscular block 312
19 Psychotropic drugs 330
20 Epilepsy, parkinsonism and allied conditions 372

SECTION 5: CARDIORESPIRATORY AND RENAL SYSTEMS
21 Cholinergic and antimuscarinic (anticholinergic) mechanisms and drugs 391
22 Adrenergic mechanisms and drugs 403
23 Arterial hypertension, angina pectoris, myocardial infarction 415
24 Cardiac arrhythmia and heart failure 448
25 Hyperlipidaemias 469
26 Kidney and genitourinary tract 478
27 Respiratory system 495

SECTION 6: BLOOD AND NEOPLASTIC DISEASE
28 Drugs and haemostasis 513
29 Cellular disorders and anaemias 529
30 Neoplastic disease and immunosuppression 541

SECTION 7: GASTROINTESTINAL SYSTEM
31 Oesophagus, stomach and duodenum 561
32 Intestines 572
33 Liver, biliary tract, pancreas 582

SECTION 8: ENDOCRINE SYSTEM, METABOLIC CONDITIONS
34 Adrenal corticosteroids, antagonists, corticotropin 593
35 Diabetes mellitus, insulin, oral antidiabetes agents, obesity 608
36 Thyroid hormones, antithyroid drugs 627
37 Hypothalamic, pituitary and sex hormones 637
38 Vitamins, calcium, bone 660

Index 671

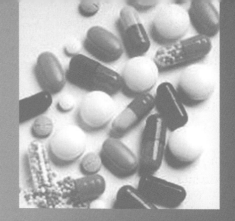

Section 1

GENERAL

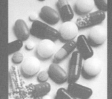

1

Clinical pharmacology

SYNOPSIS

Clinical pharmacology comprises all aspects of the scientific study of drugs in humans. Its objective is to optimise drug therapy and it is justified in so far as it is put to practical use.

Over the centuries humans have sought relief from discomfort in 'remedies' concocted from parts of plants, animals and other sources; numerous formularies attest to their numbers and complexity. Then a more critical view emerged, recognising the need for proper investigation of medications. In 1690, John Locke[1] was moved to write '… we should be able to tell beforehand that rhubarb will purge, hemlock kill, and opium make a man sleep …'.

The early years of the 20th century saw the use of specific chemical substances to achieve particular biological effects, i.e. the exact science of drug action, which is pharmacology. Subsequently the discipline underwent a major expansion resulting from technology that allowed the understanding of molecular action and the capacity to exploit this. The potential consequences for drug therapy are enormous. All cellular mechanisms (normal and pathological), in their immense complexity are, in principle, identifiable. What seems almost an infinity of substances, transmitters, local hormones, cell growth factors, can be made, modified and tested to provide agonists, partial agonists, inverse agonists and antagonists. And the unravelling of the human genome opens the way for interference with disease processes in ways that were never thought possible.

Increasingly large numbers of substances will deserve to be investigated and used for altering physiology to the advantage of humans. And with all these developments and their potential for good, comes capacity for harm, whether inherent in the substances or as a result of human misapplication. Successful use of the power conferred (by biotechnology in particular) requires understanding of the growing evidence base of the true consequences of interference. The temporary celebrity of new drugs is not a new phenomenon. Jean Nicholas Corvisart (Emperor Napoleon's favourite physician) reputedly expressed the issue in the dictum: 'Here is a new remedy; take it fast, as long as it still works'.

Clinical pharmacology provides the scientific basis for:
- the general aspects of rational, safe and effective drug therapy
- drug therapy of individual diseases
- the safe introduction of new medicines.

The drug and information 'explosion' of the past six decades combined with medical need has called into being a new discipline, clinical pharmacology[2]. The discipline finds recognition as both a health-care and an academic specialty; indeed, no medical school can be considered complete without a department or sub-department of Clinical Pharmacology.

---

[1]Locke J 1690 An essay concerning human understanding. Clarendon Press, Oxford, Book iv, Chapter iii, p. 556. The English philosopher John Locke (1632–1704) argued that all human knowledge came only from experience and sensations.

[2]The term was first used by Paul Martini (1889–1964). He addressed issues that are now integral parts of clinical trials, including the use of placebo, control groups, sample size, relationship between dose and response, probability of efficacy. His monograph, 'Methodology of therapeutic investigation' (Springer, Berlin, 1932), was published in German and went largely unnoticed by English speakers. (Shelly J H, Baur M P 1999 Paul Martini: the first clinical pharmacologist? Lancet 353:1870–1873).

A signal pioneer was Harry Gold[3] (1899–1972) of Cornell University, USA, whose influential studies in the 1930s showed the qualities needed to be a clinical pharmacologist. In 1952, he wrote in a seminal article:

> … a special kind of investigator is required, one whose training has equipped him not only with the principles and technics of laboratory pharmacology but also with knowledge of clinical medicine …
>
> Clinical scientists of all kinds do not differ fundamentally from other biologists; they are set apart only to the extent that there are special difficulties and limitations, ethical and practical, in seeking knowledge from man.[4]

Willingness to learn the principles of pharmacology, and how to apply them in individual circumstances of infinite variety is vital to success without harm: to maximise benefit and minimise risk. All of these issues are the concern of clinical pharmacology and are the subject of this book.

More detailed aspects comprise:

1. Pharmacology
   - *Pharmacodynamics*: how drugs, alone and in combination, affect the body (young, old, well, sick).
   - *Pharmacokinetics*: absorption, distribution, metabolism, excretion or, how the body, well or sick, affects drugs.
2. Therapeutic evaluation
   - Whether a drug is of value.
   - How it may best be used.
   - Formal therapeutic trials.
   - Surveillance studies for both efficacy and safety (adverse effects) – pharmacoepidemiology and pharmacovigilance.
3. Control
   - Rational prescribing and formularies.
   - Official regulation of medicines.
   - Social aspects of the use and misuse of medicines.
   - Pharmacoeconomics.

Clinical pharmacology finds expression in concert with other clinical specialties. Therapeutic success with drugs is becoming more and more dependent on the user having at least an outline understanding of both pharmacodynamics and pharmacokinetics. This outline is quite simple and easy to acquire. However humane and caring doctors may be, they cannot dispense with scientific skill. Knowledge of clinical pharmacology underpins decisions in therapeutics, which is concerned with the prevention, suppression or cure of disease and, from the point of view of society, is the most vital aspect of medicine.

Pharmacology is the same science whether it investigates animals or humans. The need for it grows rapidly as not only scientists, but now the whole community, can see its promise of release from distress and premature death over yet wider fields. The concomitant dangers of drugs (fetal deformities, adverse reactions, dependence) only add to the need for the systematic and ethical application of science to drug development, evaluation, and use, i.e. clinical pharmacology.

---

[3]Gold H 1952 The proper study of mankind is man. American Journal of Medicine 12:619. The title is taken from 'An essay on man' by Alexander Pope (English poet, 1688–1744) which begins with the lines: 'Know then thyself, presume not God to scan,/The proper study of mankind is man'. Indeed, the whole passage is worth accessing, for it reads as if it were relevant to modern clinical pharmacology and drug therapy.
[4]Self-experimentation has always been a feature of clinical pharmacology. A survey of 250 members of the Dutch Society of Clinical Pharmacology evoked 102 responders of whom 55 had done experiments on themselves (largely for convenience) (van Everdingen J J, Cohen A F 1990 Self-experimentation by doctors. Lancet 336:1448). A spectacular example occurred at the 1983 meeting of the American Urological Association at Las Vegas, USA, during a lecture on pharmacologically induced penile erection, when the lecturer stepped out from behind the lectern to demonstrate personally the efficacy of the technique (Zorgniotti A W 1990 Self-experimentation. Lancet 336:1200).

GUIDE TO FURTHER READING

Baber N S, Ritter J M, Aronson J K 2004 Medicines regulation and clinical pharmacology. British Journal of Clinical Pharmacology 58(6):569–570 (and other articles in this issue)

Brater D C, Daly W J 2000 Clinical pharmacology in the middle ages: principles that presage the 21st century. Clinical Pharmacology and Therapeutics 67:447–450

Breckenridge A M 1999 Clinical pharmacology and drug regulation. British Journal of Clinical Pharmacology 47:11–12

Dollery C T 2006 Clinical pharmacology – the first 75 years and a view of the future. British Journal of Clinical Pharmacology 61:650–665

Laurence D R 1989 Ethics and law in clinical pharmacology. British Journal of Clinical Pharmacology 27:715–722

Rawlins M D 2005 Pharmacopolitics and deliberative democracy. Clinical Medicine 5:471–475

Reidenberg M M 1999 Clinical pharmacology: the scientific basis of therapeutics. Clinical Pharmacology and Therapeutics 66:2–8

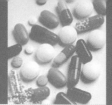

2

Topics in drug therapy

SYNOPSIS

Drug therapy involves considerations beyond the strictly scientific pharmacological aspects of medicines. These include numerous issues relating to prescribers themselves and to patients.

- The therapeutic situation
- Benefits and risks
- Public view of drugs and prescribers
- Physician-induced (iatrogenic) disease
- Drug-induced injury
- Complementary, alternative and traditional medicine
- Placebo medicines
- Prescribing, drug consumption and economics
- Compliance – patient and doctor
- Underdosing
- Pharmaco-economics
- Self-medication

Appendix: The prescription; weights and measures

THE THERAPEUTIC SITUATION

'The desire to take medicines is perhaps the greatest feature that distinguishes humans from animals' (Sir William Osler, 1849–1919).

The use of drugs[1] to increase human happiness by elimination or suppression of diseases and symptoms and to improve the quality of life in other ways is a serious matter. Overall, the major benefits of modern drugs are on quality of life (measured with difficulty), and exceed those on quantity of life (measured with ease).[2] This chapter comprises a series of essays on what we think are important topics.

Medicines are part of our way of life from birth, when we enter the world with the aid of drugs, to death where drugs assist (most of) us to depart with minimal distress and perhaps even with a remnant of dignity. In between these events, we use drugs to cure, suppress and prevent disease, and to regulate our fertility. We tend to take such usages for granted. But the average person in the USA can expect to have about 12 years of bad health in an average lifespan.[3] And medicines play a major role in this. 'At any time, 40–50% of adults [UK] are taking a prescribed medicine.'[4]

EVOLUTION OF THERAPEUTICS

Readers of this book will become aware that the medicines now available to prescribers emanate from a long process of evaluation (Chapters 3–6). The

---

[1]A World Health Organization Scientific Group has defined a drug as 'any substance or product that is used or, intended to be used, to modify or explore physiological systems or pathological states for the benefit of the recipient'. WHO 1966 Technical Report Series no. 341:7. A less restrictive definition is 'a substance that changes a biological system by interacting with it'.

A drug is a single chemical substance that forms the active ingredient of a *medicine* (a substance or mixture of substances used in restoring or preserving health). A medicine may contain many other substances to deliver the drug in a stable form, acceptable and convenient to the patient. The terms are used more or less interchangeably in this book. To use the word 'drug' intending only a harmful, dangerous or addictive substance is to abuse a respectable and useful word.

[2]Consider the worldwide total of suffering relieved and prevented each day by anaesthetics (local and general) and by analgesics, not forgetting dentistry which, because of these drugs, no longer strikes terror into even the most stoical as it did for centuries.

[3]Quoted in: USA Public Health Service 1995.

[4]George C F 1994 What do patients need to know about prescribed drugs? Prescribers' Journal 34:7. A moment's reflection will bring home to us that this is an astounding statistic, which goes a long way to account for the aggressive promotional activities of the highly competitive international pharmaceutical industry; the markets for medicines are colossal.

science of pharmacology provides the information base for the creation of new drugs and the understanding of how they act, how unwanted and toxic effects occur, and how they are best used. Increasingly, the disciplines of pharmacogenetics and pharmacogenomics will provide the means to match individual patients with drugs that give them best effect for least harm (Chapters 7–10). The general account of drugs (Chapters 11–38) and their use in a spectrum of conditions indicates the vast resource open to modern physicians. A picture emerges of progressive appraisal (punctuated by learning from mistakes) within regulated systems to produce a large number of medicines that meet set standards of safety and efficacy. The scenario is comparatively recent.

From the earliest times, alleviating effects of disease and trauma was a major concern of human beings. Records of the ancient civilisations of Mesopotamia (now Iraq), India, China, Mexico and Egypt, from about 3000 BC, describe practices of diagnosis and treatment predicated on differing, often complex, concepts of disease: the supernatural, religious theories (sin, punishment of sin, uncleanliness), omens, deities and rites. Among many modes of therapy, a reliance on diet and use of herbs (the Mexicans knew of 1200 medicinal plants) figured prominently.

The Greeks (approximately 500 BC to AD 500) replaced the supernatural with thinking that was rational, scientific and naturalistic. The core concept of the *Hippocratic corpus* (collected contributions of many writers but attributed to Hippocrates) was that health was an equilibrium, and disease a disequilibrium, of the four constituent fluids or 'humours' of the body. They comprised yellow bile and phlegm (exuded in illness), blood (associated with life) and black bile (a later addition, possibly altered blood in vomit and excreta). These humours were in symmetry with four fundamental qualities of nature – hot, wet, dry and cold – and gave rise to the system of *allopathy*, i.e. treating the first condition (the disease) by producing a second condition that was antagonistic to it. An illness involving yellow bile, regarded as 'hot' and dry', thus required a 'cold' and 'wet' medication (cf. *homoeopathy*; see p. 16). Disease as a disequilibrium of humours was correctable by evacuation techniques to re-establish the balance, and hence came venesection, cathartics, sweating and emetics. The remarkable Galen of Pergamum (AD 130–201) propagated Hippocratic principles so effectively that they dominated medical thinking to the Middle Ages and beyond. In effect, medicine through this time was stagnant. Life was 'solitary, poor, nasty, brutish and short',[5] and medical care did little to help.

The unravelling of the structure and later the function of the human body was part of the scientific resurgence of the Renaissance. Amongst many discoveries, William Harvey (1578–1657) explained the circulation of the blood, and Antoine Lavoisier (1743–1794) the crucial nature of oxygen. The human body, hitherto a mystery, appeared more like a machine – that could experience faults. But faults were interpreted in various ways. William Cullen of Edinburgh (1712–1790) evolved a system within which a 'nervous force' was the phenomenon underlying life and disease. His pupil, John Brown (1735–1778), went further and revived an ancient belief that every disease resulted from *sthenia* (over-stimulation) or *asthenia* (failure to respond to stimulation).[6]

It was only in the 19th century that medicine freed itself from a muddle of theories and systems. Microscopy revealed the cell as the basic construction unit of the body, vague theories of disease gave way to specific entities with recognisable pathology, most notably in the case of infection with microorganisms ('germ theory'). The one major dimension of medicine that remained underdeveloped was therapeutics. An abundance of preparations in pharmacopoeias compared with a scarcity of genuinely effective therapies gave to a state of 'therapeutic nihilism', expressed trenchantly by Oliver Wendell Holmes (1809–1894)[7]:

> Throw out opium …; throw out a few specifics …; throw out wine, which is a food, and the vapours which produce the miracle of anaesthesia, and I firmly believe that if the whole materia medica, as now used, could be sunk to the bottom of the sea, it would be all the better for mankind, – and all the worse for the fishes

[5]Thomas Hobbes (1588–1679), political philosopher; in: Leviathan 1651.
[6]Quoted in: Ackerknecht E H 1982 A short history of medicine. Johns Hopkins University Press, Baltimore, p. 129.
[7]Medical Essays (1891). American physician and poet, and Dean of Harvard Medical School; he introduced the term *anaesthesia* instead of 'suspended animation' or 'etherisation'. Address delivered before the Massachusetts Medical Society, 30 May 1860 (Oliver Wendell Holmes. Medical Essays. Kessinger Publishing, p. 140).

The 20th century saw this position alter beyond recognition (see before).

> Drug therapy involves a great deal more than matching the name of the drug to the name of a disease; it requires knowledge, judgement, skill and wisdom, but above all a sense of responsibility.

TREATING PATIENTS WITH DRUGS

A book can provide knowledge and contribute to the formation of judgement, but it can do little to impart skill and wisdom, which are the products of example of teachers and colleagues, of experience and of innate and acquired capacities. But:

> It is evident that patients are not treated in a vacuum and that they respond to a variety of subtle forces around them in addition to the specific therapeutic agent.[8]

When a patient receives a drug, the response can be the resultant of numerous factors:

- The pharmacodynamic effect of the drug and interactions with any other drugs the patient may be taking.
- The pharmacokinetics of the drug and its modification in the individual by genetic influences, disease, other drugs.
- The act of medication, including the route of administration and the presence or absence of the doctor.
- What the doctor has told the patient.
- The patient's past experience of doctors.
- The patient's estimate of what has been received and of what ought to happen as a result.
- The social environment, e.g. whether it is supportive or dispiriting.

The relative importance of these factors varies according to circumstances. An unconscious patient with meningococcal meningitis does not have a personal relationship with the doctor, but patients, sleepless with anxiety because they cannot cope with their family responsibilities, may respond as much to the interaction of their own personalities with that of the doctor, as to anxiolytics.

The physician may consciously use all of the factors listed above in therapeutic practice. But it is still not enough that patients get better: it is essential to know why they do so. This is because potent drugs should be given only if their pharmacodynamic effects are needed; many adverse reactions have been shown to be due to drugs that are not needed, including some severe enough to cause hospital admission.

Drugs can do good

Medically, this good may sometimes seem trivial, as in the avoidance of a sleepless night in a noisy hotel or of social embarrassment from a profusely running nose due to seasonal pollen allergy (hay fever). Such benefits are not necessarily trivial to recipients, concerned to be at their best in important matters, whether of business, of pleasure or of passion, i.e. with quality of life.

Or the good may be literally life-saving, as in serious acute infections (pneumonia, septicaemia) or in the prevention of life-devastating disability from severe asthma, from epilepsy or from blindness due to glaucoma.

Drugs can do harm

This harm may be relatively trivial, as in hangover from a hypnotic or transient headache from glyceryl trinitrate used for angina.

The harm may be life-destroying, as in the rare sudden death following an injection of penicillin, rightly regarded as one of the safest of antibiotics, or the destruction of the quality of life that occasionally attends the use of drugs that are effective in rheumatoid arthritis (adrenocortical steroids, penicillamine) and Parkinson's disease (levodopa).

There are risks in taking medicines, just as there are risks in food and transport. There are also risks in declining to take medicines when they are needed, just as there are risks in refusing food or transport when they are needed.

Efficacy and safety do not lie solely in the molecular structure of the drug. Doctors must choose which drugs to use and must apply them correctly in relation not only to their properties, but also to those of the patients and their disease. Then patients must use the prescribed medicine correctly (see Compliance/concordance below).

[8]Sherman L J 1959 The significant variables in psychopharmaceutic research. American Journal of Psychiatry 116:208–214.

Uses of drugs/medicines

> Drugs are used in three principal ways:
> - To cure disease: primary and auxiliary
> - To suppress disease
> - To prevent disease: (prophylaxis): primary and secondary.

Cure implies *primary* therapy, as in bacterial and parasitic infections, that eliminates the disease, and the drug is withdrawn; or *auxiliary* therapy, as with anaesthetics and with ergometrine and oxytocin in obstetrics.

Suppression of diseases or symptoms is used continuously or intermittently to avoid the effects of disease without attaining cure (as in hypertension, diabetes mellitus, epilepsy, asthma), or to control symptoms (such as pain and cough) whilst awaiting recovery from the causative disease.

Prevention (prophylaxis). In *primary prevention*, the person does not have the condition and avoids getting it. For malaria, vaccinations and contraception, the decision to treat healthy people is generally easy.

In *secondary prevention*, the patient has the disease and the objective is to reduce risk factors, so to retard progression or avoid repetition of an event, e.g. aspirin and lipid-lowering drugs in atherosclerosis and after myocardial infarction, antihypertensives to prevent recurrence of stroke.

Taking account of the above, a doctor might ask the following questions before treating a patient with drugs:

1. Should I interfere with the patient at all?
2. If so, what alteration in the patient's condition do I hope to achieve?
3. Which drug is most likely to bring this about?
4. How can I administer the drug to attain the right concentration in the right place at the right time and for the right duration?
5. How will I know when I have achieved the objective?
6. What other effects might the drug produce, and are these harmful?
7. How will I decide to stop the drug?
8. Does the likelihood of benefit, and its importance, outweigh the likelihood of damage, and its importance, i.e. the benefit versus risk, or efficacy against safety?

BENEFITS AND RISKS OF MEDICINES

Modern technological medicine has been criticised, justly, for following the tradition of centuries by waiting for disease to occur and then trying to cure it rather than seeking to prevent it in the first place. Although many diseases are partly or wholly preventable by economic, social and behavioural means, these are too seldom adopted and are slow to take effect. In the meantime, people continue to fall sick, and to need and deserve treatment.

We all have eventually to die from something and, even after excessive practising of all the advice on how to live a healthy life, the likelihood that the mode of death for most of us will be free from pain, anxiety, cough, diarrhoea, paralysis (the list is endless) seems so small that it can be disregarded. Drugs already provide immeasurable solace in these situations, and the development of better drugs should be encouraged.

Doctors know the sick are thankful for drugs, just as even the most dedicated pedestrians and environmentalists struck down by a passing car are thankful for a motor ambulance to take them to hospital. The reader will find reference to the benefits of drugs in individual diseases throughout this book and further expansion is unnecessary here. But a general discussion of risk of adverse events is appropriate.

Unavoidable risks

Consider, for the sake of argument, the features that a completely risk-free drug would exhibit:

- The physician would know exactly what action is required and use the drug correctly.
- The drug would deliver its desired action and nothing else, either by true biological selectivity or by selective targeted delivery.
- The drug would achieve exactly the right amount of action – neither too little, nor too much.

These criteria may be *completely* fulfilled, for example in a streptococcal infection sensitive to penicillin in patients whose genetic constitution does not render them liable to an allergic reaction to penicillin.

These criteria are *partially* fulfilled in insulin-deficient diabetes. But the natural modulation of insulin secretion in response to need (food, exercise) does not operate with injected insulin and even sophisticated technology cannot yet exactly mimic the normal physiological responses. The criteria are still further from realisation in, for example, some cancers and schizophrenia.

Some reasons why drugs fail to meet the criteria of being risk-free include:

- *Drugs may be insufficiently selective*. As the concentration rises, a drug that acts at only one site at low concentrations begins to affect other target sites (receptors, enzymes) and recruit new (unwanted) actions; or a disease process (cancer) is so close to normal cellular mechanisms that perfectly selective cell kill is impossible.
- *Drugs may be highly selective* for one pathway but the mechanism affected has widespread functions and interference with it cannot be limited to one site only, e.g. atenolol on the β-adrenoceptor, aspirin on cyclo-oxygenase.
- *Prolonged modification* of cellular mechanisms can lead to permanent change in structure and function, e.g. carcinogenicity.
- *Insufficient knowledge of disease processes* (some cardiac arrhythmias) and of drug action can lead to interventions that, although undertaken with the best intentions, are harmful.
- *Patients are genetically heterogeneous* to a high degree and may have unpredicted responses to drugs.
- *Dosage adjustment* according to need is often unavoidably imprecise, e.g. in depression.
- *Prescribing 'without due care and attention'*.[9]

Reduction of risk

Strategies that can limit risk include those directed at achieving:

- *Better knowledge of disease* (research) – as much as 40% of useful medical advances derive from basic research that was not funded towards a specific practical outcome.
- *Site-specific effect* – by molecular manipulation.
- *Site-specific delivery* – drug targeting:
  - by topical (local) application
  - by target-selective carriers.
- Informed, careful and responsible prescribing.

Two broad categories of risk

First are those that we accept by deliberate choice. We do so even if we do not exactly know their magnitude, or we know but wish they were smaller, or, especially where the likelihood of harm is sufficiently remote though the consequences may be grave, we do not even think about the matter. Such risks include transport and sports, both of which are inescapably subject to potent physical laws such as gravity and momentum, and surgery to rectify disorders that we could tolerate or treat in other ways, e.g. much cosmetic surgery.

Second are those risks that cannot be significantly altered by individual action. We experience risks imposed by food additives (preservatives, colouring), air pollution and some environmental radioactivity. But there are also risks imposed by nature, such as skin cancer due to excess ultraviolet radiation in sunny climes, as well as some radioactivity.

It seems an obvious course to avoid unnecessary risks, but there is disagreement on what risks are truly unnecessary and, on looking closely at the matter, it is plain that many people habitually take risks in their daily and recreational life that it would be a misuse of words to describe as necessary. Furthermore, some risks, although known to exist, are, in practice, ignored other than by conforming to ordinary prudent conduct. These risks are negligible in the sense that they do not influence behaviour, i.e. they are neglected.[10]

Elements of risk

> Risk has two elements:
> - The likelihood or probability of an adverse event
> - Its severity.

In medical practice in general, concern ceases when risks fall below about 1 in 100 000 instances, when the procedure then is regarded as 'safe'. In such cases, when disaster occurs, it can be difficult indeed for individuals to accept that they 'deliberately' accepted a risk; they feel 'it should not have happened to me' and in their distress they may seek to lay blame on others where there is no fault or negligence, only misfortune (see Warnings and consent).

---

[9]This phrase is commonly used in the context of motor vehicle accidents, but applies equally well to the prescribing of drugs.

[10]Sometimes the term minimal risk is used to mean risk about equal to going about our ordinary daily lives; it includes travel on public transport, but not motor bicycling on a motorway.

The benefits of chemicals used to colour food verge on or even attain negligibility, although some cause allergy in humans. Our society permits their use.

There is general agreement that drugs prescribed for disease are themselves the cause of a significant amount of disease (adverse reactions), of death, of permanent disability, of recoverable illness and of minor inconvenience. In one major UK study the prevalence of adverse drug reactions as a cause of admission to hospital was 6.5% (see p. 117 for other examples).

Three major grades of risk

These are: *unacceptable, acceptable* and *negligible*. Where disease is life-threatening and there is reliable information on both the disease and the drug, then decisions, though they may be painful, present relatively obvious problems. But where the disease risk is remote, e.g. mild hypertension, or where drugs are to be used to increase comfort or to suppress symptoms that are, in fact, bearable, or for convenience rather than for need, then the issues of risk acceptance are less obvious.

Risks should not be weighed without reference to benefits any more than benefits should be weighed without reference to risks.

> Risks are among the facts of life. In whatever we do and in whatever we refrain from doing, we are accepting risk. Some risks are obvious, some are unsuspected and some we conceal from ourselves. But risks are universally accepted, whether willingly or unwillingly, whether consciously or not.[11]

Whenever a drug is taken a risk is taken

The risk comprises the properties of the drug, the prescriber, the patient and the environment; it is often so small that second thoughts are hardly necessary, but sometimes it is substantial. The doctor must weigh the likelihood of gain for the patient against the likelihood of loss. There are often insufficient data for a rational decision to be reached, but a decision must yet be made, and this is one of the greatest difficulties of clinical practice. Its effect on the attitudes of doctors is often not appreciated by those who have never been in this situation. The patient's protection lies in the doctor's knowledge of the drug and of the disease, and experience of both, together with knowledge of the patient.

We continue to use drugs that are capable of killing or disabling patients at doses within the therapeutic range where the judgement of overall balance of benefit and risk is favourable. This can be very difficult for the patient who has suffered a rare severe adverse reaction, to understand and to accept (see below).

In some chronic diseases that ultimately necessitate suppressive drugs, the patient may not experience benefit in the early stages. Patients with early Parkinson's disease may experience little inconvenience or hazard from the condition, and premature exposure to drugs can exact such a price in unwanted effects that they prefer the untreated state. What patients will tolerate depends on their personality, their attitude to disease, their occupation, mode of life and relationship with their doctor (see Compliance, p. 22).

PUBLIC VIEW OF DRUGS AND PRESCRIBERS

The current public view of modern medicines, ably fuelled by the mass media, is a compound of vague expectation of 'miracle' cures with outrage when anything goes wrong. It is also unreasonable to expect the public to trust the medical profession (in collaboration with the pharmaceutical industry) to the extent of leaving to them all drug matters.

The public wants benefits without risks and without having to alter its unhealthy ways of living; this is a deeply irrational position. But it is easy to understand that a person who has taken into their body a chemical with intent to relieve suffering, whether or not it is self-induced, can feel profound anger when harm ensues. Expectations are high, and now, at the beginning of the 21st century, with the manifest achievement of technology all around us, the expectation that happiness can be a part of the technological package must yet be seen as naive and unrealisable.

Patients are aware that there is justifiable criticism of the standards of medical prescribing – indeed, doctors are in the forefront of this – as well as justifiable criticism of promotional practices of the profitably rich, aggressive, international pharmaceutical industry.

There are obvious areas where some remedial action is possible:

---

[11]Pochin E E 1975 The acceptance of risk. British Medical Bulletin 31:184–190.

- *Maintaining high standards of prescribing* by doctors, including better communication with patients, i.e. doctors must learn to feel that introduction of foreign chemicals into their patients' bodies is a serious matter, which the majority do not seem to feel at present.
- Introduction of *no-fault compensation* schemes for serious drug injury (some countries already have these).
- *Informed public discussion* of the issues between the medical profession, industrial drug developers, politicians and other 'opinion formers' in society, and patients (the public).
- *Restraint in promotion by the pharmaceutical industry*, including self-control by both industry and doctors in their necessarily close relationship, which the public is inclined to regard as a conspiracy.

If restraint by both parties is not forthcoming, and it may not be, then both doctor and industry can expect the exercise of more control over them by politicians responding to public demand.

CRITICISMS OF MODERN DRUGS

Extremist critics have attracted public attention for their view that modern drug therapy, indeed modern medicine in general, does more harm than good; others, whilst admitting some benefits from drugs, insist that this is medically marginal.

These opinions rest on the undisputed fact that favourable trends in many diseases preceded the introduction of modern drugs and were due to economic and environmental changes, sanitation, nutrition and housing. They also rest on the claim that drugs have not changed expectation of life or mortality (as measured by national mortality statistics), and that drugs can cause illness (adverse reactions).

If something is to be measured then the correct criteria must be chosen. Overall mortality figures are an extremely crude and often an irrelevant measure of the effects of drugs whose major benefits are so often on quality of life rather than on its quantity.

Two examples of inappropriate measurements will suffice:

1. In the case of many infections, environmental changes have had an indisputably greater beneficial effect on health than the subsequently introduced antimicrobials. But this does not mean that environmental improvements alone are sufficient in the fight against infections. When comparisons of illnesses in the pre- and post-antimicrobial eras are made, like is not compared with like. Environmental changes achieved their results when the mortality rate from infections was high and antimicrobials were not available; antimicrobials came later, against a background of low mortality as well as of environmental change; decades separate the two parts of the comparison, and observers, diagnostic criteria and data recording changed during this long period. It is evident that determining the value of antimicrobials is not simply a matter of looking at mortality rates.

2. About 1% of the UK population has diabetes mellitus and about 1% of death certificates mention diabetes. This is no surprise because all must die and insulin is no cure[12] for this lifelong disease. A standard medical textbook of 1907 stated that juvenile-onset 'diabetes is in all cases a grave disease, and the subjects are regarded by all assurance companies as uninsurable lives: life seems to hang by a thread, a thread often cut by a very trifling accident'. Most, if not all, life insurance companies now accept young people with diabetes with no or only modest financial penalty – the premium of a person 5–10 years older. Before insulin replacement therapy was available few survived beyond 3 years[13] after diagnosis they died for lack of insulin. It is unjustified to assert that a treatment is worthless just because its mention on death certificates (whether as a prime or as a contributory cause) has not declined. The relevant criteria for juvenile-onset diabetes are change in the age at which the subjects die and the quality of life between diagnosis and death, and both of these have changed enormously.

---

[12]A cure eliminates a disease and may be withdrawn when this is achieved.

[13]Even if given the best treatment. 'Opium alone stands the test of experience as a remedy capable of limiting the progress of the disease', wrote the great Sir William Osler, successively Professor of Medicine in Pennsylvania, McGill, Johns Hopkins and Oxford Universities, in 1918, only 3 years before the discovery of insulin.

PHYSICIAN-INDUCED (IATROGENIC) DISEASE

> They used to have a more equitable contract in Egypt: for the first three days the doctor took on the patient at the patient's risk and peril: when the three days were up, the risks and perils were the doctor's.
>
> But doctors are lucky: the sun shines on their successes and the earth hides their failures.[14]

It is a salutary thought that each year medical errors kill an estimated 44 000 to 98 000 Americans (more than die in motor vehicle accidents) and injure 1 000 000.[15] Among inpatients in the USA and Australia, about half of the injuries caused by medical mismanagement result from surgery, but therapeutic mishaps and diagnostic errors are the next most common. In one survey of adverse drug events, 1% were fatal, 12% life-threatening, 30% serious and 57% significant.[16] About half of the life-threatening and serious events were preventable. Errors of prescribing account for one-half and those of administering drugs for one-quarter of these. Inevitably, a proportion of lapses result in litigation, and in the UK 20–25% of complaints received by the medical defence organisations about general practitioners follow medication errors.

The most shameful act in therapeutics, apart from actually killing a patient, is to injure a patient who is but little disabled or who is suffering from a self-limiting disorder. Such iatrogenic disease,[17] induced by misguided treatment, is far from rare.

Doctors who are temperamentally extremist will do less harm by therapeutic nihilism than by optimistically overwhelming patients with well intentioned poly-pharmacy. If in doubt whether or not to give a drug to a person who will soon get better without it, don't.

In 1917 the famous pharmacologist, Sollmann, felt able to write:

> Pharmacology comprises some broad conceptions and generalisations, and some detailed conclusions, of such great and practical importance that every student and practitioner should be absolutely familiar with them. It comprises also a large mass of minute details, which would constitute too great a tax on human memory, but which cannot safely be neglected.[18]

The doctor's aim must be not merely to give the patient what will do good, but to give only what will do good, or at least more good, than harm. The information explosion of recent decades is now under better control such that prescribers can, from their desktop computer terminals, enter the facts about their patient (age, sex, weight, principal and secondary diagnoses) and receive suggestions for which drugs should be considered, with proposed doses and precautions.

DRUG-INDUCED INJURY[19] (see also Chapter 8)

Responsibility for drug-induced injury raises important issues affecting medical practice and development of needed new drugs, as well as of law and of social justice.

Negligence and strict and no-fault liability

All civilised legal systems provide for compensation to be paid to a person injured as a result of using a product of any kind that is defective due to negligence (fault is a failure to exercise reasonable care).[20]

But there is a growing opinion that special compensation for serious personal injury, beyond the modest sums that general social security systems provide, should be automatic and not dependent on fault and proof of fault of the producer, i.e. there

---

[14]Michael de Montaigne 1533–1592. French essayist.

[15]Kohn L, Corrigan J, Donaldson M (eds) for the Committee on Quality of Health Care in America, Institute of Medicine 2000 To err is human: building a safer health system. National Academy Press, Washington, DC.

[16]Bates DW et al 1995 Incidence of adverse drug events and potential adverse drug events. Journal of the American Medical Association 274:29–34.

[17]Iatrogenic means 'physician-caused', i.e. disease consequent on following medical advice or intervention (from the Greek *iatros*, physician).

[18]Sollman T A 1917 Manual of pharmacology. Saunders, Philadelphia.

[19]This discussion is about drugs that have been properly manufactured and meet proper standards, e.g. of purity, stability, as laid down by regulatory bodies or pharmacopoeias. A manufacturing defect would be dealt with in a way no different from manufacturing errors in other products.

[20]A plaintiff (person who believes he or she has been injured) seeking to obtain compensation from a defendant (via the law of negligence) must prove three things: (1) that the defendant owed a duty of care to the plaintiff; (2) that the defendant failed to exercise reasonable care; and (3) that the plaintiff has suffered an actual injury as a result.

should be 'liability irrespective of fault', 'no-fault liability' or 'strict liability'.[21]

Many countries are now revising their laws on liability for personal injury due to manufactured products and are legislating Consumer Protection Acts (Statutes) that include medicines, for 'drugs represent the class of product in respect of which there has been the greatest pressure for surer compensation in cases of injury'.[22]

Issues that are central to the debate include:

- *Capacity to cause harm* is inherent in drugs in a way that sets them apart from other manufactured products; and harm often occurs in the absence of fault.
- *Safety*, i.e. the degree of safety that a person is entitled to expect, and adverse effects that should be accepted without complaint, must often be a matter of opinion and will vary with the disease being treated, e.g. cancer or insomnia.
- *Causation*, i.e. proof that the drug in fact caused the injury, is often impossible, particularly where it increases the incidence of a disease that occurs naturally.
- *Contributory negligence*. Should compensation be reduced in smokers and drinkers where there is evidence that these pleasure-drugs increase liability to adverse reactions to therapeutic drugs?
- *The concept of defect*, i.e. whether the drug or the prescriber or indeed the patient can be said to be 'defective' so as to attract liability, is a highly complex matter and indeed is a curious concept as applied to medicine.

A scheme that meets all the major difficulties has not yet been implemented anywhere. This is not because there has been too little thought; it is because the subject is difficult. Nevertheless, no-fault schemes operate in New Zealand, Scandanavia and France.[23] The following principles might form the basis of a workable compensation scheme for injury due to drugs:

- *New unlicensed drugs undergoing clinical trial in small numbers of subjects* (healthy or patient volunteers): the developer should be strictly liable for all adverse effects.
- *New unlicensed drugs undergoing extensive trials in patients who may reasonably expect benefit*: the producer should be strictly liable for any serious effect.
- *New drugs after licensing by an official body*: the manufacturer and the community should share liability for serious injury, as new drugs provide general benefit. An option might be to institute a defined period of formal prospective drug surveillance monitoring, in which both doctors and patients agree to participate.
- *Standard drugs in day-to-day therapeutics*:

  1. There should be a no-fault scheme, operated by or with the assent of government that has authority, through tribunals, to decide cases quickly and to make awards. This body would have authority to reimburse itself from others – manufacturer, supplier, prescriber – wherever that was appropriate. An award must not have to wait on the outcome of prolonged, vexatious, adversarial, expensive court proceedings.
  2. Patients would be compensated where:
     - causation was proven on 'balance of probability'[24]
     - the injury was serious
     - the event was rare and remote and not reasonably taken into account in making the decision to treat.

COMPLEMENTARY, ALTERNATIVE AND TRADITIONAL MEDICINE

Practitioners of complementary and alternative medicine (CAM)[25] are severely critical of modern

---

[21]The following distinction is made in some discussions of product liability. Strict liability: the producer/manufacturer provide compensation. No-fault liability or scheme: a central fund provides compensation.

[22]Royal Commission on Civil Liability and Compensation for Personal Injury 1978 HMSO, London: Cmnd. 7054. Although the Commission considered compensation for death and personal injury suffered by any person through manufacture, supply or use of products, i.e. all goods whether natural or manufactured, and included drugs and even human blood and organs, it made no mention of tobacco or alcohol.

[23]Gaine W J 2003 No-fault compensation schemes. British Medical Journal 326:997–998.

[24]This is the criterion for (UK) civil law, rather than 'beyond reasonable doubt', which is the criterion of criminal law.

[25]The definition adopted by the Cochrane Collaboration is: 'Complementary and alternative medicine (CAM) is a broad domain of healing resources that accompanies all health systems, modalities, and practices and their accompanying theories and beliefs, other than those intrinsic to the politically dominant health system of a particular society or culture in a given historical period. CAM includes all such practices and ideas self-defined by their users as preventing or treating illness or promoting health and well-being. Boundaries within CAM and between the CAM domain and that of the dominant system are not always sharp or fixed.'

drugs, and use practices according to their own special beliefs. It is appropriate therefore to discuss such medical systems here.

The term 'complementary and alternative' medicine covers a broad range of heterogeneous systems of therapy (from acupuncture to herbalism to yoga), and diagnosis (from bioresonance to pulse and tongue diagnosis). The present discussion relates largely to CAM but recognises that traditional or indigenous medicinal therapeutics has developed since before history in all societies. This comprises a mass of practices varying from the worthless to highly effective remedies, e.g. digitalis (England), quinine (South America), reserpine (India), atropine (various countries). It is the task of science to find the gems and to discard the dross,[26] and at the same time to leave intact socially valuable supportive aspects of traditional medicine.

There is no doubt that the domain of CAM has grown in popularity in recent years; a survey estimated that about 20% of the UK population had consulted a CAM practitioner in the previous year.[27] In Germany, the figure exceeds 60%, with $2.06 billion in over-the-counter sales in 2003.[28] Usage rises sharply among those with chronic, relapsing conditions such as cancer, multiple sclerosis, human immunodeficiency virus (HIV) infection, psoriasis and rheumatological diseases. It is difficult to resist the conclusion that when scientific medicine neither guarantees happiness nor wholly eliminates the disabilities of degenerative diseases in long-lived populations, and when drugs used in modern medicine cause serious harm, public disappointment naturally leads to a revival of interest in alternatives that alluringly promise efficacy with complete safety. These range from a revival of traditional medicine to adoption of the more modern cults.[29]

Features common to medical cults: are absence of scientific thinking, naive acceptance of hypotheses, uncritical acceptance of causation, e.g. reliance on anecdote or opinion (as opposed to evidence), assumption that if recovery follows treatment it is due to the treatment, and close attention to the patient's personal feelings. Lack of understanding of how therapeutic effects may be measured is also a prominent feature. An extensive analysis of recommendations of CAM therapies for specific medical conditions from seven textbook sources revealed numerous treatments recommended for the same condition, for example: addictions (120 treatments recommended), arthritis (121), asthma (119) and cancer (133), but there was lack of agreement between these authors as to the preferred therapies for specified conditions.[30] The question must arise that if numerous and heterogeneous treatments are effective for the same condition, could they not have some common feature, such as the ability of the practitioner to inspire confidence in the patient?

---

[26]Traditional medicine is fostered particularly in countries where scientific medicine is not accessible to large populations for economic reasons, and destruction of traditional medicine would leave unhappy and sick people with nothing. For this reason, governments are supporting traditional medicine and at the same time initiating scientific clinical evaluations of the numerous plants and other items employed, many of which contain biologically active substances. The World Health Organization is supportive to these programmes.

[27]Ernst E 2000 The role of complementary and alternative medicine. British Medical Journal 32:1133–1135.

[28]De Smet P A G M 2005 Herbal medicine in Europe – relaxing regulatory standards. New England Journal of Medicine 352:1176–1178.

[29]A cult is a practice that follows a dogma, tenet or principle based on theories or beliefs of its promulgator to the exclusion of demonstrable scientific experience (definition of the American Medical Association). Scientific medicine changes in accord with evidence obtained by scientific enquiry applied with such intellectual rigour as is humanly possible. But this is not the case with cults, the claims for which are characterised by absence of rigorous intellectual evaluation and unchangeability of beliefs. The profusion of medical cults prompts the question why, if each cult has the efficacy claimed by its exponents, conventional medicine and indeed the other cults are not swept away. Some practitioners use conventional medicine and, where it fails, turn to cult practices. Where such complementary practices give comfort they are not to be despised, but their role and validity should be clearly defined. No community can afford to take these cults at their own valuation; they must be tested, and tested with at least the rigour required to justify a therapeutic claim for a new drug. It is sometimes urged in extenuation that traditional and cult practices do no harm to patients, unlike synthetic drugs. But, even if that were true (which it is not), investment of scarce resources in delivering what may be ineffective, though sometimes pleasing, experiences, e.g. dance therapy, exaltation of flowers and the admittedly inexpensive urine therapy, means that resources are not available for other desirable social objectives, e.g. housing, art subsidies, medicine. We do not apologise for this diversion to consider medical cults and practices, for the world cannot afford unreason, and the antidote to unreason is reason and the rigorous pursuit of knowledge, i.e. evidence-based medicine.

[30]Ernst E (ed.) 2001 The desktop guide to complementary and alternative medicine. Harcourt, Edinburgh.

A proposition belongs to science if we can say what kind of event we would accept as refutation (and this is easy in therapeutics). A proposition (or theory) that cannot clash with any possible or even conceivable event (evidence) is outside science, and this in general applies to cults where everything is interpreted in terms of the theory of the cult; the possibility that the basis of the cult is false is not entertained. This appears to be the case with medical cults, which join freudianism, and indeed religions, as outside science (after Karl Popper). Willingness to follow where the evidence leads is a distinctive feature of conventional scientific medicine.

> A scientific approach does not mean treating a patient as a mere biochemical machine. It does not mean the exclusion of spiritual, psychological and social dimensions of human beings. But it does mean treating these in a rational manner.

Some common false beliefs of CAM practitioners are that synthetic modern drugs are toxic, but products obtained in nature are not.[31] Scientific medicine is held to accept evidence that remedies are effective only where the mechanism is understood, that it depends on adherence to rigid and unalterable dogmas, and recognises no form of evaluation other than the strict randomised controlled trial. Traditional (pre-scientific) medicine is deemed to have special virtue, and the collection and formal analysis of data on therapeutic outcomes, failures as well as successes, is deemed inessential. There is also a tenet that if patient gets better when treated in accordance with certain beliefs, this provides evidence for the truth of these beliefs (the *post hoc ergo propter hoc*[32] fallacy).

Exponents of CAM often state that comparative controlled trials of their medicines against conventional medicines are impracticable because the classic double-blind randomised controlled designs are inappropriate and in particular do not allow for the individual approach characteristic of complementary medicine. But modern therapeutic trial designs can cope with this. There remain extremists who contend that they understand scientific method, and reject it as invalid for what they do and believe, i.e. their beliefs are not, in principle, refutable. This is the position taken up by magic and religion where subordination of reason to faith is a virtue.

CAM particularly charges that conventional medicine seriously neglects patients as whole integrated human beings (body, mind, spirit) and treats them too much as machines. Conventional practitioners may well feel uneasily that there has been and still is truth in this, that with the development of specialisation some doctors have been seduced by the enormous successes of medical science and technology and have become liable to look too narrowly at their patients where a much broader (holistic) approach is required. It is evident that such an approach is likely to give particular satisfaction in psychological and psychosomatic conditions for which conventional doctors in a hurry have been all too ready to think that a prescription meets all the patients' needs.

CAM does not compete with the successful mainstream of scientific medicine. Users of CAM commonly have chronic conditions and have tried conventional medicine but found that it has not offered a satisfactory solution, or has caused adverse effects. The problems, when they occur, are often at the interface between CAM and mainstream medicine. A doctor prescribing a conventional medicine

---

[31]Black cohosh (*Cimicifuga racemosa*), taken for hot flushes and other menopausal symptoms (but no better than placebo in clinical trial), can cause serious liver disorder. Herbal teas containing pyrrolidizine alkaloids (*Senecio, Crotalaria, Heliotropium*) cause serious hepatic veno-occlusive disease. Comfrey (*Symphitum*) is similar but also causes hepatocellular tumours and haemangiomas. Sassafras (carminative, antirheumatic) is hepatotoxic. Mistletoe (*Viscum*) contains cytotoxic alkaloids. Ginseng contains oestrogenic substances that have caused gynaecomastia; long-term users may show 'ginseng abuse syndrome' comprising central nervous system excitation; arterial hypertension can occur. Liquorice (*Glycyrrhiza*) has mineralocorticoid action. An amateur 'health food enthusiast' made himself a tea from 'an unfamiliar [*to him*] plant' in his garden: unfortunately this was the familiar foxglove (*Digitalis purpurea*); he became very ill, but happily recovered. Other toxic natural remedies include lily of the valley (*Convallaria*) and horse chestnut (*Aesculus*). 'The medical herbalist is at fault for clinging to outworn historical authority and for not assessing his drugs in terms of today's knowledge, and the orthodox physician is at fault for a cynical scepticism with regard to any healing discipline other than his own' (Penn R G 1983 Adverse reactions to herbal medicines. Adverse Drug Reaction Bulletin 102:376–379). The Medicines and Healthcare products Regulatory Agency provides advice at: http://www.mhra.gov.uk.

[32]Latin: after this; therefore on account of this.

may be unaware that a patient is taking herbal medicine, and there is ample scope for unwanted herb–drug interaction by a variety of mechanisms.[33] These include:

- *CYP450 enzyme induction* – St John's wort (by reducing the plasma concentration or therapeutic efficacy of warfarin, ciclosporin, simvastatin, oral contraceptives).
- *CYP450 enzyme inhibition* – piperine (by increasing plasma concentrations of propranolol and theophylline).
- *Additive action* – St John's wort on serotonin-specific reuptake inhibitors (by increasing their unwanted effects).

More troubling is the issue of conflicting advice between CAM and mainstream drugs, as witnessed by the advice to travellers from some homoeopathic pharmacies to use their products for malaria prophylaxis in place of conventional drugs (an action that drew criticism from the Society of Homoeopaths). Regulations being introduced by European Union Directive (and voluntarily in the UK) will move towards formal registration of practitioners of some forms of CAM (notably herbal medicines), according to agreed standards of qualification.

The following will suffice to give the flavour of homoeopathy, the principal complementary medicine system involving medicines, and the kind of criticism with which it has to contend.

HOMOEOPATHY

Homoeopathy[34] is a system of medicine founded by Samuel Hahnemann (German physician, 1755–1843) and expounded by him in the 'Organon of the Rational Art of Healing'.[35] Hahnemann described his position:

> After I had discovered the weakness and errors of my teachers and books I sank into a state of sorrowful indignation, which had nearly disgusted me with the study of medicine. I was on the point of concluding that the whole art was vain and incapable of improvement. I gave myself up to solitary reflection, and resolved not to terminate

my train of thought until I had arrived at a definite conclusion on the subject.[36]

By understandable revulsion at the medicine of his time, by experimentation on himself (a large dose of quinine made him feel as though he had a malarial attack) and by search of records he 'discovered' a 'law' that is central to *homoeopathy*, and from which the name is derived (cf. *allopathy*, p. 6):

> Similar symptoms in the remedy remove similar symptoms in the disease. The eternal, universal law of Nature, that every disease is destroyed and cured through the similar artificial disease which the appropriate remedy has the tendency to excite, rests on the following proposition: that only one disease can exist in the body at any one time.

In addition to the above, Hahnemann 'discovered' that dilution potentiates the effect of drugs, but not of trace impurities (provided the dilution is shaken correctly, i.e. by 'succussion'), even to the extent that an effective dose may not contain a single molecule of the drug. It has been pointed out[37] that the 'thirtieth potency' (1 in 10^{30}), recommended by Hahnemann, provided a solution in which there would be one molecule of drug in a volume of a sphere of literally astronomical circumference.

The therapeutic efficacy of a dilution at which no drug is present (including sodium chloride prepared in this way) is explained by the belief that a spiritual energy diffused throughout the medicine by the particular way in which the dilutions are shaken (succussion) during preparation, or that the active molecules leave behind some sort of 'imprint' on solvent or excipient.[38] The absence of potentiation of the inevitable contaminating impurities is attributed to the fact that they are not incorporated by serial dilution.

Thus, writes a critic:

> We are asked to put aside the whole edifice of evidence concerning the physical nature of materials and the normal concentration–response relationships of biologically active substances in order to accommodate homoeopathic potency.[39]

---

[33]Hu Z, Yang X, Ho P C L et al 2005 Herb–drug interactions. A literature review. Drugs 65:1239–1281.

[34]Greek: *homos* = same; *patheia* = suffering.

[35]1810: trans. Wheeler C E 1913 [Organon of the rational art of healing.] Dent, London.

[36]Hahnemann S 1805 Aesculapius in the balance. Leipsic.

[37]Clark A J 1937 General pharmacology. In: Hefter's Handbuch. Springer, Berlin.

[38]Homoeopathic practitioners repeatedly express their irritation that critics give so much attention to dilution. They should not be surprised, considering the enormous implications of their claim.

[39]Cuthbert A W 1982 Pharmaceutical Journal 15 May:547.

But no hard evidence that tests the hypothesis is supplied to justify this, and we are invited, for instance, to accept that sodium chloride merely diluted is no remedy, but that 'it raises itself to the most wonderful power through a well prepared dynamisation process' and stimulates the defensive powers of the body against the disease.

Pharmacologists have felt, in the absence of conclusive evidence from empirical studies that homoeopathic medicines can reproducibly be shown to differ from placebo, that there is no point in discussing its hypotheses.[40] But empirical studies can be made without accepting any particular theory of causation; nor should the results of good studies be disregarded just because the proposed theory of action seems incredible or is unknown.

A meta-analysis of 186 double-blind and/or randomised placebo-controlled trials of homoeopathic remedies found that 89 had adequate data for analysis. The authors concluded that their results 'were not compatible with the hypothesis that the clinical effects are completely due to placebo', but also found 'insufficient evidence from these studies that homoeopathy is clearly efficacious for any single clinical condition'.[41] A subsequent analysis of 110 homoeopathic and 110 conventional medicine trials found that there was 'weak evidence for a specific effect of homeopathic remedies, but strong evidence for a specific effect of conventional interventions.' The authors concluded: 'This finding is compatible with the notion that the clinical effects of homeopathy are placebo effects.'[42] These studies evoked strong reactions from practitioners of homoeopathy and others, but they raise the possibility that patients' reactions to homoeopathy, and indeed some other forms of CAM, may rest within an understanding of the complex nature of the placebo response and, in particular, its biology (see below).

CONCLUSION

There is a single fundamental issue between conventional scientific medicine and traditional, complementary and alternative medicine (although it is often obscured by detailed debates on individual practices); the issue is: what constitutes acceptable evidence, i.e. what is the nature, quality and interpretation of evidence that can justify general adoption of modes of treatment and acceptance of hypotheses? When there is agreement that a CAM treatment works, it becomes conventional and, in respect of that treatment, there is no difference between CAM and orthodox scientific medicine.

In the meantime, we depend on the accumulation of evidence from empirical studies to justify the allocation of resources for future research.

PLACEBO MEDICINES

A placebo[43] is any component of therapy that is without specific biological activity for the condition being treated.

Placebo medicines are used for two purposes:

- As a control in scientific evaluation of drugs (see Therapeutic trials, p. 50).
- To benefit or please a patient, not by any pharmacological actions, but by psychological means.

All treatments have a psychological component, whether to please (placebo effect) or, occasionally, to vex (negative placebo or nocebo[44] effect).

---

[40]Editorial 1988 When to believe the unbelievable. Nature 333:787. A report of an investigation into experiments with antibodies in solutions that contained no antibody molecules (as in some homoeopathic medicines). The editor of *Nature* took a three-person team (one of whom was a professional magician, included to detect any trickery) on a week-long visit to the laboratory that claimed positive results. Despite the scientific seriousness of the operation, it developed comical aspects (codes of the contents of test tubes were taped to the laboratory ceiling); the *Nature* team, having reached an unfavourable view of the experiments, 'sped past the [*laboratory*] common-room filled with champagne bottles destined now not to be opened'. Full reports in this issue of *Nature* (28 July 1988), including an acrimonious response by the original scientist, are highly recommended reading, both for scientific logic and for entertainment. See also Nature (1994) 370:322.

[41]Linde K, Clausius N, Melchart D et al 1997 Are the clinical effects of homoeopathy placebo effects? A meta-analysis of placebo-controlled trials. Lancet 350:834–843.

[42]Shang A, Huwiler-Müntener K, Nartey L et al 2005 Are the clinical effects of homeopathy placebo effects? Comparative study of placebo-controlled trials of homeopathy and allopathy. Lancet 366:726–732.

[43]Latin: *placebo* = shall be pleasing or acceptable. For a comment on its historical use, see Edwards M 2005 Lancet 365:1023.

[44]Latin: *nocebo* = shall injure; the term is little used.

A placebo medicine is a vehicle for 'cure' by suggestion, and is surprisingly often successful, if only temporarily.[45] All treatments carry a placebo effect – physiotherapy, psychotherapy, surgery, entering a patient into a therapeutic trial, even the personality and style of the doctor – but the effect is most easily investigated with drugs, for the active and the inert can often be made to appear identical to allow comparisons.

The deliberate use of drugs as placebos is a confession of therapeutic failure by the doctor. Failures, however, are sometimes inevitable and an absolute condemnation of the use of placebos on all occasions would be unrealistic.

> A placebo-reactor is an individual who reports changes of physical or mental state after taking a pharmacologically inert substance.

Placebo-reactors are suggestible people who are likely to respond favourably to any treatment. They have misled doctors into making false therapeutic claims.

Negative reactors, who develop adverse effects when given a placebo, exist but, fortunately, are fewer.

Some 30–80% of patients with chronic stable angina pectoris and 30–50% with depression respond to placebos. Placebo reaction is an inconstant attribute: a person may respond at one time in one situation and not at another time under different conditions. In one study on medical students, psychological tests revealed that those who reacted to a placebo tended to be extroverted, sociable, less dominant, less self-confident, more appreciative of their teaching, more aware of their autonomic functions and more neurotic than their colleagues who did not react to a placebo under the particular conditions of the experiment.

Modern brain-scanning techniques provide evidence that the placebo effect has a physiological basis. Positron emission tomography showed that both opioid and placebo analgesia were associated with increased activity in the same cortical area of the brain, the greatest responses occurring in high placebo responders.[46] Functional magnetic resonance imaging demonstrated that strong cortical activation correlated with greater placebo-induced pain relief.[47]

It is important that all who administer drugs should be aware that their attitudes to the treatment may greatly influence the outcome. Undue scepticism may prevent a drug from achieving its effect, and enthusiasm or confidence may potentiate the actions of drugs.

Tonics are placebos. They may be defined as substances that aspire to strengthen and increase the appetite of those so weakened by disease, misery, overindulgence in play or work, or by physical or mental inadequacy, that they cannot face the stresses of life. The essential feature of this weakness is the absence of any definite recognisable defect for which there is a known remedy. As tonics are placebos, they must be harmless.[48]

PRESCRIBING, DRUG CONSUMPTION AND ECONOMICS

The reasons for taking a drug history from patients are:

- Drugs are a *cause* of disease. Withdrawal of drugs, if abrupt, can cause disease, e.g. benzodiazepines, antiepilepsy drugs.
- Drugs can *conceal* disease, e.g. adrenal steroid.

---

[45]As the following account by a mountain rescue guide illustrates: 'The incident involved a 15-year-old boy who sustained head injuries and a very badly broken leg. Helicopter assistance was unavailable and therefore we had to carry him by stretcher to the nearest landrover (several miles away) and then on to a waiting ambulance. During this long evacuation the boy was in considerable distress and we administered Entonox (a mixture of nitrous oxide and oxygen, 50% each) sparingly as we only had one small cylinder. He repeatedly remarked how much better he felt after each intake of Entonox (approximately every 20 minutes) and after 7 hours or so, we eventually got him safely into the ambulance and on his way to hospital. On going to replace the Extonox we discovered the cylinder was still full of gas due to the equipment being faulty. There was no doubt that the boy felt considerable pain relief because he thought he was receiving Entonox.'

[46]Petrovic P, Kalso E, Petersson K et al 2002 Placebo and opioid analgesia – imaging a shared neuronal network. Science 295:1737–1740.
[47]Wager T D, Rilling J K, Smith E S et al 2004 Placebo induced changes in fMRI in anticipation and experience of pain. Science 303:1162–1167.
[48]Tonics (licensed) available in the UK include: Gentian Mixture, acid (or alkaline) (gentian, a natural plant bitter substance, and dilute hydrochloric acid or sodium bicarbonate); Labiton (thiamine, caffeine, alcohol, all in low dose).

- Drugs can *interact*, producing a positive adverse effect or a negative adverse effect, i.e. therapeutic failure.
- Drugs can give *diagnostic clues*, e.g. ampicillin and amoxicillin causing rash in infectious mononucleosis – a diagnostic adverse effect, not a diagnostic test.
- Drugs can cause *false results* in clinical chemistry tests, e.g. plasma cortisol, urinary catecholamine, urinary glucose.
- Drug history can assist *choice of drugs* in the future.
- Drugs can leave *residual effects* after administration has ceased, e.g. chloroquine, amiodarone.
- Drugs available for *independent patient self-medication* are increasing in range and importance.

(See also Appendix: the prescription.)
Prescribing should be *appropriate*:[49]

> Appropriate [*prescribing is that*] which bases the choice of a drug on its effectiveness, safety and convenience relative to other drugs or treatments (e.g. surgery or psychotherapy), and considers cost only when those criteria for choice have been satisfied. In some circumstances appropriateness will require the use of more costly drugs. Only by giving appropriateness high priority will [*health payers*] be able to achieve their aim of ensuring that patients' clinical needs will be met (Report).

Prescribing that is *inappropriate* is the result of several factors:

- Giving in to patient pressure to write unnecessary prescriptions. The extra time spent in careful explanation will, in the long run, be rewarded.
- Continuing patients, especially the elderly, on courses of medicinal treatment over many months without proper review of their medication.
- Doctors may 'prescribe brand-name drugs rather than cheaper generic equivalents, even where there is no conceivable therapeutic advantage in

so doing. The fact that the brand-name products often have shorter and more memorable names than their generic counterparts' contributes to this. (Report) (See also Chapter 6.)
- 'Insufficient training in clinical pharmacology. Many of the drugs on the market may not have been available when a general practitioner was at medical school. The sheer quantity of new products may lead to a practitioner becoming over-reliant on drugs companies' promotional material, or sticking to "tried and tested" products out of caution based on ignorance' (Report).
- Failure of doctors to keep up to date (see below, Doctor compliance).

Computerising prescribing addresses some of these issues, for example by prompting regular review of a patient's medication, by instantly providing generic names from brand names, by giving ready access to formularies and prescribing guidelines.

COST-CONTAINMENT

Cost-containment in prescription drug therapy attracts increasing attention. It may involve two particularly contentious activities:

1. *Generic substitution*, where a generic formulation (see p. 71) is substituted (by a pharmacist) for the proprietary formulation prescribed by the doctor.
2. *Therapeutic substitution*, where a drug of different chemical structure is substituted for the drug prescribed by the doctor. The substitute is of the same chemical class and is deemed to have similar pharmacological properties and to give similar therapeutic benefit. Therapeutic substitution is a particularly controversial matter where it is done without consulting the prescriber, and legal issues may be raised in the event of adverse therapeutic outcome.

The following facts and opinions are worth some thought:

- UK National Health Service (NHS) spending on drugs has been 9–11% per year (of the total cost) for nearly 50 years.
- General practitioners (i.e. primary care) spend some 80% of the total cost of drugs.
- In the past 25 years, the number of NHS prescriptions has risen from 5.5 to over 13 per person.

---

[49]The text on appropriate prescribing and some quotations (designated 'Report') are based on a UK Parliamentary Report (The National Health Service Drugs Budget 1994 HMSO, London). Twelve members of Parliament took evidence from up to 100 organisations and individuals orally and/or in writing.

- The average cost per head of medicines supplied to people aged over 75 years is nearly five times that of medicines supplied to those below pensionable age (in the UK: women 62 years, men 65 years, but under revision).
- Underprescribing can be just as harmful to the health of patients as overprescribing.

It is crucially important that incentives and sanctions address quality of prescribing as well as quantity: 'it would be wrong if too great a preoccupation with the cost issue in isolation were to encourage underprescribing or have an adverse effect on patient care' (Report).

Reasons for underprescribing include: lack of information or lack of the will to use available information (in economically privileged countries there is, if anything, a surplus of information); fear of being blamed for adverse reactions (affecting doctors who lack the confidence that a knowledge of pharmacological principles confers); fear of sanctions against over-costly prescribing. Prescription frequency and cost per prescription are lower for older than for younger doctors. There is no evidence that the patients of older doctors are worse off as a result.

REPEAT PRESCRIPTIONS

About two-thirds of general (family) practice prescriptions are for repeat medication (half issued by the doctor at a consultation and half via the practice nurse or receptionist without patient contact with the doctor). Some 95% of patients' requests are acceded to without further discussion; 25% of patients who receive repeat prescriptions have had 40 or more repeats; and 55% of patients aged over 75 years are on repeat medication (with periodic review).

Many patients taking the same drug for years are doing so for the best reason, i.e. firm diagnosis for which effective therapy is available, such as epilepsy, diabetes, hypertension, but some are not.

WARNINGS AND CONSENT

Doctors have a professional duty to inform and to warn, so that patients, who are increasingly informed and educated, may make meaningful personal choices, which it is their right to do (unless they opt to leave the choice to the doctor, which it is also their right). Patients now have access to a potentially confusing quantity of detail about the unwanted effects of drugs (information sheet, the internet, the media) but without the balancing influence of data on their frequency of occurrence. It would be prudent for doctors to draw attention at least to adverse effects that are common, serious (even if uncommon), or avoidable or mitigated if recognised.

> Warnings to patients are of two kinds:
> - Warnings that will affect the patient's choice to accept or reject the treatment
> - Warnings that will affect the safety of the treatment once it has begun, e.g. risk of stopping treatment, occurrence of drug toxicity.

Just as engineers say that the only safe aeroplane is the one that stays on the ground in still air on a disused airfield or in a locked hangar, so the only safe drug is one that stays in its original package. If drugs are not safe then plainly patients are entitled to be warned of their hazards, which should be explained to them, i.e. probability, nature and severity.

There is no formal legal or ethical obligation on doctors to warn all patients of all possible adverse consequences of treatment. It is their duty to adapt the information they give (not too little, and not so much as to cause confusion) so that the best interest of each patient is served. If there is a 'real' (say 1–2%) risk inherent in a procedure of some misfortune occurring, then doctors should warn patients of the possibility that the injury may occur, however well the treatment is performed. Doctors should take into account the personality of the patient, the likelihood of any misfortune arising and what warning was necessary for each particular patient's welfare.[50]

Doctors should consider what their particular individual patients would wish to know (i.e. would be likely to attach significance to) and not only what they think (paternalistically) the patients ought to know. It is part of the professionalism of doctors to tell what is appropriate to the individual patient's interest. If things go wrong doctors must be prepared to defend what they did or, more important in the case of warnings, what they did not do, as being in their patient's best interest. Courts of law will look critically at doctors who seek to justify under-information by saying that they feared to confuse or

---

[50]Legal correspondent 1980 British Medical Journal 280:575.

frighten the patient (or that they left it to the patient to ask, as one doctor did). The increasing availability of patient information leaflets (PILs) prepared by the manufacturer indicates the increasing trend to give more information. Doctors should know what their patients have read (or not read, as is so often the case) when patients express dissatisfaction.

Evidence that extensive information on risks causes 'unnecessary' anxiety or frightens patients suggests that this is only a marginal issue and it does not justify a general policy of withholding of information.

LEGAL HAZARDS FOR PRESCRIBERS

Doctors would be less than human if, as well as trying to help their patients, they were not also concerned to protect themselves from allegations of malpractice (negligence). A lawyer specialising in the field put the legal position regarding a doctor's duty pungently:

> The provision of information to patients is treated by (English) law as but one part of the way a doctor discharges the obligation he owes to a patient to take reasonable care in all aspects of his treatment of that patient. The provision of information is a corollary of the patient's right to self-determination which is a right recognised by law. Failure to provide appropriate information will usually be a breach of duty and if that breach leads to the patient suffering injury then the basis for a claim for compensation exists.[51]

The keeping of appropriate medical records, written at the time of consultation (and which is so frequently neglected), is not only good medical practice, it is the best way of ensuring that there is an answer to unjustified allegations, made later, when memory has faded. At the very least, these should include records of warning about treatments that are potentially hazardous.

FORMULARIES, GUIDELINES AND 'ESSENTIAL' DRUGS

Increasingly, doctors recognise that they need guidance through the bountiful menu (thousands of medicines) so seductively served to them by the pharmaceutical industry. Principal sources of guidance are the pharmaceutical industry ('prescribe my drug') and governments ('spend less'), and also the developing (profit-making) managed care/insurance bodies ('spend less') and the proliferating drug bulletins offering independent, and supposedly unbiased advice ('prescribe appropriately').

Even the pharmaceutical industry, in its more sober moments, recognises that their ideal world in which doctors, advised and informed by industry alone, were free to prescribe whatever they pleased,[52] to whomsoever they pleased, for as long as they pleased with someone other than the patient paying, is an unrealisable dream of a 'never-never land'.

The industry knows that it has to learn to live with restrictions of some kinds and one of the means of restriction is the formulary, a list of formulations of medicines with varying amounts of added information. A formulary may list all nationally licensed medicines prescribable by health professionals, or list only preferred drugs.

It may be restricted to what a third-party payer will reimburse, or to the range of formulations stocked in a hospital (and chosen by a local drugs and therapeutics committee, which all hospitals or groups of hospitals should have), or the range agreed by a partnership of general practitioners or primary care health centre.

All restricted formularies are heavily motivated to keep costs down without impairing appropriate prescribing (see p. 19). They should make provision for prescribing outside their range in cases of special need with an 'escape clause'.

Thus, restricted formularies are in effect guidelines for prescribing. There is a profusion of these from national sources, hospitals, group practices and specialty organisations (epilepsy, diabetes mellitus).

'Essential' drugs

Economically disadvantaged countries may seek help to construct formularies. Technical help comes

---

[52]It is difficult for us now to appreciate the naive fervour and trust in doctors that allowed them almost unlimited rights to prescribe in the early years of the UK National Health Service (founded in 1948). Beer was a prescription item in hospitals until, decades later, an audit revealed that only 1 in 10 bottles reached a patient. More recently (1992): 'There could be fewer Christmas puddings consumed this year. The puddings were recently struck off a bizarre list of items that doctors were able to prescribe for their patients. They were removed by Health Department officials without complaint from the medics, on the grounds they had "no therapeutic or clinical value".' (Lancet [1992] 340:1531).

---

[51]Ian Dodds-Smith.

from the World Health Organization (WHO) with its Model List of Essential Medicines,[53] i.e. drugs (or representatives of classes of drugs) 'that satisfy the health care needs of the majority of the population; they should therefore be available at all times in adequate amounts and in the appropriate dosage forms'. Countries seeking such advice can use the list as a basis for their own choices (the WHO also publishes model prescribing information).[54] The list, updated regularly, contains about 300 items.

The pharmaceutical industry dislikes the concept of drugs classed as essential as others, by implication, are judged inessential. But the WHO programme has attracted much interest and approval (see WHO Technical Report Series: The use of essential drugs: current edition).

COMPLIANCE

Successful therapy, especially if it is long term, comprises a great deal more than choosing a standard medicine. It involves patient and doctor compliance.[55] The latter is liable to be overlooked (by doctors), for doctors prefer to dwell on the deficiencies of their patients rather than of themselves.

PATIENT COMPLIANCE

Patient compliance is the extent to which the actual behaviour of the patient coincides with medical advice and instructions; it may be complete, partial, erratic, nil, or there may be over-compliance. To make a diagnosis and to prescribe evidence-based effective treatment is a satisfying experience for doctors, but too many assume that patients will gratefully or accurately do what they are told, i.e. obtain the medicine and consume it as instructed. This assumption is wrong.

The rate of non-presentation (or redemption) of prescriptions in the UK is around 5%, but is up to 20% or even more in the elderly (who pay no prescription charge). Where lack of money to pay for the medicine is not the cause, this is due to lack of motivation.

Having obtained the medicine, some 25–50% (sometimes even more) of patients either fail to follow the instruction to a significant extent (taking 50–90% of the prescribed dose), or they do not take it at all.

Patient non-compliance is identified as a major factor in therapeutic failure in both routine practice and in scientific therapeutic trials; but, sad to say, doctors are too often non-compliant about remedying this. All patients are potential non-compliers;[56] clinical criteria cannot reliably predict good compliance, but non-compliance often can be predicted.

In addition to therapeutic failure, undetected non-compliance may lead to rejection of the best drug when it is effective, leading to substitution by second-rank medcines.

Non-compliance may occur because:

- the patient has not understood the instructions, so cannot comply,[57] or
- understands the instructions, but fails to carry them out.

Prime factors for poor patient compliance are:

- *Frequency and complexity of the drug regimen.* Many studies attest to polypharmacy as an inhibitor of compliance, i.e. more than three

---

[53]Available on the WHO website: http://www.who.org.
[54]There is an agency for WHO publications in all UN countries.
[55]The term compliance meets objection as having undertones of obsolete, authoritarian attitudes, implying 'obedience' to doctors' 'orders'. The words adherence or concordance are preferred by some, the latter because it expresses the duality of drug prescribing (by the doctor) and taking (by the patient), i.e. a therapeutic alliance. We retain compliance, pointing out that it applies equally to those doctors who neither keep up to date, nor follow prescribing instructions, and to patients who fail, for whatever reason, to keep to a drug regimen.

[56]Even where the grave consequences of non-compliance are understood (glaucoma: blindness) (renal transplant: organ rejection), significant non-compliance has been reported in as many as 20% of patients; psychologists will be able to suggest explanations for this.
[57]Cautionary tales:
– A 62-year-old man requiring a metered-dose inhaler (for the first time) was told to 'spray the medicine to the throat'. He was found to have been conscientiously aiming and firing the aerosol to his anterior neck around the thyroid cartilage, four times a day for 2 weeks (Chiang A A, Lee J C 1994 New England Journal of Medicine 330:1690).
– A patient thought that 'sublingual' meant able to speak two languages; another that tablets cleared obstructed blood vessels by exploding inside them (E A Kay) – reference, no doubt, to colloquial use of the term 'clot-busting drugs' (for thrombolytics).
– These are extreme examples; most are more subtle and less detectable. Doctors may smile at the ignorant naivety of patients, but the smile should give way to a blush of shame at their own deficiencies as communicators.

drugs taken concurrently or more than three drug-taking occasions in the day (the ideal of one occasion only is often unattainable).

- *Unintentional non-compliance*, or forgetfulness,[58] may be addressed by associating drug-taking with cues in daily life (breakfast, bedtime), by special packaging (e.g. calendar packs) and by enlisting the aid of others (e.g. carers, teachers).
- *'Intelligent' or wilful non-compliance*.[59] Patients decide they do not need the drug (asymptomatic disease) or they do not like the drug (unwanted effects), or take 2–3-day 'drug holidays'.
- *Illness*. This includes cognitive impairment and psychological problems, with depression being a particular problem.
- *Lack of information*. Oral instructions alone are not enough; one-third of patients are unable to recount instructions immediately on leaving the consulting room. Lucid and legible labelling of containers is essential, as well as patient-friendly information leaflets, which are increasingly available via doctors and pharmacists, and as package inserts.
- *Poor patient–doctor relationship and lack of motivation* to take medicines as instructed offer a major challenge to the prescriber whose diagnosis and prescription may be perfect, yet loses efficacy by patient non-compliance. Unpleasant disease symptoms, particularly

where these are recurrent and known by previous experience to be quickly relieved, provide the highest motivation (i.e. self-motivation) to comply. But particularly where the patient does not feel ill, adverse effects are immediate, and benefits are perceived to be remote, e.g. in hypertension, where they may be many years away in the future, doctors must consciously address themselves to motivating compliance. The best way to achieve compliance is to cultivate the patient–doctor relationship. Doctors cannot be expected actually to like all their patients, but it is a great help (where liking does not come naturally) if they make a positive effort to understand how individual patients must feel about their illnesses and their treatments, i.e. to empathise with their patients. This is not always easy, but its achievement is the action of the true professional, and indeed is part of their professional duty of care.

Suggestions for doctors to enhance patient compliance

- Form a non-judgemental alliance or partnership with the patient, giving the patient an opportunity to ask questions.
- Plan a regimen with the minimum number of drugs and drug-taking occasions, adjusted to fit the patient's lifestyle. Use fixed-dose combinations, sustained-release (or injectable depot) formulations, or long $t_{1/2}$ drugs as appropriate; arrange direct observation of each dose in exceptional cases.
- Provide clear oral and written information adapted to the patient's understanding and medical and cultural needs.
- Use patient-friendly packaging, e.g. calendar packs, where appropriate; or monitored-dose systems, e.g. boxes compartmented and labelled.
- See the patient regularly and not so infrequently that the patient feels the doctor has lost interest.
- Enlist the help of family members, carers, friends.
- Use computer-generated reminders for repeat prescriptions.

Directly observed therapy (DOT) (where a reliable person supervises each dose). In addition to the areas where supervision is obviously in the inter-est of patients, e.g. a child, DOT is employed (even

[58]Where non-compliance, whether intentional or unintentional, is medically serious it becomes necessary to bypass self-administration (unsupervised) and to resort to directly observed (supervised) oral administration or to injection (e.g. in schizophrenia).

[59]Of the many causes of failure of patient compliance, the following case must be unique: On a transatlantic flight the father of an asthmatic boy was seated in the row behind two doctors. He overheard one of the doctors expressing doubt about the long-term safety in children of inhaled corticosteroids. He interrupted the conversation, explaining that his son took this treatment; he had a lengthy conversation with one of the doctors, who gave his name. Consequently, on arrival, he faxed his wife at home to stop the treatment of their son immediately. She did so, and 2 days later the well controlled patient had a brisk relapse that responded to urgent treatment by the family doctor (who had been conscientiously following guidelines recently published in an authoritative journal). The family doctor later ascertained that the doctor in the plane was a member of the editorial team of the journal that had so recently published the guidelines that were favourable to inhaled corticosteroid (Cox S 1994 Is eavesdropping bad for your health? British Medical Journal 309:718).

imposed) among free-living uncooperative patients who may be a menace to the community, such as those with multiple drug-resistant tuberculosis.

What every patient needs to know[60]

- An account of the disease and the reason for prescribing
- The name of the medicine
- The objective:
  – to treat the disease and/or
  – to relieve symptoms, i.e. how important the medicine is, whether the patient can judge its efficacy and when benefit can be expected to occur
- How and when to take the medicine
- Whether it matters if a dose is missed and what, if anything, to do about it (see p. 26)
- For how long the medicine is likely to be needed
- How to recognise adverse effects and any action that should be taken, including effects on car driving
- Any interaction with alcohol or other medicines.

A remarkable instance of non-compliance, with hoarding, was that of a 71-year-old man who attempted suicide and was found to have in his home 46 bottles containing 10 685 tablets. Analysis of his prescriptions showed that over a period of 17 months he had been expected to take 27 tablets of several different kinds daily.[61]

From time to time there are campaigns to collect all unwanted drugs from homes in an area. Usually the public are asked to deliver the drugs to their local pharmacies. In one UK city (population 600 000),

500 000 'solid dose units' (tablets, capsules, etc.) were handed in (see below, Opportunity cost); such quantities have even caused local problems for safe waste disposal.

Factors that are *insignificant* for compliance are: age[62] (except at extremes), sex, intelligence (except at extreme deficiency) and educational level (probably).

Over-compliance. Patients (up to 20%) may take more drug than is prescribed, even increasing the dose by 50%. In diseases where precise compliance with frequent or complex regimens is important, for example in glaucoma where sight is at risk, there have been instances of obsessional patients responding to their doctors' overemphatic instructions by clock-watching in a state of anxiety to avoid the slightest deviance from timed administration of the correct dose, to the extent that their daily (and nightly) life becomes dominated by this single purpose.

Evaluation of patient compliance. Merely asking patients whether they have taken the drug as directed is not likely to provide reliable evidence[63]. It is safest to assume that any event that can impair compliance, will sometimes happen.

Estimations of compliance come from a variety of measures. DOT (above) is the most accurate, and identification of the drug or metabolites in plasma (or an artificial biological marker in the case of a clinical trial) is persuasive at least of recent compliance.

Requiring patients to produce containers when they attend the doctor, who counts the tablets, seems to do little more than show the patient that the doctor cares about the matter (which is useful); a tablet absent from a container has not necessarily entered the patient's body. On the other hand, although patients are known to practise deliberate deception, to maintain effective deception successfully

---

[60]After: Drug and Therapeutics Bulletin 1981; 19:73. *Patient information leaflets.* In economically privileged countries, original or patient-pack dispensing is becoming the norm, i.e. patients receive an unopened pack just as it left the manufacturer. The pack contains a Patient Information Leaflet (PIL) (which therefore accompanies each repeat prescription). Regulatory authorities increasingly determine its content. In this litigous age, requirements to be comprehensive and, to protect both manufacturer and regulatory authority, impair the patient-friendliness of PILs. But studies have shown that patients who receive leaflets are more satisfied than those who do not. Doctors need to have copies of these leaflets so that they can discuss with their patients what they are (or are not) reading.

[61]Smith S E, Stead K C 1974 Non-compliance or misprescribing? Lancet i:937 (letter).

[62]But the elderly are commonly taking several drugs – a major factor in non-compliance – and monitoring compliance in this age group becomes particularly important. The oversixties in the UK are, on average, each receiving two or three medications.

[63]Hippocrates (460–377 BC) noted that patients are liars regarding compliance. The way the patient is questioned may be all important, e.g. 'Were you able to take the tablets?' may get a truthful reply, whereas 'Did you take the tablets?' may not, because the latter question may be understood by the patient as implying personal criticism (Pearson R M 1982 Who is taking their tablets? British Medical Journal 285:757).

over long periods requires more effort than most patients are likely to make. Memory aids, such as drug diaries, monitored-dosage systems (e.g. compartmented boxes) and electronic containers that record times of opening are helpful.

Some pharmacodynamic effects, e.g. heart rate with a β-adrenoceptor blocker, provide a physiological marker as an indicator of the presence of drug in the body.

Compliance in new drug development

Non-compliance, discovered or undiscovered, can invalidate therapeutic trials (where compliance monitoring is essential). In new drug development trials the diluting effect of undetected non-compliance (prescribed doses are increased) can result in unduly high doses being initially recommended (licensed) (with toxicity in good compliers after marketing), so that the standard dose has soon to be urgently reduced (this has probably occurred with some new nonsteroidal anti-inflammatory drugs).

DOCTOR COMPLIANCE

Doctor compliance is the extent to which the behaviour of doctors fulfils their professional duty:

- not to be ignorant
- to adopt new advances when they are sufficiently proved (which doctors are often slow to do)
- to prescribe accurately[64]
- to tell patients what they need to know
- to warn, i.e. to recognise the importance of the act of prescribing.

In one study in a university hospital, where standards might be expected to be high, there was an error of drug use (dose, frequency, route) in 3% of prescriptions and an error of prescription writing (in relation to standard hospital instructions) in 30%. Many errors were trivial, but many could have resulted in overdose, serious interaction or under-treatment.

In other hospital studies, error rates in drug administration of 15–25% have been found, rates rising rapidly where four or more drugs are being given concurrently, as is often the case; studies of hospital inpatients show that each receives about six drugs, and up to 20 during a stay is not rare. Merely providing information (on antimicrobials) did not influence prescribing, but gently asking physicians to justify their prescriptions caused a marked fall in inappropriate prescribing.

On a harsher note, in recent years doctors who gave drugs, about which they later admitted ignorance (e.g. route of administration and/or dose), stood charged with manslaughter[65] and were convicted. Shocked by this, fellow doctors have written to the medical press offering understanding sympathy to these, sometimes junior, colleagues: 'There, but for the grace of God, go I'.[66] But the public response is not sympathetic. Doctors put themselves forward as trained professionals who offer a service of responsible, competent provision of drugs that they have the legal right to prescribe. The public is increasingly inclined to hold them to that claim, and, where doctors seriously fail, to exact retribution.[67]

If you do not know about a drug, find out before you act, or take the personal consequences, which, increasingly, may be very serious indeed.

UNDERDOSING

Use of suboptimal doses of drugs in serious disease occurs, sacrificing therapeutic efficacy to avoid serious adverse effects. Instances are commonest with drugs of low therapeutic index (see Index), i.e. where the effective and toxic dose ranges are close, or even overlap, e.g. heparin, anticancer drugs, aminoglycoside antimicrobials. In these cases dose adjustment

---

[64]Accuracy includes legibility: a doctor wrote Intal (sodium cromoglycate) for an asthmatic patient; the pharmacist read it as Inderal (propranolol) – the patient died. See also, Names of drugs (Chapter 6).

[65]Unlawful killing in circumstances that do not amount to murder (which requires an intention to kill), e.g. causing death by negligence that is much more serious than mere carelessness; reckless breach of the legal duty of care.

[66]Attributed to John Bradford, an English preacher and martyr (16th century), on seeing a convicted criminal pass by.

[67]A doctor wrote a prescription for isosorbide dinitrate 20 mg 6-hourly, but because of the illegibility of the handwriting the pharmacist dispensed felodipine in the same dose (maximum daily dose 10 mg). The patient died and a court ordered the doctor and pharmacist to pay compensation of $450 000 to the family. Charatan F 1999 Family compensated for death after illegible prescription. British Medical Journal 319:1456.

to obtain maximum benefit with minimum risk requires both knowledge and attentiveness.

THE CLINICAL IMPORTANCE OF MISSED DOSE(S)

Even the most conscientious of patients will miss a dose or doses occasionally. Patients should therefore be told whether this matters and what they should do about it, if anything.

Missed dose(s) may lead to:
- loss of therapeutic efficacy (acute disease)
- resurgence (chronic disease)
- rebound or withdrawal syndrome.

Loss of therapeutic efficacy involves the *pharmacokinetic properties* of drugs. With some drugs of short $t_{1/2}$, the issue is simply a transient drop in plasma concentration below a defined therapeutic concentration. The issues are more complex where therapeutic effect may not decline in parallel with plasma concentration, as with recovery of negative feedback homoeostatic mechanisms (adrenocortical steroids).

A single missed dose may be important with some drugs, e.g. oral contraceptives, but with others (long $t_{1/2}$), omission of several doses is tolerated without any serious decline in efficacy, e.g. thyroxine (levothyroxine).

These pharmacokinetic considerations are complex and important, and are, or should be, taken into account by drug manufacturers in devising dosage schedules and informative data sheets. Manufacturers should aim at one or two doses per day (not more), and this is generally best achieved with drugs with relatively long biological effect $t_{1/2}$ or, where the biological effect $t_{1/2}$ is short, by using sustained-release formulations.

Discontinuation syndrome (recurrence of disease, rebound, or withdrawal syndrome) may occur due to a variety of mechanisms (see Index).

PHARMACOECONOMICS

Even the richest societies cannot satisfy the appetite of their citizens for health care based on their real needs, on their wants and on their (often unrealistic) expectations.

Health-care resources are rationed[68] in one way or another, whether according to national social policies or to individual wealth. The debate on supply is not about whether there should be rationing, but about what form rationing should take; whether it should be explicit or concealed (from the public).

Doctors prescribe, patients consume and, increasingly throughout the world, third (purchasing) parties (government, insurance companies) pay the bill with money they have obtained from increasingly reluctant healthy members of the public.

The purchasers of health care are now engaged in serious exercises to contain drug costs in the short term without impairing the quality of medical care, or damaging the development of useful new drugs (which is an enormously expensive and long-term process). This can be achieved successfully only if reliable data are available on costs and benefits, both absolute and relative. The difficulties of generating such data, not only during development, but later under conditions of actual use, are enormous and are addressed by a special breed of professionals: the health economists.

Economics is the science of the distribution of wealth and resources. Prescribing doctors, who have a duty to the community as well as to individual patients, cannot escape involvement with economics.

THE ECONOMISTS' OBJECTIVE

The objective is to define needs, thereby enabling the deployment of resources according to priorities set by society, which has an interest in fairness between its members.

Resources can be distributed by the outcome of an unregulated power struggle between professionals and associations of patients and public pressure groups – all, no doubt, warm-hearted towards deserving cases of one kind or another, but none able to view the whole scene. Alternatively, distribution can occur by a planned evaluation that allows division of the resources based on some visible attempt at fairness.

A health economist[69] writes:

---

[68]The term rationing is used here to embrace the allocation of priorities as well as the actual withholding of resources (in this case, drugs).
[69]Professor Michael Drummond.

The economist's approach to evaluating drug therapies is to look at a group of patients with a particular disorder and the various drugs that could be used to treat them. The costs of the various treatments and some costs associated with their use (together with the costs of giving no treatment) are then considered in terms of impact on health status (survival and quality of life) and impact on other health care costs (e.g. admissions to hospital, need for other drugs, use of other procedures).

Economists are often portrayed as people who want to focus on cost, whereas in reality they see everything in terms of a balance between costs and benefits.

Four economic concepts have particular importance to the thinking of every doctor who makes a decision to prescribe, i.e. to distribute resources:

- *Opportunity cost* means that which has to be sacrificed in order to carry out a certain course of action, i.e. costs are benefits foregone elsewhere. Money spent on prescribing is not available for another purpose; wasteful prescribing is as an affront to those who are in serious need, e.g. institutionalised mentally handicapped citizens who everywhere would benefit from increased resources.
- *Cost–effectiveness analysis* is concerned with how to attain a given objective at minimal financial cost, e.g. prevention of post-surgical venous thromboembolism by heparins, warfarin, aspirin, external pneumatic compression. Analysis includes the cost of materials, adverse effects, any tests, nursing and doctor time, duration of stay in hospital (which may greatly exceed the cost of the drug).
- *Cost–benefit analysis* is concerned with issues of whether (and to what extent) to pursue objectives and policies; it is thus a broader activity than cost–effectiveness analysis and puts monetary values on the quality as well as on the quantity (duration) of life.
- *Cost–utility analysis* is concerned with comparisons between programmes, such as an antenatal drug treatment, which saves a young life, or a hip replacement operation, which improves mobility in a man of 60 years. Such differing issues are also the basis for comparison by computing quality-adjusted life-years (see below).

An allied measure is the *cost–minimisation analysis*, which finds the least costly programme among those shown or assumed to be of equal benefit. Economic analysis requires that both quantity and quality of life be measured. The former is easy, the latter is hard to determine.

In the UK the National Institute for Health and Clinical Excellence (NICE) appraises the clinical effectiveness and cost effectiveness of drugs, devices and diagnostic tools, and advises health-care professionals in the NHS on their use. The NHS is legally obliged to make resources available to implement NICE guidance, so avoiding differential treatment according to a patient's area of residence – so-called 'postcode prescribing'.

QUALITY OF LIFE

Everyone is familiar with the measurement of the benefit of treatment in saving or extending life, i.e. life expectancy: the measure is the *quantity* of life (in years). But it is evident that life may be extended and yet have a low quality, even to the point that it is not worth having at all. It is therefore useful to have a unit of health measurement that combines the quantity of life with its *quality*, to place individual and social decision-making on a sounder basis than mere intuition. Economists met this need by developing the *quality-adjusted life-year* (QALY) whereby estimations of years of life expectancy are modified according to estimations of quality of life.

Quality of life has four principal dimensions:[70]

1. Physical mobility.
2. Freedom from pain and distress.
3. Capacity for self-care.
4. Ability to engage in normal work and social interactions.

The approach for determining quality of life is by questionnaire, to measure what the subject perceives as personal health. The assessments are refined to provide improved assessment of the benefits and risks of medicines to the individual and to society. The challenge is to ensure that these are sufficiently robust to make resource allocation decisions between, for example, the rich and the poor, the educated and the uneducated, the old and the young, as well as between groups of patients with very different diseases. Plainly, quality of life is a major aspect of what is called outcomes research.

---

[70]Williams A 1983 In: Smith G T (ed.) Measuring the social benefits of medicine. Office of Health Economics, London.

SELF-MEDICATION

To feel unwell is common, although the frequency varies with social and cultural circumstances. People commonly experience symptoms or complaints, and commonly want to take remedial action. In one study of adults randomly selected from a large population, 9 out of 10 had one or more complaints in the 2 weeks before interview; in another of pre-menopausal women, a symptom occurred as often as 1 day in 3; in both studies a medicine was taken for more than half of these occurrences.

SELF-MEDICATION AND CONSUMER RIGHTS

> Increasingly, educated and confident consumers are aware of five consumer rights (United Nations charter):
> - access (to a wide range of products)
> - choice (self-determination)
> - information (on which to base choice)
> - redress (when things go wrong)
> - safety (appropriate to the use of the product).

Modern consumers (patients) wish to take a greater role in the maintenance of their own health and are often competent to manage (uncomplicated) chronic and recurrent illnesses (not merely short-term symptoms) after proper medical diagnosis and with only occasional professional advice, e.g. use of histamine H_2-receptor blockers, topical corticosteroids and antifungals, and oral contraceptives. They are understandably unwilling to submit to the inconvenience of visiting a doctor for what they rightly feel they can manage for themselves, given adequate information. Legislation in the USA permits the advertising of prescription drugs direct to consumer (DTC). Advertising has spurred millions of people to take cyclo-oxygenase-2 (COX-2) inhibitors, even when not indicated (see rofecoxib, pp. 256–257).

Increased consumer autonomy leads to satisfied:

- consumers (above)
- governments (lower drug bill)
- industry (profits)
- doctors (reduced workload).

The pharmaceutical industry enthusiastically estimates that extending the use of self-medication to all potentially self-treatable illnesses could save 100 to 150 million general practitioner consultations per year in the UK (population 60 million). But there will also be added costs as pharmacists extend their responsibilities for supply and information.

Regulatory authorities are increasingly receptive to switching hitherto prescription-only medicines (POM) for self-medication (over-the-counter, OTC, sale) via pharmacies (P) or via any retail outlet (general sale). The operation is known as POM-OTC or POM-P 'switch'. It requires particularly exacting standards of safety.

> **Self-medication is appropriate for:**
> - short-term relief of symptoms where accurate diagnosis is unnecessary
> - uncomplicated cases of some chronic and recurrent disease (a medical diagnosis having been made and advice given).

Safety in self-medication (an overriding requirement) depends on four items:

1. *The drug* – its inherent properties, dose and duration of use, including its power to induce dependence.
2. *The formulation* – devised with unsupervised use in mind, e.g. low dose.
3. *Information* – available with all purchases (printed) and rigorously reviewed (by panels of potential users) for user-friendliness and adequacy for a wide range of education and intellectual capacity.
4. *Patient compliance.*

> Doctors must recognise the increasing importance of questioning about self-medication when taking a drug history (see p. 18).

GUIDE TO FURTHER READING

Barach P, Small S D 2000 Reporting and preventing medical mishaps: lessons from non-medical near miss reporting systems. British Medical Journal 320:759–763
The whole issue (18 March 2000) should be consulted for its extensive coverage of the subject of medical error
Berndt E R 2005 To inform or persuade? Direct-to-consumer advertising of prescription drugs. New England Journal of Medicine 352(4):325–328

Blake D R 2003 Alternative prescribing and negligence. British Medical Journal 326:455

Buetow S, Elwyn G 2007 Patient safety and patient error. Lancet 369:158–161

Cohen J P, Paquette C, Cairns C P 2005 Switching prescription drugs to over the counter. British Medical Journal 330:39–41

De Smet P A G M 2004 Health risks of herbal remedies. Clinical Pharmacology and Therapeutics 76(1):1–17

Jones G 2003 Prescribing and taking medicines. British Medical Journal 327:819 (and other related articles in issue no. 7419 [11 October 2003] of this journal)

Kandela P 1999 Sketches from *The Lancet*: Doctors' handwriting. Lancet 353:1109

Kessels R P C 2003 Patients' memory for medical information. Journal of the Royal Society of Medicine 96(5):219–222

Loudon I 2006 A brief history of homeopathy. Journal of the Royal Society of Medicine 99:607–610

Mason S, Tovey P, Long A F 2002 Evaluating complementary medicine: methodological challenges of randomised controlled trials. British Medical Journal 325:832–834

Meltzer M I 2001 Introduction to health economics for physicians. Lancet 358:993–998 (and subsequent papers in this quintet)

Moynihan R, Bero L, Ross-Degnan D et al 2000 Coverage by the news media of the benefits and risks of medications. New England Journal of Medicine 342(22):1645–1650

Neale G, Chapman E J, Hoare J, Olsen S 2006 Recognising adverse events and critical incidents in medical practice in a district general hospital. Clinical Medicine 6(4):157–162

Osterberg L, Blaschke T 2005 Adherence to medication. New England Journal of Medicine 353(5):487–497

Rawlins M D 2004 NICE work – providing guidance to the British National Health Service. New England Journal of Medicine 351(3):1381–1385

Simpson S H, Eurich D T, Majumdar S R et al 2006 A meta-analysis of the association between adherence to drug therapy and mortality. British Medical Journal 333:15

Vincent C 2003 Understanding and responding to adverse events. New England Journal of Medicine 348(11):1051–1056

APPENDIX: THE PRESCRIPTION

The prescription is the means by which patients receive medicines that are considered unsafe for sale directly to the public. Its format is officially regulated to ensure precision in the interests of safety and efficacy, and to prevent fraudulent misuse; full details appear in national formularies, and prescribers have a responsibility to comply with these.

Prescriptions of pure drugs or of formulations from the *British National Formulary* (BNF)[71] are satisfactory for almost all purposes. The composition of many of the preparations in the BNF is laid down in official pharmacopoeias, e.g. British Pharmacopoeia (BP). There are also many national and international pharmacopoeias.

Traditional extemporaneous prescription-writing art, defining drug, base, adjuvant, corrective, flavouring and vehicle, is obsolete, as is the use of the Latin language. Certain convenient Latin abbreviations do survive for lack of convenient English substitutes. They appear below, without approval or disapproval.

> The elementary requirements of a prescription are that it should state what is to be given to whom and by whom prescribed, and give instructions on how much should be taken, how often, by what route and for how long, or the total quantity to be supplied, as below.

1. **Date.**
2. **Address of doctor.**
3. **Name and address of patient**: date of birth is also desirable for safety reasons; in the UK it is a legal requirement for children aged under 12 years.
4. **R** – This is a traditional esoteric symbol[72] for the word 'Recipe' – 'take thou', which is addressed to the pharmacist. It is pointless; but as many doctors gain a harmless pleasure from writing it with a flourish before the name of a proprietary preparation of whose exact nature they may be ignorant, it is likely to survive as a sentimental link with the past.
5. **Name and dose of the medicine.**
   Abbreviations. Only abbreviate where there is an official abbreviation. Never use unofficial abbreviations or invent your own; *it is not safe to do so.*
   Quantities (after BNF):
   – 1 gram or more: write 1 g, etc.
   – less than 1 g: write as milligrams: 500 mg, not 0.5 g
   – less than 1 mg: write as micrograms, e.g. 100 micrograms, not 0.1 mg

---

[71]Supplied free to all doctors practising in the UK National Health Service.
[72]Derived from the eye of Horus, ancient Egyptian sun god.

– for decimals, a zero should precede the decimal point where there is no other figure, e.g. 0.5 mL, not .5 mL; for a range, 0.5–1 g
– do not abbreviate microgram, nanogram or unit
– use millilitre (ml or mL), not cubic centimetre (cc)
– for home/domestic measures, see below.

State dose and dose frequency; for 'as required', specify minimum dose interval or maximum dose per day.

6. **Directions to the pharmacist**, if any: 'mix', 'make a solution'. Write the total quantity to be dispensed (if this is not stated in 5 above); or duration of supply.
7. **Instruction for the patient**, to be written on container by the pharmacist. Here brevity, clarity and accuracy are especially important. It is dangerous to rely on the patient remembering oral instructions. The BNF provides a list of recommended 'cautionary and advisory labels for dispensed medicines', representing a balance between 'the unintelligibly short and the inconveniently long', for example: 'Do not stop taking this medicine except on your doctor's advice'.

Pharmacists nowadays use their own initiative in giving advice to patients.
8. **Signature of doctor**.

Example of a prescription for a patient with an annoying unproductive cough:

1, 2, 3, as above
4. R
5. Codeine Linctus, BNF, 5 mL
6. Send 60 mL
7. Label: Codeine Linctus (or NP). Take 5 mL twice a day and on retiring
8. Signature of doctor.

Computer-issued prescriptions must conform to recommendations of professional bodies. Computer-generated facsimile signatures do not meet the legal requirement.

If altered by hand (undesirable), the alteration must be signed.

Medicine containers. Reclosable child-resistant containers and blister packs are now standard, as is dispensing in manufacturers' original sealed packs containing a patient information leaflet. These add to immediate cost but may save money in the end (increased efficiency of use, and safety).

Unwanted medicines. Patients should be encouraged to return these to the original supplier for disposal.

Drugs liable to cause dependence or be the subject of misuse. Doctors have a particular responsibility to ensure that: (1) they do not create dependence, (2) the patient does not increase the dose and create dependence, (3) they do not become an unwitting source of supply to addicts. To many such drugs, special prescribing regulations apply (see BNF).

Abbreviations (see also Weights and measures, below)

b.d.: bis in die	twice a day (b.i.d. is also used)
BNF	British National Formulary
BP	British Pharmacopoeia
BPC	British Pharmaceutical Codex
i.m.: intramuscular	by intramuscular injection
IU	International Unit
i.v.: intravenous	by intravenous injection
NP: nomen proprium	proper name
o.d.: omni die	every day
o.m.: omni mane	every morning
o.n.: omni nocte	every night
p.o.: per os	by mouth
p.r.: per rectum	by the anal/rectal route
p.r.n.: pro re nata	as required. It is best to add the maximum frequency of repetition, e.g. aspirin and codeine tablets, 1 or 2 p.r.n., 4-hourly
p.v.: per vaginam	by the vaginal route
q.d.s.: quater die sumendus	four times a day (q.i.d. is also used)
rep: repetatur	let it be repeated, as in rep. mist(ura), repeat the mixture
s.c.: subcutaneous	by subcutaneous injection
stat: statim	immediately
t.d.s.: ter (in) die sumendus	three times a day (t.i.d. is also used)

WEIGHTS AND MEASURES

In this book doses are given in the metric system, or in international units (IU) when metric doses are impracticable.

Equivalents:

1 litre (l or L) = 1.76 pints
1 kilogram (kg) = 2.2 pounds (lbs).

Abbreviations:

1 gram (g)
1 milligram (mg) $(1 \times 10^{-3} g)$
1 microgram[73] $(1 \times 10^{-6} g)$
1 nanogram[73] $(1 \times 10^{-9} g)$
1 decilitre (dL) $(1 \times 10^{-1} L)$
1 millilitre (mL) $(1 \times 10^{-3} L)$.

Home/domestic measures. A standard 5-mL spoon and a graduated oral syringe are available. Otherwise the following approximations will serve:

1 tablespoonful = 14 ml (or mL)
1 dessertspoonful = 7 ml (or mL)
1 teaspoonful = 5 ml (or mL).

PERCENTAGES, PROPORTIONS, WEIGHT IN VOLUME

Some solutions of drugs (e.g. local anaesthetics, epinephrine/adrenaline) for parenteral use are labelled in a variety of ways: percentage, proportion, or weight in volume (e.g. 0.1%, 1 : 1000, 1 mg/mL). In addition, dilutions may have to be made by doctors at the time of use. Such drugs are commonly dangerous in overdose and great precision is required, especially as any errors are liable to be by a factor of 10 and can be fatal. Doctors who do not feel confident with such calculations (because they do not do them frequently) should feel no embarrassment,[74] but should recognise that they have a responsibility to check their results with a competent colleague or pharmacist before proceeding.

---

[73]Spell out in full in prescriptions.

[74]Called to an emergency tension pneumothorax on an intercontinental flight, two surgeons, who chanced to be passengers, were provided with lidocaine 100 mg in 10 mL (in the aircraft medical kit). They were accustomed to thinking in percentages for this drug and 'in the heat of the moment' neither was able to make the conversion. Chest surgery was conducted successfully with an adapted wire coat-hanger as a trocar ('sterilised' in brandy), using a urinary catheter. The patient survived the flight and recovered in hospital. Wallace W A 1995 Managing in-flight emergencies: a personal account. British Medical Journal 311:374.

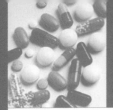

3

Discovery and development of drugs

SYNOPSIS

- Preclinical drug development. Discovery of new drugs in the laboratory is an exercise in prediction
- Techniques of discovery. Sophisticated molecular modelling allows precise design of potential new therapeutic substances and new technologies have increased the rate of development of potential medicines
- Studies in animals
- Ethical issues
- Need for animal testing
- Prediction. Failures of prediction occur and a drug may be abandoned at any stage, including after marketing. New drug development is a colossally expensive and commercially driven activity
- Orphan drugs and diseases.

PRECLINICAL DRUG DEVELOPMENT

The development of new medicines (drugs) is an exercise in *extrapolation* from laboratory studies in vitro and in vivo (animals), in order to predict what the agent will do in humans. Medicinal therapeutics rests on the two great supporting pillars of pharmacology:

- *Selectivity*– the desired effect alone is obtained: 'We must learn to aim, learn to aim with chemical substances' (Paul Ehrlich).[1]
- *Dose*– '… The dose alone decides that something is no poison' (Paracelsus).[2]

For decades, the rational discovery of new medicines has depended on modifications of the molecular structures of increasing numbers of known natural chemical mediators. Often the exact molecular basis of drug action is unknown, and this book contains frequent examples of old drugs whose mechanism of action remains mysterious. The evolution of *molecular medicine* (including recombinant DNA technology) in the past 30 years has led to a new pathway of drug discovery: *pharmacogenomics*.[3] This broad term encompasses all genes in the genome that may determine drug response, desired and undesired. Completion of the Human Genome Project in 2001 yielded a minimum of 30 000 potential drug targets, although the function of many of these genes remains unknown. In the future, drugs may be designed according to individual genotypes, thereby enhancing safety as well as efficacy.

The chances of discovering a truly novel medicine, i.e. one that does something valuable that had previously not been possible (or that does safely what could previously have been achieved only with substantial risk), are increased when the development programme is founded on precise knowledge, at molecular level, of the biological processes it is desired to change. The commercial rewards of a successful product are potentially enormous and

---

[1]Paul Ehrlich (1845–1915), a German scientist, pioneered the scientific approach to drug discovery. The 606th organic arsenical that he tested against spirochaetes (in animals) became a successful medicine (Salvarsan 1910); it and a minor variant were used against syphilis until superseded by penicillin in 1945.

[2]Paracelsus (1493–1541) was a controversial figure who has been portrayed as both ignorant and superstitious. He had no medical degree; he burned the classical medical works

(Galen, Avicenna) before his lectures in Basle (Switzerland) and had to leave the city following a dispute about fees with a prominent churchman. He died in Salzburg (Austria), either as a result of a drunken debauch or because he was thrown down a steep incline by 'hitmen' employed by jealous local physicians. But he was right about the dose.

[3]An example of the opportunity created by pharmacogenomics comes in the announcement by a major pharmaceutical company of plans to search the entire human genome for genetic evidence of intolerance to one of its drugs. If achieved, adverse reactions to the drug would be virtually eliminated.

provide a massive incentive for developers to invest and risk huge sums of money.

Studies of signal transduction, the fundamental process by which cells talk to one another as intracellular proteins transmit signals from the surface of the cell to the nucleus inside, have opened an entirely new approach to the development of therapeutic agents that can target discrete steps in the body's elaborate pathways of chemical reactions. The opportunities are endless.[4]

The molecular approach to drug discovery should enable a 'molecular dissection' of any disease process. There are two immediate consequences:

- More potential drugs and therapeutic targets will be produced than can be experimentally validated in animals and humans. A further risk is that this 'production line' approach could lead to a loss of integration of the established specialities (chemistry, biochemistry, pharmacology) and to an overall lack of understanding of how physiological and pathophysiological processes contribute to the interaction of drug and disease.
- New drugs could be targeted at selected groups of patients based on their genetic make-up. This concept of 'the right medicine for the right patient' is the basis of *pharmacogenetics* (see p. 105), the genetically determined variability in drug response.

Pharmacogenetics has gained momentum from recent advances in molecular genetics and genome sequencing, due to:

- Rapid screening for specific gene polymorphisms (see p. 106)
- Knowledge of the genetic sequences of target genes such as those coding for enzymes, ion channels, and other receptor types involved in drug response

There are high expectations of pharmacogenetics and its progeny, pharmacoproteomics (understanding of and drug effects on protein variants). They include:

- The identification of subgroups of patients with a disease or syndrome based on their genotype
- Targeting of specific drugs for patients with specific gene variants

Consequences of these expectations include: smaller clinical trial programmes, better understanding of the pharmacokinetics and dynamics according to genetic variation, and simplified monitoring of adverse events after marketing.

New drug development proceeds thus:

- Idea or hypothesis.
- Design and synthesis of substances.
- Studies on tissues and whole animal (preclinical studies).
- Studies in humans (clinical studies) (see Chapter 4).
- Granting of an official licence to make therapeutic claims and to sell (see Chapter 5).
- Post-licensing (marketing) studies of safety and comparisons with other medicines.

The (critical) phase of progress from the laboratory to humans is termed *translational science*. It was defined as 'the application of biomedical research (pre-clinical and clinical), conducted to support drug development, which aids in the identification of the appropriate patient for treatment (patient selection), the correct dose and schedule to be tested in the clinic (dosing regimen) and the best disease in which to test a potential agent'.[5]

It will be obvious from the account that follows that drug development is an extremely arduous, highly technical and enormously expensive operation. Successful developments (1% of compounds that proceed to full test eventually become licensed medicines) must carry the cost of the failures (99%).[6]

---

[4]Culliton B J 1994 Nature Medicine 1:1 (editorial).

[5]Johnstone D 2006 pA2 (British Pharmacological Society), Volume 4, Issue 2.
[6]The cost of development of a new chemical entity (NCE) (a novel molecule not previously tested in humans) from synthesis to market (general clinical use) is estimated at US$500 million; the process may take as long as 15 years (including up to 10 years for clinical studies), which is relevant to duration of patent life and so to ultimate profitability; if the developer does not see profit at the end of the process, the investment will not be made. The drug may fail at any stage, including the ultimate, i.e. at the official regulatory body after all the development costs have been incurred. It may also fail (due to adverse effects) within the first year after marketing, which constitutes a catastrophe (in reputation and finance) for the developer as well as for some of the patients. Pirated copies of full regulatory dossiers have substantial black market value to competitor companies, who have used them to leapfrog the original developer to obtain a licence for their unresearched copied molecule. Dossiers may be enormous, even one million pages or the electronic equivalent, the latter being very convenient as it allows instant searching.

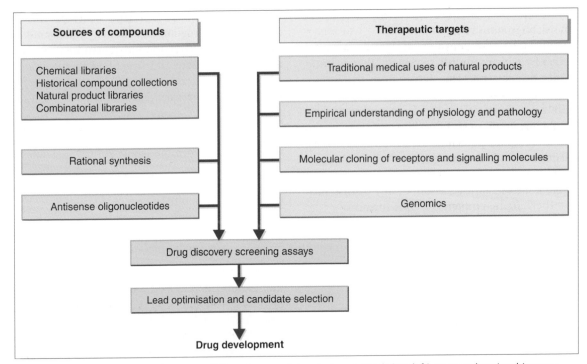

Fig. 3.1 Drug discovery sources in context. Different types of chemical compounds (top left) are tested against bioassays that are relevant to therapeutic targets, which are derived from several possible sources of information (right). The initial lead compounds discovered by the screening process are optimised by analogue synthesis and tested for appropriate pharmacokinetic properties. The candidate compounds then enter the development process involving regulatory toxicology studies and clinical trials.

It is also obvious that such programmes are likely to be carried to completion only when the organisations and the individuals within them are motivated overall by the challenge to succeed and to serve society, as well as to make money. A professor of clinical pharmacology wrote:

> Let us get one thing straight: the drug industry works within a system that demands it makes a profit to satisfy shareholders. Indeed, it has a fiduciary[7] duty to do so. The best way to make a lot of money is to invent a drug that produces a dramatically beneficial clinical effect, is far more effective than existing options, and has few unwanted effects. Unfortunately most drugs fall short of this ideal.[8]

TECHNIQUES OF DISCOVERY

(See Figure 3.1)

The *newer technologies*, the impact of which has yet to be fully felt, include the following.

Molecular modelling aided by three-dimensional computer graphics (including virtual reality) allows the design of structures based on new and known molecules to enhance their desired, and to eliminate their undesired, properties to create highly selective targeted compounds. In principle all molecular structures capable of binding to a single high-affinity site can be modelled.

Combinatorial chemistry involves the random mixing and matching of large numbers of chemical building blocks (amino acids, nucleotides, simple chemicals) to produce 'libraries' of all possible combinations. This technology can generate billions of new compounds that are initially evaluated using automated

[7]Held or given in trust (OED).
[8]Vallance P 2005 Developing an open relationship with the drug industry. Lancet 366:1062–1064.

robotic high-throughput screening devices that can handle thousands of compounds a day.[9] If the screen records a positive response, the compound is further investigated using traditional laboratory methods, and the molecule is manipulated to enhance selectivity and/or potency.

Proteins as medicines: biotechnology. The targets of most drugs are proteins (cell receptors, enzymes) and it is only lack of technology that has hitherto prevented the exploitation of proteins (and peptides) as medicines. This technology is now available, although there are practical problems in getting the proteins to the target site in the body (they are digested when swallowed and cross cell membranes with difficulty). Biotechnology involves the use of recombinant DNA technology/genetic engineering to clone and express human genes, for example in microbial (*Escherichia coli* or yeast) cells so that they manufacture proteins that medicinal chemists have not been able to synthesise. Such techniques can deliver hormones and autacoids in commercial amounts (such as insulin and growth hormone, erythropoietins, cell growth factors and plasminogen activators, interferons, vaccines and immune antibodies).

Transgenic animals (that breed true for the gene) are also being developed as models for human disease as well as for production of medicines.

The *polymerase chain reaction* (PCR) is a method of gene amplification that does not require living cells; it takes place in vitro and can produce (in a cost-effective way) commercial quantities of pure potential medicines.

Genetic medicines. Synthetic oligonucleotides are being developed to target sites on DNA sequences or genes (double-stranded DNA: triplex approach) or messenger RNA (the antisense approach), so that the production of disease-related proteins is blocked. These oligonucleotides offer prospects of treatment for cancers and viruses without harming healthy tissues.[10,11]

Gene therapy of human genetic disorders is 'a strategy in which nucleic acid, usually in the form of DNA, is administered to modify the genetic repertoire for therapeutic purposes', e.g. cystic fibrosis. 'The era of "the gene as drug" is clearly upon us' (R G Crystal). Significant problems remain; in particular the methods of delivery. Three methods are available: an injection of 'naked' DNA; using a virus as carrier with DNA incorporated into its genome; or DNA encapsulated within a liposome.

Immunopharmacology. Understanding of the molecular basis of immune responses has allowed the definition of mechanisms by which cellular function is altered by a legion of local hormones or autacoids in, for example, infections, cancer, autoimmune diseases, organ transplant rejection. These processes present targets for therapeutic intervention – hence the rise of immunopharmacology.

Positron emission tomography (PET) allows non-invasive pharmacokinetic and pharmacodynamic measurements in previously inaccessible sites, e.g. the brain in intact humans and animals.

Older approaches to the discovery of new medicines that continue in use include:

- *Animal models of human disease* or an aspect of it of varying relevance to humans.
- *Natural products*: modern technology for screening has revived interest and intensified the search. Multinational pharmaceutical companies now scour the world for leads from microorganisms (in soil or sewage or even from insects entombed in amber 40 million years ago), fungi, plants and animals. Developing countries in the tropics (with their luxuriant natural resources) are prominent targets in this search and have justly complained of

---

[9]It is too early to say what success these programmes may have but automation of assays, possibly coupled to similar automation of syntheses, promises to speed up the search for new leads which is the rate-limiting step in the introduction of really novel therapeutic agents. Their value in medicine will depend upon the significance of the control mechanism concerned in the pathogenesis of a disease process. Critics fear that the result may well be large numbers of drugs in search of a disease to treat' (Dollery C T 1994 Harveian Oration: Medicine and the pharmacological revolution. Journal of the Royal College of Physicians of London 28:59–69).

[10]Cohen J S, Hogan M E 1994 The new genetic medicines. Scientific American 271:76–82.
[11]Lesko L, Woodcock J 2004 Translation of pharmacogenomics and pharmacogenetics: a regulatory perspective. Nature Reviews. Drug Discovery 3:763–769.

exploitation ('gene robbery'). Many now require formal profit-sharing agreements to allow such searches.

- *Traditional medicine*, which is being studied for possible leads to usefully active compounds.
- *Modifications of the structures of known drugs*: these are obviously likely to produce more agents with similar basic properties, but may deliver worthwhile improvements. It is in this area that the 'me too' and 'me again' drugs are developed (sometimes for purely commercial reasons).
- *Random screening* of synthesised and natural products.
- New *uses for drugs already in general use* as a result of intelligent observation and serendipity,[12] or advancing knowledge of molecular mechanisms, e.g. aspirin for antithrombotic effect.

DRUG QUALITY

It is easy for an investigator or prescriber, interested in pharmacology, toxicology and therapeutics, to forget the fundamental importance of chemical and pharmaceutical aspects. An impure, unstable drug or formulation is useless. Pure drugs that remain pure drugs after 5 years of storage in hot, damp climates are vital to therapeutics. The record of manufacturers in providing this is impressive.

STUDIES IN ANIMALS[13]

Generally, the following are undertaken:

Pharmacodynamics – to investigate the *actions* relating to the proposed therapeutic use. In addition, there is a need to investigate potential undesirable pharmacodynamic effects of the substance on physiological functions.

Pharmacokinetics – the study of the *fate* of the active substance and its metabolites, within the organism (absorption, distribution, metabolism and excretion of these substances). The programme should be designed to allow comparison and extrapolation between animal and human.

Toxicology – to reveal physiological and/or histopathological changes induced by the drug, and to determine how these changes relate to dose.[14] These involve:

- Acute toxicity: single-dose studies that allow qualitative and quantitative assessment of toxic reactions.
- Chronic and subchronic toxicity: repeat-dose studies to characterise the toxicological profile of a drug following repeated administration. This includes the identification of potential target organs and exposure–response relationships, and may include the potential for reversibility of effects.

Generally, it is desirable that tests be performed in two relevant species, based on the pharmacokinetic profile, one a rodent and one a non-rodent. The duration of the studies depends on the conditions of clinical use and is defined by Regulatory Agencies (Tables 3.1 & 3.2).

Genotoxicity – to reveal the changes that a drug may cause in the genetic material of individuals or cells. Mutagenic substances present a hazard to health because exposure carries the risk of inducing germline mutation (with the possibility of inherited disorders) and somatic mutations (including those leading to cancer). A standard battery of investigations includes: a test for gene mutation in bacteria (e.g. the Ames test); an in vitro test with cytogenetic

---

[12]Serendipity is the faculty of making fortunate discoveries by general sagacity or by accident; the word derives from a fairytale about three princes of Serendip (Sri Lanka) who had this happy faculty.

[13]Mouse, rat, hamster, guinea-pig, rabbit, cat, dog, monkey are used (but not all for any one drug). Non-clinical (pharmacotoxicological) studies must be carried out in conformity with the provisions of internationally agreed standards known as Good Laboratory Practice (GLP). In Europe, regulations ensure that all tests on animals

are conducted in accordance with Council Directive 86/609/EEC. Studies in animals can be substituted by validated in vitro tests provided that the test results are of comparable quality and usefulness for the purpose of safety evaluation. The pharmacological and toxicological tests must demonstrate the potential toxicity of the product and any dangerous or undesirable toxic effects that may occur under the proposed conditions of use in human beings; these should be evaluated in relation to the pathological condition concerned.
The studies must also demonstrate the pharmacological properties of the product, in both qualitative and quantitative relationship to the proposed use in human beings.

[14]Details can be found at: http://www.emea.eu.int.

Table 3.1 Single and repeated dose toxicity requirements to support studies in healthy normal volunteers (Phase 1) and in patients (Phase 2) in the European Union (EU), and Phases 1, 2 and 3 in the USA and Japan[1]

Duration of clinical trial	Minimum duration of repeated-dose toxicity studies	
	Rodents	Non-rodents
Single dose	2 weeks[2]	2 weeks
Up to 2 weeks	2 weeks	2 weeks
Up to 1 month	1 month	1 month
Up to 3 months	3 months	3 months
Up to 6 months	6 months	6 months
>6 months	6 months	Chronic[3]

[1]In Japan, if there are no Phase 2 clinical trials of equivalent duration to the planned Phase 3 trials, conduct of longer-duration toxicity studies is recommended as given in Table 3.2.
[2]In the USA, specially designed single-dose studies with extended examinations can support single-dose clinical studies.
[3]Regulatory authorities may request a 12-month study or accept a 6-month study, determined on a case-by-case basis.

Table 3.2 Repeated-dose toxicity requirements to support Phase 3 studies in the EU, and marketing in all regions[1]

Duration of clinical trial	Minimum duration of repeated-dose toxicity studies	
	Rodents	Non-rodents
Up to 2 weeks	1 month	1 month
Up to 1 month	3 months	3 months
Up to 3 months	6 months	3 months
>3 months	6 months	Chronic[2]

[1]When a chronic non-rodent study is recommended if clinical use more than 1 month.
[2]Regulatory authorities may request a 12-month study or accept a 6-month study, determined on a case-by-case basis.

evaluation of chromosomal damage with mammalian cells *or* an in vitro mouse lymphoma thymidine kinase (tk) assay; an in vivo test for chromosomal damage using rodent haematopoietic cells (e.g. the mouse micronucleus test).

Carcinogenicity – to reveal carcinogenic effects. These studies are performed for any medicinal product if its expected clinical use is prolonged (about 6 months), either continuously or repeatedly. These studies are also recommended if there is concern about their carcinogenic potential, e.g. from a product of the same class or similar structure, or from evidence in repeated-dose toxicity studies. Studies with unequivocally genotoxic compounds are not needed, as they are presumed to be trans-species carcinogens, implying a hazard to humans.

Reproductive and developmental toxicity – these tests study effects on adult male or female reproductive function, toxic and teratogenic effects at all stages of development from conception to sexual maturity and latent effects, when the medicinal product under investigation has been administered to the female during pregnancy. Embryo/fetal toxicity studies are normally conducted on two mammalian species, one a non-rodent. If the metabolism of a drug in particular species is known to be similar to that in humans, it is usual to include this species. Studies in juvenile animals may also be required prior to developing drugs for use in children.

Local tolerance – to ascertain whether drugs are tolerated at sites in the body at which they may come into contact in clinical use. The testing strategy is such that any mechanical effects of administration or purely physicochemical actions of the product can be distinguished from toxicological or pharmacodynamic ones.

Biotechnology-derived pharmaceuticals – present a special case and the standard regimen of toxicology studies is not appropriate. The choice of species used depends on the expression of the relevant receptor. If no suitable species exists, homologous proteins or transgenic animals expressing the human receptor may be studied and additional immunological studies are required.

ETHICS AND LEGISLATION

Controversy surrounding the use of animals in scientific research is not new. The renowned Islamic physician Avicenna (980–1037) was aware of the issues for he held that 'the experimentation must be done with the human body, for testing a drug on a lion or a horse might not prove anything about its effect on man'.[15] Leonardo da Vinci (1452–1519)

[15]Bull J P 1959 The historical development of clinical therapeutic trials. Journal of Chronic Diseases 10:218–248.

predicted that one day experimentation on animals would be judged a crime, but Descartes[16] asserted that 'Animals do not speak, therefore they do not think, therefore they do not feel.' Later, Jeremy Bentham (1748–1832), the founding father of utilitarian philosophy, asked of animals: 'The question is not, Can they reason? nor Can they talk? but Can they suffer?'.

In our present world, billions of animals are raised to provide food and many to be used for scientific experiments. The arguments that evolve from this activity centre on the extent to which non-human animals can be respected as sentient beings of moral worth, albeit with differences between species. In recent years, a boisterous animal rights movement, asserting the moral status of animals, has challenged their use as experimental subjects.[17] Mainstream medical and scientific opinion around the world accepts that animal research continues to be justified, subject to important protections. This position is based on the insight that research involving animals has contributed hugely to advances in biological knowledge that have in turn allowed modern therapeutics to improve human morbidity and mortality. Animal models contribute enormously to the understanding of human physiology and disease because we share so many biological characteristics. A medicine when introduced into the organism is exposed to a vast array of conditions that we do not fully understand and are unable to reproduce outside the living body. The study of a drug in the whole organism gives more information, more rapidly.

Safety testing in animals is at present the only reliable way to evaluate risks before undertaking clinical trials of potentially useful medicines in humans. The investigation of reproductive effects and potential carcinogenicity would not be undertaken in humans for both ethical and practical reasons. Animal testing eliminates many unsafe test materials before clinical testing on humans, and minimises the risk of possible adverse effects when people are exposed to potential new medicines. In other words, experiments in animal models provide a critical safety check on candidate drugs; potentially hazardous or ineffective drugs can be eliminated and for those drugs that do progress to clinical trials, target organs identified in animal studies can be monitored.

Animal research has contributed to virtually every area of medical research, and almost all of the best known drug and surgical treatments of the past and present owe their origins in some way to evidence from animals. The antibacterial effectiveness of penicillin was as proved in tests on mice. Insulin came about because of research on rabbits and dogs in the 1920s. Poliomyelitis epidemics, which until the 1950s killed and paralysed millions of children, were consigned to history by vaccines resulting from studies on a range of laboratory animals, including monkeys. Major heart surgery, such as coronary artery bypass grafts and heart transplants, was developed through research on dogs and pigs. The BCG vaccine for tuberculosis was developed through research on rats and mice. Meningitis due to *Haemophilus influenzae* type b, formerly common especially in children, is now almost unknown in the UK because of a vaccine developed through work on mice and rabbits. Almost all of the highly effective drug treatments we currently use were developed using animals: β-adrenoceptor blockers, angiotensin-converting enzyme inhibitors, cytotoxics, analgesics, psychotropics, and so on.

Given this evidence, there is broad public support for the position that experiments on animals is a regrettable necessity that should be limited to what is deemed essential while alternatives are developed. In the UK, for example, this reservation is expressed in progressively more stringent legislation. The Animals (Scientific Procedures) Act 1986 makes it an offence to carry out any scientific procedure on animals except under licence, the requirements of which include that:

■ Animals are only used as a last resort.
■ Every practical step is taken to avoid distress or suffering.
■ The smallest possible number of animals is used.
■ The potential benefits have to be weighed against the cost to the animals; the simplest or least sentient species is used.
■ The work is realistic and achievable, and the programme designed in the way most likely to produce satisfactory results.

---

[16]René Descartes (1596–1650), French philosopher, mathematician and scientist, acknowledged as one of the chief architects of the modern age.

[17]The publication of *Animal Liberation* (New York: New York Review/Random House) by Peter Singer in 1975 is widely regarded as having provided its moral foundation.

PREDICTION

It is frequently pointed out that regulatory guidelines are not rigid requirements to be universally applied. But whatever the intention, they do tend to be treated as minimum requirements, if only because research directors fear to risk holding up their expensive coordinated programmes with disagreements that result in their having to go back to the laboratory, with consequent delay and financial loss. Knowledge of the *mode of action* of a potential new drug obviously greatly enhances prediction from animal studies of what will happen in humans. Whenever practicable, such knowledge should be obtained; sometimes this is quite easy, but sometimes it is impossible. Many drugs have been introduced safely without such knowledge, the later acquisition of which has not always made an important difference to their use (e.g. antimicrobials). Pharmacological studies are integrated with those of the toxicologist to build up a picture of the undesired as well as the desired drug effects.

In *pharmacological testing*, the investigators know what they are looking for and choose the experiments to gain their objectives.

In *toxicological testing*, the investigators have a less clear idea of what they are looking for; they are screening for risk, unexpected as well as predicted, and certain major routines must be done. Toxicity testing is therefore liable to become mindless routine to meet regulatory requirements to a greater extent than the pharmacological studies. The predictive value of special toxicology (above) is particularly controversial. All drugs are poisons if enough is given, and the task of the toxicologist is to find out whether, where and how a compound acts as a poison to animals, and to give an opinion on the significance of the data in relation to risks likely to be run by human beings. This will remain a nearly impossible task until molecular explanations of all effects can be provided.

Toxicologists are in an unenviable position. When a useful drug is safely introduced, they are considered to have done no more than their duty. When an accident occurs, they are invited to explain how this failure of prediction came about. When they predict that a chemical is unsafe in a major way for humans, this prediction is never tested.

ORPHAN DRUGS AND DISEASES

A free-market economy is liable to leave untreated, rare diseases, e.g. some cancers (in all countries), and some common diseases, e.g. parasitic infections (in poor countries).

When a drug is not developed into a usable medicine because the developer will not recover the costs, it is known as an orphan drug, and the disease is an orphan disease; the sufferer is a health orphan.[18] Drugs for rare diseases inevitably must often be licensed on less than ideal amounts of clinical evidence. The remedy for these situations lies in government itself undertaking drug development (which is likely to be inefficient) or in government-offered incentives, such as tax relief, subsidies, exclusive marketing rights, to pharmaceutical companies and, in the case of poor countries, international aid programmes; such programmes are being implemented.[19]

GUIDE TO FURTHER READING

Banks R E, Dunn M J, Hochstrasser D F et al 2000 Proteomics: new perspectives, new biomedical opportunities. Lancet 356:1749–1756

Beeley N, Berger A 2000 A revolution in drug discovery: combinatorial chemistry still needs logic to drive science forward. British Medical Journal 321:581–582

Dolan K 1999 Ethics, animals and science. Blackwell Science, London

Dollery C T 1999 Drug discovery and development in the molecular era. British Journal of Clinical Pharmacology 47(1):5–6

Evans W E, Relling M V 2004 Moving towards individualized medicine with pharmacogenomics. Nature 429:464–468

Fears R, Roberts D, Poste G 2000 Rational or rationed medicine? The promise of genetics for improved clinical practice. British Medical Journal 320:933–935

Gale E A M 2001 Lessons from the glitazones: a story of drug development. Lancet 357:1870–1875

---

[18]The cost of treating a patient with the rare genetic Gaucher's liposome storage disease with genetically engineered enzyme is US$145 000–400 000 per annum, according to severity. Who can and will pay? More such situations will occur.

[19]Official recognition of orphan drug status is accorded in the USA (population 240 million) where the relevant disease affects fewer than 200 000 people; in Japan (population 121 million) for fewer than 50 000 people.

Grahame-Smith D G 1999 How will knowledge of the human genome affect drug therapy? British Journal of Clinical Pharmacology 47(1):7–10

Lesko L J 2007 Personalized Medicine: elusive dream or imminent reality?. Clinical Pharmacology & Therapeutics 81(6):807–816

Meyer U A 2004 Pharmacogenetics – five decades of therapeutic lessons from genetic diversity. Nature Reviews/Genetics 5(9):669–676

Pound P, Ebrahim S, Sandercock P et al 2004 Where is the evidence that animal research benefits humans? British Medical Journal 328:514–517

Roses A D 2000 Pharmacogenetics and future drug development and delivery. Lancet 355:1358–1361

Sykes R 1998 Being a modern pharmaceutical company. British Medical Journal 317:1172–1180

Trouiller P, Olliaro P, Torreele E et al 2002 Drug development for neglected diseases: a deficient market and a public-health policy failure. Lancet 359:2188–2194

Weinshilboum R, Wang L 2004 Pharmacogenomics: bench to bedside. Nature Reviews/Drug Discovery 3(9):739–748

Wolf C R, Smith G, Smith R L 2000 Pharmacogenetics. British Medical Journal 320:987–990

4

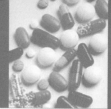

Evaluation of drugs in humans

SYNOPSIS

This chapter is about evidence-based drug therapy.

New drugs are progressively introduced by clinical pharmacological studies in rising numbers of healthy and/or patient volunteers until sufficient information has been gained to justify formal therapeutic studies. Each of these is usually a randomised controlled trial, in which a precisely framed question is posed and answered by treating equivalent groups of patients in different ways.

The key to the ethics of such studies is informed consent from patients, efficient scientific design and review by an independent research ethics committee. The key interpretative factors in the analysis of trial results are calculations of confidence intervals and statistical significance. Potential clinical significance develops within the confines of controlled clinical trials. This is best expressed by stating not only the percentage differences, but also the absolute difference or its reciprocal, the number of patients who have to be treated to obtain one desired outcome. The outcome might include both efficacy and safety.

Surveillance studies and the reporting of spontaneous adverse reactions respectively determine the clinical profile of the drug and detect rare adverse events. Further trials to compare new medicines with existing medicines are also required. These form the basis of cost–effectiveness comparisons.

Topics include:
- Experimental therapeutics
- Ethics of research
- Rational introduction of a new drug
- Need for statistics
- Types of trial: design, size
- Meta-analysis
- Pharmacoepidemiology

grows. There are two main groups: healthy volunteers and volunteer patients (plus, rarely, nonvolunteer patients). Studies in healthy normal volunteers can help to determine the safety, tolerability, pharmacokinetics and, for some drugs (e.g. anticoagulants and anaesthetic agents), their dynamic effect. For most drugs, the dynamic effect and hence therapeutic potential can be investigated only in patients, e.g. drugs for parkinsonism and antimicrobials. These two groups of subjects for drug testing are complementary, not mutually exclusive in drug development. Introduction of novel agents into both groups poses ethical and scientific problems (see below). There are four main reasons why doctors should have grounding in the knowledge and application of the principles of experimental therapeutics:

1. The optimal selection of a specific dose of a drug for a specific patient should be based on good clinical research. To some extent, every new administration to a patient is an exercise in experimental therapeutics.
2. Increasingly, doctors are personally involved.
3. Good therapeutic research alters clinical practice.
4. Such study provides an exercise in ethical and logical thinking.

Plainly, doctors cannot read in detail and evaluate for themselves all the published studies (often hundreds) that *might* influence their practice. They therefore turn to specialist research articles and abstracts[1] including meta-analyses (see p. 54) for guidance, but readers must approach these critically.

Modern medicine is sometimes accused of callous application of science to human problems and of subordinating the interest of the individ-

EXPERIMENTAL THERAPEUTICS

As the number of potential medicines produced increases, the problem of whom to test them on

---

[1]There are whole journals devoted to reviews. Some merely report uncritically the opinions of the original authors, but high-quality critical reviews are to be treasured.

ual to those of the group (society).[2] Official regulatory bodies rightly require scientific evaluation of drugs. Drug developers need to satisfy the official regulators and they also seek to persuade an increasingly sophisticated medical profession to prescribe their products. Patients, too, are far more aware of the comparative advantages and limitations of their medicines than they used to be. For these reasons, scientific drug evaluation as described here is likely to increase in volume and the doctors involved will be held responsible for the ethics of what they do, even if they played no personal part in the study design. Therefore, we provide a brief discussion of some relevant ethical aspects (and particularly of the randomised controlled trial).

RESEARCH INVOLVING HUMAN SUBJECTS

'The definition of research continues to present difficulties. The distinction between medical research and innovative medical practice derives from the *intent*. In medical *practice* the sole intention is to benefit the *individual patient* consulting the clinician, not to gain knowledge of general benefit, though such knowledge may incidentally emerge from the clinical experience gained. In medical *research* the primary intention is to advance knowledge so that *patients in general* may benefit; the individual patient may or may not benefit directly.'[3] Consider also the process of *audit*, which is used extensively to assess performance, e.g. by individual health-care workers, by departments within hospitals or between hospitals. Audit is a systematic examination designed

to determine the degree to which an action or set of actions achieves predetermined objectives. It can be used to address, for example, the delivery of service to patients passing through selected areas of a health-care system with the objective of identifying under-performance and improving standards in the future; there is no added intervention in the care that patients receive.

A distinction has been made between research that is *therapeutic*, i.e. which may actually have a therapeutic effect or provide information that can be used to help the participating subjects, and that which is *non-therapeutic*, i.e. which provides information that cannot be of direct use to them, e.g. healthy volunteers always and patients sometimes. This is a somewhat artificial separation, because some trials that are 'therapeutic', i.e. involve use of new potential medicines, may, by including a placebo in their design, confer no therapeutic benefit for some participants nor may the new trial medicine be given for sufficient time to judge its long term clinical benefit. Research may also be *experimental* (involving psychologically intrusive or physically invasive intervention) or solely *observational* (sometimes called non-interventional) (including epidemiology).

Ethics of research in humans[4]

Some dislike the word 'experiment' in relation to humans, thinking that its mere use implies a degree of impropriety in what is done. It is better that all should recognise from the true meaning of the word, 'to ascertain or establish by trial',[5] that the benefits of modern medicine derive almost wholly from experimentation and that some risk is inseparable from much medical advance.

The issue of (adequately informed) *consent* is a principal concern for Research Ethics Committees (also called Institutional Review Boards). People

---

[2]Guidance to researchers in this matter is clear. The World Medical Association declaration of Helsinki (Edinburgh revision 2000) states that '… considerations related to the well-being of the human subject should take precedence over the interests of science and society.' The General Assembly of the United Nations adopted in 1966 the International Covenant on Civil and Political Rights, of which Article 7 states, 'In particular, no one shall be subjected without his free consent to medical or scientific experimentation.' This means that subjects are entitled to know that they are being entered into research even though the research be thought to be 'harmless'. But there are people who cannot give (informed) consent, e.g. the demented. The need for special procedures for such is now recognised, for there is a consensus that, without research, they and the diseases from which they suffer will become therapeutic 'orphans'.

[3]Report: Royal College of Physicians of London 1996 Guidelines on the practice of ethics committees in medical research involving human subjects. RCP, London.

[4]For extensive practical detail, see International ethical guidelines for biomedical research involving human subjects. Council for International Organisations of Medical Sciences (CIOMS) in collaboration with the World Health Organization (WHO). 2002, CIOMS, Geneva (WHO publications are available in all UN member countries). See also: Guideline for Good Clinical Practice, International Conference on Harmonisation Tripartite Guideline. EU Committee on Proprietary Medicinal Products (CPMP/ICH/135/95). Smith T 1999 Ethics in medical research. A handbook of good practice. Cambridge University Press, Cambridge.

[5]*Oxford English Dictionary*. See also: Edwards M 2004 Historical keywords. Trial Lancet 364:1659.

have the right to choose for themselves whether or not they will participate in research, i.e. they have the right to self-determination (expressing the ethical principle of *autonomy*). They should be given whatever information is necessary for making an adequately informed choice (consent) with the right to withdraw at any stage. Consent procedures, especially information on risks, loom larger in research (particularly where it is non-therapeutic) than they do in medical practice.

The moral obligation of all doctors lies in ensuring that in their desire to help patients (the ethical principal of *beneficence*) they should never allow themselves to put the individual who has sought their aid at any disadvantage (the ethical principal of *non-maleficence*) for 'the scientist or physician has no right to choose martyrs for society'.[6]

It is proper to perform a therapeutic trial only when doctors (and patients) have genuine uncertainty as to which treatment is best.[7] Sometimes (and uncommonly) there is a real feeling that a new drug will turn out to be the more valuable medicine. Much more often, the probability is that a new drug will be broadly equivalent to current therapy with possible advantages for some patients. Indeed, much of the testing of new drugs is undertaken in the search for small advantages such as better therapeutic efficacy or tolerability in some sections of the population, for example due to age, genetics or race. Indeed, the definition of such differences is essential for the effective selection of drugs in medical practice.

It is, of course, more difficult to justify a new treatment when existing treatments are good than when they are bad, and this difficulty is likely to grow. The need of future patients who may benefit from the results of a study must be balanced against the needs of patients who are actually taking part, some of whom will receive a new (and possibly less effective) treatment. A fair judgement requires the exercise of the ethical principle of *justice*.[8]

The ethics of the randomised and placebo controlled trial

History, including recent history, is replete with examples of even the best-intentioned doctors being wrong about the efficacy and safety of (new) treatments. This situation can and should be remedied by the ethical employment of science.

The use of a placebo (or dummy) raises both ethical and scientific issues (see *placebo medicines* and the *placebo effect*, Chapter 1). There are clear-cut cases when placebo use would be ethically unacceptable and scientifically unnecessary, e.g. drug trials in epilepsy and tuberculosis, when the control groups comprise patients receiving the best available therapy.

The pharmacologically inert (placebo) treatment arm of a trial is useful:

- To distinguish the *pharmacodynamic effects* of a drug from the psychological effects of the act of medication and the circumstances surrounding it, e.g. increased interest by the doctor, more frequent visits, for these latter may have their placebo effect. Placebo responses have been reported in 30–50% of patients with depression and in 30–80% with chronic stable angina pectoris.
- To distinguish *drug effects* from natural fluctuations in disease that occur with time, e.g. with asthma or hay fever, and other external factors, provided active treatment, if any, can be ethically withheld. This is also called the 'assay sensitivity' of the trial.
- To avoid *false conclusions*. The use of placebos is valuable in Phase I healthy volunteer studies of novel drugs to help determine whether minor but frequently reported adverse events are drug related or not. Although a placebo treatment can pose ethical problems, it is often preferable to the continued use of treatments of unproven efficacy or safety. The ethical dilemma of subjects suffering as a result of receiving a placebo (or ineffective drug) can be overcome by designing clinical trials that provide mechanisms to allow them to be withdrawn ('escape') when defined criteria are reached, e.g. blood pressure above levels that represent treatment failure. Similarly, placebo (or new drug) can be added against a background of established therapy; this is called the 'add on' design.

[6]Kety S. Quoted by Beecher H K 1959 Journal of the American Medical Association 169:461.

[7]This is the uncertainty principle: the concept that patients entering a randomised therapeutic trial will have equal potential for benefit and risk is referred to as equipoise.

[8]The 'four principles' approach (above) is widely utilised in biomedical ethics. A full description and an analysis of the contribution of this and other ethical theories to decision-making in clinical, including research, practice can be found in: Beauchamp T L, Childress J F 2001 Principles of biomedical ethics, 5th edn. Oxford University Press, Oxford.

- To provide a result using *fewer research subjects*. The difference in response when a test drug is compared with a placebo is likely to be greater than that when a test drug is compared with the best current, i.e. active, therapy (see p. 48).

Investigators who propose to use a placebo, or otherwise withhold effective treatment, should specifically justify their intention. The variables to consider are:

- The severity of the disease.
- The effectiveness of standard therapy.
- Whether the novel drug under test aims to give only symptomatic relief, or has the potential to prevent or slow up an irreversible event, e.g. stroke or myocardial infarction.
- The length of treatment.
- The objective of the trial (equivalence, superiority or non-inferiority; see p. 51). Thus it may be quite ethical to compare a novel analgesic against placebo for 2 weeks in the treatment of osteoarthritis of the hip (with escape analgesics available). It would not be ethical to use a placebo alone as comparator in a 6-month trial of a novel drug in active rheumatoid arthritis, even with escape analgesia.

The precise use of the placebo will depend on the study design, e.g. whether *cross-over*, when all patients receive placebo at some point in the trial, or *parallel group*, when only one cohort receives placebo. Generally, patients easily understand the concept of distinguishing between the imagined effects of treatment and those due to a direct action on the body. Provided research subjects are properly informed and give consent freely, they are not the subject of deception in any ethical sense; but a patient given a placebo in the absence of consent is deceived and research ethics committees will, rightly, decline to agree to this (but see Lewis et al 2002, p. 60).

Injury to research subjects[9]

The question of compensation for accidental (physical) injury due to participation in research is a vexed one. Plainly there are substantial differences between the position of healthy volunteers (whether or not they are paid) and that of patients who may benefit and, in some cases, who may be prepared to accept even serious risk for the chance of gain. There is no simple answer. But the topic must always be addressed in any research carrying risk, including the risk of withholding known effective treatment. The CIOMS/WHO Guidelines[4] state:

Research subjects who suffer physical injury as a result of their participation are entitled to such financial or other assistance as would compensate them equitably for any temporary or permanent impairment or disability. In the case of death, their dependents are entitled to material compensation. The right to compensation may not be waived.

Therefore, when giving their informed consent to participate, research subjects should be told whether there is provision for compensation in case of physical injury, and the circumstances in which they or their dependants would receive it.

Payment of subjects in clinical trials

Healthy volunteers are usually paid to take part in a clinical trial. The rationale is that they will not benefit from treatment received and should be compensated for discomfort and inconvenience. There is a fine dividing line between this and a financial inducement, but it is unlikely that more than a small minority of healthy volunteer studies would now take place without a 'fee for service' provision, including 'out of pocket' expenses. It is all the more important that the sums involved are commensurate with the invasiveness of the investigations and the length of the studies. The monies should be declared and agreed by the ethics committee.

There is an intuitive abreaction by physicians to pay patients (compared with healthy volunteers), because they feel the accusation of inducement

---

[9]Injury to participants in clinical trials is uncommon and serious injury is rare. In March 2006, eight healthy young men entered a trial of a humanised monoclonal antibody designed to be an agonist of a particular receptor on T lymphocytes that stimulates their production and activation. This was the first administration to humans; preclinical testing in rabbits and monkeys at doses up to 500 times those received by the volunteers apparently showed no ill effect. Six of the volunteers quickly became seriously ill and required admission to an intensive care facility with multi-organ failure due to a 'cytokine release syndrome', in effect a massive attack on the body's own tissues. All the volunteers recovered but with some with disability. This toxicity in humans, despite apparent safety in animals, may be due to the specifically humanised nature of the monoclonal antibody. Testing of perceived high-risk new medicines is likely to be subject to particularly stringent regulation in future. See Wood A J J, Darbyshire J 2006 Injury to research volunteers – the clinical research nightmare. New England Journal of Medicine 354:1869–1871.

or persuasion could be levelled at them, and because they assuage any feeling of taking advantage of the doctor–patient relationship by the hope that the medicines under test may be of benefit to the individual. This is not an entirely comfortable position.[10]

RATIONAL INTRODUCTION OF A NEW DRUG TO HUMANS

When studies in animals predict that a new molecule may be a useful medicine, i.e. effective and safe in relation to its benefits, then the time has come to put it to the test in humans. Most doctors will be involved in clinical trials at some stage of their career and need to understand the principles of drug development. When a new chemical entity offers a possibility of doing something that has not been done before or of doing something familiar in a different or better way, it can be seen to be worth testing. But where it is a new member of a familiar class of drug, potential advantage may be harder to detect. Yet these 'me too' drugs are often worth testing. Prediction from animal studies of modest but useful clinical advantage is particularly uncertain and, therefore, if the new drug seems reasonably effective and safe in animals it is rational to test it in humans. From the commercial standpoint, the investment in the development of a new drug can be in the order of £500 million, but will be substantially less for a 'me too' drug entering an already developed and profitable market.

PHASES OF CLINICAL DEVELOPMENT

Human experiments progress in a commonsense manner that is conventionally divided into four phases. These phases are divisions of convenience in what is a continuous expanding process. It begins with a small number of subjects (healthy subjects and volunteer patients) closely observed in laboratory settings, and proceeds through hundreds of patients, to thousands before the drug is agreed to be a medicine by a national or international regulatory authority. It is then licensed for general prescribing (though this is by no means the end of the evaluation). The process may be abandoned at any stage for a variety of reasons, including poor tolerability or safety, inadequate efficacy and commercial pressures. The phases are:

- *Phase 1. Human pharmacology* (20 to 50 subjects)
  –healthy volunteers or volunteer patients, according to the class of drug and its safety
  –pharmacokinetics (absorption, distribution, metabolism, excretion)
  –pharmacodynamics (biological effects) where practicable, tolerability, safety, efficacy.
- *Phase 2. Therapeutic exploration* (50 to 300 subjects)
  –patients
  –pharmacokinetics and pharmacodynamic dose-ranging, in carefully controlled studies for efficacy and safety,[11] which may involve comparison with placebo.
- *Phase 3. Therapeutic confirmation* (randomised controlled trials; 250 to 1000+ subjects)
  –patients
  –efficacy on a substantial scale; safety; comparison with existing drugs.
- *Phase 4. Therapeutic use* (pharmacovigilance, post-licensing studies) (2000 to 10 000+ subjects)
  –surveillance for safety and efficacy: further formal therapeutic trials, especially comparisons with other drugs, marketing studies and pharmacoeconomic studies.

OFFICIAL REGULATORY GUIDELINES AND REQUIREMENTS[12]

For studies in humans (see also Chapter 5) these ordinarily include:

- Studies of *pharmacokinetics* and (when other manufacturers have similar products) of

---

[10]Freedman B 1987 Equipoise and the ethics of clinical research. New England Journal of Medicine 317:141–145.

[11]Moderate to severe adverse events have occurred in about 0.5% of healthy subjects. See Orme M et al 1989 British Journal of Clinical Pharmacology 27:125; Sibille M et al 1992 European Journal of Clinical Pharmacology 42:393.

[12]Guidelines for the conduct and analysis of a range of clinical trials in different therapeutic categories are released from time to time by the Committee on Medicinal Products (CMP) of the European Commission. These guidelines apply to drug development in the European Union. Other regulatory authorities issue guidance, e.g. the Food and Drug Administration in the USA, the Ministry of Health, Labour and Welfare in Japan. There has been considerable success in aligning different guidelines across the world through the International Conferences on Harmonisation (ICH). The source for CMP guidelines is info@mkra.gsi.gov.uk or EuroDirect Publications Officer, Medicines and Healthcare Products Agency, Room 10–238, Market Towers, 1 Nine Elms Lane, London SW8 5NQ, UK.

bioequivalence (equal bioavailability) with alternative products.

- *Therapeutic trials* (reported in detail) that substantiate the safety and efficacy of the drug under likely conditions of use, e.g. a drug for long-term use in a common condition will require a total of at least 1000 patients (preferably more), depending on the therapeutic class, of which at least 100 have been treated continuously for about 1 year.

- *Special groups*. If the drug will be used in, for example, the elderly, then elderly people should be studied if there are reasons for thinking they may react to or handle the drug differently. The same applies to children and to pregnant women (who present a special problem), and who, if they are not studied, may be excluded from licensed uses and so become health 'orphans'. Studies in patients having disease that affects drug metabolism and elimination may be needed, such as patients with impaired liver or kidney function.

- *Fixed-dose combination* products will require explicit justification for each component.

- *Interaction studies* with other drugs likely to be taken simultaneously. Plainly, all possible combinations cannot be evaluated; an intelligent choice, based on knowledge of pharmacodynamics and pharmacokinetics, is made.

- The application for a licence for general use (marketing application) should include a draft Summary of Product Characteristics for prescribers. A Patient Information Leaflet must be submitted. These should include information on the form of the product (e.g. tablet, capsule, sustained-release, liquid), its uses, dosage (adults, children, elderly where appropriate), contraindications (strong recommendation), warnings and precautions (less strong), side-effects/adverse reactions, overdose and how to treat it.

The emerging discipline of *pharmacogenomics* seeks to identify patients who will respond beneficially or adversely to a new drug by defining certain genotypic profiles. Individualised dosing regimens may be evolved as a result. This tailoring of drugs to individuals is consuming huge resources from drug developers but has yet to establish a place in routine drug development.

THERAPEUTIC INVESTIGATIONS

> There are three key questions to be answered during drug development:
> - Does it work?
> - Is it safe?
> - What is the dose?

With few exceptions, none of these is easy to answer definitively within the confines of a pre-registration clinical trials programme. Effectiveness and safety have to be balanced against each other. What may be regarded as 'safe' for a new oncology drug in advanced lung cancer would not be so regarded in the treatment of childhood eczema. The use of the term 'dose', without explanation, is irrational as it implies a single dose for all patients. Pharmaceutical companies cannot be expected to produce a large array of different doses for each medicine, but the maxim to use the smallest effective dose that results in the desired effect holds true. Some drugs require titration, others have a wide safety margin so that one 'high' dose may achieve optimal effectiveness with acceptable safety. There are two classes of endpoint or outcome of a therapeutic investigation:

- The *therapeutic* effect itself (sleep, eradication of infection), i.e. the outcome.
- A *surrogate* effect, a short-term effect that can be reliably correlated with long-term therapeutic benefit, e.g. blood lipids or glucose or blood pressure. A surrogate endpoint might also be a pharmacokinetic parameter, if it is indicative of the therapeutic effect, e.g. plasma concentration of an antiepileptic drug.

Use of surrogate effects presupposes that the disease process is fully understood. They are best justified in diseases for which the true therapeutic effect can be measured only by studying large numbers of patients over many years. Such long-term outcome studies are indeed always preferable but may be impracticable on organisational, financial and sometimes ethical grounds prior to releasing new drugs for general prescription. It is in areas such as these that the techniques of large-scale surveillance for efficacy, as well as for safety, under conditions of ordinary use (below), would be needed to supplement the necessarily smaller and shorter formal therapeutic trials employing surrogate effects. Surrogate endpoints are of particular value in early drug development to select candidate drugs from a range of agents.

Therapeutic evaluation

The *aims* of therapeutic evaluation are three-fold:

1. To assess the efficacy, safety and quality of new drugs to meet unmet clinical needs
2. To expand the indications for the use of current drugs (or generic drugs[13]) in clinical and marketing terms
3. To protect public health over the lifetime of a given drug.

The process of therapeutic evaluation may be divided into pre- and post-registration phases (Table 4.1), the purposes of which are set out below.

When a new drug is being developed, the first therapeutic trials are devised to find out the best that the drug can do under conditions ideal for showing efficacy, e.g. uncomplicated disease of mild to moderate severity in patients taking no other drugs, with carefully supervised administration by specialist doctors. Interest lies particularly in patients who complete a full course of treatment. If the drug is ineffective in these circumstances there is no point in proceeding with an expensive development programme. Such studies are sometimes called *explanatory trials* as they attempt to 'explain' why a drug works (or fails to work) in ideal conditions.

If the drug is found useful in these trials, it becomes desirable next to find out how closely the ideal may be approached in the rough and tumble of routine medical practice: in patients of all ages, at all stages of disease, with complications, taking other drugs and relatively unsupervised. Interest continues in all patients from the moment they are entered into the trial and it is maintained if they fail to complete, or even to start, the treatment; the need is to know the outcome in all patients deemed suitable for therapy, not only in those who successfully complete therapy.[14]

The reason some drop out may be related to aspects of the treatment and it is usual to analyse these according to the clinicians' *initial* intention (*intention-to-treat analysis*), i.e. investigators are not allowed to risk introducing bias by exercising their own judgement as to who should or should not be excluded from the analysis. In these real-life, or 'naturalistic', conditions the drug may not perform so well, e.g. minor adverse effects may now cause patient non-compliance, which had been avoided by supervision and enthusiasm in the early trials. These naturalistic studies are sometimes called '*pragmatic*' trials.

The *methods* used to test the therapeutic value depend on the stage of development, who is conducting the study (a pharmaceutical company, or an academic body or health service at the behest of a regulatory authority), and the *primary endpoint* or *outcome* of the trial. The methods include:

- Formal therapeutic trials.
- Equivalence and non-inferiority trials.
- Safety surveillance methods.

Formal therapeutic trials are conducted during Phase 2 and Phase 3 of pre-registration development, and in the post-registration phase to test the drug in new indications. *Equivalence* trials aim to show the

Table 4.1 Process of therapeutic evaluation				
	Pre-registration		Post-registration	
	Pharmaceutical company	Regulatory authority	Pharmaceutical company	Regulatory authority
Purpose of therapeutic evaluation	To select best candidate for development and registration	To satisfy the regulatory authority on efficacy, safety and quality	To promote drug to expand the market	To add to indications (by variation to licence) and to add evolving safety information

[13]A drug for which the original patent has expired, so that any pharmaceutical company may market it in competition with the inventor. The term 'generic' has come to be synonymous with the non-proprietary or approved name (see Chapter 6).

[14]Information on both categories (method effectiveness and use effectiveness) is valuable (Sheiner L B, Rubin D B 1995 Intention-to-treat analysis and the goals of clinical trials. Clinical Pharmacology and Therapeutics 57(1)6–15).

therapeutic equivalence of two treatments, usually the new drug under development and an existing drug used as a standard active comparator. Equivalence trials may be conducted before or after registration for the first therapeutic indication of the new drug (see p. 50 for further discussion). *Safety surveillance methods* use the principles of pharmaco-epidemiology (see p. 57) and are concerned mainly with evaluating adverse events and especially rare events, which formal therapeutic trials are unlikely to detect.

NEED FOR STATISTICS

In order truly to know whether patients treated in one way are benefited more than those treated in another, it is essential to use numbers. Statistics has been defined as 'a body of methods for making wise decisions in the face of uncertainty'.[15] Used properly, they are tools of great value for promoting efficient therapy. More than 100 years ago Francis Galton saw this clearly:

> The human mind is … a most imperfect apparatus for the elaboration of general ideas … In our general impressions far too great weight is attached to what is marvellous … Experience warns us against it, and the scientific man takes care to base his conclusions upon actual numbers … to devise tests by which the value of beliefs may be ascertained.[16]

CONCEPTS AND TERMS

Hypothesis of no difference

When it is suspected that treatment A may be superior to treatment B and the truth is sought, it is convenient to start with the proposition that the treatments are equally effective – the 'no difference' hypothesis (*null hypothesis*). After two groups of patients have been treated and it has been found that improvement has occurred more often with one treatment than with the other, it is necessary to decide how likely it is that this difference is due to a real superiority of one treatment over the other.

To make this decision we need to understand two major concepts, *statistical significance* and *confidence intervals*.

A statistical significance test[17] such as the Student's *t* test or the chi squared (χ^2) test will tell how often an observed difference would occur due to chance (random influences) if there is, in reality, no difference between the treatments. Where the statistical significance test shows that an observed difference would occur only five times if the experiment were repeated 100 times, this is often taken as sufficient evidence that the null hypothesis is *unlikely* to be true. Therefore, the conclusion is that there is (probably) a real difference between the treatments. This level of probability is generally expressed in therapeutic trials as: 'the difference was statistically significant', or 'significant at the 5% level' or '$P = 0.05$' (*P* is the probability based on chance alone). Statistical significance simply means that the result is *unlikely* to have occurred if there was *no* genuine treatment difference, i.e. there probably *is* a difference.

If the analysis reveals that the observed difference, or greater, would occur only once if the experiment were repeated 100 times, the results are generally said to be 'statistically highly significant', or 'significant at the 1% level' or '$P = 0.01$'.

Confidence intervals. The problem with the *P* value is that it conveys no information on the *amount* of the differences observed or on the *range* of possible differences between treatments. A result that a drug produces a uniform 2% reduction in heart rate may well be statistically significant but it is clinically meaningless. What doctors are interested to know is the *size* of the difference, and what degree of assurance (confidence) they may have in the *precision* (reproducibility) of this estimate. To obtain this it is necessary to calculate a confidence interval (see Figs 4.1 & 4.2).[18]

A confidence interval expresses a range of values that contains the true value with 95% (or other chosen percentage) certainty. The range may be broad, indicating uncertainty, or narrow, indicating (relative) certainty. A wide confidence interval occurs

[15]Wallis W A, Roberts H V 1957 Statistics, a new approach. Methuen, London.

[16]Galton F 1879 Generic images. Proceedings of the Royal Institution.

[17]Altman D G, Gore S M, Gardner M J, Pocock S J 1983 Statistical guidelines for contributors to medical journals. British Medical Journal 286:1489–1493.

[18]Gardner M J, Altman D G 1986 Confidence intervals rather than P values: estimation rather than hypothesis testing. British Medical Journal 292:746–750.

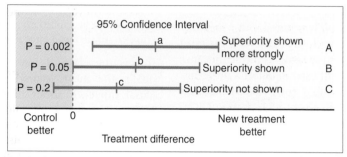

Fig. 4.1 Relationship between significance tests and confidence intervals for the comparisons between a new treatment and control. The treatment differences a, b, c are all in favour of 'New treatment', but superiority is shown only in A and B. In C, superiority has not been shown. This may be because the effect is small and not detected. The result, nevertheless, is compatible with equivalence or non-inferiority. Adequate precision and power are assumed for all the trials.

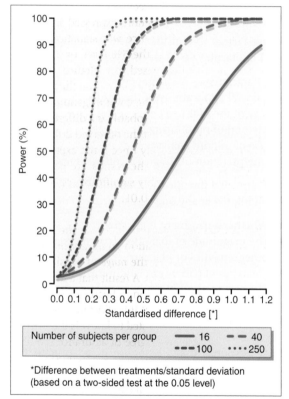

*Difference between treatments/standard deviation (based on a two-sided test at the 0.05 level)

Fig. 4.2 Power curves – an illustrative method of defining the number of subjects required in a given study. In practice, the actual number would be calculated from standard equations. In this example the curves are constructed for 16, 40, 100 and 250 subjects per group in a two-limb comparative trial. The graphs can provide three pieces of information: (1) the number of subjects that need to be studied, given the power of the trial and the difference expected between the two treatments; (2) the power of a trial, given the number of subjects included and the difference expected; and (3) the difference that can be detected between two groups of subjects of given number, with varying degrees of power. (With permission from Baber N, Smith R N, Griffin J P, O'Grady J, D'Arcy P F (eds) 1998 Textbook of pharmaceutical medicine, 3rd edn. Queen's University of Belfast Press, Belfast.)

when numbers are small or differences observed are variable and points to a lack of information, whether the difference is statistically significant or not; it is a warning against placing much weight on (or confidence in) the results of small or variable studies. Confidence intervals are extremely helpful in interpretation, particularly of small studies, as they show the degree of uncertainty related to a result. Their use in conjunction with non-significant results may be especially enlightening.[19]

A finding of 'not statistically significant' can be interpreted as meaning there is no clinically useful difference only if the confidence intervals for the results are also stated in the report and are narrow. If the confidence intervals are wide, a real difference may be missed in a trial with a small number of subjects, i.e. absence of evidence that there is a difference is not the same as showing that there is no difference. Small numbers of patients inevitably give low precision and low power to detect differences.

Types of error

The above discussion provides us with information on the likelihood of falling into one of the two principal kinds of error in therapeutic experiments, for the hypothesis that there is no difference between treatments may either be accepted incorrectly or rejected incorrectly.

Type I error (α) is the finding of a difference between treatments when in reality they do not differ, i.e. *rejecting* the null hypothesis incorrectly. Investigators decide the degree of this error which they are pre-

[19]Altman D G, Gore S M, Gardner M J, Pocock S J 1983 Statistical guidelines for contributors to medical journals. British Medical Journal 286:1489–1493.

pared to tolerate on a scale in which 0 indicates complete rejection of the null hypothesis and 1 indicates its complete acceptance; clearly the level for α must be set near to 0. This is the same as the significance level of the statistical test used to detect a difference between treatments. Thus α (or $P = 0.05$) indicates that the investigators will accept a 5% chance that an observed difference is not a real difference.

Type II error (β) is the finding of no difference between treatments when in reality they do differ, i.e. *accepting* the null hypothesis incorrectly. The probability of detecting this error is often given wider limits, e.g. β = 0.1–0.2, which indicates that the investigators are willing to accept a 10–20% chance of missing a real effect. Conversely, the *power* of the study $(1 - β)$ is the probability of avoiding this error and detecting a real difference, in this case 80–90%.

It is up to the investigators to decide the target difference[20] and what probability level (for either type of error) they will accept if they are to use the result as a guide to action.

Plainly, trials should be devised to have adequate *precision* and *power*, both of which are consequences of the size of study. It is also necessary to make an estimate of the likely size of the difference between treatments, i.e. the target difference. Adequate power is often defined as giving an 80–90% chance of detecting (at 1–5% statistical significance, $P = 0.01$–0.05) the defined useful target difference (say 15%). It is rarely worth starting a trial that has less than a 50% chance of achieving the set objective, because the power of the trial is too low.

TYPES OF THERAPEUTIC TRIAL

A therapeutic trial is:

a carefully, and ethically, designed experiment with the aim of answering some precisely framed question. In its most rigorous form it demands equivalent groups of patients concurrently treated in different ways or in randomised sequential order in crossover designs. These groups are constructed by the random allocation of patients to one or other treatment … In principle the method has

application with any disease and any treatment. It may also be applied on any scale; it does not necessarily demand large numbers of patients.[21]

This is the classical randomised controlled trial (RCT), the most secure method for drawing a causal inference about the effects of treatments. Randomisation attempts to control biases of various kinds when assessing the effects of treatments. RCTs are employed at all phases of drug development and in the various types and designs of trials discussed below. Fundamental to any trial are:

- A hypothesis.
- Definition of the primary endpoint.
- The method of analysis.
- A protocol.

Other factors to consider when designing or critically appraising a trial are the:

- Characteristics of the patients.
- General applicability of the results.
- Size of the trial.
- Method of monitoring.
- Use of interim analyses.[22]
- Interpretation of subgroup comparisons.

The aims of a therapeutic trial, not all of which can be attempted at any one occasion, are to decide:

- Whether a treatment is effective.
- The magnitude of that effect (compared with other remedies or placebo).
- The types of patients in whom it is effective.
- The best method of applying the treatment (how often, and in what dosage if it is a drug).
- The disadvantages and dangers of the treatment.

Dose–response trials. Response in relation to the dose of a new investigational drug may be explored in all phases of drug development. Dose–response trials serve a number of objectives, of which the following are of particular importance:

- Confirmation of efficacy (hence a therapeutic trial).

---

[20]The Target Difference. Differences in trial outcomes fall into three grades: (1) that the doctor will ignore, (2) that will make the doctor wonder what to do (more research needed), and (3) that will make the doctor act, i.e. change prescribing practice.

[21]Bradford Hill A 1977 Principles of medical statistics. Hodder and Stoughton, London. If there is a 'father' of the modern scientific therapeutic trial, it is he.

[22]Particularly in large-scale outcome trials, an independent data monitoring committee is given access to the results as these are accumulated; the committee is empowered to discontinue a trial if the results show significant advantage or disadvantage to one or other treatment.

- Investigation of the shape and location of the dose–response curve.
- The estimation of an appropriate starting dose.
- The identification of optimal strategies for individual dose adjustments.
- The determination of a maximal dose beyond which additional benefit is unlikely to occur.

Superiority, equivalence and non-inferiority in clinical trials. The therapeutic efficacy of a novel drug is most convincingly established by demonstrating superiority to placebo, or to an active control treatment, or by demonstrating a dose–response relationship (as above).

In some cases, however, the purpose of a comparison is to show not necessarily superiority, but either equivalence or non-inferiority. The objectives of such trials are to avoid the use of a placebo, to explore possible advantages of safety, dosing convenience and cost, and to present an alternative or 'second-line' therapy.

Examples of possible outcome in a 'head to head' comparison of two active treatments appear in Figure 4.1.

There are in general, two types of equivalence trials in clinical development: *bio*-equivalence and *clinical* equivalence. In the former, certain pharmacokinetic variables of a new formulation have to fall within specified (and regulated) margins of the standard formulation of the same active entity. The advantage of this type of trial is that, if bioequivalence is 'proven', then proof of clinical equivalence is not required. Proof of clinical equivalence of a generic product to the marketed product can be much more difficult to demonstrate.

DESIGN OF TRIALS

Techniques to avoid bias

The two most important techniques are:

- Randomisation.
- Blinding.

Randomisation Introduces a deliberate element of chance into the assignment of treatments to the subjects in a clinical trial. It provides a sound statistical basis for the evaluation of the evidence relating to treatment effects, and tends to produce treatment groups that have a balanced distribution of prognostic factors, both known and unknown. Together

with blinding, it helps to avoid possible bias in the selection and allocation of subjects.

Randomisation may be accomplished in simple or more complex ways, such as:

- Sequential assignments of treatments (or sequences in crossover trials).
- Randomising subjects in blocks. This helps to increase comparability of the treatment groups when subject characteristics change over time or there is a change in recruitment policy. It also gives a better guarantee that the treatment groups will be of nearly equal size.
- By dynamic allocation, in which treatment allocation is influenced by the current balance of allocated treatments.[23]

Blinding. The fact that both doctors and patients are subject to bias due to their beliefs and feelings has led to the invention of the double-blind technique, which is a control device to prevent bias from influencing results. On the one hand, it rules out the effects of hopes and anxieties of the patient by giving both the drug under investigation and a placebo (dummy) of identical appearance in such a way that the subject (the first 'blind' person) does not know which he or she is receiving. On the other hand, it also rules out the influence of preconceived hopes of, and unconscious communication by, the investigator or observer by keeping him or her (the second 'blind' person) ignorant of whether he or she is prescribing a placebo or an active drug. At the

---

[23]Note also patient preference trials. Conventionally, patients are invited to participate in a clinical trial, give consent and are then randomised to a particular treatment group. In special circumstances, randomisation takes place first, the patients are informed of the treatment to be offered and are allowed to opt for this or another treatment. This is called pre-consent randomisation or 'pre-randomisation'. In a trial of simple mastectomy versus lumpectomy with or without radiotherapy for early breast cancer, recruitment was slow because of the disfiguring nature of the mastectomy option. A policy of pre-randomisation was then adopted, letting women know the group to which they would be allocated should they consent. Recruitment increased six-fold and the trial was completed, providing sound evidence that survival was as long with the less disfiguring option (Fisher B, Bauer M, Margolese R et al 1985 Five-year results of a randomised clinical trial comparing total mastectomy and segmental mastectomy with and without radiotherapy in the treatment of breast cancer. New England Journal of Medicine 312:665–673). However, the benefit of enhanced recruitment may be limited by potential for introducing bias.

same time, the technique provides another control, a means of comparison with the magnitude of placebo effects. The device is both philosophically and practically sound.[24]

A non-blind trial is called an *open trial*.

The double-blind technique should be used wherever possible, and especially for occasions when it might at first sight seem that criteria of clinical improvement are objective when in fact they are not. For example, the range of voluntary joint movement in rheumatoid arthritis has been shown to be influenced greatly by psychological factors, and a moment's thought shows why, for the amount of pain patients will put up with is influenced by their mental state.

Blinding should go beyond the observer and the observed. None of the investigators should be aware of treatment allocation, including those who evaluate endpoints, assess compliance with the protocol and monitor adverse events. Breaking the blind (for a single subject) should be considered only when the subject's physician deems knowledge of the treatment assignment essential in the subject's best interests.

Sometimes the double-blind technique is not possible, because, for example, side-effects of an active drug reveal which patients are taking it or tablets look or taste different; but it never carries a disadvantage ('only protection against biased data'). It is not, of course, used with new chemical entities fresh from the animal laboratory, whose dose and effects in humans are unknown, although the subject may legitimately be kept in ignorance (single blind) of the time of administration. Single-blind techniques have a place in therapeutics research, but only when the double-blind procedure is impracticable or unethical.

Ophthalmologists are understandably disinclined to refer to the double-blind technique; they call it double-masked.

SOME COMMON DESIGN CONFIGURATIONS

Parallel group design

This is the most common clinical trial design for confirmatory therapeutic (Phase 3) trials. Subjects are randomised to one of two or more treatment 'arms'.

These treatments will include the investigational drug at one or more doses, and one or more control treatments such as placebo and/or an active comparator. Parallel group designs are particularly useful in conditions that fluctuate over a short term, e.g. migraine or irritable bowel syndrome, but are also used for chronic stable diseases such as Parkinson's disease and types of cancer. The particular advantages of the parallel group design are simplicity, the ability to approximate more closely the likely conditions of use, and the avoidance of 'carry-over effects' (see below).

Cross-over design

In this design, each subject is randomised to a sequence of two or more treatments, and hence acts as his or her own control for treatment comparisons. The advantage of this design is that subject-to-subject variation is eliminated from treatment comparison so that number of subjects is reduced.

In the basic cross-over design each subject receives each of the two treatments in a randomised order. There are variations to this in which each subject receives a subset of treatments or ones in which treatments are repeated within the same subject (to explore the reproducibility of effects).

The main disadvantage of the cross-over design is carry-over, i.e. the residual influence of treatments on subsequent treatment periods. This can be avoided to some extent by separating treatments with a 'wash-out' period and, more importantly, by selecting treatment lengths based on a knowledge of the disease and the new medication. The cross-over design is best suited for chronic stable diseases e.g. hypertension, chronic stable angina pectoris, where the baseline conditions are attained at the start of each treatment arm. The pharmacokinetic characteristics of the new medication are also important, the principle being that the plasma concentration at the start of the next dosing period is zero and no dynamic effect can be detected.

Factorial designs

In the factorial design, two or more treatments are evaluated simultaneously through the use of varying combinations of the treatments. The simplest example is the 2×2 factorial design in which subjects are randomly allocated to one of four possible combinations of two treatments A and B. These are: A alone, B alone, A + B, neither A nor

[24]Modell W, Houde R W 1958 Factors influencing clinical evaluation of drugs; with special reference to the double-blind technique. Journal of the American Medical Association 167:2190–2199.

B (placebo). The main uses of the factorial design are to:

- make efficient use of clinical trial subjects by evaluating two treatments with the same number of individuals
- examine the interaction of A with B
- establish dose–response characteristics of the combination of A and B when the efficacy of each has been previously established.

Multicentre trials

Multicentre trials are carried out for two main reasons. First, they are an efficient way of evaluating a new medication, by accruing sufficient subjects in a reasonable time to satisfy trial objectives. Second, multicentre trials may be designed to provide a better basis for the subsequent generalisation of their findings. Thus they provide the possibility of recruiting subjects from a wide population and of administering the medication in a broad range of clinical settings. Multicentre trials can be used at any phase in clinical development, but are especially valuable when used to confirm therapeutic value in Phase 3.

The main potential problem with a multicentre clinical trial is that heterogeneity of treatment effects between centres may create difficulty in arriving at a single interpretation. This is not as big a problem as is sometimes painted, and large-scale multicentre trials using minimised data collection techniques and simple endpoints have been of immense value in establishing modest but real treatment effects that apply to a large number of patients, e.g. drugs that improve survival after myocardial infarction.

N-of-1 trials

Patients give varied treatment responses and the average effect derived from a population sample may not be helpful in expressing the size of benefit or harm for an individual. In the future pharmacogenomics may provide an answer, but in the meantime the best way to settle doubt as to whether a test drug is effective for an individual patient is the *n-of-1 trial*. This is a cross-over design in which each patient receives two or more administrations of drug or placebo in random manner; the results from individuals can then be displayed. Two conditions apply. First, the disease in which the drug is being tested must be chronic and stable. Second, the treatment effect must wear off rapidly. N-of-1 trials are

not used routinely in drug development and, if so, only at the Phase 3 stage.[25,26]

Historical controls

Any temptation simply to give a new treatment to all patients and to compare the results with the past (historical controls) is almost always unacceptable, even with a disease such as leukaemia. The reasons are that standards of diagnosis and treatment change with time, and the severity of some diseases (infections) fluctuates. The general provision stands that controls must be concurrent and concomitant. An exception to this rule is the case–control study (see p. 58).

SIZE OF TRIALS

Before the start of any controlled trial it is necessary to decide the number of patients that will be needed to deliver an answer, for ethical as well as practical reasons. This is determined by four factors:

1. The *magnitude* of the difference sought or expected on the primary efficacy endpoint (the target difference). For between-group studies, the focus of interest is the mean difference that constitutes a clinically significant effect.
2. The *variability* of the measurement of the primary endpoint as reflected by the standard deviation of this primary outcome measure. The magnitude of the expected difference (above) divided by the standard deviation of the difference gives the *standardised difference* (Fig. 4.2).
3. The defined *significance* level, i.e. the level of chance for accepting a Type I (α) error. Levels of 0.05 (5%) and 0.01 (1%) are common targets.
4. The *power* or desired probability of detecting the required mean treatment difference, i.e. the level of chance for accepting a Type II (β) error. For most controlled trials, a power of 80–90% (0.8–0.9) is frequently chosen as adequate, although higher power is chosen for some studies.

It will be intuitively obvious that a *small* difference in the effect that can be detected between two treatment groups, or a *large* variability in the measurement of

[25]Senn S 1997 N-of-1 trials. Statistical issues in drug development. John Wiley, Chichester, p. 249–255.
[26]Jull A, Bennet D 2005 Do N-of-1 trials really tailor treatment? Lancet 365:1992–1994.

the primary endpoint, or a *high* significance level (low *P* value) or a large power requirement, all act to increase the required sample size. Figure 4.2 gives a graphical representation of how the power of a clinical trial relates to values of clinically relevant standardised difference for varying numbers of trial subjects (shown by the individual curves). It is clear that the larger the number of subjects in a trial, the smaller is the difference that can be detected for any given power value.

The aim of any clinical trial is to have small Type I and II errors, and consequently sufficient power to detect a difference between treatments, if it exists. Of the four factors that determine sample size, the power and significance level are chosen to suit the level of risk felt to be appropriate; the magnitude of the effect can be estimated from previous experience with drugs of the same or similar action; the variability of the measurements is often known from published experiments on the primary endpoint, with or without drug. These data will, however, not be available for novel substances in a new class, and frequently the sample size in the early phase of development is chosen on a more arbitrary basis. As an example, a trial that would detect, at the 5% level of statistical significance, a treatment that raised a cure rate from 75% to 85% would require 500 patients for 80% power.

Fixed-sample size and sequential designs

Defining when a clinical trial should end is not as simple as it first appears. In the standard clinical trial the end is defined by the passage of all of the recruited subjects through the complete design. However, it is results and decisions based on the results that matter, not the number of subjects. The result of the trial may be that one treatment is superior to another or that there is no difference. These trials are of *fixed sample size*. In fact, patients are recruited sequentially, but the results are analysed at a fixed time-point.

The results of this type of trial may be disappointing if they miss the agreed and accepted level of significance.

It is not legitimate, having just failed to reach the agreed level (say, *P*=0.05), to take in a few more patients in the hope that they will bring *P* value down to 0.05 or less, for this is deliberately not allowing chance and the treatment to be the sole factors involved in the outcome, as they should be.

An alternative (or addition) to repeating the fixed-sample size trial is to use a *sequential design* in which the trial is run until a useful result is reached.[27] These adaptive designs, in which decisions are taken on the basis of results to date, can assess results on a continuous basis as data for each subject become available or, more commonly, on groups of subjects (group sequential design). The essential feature of these designs is that the trial is terminated when a *predetermined* result is attained and not when the investigator looking at the results thinks it appropriate. Reviewing results in a continuous or interim basis requires *formal interim analysis* and there are specific statistical methods for handling the data, which need to be agreed in advance. Group sequential designs are especially successful in large long-term trials of mortality or major non-fatal endpoints when safety must be monitored closely.

Interim analyses can reduce the power of statistical significance tests to a serious degree if they are scheduled to occur more than, say, about four times in a trial. Such sequential designs recognise the reality of medical practice and provide a reasonable balance between statistical, medical and ethical needs. It is a necessity to have expert statistical advice when undertaking such trials; poorly designed and executed studies cannot be salvaged after the event.

SENSITIVITY OF TRIALS

Definitive therapeutic trials are expensive and tedious, and may be so prolonged that aspects of treatment have been superseded by the time a result is obtained. A single trial, however well designed, executed and analysed, can answer only the question addressed. The regulatory authorities give guidance as to the number and design of trials that, if successful, would lead to a therapeutic claim. But changing clinical practice in the longer term depends on many other factors, of which confirmatory trials in other centres by different investigators under different conditions are an important part.

META-ANALYSIS

The two main outcomes for therapeutic trials are to influence clinical practice and, where appropriate, to make a successful claim for a drug with the regulatory

---

[27]Whitehead J 1992 The design analysis of sequential clinical trials, 2nd edn. Ellis Horwood, Chester.

authorities. Investigators are eternally optimistic and frequently plan their trials to look for large effects. Reality is different. The results of a planned (or unplanned) series of clinical trials may vary considerably for several reasons, but most significantly because the studies are too small to detect a treatment effect. In common but serious diseases such as cancer or heart disease, however, even small treatment effects can be important in terms of their total impact on public health. It may be unreasonable to expect dramatic advances in these diseases; we should be looking for small effects. Drug developers, too, should be interested not only in whether a treatment works, but also how well and for whom.

The collecting together of a number of trials with the same objective in a *systematic review*[28] and analysing the accumulated results using appropriate statistical methods is termed *meta-analysis*. The principles of a meta-analysis are that:

- It should be comprehensive, i.e. include data from all trials, published and unpublished.
- Only randomised controlled trials should be analysed, with patients entered on the basis of 'intention to treat'.[29]
- The results should be determined using clearly defined, disease-specific endpoints (this may involve a re-analysis of original trials).

There are strong advocates and critics of the concept, its execution and interpretation. Arguments that have been advanced against meta-analysis are:

- An effect of reasonable size ought to be demonstrable in a single trial.
- Different study designs cannot be pooled.
- Lack of accessibility of all relevant studies.
- Publication bias ('positive' trials are more likely to be published).

---

[28]A review that strives comprehensively to identify and synthesise all the literature on a given subject (sometimes called an overview). The unit of analysis is the primary study, and the same scientific principles and rigour apply as for any study. If a review does not state clearly whether and how all relevant studies were identified and synthesised, it is not a systematic review (The Cochrane Library 1998).

[29]Reports of therapeutic trials should contain an analysis of all patients entered, regardless of whether they dropped out or failed to complete, or even started the treatment for any reason. Omission of these subjects can lead to serious bias (Laurence D R, Carpenter J 1998 A dictionary of pharmacological and allied topics. Elsevier, Amsterdam).

In practice, the analysis involves calculating an *odds ratio* for each trial included in the meta-analysis. This is the ratio of the number of patients experiencing a particular endpoint, e.g. death, and the number who do not, compared with the equivalent figures for the control group. The number of deaths *observed* in the treatment group is then compared with the number to be *expected* if it is assumed that the treatment is ineffective, to give the *observed minus expected* statistic. The treatment effects for all trials in the analysis are then obtained by summing all the 'observed minus expected' values of the individual trials to obtain the overall odds ratio. An odds ratio of 1.0 indicates that the treatment has no effect, an odds ratio of 0.5 indicates a halving and an odds ratio of 2.0 indicates a doubling of the risk that patients will experience the chosen endpoint.

From the position of drug development, the general requirement that scientific results have to be repeatable has been interpreted in the past by the Food and Drug Administration (the regulatory agency in the USA) to mean that two well controlled studies are required to support a claim. But this requirement is itself controversial and its relation to a meta-analysis in the context of drug development is unclear.

In clinical practice, and in the era of cost-effectiveness, the use of meta-analysis as a tool to aid medical decision-making and underpinning 'evidence-based medicine' is here to stay.

Figure 4.3 shows detailed results from 11 trials in which antiplatelet therapy after myocardial infarction was compared with a control group. The number of vascular events per treatment group is shown in the second and third columns, and the odds ratios with the point estimates (the value most likely to have resulted from the study) are represented by black squares and their 95% confidence intervals (CI) in the fourth column.

The size of the square is proportional to the number of events. The diamond gives the point estimate and CI for overall effect.

RESULTS: IMPLEMENTATION

The way in which data from therapeutic trials are presented can influence doctors' perceptions of the advisability of adopting a treatment in their routine practice.

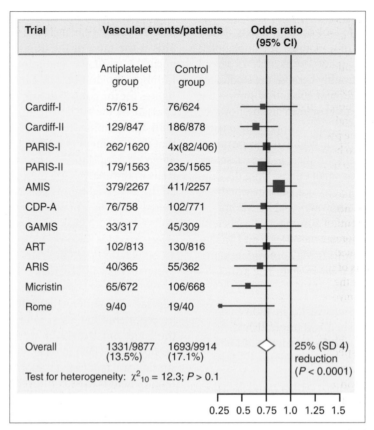

Fig. 4.3 A clear demonstration of benefits from meta-analysis of available trial data, when individual trials failed to provide convincing evidence. (Reproduced with permission of Collins R 2001 Lancet 357:373–380.)

Relative and absolute risk

The results of therapeutic trials are commonly expressed as the percentage reduction of an unfavourable (or percentage increase in a favourable) outcome, i.e. as the *relative risk*, and this can be very impressive indeed until the figures are presented as the number of individuals actually affected per 100 people treated, i.e. as the *absolute risk*.

Where a baseline risk is *low*, a statement of relative risk alone is particularly misleading as it implies large benefit where the actual benefit is small. Thus a reduction of risk from 2% to 1% is a 50% relative risk reduction, but it saves only one patient for every 100 patients treated. But where the baseline is high, say 40%, a 50% reduction in relative risk saves 20 patients for every 100 treated.

To make clinical decisions, readers of therapeutic studies need to know: how many patients must be treated[30] (and for how long) to obtain one desired result (*number needed to treat*). This is the inverse (or reciprocal) of absolute risk reduction.

Relative risk reductions can remain high (and thus make treatments seem attractive) even when susceptibility to the events being prevented is low (and the corresponding numbers needed to be treated are large). As a result, restricting the reporting of efficacy

[30]See Cooke R J, Sackett D L 1995 The number needed to treat: a clinically useful treatment effect. British Medical Journal 310:452.

to just relative risk reductions can lead to great – and at times excessive – zeal in decisions about treatment for patients with low susceptibilities.[31]

A real-life example follows:

> Antiplatelet drugs reduce the risk of future non-fatal myocardial infarction by 30% [*relative risk*] in trials of both primary and secondary prevention. But when the results are presented as the number of patients who need to be treated for one nonfatal myocardial infarction to be avoided [*absolute risk*] they look very different.
>
> In secondary prevention of myocardial infarction, 50 patients need to be treated for 2 years, while in primary prevention 200 patients need to be treated for 5 years, for one nonfatal myocardial infarction to be prevented. In other words, it takes 100 patient-years of treatment in primary prevention to produce the same beneficial outcome of one fewer nonfatal myocardial infarction.[32]

Whether a low incidence of adverse drug effects is acceptable becomes a serious issue in the context of absolute risk. Non-specialist doctors, particularly those in primary care, need and deserve clear and informative presentation of therapeutic trial results that measure the overall impact of a treatment on the patient's life, i.e. on clinically important outcomes such as morbidity, mortality, quality of life, working capacity, fewer days in hospital. Without it, they cannot adequately advise patients, who may themselves be misled by inappropriate use of statistical data in advertisements or on internet sites.

Important aspects of therapeutic trial reports
- Statistical significance and its clinical importance
- Confidence intervals
- Number needed to treat, or absolute risk

---

[31]Sackett D L, Cooke R J 1994 Understanding clinical trials: what measures of efficacy should journal articles provide busy clinicians? British Medical Journal 309:755.

[32]For example, drug therapy for high blood pressure carries risks, but the risks of the disease vary enormously according to severity of disease: 'Depending on the initial absolute risk, the benefits of lowering blood pressure range from preventing one cardiovascular event a year for about every 20 people treated, to preventing one event for about every 5000–10 000 people treated. The level of risk at which treatment should be started is debatable' (Jackson R, Barham P, Bills J et al 1993 Management of raised blood pressure in New Zealand: a discussion document. British Medical Journal 307:107–110).

PHARMACOEPIDEMIOLOGY

Pharmacoepidemiology is the study of the use and effects of drugs in large numbers of people. Some of the principles of pharmacoepidemiology are used to gain further insight into the efficacy, and especially the safety, of new drugs once they have passed from limited exposure in controlled therapeutic pre-registration trials to the looser conditions of their use in the community. Trials in this setting are described as *observational* because the groups to be compared are assembled from subjects who are, or who are not (the controls), taking the treatment in the ordinary way of medical care. These (Phase 4) trials are subject to greater risk of selection bias[33] and confounding[34] than *experimental* studies (randomised controlled trials) where entry and allocation of treatment are strictly controlled (increasing internal validity). Observational studies, nevertheless, come into their own when sufficiently large randomised trials are logistically and financially impracticable. The following approaches are used.

Observational cohort[35] studies

Patients receiving a drug are followed up to determine the outcomes (therapeutic or adverse). This is usually forward-looking (prospective) research. A cohort study does not require a suspicion of causality; subjects can be followed 'to see what happens' (event recording). *Prescription event monitoring* (below) is an example, and there is an increasing tendency to recognise that most new drugs should be monitored in this way when prescribing becomes general. Major difficulties include the selection of an appropriate control group, and the need for large numbers of subjects and for prolonged surveillance. This sort of study is scientifically inferior to the *experimental* cohort study (the randomised controlled trial) and is cumbersome for research on drugs.

---

[33]A systematic error in the selection or randomisation of patients on admission to a trial such that they differ in prognosis, i.e. the outcome is weighted one way or another by the selection, not by the trial.

[34]When the interpretation of an observed association between two variables may be affected by a strong influence from a third variable (which may be hidden or unknown). Examples of confounders would be concomitant drug therapy or differences in known risk factors, e.g. smoking, age, sex.

[35]Used here for a group of people having a common attribute, e.g. they have all taken the same drug.

Investigation of the question of thromboembolism and the combined oestrogen–progestogen contraceptive pill by means of an observational cohort study required enormous numbers of subjects[36] (the adverse effect is, fortunately, uncommon) followed over years. An investigation into cancer and the contraceptive pill by an observational cohort would require follow-up for 10–15 years. Happily, epidemiologists have devised a partial alternative: the case–control study.

Case–control studies

This reverses the direction of scientific logic from a forward-looking, 'what happens next' (*prospective*) to a backward-looking, 'what has happened in the past' (*retrospective*)[37] investigation. The case–control study requires a definite hypothesis or suspicion of causality, such as an adverse reaction to a drug. The investigator assembles a group of patients who have the condition. A control group of people who have not had the reaction is then assembled (matched, e.g. for sex, age, smoking habits) from hospital admissions for other reasons, primary care records or electoral rolls. A complete drug history is taken from each group, i.e. the two groups are 'followed up' backwards to determine the proportion in each group that has taken the suspect agent. Case–control studies do not prove causation.[38] They reveal associations and it is up to investigators and critical readers to decide the most plausible explanation.

A case–control study has the advantage that it requires a much smaller number of cases (hundreds) of disease and can thus be done quickly and cheaply. It has the disadvantage that it follows up subjects backwards and there is always suspicion of the intrusion of unknown and so unavoidable biases in the selection of both patients and controls. Here again, inde-

pendent repetition of the studies, if the results are the same, greatly enhances confidence in the outcome.

SURVEILLANCE SYSTEMS: PHARMACOVIGILANCE

When a drug reaches the market, a good deal is known about its therapeutic activity but rather less about its safety when used in large numbers of patients with a variety of diseases, for which they are taking other drugs. The term *pharmacovigilance* refers to the process of identifying and responding to issues of drug safety through the detection in the community of drug effects, usually adverse. Over a number of years increasingly sophisticated systems have been developed to provide surveillance of drugs in the post-marketing phase. For understandable reasons, they are strongly supported by governments. The position has been put thus:

Four kinds of logic can be applied to drug safety monitoring:

- to attempt to follow a complete cohort of (new) drug users for as long as it is deemed necessary to have adequate information
- to perform special studies in areas which may be predicted to give useful information
- to try to gain experience from regular reporting of suspected adverse drug reactions from health professionals during the regular clinical use of the drug
- to examine disease trends for drug-related causality.[39]

Drug safety surveillance relies heavily on the techniques of pharmacoepidemiology, which include the following.

Voluntary reporting. Doctors, nurses and pharmacists are supplied with cards on which to record suspected adverse reaction to drugs. In the UK, this is called the 'Yellow Card' system and the Commission for Human Medicines collates the results and advises the Medicines and Healthcare products Regulatory Agency of the government. It is recommended that for:

- newer drugs: all suspected reactions should be reported, i.e. any adverse or any unexpected

---

[36]The Royal College of General Practitioners (UK) recruited 23 000 women takers of the pill and 23 000 controls in 1968 and issued a report in 1973. It found an approximately doubled incidence of venous thrombosis in combined-pill takers (the dose of oestrogen was reduced because of this study).

[37]For this reason such studies have been named *trohoc* (cohort spelled backwards) studies (Feinstein A 1981 Journal of Chronic Diseases 34:375).

[38]Experimental cohort studies (i.e. randomised controlled trials) are on firmer ground with regard to causation as there should be only one systematic difference between the groups (i.e. the treatment being studied). In case–control studies the groups may differ systematically in several ways.

[39]Edwards I R 1998 A perspective on drug safety. In: Edwards I R (ed.) Drug safety. Adis International, Auckland, p. xii.

event, however minor, that could conceivably be attributed to the drug

- established drugs: all serious suspected reactions should be reported, even if the effect is well recognised.

Inevitably the system depends on the intuitions and willingness of those called on to respond. Surveys suggest that no more than 10% of serious reactions are reported. Voluntary reporting is effective for identifying reactions that develop shortly after starting therapy, i.e. at providing early warnings of drug toxicity. Thus, it is the first line in post-marketing surveillance. Reporting is particularly low, however, for reactions with long latency, such as tardive dyskinesia from chronic neuroleptic use. As the system has no limit of quantitative sensitivity, it may detect the rarest events, e.g. those with an incidence of 1 : 5000–1 : 10 000. Voluntary systems are, however, unreliable for estimating the *incidence* of adverse reactions as this requires both a high rate of reporting (the numerator) and a knowledge of the rate of drug usage (the denominator).

Prescription event monitoring. This is a form of observational cohort study. Prescriptions for a drug (say, 20 000) are collected (in the UK this is made practicable by the existence of a National Health Service in which prescriptions are sent to a single central authority for pricing and payment of the pharmacist). The prescriber is sent a questionnaire and asked to report all events that have occurred (not only suspected adverse reactions) with no judgement regarding causality. Thus 'a broken leg is an event. If more fractures were associated with this drug they could have been due to hypotension, CNS effects or metabolic disease'.[40] By linking general practice and hospital records and death certificates, both prospective and retrospective studies can be done and unsuspected effects detected. Prescription event monitoring can be used routinely on newly licensed drugs, especially those likely to be widely prescribed in general practice, and it can also be implemented quickly in response to a suspicion raised, e.g. by spontaneous reports.

Medical record linkage allows computer correlation in a population of life and health events (birth, marriage, death, hospital admission) with history of drug use. It is being developed as far as resources permit. It includes prescription event monitoring (above). The largest UK medical record linkage is the General Practitioner Research Data Base at the Medicines Healthcare Products Regulatory Agency.

Population statistics e.g. birth defect registers and cancer registers. These are insensitive unless a drug-induced event is highly remarkable or very frequent. If suspicions are aroused then case–control and observational cohort studies will be initiated.

STRENGTH OF EVIDENCE

A number of types of clinical investigation are described in this chapter, and elsewhere in the book. When making clinical decisions about a course of therapeutic action, it is obviously relevant to judge the strength of evidence generated by different types of study. This has been summarised as follows, in rank order:[41]

1. Systematic reviews and meta-analysis.
2. Randomised controlled trials with definitive results (confidence intervals that do not overlap the threshold of the clinically significant effect).[42]
3. Randomised controlled trials with non-definitive results (a difference that suggests a clinically significant effect but with confidence intervals overlapping the threshold of this effect).
4. Cohort studies.
5. Case–control studies.
6. Cross-sectional surveys.
7. Case reports.

[40]Inman W H W, Rawson N S B, Wilton L V 1986 Prescription-event monitoring. In: Inman W H W (ed.) Monitoring for drug safety, 2nd edn. MTP, Lancaster, p. 217.

[41]Guyatt G H, Sackett D L, Sinclair J C et al 1995 Users' guides to the medical literature. IX. A method for grading health care recommendations. Evidence-Based Medicine Working Group. Journal of the American Medical Association 274:1800–1804.

[42]The reporting of randomised controlled trials has been systemised so that only high-quality studies will be considered. See Moher D, Schulz K F, Altman D G 2001 CONSORT Group. The CONSORT statement: revised recommendations for improving the quality of reports of parallel group randomised trials. Lancet 357:1191–1194.

IN CONCLUSION[43]

Drug development is a high risk business. Early hopes and expectations can later be shattered by the realities of clinical practice, when the risks as well as the benefits of a medicine emerge with the passage of time.

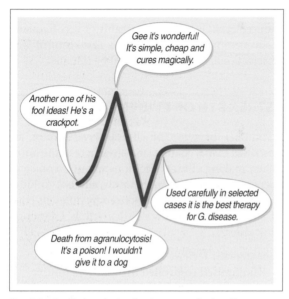

Fig. 4.4 Oscillations in the development of a drug.[44]

GUIDE TO FURTHER READING

Biomarkers Definitions Working Group 2001 Biomarkers and surrogate endpoints: preferred definitions and conceptual framework. Clinical Pharmacology and Therapeutics 69(3):89–95

Bland J M, Altman D G 2000 Statistical notes: the odds ratio. British Medical Journal 320:1468

Chatellier G, Zapletal E, Lemaitre D, Menard J, Degoulet P 1996 The number needed to treat: a clinically useful nomogram in its proper context. British Medical Journal 312:426–429

Doll R 1998 Controlled trials: the 1948 watershed. British Medical Journal 317:1217–1220 (and following articles)

Egger M, Smith G D, Phillips A N 1997 Meta-analysis: principles and procedures. British Medical Journal 315:1533–1537 (see also other articles in the series entitled 'Meta-analysis')

Emanuel E J, Miller F G 2001 The ethics of placebo-controlled trials – a middle ground. New England Journal of Medicine 345(12):915–919

Greenhalgh T 1997 Papers that report drug trials. British Medical Journal 315:480–483 (see also other articles in the series entitled 'How to read a paper')

Kaptchuk T J 1998 Powerful placebo: the dark side of the randomised controlled trial. Lancet 351:1722–1725

Khan K S, Kunz R, Kleijnen J, Antes G 2003 Five steps to conducting a systematic review. Journal of the Royal Society of Medicine 96(3):118–121

Lewis J A, Jonsson B, Kreutz G et al 2002 Placebo-controlled trials and the Declaration of Helsinki. Lancet 359:1337–1340

Miller F G, Rosenstein D L 2003 The therapeutic orientation to clinical trials. New England Journal of Medicine 348(14):1383–1386

Rochon P A, Gurwitz J H, Sykora K et al 2005 Reader's guide to critical appraisal of cohort studies: 1. Role and design. British Medical Journal 330:895–897

Rothwell P M 2005 External validity of randomised controlled trials: 'to whom do the results of this trial apply?' Lancet 365:82–93

Rothwell P M 2005 Treating individuals 2. Subgroup analysis in randomised controlled trials: importance, indications, and interpretation. Lancet 365: 176–186

Silverman W A, Altman D G 1996 Patients' preferences and randomised trials. Lancet 347:171–174

Vlahakes G J 2006 Editorial: The value of phase 4 clinical testing. New England Journal of Medicine 354(4):413–415

Waller P C, Jackson P R, Tucker G T, Ramsay L E 1994 Clinical pharmacology with confidence [intervals]. British Journal of Clinical Pharmacology 37(4):309

Williams R L, Chen M-L, Hauck W W 2002 Equivalence approaches. Clinical Pharmacology and Therapeutics 72(3):229–237

---

[43]'Quick, let us prescribe this new drug while it remains effective'. Richard Asher.

[44]By courtesy of Dr Robert H. Williams and the editor of the Journal of the American Medical Association.

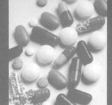

5

Official regulation of medicines

SYNOPSIS

This chapter describes the background to why it became necessary to regulate the use and supply of drugs, and the ways in which these processes are managed.

- Basis for regulation: safety, efficacy, quality, supply
- Present medicines regulatory system
- Present-day requirements
  - Counterfeit drugs
  - Complementary and alternative medicine
  - Medicines regulation: the future

BASIS FOR REGULATION

Neither patients nor doctors are in a position to decide for themselves, across the range of medicines that they use, which ones are *pure* and *stable*, and *effective* and *safe*. They need assurance that the medicines they are offered fulfil these requirements and are supported by information that permits optimal use. The information about and the usage of medicines gets out of date, and there is an obligation on licence holders continually to review their licence with particular regard to safety. Marketing Authorisation Holders (MAHs), i.e. pharmaceutical companies, can also change the efficacy claims to their licence (e.g. new indications, extension of age groups) or change the safety information (e.g. add new warnings, or contraindications). The quality aspects may also need to be revised as manufacturing practices change. MAHs have strong profit motives for making claims about their drugs. Only governments can provide the assurance about all those aspects in the life of a medicine (in so far as it can be provided).

The principles of official (statutory) medicines regulation are that:

- No medicines will be marketed without prior licensing by the government.
- A licence will be granted on the basis of scientific evaluation of:

1. *Safety*, in relation to its use: evaluation at the point of marketing is provisional in the sense that it is followed in the community by a pharmacovigilance programme.
2. *Efficacy* (now often including quality of life).
3. *Quality*, i.e. purity, stability (shelf-life).
4. *Supply*, i.e. whether the drug is suitable to be unrestrictedly available to the public or whether it should be confined to sales through pharmacies or on doctors' prescriptions; and what printed information should accompany its sale (labelling, leaflets).

- A licence shall specify the clinical indications that may be promoted and shall be for a limited period (5 years), which is renewable on application. A regulatory authority may review the risk:benefit ratio or safety of a drug at any time and restrict the licensing, or remove the drug from the market for good cause.[1]
- A licence may be varied (altered) by an application from the pharmaceutical company to update efficacy, safety and quality sections; safety and (less commonly) efficacy variations may be initiated by the regulatory authority.

Plainly manufacturers and developers are entitled to be told what substances are regulated and what are not[2], and what kinds and amounts of data are likely

---

[1] As from 2006, the European Community regulations requires one renewal at 5 years and a second at 10 years only if safety issues demand it, with safety update reviews every 3 years after licensing.

[2] It is obviously impossible to list substances that will be regulated if anybody should choose one day to synthesise them. Therefore regulation is based on the supply of 'medicinal products', i.e. substances are regulated according to their proposed use; and they must be defined in a way that will resist legal challenge (hence the stilted regulatory language). The following terms have gained informal acceptance for 'borderline substances' (which may or may not be regulated): nutriceutical – a food or part of a food that provides medicinal benefits; cosmeceutical – a cosmetic that also has medicinal use.

to persuade a regulatory authority to grant a marketing application (licence) and for what medical purpose. In summary, medicines regulation aims to provide an objective, rigorous and transparent assessment of efficacy, safety and quality in order to protect and promote public health but not to impede the pharmaceutical industry. Inevitably, an interesting tension exists between regulators and regulated.[3]

HISTORICAL BACKGROUND

The beginning of substantial government intervention in the field of medicines paralleled the proliferation of synthetic drugs in the early 20th century when the traditional and familiar pharmacopoeia[4] expanded slowly and then, in mid-century, with enormous rapidity. The first comprehensive regulatory law that required pre-marketing testing was passed in the USA in 1938, following the death of about 107 people due to the use of diethylene glycol (a constituent of antifreeze) as a solvent for a stable liquid formulation of sulphanilamide for treating common infections.[5]

Other countries did not take on board the lesson provided by the USA and it took *the thalidomide disaster*[6,7] to make governments all over the world initiate comprehensive control over all aspects of drug introduction, therapeutic claims and supply.

---

[3]However much doctors may mock the bureaucratic 'regulatory mind', regulation provides an important service and it is expedient that doctors should have some insight into its working and some of the very real problems faced by public servants and their advisory committees who are trying to do good without risking losing their jobs and reputations.

[4]Pharmacopoeia: a book (often official) listing drugs and, for example, their standards of purity, manufacture, assay and directions for use.

[5]Report of the Secretary of Agriculture submitted in response to resolutions in the House of Representatives and Senate (USA) 1937 Journal of the American Medical Association 111:583, 919. Recommended reading. A similar episode occurred as recently as 1990–1992 (Hanif M, Mobarak M R, Ronan A et al 1995 Fatal renal failure caused by diethylene glycol in paracetamol elixir: the Banglandesh epidemic. British Medical Journal 311:88–91). Note: diethylene glycol is cheap.

[6]Mellin G W, Katzenstein M 1962 The saga of thalidomide. Neuropathy to embryopathy, with case reports of congenital anomalies. New England Journal of Medicine 267:1184–1192, 1238–1244.

[7]Dally A 1998 Thalidomide: was the tragedy preventable? Lancet 351:1197–1199.

In 1960–1961 in (West) Germany, the incidence of phocomelia in newborns was noted. The term means 'seal extremities' and is a deformity in which the long bones of the limbs are defective and substally normal or rudimentary hands and feet arise on, or nearly on, the trunk, like the flippers of a seal; other abnormalities may occur. Phocomelia is ordinarily exceedingly rare. Case–control and prospective observational cohort studies in antenatal clinics where women had yet to give birth provided evidence incriminating a sedative and hypnotic called thalidomide; it was recommended for use in pregnant women, although it had not been tested on pregnant animals. The worst had happened: a trivial new drug was the cause of the most grisly disaster in the short history of modern scientific drug therapy. Many thalidomide babies died, but many live on with deformed limbs, eyes, ears, heart and alimentary and urinary tracts. The world total of survivors was probably about 10 000.

In the UK, two direct consequences were the development of a spontaneous adverse drug reaction reporting scheme (the Yellow Card system) and legislation to provide regulatory control on the safety, quality and efficacy of medicines through the systems of standards, authorisation, pharmacovigilance (see p. 58) and inspection (Medicines Act 1968). A further landmark was the establishment of the Committee on Safety of Medicines in 1971 (from 2006 renamed the Commission on Human Medicines) to advise the Licensing Authority in the UK. In 1995, the new European regulatory system was introduced (see below).

Despite these protective systems, other drug disasters occurred. In 1974 the (β-blocking agent *practolol* was withdrawn because of a rare but severe syndrome affecting the eyes and other mucocutaneous regions in the body (not detected by animal tests), and in 1982 *benoxaprofen*, a non-steroidal anti-inflammatory drug, was found to cause serious adverse effects including onycholysis and photosensitivity in elderly patients. More recent examples that have gained wide public notice include the association of serotonin-specific reuptake inhibitors with the occurrence of suicide and that of *cyclo-oxygenase I and II inhibitors* with cardiovascular disease.

CURRENT MEDICINES REGULATORY SYSTEMS

All countries where medicines are licensed for use have a regulatory system. When a pharmaceutical company seeks worldwide marketing rights, its programmes *must* satisfy the Food and Drug Administration (FDA) of the USA, the European Medicines Agency[8] (EMA) and the Japanese Pharmaceutical Affairs Bureau. The national regulatory bodies of the individual European Union members remain in place but work with the EMA, which acts as a single source of authority. National licences can still be granted through individual member states, which maintain particular responsibility for their own public health issues. Significant harmonisation of practices and procedures at a global level was also achieved through the International Conferences on Harmonisation (ICH) involving Europe, Japan and the USA.

In the European Union drugs can be licensed in three ways:

1. The *centralised procedure* allows applications to be made directly to the EMA; applications are allocated for assessment to one member state (the rapporteur) assisted by a second member state (co-rapporteur). Approval of the licence is then binding on all member states. This approach is mandatory for biotechnology products and for certain new medicinal products.
2. The *mutual recognition (or decentralised) procedure* allows applicants to nominate one member state (known as a reference member state), which assesses the application and seeks opinion from the other (concerned) member states. Granting the licence will ensure simultaneous mutual recognition in these other states, provided agreement is reached among them. There is an arbitration procedure to resolve disputes.
3. A product to be marketed in a single country can have its licence applied for through the *national route*.

The European systems are conducted according to strict timelines and written procedures. Once a medicine has been licensed for sale by one of the above procedures, its future regulatory life remains within that procedure. Licences have to be reviewed every 6 months for the first 2 years, then annually until 5 years. Thereafter, there may be a second renewal at 10 years, if safety issues demand.[1] The renewal of a licence is primarily the responsibility of the pharmaceutical company, but requires approval from the reg-ulatory authority. This provides the opportunity for companies to review, in particular, the safety aspects to keep the licence in line with current clinical practice. Any major changes to licences must be made by variation of the original licence (safety, efficacy or quality; see below) and supported by data, which for a major indication can be substantial.

REQUIREMENTS

AUTHORISATION FOR CLINICAL TRIALS IN THE UK

The EU Clinical Trial Directive 2001/20/EC harmonised the laws and administrative procedures relating to the regulation of clinical trials across Europe and replaced the previous legislation in each of the separate member states. It is implemented in the UK through the Medicines for Human Use (Clinical Trials) Regulations.[9] All clinical trials, including human volunteer trials, require regulatory approval through a Clinical Trial Authorisation (CTA) application that must include summaries of preclinical, clinical and pharmaceutical data. For most trials a response must be provided by the regulatory authority within 30 days, with a maximum of up to 60 days. There is a complementary process to allow for amendments to the original application, and there is a requirement to notify each involved regulatory agency when the trial is completed.

REGULATORY REVIEW OF A NEW DRUG APPLICATION

A drug regulatory authority requires the following:

- *Preclinical tests*
    - tests carried out in animals to allow some prediction of potential efficacy and safety in humans (see Chapter 4)
    - chemical and pharmaceutical quality checks, e.g. purity, stability, formulation.
- *Clinical (human) tests (Phases 1, 2, 3).*
- *Knowledge of the environmental impact of pharmaceuticals.* Regulatory authorities expect manufacturers to address this concern in their application to market new chemical entities. Aspects include manufacture (chemical pollution), packaging (waste disposal), pollution

---

[8]Formerly the European Medicines Evaluation Agency (EMEA).

[9]2004 Statutory Instrument No. 1031. The Stationary Office, UK.

in immediate use, e.g. antimicrobials and, more remotely, drugs or metabolites entering the food chain or water where use may be massive, e.g. hormones.

The full process of regulatory review of a truly novel drug (new chemical entity) may take months.

Regulatory review

Using one of the regulatory systems described above, an authority normally conducts a review in two stages:

1. Examination of preclinical data to determine whether the drug is safe enough to be tested for (predicted) human therapeutic efficacy.[10]
2. Examination of the clinical studies to determine whether the drug has been shown to be therapeutically effective with safety appropriate to its use.[11]

If the decision is favourable, the drug is granted a marketing authorisation (for 5 years: renewable), which allows it to be marketed for *specified therapeutic uses*. The authority must satisfy itself of the adequacy of the information to be provided to prescribers in a Summary of Product Characteristics (SPC) and also a Patient Information Leaflet (PIL).

The PIL must also be approved by the licensing authority, be deemed fairly to represent the SPC, and be comprehensive and understandable to patients and carers. Where a drug has special advantage, but also has special risk, restrictions on its promotion and use can be imposed, e.g. isotretinoin and clozapine (see Index).

Central to the decision to grant a marketing authorisation is the assessment procedure undertaken by professional medical, scientific, statistical and pharmaceutical staff at one of the national agencies. In the UK these are employed as civil servants within the Medicines Healthcare products Regulatory Agency (MHRA) and are advised by various independent expert committees.[12]

When a novel drug is granted a marketing authorisation it is recognised as a medicine by independent critics and there is rejoicing amongst those who have spent many years developing it. But the testing is not over: the most stringent test of all is about to begin. It will be used in all sorts of people of all ages and sizes, and having all sorts of other conditions. Its use can no longer be supervised so closely as hitherto. Doctors will prescribe it and patients will use it correctly and incorrectly. It will have effects that have not been anticipated. It will be taken in overdose. It has to find its place in therapeutics, through extended comparisons with other drugs available for the same diseases.

Drugs used to prevent a long-term morbidity, e.g. stroke in hypertensive patients, can be proven effective only in *outcome* trials that are usually considered too expensive even to start until marketing of the drug is guaranteed. The effect of a drug at preventing rare occurrences requires many thousands of patients, more than are usually studied during development. Similarly rare adverse events cannot be detected prior to marketing, and it would be unethical to expose large numbers of trial patients to a novel drug for purely safety reasons.[13]

Post-licensing responsibilities

The pharmaceutical company is predominantly interested in gaining as widespread usage as fast as possible, based on the efficacy of the drug demonstrated in pre-registration trials. The regulatory authorities are more concerned with the safety profile of the drug and protection of public health. The most important source of safety data once the drug is in clinical use is spontaneous reporting of adverse events, which will generate 'signals' and raise suspicion of infrequent but potentially serious adverse events caused by the drug.[14] Proving the causal link from sporadic signals can be extremely difficult, and is entirely dependent on the number and quality of these spontaneous reports. In the UK, these reports are captured through the Yellow Card system (see p. 58), which may be completed by doctors, nurses or pharmacists and, most recently, by patients. Other countries have their

---

[10]The Licensing Authority consists of the responsible Minister(s) and the Medicines Control Agency (MCA) – the executive arm in the Department of Health: the Medicines and Healthcare products Regulatory Agency.

[11]Common sense dictates that what, in regulatory terms, is 'safe' for leukaemia would not be 'safe' for anxiety.

[12]Breckenridge A M 2004 The changing scene of the regulation of medicines in the UK. British Journal of Clinical Pharmacology 58:571–574.

[13]After marketing, doctors should use a new drug only when they believe it an improvement (in efficacy, safety, convenience or cost) on the older alternatives.

[14]Waller P C, Bahri P 2002 Regulatory pharmacovigilance in the EU. In: Mann R, Andrews E (eds). Pharmacovigilance. John Wiley, Chichester, p. 183–194.

own systems. The importance of encouraging accurate spontaneous reporting of adverse events cannot be overemphasised.

Post-marketing (Phase 4) studies are not generally regulated by legislation, although in the EU, in exceptional circumstances, they may be a condition of the marketing authorisation. Voluntary guidelines are in use for post-marketing studies agreed between industry and the regulatory authorities. All company-sponsored trials that are relevant to the safety of a marketed medicine are included; they clearly state that such studies should not be conducted for the purposes of promotion. Other studies investigating the safety of a medicine that are not directly sponsored by the manufacturer may be identified from various organisations, e.g. the Drug Safety Research Unit (Southampton, UK) using Prescription Event Monitoring (PEM), the Medicines Monitoring Unit (MEMO) (Tayside, UK), and the use of computerised record linkage schemes (in place in the USA for many years) such as the UK General Practice Research Database at the MHRA. All these systems have the important capacity to obtain information on very large numbers of patients (10 000 to 20 000) in *observational cohort* studies and *case–control* studies, complementing the spontaneous reporting system (see Chapter 4).

In the UK, many new drugs are highlighted as being under special consideration by the regulatory authorities, by marking the drug with a symbol, the inverted black triangle (▼), in formularies. The regulatory authority communicates emerging data on safety of drugs to doctors through letters or papers in journals, through specialist journals, e.g. *Current Problems in Pharmacovigilance*, in the UK, and for very significant issues by direct ('Dear Doctor') letters and fax messages.

Two other important regulatory activities that affect marketed drugs are:

- Variations to licences.
- Reclassifications.

Variations are substantial changes instigated usually by pharmaceutical companies, but sometimes by the regulatory authority, to the efficacy, safety or quality aspects of the medicine. Most significant variations involve additions to indications or dosing regimens, or to the warnings and contraindication sections of the SPC. They need to be supported by evidence and undergo formal assessment.

Reclassification means change in the legal status of a medicine and is the process by which a prescription-only medicine can be converted to one that is available directly to the public through pharmacies and shops. It follows a rigorous assessment process with a particular stress on safety aspects of the medicine; it involves advice from the Commission on Human Medicines and requires a change in secondary legislation. The purpose of reclassification is to allow easier access of the general public to effective and safe medicines. In the UK, emergency contraception ('morning after' pill), simvastatin and omeprazole have been reclassifications to be available from pharmacies without prescription.

DISCUSSION

It may be wondered why post-licensing/marketing surveillance and pharmacovigilance should be necessary. Common sense would seem to dictate that safety and efficacy of a drug should be fully defined before it is granted marketing authorisation. Pre-licensing trials with very close supervision are commonly limited to hundreds of patients and this is unavoidable, chiefly because this close supervision is impracticable on a large scale for a very long time. Post-licensing studies are increasingly regarded as essential to complete the definitive evaluation of drugs under conditions of ordinary use on a large scale, these programmes being preferable to attempts to enlarge and prolong formal therapeutic trials.

It would also seem sensible to require developers to prove that a new drug is not only effective but is actually *needed* in medicine before it is licensed. Strong voices are now arguing that a *risk:benefit* assessment of new (candidate) medicines against old medicines should be part of a regulatory application.[15,16] It is argued that a novel drug finds its place only after several, sometimes many, years, and to delay licensing is simply impracticable on financial grounds. Thus a 'need clause' in licensing is not generally practicable if drug developers are to stay in that business. This is why *comparative* therapeutic studies of a new drug with existing drugs are not

[15]Garratini S, Bertile V 2004 Risk:benefit assessment of old medicines. British Journal of Clinical Pharmacology 58:581–586.
[16]Motola D, De Ponti F, Rossi P et al 2005 Therapeutic innovation in the European Union: analysis of the drugs approved by the EMEA between 1995 and 2003. British Journal of Clinical Pharmacology 59(4):457–478.

required for licensing in countries having a research-based pharmaceutical industry. A 'need clause' is, however, appropriate for economically deprived countries (see World Health Organization Essential Drugs Programme); indeed, such countries have no alternative.

The licensing authority in the UK is not concerned with the pricing of drugs or their cost-effectiveness. The cost of medicines does, however, concern all governments, as part of the rising costs of national health services. A serious attempt to control costs on drug usage by the introduction of national guidelines on disease management (including the use of individual drugs) and the appraisal of new and established medicines for cost-effectiveness now operate through a government-funded body called the National Institute for Health and Clinical Excellence (NICE). Where relevant, elements of guidance notes are issued by NICE appear within this book.

Licensed medicines for unlicensed indications

Doctors may generally prescribe any medicine for any legitimate medical purpose.[17] But if they use a drug for an indication that is not formally included in the product licence ('off-label' use) they would be wise to think carefully and to keep particularly good records for, if a patient is dissatisfied, prescribers may find themselves having to justify the use in a court of law. (Written records made at the time of a decision carry substantial weight, but records made later, when trouble is already brewing, lose much of their power to convince, and records that have been altered later are quite fatal to any defence.) Manufacturers are not always willing to go to the trouble and expense of the rigorous clinical studies required to extend their licence unless a new use is likely to generate significant profits. They are prohibited by law from promoting an unlicensed use. Much prescribing for children is in fact 'off licence' because clinical trials are usually conducted in adults and information sufficient for regulatory purposes in children does not exist. Paediatricians have to use adult data, scaled by body-weight or surface area, together with their clinical experience; this deficiency is being actively addressed in Europe and the USA.

Unlicensed medicines and accelerated licensing

Regulatory systems make provision for the supply of an unlicensed medicine, e.g. one that has not yet completed its full programme of clinical trials, for patients who, on the judgement of their doctors, have no alternative amongst licensed drugs. The doctor must apply to the manufacturer, who may supply the drug for that particular patient and at the doctor's own responsibility. Various terms are used, e.g. supply on a 'named patient' basis (UK); 'compassionate' drug use (USA). It is illegal to exploit this sensible loophole in supply laws to conduct research. Precise record-keeping of such use is essential. But there can be desperate needs involving large numbers of patients, e.g. AIDS, and regulatory authorities may respond by licensing a drug before completion of the usual range of studies (making it clear that patients must understand the risks they are taking). Unfortunately such well intentioned practice discourages patients from entering formal trials and may, in the long run, actually delay the definition of life-saving therapies.

Decision-taking

> It must be remembered always that, although there are risks in taking drugs, there are also risks in not taking drugs, and there are risks in not developing new drugs.

The responsibility to protect public health on the one hand, yet to allow timely access to novel medicines on the other, is one shared by drug regulators, expert advisory bodies and developers. It is complicated by an ever-increasing awareness of the risks and benefits (real or perceived) of medicines by the general public. Some new medicines are registered with the high expectation of effectiveness and with very little safety information; rare and unpredictable adverse events may take years to appear with sufficient conviction that causality is accepted. In taking decisions about drug regulation, it has been pointed out that there is uncertainty in three areas:[18]

- Facts.
- Public reaction to the facts.
- Future consequences of decisions.

---

[17]In many countries this excludes supply of drugs such as heroin or cocaine for controlled/supervised maintenance of drug addicts. In the UK such supply is permitted to doctors.

[18]Lord Ashby 1976 Proceedings of the Royal Society of Medicine 69:721.

Regulators are influenced not only to avoid risk but also to avoid regret later (*regret avoidance*), and this consideration has a profound effect whether or not the decision-taker is conscious of it; it promotes defensive regulation. Regulatory authorities are frequently accused of being too cautious, and responsible, at least in part, for the stagnation in new drug development.

It is self-evident that it is much harder to detect and quantitate a good that is not done than it is to detect and quantitate a harm that is done. Therefore, although it is part of the decision-taker's job to facilitate the doing of good, the avoidance of harm looms larger. Attempts to blame regulators for failing to do good due to regulatory procrastination, the 'drug lag'[19], do not induce the same feelings of horror in regulators and their advisory committees as are induced by the prospect of finding they have approved a drug that has, or may have, caused serious injury and that the victims are about to appear on television.[20] The bitterness of people injured by drugs, whether or not there is fault, could be much reduced by the institution of simple non-adversarial arrangements for compensation. This is not to ridicule the regulators and their advisers. They are doing their best, and commonly make good and sensible decisions that receive no congratulations.

COUNTERFEIT DRUGS

Fraudulent medicines make up as much as 6% of pharmaceutical sales worldwide. They present a serious health (and economic) problem in countries with weak regulatory authorities and lacking money to police drug quality. In these countries counterfeit medicines may comprise 20–50% of available products. The trade may involve false labelling of legally manufactured products, in order to play one national market against another; also low-quality manufacture of correct ingredients; wrong ingredients, including added ingredients (such as corticosteroids added to herbal medicine for arthritis); no active ingredient; false packaging. The trail from raw material to appearance on a pharmacy shelf may involve as many

as four countries, with the final stages (importer, wholesaler) quite innocent, so well has the process been obscured. Developed countries have inspection and enforcement procedures to detect and take appropriate action on illegal activities.

COMPLEMENTARY AND ALTERNATIVE MEDICINE

(See also p. 13.)

The broad term complementary and alternative medicine (CAM) covers a range of widely varied diagnostic and therapeutic practices; it includes herbal and traditional (mainly Chinese) medicines, homoeopathic remedies and dietary supplements.[21] The public demand for these substances is substantial and the financial interests are huge: annual USA sales of herbal medicines reached an estimated US$4 billion in 1998. The efficacy, safety and quality of herbal[22] and homoeopathic[23] preparations have been critically reviewed. Physicians need to be aware that their patients may be taking CAM preparations, not least because of the risk of adverse reactions and drug–drug interactions, e.g. enzyme induction with St John's Wort (*Hypericum perforatum*).[24]

In the UK, largely for historical reasons, the regulation of CAM is problematic and rife with inconsistencies. Some herbal medicines are licensed as such; some are exempt from licensing; some are sold as food supplements; and some products are available in all three categories. Herbal products were granted a Product Licence of Right (PLR) when the licensing system was introduced in the 1970s. Proof of efficacy, safety and quality (mandatory for 'regular' chemical and biologically developed medicinal products) is usually absent. European legislation is currently being introduced for CAM using a modified licensing procedure; manufacturers will be obliged to report adverse reactions.

---

[19]Nevertheless, regulatory authorities have responded by providing a facility for 'fast-tracking' drugs for which clinical need may be urgent, e.g. AIDS (see above).

[20]The very last thing a drug regulator wishes to be able to say is, 'I awoke one morning and found myself famous' – Lord Byron (1788–1824) on the publication of his poem, Childe Harold's Pilgrimage.

---

[21]Baber N S 2003 Complementary medicine, clinical pharmacology and therapeutics (editorial). British Journal of Clinical Pharmacology 55:225.

[22]Barnes J 2003 Quality, efficacy and safety of complementary medicines; fashions, facts and the future. British Journal of Clinical Pharmacology Part I: Regulation and Quality 55: 226–233; Part II: Efficacy and Safety 55:331–340.

[23]Ernst E 2002 A systematic review of systematic reviews of homeopathy. British Journal of Clinical Pharmacology 54:577–582.

[24]Henderson L, Yue Q Y, Bergquist C et al 2002 St John's Wort (*Hypericum perforatum*): drug interactions and clinical outcomes. British Journal of Clinical Pharmacology 54:349–356.

MEDICINES REGULATION: THE FUTURE

In the UK, the principal responsibilities of medicine regulation, i.e. for safe and effective medicines of high quality, will remain the same but the following themes will provide special attention:

- The promotion and protection of public health: the obligations to ministers, the public and industry are unchanged but regulators will operate in an environment in which the public increasingly expects more effective medicines without sacrifice of safety. Some results of this are already apparent.
- A wider and more rapid international pharmacovigilance.[25]
- Greater transparency in regulatory decision-making.
- The results of assessed applications for new medicines will see a shift from complex technical to patient-oriented documents with clear expressions of risk and benefit.
- A widening of the availability of medicines for chronic disorders through pharmacies, by nurses and other non-medical professionals, and directly to the public.
- Attention to the regulation of medicines for special populations, e.g. the licensing of old and new medicines for children.
- The regulation of complementary medicines.

GUIDE TO FURTHER READING

Baber N 1994 International conference on harmonization of technical requirements for registration of pharmaceuticals. British Journal of Clinical Pharmacology 37:401–404

Brass E P 2001 Changing the status of drugs from prescription to over-the-counter availability. New England Journal of Medicine 345(11):810–816

Collier J 1999 Paediatric prescribing: using unlicensed drugs and medicines outside their licensed indications. British Journal of Clinical Pharmacology 48(1):5–8

Conroy S, Choonara I, Impicciatore P et al 2000 Survey of unlicensed and off label drug use in paediatric wards in European countries. British Medical Journal 320:79–82

Gale E A M, Clark A 2000 A drug on the market? Lancet 355:61–63

Moynihan R 2002 Alosetron: a case study in regulatory capture, or a victory for patients' rights?. British Medical Journal 325:592–595

Permanand G, Mossialos E, McKee M 2006 Regulating medicines in Europe: the European Medicines Agency, marketing authorisation, transparency and pharmacovigilance. Clinical Medicine 6(1):87–90

Reichert J M 2000 New biopharmaceuticals in the USA: trends in development and marketing approvals 1995–1999. Trends in Biotechnology 18(9):364–369

Rudolf P M, Bernstein I B G 2004 Counterfeit drugs. New England Journal of Medicine 350(14):1384–1386

Zarin D A, Tse T, Ide N C 2005 Trial registration at ClinicalTrials.gov between May and October 2005. New England Journal of Medicine 353(26): 2779–2787

---

[25]Waller P C, Evan S J W 2003 A model for the future conduct of pharmacovigilance. Pharmacoepidemiology and Drug Safety 12:17–19.

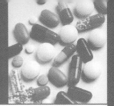

6

Classification and naming of drugs

SYNOPSIS

In any science there are two basic requirements, classification and nomenclature (names):

- Classification – drugs cannot be classified and named according to a single rational system because the requirements of chemists, pharmacologists and doctors differ
- Nomenclature – nor is it practicable always to present each drug under a single name because the formulations in which they are presented as prescribable medicines may vary widely and commercial considerations are too often paramount

Generic (non-proprietary) names should be used as far as possible when prescribing except where pharmaceutical bioavailability differences have overriding importance.

The wider availability of proprietary medicines through pharmacy sale and direct to the public has the potential for greater confusion to consumers (patients) and doctors.

CLASSIFICATION

It is evident from the way this book is organised that there is no homogeneous system for classifying drugs that suits the purpose of every user. Drugs are commonly categorised according to the convenience of who is discussing them: clinicians, pharmacologists or medicinal chemists.

Drugs may be classified by:

- *Body system*, e.g. alimentary, cardiovascular.
- *Therapeutic use*, e.g. receptor blockers, enzyme inhibitors, carrier molecules, ion channels.
- Mode or site of action
  - *molecular interaction*, e.g. glucoside, alkaloid, steroid
  - *cellular site*, e.g. loop diuretic, catecholamine uptake inhibitor (imipramine).
- *Molecular structure*, e.g. glycoside, alkaloid, steroid.[1]

NOMENCLATURE (NAMES)

Any drug may have names in all three of the following classes:

1. The *full chemical name*.
2. A *non-proprietary (official, approved, generic) name* used in pharmacopoeias and chosen by official bodies; the World Health Organization (WHO) chooses recommended International Non-proprietary Names (rINNs). The harmonisation of names began 50 years ago, and most countries have used rINNs for many years. The USA is an exception, but even here most USA National Names are the same as their rINN counterparts. In the UK, since 1 December 2003, where there is a difference between the rINN and the British Approved Name (BAN), the rINN is the correct name. This is a requirement in both European and UK legislation, and applies to all health-care professionals who prescribe, dispense or administer medicines. In most cases the changes are minor, for example amoxycillin (BAN) and amoxicillin (rINN). Some differences are more substantial, e.g. bendrofluazide and bendroflumethiazide, and in a few cases the name is changed completely, e.g. benzhexol to trihexyphenidyl. There are two exceptions to the policy: adrenaline (rINN epinephrine) and noradrenaline (rINN norepinephrine). Manufacturers are advised to use both names on the product packaging and information literature. Prescribers and dispensers are recommended to retain the BANs adrenaline and noradrenaline.

---

[1]The ATC Classification System developed by the Nordic countries and widely used in Europe meets most classification requirements. Drugs are classified according to their Anatomical, Therapeutic and Chemical characteristics into five levels of specificity, the fifth being that for the single chemical substance.

In general we use rINNs in this book and aim to minimise some unavoidable differences with, where appropriate, alternative names in the text and index (in brackets).

3. A *proprietary (brand) name* that is the commercial property of a pharmaceutical company or companies. In this book proprietary names are distinguished by an initial capital letter.

Example: One drug – three names
1. 3-(10,11-dihydro-5H-dibenz[b.*f*]-azepin-5-yl) propyldimethylamine
2. imipramine
3. Tofranil (UK), Melipramine, Novopramine, Pryleugan, Surplix, etc. (various countries)

The *full chemical name* describes the compound for chemists. It is obviously unsuitable for prescribing.

A *non-proprietary* (generic,[2] approved) *name* is given by an official (pharmacopoeia) agency, e.g. WHO.

> Three principles remain supreme and unchallenged in importance: the need for distinction in sound and spelling, especially when the name is handwritten; the need for freedom from confusion with existing names, both non-proprietary and proprietary, and the desirability of indicating relationships between similar substances.[3]

The generic names *diazepam, nitrazepam* and *flurazepam* are all of benzodiazepines. Their proprietary names are Valium, Mogadon and Dalmane respectively. Names ending in *-olol* are adrenoceptor blockers; those ending in *-pril* are angiotensin-converting enzyme (ACE) inhibitors; and those in *-floxacin* are quinolone antimicrobials. Any pharmaceutical company may manufacture a drug that has a well established use and is no longer under patent restriction, in accordance with official pharmacopoeial quality criteria, and may apply to the regulatory authority for a licence to market. The task of authority is to ensure that these *generic* or *multi-source pharmaceuticals* are

interchangeable, i.e. they are pharmaceutically and biologically equivalent, so that a formulation from one source will be absorbed and give the same blood concentrations and have the same therapeutic efficacy as that from another. (Further formal therapeutic trials are not demanded for these well established drugs.) A prescription for a generic drug formulation may be filled for any officially licensed product that the dispensing pharmacy has chosen to purchase (on economic criteria; see 'generic substitution' below).[4]

The *proprietary name* is a trademark applied to particular formulation(s) of a particular substance by a particular manufacturer. Manufacture is confined to the owner of the trademark or to others licensed by the owner. It is designed to maximise the difference between the names of similar drugs marketed by rivals for obvious commercial reasons. To add confusion, some companies give their proprietary products the same names as their generic products in an attempt to capture the prescription market, both proprietary and generic, and some market lower-priced generics of their own proprietaries. When a prescription is written for a proprietary product, pharmacists under UK law must dispense that product only. But, by agreement with the prescribing doctor, they may substitute an approved generic product (*generic substitution*). What is not permitted is the substitution of a different molecular structure deemed to be pharmacologically and therapeutically equivalent (*therapeutic substitution*).

NON-PROPRIETARY NAMES

The principal reasons for advocating the habitual use of non-proprietary (generic) names in prescribing are described below.

Clarity. Non-proprietary names give information on the class of drug; for example, nortriptyline and amitriptyline are plainly related, but their proprietary names, Allegron and Triptafen, are not. It is not unknown for prescribers, when one drug has failed, unwittingly to add or substitute another drug of the same group (or even the same drug), thinking that different proprietary names must mean different classes of drugs. Such occurrences underline the wisdom of prescribing generically, so that group

---

[2]The generic name is now widely accepted as being synonymous with the non-proprietary name. Strictly 'generic' (L. *genus*, race, a class of objects) should refer to a group or class of drug, e.g. benzodiazepines, but by common usage the word is now taken to mean the non-proprietary name of individual members of a group, e.g. diazepam.

[3]Trigg R B 1998 Chemical nomenclature. Kluwer Academic, Dordrecht, p. 208–234.

[4]European Medicines Agency and US Food and Drug Agency guidelines are available and give pharmacokinetic limits that must be met.

similarities are immediately apparent, but highlight the requirement for brand names to be as distinct from one another as possible. Relationships cannot, and should not, be shown by brand names.

Economy. Drugs sold under non-proprietary names are usually, but not always, cheaper than those sold under proprietary names.

Convenience. Pharmacists may supply whatever version they stock,[5] whereas if a proprietary name is used they are obliged to supply that preparation alone. They may have to buy in the preparation named even though they have an equivalent in stock. Mixtures of drugs are sometimes given non-proprietary names, having the prefix *co-* to indicate more than one active ingredient, e.g. co-amoxiclav for Augmentin, but many are not because they exist for commercial advantage rather than for therapeutic need.[6] No prescriber can be expected to write out the ingredients, so proprietary names are used in many cases, there being no alternative. International travellers with chronic illnesses will be grateful for rINNs (see above), as proprietary names often differ from country to country. The reasons are linguistic as well as commercial (see below).

PROPRIETARY NAMES

The principal non-commercial reason for advocating the use of proprietary names in prescribing is consistency of the product, so that problems of quality, especially of bioavailability, are reduced. There is substance in this argument, though it is often exaggerated.

It is reasonable to use proprietary names when dosage, and therefore pharmaceutical bioavailability, is critical, so that small variations in the amount of drug available for absorption may have a big effect on the patient, e.g. drugs with a low therapeutic ratio, digoxin, hormone replacement therapy, adrenocortical steroids (oral), antiepileptics, cardiac antiarrhythmics, warfarin. In addition, with the introduction of complex formulations, e.g. sustained release, it is important clearly

to identify these, and the use of proprietary names has a role.

The present situation is that the pharmaceutical industry spends an enormous amount of money promoting its many names for the same article, and the community, as represented in the UK by the Department of Health, spends a relatively small sum trying to persuade doctors to use non-proprietary names. Ordinary doctors who prescribe for their ordinary patients are the targets of both sides. Fortunately, the position is eased by the now widespread use of computer programs for prescribing, which prompt the doctor to use non-proprietary names.

Generic names are intentionally longer than trade names to minimise the risk of confusion, but the use of accepted prefixes and stems for generic names works well and the average name length is four syllables, which is manageable. The search for proprietary names is a 'major problem' for pharmaceutical companies, increasing, as they are, their output of new preparations. A company may average 30 new preparations (not new chemical entities) a year, another warning of the urgent necessity for the doctor to cultivate a sceptical habit of mind. The names that 'look and sound medically seductive' are being picked out. 'Words that survive scrutiny will go into a stock-pile and await inexorable proliferation of new drugs'.[7] One firm (in the USA) commissioned a computer to produce a dictionary of 42 000 nonsense words of an appropriately scientific look and sound.

A more recent cause for confusion for patients (consumers) in purchasing proprietary medicines is the use by manufacturers of a well established 'brand' name that is associated in the mind of the purchaser with a particular therapeutic effect, e.g. analgesia, when in fact the product may contain a quite different pharmacological entity. By a subtle change or addition to the brand name of the original medicine, the manufacturer aims to establish 'brand loyalty'. This unsavoury practice is called

---

[5]This can result in supply of a formulation of appearance different from that previously used. Patients naturally find this disturbing.

[6]This is a practice confined largely to the UK. It is unknown in Europe, and not widely practised in the USA.

[7]Pharmaceutical companies increasingly operate worldwide and are liable to find themselves embarrassed by unanticipated verbal associations. For example, names marketed (in some countries), such as Bumaflex, Kriplex, Nokhel and Snootie, conjure up in the minds of native English-speakers associations that may inhibit both doctors and patients from using them (see Jack & Soppitt 1991 in Guide to Further Reading).

'umbrella branding'. It is also important to doctors to be aware of what over-the-counter (OTC) medicines their patients are taking, as proprietary products that were at one time familiar to them may contain other ingredients, with the increased risk of adverse events and drug interactions.

For the practising doctor (in the UK) the *British National Formulary* provides a regularly updated and comprehensive list of drugs in their non-proprietary (generic) and proprietary names. 'The range of drugs prescribed by any individual is remarkably narrow, and once the decision is taken to "think generic" surely the effort required is small'.[8] And, we would add, worthwhile.

Confusing names. The need for both clear thought and clear handwriting is shown by medicines of totally different class that have similar names. Serious events have occurred as a result of the confusion of names and dispensing the wrong drug, e.g. Lasix (furosemide) for Losec (omeprazole) (death); AZT (intending zidovudine) was misinterpreted in the pharmacy and azathiorine was dispensed (do not use abbreviations for drug names); Daonil (glibenclamide) for De-nol (bismuth chelate) and for

Danol (danazol). It will be noted that non-proprietary names are less likely to be confused with other classes of drugs.

GUIDE TO FURTHER READING

Aronson J K 2000 Where name and image meet – the argument for adrenaline. British Medical Journal 320:506–509

Chief Medical Officer, Department of Health, Medicines and Healthcare Products Regulatory Agency 2004 Change in names of certain medicinal substances. Professional letter of 17 March 2004: 1–6 (available to download as PL CMO (2004)1: change in names of certain medicinal substances from http//www.dh.gov.uk)

Furberg C D, Herrington D M, Psaty B M 1999 Are drugs within a class interchangeable? Lancet 354:1201–1204 (and correspondence: are drugs interchangeable? 2000 Lancet 355:316–317)

George C F 1996 Naming of drugs: pass the epinephrine please. British Medical Journal 312:1315 (and correspondence in British Medical Journal [1996] 313:688–689)

Jack D B, Soppitt A L 1991 Give a drug a bad name. British Medical Journal 303:1606–1608

---

[8]Editorial 1977 British Medical Journal 4:980 (and subsequent correspondence).

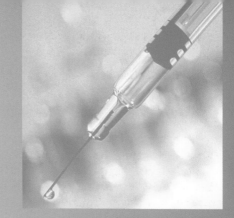

Section 2

FROM PHARMACOLOGY TO TOXICOLOGY

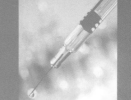

7

General pharmacology

SYNOPSIS

How drugs act and interact, how they enter the body, what happens to them inside the body, how they are eliminated from it; the effects of genetics, age and disease on drug action – these topics are important. Although they will generally not be in the front of the conscious mind of the prescriber, an understanding of them will enhance rational decision taking.

Knowledge of the requirements for success and the explanations for failure and for adverse events will enable the doctor to maximise the benefits and minimise the risks of drug therapy. It is self-evident that knowledge of pharmacodynamics is essential to the choice of drug therapy. But the well chosen drug may fail to produce benefit or may be poisonous because too little or too much is present at the site of action for too short or too long a time. Drug therapy can fail for pharmacokinetic as well as for pharmacodynamic reasons.

Pharmacodynamics

- Qualitative aspects: receptors, enzymes, selectivity
- Quantitative aspects: dose–response, therapeutic efficacy, potency, tolerance

Pharmacokinetics

- Time course of drug concentration: drug passage across cell membranes; order of reaction; plasma half-life and steady-state concentration; therapeutic drug monitoring
- Individual processes: absorption, distribution, metabolism, elimination
- Drug dosage: dosing schedules
- Chronic pharmacology: the consequences of prolonged drug administration and drug discontinuation syndromes
- Individual or biological variation: variability due to inherited influences, environmental and host influences
- Drug interactions: outside the body, at site of absorption, at transporters, enzymes and receptors

> Pharmacodynamics is what drugs do to the body; pharmacokinetics is what the body does to drugs.

The practice of drug therapy entails more than remembering an apparently arbitrary list of actions or indications. Scientific incompetence in the modern doctor is inexcusable and, contrary to some assertions, scientific competence is wholly compatible with a humane approach.

PHARMACODYNAMICS

> Understanding how drugs act is not only an objective of the pharmacologist who seeks to develop new and better therapies, it is also the basis of intelligent use of medicines.

QUALITATIVE ASPECTS

The starting point is to consider what drugs do and how they do it, i.e. the nature of drug action. The body functions through control systems that involve chemotransmitters or local hormones, receptors, enzymes, carrier molecules and other specialised macromolecules such as DNA.

Most medicinal drugs act by altering the body's control systems and, in general, they do so by binding to some specialised constituent of the cell, selectively to alter its function and consequently that of the physiological or pathological system to which it contributes. Such drugs are structurally specific in that small modifications to their chemical structure may profoundly alter their effect.

MECHANISMS

An overview of the mechanisms of drug action shows that drugs act on *specific receptors* in the cell membrane and interior by:

- *Ligand-gated ion channels*, i.e. receptors coupled directly to membrane ion channels; neurotransmitters act on such receptors in the postsynaptic membrane of a nerve or muscle cell and give a response within milliseconds.
- *G-protein-coupled receptor systems*, i.e. receptors bound to the cell membrane and coupled to intracellular effector systems by a *G-protein*. For instance, catecholamines (*the first messenger*) activate β-adrenoceptors through a coupled G-protein system. This increases the activity of intracellular adenylyl cyclase, increasing the rate of formation of cyclic AMP (*the second messenger*), a modulator of the activity of several enzyme systems that cause the cell to act. The process takes seconds.
- *Protein kinase receptors*, so called because the structure incorporates a protein kinase, are targets for peptide hormones involved in the control of cell growth and differentiation, and the release of inflammatory mediators over a course of hours.
- *Cytosolic (nuclear) receptors*, i.e. within the cell itself, regulate DNA transcription and, thereby, protein synthesis, e.g. by steroid and thyroid hormones, a process that takes hours or days.

Drugs also act on *processes within or near the cell* by:

- *Enzyme inhibition*, e.g. platelet cyclo-oxygenase by aspirin, cholinesterase by pyridostigmine, xanthine oxidase by allopurinol.
- Inhibition or induction of *transporter processes* that carry substances into, across and out of cells, e.g. blockade of anion transport in the renal tubule cell by probenecid is used to protect against the nephrotoxic effects of cidofovir (used for cytomegalovirus retinitis).
- *Incorporation into larger molecules*, e.g. 5-fluorouracil, an anticancer drug, is incorporated into messenger RNA in place of uracil.
- In the case of successful antimicrobial agents, *altering metabolic processes* unique to microorganisms, e.g. penicillin interferes with formation of the bacterial cell wall; or by showing enormous quantitative differences in affecting a process common to both humans and microbes, e.g. inhibition of folic acid synthesis by trimethoprim.

Outside the cell drugs act by:

- Direct *chemical interaction*, e.g. chelating agents, antacids.

- *Osmosis*, as with purgatives, e.g. magnesium sulfate, and diuretics, e.g. mannitol, which are active because neither they nor the water in which they are dissolved is absorbed by the cells lining the gut and kidney tubules respectively.

RECEPTORS

Most receptors are protein macromolecules. When the agonist binds to the receptor, the proteins undergo an alteration in conformation, which induces changes in systems within the cell that in turn bring about the response to the drug over differing time courses. Many kinds of effector response exist, but those indicated above are the four basic types.

Radioligand binding studies[1] have shown that the receptor numbers do not remain constant but change according to circumstances. When tissues are continuously exposed to an agonist, the number of receptors decreases (*down-regulation*) and this may be a cause of *tachyphylaxis* (loss of efficacy with frequently repeated doses), e.g. in asthmatics who use adrenoceptor agonist bronchodilators excessively. Prolonged contact with an antagonist leads to formation of new receptors (*up-regulation*). Indeed, one explanation for the worsening of angina pectoris or cardiac ventricular arrhythmia in some patients following abrupt withdrawal of a β-adrenoceptor blocker is that normal concentrations of circulating catecholamines now have access to an increased (up-regulated) population of β-adrenoceptors (see Chronic pharmacology, p. 103).

Agonists. Drugs that activate receptors do so because they resemble the natural transmitter or hormone, but their value in clinical practice often rests on their greater capacity to resist degradation and so to act for longer than the natural substances (endogenous ligands) they mimic; for this reason, bronchodilatation produced by salbutamol lasts longer than that induced by adrenaline (epinephrine).

Antagonists (blockers) of receptors are sufficiently similar to the natural agonist to be 'recognised' by

[1]The extraordinary discrimination of this technique is shown by the calculation that the total β-adrenoceptor protein in a large cow amounts to 1 mg (Maguire M E, Ross E M, Gilman A G et al 1977 β-Adrenergic receptor: ligand binding properties and the interaction with adenylyl cyclase. Advances in Cyclic Nucleotide Research 8:1–83).

the receptor and to occupy it without activating a response, thereby preventing (blocking) the natural agonist from exerting its effect. Drugs that have no activating effect whatever on the receptor are termed *pure antagonists*. A receptor occupied by a low-efficacy agonist is inaccessible to a subsequent dose of a high-efficacy agonist, so that, in this specific situation, a low-efficacy agonist acts as an antagonist. This can happen with opioids.

Partial agonists. Some drugs, in addition to blocking access of the natural agonist to the receptor, are capable of a low degree of activation, i.e. they have both antagonist and agonist action. Such substances show *partial agonist activity* (PAA). The β-adrenoceptor antagonists pindolol and oxprenolol have partial agonist activity (in their case it is often called *intrinsic sympathomimetic activity*, ISA), whilst propranolol is devoid of agonist activity, i.e. it is a pure antagonist.

A patient may be as extensively 'β-blocked' by propranolol as by pindolol, i.e. with eradication of exercise tachycardia, but the resting heart rate is lower on propranolol; such differences can have clinical importance.

Inverse agonists. Some substances produce effects that are specifically opposed to those of the agonist. The agonist action of benzodiazepines on the benzodiazepine receptor in the central nervous system produces sedation, anxiolysis, muscle relaxation and controls convulsions; substances called β-carbolines, which also bind to this receptor, cause stimulation, anxiety, increased muscle tone and convulsions; they are *inverse agonists*. Both types of drug act by modulating the effects of the neurotransmitter γ-aminobutyric acid (GABA).

Receptor binding (and vice versa). If the forces that bind drug to receptor are weak (hydrogen bonds, van der Waals' bonds, electrostatic bonds), the binding will be easily and rapidly reversible; if the forces involved are strong (covalent bonds), then binding will be effectively irreversible.

An antagonist that binds *reversibly* to a receptor can by definition be displaced from the receptor by mass action (see p. 84) of the agonist (and vice versa). A sufficient increase of the concentration of agonist above that of the antagonist restores the response. β-blocked patients who increase their low heart rate with exercise are demonstrating a rise in sympathetic drive and releasing enough catecholamine (agonist) to overcome the prevailing degree of receptor blockade.

Raising the dose of β-adrenoceptor blocker will limit or abolish exercise-induced tachycardia, showing that the degree of blockade is enhanced as more drug becomes available to compete with the endogenous transmitter.

As agonist and antagonist compete to occupy the receptor according to the law of mass action, this type of drug action is termed *competitive antagonism*.

When receptor-mediated responses are studied either in isolated tissues or in intact humans, a graph of the logarithm of the dose given (horizontal axis) plotted against the response obtained (vertical axis) commonly gives an S-shaped (sigmoid) curve, the central part of which is a straight line. If the measurements are repeated in the presence of an antagonist, and the curve obtained is parallel to the original but displaced to the right, then antagonism is said to be competitive and the agonist to be *surmountable*.

Drugs that bind *irreversibly* to receptors include phenoxybenzamine (to the α-adrenoceptor). Because the drug fixes to the receptor, increasing the concentration of agonist does not fully restore the response, and antagonism of this type is described as *insurmountable*.

The log dose–response curves for the agonist in the absence of, and in the presence of, a non-competitive antagonist are not parallel. Some toxins act in this way; for example, α-bungarotoxin, a constituent of some snake and spider venoms, binds irreversibly to the acetylcholine receptor and is used as a tool to study it.

Restoration of the response after irreversible binding requires elimination of the drug from the body and synthesis of new receptor, and for this reason the effect may persist long after drug administration has ceased. Irreversible agents find little place in clinical practice.

Physiological (functional) antagonism

An action on the same receptor is not the only mechanism by which one drug may oppose the effect of another. Extreme bradycardia following overdose of a β-adrenoceptor blocker can be relieved by atropine, which accelerates the heart by blockade of the parasympathetic branch of the autonomic nervous system, the cholinergic tone of which (vagal tone) operates continuously to slow it.

Adrenaline (epinephrine) and theophylline counteract bronchoconstriction produced by histamine released from mast cells in anaphylactic shock by relaxing bronchial smooth muscle (β_2-adrenoceptor effect). In both cases, a second drug overcomes the pharmacological effect, by a different physiological mechanism, i.e. there is *physiological* or *functional* antagonism.

ENZYMES

Interaction between drug and enzyme is in many respects similar to that between drug and receptor. Drugs may alter enzyme activity because they resemble a natural substrate and hence compete with it for the enzyme. For example, enalapril is effective in hypertension because it is structurally similar to the part of angiotensin I that is attacked by angiotensin-converting enzyme (ACE); enalapril prevents formation of the pressor angiotensin II by occupying the active site of the enzyme and so inhibiting its action.

Carbidopa competes with levodopa for dopa decarboxylase, and the benefit of this combination in Parkinson's disease is reduced metabolism of levodopa to dopamine in the blood (but not in the brain because carbidopa does not cross the blood–brain barrier).

Ethanol prevents metabolism of methanol to its toxic metabolite, formic acid, by competing for occupancy of the enzyme alcohol dehydrogenase; this is the rationale for using ethanol in methanol poisoning. The above are examples of competitive (*reversible*) inhibition of enzyme activity.

Irreversible inhibition occurs with organophosphorus insecticides and chemical warfare agents (see p. 395), which combine covalently with the active site of acetylcholinesterase; recovery of cholinesterase activity depends on the formation of new enzyme. Covalent binding of aspirin to cyclooxygenase (COX) inhibits the enzyme in platelets for their entire lifespan because platelets have no system for synthesising new protein; this is why low doses of aspirin are sufficient for antiplatelet action.

SELECTIVITY

The pharmacologist who produces a new drug and the doctor who gives it to a patient share the desire that it should possess a selective action so that additional and unwanted (adverse) effects do not complicate the management of the patient.

Approaches to obtaining selectivity of drug action include the following.

Modification of drug structure. Many drugs have in their design a structural similarity to some natural constituent of the body, e.g. a neurotransmitter, a hormone, a substrate for an enzyme; replacing or competing with that natural constituent achieves selectivity of action. Enormous scientific effort and expertise go into the synthesis and testing of analogues of natural substances in order to create drugs capable of obtaining a specified effect and that alone (see Therapeutic index, p. 79). The approach is the basis of modern drug design and it has led to the production of adrenoceptor antagonists, histamine receptor antagonists and many other important medicines.

But there are biological constraints to selectivity. Anticancer drugs that act against rapidly dividing cells lack selectivity because they also damage other tissues with a high cell replication rate, such as bone marrow and gut epithelium.

Selective delivery (drug targeting). Simple topical application, e.g. skin and eye, and special drug delivery systems, e.g. intrabronchial administration of β_2-adrenoceptor agonist or corticosteroid (inhaled, pressurised, metered aerosol for asthma) can achieve the objective of target tissue selectivity. Selective targeting of drugs to less accessible sites of disease offers considerable scope for therapy as technology develops, e.g. attaching drugs to antibodies selective for cancer cells.

Stereoselectivity. Drug molecules are three-dimensional and many drugs contain one or more *asymmetrical* or *chiral*[2] centres in their structures, i.e. a single drug can be, in effect, a mixture of two non-identical mirror images (like a mixture of left- and right-handed gloves). The two forms, which are known as *enantiomorphs*, can exhibit very different pharmacodynamic, pharmacokinetic and toxicological properties.

For example, (1) the S form of warfarin is four times more active than the R form,[3] (2) the peak

---

[2]Greek: *cheir* = a hand.
[3]R (rectus) and S (sinister) refer to the sequential arrangement of the constituent parts of the molecule around the chiral centre.

plasma concentration of S fenoprofen is four times that of R fenoprofen after oral administration of RS fenoprofen, and (3) the S, but not the R, enantiomorph of thalidomide is metabolised to primary toxins.

Many other drugs are available as mixtures of enantiomorphs (racemates). Pharmaceutical development of drugs as single enantiomers rather than as racemic mixtures offers the prospect of greater selectivity of action and lessens risk of toxicity.

QUANTITATIVE ASPECTS

That a drug has a desired qualitative action is obviously all important, but is not by itself enough. There are also quantitative aspects, i.e. the right amount of action is required, and with some drugs the dose has to be adjusted very precisely to deliver this, neither too little nor too much, to escape both inefficacy and toxicity, e.g. digoxin, lithium, gentamicin. Whilst the general correlation between dose and response may evoke no surprise, certain characteristics of the relation are fundamental to the way drugs are used, as described below.

DOSE–RESPONSE RELATIONSHIPS

Conventionally, the horizontal axis shows the dose and the response appears on the vertical axis. The slope of the dose–response curve defines the extent to which a desired response alters as the dose is changed. A steeply rising and prolonged curve indicates that a small change in dose produces a large change in drug effect over a wide dose range, e.g. with the loop diuretic, furosemide (used in doses from 20 mg to over 250 mg/day). By contrast, the dose–response curve for thiazide diuretics soon reaches a plateau, and the clinically useful dose range for bendroflumethiazide, for example, extends from 5 to 10 mg; increasing the dose beyond this produces no added diuretic effect, although it adds to toxicity.

Dose–response curves for wanted and unwanted effects can illustrate and quantify selective and non-selective drug action (see Fig. 7.1 below).

POTENCY AND EFFICACY

A clear distinction between potency and efficacy is pertinent, particularly in relation to claims made for usefulness in therapeutics.

Potency is the amount (weight) of drug in relation to its effect, e.g. if weight-for-weight drug A has a greater effect than drug B, then drug A is more potent than drug B, although the maximum therapeutic effect obtainable may be similar with both drugs.

The diuretic effect of bumetanide 1 mg is equivalent to that of furosemide 50 mg; thus bumetanide is more potent than furosemide but both drugs achieve about the same maximum effect. The difference in weight of drug administered is of no clinical significance unless it is great.

Pharmacological efficacy refers to the strength of response induced by occupancy of a receptor by an agonist (intrinsic activity); it is a specialised pharmacological concept. But clinicians are concerned with therapeutic efficacy, as follows.

Therapeutic efficacy, or effectiveness, is the capacity of a drug to produce an effect and refers to the maximum such effect. For example, if drug A can produce a therapeutic effect that cannot be obtained with drug B, however much of drug B is given, then drug A has the higher *therapeutic efficacy*. Differences in therapeutic efficacy are of great clinical importance.

Amiloride (*low* efficacy) can at best effect excretion of no more than 5% of the sodium load filtered by the glomeruli; there is no point in increasing the dose beyond that which achieves this, as this is its maximum diuretic effect. Bendroflumethiazide (*moderate* efficacy) can effect excretion of no more than 10% of the filtered sodium load no matter how large the dose. Furosemide can effect excretion of 25% and more of filtered sodium; it is a *high-efficacy* diuretic.

Therapeutic index. With progressive increases in dose, the desired response in the patient usually rises to a maximum beyond which further increases elicit no greater benefit but induce unwanted effects. This is because most drugs do not have a single dose–response curve, but a different curve for each action, wanted as well as unwanted. Increases in dose beyond that which gives the maximum wanted response recruit only new and unwanted actions.

A sympathomimetic bronchodilator might exhibit one dose–response relation for decreasing airway resistance (wanted) and another for increase in heart rate (unwanted). Clearly, the usefulness of any drug relates closely to the extent to which such dose–response relations overlap.

Ehrlich (see p. 175) introduced the concept of the therapeutic index or ratio as the maximum tolerated dose divided by the minimum curative dose, but the index is never calculated thus as such single doses cannot be determined accurately in humans. More realistically, a dose that has some unwanted effect in 50% of humans, e.g. in the case of an adrenoceptor agonist bronchodilator a specified increase in heart rate, is compared with that which is therapeutic in 50% (ED_{50}), e.g. a specified decrease in airways resistance.

In practice, such information is not available for many drugs but the therapeutic index does embody a concept that is fundamental in comparing the usefulness of one drug with another, namely, *safety in relation to efficacy*. Figure 7.1 expresses the concept diagrammatically.

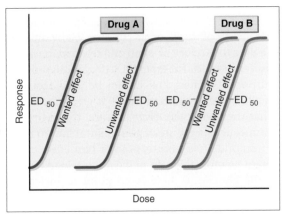

Fig. 7.1 Dose–response curves for two hypothetical drugs. For drug A, the dose that brings about the maximum wanted effect is less than the lowest dose that produces the unwanted effect. The ratio ED_{50} (unwanted effect)/ED_{50} (wanted effect) indicates that drug A has a large therapeutic index; it is thus highly *selective* in its wanted action. Drug B causes unwanted effects at doses well below producing its maximum benefit. The ratio ED_{50} (unwanted effect)/ED_{50} (wanted effect) indicates that the drug has a small therapeutic index: it is thus *non-selective*.

TOLERANCE

Continuous or repeated administration of a drug is often accompanied by a gradual diminution of the effect it produces. A state of *tolerance* exists when it becomes necessary to increase the dose of a drug to get an effect previously obtained with a smaller dose, i.e. reduced sensitivity. By contrast, the term *tachyphylaxis* describes the phenomenon of progressive lessening of effect (refractoriness) in response to frequently administered doses (see Receptors, p. 76); it tends to develop more rapidly than tolerance.

The use of opioids readily illustrates tolerance, as witnessed by the huge doses of morphine that may be necessary to maintain pain relief in terminal care; the effect is due to reduced pharmacological efficacy (see p. 79) at receptor sites or to down-regulation of receptors. Tolerance is acquired rapidly with nitrates used to prevent angina, possibly mediated by the generation of oxygen free radicals from nitric oxide; it can be avoided by removing transdermal nitrate patches for 4–8 h, e.g. at night, to allow the plasma concentration to fall.

Accelerated metabolism by enzyme induction (see p. 97) also leads to tolerance, as experience shows with alcohol, taken regularly as opposed to sporadically. There is commonly cross-tolerance between drugs of similar structure.

Failure of certain individuals to respond to normal doses of a drug, e.g. resistance to warfarin, vitamin D, constitutes a form of natural tolerance (see Pharmacogenetics, p. 105).

BIOASSAY AND STANDARDISATION

Biological assay (bioassay) is the process by which the activity of a substance (identified or unidentified) is measured on living material: e.g. contraction of bronchial, uterine or vascular muscle. It is used only when chemical or physical methods are not practicable as in the case of a mixture of active substances, or of an incompletely purified preparation, or where no chemical method has been developed. The activity of a preparation is expressed relative to that of a standard preparation of the same substance.

Biological standardisation is a specialised form of bioassay. It involves matching of material of unknown potency with an international or national standard with the objective of providing a preparation for use in therapeutics and research. The results are expressed as *units* of a substance rather than its weight, e.g. insulin, vaccines.

PHARMACOKINETICS

To initiate a desired drug action is a *qualitative* choice but, when the qualitative choice is made, considerations of *quantity* immediately arise; it is possible to have too much or too little of a good thing. To obtain the right effect at the right intensity, at the right time, for the right duration, with minimal risk of unpleasantness or harm, is what pharmacokinetics is about.

Dosage regimens of long-established drugs grew from trial and error. Doctors learned by experience the dose, the frequency of dosing and the route of administration that was most likely to benefit and least likely to harm. But this empirical ('suck it and see') approach is no longer tenable. We now have an understanding of how drugs cross membranes to enter the body, how they are distributed round it in the blood and other body fluids, how they are bound to plasma proteins and tissues (which act as stores), and how they are eliminated from the body. Quantification of these processes paves the way for efficient development of dosing regimens.

> **Pharmacokinetics**[4] is concerned with the rate at which drug molecules cross cell membranes to enter the body, to distribute within it and to leave the body, as well as with the structural changes (metabolism) to which they are subject within it.

The discussion covers the following topics:

- Drug passage across cell membranes.
- Order of reaction or process (first and zero order).
- Time course of drug concentration and effect:
  – plasma half-life and steady-state concentration
  – therapeutic monitoring.
- The individual processes: absorption, distribution, metabolism (biotransformation), elimination.

DRUG PASSAGE ACROSS CELL MEMBRANES

Certain concepts are fundamental to understanding how drug molecules make their way around the body to achieve their effect. The first concerns the modes by which drugs cross cell membranes and cells.

Our bodies are labyrinths of fluid-filled spaces. Some, such as the lumina of the kidney tubules or intestine, are connected to the outside world; the blood, lymph and cerebrospinal fluid are enclosed. Sheets of cells line these spaces, and the extent to which a drug can cross epithelia or endothelia is

fundamental to its clinical use, determining whether a drug can be taken orally for systemic effect, and whether within the glomerular filtrate it will be reabsorbed or excreted in the urine.

Cell membranes are essentially bilayers of lipid molecules with 'islands' of protein, and they preserve and regulate the internal environment. *Lipid-soluble* substances diffuse readily into cells and therefore throughout body tissues. Adjacent epithelial or endothelial cells are linked by tight junctions, some of which are traversed by water-filled channels that allow the passage of water-soluble substances of small molecular size.

The jejunum and proximal renal tubule contain many such channels and are *leaky epithelia*, whereas the tight junctions in the stomach and urinary bladder do not have these channels and water cannot pass; they are termed *tight epithelia*. Special protein molecules within the lipid bilayer allow specific substances to enter or leave the cell preferentially, i.e. *energy-utilising transporter processes*, described later. The natural processes of passive diffusion, filtration and carrier-mediated transport determine the passage of drugs across membranes and cells and their distribution round the body.

PASSIVE DIFFUSION

This is the most important means by which a drug enters the tissues and distributes through them. It refers simply to the natural tendency of any substance to move passively from an area of high concentration to one of low concentration. In the context of an individual cell, the drug moves at a rate proportional to the concentration difference across the cell membrane, i.e. it shows first-order kinetics (see p. 84); cellular energy is not required, which means that the process does not become saturated and is not inhibited by other substances.

The extent to which drugs are soluble in *water* or *lipid* is central to their capacity to cross cell membranes and depends on environmental pH and the structural properties of the molecule.

> Lipid solubility is promoted by the presence of a benzene ring, a hydrocarbon chain, a steroid nucleus or halogen (–Br, –Cl, –F) groups. Water solubility is promoted by the presence of alcoholic (–OH), amide (–CO·NH$_2$) or carboxylic (–COOH) groups, or the formation of glucuronide and sulphate conjugates.

---

[4]Greek: *pharmacon* = drug; *kinein* = to move.

It is useful to classify drugs in a physicochemical sense into:

- Those that are *variably* ionised according to environmental pH (electrolytes) (lipid soluble or water soluble).
- Those that are *incapable* of becoming ionised whatever the environmental pH (un-ionised, non-polar substances) (lipid soluble).
- Those that are *permanently* ionised whatever the environmental pH (ionised, polar substances) (water soluble).

DRUGS THAT IONISE ACCORDING TO ENVIRONMENTAL pH

Many drugs are *weak electrolytes*, i.e. their structural groups ionise to a greater or lesser extent, according to environmental pH. Most such molecules are present partly in the ionised and partly in the un-ionised state. The degree of ionisation influences lipid solubility (and hence diffusibility) and so affects absorption, distribution and elimination.

Ionisable groups in a drug molecule tend either to lose a hydrogen ion (acidic groups) or to add a hydrogen ion (basic groups). The extent to which a molecule has this tendency to ionise is given by the dissociation (or ionisation) constant (K_a), expressed as the pK_a, i.e. the negative logarithm of the K_a (just as pH is the negative logarithm of the hydrogen ion concentration). In an acidic environment, i.e. one already containing many free hydrogen ions, an acidic group tends to retain a hydrogen ion and remains un-ionised; a relative deficit of free hydrogen ions, i.e. a basic environment, favours loss of the hydrogen ion from an acidic group, which thus becomes ionised. The opposite is the case for a base. The issue may be summarised:

- Acidic groups become less ionised in an acidic environment.
- Basic groups become less ionised in a basic (alkaline) environment and vice versa.

This in turn influences *diffusibility* because:

- Un-ionised drug is lipid soluble and diffusible.
- Ionised drug is lipid insoluble and non-diffusible.

Quantifying the degree of ionisation helps to express the profound effect of environmental pH. Recall that when the pH of the environment is the same as the pK_a of a drug within it, then the ratio of un-ionised to ionised molecules is 1 : 1. But for every unit by which pH is changed, the ratio of un-ionised to ionised molecules changes 10-fold. Thus, when the pH is 2 units less than the pK_a, molecules of an acid become 100 times more un-ionised and when the pH is 2 units more than the pK_a, molecules of an acid become 100 more ionised. Such pH change profoundly affects drug kinetics.

pH variation and drug kinetics. The *pH partition hypothesis* expresses the separation of a drug across a lipid membrane according to differences in environmental pH. There is a wide range of pH in the gut (pH 1.5 in the stomach, 6.8 in the upper and 7.6 in the lower intestine). But the pH inside the body is maintained within a limited range (pH 7.46 ± 0.04), so that only drugs that are substantially un-ionised at this pH will be lipid soluble, diffuse across tissue boundaries and so be widely distributed, e.g. into the CNS. Urine pH varies between the extremes of 4.6 and 8.2, and the prevailing pH affects the amount of drug reabsorbed from the renal tubular lumen by passive diffusion.

In the stomach, aspirin (acetylsalicylic acid, pK_a 3.5) is un-ionised and thus lipid soluble and diffusible. When aspirin enters the gastric epithelial cells (pH 7.4) it will ionise, become less diffusible and so will localise there. This *ion trapping* is one mechanism whereby aspirin is concentrated in, and so harms, the gastric mucosa. In the body aspirin is metabolised to salicylic acid (pK_a 3.0), which at pH 7.4 is highly ionised and thus remains in the extracellular fluid. Eventually the molecules of salicylic acid in the plasma are filtered by the glomeruli and pass into the tubular fluid, which is generally more acidic than plasma and causes a proportion of salicylic acid to become un-ionised and lipid soluble so that it diffuses back into the tubular cells. Alkalinising the urine with an intravenous infusion of sodium bicarbonate causes more salicylic acid to become ionised and lipid insoluble so that it remains in the tubular fluid, and is then eliminated in the urine. Treatment for salicylate (aspirin) overdose utilises this effect.

Conversely, acidifying the urine increases the elimination of the base amfetamine (pK_a 9.9) (see Acidification of urine, Chapter 9, p. 134).

DRUGS THAT ARE INCAPABLE OF BECOMING IONISED

These include digoxin and steroid hormones such as prednisolone. Effectively lacking any ionisable groups, they are unaffected by environmental pH, are lipid soluble and so diffuse readily across tissue boundaries. These drugs are also referred to as *non-polar*.

PERMANENTLY IONISED DRUGS

Drugs that are permanently ionised contain groups that dissociate so strongly that they remain ionised over the range of the body pH. Such compounds are termed *polar*, for their groups are either negatively charged (acidic, e.g. heparin) or positively charged (basic, e.g. ipratropium, tubocurarine, suxamethonium) and all have a very limited capacity to cross cell membranes. This is a disadvantage with heparin, which the gut does not absorb so that it is given parenterally. Conversely, heparin is a useful anticoagulant in pregnancy because it does not cross the placenta (which the orally effective warfarin does and is liable to cause fetal haemorrhage as well as being teratogenic).

The following are particular examples of the relevance of drug passage across membranes.

Brain and cerebrospinal fluid (CSF). The capillaries of the cerebral circulation differ from those in most other parts of the body in that they lack the filtration channels between endothelial cells through which substances in the blood normally gain access to the extracellular fluid. Tight junctions between adjacent capillary endothelial cells, together with their basement membrane and a thin covering from the processes of astrocytes, separate the blood from the brain tissue, forming the *blood–brain barrier*. Compounds that are *lipid insoluble* do not cross it readily, e.g. atenolol, compared with propranolol (lipid soluble), and unwanted CNS effects are more prominent with the latter. Therapy with methotrexate (lipid insoluble) may fail to eliminate leukaemic deposits in the CNS.

Conversely *lipid-soluble* substances enter brain tissue with ease; thus diazepam (lipid soluble) given intravenously is effective within 1 min for status epilepticus, and effects of alcohol (ethanol) by mouth are noted within minutes; the level of general anaesthesia can be controlled closely by altering the concentration of inhaled anaesthetic gas (lipid soluble).

Placenta. Maternal blood bathes the chorionic villi, which consist of a layer of trophoblastic cells

that enclose fetal capillaries. Their large surface area and the high placental blood flow (500 mL/min) are essential for gas exchange, uptake of nutrients and elimination of waste products. Thus a lipid barrier separates the fetal and maternal bloodstreams, allowing the passage of lipid-soluble substances but excluding water-soluble compounds, especially those with a molecular weight exceeding 600.[5]

This exclusion is of particular importance with short-term use, e.g. tubocurarine (mol. wt. 772) (lipid insoluble) or gallamine (mol. wt. 891) used as a muscle relaxant during caesarean section do not affect the infant; with prolonged use, however, all compounds will eventually enter the fetus to some extent (see Index).

FILTRATION

Aqueous channels in the tight junctions between adjacent epithelial cells allow the passage of some water-soluble substances. Neutral or uncharged, i.e. non-polar, molecules pass most readily because the pores are electrically charged. Within the alimentary tract, channels are largest and most numerous in jejunal epithelium, and filtration allows for rapid equilibration of concentrations and consequently of osmotic pressures across the mucosa. Ions such as sodium enter the body through the aqueous channels, the size of which probably limits passage to substances of low molecular weight, e.g. ethanol (mol. wt. 46). Filtration seems to play at most a minor role in drug transfer within the body except for glomerular filtration, which is an important mechanism of drug excretion.

CARRIER-MEDIATED TRANSPORT

The membranes of many cells incorporate carrier-mediated transporter processes that control the entry and exit of endogenous molecules, and show a high degree of specificity for particular compounds because they have evolved from biological needs for the uptake of essential nutrients or elimination of metabolic products. Drugs that bear some structural resemblance to natural constituents of the body are likely to utilise these mechanisms.

---

[5]Most drugs have a molecular weight of less than 600 (e.g. diazepam 284, morphine 303) but some have more (erythromycin 733, digoxin 780).

Some carrier-mediated transport processes operate passively, i.e. do not require cellular energy, and this is *facilitated diffusion*, e.g. vitamin B_{12} absorption. Other, energy-requiring processes move substrates into or out of cells against a concentration gradient very effectively, i.e. by *active transport*; they are subject to saturation, inhibition and induction (see p. 97).

THE ORDER OF REACTION OR PROCESS

In the body, drug molecules reach their sites of action after crossing cell membranes and cells, and many are metabolised in the process. The rate at which these movements or changes take place is subject to important influences called the *order of reaction* or process. In biology generally, two orders of such reactions are recognised, and are summarised as follows:

- First-order processes by which a constant *fraction* of drug is transported/metabolised in unit time.
- Zero-order processes by which a constant *amount* of drug is transported/metabolised in unit time.

FIRST-ORDER (EXPONENTIAL) PROCESSES

In the majority of instances, the rates at which absorption, distribution, metabolism and excretion of a drug occur are directly proportional to its concentration in the body. In other words, transfer of drug across a cell membrane or formation of a metabolite is high at high concentrations and falls in direct proportion to be low at low concentrations (an exponential relationship).

This is because the processes follow the Law of Mass Action, which states that the rate of reaction is directly proportional to the active masses of reacting substances. In other words, at high concentrations there are more opportunities for crowded molecules to interact with one another or to cross cell membranes than at low, uncrowded concentrations. Processes for which the rate of reaction is proportional to the concentration of participating molecules are *first order*.

In doses used clinically, most drugs are subject to first-order processes of absorption, distribution, metabolism and elimination, and this knowledge is useful. The current chapter later describes how the rate of elimination of a drug from the plasma falls as the concentration in plasma falls, and the time for any plasma concentration to fall by 50% ($t_{1/2}$, the plasma half-life) is always the same. Thus it becomes possible to quote a constant value for the $t_{1/2}$ of the drug. This occurs because rate and concentration are in proportion, i.e. the process obeys first-order kinetics.

Knowing that first-order conditions apply to a drug allows the performance of accurate calculations that depend on its $t_{1/2}$, i.e. time to achieve steady-state plasma concentration, time to elimination, and the construction of dosing schedules.

ZERO-ORDER PROCESSES (SATURATION KINETICS)

As the amount of drug in the body rises, metabolic reactions or processes that have limited capacity become saturated. In other words, the rate of the process reaches a maximum amount at which it stays constant, e.g. due to limited activity of an enzyme, and any further increase in rate is impossible despite an increase in the dose of drug. In these circumstances, the rate of reaction is no longer proportional to dose, and exhibits *rate-limited* or *dose-dependent*[6] or *zero-order* or *saturation* kinetics. In practice, enzyme-mediated metabolic reactions are the most likely to show rate limitation because the amount of enzyme present is finite and can become saturated. Passive diffusion does not become saturated. There are some important consequences of zero-order kinetics.

Alcohol (ethanol) (see also p. 148) is a drug whose kinetics has considerable implications for society as well as for the individual, as follows.

Alcohol is subject to first-order kinetics with a $t_{1/2}$ of about 1 h at plasma concentrations below 10 mg/dL (attained after drinking about two-thirds of a unit [glass] of wine or beer). Above this concentration the main enzyme (alcohol dehydrogenase) that converts the alcohol into acetaldehyde approaches and then reaches saturation, at which point alcohol metabolism cannot proceed any faster than about 10 mL or 8 g/h for a 70-kg man. If the subject continues to

---

[6]We quote all of these terms for they appear in the relevant literature. *Note:* because the *rate* of a reaction is constant when it is zero order, it is dose *independent*, but as zero order is approached, with increasing dose the *kinetics* alter, and thus are called dose *dependent*.

drink, the blood alcohol concentration rises dispro-portionately, for the rate of metabolism remains the same, as alcohol shows zero-order kinetics.

An illustration. Consider a man of average size whose life is unhappy to a degree where he drinks about half (375 mL) a standard bottle of whisky (40% alcohol), i.e. 150 mL alcohol, over a short period, absorbs it and goes drunk to bed at midnight with a blood alcohol concentration of about 250 mg/dL. *If* alcohol metabolism were subject to first-order kinetics, with a $t_{\frac{1}{2}}$ of 1 h throughout the whole range of social consumption, the subject would halve his blood alcohol concentration each hour (see Fig. 7.2). It is easy to calculate that, when he drives his car to work at 08.00 hours the next morning, he has a negligible blood alcohol concentration (less than 1 mg/dL) though, no doubt, a hangover might reduce his driving skill.

But at these high concentrations, alcohol is sub-ject to *zero-order* kinetics and so, metabolising about 10 mL alcohol per hour, after 8 h the subject has elim-inated only 80 mL, leaving 70 mL in his body and giving a blood concentration of about 120 mg/dL. At this level, his driving skill is seriously impaired. The subject has an accident on his way to work despite his indignant protests that he last touched a drop before midnight. Banned from the road, on his train journey to work he has leisure to reflect on the dif-ference between first-order and zero-order kinetics.

In practice. The instance above describes an imag-ined event but similar cases occur in everyday therapeutics. Phenytoin, at low dose, exhibits a first-order elimination process and there is a directly

proportional increase in the steady-state plasma concentration with increase in dose. But gradu-ally the enzymatic elimination process approaches and reaches saturation, the process becoming con-stant and zero order. While the dosing rate can be increased, the metabolism rate cannot, and the plasma concentration rises steeply and *disproportion-ately*, with danger of toxicity. Salicylate metabolism also exhibits saturation kinetics but at high thera-peutic doses. Clearly saturation kinetics is a signifi-cant factor in delay of recovery from drug overdose, e.g. with aspirin or phenytoin.

Order of reaction and $t_{\frac{1}{2}}$. When a drug is subject to first-order kinetics, the $t_{\frac{1}{2}}$ is a constant character-istic, i.e. a constant value can be quoted through-out the plasma concentration range (accepting that there will be variation in $t_{\frac{1}{2}}$ between individuals), and this is convenient. But if the rate of a process is not directly proportional to plasma concentra-tion, then the $t_{\frac{1}{2}}$ cannot be constant. Consequently, no single value for $t_{\frac{1}{2}}$ describes overall elimination when a drug exhibits zero-order kinetics. In fact, $t_{\frac{1}{2}}$ decreases as plasma concentration falls and the cal-culations on elimination and dosing that are so easy with first-order elimination (see below) become more complicated.

Zero-order absorption processes apply to iron, to depot intramuscular formulations and to drug implants, e.g. antipsychotics and sex hormones.

TIME COURSE OF DRUG CONCENTRATION AND EFFECT

PLASMA HALF-LIFE AND STEADY-STATE CONCENTRATION

The manner in which plasma drug concentration rises or falls when dosing begins, alters or ceases follows certain simple rules, which provide a means for rational control of drug effect. Central to under-standing these is the concept of *half-life* ($t_{\frac{1}{2}}$) or half-time.

Decrease in plasma concentration after an intravenous bolus injection

Following an intravenous bolus injection (a sin-gle dose injected in a period of seconds as distinct from a continuous infusion), plasma concentration

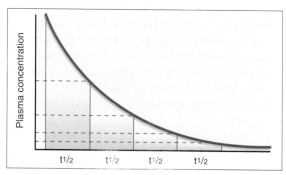

Fig. 7.2 Changes in plasma concentration following an intravenous bolus injection of a drug in the elimination phase (the distribution phase, see text, is not shown). As elimination is a first-order process, the time for any concentration point to fall by 50% ($t_{\frac{1}{2}}$) is always the same.

rises quickly as drug enters the blood to reach a peak. There is then a sharp drop as the drug distributes round the body (distribution phase), followed by a steady decline as drug is removed from the blood by the liver or kidneys (elimination phase). If the elimination processes are first order, the time taken for any concentration point in the elimination phase to fall to half its value (the $t_{1/2}$) is always the same; see Figure 7.2. Note that the drug is virtually eliminated from the plasma in five $t_{1/2}$ periods.

> The $t_{1/2}$ is the one pharmacokinetic value of a drug that it is most useful to know.

Increase in plasma concentration with constant dosing

With a constant rate infusion, the amount of drug in the body and with it the plasma concentration rise until a state is reached at which the rate of administration to the body is exactly equal to the rate of elimination from it: this is called the *steady state*. The plasma concentration is then on a plateau, and the drug effect is stable. Figure 7.3 depicts the smooth changes in plasma concentration that result from a constant intravenous infusion. Clearly, giving a

drug by regularly spaced oral or intravenous doses will result in plasma concentrations that fluctuate between peaks and troughs, but in time all of the peaks will be of equal height and all of the troughs will be of equal depth; this is also called a steady-state concentration, as the mean concentration is constant.[7]

Time to reach steady state

It is important to know *when* a drug administered at a constant rate achieves a steady-state plasma concentration, for maintaining the same dosing schedule then ensures a constant amount of drug in the body and the patient will experience neither acute toxicity nor decline of effect. The $t_{1/2}$ provides the answer. Taking *ultimate* steady state attained as 100%:

in $1 \times t_{1/2}$, the concentration will be (100/2) 50%
in $2 \times t_{1/2}$, (50 + 50/2) 75%
in $3 \times t_{1/2}$, (75 + 25/2) 87.5%
in $4 \times t_{1/2}$, (87.5 + 12.5/2) 93.75%
in $5 \times t_{1/2}$, (93.75 + 6.25/2) 96.875% of the ultimate steady state.

> When a drug is given at a constant rate (continuous or repeated administration), the time to reach steady state depends *only* on the $t_{1/2}$ and, for all practical purposes, after $5 \times t_{1/2}$ periods the amount of drug in the body is constant and the plasma concentration is at a plateau (a–b in Fig. 7.3).

Change in plasma concentration with change or cessation of dosing

The same principle holds for *change* from any steady-state plasma concentration to a *new* steady state brought about by increase or decrease in the rate of drug administration. Provided the kinetics remain first order, increasing or decreasing the rate of drug administration (b and c in Fig. 7.3) gives rise to a new steady-state concentration in a time equal to $5 \times t_{1/2}$ periods.

Similarly, starting at any steady-state plasma concentration (100%), discontinuing the dose (d in

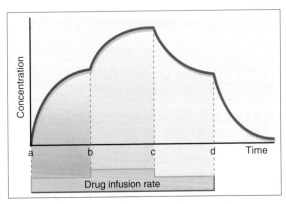

Fig. 7.3 Changes in plasma concentration during the course of a constant-rate intravenous infusion. (a) The infusion commences and plasma concentration rises to reach a steady-state (plateau) in about $5 \times t_{1/2}$ periods. (b) The infusion rate is increased by 50% and the plasma concentration rises further to reach a new steady state that is 50% higher than the original steady state; the process takes another $5 \times t_{1/2}$ periods. (c) The infusion is decreased to the original rate and the plasma concentration returns to the original steady state in $5 \times t_{1/2}$ periods. (d) The infusion is discontinued and the plasma concentration falls to virtually zero in $5 \times t_{1/2}$ periods.

---

[7] The peaks and troughs can be of practical importance with drugs of low therapeutic index, e.g. aminoglycoside antibiotics; it may be necessary to monitor both for safe and effective therapy.

Fig. 7.3) will cause the plasma concentration to fall to virtually zero in $5 \times t_{1/2}$ periods, as described in Figure 7.2.

Note that the difference between the rate of drug administration (input) and the rate of elimination (output) determines the actual *level* of any steady-state plasma concentration (as opposed to the *time taken* to reach it). If drug elimination remains constant and administration increases by 50%, in time the plasma concentration will reach a new steady-state concentration, which will be 50% greater than the original.

The relation between $t_{1/2}$ and time to reach steady-state plasma concentration applies to all drugs that obey first-order kinetics. This holds as much to dobutamine ($t_{1/2}$ 2 min), when it is useful to know that an alteration of infusion rate will reach a plateau within 10 min, as to digoxin ($t_{1/2}$ 36 h), when a constant daily oral dose will give a steady-state plasma concentration only after 7.5 days. This book quotes plasma $t_{1/2}$ values where they are relevant. Inevitably, natural variation within the population produces a range in $t_{1/2}$ values for any drug and the text quotes only single average $t_{1/2}$ values while recognising that the population range may be as much as 50% from the stated figure in either direction.

Some $t_{1/2}$ values are listed in Table 7.1 to illustrate their range and implications for dosing in clinical practice.

Biological effect $t_{1/2}$ is the time in which the biological effect of a drug declines by one-half. With drugs that act competitively on receptors (α- and β-adrenoceptor agonists and antagonists) the biological effect $t_{1/2}$ can be estimated with reasonable accuracy. Sometimes the biological effect $t_{1/2}$ cannot be provided, e.g. with antimicrobials when the number of infecting organisms and their sensitivity determine the outcome.

THERAPEUTIC DRUG MONITORING

Patients differ greatly in the dose of drug required to achieve the same response. The dose of warfarin that maintains a therapeutic concentration may vary as much as five-fold between individuals. This is a consequence of variation in rates of drug metabolism, disposition and tissue responsiveness, and it raises the question of how optimal drug effect can be achieved quickly for the individual patient.

In principle, drug effect relates to free (unbound) concentration at the tissue receptor site, which in turn reflects (but is not necessarily the same as) the concentration in the plasma. For many drugs, correlation between plasma concentration and effect is indeed better than that between dose and effect. Yet monitoring therapy by measuring drug in plasma is of practical use only in selected instances. The underlying reasons repay some thought.

Plasma concentration may not be worth measuring where dose can be titrated against a quickly and easily measured effect such as blood pressure (antihypertensives), body-weight (diuretics), INR (oral anticoagulants) or blood sugar (hypoglycaemics).

Plasma concentration has no correlation with effect with drugs that act irreversibly (named 'hit and run drugs' because their effect persists long after the drug has left the plasma). Such drugs destroy or inactivate target tissue (enzyme, receptor) and restoration of effect occurs only after days or weeks, when resynthesis takes place, e.g. some monoamine oxidase inhibitors, aspirin (on platelets), some anticholinesterases and anticancer drugs.

Plasma concentration may correlate poorly with effect. When a drug is metabolised to several products, active to varying degree or inactive, the assay of the parent drug alone is unlikely to reflect its activity, e.g. some benzodiazepines. Similarly binding of basic drugs, e.g. lidocaine, to acute phase proteins, e.g. α_1-acid glycoprotein, spuriously increases the total concentration in plasma. The best correlation is likely to be achieved by measurement of free

Table 7.1 Plasma $t_{1/2}$ of some drugs	
Drug	$t_{1/2}$
adenosine	<2 s
dobutamine	2 min
benzylpenicillin	30 min
amoxicillin	1 h
paracetamol	2 h
midazolam	3 h
tolbutamide	6 h
atenolol	7 h
dosulepin	25 h
diazepam	40 h
piroxicam	45 h
ethosuximide	54 h

(active) drug in plasma water, but this is technically more difficult and total drug in plasma is usually monitored in routine clinical practice.

Plasma concentration may correlate well with effect. Plasma concentration monitoring has proved useful:

- As a guide to the effectiveness of therapy, e.g. plasma gentamicin and other antimicrobials against sensitive bacteria, plasma theophylline for asthma, plasma ciclosporin to avoid transplant rejection, lithium for mood disorder.
- To reduce the risk of adverse drug effects when therapeutic doses are close to toxic doses (low therapeutic index), e.g. otic damage with aminoglycoside antibiotics; adverse CNS effects of lithium, nephrotoxicity with ciclosporin.
- When the desired effect is suppression of infrequent sporadic events such as epileptic seizures or episodes of cardiac arrhythmia.
- To check patient compliance on a drug regimen, when there is failure of therapeutic effect at a known effective dose, e.g. antiepilepsy drugs.
- To diagnose and manage drug overdose.
- When lack of therapeutic effect and toxicity may be difficult to distinguish. Digoxin is both a treatment for, and sometimes the cause of, cardiac supraventricular tachycardia; a plasma digoxin measurement will help to distinguish whether an arrhythmia is due to too little or too much digoxin.

Interpreting plasma concentration measurements. Recommended plasma concentrations for drugs appear throughout this book where these are relevant but the following points ought to be kept in mind:

- The target therapeutic concentration range for a drug is a guide to optimise dosing together with other clinical indicators of progress.
- Take account of the time needed to reach steady-state dosing conditions (see above). Additionally, some drugs alter their own rates of metabolism by enzyme induction, e.g. carbamazepine and phenytoin, and it is best to allow 2–4 weeks between change in dose and meaningful plasma concentration measurement.
- As a general rule, when a drug has a short $t_{1/2}$ it is desirable to know both peak (15 min after an intravenous dose) and trough (just before the next

dose) concentrations to provide efficacy without toxicity, as with gentamicin ($t_{1/2}$ 2.5 h). For a drug with a long $t_{1/2}$, it is usually best to sample just before a dose is due; effective immunosuppression with ciclosporin ($t_{1/2}$ 27 h) is obtained with trough concentrations of 50–200 micrograms/L when the drug is given by mouth.

INDIVIDUAL PHARMACOKINETIC PROCESSES

Drug absorption into, distribution around, metabolism by and eliminated from the body are reviewed.

ABSORPTION

Commonsense considerations of anatomy, physiology, pathology, pharmacology, therapeutics and convenience determine the routes by which drugs are administered. Usually these are:

- *Enteral*: by mouth (swallowed) or by sublingual or buccal absorption; by rectum.
- *Parenteral*: by intravenous injection or infusion, intramuscular injection, subcutaneous injection or infusion, inhalation, topical application for local (skin, eye, lung) or for systemic (transdermal) effect.
- *Other routes*, e.g. intrathecal, intradermal, intranasal, intratracheal, intrapleural, are used when appropriate.

The features of the various routes, their advantages and disadvantages are relevant.

ABSORPTION FROM THE GASTROINTESTINAL TRACT

The *small intestine* is the principal site for absorption of nutrients and it is also where most orally administered drugs enter the body. This part of the gut has an enormous surface area due to the intestinal villi, and an epithelium through which fluid readily filters in response to osmotic differences caused by the presence of food. Disturbed alimentary motility can reduce drug absorption, i.e. if gastric emptying is slowed by food, or intestinal transit is accelerated by gut infection. Additionally, it is becoming apparent that uptake and efflux transporters in enterocytes (see p. 97) play a substantial role in controlling the absorption of certain drugs, e.g. digoxin, ciclosporin. Many sustained-release formulations probably depend on absorption from the colon.

Absorption of ionisable drugs from the *buccal mucosa* responds to the prevailing pH, which is 6.2–7.2. Lipid-soluble drugs are rapidly effective by this route because blood flow through the mucosa is abundant; these drugs enter directly into the systemic circulation, avoiding the possibility of first-pass (presystemic) inactivation by the liver and gut (see below).

The *stomach* does not play a major role in absorbing drugs, even those that are acidic and thus un-ionised and lipid soluble at gastric pH, because its surface area is much smaller than that of the small intestine and gastric emptying is speedy ($t_{1/2}$ 30 min).

ENTEROHEPATIC CIRCULATION

This system is illustrated by the bile salts which are formed in the liver, then conserved by circulating round liver, intestine and portal blood about eight times a day. Several drugs form conjugates with glucuronic acid in the liver and enter the bile. Too polar (ionised) to be reabsorbed, the glucuronides remain in the gut, are hydrolysed by intestinal enzymes and bacteria, and the parent drug, thus released, is reabsorbed and reconjugated in the liver. Enterohepatic recycling appears to help sustain the plasma concentration and thus the effect of sulindac, pentaerithrityl tetranitrate and ethinylestradiol (in many oral contraceptives).

SYSTEMIC AVAILABILITY AND BIOAVAILABILITY

A drug that is injected intravenously enters the systemic circulation and thence gains access to the tissues and to receptors, i.e. 100% is available to exert its therapeutic effect. If the same quantity of the drug is swallowed, it does not follow that the entire amount will reach first the portal blood and then the systemic blood, i.e. its availability for therapeutic effect via the systemic circulation may be less than 100%. The anticipated response to a drug must take account of its availability to the systemic circulation.

While considerations of reduced availability attach to any drug given by any route other than intravenously, and intended for systemic effect, in practice the issue concerns enteral administration. The extent of systemic availability is ordinarily calculated by relating the area under the plasma concentration–time curve (AUC) after a single oral dose to that obtained after intravenous administration of the same amount (by which route a drug is 100% systemically available). Calculation of AUCs after oral doses also allows a comparison of the bioavailability of different pharmaceutical formulations of the same drug. Factors influencing systemic availability present in three main ways, as described below.

Pharmaceutical factors[8]

The amount of drug released from a dose form (and so becoming available for absorption) is referred to as its *bioavailability*. This is highly dependent on its pharmaceutical formulation. With tablets, for example, particle size (surface area exposed to solution), diluting substances, tablet size and pressure used in the tabletting process can affect disintegration and dissolution and so the bioavailability of the drug. Manufacturers must test their products to ensure that their formulations release the same amount of drug at the same speed from whatever manufactured batch or brand the patient may be taking.

Differences in bioavailability are prone to occur with *modified-release* (m/r) formulations, i.e. where the rate or place of release of the active ingredients has been modified (also called *sustained*, *controlled* or *delayed* release) (see p. 102). Modified-release preparations from different manufacturers may differ in their bioavailability profiles despite containing the same amount of drug, i.e. there is neither *bioequivalence* nor *therapeutic equivalence*, and the problem is particularly acute where the therapeutic ratio is narrow. In this case, 'brand name prescribing', i.e. using only a particular brand name for a particular patient is justified, e.g. for m/r preparations of theophylline, lithium, nifedipine and diltiazem.

---

[8]Some definitions of enteral dose forms: *Tablet:* a solid dose form in which the drug is compressed or moulded with pharmacologically inert substances (excipients); variants include sustained-release and coated tablets. *Capsule:* the drug is provided in a gelatin shell or container. *Mixture:* a liquid formulation of a drug for oral administration. *Suppository:* a solid dose-form shaped for insertion into rectum (or vagina, when it may be called a pessary); it may be designed to dissolve or it may melt at body temperature (in which case there is a storage problem in countries where the environmental temperature may exceed 37°C); the vehicle in which the drug is carried may be fat, glycerol with gelatin, or macrogols (polycondensation products of ethylene oxide) with gelatin. *Syrup:* the drug is provided in a concentrated sugar (fructose or other) solution. *Linctus:* a viscous liquid formulation, traditional for cough.

Physicians tend to ignore pharmaceutical formulation as a factor in variable or unexpected responses because they do not understand it and feel entitled to rely on reputable manufacturers and official regulatory authorities to ensure provision of reliable formulations. Good pharmaceutical companies reasonably point out that, having a reputation to lose, they take much trouble to make their preparations consistently reliable. This is a matter of great importance when dosage must be precise (anticoagulants, antidiabetics, adrenal corticosteroids). The following account by the physician Lauder Brunton in 1897 indicates that the phenomenon of variable bioavailability is not recent:

> A very unfortunate case occurred some time ago in a doctor who had prescribed aconitine to a patient and gradually increased the dose. He thought he was quite certain that he knew what he was doing. The druggist's supply of aconitine ran out, and he procured some new aconitine from a different maker. This turned out to be many times stronger than the other, and the patient unfortunately became very ill. The doctor said, 'It cannot be the medicine', and to show that this was true, he drank off a dose himself with the result that he died. So you must remember the difference in the different preparations of aconitine[9]

i.e. they had different *bioavailability* and so lacked *therapeutic equivalence*.

Biological factors

Biological factors related to the gut include limitation of drug absorption by drug transporter systems (see p. 97), destruction of drug by gastric acid, e.g. benzylpenicillin, and impaired absorption due to rapid intestinal transit, which is important for all drugs that are absorbed slowly. Drugs may also bind to food constituents, e.g. tetracyclines to calcium (in milk), and to iron, or to other drugs (e.g. acidic drugs to colestyramine), and the resulting complex is not absorbed.

Presystemic (first pass) elimination

Some drugs readily enter gut mucosal cells, yet appear in low concentration in the systemic circulation. The reason lies in the considerable extent to which such drugs are metabolised in a single passage through the gut mucosa and (principally) the liver. As little as 10–20% of the parent drug may enter the systemic circulation unchanged. By contrast, after intravenous administration, 100% becomes systemically available and the patient experiences higher concentrations with greater, but more predictable, effect. Dosing, particularly *initial* doses, must take account of discrepancy in anticipated plasma concentrations between the intravenous and oral routes. The difference is less if a drug produces active metabolites.

Once a drug is in the systemic circulation, irrespective of which route is used, about 20% is subject to the hepatic metabolic processes in each circulation time because that proportion of cardiac output passes to the liver.

As the degree of presystemic elimination differs much between drugs and individuals, the phenomenon of first-pass elimination adds to variation in systemic plasma concentrations, and thus particularly in initial response to the drugs that are subject to this process. In drug overdose, decreased presystemic elimination with increased bioavailability may account for the rapid onset of toxicity with antipsychotic drugs.

Drugs for which *presystemic elimination* is significant include:[10]

Analgesics	Adrenoceptor blockers	Others
dextropropoxyphene	labetalol	clomethiazole
morphine	propranolol	chlorpromazine
pentazocine	metoprolol	isosorbide dinitrate
pethidine	oxprenolol	nortriptyline

In severe hepatic cirrhosis with both impaired liver cell function and well developed channels shunting blood into the systemic circulation without passing through the liver, first-pass elimination reduces and systemic availability is increased. The result of these changes is an increased likelihood of exaggerated response to normal doses of drugs having high hepatic clearance and, on occasion, frank toxicity.

---

[9]The doctor would have died from cardiac arrhythmia and/or cerebral depression. Aconitine is a plant alkaloid and has no place in medicine.

[10]For a more detailed list, see Wilkinson G R 2005 Drug metabolism and variability among patients in drug response. New England Journal of Medicine 352:2211–2221.

Drugs that exhibit the hepatic first-pass phenomenon do so because of the rapidity with which they are metabolised. The rate of delivery to the liver, i.e. blood flow, is then the main determinant of its rate of metabolism. Many other drugs are completely metabolised by the liver but at a slower rate and consequently loss in the first pass through the liver is unimportant. Dose adjustment to account for presystemic elimination is unnecessary, e.g. for diazepam, phenytoin, theophylline, warfarin.

ADVANTAGES AND DISADVANTAGES OF ENTERAL ADMINISTRATION

By swallowing

For systemic effect. *Advantages* are convenience and acceptability.

Disadvantages are that absorption may be delayed, reduced or even enhanced after food, or slow or irregular after drugs that inhibit gut motility (antimuscarinic, opioid). Differences in presystemic elimination are a cause of variation in drug effect between patients. Some drugs are not absorbed (gentamicin) and some drugs are destroyed in the gut (insulin, oxytocin, some penicillins). Tablets taken with too small a quantity of liquid and in the supine position, can lodge in the oesophagus with delayed absorption[11] and may even cause ulceration (sustained-release potassium chloride and doxycycline tablets), especially in the feeble elderly and those with an enlarged left atrium which impinges on the oesophagus.[12]

For effect in the gut. *Advantages* are that the drug is placed at the site of action (neomycin, anthelminthics), and with non-absorbed drugs the local concentration can be higher than would be safe in the blood.

Disadvantages are that drug distribution may be uneven, and in some diseases of the gut the whole thickness of the wall is affected (severe bacillary dysentery, typhoid) and effective blood concentrations (as well as luminal concentrations) may be needed.

Sublingual or buccal for systemic effect

Advantages are that the effect is quick, e.g. with glyceryl trinitrate as an aerosol spray, or as sublingual tablets that are chewed, giving greater surface area for solution. Spitting out the tablet will terminate the effect.

Disadvantages are the inconvenience if use has to be frequent, irritation of the mucous membrane and excessive salivation, which promotes swallowing, so losing the advantages of bypassing presystemic elimination.

Rectal administration

For systemic effect (suppositories or solutions). The rectal mucosa has a rich blood and lymph supply and, in general, dose requirements are either the same or slightly greater than those needed for oral use. Drugs chiefly enter the portal system, but those that are subject to hepatic first-pass elimination may escape this if they are absorbed from the lower rectum, which drains directly to the systemic circulation. The degree of presystemic elimination thus depends on distribution within the rectum and this is somewhat unpredictable.

Advantages are that a suppository can replace a drug that irritates the stomach (aminophylline, indometacin); the route is suitable in vomiting, motion sickness, migraine or when a patient cannot swallow, and when cooperation is lacking (sedation in children).

Disadvantages are psychological in that the patient may be embarrassed or may like the route too much; rectal inflammation may occur with repeated use and absorption can be unreliable, especially if the rectum is full of faeces.

For local effect, e.g. in proctitis or colitis, is an obvious use. A survey in the UK showed that a substantial proportion of patients did not remove the wrapper before inserting the suppository.

ADVANTAGES AND DISADVANTAGES OF PARENTERAL ADMINISTRATION

(for systemic and local effect)

Intravenous (bolus or infusion)

An intravenous bolus, i.e. rapid injection, passes round the circulation being progressively diluted each

---

[11]A woman's failure to respond to antihypertensive medication was explained when she was observed to choke on drinking. Investigation revealed a large pharyngeal pouch that was full of tablets and capsules. Her blood pressure became easy to control when the pouch was removed. Birch D J, Dehn T C B 1993 British Medical Journal 306:1012.

[12]Ideally solid-dose forms should be taken while standing up and washed down with 150 mL (a tea-cup) of water; even sitting (higher intra-abdominal pressure) impairs passage. At least, patients should be told to sit and take three or four mouthfuls of water (a mouthful = 30 mL) or a cupful. Some patients do not even know they should take water.

time; it is delivered principally to the organs with high blood flow (brain, liver, heart, lung, kidneys).

Advantages are that the intravenous route gives swift, effective and highly predictable blood concentration and allows rapid modification of dose, i.e. immediate cessation of administration is possible if unwanted effects occur during administration. The route is suitable for administration of drugs that are not absorbed from the gut or are too irritant (anti-cancer agents) to be given by other routes.

Disadvantages are the hazard if drug administration too rapid, as plasma concentration may rise at a rate such that normal mechanisms of distribution and elimination are outpaced. Some drugs will act within one arm-to-tongue (brain) circulation time, which is 13 ± 3 s; with most drugs an injection given over four or five circulation times seems sufficient to avoid excessive plasma concentrations. Local venous thrombosis is liable to occur with prolonged infusion and with bolus doses of irritant formulations, e.g. diazepam, or microparticulate components of infusion fluids, especially if small veins are used. Infection of the intravenous catheter and the small thrombi on its tip are also a risk during prolonged infusions.

Intramuscular injection

Blood flow is greater in the muscles of the upper arm than in the gluteal mass and thigh, and increases with physical exercise.[13]

Advantages are that the route is reliable, suitable for irritant drugs, and depot preparations (neuroleptics, hormonal contraceptives) are suitable for administration at monthly or longer intervals. Absorption is more rapid than following subcutaneous injection (soluble preparations are absorbed within 10–30 min).

Disadvantages are that the route is not acceptable for self-administration, it may be painful, and if any adverse effects occur with a depot formulation, it may not be removable.

Subcutaneous injection

Advantages are that the route is reliable and is acceptable for self-administration.

Disadvantages are poor absorption in peripheral circulatory failure. Repeated injections at one site can cause lipoatrophy, resulting in erratic absorption (see Insulin, Chapter 35).

By inhalation

As a gas, e.g. volatile anaesthetics.

As an aerosol, e.g. β_2-adrenoceptor agonist bronchodilators. Aerosols are particles dispersed in a gas, the particles being small enough to remain in suspension for a long time instead of sedimenting rapidly under the influence of gravity; the particles may be liquid (fog) or solid (smoke).

As a powder, e.g. sodium cromoglicate. Particle size and air-flow velocity are important. Most particles greater than 5 micrometres in diameter impact in the upper respiratory areas; particles of about 2 micrometres reach the terminal bronchioles; a large proportion of particles less than 1 micrometre are exhaled. Air-flow velocity diminishes considerably as the bronchi progressively divide, promoting drug deposition peripherally.

Advantages are the rapid uptake or elimination of drugs as gases, giving the close control that has marked the use of this route in general anaesthesia from its earliest days. Self-administration is practicable. Aerosols and powders provide high local concentration for action on bronchi, minimising systemic effects.

Disadvantages are that special apparatus is needed (some patients find pressurised aerosols difficult to use to best effect) and a drug must be non-irritant if the patient is conscious. Obstructed bronchi (mucous plugs in asthma) may cause therapy to fail.

Topical application

For local effect, e.g. to skin, eye, lung, anal canal, rectum, vagina.

Advantage is the provision of high local concentration without systemic effect (usually[14]).

---

[13]Usually these influences are unimportant, but one football-playing patient who received an intramuscular injection of a sustained-release phenothiazine developed an extrapyramidal disorder towards the end of the game, presumably due to too rapid absorption of the drug following muscular exercise.

[14]*A cautionary tale.* A 70-year-old man reported left breast enlargement and underwent mastectomy; histological examination revealed benign gynaecomastia. Ten months later the right breast enlarged. Tests of endocrine function were normal but the patient himself was struck by the fact that his wife had been using a vaginal cream (containing 0.01% dienestrol), initially for atrophic vaginitis but

Disadvantage is that absorption can occur, especially when there is tissue destruction so that systemic effects result, e.g. adrenal corticosteroids and neomycin to the skin, atropine to the eye. Ocular administration of a β-adrenoceptor blocker may cause systemic effects (bypassing first-pass elimination) and such eye-drops are contraindicated in asthma or chronic lung disease.[15] There is extensive literature on this subject characterised by expressions of astonishment that serious effects, even death, can occur.

For systemic effect. Transdermal delivery systems release drug through a rate-controlling membrane into the skin and so into the systemic circulation. This avoids the fluctuations in plasma concentration associated with other routes of administration, as is first-pass elimination in the liver. Glyceryl trinitrate and postmenopausal hormone replacement therapy may be given this way, in the form of a sticking plaster attached to the skin[16] or as an ointment (glyceryl trinitrate). One treatment for migraine is a nasal spray containing sumatriptan.

DISTRIBUTION

If a drug is required to act throughout the body or to reach an organ inaccessible to topical administration, it must get into the blood and other body compartments. Most drugs distribute widely, in part dissolved in body water, in part bound to plasma proteins, in part to tissues. Distribution is often uneven, for drugs may bind selectively to plasma or tissue proteins or be localised within particular organs. Clearly, the site of localisation of a drug is likely to influence its action, e.g. whether it crosses the blood–brain barrier to enter the brain; the extent (amount) and strength (tenacity) of protein or tissue binding (stored drug) will affect the time it spends in the body and thereby its duration of action.

DISTRIBUTION VOLUME

The pattern of distribution from plasma to other body fluids and tissues is a characteristic of each drug that enters the circulation, and it varies between drugs. Precise information on the concentration of drug attained in various tissues and fluids is usually not available for humans.[17] What is sampled readily in humans is *blood plasma*, the drug concentration in which, taking account of the dose given, is a measure of whether a drug tends to remain in the circulation or to distribute from the plasma into the tissues. In other words:

- If a drug remains mostly in the plasma, its distribution volume will be small.
- If a drug is present mainly in other tissues, the distribution volume will be large.

Such information can be useful. In drug overdose, if a major proportion of the total body load is known to be in the plasma, i.e. the distribution volume is small, then haemodialysis/filtration is likely to be a useful option (as is the case with severe salicylate poisoning), but it is an inappropriate treatment for overdose with dosulepin (see Table 7.2).

---

latterly the cream had been used to facilitate sexual intercourse which took place two or three times a week. On the assumption that penile absorption of oestrogen was responsible for the disorder, exposure to the cream was terminated. The gynaecomastia in the remaining breast then resolved (DiRaimondo C V, Roach A C, Meador C K 1980 Gynecomastia from exposure to vaginal estrogen cream. New England Journal of Medicine 302:1089–1090).

[15]Two drops of 0.5% timolol solution, one to each eye, can equate to 10 mg by mouth.

[16]But transdermal delivery systems may have an unexpected outcome for, not only may the sticking plaster drop off unnoticed, it may find its way on to another person. A hypertensive father rose one morning and noticed that his clonidine plaster was missing from his upper arm. He could not find it and applied a new plaster. His 9-month-old child, who had been taken into the paternal bed during the night because he needed comforting, spent an irritable and hypoactive day, refused food, but drank and passed more urine than usual. The missing clonidine patch was discovered on his back when he was being prepared for his bath. No doubt this was accidental, but children also enjoy stick-on decoration and the possibility of poisoning from misused, discarded or new (e.g. strong opioid, used in palliative care) drug plasters means that these should be kept and disposed of as carefully as oral formulations (Reed M T, Hamburg E L 1986 Person-to-person transfer of transdermal drug-delivery systems: a case report. New England Journal of Medicine 314:1120–1121).

[17]But positive emission tomography (PET) offers a prospect of obtaining similar information. With PET, a positron emitting isotope, e.g. ^{15}O, is substituted for a stable atom without altering the chemical behaviour of the molecule. The radiation dose is very low but can be imaged tomographically using photomultiplier–scintillator detectors. PET can be used to monitor effects of drugs on metabolism in the brain, e.g. 'on' and 'off' phases in parkinsonism. There are many other applications.

Table 7.2 Apparent distribution volume of some drugs (values are in litres for a 70-kg person who would displace about 70 L)*

Drug	Distribution volume	Drug	Distribution volume
Evans blue	3 (plasma volume)	atenolol	77
heparin	5	diazepam	140
salicylate	9	pethidine	280
inulin	15 (extracellular water)	digoxin	420
gentamicin	18	nortriptyline	1000
furosemide	21	dosulepin	4900
amoxicillin	28	chloroquine	13 000
antipyrine	43 (total body water)		

*Litres per kilogram are commonly used, but give a less vivid image of the implication of the term 'apparent', e.g. chloroquine.

The principle for measuring the distribution volume is essentially that of using a dye to find the volume of a container filled with liquid. The weight of added dye divided by the concentration of dye once mixing is complete gives the distribution volume of the dye, which is the volume of the container. Similarly, the distribution volume of a drug in the body may be determined after a single intravenous bolus dose by dividing the dose given by the concentration achieved in plasma.[18]

The result of this calculation, the distribution volume, in fact only rarely corresponds with a physiological body space such as extracellular water or total body water, for it is a measure of the volume a drug would apparently occupy knowing the dose given and the plasma concentration achieved, and assuming the entire volume is at that concentration. For this reason, the term *apparent* distribution volume is often preferred. Indeed, the apparent distribution volume of some drugs that bind extensively to extravascular tissues, which is based on the resulting low plasma concentration, is many times total body volume.

> The distribution volume of a drug is the volume in which it appears to distribute (or which it would require) if the concentration throughout the body were equal to that in plasma, i.e. as if the body were a single compartment.

The list in Table 7.2 illustrates a range of apparent distribution volumes. The names of those substances that distribute within (and have been used to measure) physiological spaces are printed in italics.

Selective distribution within the body occurs because of special affinity between particular drugs and particular body constituents. Many drugs bind to proteins in the plasma; phenothiazines and chloroquine bind to melanin-containing tissues, including the retina, which may explain the occurrence of retinopathy. Drugs may also concentrate selectively in a particular tissue because of specialised transport mechanisms, e.g. iodine in the thyroid.

PLASMA PROTEIN AND TISSUE BINDING

Many natural substances circulate around the body partly free in plasma water and partly bound to plasma proteins; these include cortisol, thyroxine, iron, copper and, in hepatic or renal failure, byproducts of physiological intermediary metabolism.

Drugs, too, circulate in the protein-bound and free states, and the significance is that the free fraction is pharmacologically active whereas the protein-bound component is a reservoir of drug that is inactive because of this binding. Free and bound fractions are in equilibrium, and free drug removed from the plasma by metabolism, renal function or dialysis is replaced by drug released from the bound fraction.

[18] Clearly a problem arises in that the plasma concentration is not constant but falls after the bolus has been injected. To get round this, use is made of the fact that the relation between the logarithm of plasma concentration and the time after a single intravenous dose is a straight line. The log concentration–time line extended back to zero time gives the theoretical plasma concentration at the time the drug was given. In effect, the assumption is made that drug distributes instantaneously and uniformly through a single compartment, the distribution volume. This mechanism, although seeming artificial, does usefully characterise drugs according to the extent to which they remain in or distribute out from the circulation.

Albumin is the main binding protein for many natural substances and drugs. Its complex structure has a net negative charge at blood pH and a high *capacity* but low (weak) *affinity* for many basic drugs, i.e. a lot is bound but it is readily released. Two particular sites on the albumin molecule bind acidic drugs with high affinity (strongly), but these sites have low capacity. Saturation of binding sites on plasma proteins in general is unlikely in the doses in which most drugs are used.

Other binding proteins in the blood include lipoprotein and α_1-acid glycoprotein, both of which carry basic drugs such as quinidine, chlorpromazine and imipramine. Thyroxine and sex hormones are bound in the plasma to specific globulins.

Disease may modify protein binding of drugs to an extent that is clinically relevant, as Table 7.3 shows. In *chronic renal failure*, hypoalbuminaemia and retention of products of metabolism that compete for binding sites on protein are both responsible for the decrease in protein binding of drugs. Most affected are acidic drugs that are highly protein bound, e.g. phenytoin, and initiating or modifying the dose of such drugs for patients with renal failure requires special attention (see also Prescribing in renal disease, p. 489).

Chronic liver disease also leads to hypoalbuminaemia and an increase of endogenous substances such as bilirubin that may compete for binding sites on protein. Drugs that are normally extensively protein bound should be used with special caution, for increased free concentration of diazepam, tolbutamide and phenytoin have been demonstrated in patients with this condition (see also Prescribing for patients with liver disease, p. 583).

The free, unbound, and therefore pharmacologically active percentages of some drugs are listed in Table 7.3 to illustrate the range and, in some cases, changes recorded in disease.

Tissue binding. Some drugs distribute readily to regions of the body other than plasma, as a glance at Table 7.2 will show. These include many lipid-soluble drugs, which may enter fat stores, e.g. most benzodiazepines, verapamil and lidocaine. There is less information about other tissues, e.g. muscle, than about plasma protein binding because solid tissue samples require invasive biopsy. Extensive binding to tissues delays elimination from the body and accounts for the long $t_{1/2}$ of chloroquine and amiodarone.

Table 7.3 Examples of plasma protein binding of drugs and effects of disease

Drug	% Unbound (free)
warfarin	1
diazepam	2 (6% in liver disease)
furosemide	2 (6% in nephrotic syndrome)
tolbutamide	2
amitriptyline	5
phenytoin	9 (19% in renal disease)
triamterene	19 (40% in renal disease)
trimethoprim	30
theophylline	35 (71% in liver disease)
morphine	65
digoxin	75 (82% in renal disease)
amoxicillin	82
ethosuximide	100

METABOLISM

The body treats most drugs as foreign substances (xenobiotics) and subjects them to various mechanisms for eliminating chemical intruders.

Metabolism is a general term for chemical transformations that occur within the body and its processes change drugs in two major ways by:

- reducing lipid solubility
- altering biological activity.

REDUCING LIPID SOLUBILITY

> Metabolic reactions tend to make a drug molecule progressively more water soluble and so favour its elimination in the urine.

Drug-metabolising enzymes developed during evolution to enable the body to dispose of lipid-soluble substances such as hydrocarbons, steroids and alkaloids that are ingested with food.[19] Some environmental chemicals may persist indefinitely in our fat deposits, e.g. dicophane (DDT), with consequences that are currently unknown.

---

[19]Fish lose lipid-soluble substances through the gills. They do not need such effective metabolising enzymes and they have not got them.

ALTERING BIOLOGICAL ACTIVITY

The end-result of metabolism usually is the abolition of biological activity, but various steps in between may have the following consequences:

1. Conversion of a pharmacologically *active* to an *inactive* substance – this applies to most drugs.
2. Conversion of one pharmacologically *active* to another *active* substance – this has the effect of prolonging drug action, as shown below.

Active drug	Active metabolite
amitriptyline	nortriptyline
codeine	morphine
chloroquine	hydroxychloroquine
diazepam	oxazepam
spironolactone	canrenone

3. Conversion of a pharmacologically *inactive* to an *active* substance (then called a prodrug). The process then follows 1 or 2, above.

Inactive substance	Active metabolite(s)	Comment
aciclovir	aciclovir triphosphate	see p. 225
colecalciferol	calcitriol and alfacalcidol	highly active metabolites of vitamin D₃; see p. 663
cyclophospha-mide	phosphoramide mustard	another metabolite, acrolein, causes the bladder toxicity; see p. 544
perindopril	perindoprilat	less risk of first dose hypotension (applies to all ACE inhibitors except captopril)
levodopa	dopamine	levodopa, but not dopamine, can cross the blood–brain barrier
sulindac	sulindac sulphide	possibly reduced gastric toxicity
sulfasalazine	5-aminosalicylic acid	see p. 577
zidovudine	zidovudine triphosphate	see p. 228

THE METABOLIC PROCESSES

The liver is by far the most important drug-metabolising organ, although a number of tissues, including the kidney, gut mucosa, lung and skin, also contribute. It is useful to think of drug metabolism in two broad phases.

Phase I metabolism brings about a change in the drug molecule by oxidation, reduction or hydrolysis and usually introduces or exposes a chemically active site on it. The new metabolite often has reduced biological activity and different pharmacokinetic properties, e.g. a shorter $t_{\frac{1}{2}}$.

The principal group of reactions is the *oxidations*, in particular those undertaken by the (microsomal) *mixed-function oxidases* which, as the name indicates, are capable of metabolising a wide variety of compounds. The most important of these is a large 'superfamily' of haem proteins, the *cytochrome P450 enzymes*, which metabolise chemicals from the environment, the diet and drugs. By a complex process, the drug molecule incorporates one atom of molecular oxygen (O_2) to form a (chemically active) hydroxyl group and the other oxygen atom converts to water.

The following explanation provides a background to the P450 nomenclature that accompanies accounts of the metabolism of several individual drugs in this book. The many cytochrome P450 isoenzymes[20] are indicated by the letters CYP (from cytochrome P450) followed by a number denoting a family group, then a subfamily letter, and then a number for the individual enzyme within the family: for example, CYP 2E1 is an isoenzyme that catalyses a reaction involved in the metabolism of alcohol, paracetamol, estradiol and ethinylestradiol.

The enzymes of families CYP 1, 2 and 3 metabolise 70–80% of clinically used drugs as well as many other foreign chemicals and, within these, CYP 3A, CYP 2D and CYP 2C are the most important.[21] The very size and variety of the P450 superfamily ensures that we do not need new enzymes for every existing or yet-to-be synthesised drug. Induction and

---

[20] An isoenzyme is one of a group of enzymes that catalyse the same reaction but differ in protein structure.

[21] Wolf C R, Smith G, Smith R L 2000 Pharmacogenetics. British Medical Journal 320:987–990.

inhibition of P450 enzymes is a fruitful source of drug–drug interactions.[22]

Each P450 enzyme protein is encoded by a separate gene (57 have been identified in humans), and variation in genes leads to differences between individuals, and sometimes between ethnic groups, in the ability to metabolise drugs. Persons who exhibit *polymorphisms* (see p. 105) inherit diminished or increased ability to metabolise substrate drugs, predisposing to toxicity or lack of efficacy.

Phase I oxidation of some drugs results in the formation of *epoxides*, which are short-lived and highly reactive metabolites that bind irreversibly through covalent bonds to cell constituents and are toxic to body tissues. Glutathione is a tripeptide that combines with epoxides, rendering them inactive, and its presence in the liver is part of an important defence mechanism against hepatic damage by halothane and paracetamol.

Note that some drug oxidation reactions do not involve the P450 system: several biologically active amines are inactivated by monoamine oxidase (see p. 339) and methylxanthines (see p. 169); mercaptopurine by xanthine oxidase (see p. 272); ethanol by alcohol dehydrogenase (see p. 149).

Hydrolysis (Phase I) reactions create active sites for subsequent conjugation of, e.g. aspirin, lidocaine.

Phase II metabolism involves combination of the drug with one of several polar (water soluble) endogenous molecules (products of intermediary metabolism), often at the active site (hydroxyl, amino, thiol) created by Phase I metabolism. The kidney readily eliminates the resulting water-soluble conjugate, or the bile if the molecular weight exceeds 300. Morphine, paracetamol and salicylates form conjugates with glucuronic acid (derived from glucose); oral contraceptive steroids form sulphates; isoniazid, phenelzine and dapsone are acetylated. Conjugation with a more polar molecule is also an elimination mechanism for natural substances, e.g. bilirubin as glucuronide, oestrogens as sulphates.

Phase II metabolism almost invariably terminates biological activity.

Transporters.[23] It is convenient here to introduce the subject of *carrier mediated transporter processes* whose physiological functions include the passage of amino acids, lipids, sugars, hormones and bile acids across cell membranes, and the protection of cells against environmental toxins.

There is an emerging understanding that membrane transporters have a key role in the overall disposition of drugs to their targeted organs. There are broadly two types: *uptake transporters*, which facilitate, for example, the passage of organic anions and cations into cells, and *efflux transporters*, which transport substances out of cells, often against high concentration gradients. Some transporters possess both influx and efflux properties.

Most efflux transporters are members of the ATP-binding cassette (ABC) superfamily that utilises energy derived from the hydrolysis of ATP; they include the P-glycoprotein family that expresses multidrug resistance protein 1 (MDR1) (see p. 549).

Their varied locations illustrate the potential for transporters widely to affect the distribution of drugs, namely in:

- Enterocytes of the small intestine, controlling absorption and thus bioavailability, e.g. of ciclosporin, digoxin.
- Liver cells, controlling uptake from the blood and excretion into the bile, e.g. of pravastatin.
- Renal tubular cells, controlling uptake from the blood, secretion into tubular fluid (and thus excretion) of organic anions, e.g. β-lactam antibiotics, diuretics, non-steroidal anti-inflammatory drugs.
- Brain capillary endothelial cells, controlling passage across the blood–brain barrier, e.g. of levodopa (but not dopamine) for benefit in Parkinson's disease (see p. 381).

In time, it is likely that drug occupancy of transporter processes will provide explanations for drug-induced toxicities and for a number of drug–drug interactions.

ENZYME INDUCTION

The mechanisms that the body evolved over millions of years to metabolise foreign substances

---

[22]In this expanding field, useful lists of substrate drugs for P450 enzymes with inducers and inhibitors can be found in periodic reviews, e.g. Wilkinson G R 2005 Drug metabolism and variability among patients in drug response. New England Journal of Medicine 352:2211–2221.

[23]Parts of this section are based on the review by Ho R H, Kim R B 2005 Transporters and drug therapy: implications for drug disposition and disease. Clinical Pharmacology and Therapeutics 78:260–277.

now enable it to meet the modern environmental challenges of tobacco smoke, hydrocarbon pollutants, insecticides and drugs. At times of high exposure, our enzyme systems respond by increasing in amount and so in activity, i.e. they become *induced*; when exposure falls off, enzyme production lessens.

For example, a first alcoholic drink taken after a period of abstinence from alcohol may have a noticeable effect on behaviour, but the same drink taken at the end of 2 weeks of regular imbibing may pass almost unnoticed because the individual's liver enzyme activity is increased (induced), and alcohol is metabolised more rapidly, having less effect, i.e. tolerance is acquired.

Inducing substances in general share some important properties: they tend to be lipid soluble, are substrates, though sometimes only minor ones, e.g. DDT, for the enzymes they induce, and generally have a long $t_{1/2}$. The time for onset and offset of induction depends on the rate of enzyme turnover, but significant induction generally occurs within a few days and it passes off over 2–3 weeks following withdrawal of the inducer.

Thus, certain drugs can alter the capacity of the body to metabolise other substances including drugs, especially in long-term use; this phenomenon has implications for drug therapy. More than 200 substances induce enzymes in animals but the list of proven enzyme inducers in humans is more restricted, as set out below.

Substances that cause enzyme induction in humans
• barbecued meats   • nevirapine
• barbiturates   • phenobarbital
• Brussels sprouts   • phenytoin
• carbamazepine   • primidone
• DDT (dicophane, and   • rifampicin
other insecticides)   • St John's Wort
• ethanol (chronic use)   • sulfinpyrazone
• glutethimide   • tobacco smoke
• griseofulvin
• meprobamate

Enzyme induction is relevant to drug therapy because:

- Clinically important drug–drug (and drug–herb[24]) *interactions* may result, for example, in failure of oral contraceptives, loss of anticoagulant control, failure of cytotoxic chemotherapy.
- *Disease* may result. Antiepilepsy drugs accelerate the breakdown of dietary and endogenously formed vitamin D, producing an inactive metabolite – in effect a vitamin D deficiency state, which can result in osteomalacia. The accompanying hypocalcaemia can increase the tendency to fits and a convulsion may lead to fracture of the demineralised bones.
- *Tolerance* to drug therapy may result in and provide an explanation for suboptimal treatment, e.g. with an antiepilepsy drug.
- *Variability* in response to drugs is increased. Enzyme induction caused by heavy alcohol drinking or heavy smoking may be an unrecognised cause for failure of an individual to achieve the expected response to a normal dose of a drug, e.g. warfarin, theophylline.
- *Drug toxicity* may occur. A patient who becomes enzyme induced by taking rifampicin is more likely to develop liver toxicity after paracetamol overdose by increased production of a hepatotoxic metabolite. (Such a patient will also present with a deceptively low plasma concentration of paracetamol due to accelerated metabolism; see p. 258).

ENZYME INHIBITION

The consequences of inhibiting drug metabolism can be more profound and more selective than enzyme induction because the outcome is prolongation of action of a drug or metabolite. Consequently, enzyme inhibition offers more scope for therapy (Table 7.4).

Enzyme inhibition by drugs is also the basis of a number of clinically important drug interactions (see p. 112).

ELIMINATION

The body eliminates drugs following their part or complete conversion to water-soluble metabolites

---

[24]Tirona R G, Bailey D G 2006 Herbal product–drug interactions mediated by induction. British Journal of Clinical Pharmacology 61:677–681.

Table 7.4 Some drugs that act by enzyme inhibition

Drug	Enzyme inhibited	In treatment of
acetazolamide	carbonic anhydrase	glaucoma
allopurinol	xanthine oxidase	gout
benserazide	DOPA decarboxylase	Parkinson's disease
disulfiram	aldehyde dehydrogenase	alcoholism
enalapril	angiotensin converting enzyme	hypertension, cardiac failure
moclobemide	monoamine oxidase, A type	depression
non-steroidal anti-inflammatory drugs	cyclo-oxygenase	pain, inflammation
selegiline	monoamine oxidase, B type	Parkinson's disease

or, in some cases, without their being metabolised. To avoid repetition the following account refers to drug whereas the processes deal with both drug and metabolites.

RENAL ELIMINATION

The following mechanisms are involved.

Glomerular filtration. The rate at which a drug enters the glomerular filtrate depends on the concentration of free drug in plasma water and on its molecular weight. Substances having a molecular weight in excess of 50 000 do not cross into the glomerular filtrate, whereas those of molecular weight less than 10 000 (which includes almost all drugs)[25] pass easily through the pores of the glomerular membrane.

Renal tubular transport. Uptake and efflux transporters in proximal renal tubule cells transfer organic anions and cations between the plasma and the tubular fluid (see p. 97).

Renal tubular diffusion. The glomerular filtrate contains drug at the same concentration as it is free in the plasma, but the fluid is concentrated progressively as it flows down the nephron so that a gradient develops, drug in the tubular fluid becoming more concentrated than in the blood perfusing the nephron. As the tubular epithelium has the properties of a lipid membrane, the extent to which a drug diffuses back into the blood will depend on its lipid solubility, i.e. on its pK_a in the case of an electrolyte, and on the pH of tubular fluid. If the fluid becomes more alkaline, an acidic drug ionises, becomes less lipid soluble and its reabsorption diminishes, but

a basic drug becomes un-ionised (and therefore more lipid soluble) and its reabsorption increases. Manipulation of urine pH gains useful expression with sodium bicarbonate given to alkalinise the urine for salicylate overdose.

FAECAL ELIMINATION

When any drug, intended for systemic effect, is taken by mouth, a proportion may remain in the bowel and be excreted in the faeces. Some drugs are intended not be absorbed from the gut, as an objective of therapy, e.g. neomycin. The cells of the intestinal epithelium contain several carrier-mediated transporters that control the absorption of drugs. The efflux transporter MDR1, for example, drives drug from the enterocyte into the gut lumen, limiting its bioavailability (see p. 89). Drug in the blood may also diffuse passively into the gut lumen, depending on its pK_a and the pH difference between blood and gut contents. The effectiveness of activated charcoal by mouth for drug overdose depends partly on its adsorption of such diffused drug, and subsequent eliminated in the faeces (see p. 130).

Biliary excretion. Transporters regulate the uptake of organic cations and anions from portal blood to hepatocyte, and thence to the bile (see p. 97). The bile canaliculi tend to reabsorb small molecules and in general, only compounds having a molecular weight greater than 300 pass into bile. (See also Enterohepatic circulation, p. 89.)

PULMONARY ELIMINATION

The lungs are the main route of elimination (and of uptake) of volatile anaesthetics. Apart from this, they play only a trivial role in drug elimination. The route, however, acquires notable medicolegal

---

[25]Most drugs have a molecular weight of less than 1000.

significance when ethanol concentration is measured in the air expired by vehicle drivers involved in road traffic accidents (via the breathalyser).

CLEARANCE

Elimination of a drug from the plasma is quantified in terms of its clearance. The term has the same meaning as the familiar renal creatinine clearance, which is a measure of removal of endogenous creatinine from the plasma. Clearance values can provide useful information about the biological fate of a drug. There are pharmacokinetic methods for calculating *total body* and *renal* clearance, and the difference between these represents *hepatic* clearance. The renal clearance of a drug eliminated only by filtration by the kidney obviously cannot exceed the glomerular filtration rate (adult male 124 mL/min, female 109 mL/min). If a drug has a renal clearance in excess of this, then the kidney tubules must actively secrete it, e.g. benzylpenicillin (renal clearance 480 mL/min).

BREAST MILK

Most drugs that are present in a mother's plasma appear to some extent in her milk, although the amounts are so small that loss of drug in milk is of no significance as a mechanism of elimination.[26] Even small amounts, however, may sometimes be of significance for the suckling child, whose drug metabolic and eliminating mechanisms are immature.

Whilst most drugs taken by the mother pose no hazard to the child, exceptions to this observation occur because some drugs are inherently toxic, or transfer to milk in significant amounts, or there is a record of adverse effects, as below.

DRUGS AND BREAST FEEDING[27]

- *Alimentary tract.* Sulfasalazine may cause adverse effects and mesalazine appears preferable.
- *Anti-asthma.* The neonate eliminates theophylline and diprophylline slowly; observe the infant for irritability or disturbed sleep.
- *Anticancer.* Regard as unsafe because of inherent toxicity.

---

[26]But after mercury poisoning breast milk is a major route of elimination.
[27]Bennett P N (ed.) 1996 Drugs and human lactation. Elsevier, Amsterdam.

- *Antidepressants.* Avoid doxepin, a metabolite of which may cause respiratory depression.
- *Anti-arrhythmics (cardiac).* Amiodarone is present in high and disopyramide in moderate amounts.
- *Antiepilepsy.* General note of caution: observe the infant for sedation and poor suckling. Primidone, ethosuximide and phenobarbital are present in milk in high amounts; phenytoin and sodium valproate less so.
- *Anti-inflammatory.* Regard aspirin (salicylates) as unsafe (possible association with Reye's syndrome).
- *Antimicrobials.* Metronidazole is present in milk in moderate amounts; avoid prolonged exposure. Avoid nalidixic acid and nitrofurantoin where glucose-6-phosphate dehydrogenase deficiency is prevalent. Avoid clindamycin, dapsone, lincomycin, sulphonamides. Regard chloramphenicol as unsafe.
- *Antipsychotics.* Phenothiazines, butyrophenones and thioxanthenes are best avoided unless the indications are compelling: amounts in milk are small but animal studies suggest adverse effects on the developing nervous system. In particular, moderate amounts of sulpiride enter milk. Avoid lithium if possible.
- *Anxiolytics and sedatives.* Benzodiazepines are safe if use is brief but prolonged use may cause somnolence or poor suckling.
- *β-Adrenoceptor blockers.* Neonatal hypoglycaemia may occur. Sotalol and atenolol are present in the highest amounts in this group.
- *Hormones.* Oestrogens, progestogens and androgens suppress lactation in high dose. Oestrogen–progestogen oral contraceptives are present in amounts too small to be harmful, but may suppress lactation if it is not well established.
- *Miscellaneous.* Bromocriptine suppresses lactation. Caffeine may cause infant irritability in high doses.

DRUG DOSAGE

Drug dosage can be of five main kinds.

Fixed dose. The effect that is desired can be obtained at well below the toxic dose (many mydriatics, analgesics, oral contraceptives, antimicrobials) and enough drug can be given to render individual variation clinically insignificant.

Variable dose – with crude adjustments. Here fine adjustments make comparatively insignificant differences and the therapeutic endpoint may be hard to measure (depression, anxiety), may change only slowly (thyrotoxicosis), or may vary because of pathophysiological factors (analgesics, adrenal corticosteroids for suppressing disease).

Variable dose – with fine adjustments. Here a vital function (blood pressure, blood sugar level), which often changes rapidly in response to dose changes and can easily be measured repeatedly, provides the endpoint. Adjustment of dose must be accurate. Adrenocortical *replacement* therapy falls into this group, whereas adrenocortical *pharmacotherapy* falls into the group above.

Maximum tolerated dose is used when the ideal therapeutic effect cannot be achieved because of the occurrence of unwanted effects (anticancer drugs; some antimicrobials). The usual way of finding this is to increase the dose until unwanted effects begin to appear and then to reduce it slightly, or to monitor the plasma concentration.

Minimum tolerated dose. This concept is less common than the one above, but it applies to long-term adrenocortical steroid therapy against inflammatory or immunological conditions, e.g. in asthma and some cases of rheumatoid arthritis, when the dose that provides symptomatic relief may be so high that serious adverse effects are inevitable if it is continued indefinitely. The compromise is incomplete relief on the grounds of safety. This can be difficult to achieve.

DOSING SCHEDULES

Dosing schedules are simply schemes aimed at achieving a desired effect whilst avoiding toxicity. The following discussion assumes that drug effect relates closely to plasma concentration, which in turn relates closely to the amount of drug in the body. The objectives of a dosing regimen where continuing effect is required are:

To specify an initial dose that attains the desired effect rapidly without causing toxicity. Often the dose that is capable of initiating drug effect is the same as that which maintains it. On repeated dosing however, it takes $5 \times t_{1/2}$ periods to reach steady-state concentration in the plasma and this lapse of time may be undesirable. The effect may be achieved earlier by giving an initial dose that is larger than the maintenance dose; the initial dose is then called the *priming* or *loading* dose, i.e. the dose that will acheive a therapeutic effect in an individual whose body does not already contain the drug.

To specify a maintenance dose: amount and frequency. Intuitively, the maintenance dose might be half of the initial/priming dose at intervals equal to its plasma $t_{1/2}$, for this is the time by which the plasma concentration that achieves the desired effect declines by half. Whether or not this approach is satisfactory or practicable, however, depends very much on the $t_{1/2}$ itself, as is illustrated by the following cases:

1. *Half-life 6–12 h.* In this instance, replacing half the initial dose at intervals equal to the $t_{1/2}$ can indeed be a satisfactory solution because dosing every 6–12 h is acceptable.
2. *Half-life greater than 24 h.* With once-daily dosing (which is desirable for compliance), giving half the priming dose every day means that more drug is entering the body than is leaving it each day, and the drug will accumulate to give unwanted effects. The solution is to replace only the amount of drug that leaves the body in 24 h, calculated from the inital dose, dose interval, and $t_{1/2}$.
3. *Half-life less than 3 h.* Dosing at intervals equal to the $t_{1/2}$ would be so frequent as to be unacceptable. The answer is to use continuous intravenous infusion if the $t_{1/2}$ is very short, e.g. dopamine $t_{1/2}$ 2 min (steady-state plasma concentration will be reached in $5 \times t_{1/2} = 10$ min), or, if the $t_{1/2}$ is longer, e.g. lidocaine ($t_{1/2}$ 90 min), to use a priming dose as an intravenous bolus followed by a constant intravenous infusion. Intermittent administration of a drug with short $t_{1/2}$ is nevertheless reasonable provided large fluctuations in plasma concentration are acceptable, i.e. that the drug has a large therapeutic index. Benzylpenicillin has a $t_{1/2}$ of 30 min but is effective in a 6-hourly regimen because the drug is so non-toxic that it is possible safely to give a dose that achieves

a plasma concentration many times in excess of the minimum inhibitory concentration for sensitive organisms.

DOSE CALCULATION BY BODY-WEIGHT AND SURFACE AREA

A uniform, fixed drug dose is likely to be ineffective or toxic in several circumstances, e.g. cytotoxic chemotherapy, aminoglycoside antibiotics. It is usual then to calculate the dose according to body-weight. Adjustment according to body surface area is also used and may be more appropriate, for this correlates better with many physiological phenomena, e.g. metabolic rate.

The relationship between body surface area and weight is curvilinear, but a reasonable approximation is that a 70-kg human has a body surface area of $1.8 \, m^2$. A combination of body-weight and height gives a more precise value for surface area (obtained from standard nomograms) and other more sophisticated methods.[28]

The issue takes on special significance for children, if the only dose known is that for the adult; adjustment is then commonly made by body-weight, or body surface area, amongst other factors (see p. 109).

PROLONGATION OF DRUG ACTION

Giving a larger dose is the most obvious way to prolong a drug action but this is not always feasible, and other mechanisms are used:

- *Vasoconstriction* will reduce local blood flow so that distribution of drug away from an injection site is retarded, e.g. combination with epinephrine (adrenaline) prolongs local anaesthetic action.
- *Slowing of metabolism* may usefully extend drug action, as when a dopa decarboxylase inhibitor, e.g. carbidopa, is combined with levodopa (as co-careldopa) for parkinsonism.
- *Delayed excretion* is seldom practicable, the only important example being the use of probenecid to block renal tubular excretion of penicillin for single dose treatment of gonorrhoea.

- *Altered molecular structure* can prolong effect, e.g. the various benzodiazepines.
- *Pharmaceutical formulation*. Manipulating the form in which a drug is presented by modified-release[29] systems can achieve the objective of an even as well as a prolonged effect.

Sustained-release (oral) preparations can reduce the frequency of medication to once a day, and compliance becomes easier for the patient. The elderly can now receive most long-term medication as a single morning dose. In addition sustained-release preparations may avoid bowel toxicity due to high local concentrations, e.g. ulceration of the small intestine with potassium chloride tablets, and may also avoid the toxic peak plasma concentrations that can occur when dissolution of the formulation, and so absorption of the drug, is rapid. Some sustained-release formulations also contain an immediate-release component to provide rapid, as well as sustained, effect.

Depot (injectable) preparations are more reliable because the environment in which they are deposited is more constant than can ever be the case in the alimentary tract, and medication can be given at longer intervals, even weeks. In general, such preparations are pharmaceutical variants, e.g. microcrystals, or the original drug in oil, wax, gelatin or synthetic media. They include phenothiazine neuroleptics, the various insulins and penicillins, preparations of vasopressin, and medroxyprogesterone (intramusclar, subcutaneous). Tablets of hormones can be implanted subcutaneously. The advantages of infrequent administration and better patient compliance in a variety of situations are obvious.

REDUCTION OF ABSORPTION TIME

A soluble salt of the drug may be effective by being rapidly absorbed from the site of administration. In the case of subcutaneous or intramusclar injections, the same objective may be obtained with hyaluronidase, an enzyme that depolymerises hyaluronic acid,

---

[28]For example, Livingston E H, Lee S 2001 Body surface area prediction in normal-weight and obese patients. American Journal of Physiology Endocrinology and Metabolism 281:586–591.

[29]The term *modified* covers several drug delivery systems. *Delayed release*: available other than immediately after administration (mesalazine in the colon); *sustained release*: slow release as governed by the delivery system (iron, potassium); *controlled release*: at a constant rate to maintain unvarying plasma concentration (nitrate, hormone replacement therapy).

a constituent of connective tissue that prevents the spread of foreign substances, e.g. bacteria, drugs. Hyaluronidase combined with an intramusclar injection, e.g. a local anaesthetic, or a subcutaneous infusion leads to increased permeation with more rapid absorption. Hyaluronidase also promotes resorption of tissue accumulation of blood and fluid.

FIXED-DOSE DRUG COMBINATIONS

This section refers to combinations of drugs in a single pharmaceutical formulation. It does not mean concomitant drug therapy, e.g. in infections, hypertension and in cancer, when several drugs are given separately. Therapeutic aims should be clear. Combinations are logical if there is good reason to consider that the patient needs all the drugs in the formulation and that the doses are appropriate and will not need adjustment separately. Fixed-dose drug combinations are appropriate for:

- *Convenience*, with improved patient compliance, is appropriate with two drugs used at constant dose, long term, for an asymptomatic condition, e.g. a thiazide plus an ACE inhibitor in mild or moderate hypertension.
- *Enhanced effect*. Single-drug treatment of tuberculosis leads to the emergence of resistant mycobacteria and is prevented or delayed by using two or more drugs simultaneously. Combining isoniazid with rifampicin (Rifinah, Rimactazid) ensures that single drug treament cannot occur; treatment has to be two drugs or no drug at all. An oestrogen and progestogen combination provides effective oral contraception, for the same reason.
- *Minimisation of unwanted effects*. Levodopa combined with benserazide (Madopar) or with carbidopa (Sinemet) slows its metabolism outside the CNS so that smaller amounts of levodopa can be used, reducing its adverse effects.

CHRONIC PHARMACOLOGY

The pharmacodynamics and pharmacokinetics of many drugs differ according to whether their use is in a single dose, or over a brief period (acute pharmacology), or long term (chronic pharmacology). An increasing proportion of the population take drugs continuously for large portions of their lives

as tolerable suppressive and prophylactic remedies for chronic or recurrent conditions are developed; e.g. for arterial hypertension, diabetes mellitus, mental diseases, epilepsies. In general, the dangers of a drug therapy are not markedly greater if therapy lasts for years rather than months, but long-term treatment can introduce significant hazard into patients' lives unless management is skilful.

INTERFERENCE WITH SELF-REGULATING SYSTEMS

When self-regulating physiological systems (generally controlled by negative feedback systems, e.g. endocrine, cardiovascular) are subject to interference, their control mechanisms respond to minimise the effects of the interference and to restore the previous steady state or rhythm; this is *homeostasis*. The previous state may be a normal function, e.g. ovulation (a rare example of a positive feedback mechanism), or an abnormal function, e.g. high blood pressure. If the body successfully restores the previous steady state or rhythm then the subject has become tolerant to the drug, i.e. needs a higher dose to produce the desired previous effect.

In the case of hormonal contraceptives, persistence of suppression of ovulation occurs and is desired, but persistence of other effects, e.g. on blood coagulation and metabolism, is not desired.

In the case of arterial hypertension, tolerance to a single drug commonly occurs, e.g. reduction of peripheral resistance by a vasodilator is compensated by an increase in blood volume that restores the blood pressure; this is why a diuretic is commonly used together with a vasodilator in therapy.

Feedback systems. The endocrine system serves fluctuating body needs. Glands are therefore capable either of increasing or decreasing their output by means of negative (usually) feedback systems. An administered hormone or hormone analogue activates the receptors of the feedback system so that high doses cause suppression of natural production of the hormone. On withdrawal of the administered hormone, restoration of the normal control mechanism takes time, e.g. the hypothalamic–pituitary–adrenal cortex system can take months to recover full sensitivity, and sudden withdrawal of administered corticosteroid can result in an acute deficiency state that may be life endangering.

Regulation of receptors. The number (density) of receptors on cells (for hormones, autacoids or local hormones, and drugs), the number occupied (receptor occupancy) and the capacity of the receptor to respond (affinity, efficacy) can change in reponse to the concentration of the specific binding molecule or ligand,[30] whether this be agonist or antagonist (blocker). The effects always tend to restore cell function to its normal or usual state. Prolonged high concentrations of agonist (whether administered as a drug or over-produced in the body by a tumour) cause a reduction in the number of receptors available for activation (*down-regulation*); changes in receptor occupancy and affinity and the prolonged occupation of receptors antagonists lead to an increase in the number of receptors (*up-regulation*). At least some of this may be achieved by receptors moving inside the cell and out again (internalisation and externalisation).

Down-regulation and the accompanying receptor changes may explain the 'on–off' phenomenon in Parkinson's disease (see p. 384) and the action of luteinising hormone releasing hormone (LHRH) super-agonists in reducing follicle stimulating hormone (FSH) concentrations for treating endocrine-sensitive prostate cancer.

Up-regulation. The occasional exacerbation of ischaemic cardiac disease on sudden withdrawal of a β-adrenoceptor blocker may be explained by up-regulation during its administration, so that, on withdrawal, an above-normal number of receptors suddenly becomes accessible to the normal chemotransmitter, i.e. noradrenaline (norepinephrine).

Up-regulation with rebound sympathomimetic effects may be innocuous to a moderately healthy cardiovascular system, but the increased oxygen demand of these effects can have serious consequences where ischaemic disease is present and increased oxygen need cannot be met (angina pectoris, arrhythmia, myocardial infarction). Unmasking of a disease process that has worsened during prolonged suppressive use of the drug, i.e. resurgence, may also contribute to such exacerbations.

The rebound phenomenon is plainly a potential hazard and the use of a β-adrenoceptor blocker in the presence of ischaemic heart disease would be safer if rebound could be eliminated. β-Adrenoceptor blockers that are not pure antagonists but have some agonist (sympathomimetic ischaemic) activity, i.e. partial agonists, may prevent the generation of additional adrenoceptors (up-regulation). Indeed there is evidence that rebound is less or is absent with pindolol, a partial agonist β-adrenoceptor blocker.

Sometimes a distinction is made between *rebound* (recurrence at intensified degree of the symptoms for which the drug was given) and *withdrawal syndrome* (appearance of new additional symptoms). The distinction is quantitative and does not imply different mechanisms.

Rebound and withdrawal phenomena occur erratically. In general, they are more likely with drugs having a short $t_{1/2}$ (abrupt drop in plasma concentration) and pure agonist or antagonist action. They are less likely to occur with drugs having a long $t_{1/2}$ and (probably) with those having a mixed agonist–antagonist (partial agonist) action on receptors.

ABRUPT WITHDRAWAL

Clinically important consequences occur, and might occur for a variety of reasons, e.g. a patient interrupting drug therapy to undergo surgery. The following are examples:

- *Cardiovascular system*: β-adrenoceptor blockers, antihypertensives (especially clonidine).
- *Nervous system*: all depressants (hypnotics, sedatives, alcohol, opioids), antiepileptics, antiparkinsonian agents, tricyclic antidepressants.
- *Endocrine system*: adrenal corticosteroids.
- *Immune inflammation*: adrenal corticosteroids.

Resurgence of chronic disease, which has progressed in severity although its consequences have been wholly or partly suppressed, i.e. a catching-up phenomenon, is a possible outcome of discontinuing effective therapy, e.g. levodopa in Parkinson's disease. Corticosteroid withdrawal in autoimmune disease may cause both resurgence and rebound.

Drug discontinuation syndromes, i.e. rebound, withdrawal and resurgence (defined above) are phenomena that are to be expected. The exact mechanisms may remain obscure but clinicians have no reason to be surprised when they occur, and in the case of rebound they may wish to use gradual withdrawal wherever drugs are used to modify complex self-adjusting systems, and to suppress (without cure) chronic diseases.

[30]Latin: *ligare* = to bind.

OTHER ASPECTS OF CHRONIC DRUG USE

Metabolic changes over a long period may induce disease, e.g. thiazide diuretics (diabetes mellitus), adrenocortical hormones (osteoporosis), phenytoin (osteomalacia). Drugs may also enhance their own metabolism, and that of other drugs (enzyme induction).

Specific cell injury or cell functional disorder occur with individual drugs or drug classes, e.g. tardive dyskinesia (dopamine receptor blockers), retinal damage (chloroquine, phenothiazines), retroperitoneal fibrosis (methysergide), non-steroidal anti-inflammatory drugs (nephropathy). Cancer may occur, e.g. with oestrogens (endometrium) and with immunosuppressive (anticancer) drugs.

Drug holidays. The term means the deliberate interruption of long-term therapy in order to restore sensitivity (which has been lost) or to reduce the risk of toxicity. Plainly, the need for holidays is a substantial disadvantage for any drug. Patients sometimes initiate their own drug holidays (see Patient compliance, concordance p. 22).

Dangers of intercurrent illness are particularly notable with anticoagulants, adrenal corticosteroids and immunosuppressives.

Dangers of interactions with other drugs, herbs or food: see index for individual drugs.

CONCLUSIONS

Drugs not only induce their known listed primary actions, but:

- evoke compensatory responses in the complex interrelated physiological systems they perturb, and these systems need time to recover on withdrawal of the drug (gradual withdrawal is sometimes mandatory and never harmful)
- induce metabolic changes that may be trivial in the short term, but serious if they persist for a long time
- may produce localised effects in specially susceptible tissues and induce serious cell damage or malfunction
- increase susceptibility to intercurrent illness and to interaction with other drugs that may be taken for new indications.

That such consequences occur with prolonged drug use need evoke no surprise. But a knowledge of physiology, pathology and pharmacology, combined with awareness that the unexpected can occur, will allow patients who require long-term therapy may be managed safely, or at least with minimum risk of harm, and enabled to live happy lives.

INDIVIDUAL OR BIOLOGICAL VARIATION

PRESCRIBING FOR SPECIAL RISK GROUPS

That individuals respond differently to drugs, both from time to time and from other individuals, is a matter of everyday experience. Doctors need to accommodate for individual variation, for it may explain both adverse response to a drug and failure of therapy. Sometimes there are obvious physical characteristics such as age, race (genetics) or disease that warn the prescriber to adjust drug dose, but there are no external features that signify, e.g. pseudocholinesterase deficiency, which causes prolonged paralysis after suxamethonium. An understanding of the reasons for individual variation in response to drugs is relevant to all who prescribe. Both pharmacodynamic and pharmacokinetic effects are involved, and the issues fall in two general categories: inherited influences and environmental and host influences.

INHERITED INFLUENCES: PHARMACOGENETICS

Human beings are 99.9% genetically identical. The differences that reside in the remaining 0.1% determine our experience of health and disease, and our reactions to the environment, including drugs. Think how individuals in a population might respond to a fixed dose of a drug: some would show less than the usual response, most would show the usual response and some would show more than the usual response. This type of variation is described as *continuous* and, presented graphically, the result would appear as a normal or gaussian (bell shaped) distribution curve, similar to the type of curve that describes the distribution of height, weight or metabolic rate in a population. The curve is the result of a multitude of factors, some genetic (multiple genes) and some environmental, that contribute collectively to the response of the individual to the drug; they include race, sex, diet, weight, environmental and body temperature, circadian rhythm, pharmacokinetics and receptor density, but no single factor has a predominant effect.

Less commonly, variation is *discontinuous* when some people respond disparately from the majority, a condition that occurs most commonly when a single gene controls the response. These differences arise because of various combinations of alleles[31] at the same chromosome locus, and result is a *genetic polymorphism*.[32]

The P450 enzymes (see p. 96) provide an illustration. All of the genes that encode for families 1–3 are polymorphic and their capacity to metabolise drugs depends on the functional importance and frequency of the variant alleles, which often differ with ethnic group and:

'In general, four phenotypes can be identified: *poor metabolisers* who lack the functional enzyme, *intermediate metabolisers*, who are heterozygous for one deficient allele or carry two alleles that cause reduced activity, *extensive metabolisers* who have two normal alleles, and *ultra-rapid metabolisers* who have multiple gene copies, a trait that is dominantly inherited.'[33]

Clearly, any single dose of a drug used within the general population can elicit a variety of responses among individuals, provided the P450 system is significantly involved in terminating its activity.

Pharmacogenetics is the study of genetically determined variation in response to drugs. These commonly have a biochemical basis. Single genes encode for particular enzymes, and variant alleles produce enzymes of differing metabolic capacity that induce increased, decreased and bizarre (idiosyncratic) responses to drugs, i.e. *pharmacogenetic polymorphisms*. But variation also occurs from genes that encode for other proteins that influence drug responses, e.g. the drug transporters, which profoundly influence drug disposition (see p. 97), and the targets of drug action, the receptors; new polymorphisms of both these entities are recognised (see below).

As the components of the human genome and their functions are uncovered, the responses to drugs of particular molecular structures become predictable in individuals. New dimensions offered by pharmacogenetics, allied with pharmacogenomics and pharmacoproteomics (see p. 32), allow the prospect of identifying individuals who are susceptible to unwanted effects, i.e. part of a 'discontinuous variation', so to maximise benefit and minimise risk. The advantage is economic as well as clinical, for targeting of drugs only to those most likely to benefit and avoiding people who will not to respond or experience adverse effects has important implications for the use of health resources.[34]

A few illustrative examples of pharmacological polymorphisms are set out below.[35]

Psychosis. Many antipsychotic drugs are substrates for CYP 2D6. Poor metabolisers[36] experienced more

---

[31]Any one of a series of two or more different genes that may occupy the same locus on a specific chromosome. As autosomal chromosomes are paired, each autosomal gene is represented twice in normal somatic cells. If the same allele occupies both units of the locus, the individual or cell is homozygous for this allele. If the alleles are different, the individual or cell is heterozygous for both alleles (*Steadman's Medical Dictionary*).

[32]The occurrence in the same population of multiple discrete allelic states of which at least two have high frequency (conventionally of 1% or more) (*Steadman's Medical Dictionary*).

[33]Ingelman-Sundberg M 2004 Pharmacogenetics of cytochrome P450 and its application in drug therapy: the past, present and future. Trends in Pharmacological Sciences 25:193–200.

[34]O'Shaughnessy K M 2006 HapMap, pharmacogenomics, and the goal of personalised prescribing. British Journal of Clinical Pharmacology 61:783–786.

[35]Data from various sources, including the review by M Ingelman-Sundberg (footnote 33).

[36]The poor oxidiser state was first revealed in the laboratory of R L Smith, Professor of Biochemical Pharmacology, St Mary's Hospital Medical School, London, who was investigating the variable dose requirements of patients receiving the two antihypertensive drugs debrisoquine and bethanidine. He writes: 'I took 40 mg of debrisoquine sulphate; within two hours my blood pressure crashed to 70/50 mmHg and I was unable to stand for four hours due to incapacitating postural hypotension … it was two days until the blood pressure returned to normal. Analysis of my urine revealed that nearly all the dose was excreted as unchanged drug, whereas other subjects who showed little if any cardiovascular response to the same dose of debrisoquine, coverted it to the 4-hydroxy metabolite. However, the drama of the clinical response to a single dose of debrisoquine catalysed a search for its explanation and culminated in the uncovering of the first example of a genetic polymorphism of drug oxidation'.

adverse effects (parkinsonism, sedation) than did ultra-rapid metabolisers (see also Chapter 19).

Depression. Tricyclic antidepressants depend almost entirely on metabolism by CYP 2D6 to terminate their action. Ultra-rapid metabolisers needed a 10-fold larger dose of nortriptyline than did poor metabolisers to achieve the same plasma concentration. Correspondingly, failure to respond to nortriptyline is 10-fold more common in ultra-rapid than in poor metabolisers (see also Chapter 19 p. 334).

Peptic ulcer. Plasma concentrations of the proton pump inhibitor, omeprazole, are very dependent on the patient's CYP 2C19 phenotype. Ulcer cure rates reflect differences in capacity to metabolise omeprazole 20 mg/day, and were low in extensive, intermediate in intermediate and complete in poor metabolisers. Higher doses provided effective therapy for all groups.

Cancer. The anti-oestrogen, tamoxifen, is metabolised to its active form by CYP 2D6. Poor metabolisers with breast cancer experience a lesser therapeutic response than other patients.

Pseudocholinesterase deficiency. Plasma pseudocholinesterase terminates the neuromuscular blocking action of suxamethonium. 'True' cholinesterase (acetylcholinesterase) hydrolyses acetylcholine released by nerve endings, whereas various tissues and plasma contain other non-specific, hence 'pseudo', esterases. Affected individuals form so little plasma pseudocholinesterase that metabolism of suxamethonium is seriously reduced.

The deficiency characteristically declares itself when a patient fails to breathe spontaneously after surgical anaesthesia and requires assisted ventilation for hours. It is prudent to check relatives of an affected individual. The prevalence of pseudocholinesterase deficiency in the UK population is about 1 in 2500.

Resistance to suxamethonium. This rare condition is characterised by increased pseudocholinesterase activity and failure of normal doses of suxamethonium to cause muscular relaxation.

Acetylation is an important route of metabolism for many drugs that possess an amide ($-NH_2$) group. Most individuals are either rapid or slow acetylators

but the proportion varies greatly between races, e.g. some 90% of Japanese are rapid acetylators whereas in Western populations the proportion is 50% or less. Sulfasalazine (salicylazosulfapyridine) (used for rheumatoid arthritis) causes adverse effects probably because of slow acetylation of the sulfapyridine component. Dapsone appears to cause more red cell haemolysis in slow acetylators; rapid acetylators may need higher doses to control dermatitis herpetiformis and leprosy.

Glucose-6-phosphate dehydrogenase (G6PD) deficiency. G6PD activity is important to the integrity of the red blood cell. Individuals who are G6PD deficient may suffer from acute haemolysis following exposure to certain oxidant substances, including drugs.

The condition is common in African, Mediterranean, Middle Eastern and South East Asian races and in their descendants, and throughout the world affects some 100 million people. As deficiency may result from inheritance of any one of numerous variants of G6PD, affected individuals exhibit differing susceptibility to haemolysis, i.e. a substance that affects one G6PD-deficient subject adversely may be harmless in another. It is usually dose related. The following guidelines apply:[37]

- Drugs that carry a *definite* risk of haemolysis in most G6PD-deficient subjects include: dapsone (and other sulphones), methylene blue, niridazole, nitrofurantoin, pamaquin, primaquine, quinolone antimicrobials, some sulphonamides.
- Drugs that carry a *possible* risk of haemolysis in some G6PD-deficient subjects include: aspirin (when dosage exceeds 1 g/day), menadione, probenecid, quinidine, chloroquine and quinine (both are acceptable in acute malaria) rasburicase.

Affected individuals are also found to be susceptible to exposure to nitrates, anilines and naphthalenes (found in moth-balls). Some individuals, particularly children, experience haemolysis after eating the raw broad bean, *Vicia faba*, and hence the term 'favism'.[38]

---

[37]Data based on *British National Formulary,* 2007.

[38]A danger described by the Greek philosopher Pythagoras (570–495 BC) in perhaps the first recognition of an inter-individual difference in response to a xenobiotic (Nebert D W 1999 Clinical Genetics 56:345–347).

Anticoagulation with coumarins. Variant alleles of CYP 2C9 lead to polymorphisms that result in slow metabolism (and risk of toxicity) of warfarin (also tolbutamide and losartan).

By contrast, a rare variant of the enzyme that converts vitamin K to its reduced and active form (normally inhibited by coumarins) results in patients requiring 20 times or more of the usual dose to obtain an adequate response to warfarin. A similar condition also occurs in rats and has practical importance as warfarin, a coumarin, is used as a rat poison (rats with the gene are dubbed 'super-rats' by the mass media).

Anticoagulation with heparin. Patients with congenital deficiency of antithrombin (an inhibitor of activated coagulation proteases) require large doses of heparin for anticoagulant effect. The action of heparin depends on the presence of antithrombin in the plasma.

Transporter polymorphisms[37] (with resulting effects) include those of: the serotonin (5-hydroxytriptamine) transporter (antidepressant response); sodium or potassium transporters (cardiac arrhythmias from drug-induced long-QTc syndrome; MDR1 (P-glycoprotein) (numerous drugs).

Elsewhere in this book see: Malignant hyperthermia (p. 328), Porphyria (p. 120), Alcohol (p. 152). Bacterial resistance to drugs is genetically determined and is of great clinical importance.

ENVIRONMENTAL AND HOST INFLUENCES

A multitude of factors related to both individuals and their environment contribute to differences in drug response. Some of the more relevant influences are:

AGE

The neonate, infant and child[39]

Young human beings differ greatly from adults, not merely in size but also in the proportions and constituents of their bodies and the functioning of their physiological systems. These differences influence the way the body handles and responds to drugs:

- Rectal absorption is efficient with an appropriate formulation, e.g. of diazepam and theophyllines; this route may be preferred with an uncooperative infant.
- The intramuscular or subcutaneous routes tend to give unpredictable plasma concentrations, e.g. of digoxin or gentamicin, because of the relatively low proportion of skeletal muscle and fat. Intravenous administration is preferred in the seriously ill newborn.
- Drugs or other substances that come in contact with the skin are readily absorbed as the skin is well hydrated and the stratum corneum is thin; overdose toxicity may result, e.g. with hexachlorophene used in dusting powders and emulsions to prevent infection.

An understandable reluctance to test drugs extensively in children means that reliable information is often lacking. Many drugs do not have a licence to be used for children, and their prescription must be 'off licence', a practice that is recognised as necessary, if not actually promoted, by the UK drug regulatory authorities.[40]

Distribution. Total body water in the neonate amounts to 80%, compared with 65% of bodyweight in older children. Consequently:

- Weight-related priming doses of aminoglycosides, aminophylline, digoxin and furosemide need to be larger for neonates than for older children.
- Less extensive binding of drugs to plasma proteins is generally without clinical importance but there is a risk of kernicterus in the jaundiced neonate following displacement of bilirubin from protein binding sites by vitamin K, X-ray contrast media or indometacin.

Metabolism. Drug-inactivating enzyme systems are present at birth but are functionally immature (particularly in the preterm baby), especially for oxidation and conjugation with glucuronic acid. Inadequate conjugation and thus inactivation of chloramphenicol

---

[39]A neonate is under 1 month and an infant is 1–12 months of age.

[40]Stephenson T 2006 The medicines for children agenda in the UK. British Journal of Clinical Pharmacology 61:716–719.

by neonates causes the fatal 'grey' syndrome. After the initial weeks of life, because their drug metabolic capacity increases rapidly, young children may require a higher weight-related dose than adults.

Elimination. Glomerular filtration, tubular secretion and reabsorption are low in the neonate (even lower in preterm babies), reaching adult values in relation to body surface area only at 2–5 months. Drugs that the kidney excretes, e.g. aminoglycosides, penicillins, diuretics, are given in reduced dose; after about 6 months, body-weight or surface area related daily doses are the same for all ages.

Pharmacodynamic responses. There is scant information about developmental effects of interaction between drugs and receptors. Other sources suggest possible effects, e.g. thalidomide causes phocomelia only in the forming limb (see p. 62); tetracyclines stain only developing enamel; young children are particularly sensitive to liver toxicity from valproate.

Dosage in the young. No single rule or formula suffices for all cases. Computation by body-weight may overdose an obese child, for whom calculation of ideal weight from age and height is preferred. Doses based on body surface area are generally more accurate, and preferably should take into account both body-weight and height.[41] The fact that the surface area of a 70-kg adult human is $1.8\,\text{m}^2$ (see p. 102) may then be used for adjustment, as follows:

$$\text{Approximate dose} = \text{Surface area of child}(\text{m}^2)\ /1.8 \times \text{adult dose}$$

General guidance is available from formularies, e.g. the *British National Formulary*, and specialist publications.[42,43]

The elderly

The incidence of adverse drug reactions rises with age in the adult, especially after 65 years, because of:

- The increasing number of drugs that they need because they tend to have multiple diseases.
- Poor compliance with dosing regimens.
- Bodily changes of aging that require modified dosage regimens.

Absorption of drugs administered orally may be slightly slower because of reduced gastrointestinal blood flow and motility but the effect is rarely important.

Distribution reflects the following changes:

- Lean body mass is less and standard adult doses provide a greater amount of drug per kilogram.
- Body fat increases and may act as a reservoir for lipid-soluble drugs.
- Total body water is less and, in general, water-soluble drugs have a lower distribution volume. Standard doses of drugs, especially the priming doses of those that are water soluble, may thus exceed the requirement.
- Plasma albumin concentration maintains well in the healthy elderly but may fall with chronic disease, giving scope for a greater proportion of unbound (free) drug, which may be important when priming doses are given.

Metabolism reduces as liver mass and liver blood flow decline. Consequently:

- Metabolic inactivation of drugs is slower, mostly for Phase I (oxidation) reactions; the capacity for Phase II (conjugation) is better preserved.
- Drugs normally extensively eliminated in first pass through the liver appear in higher concentration in the systemic circulation and persist in it for longer. There is thus particular need initially to use lower doses of most neuroleptics, tricyclic antidepressants and cardiac antiarrhythmic agents.
- Capacity for hepatic enzyme induction appears less.

Elimination. Renal blood flow, glomerular filtration and tubular secretion decrease with age above 55 years, a decline that is not signalled by raised serum creatinine concentration because production of this metabolite is diminished by the age-associated diminution of muscle mass. Indeed, in the elderly, serum creatinine may be within the concentration range for normal young adults even when

---

[41]For example, Insley J 1996 A paediatric vade-mecum, 13th edn. Arnold, London.

[42]Neonatal and Paediatric Pharmacists Group, Royal College of Paediatrics and Child Health 2001 Pocket medicines for children. Royal College of Paediatrics and Child Health Publications, London.

[43]For practical advice, see World Health Organization 2005 Pocket book of hospital care for children. WHO, Geneva.

the creatinine clearance is 50 mL/min (compared with 127 mL/min in adult males). Particular risk of adverse effects arises with drugs that are eliminated mainly by the kidney and that have a small therapeutic ratio, e.g. aminoglycosides, chlorpropamide, digoxin, lithium.

Pharmacodynamic response may alter with age, to produce either a greater or a lesser effect than is anticipated in younger adults, for example:

- Drugs that act on the CNS appear to produce an exaggerated response in relation to that expected from the plasma concentration, and sedatives and hypnotics may have a pronounced hangover effect. These drugs are also more likely to depress respiration because of reduced vital capacity and maximum breathing capacity in the elderly.
- Response to β-adrenoceptor agonists and antagonists may attenuate in old age, possibly through reduced affinity for adrenoceptors.
- Baroreceptor sensitivity reduces leading to the potential for orthostatic hypotension with drugs that reduce blood pressure.

These pharmacokinetic and pharmacodynamic differences, together with broader issues particular to the elderly, find expression in the choice and use of drugs for this age group, as follows.

Rules of prescribing for the elderly[44]

1. Think about the necessity for drugs. Is the diagnosis correct and complete? Is the drug really necessary? Is there a better alternative?
2. Do not prescribe drugs that are not useful. Think carefully before giving an old person a drug that may have major side-effects, and consider alternatives.
3. Think about the dose. Is it appropriate to possible alterations in the patient's physiological state? Is it appropriate to the patient's renal and hepatic function at the time?
4. Think about drug formulation. Is a tablet the most appropriate form of drug or would an injection, a suppository or a syrup be better? Is the drug suitably packaged for the elderly patient, bearing in mind any disabilities?

5. Assume any new symptoms may be due to drug side-effects or, more rarely, to drug withdrawal. Rarely (if ever) treat a side-effect of one drug with another.
6. Take a careful drug history. Bear in mind the possibility of interaction with substances the patient may be taking without your knowledge, such as herbal or other non-prescribed remedies, old drugs taken from the medicine cabinet or drugs obtained from friends.
7. Use fixed combinations of drugs only when they are logical and well studied, and they either aid compliance or improve tolerance or efficacy. Few fixed combinations meet this standard.
8. When adding a new drug to the therapeutic regimen, see whether another can be withdrawn.
9. Attempt to check whether the patient's compliance is adequate, e.g. by counting remaining tablets. Has the patient (or relatives) been properly instructed?
10. Remember that stopping a drug is as important as starting it.

The old (80 + years) are particulary intolerant of neuroleptics (given for confusion) and of diuretics (given for ankle swelling that is postural and not due to heart failure), which cause adverse electrolyte changes. Both classes of drug may result in admission to hospital of semi-comatose 'senior citizens' who deserve better treatment from their juniors.

PREGNANCY

As pregnancy evolves, profound changes occur in physiology, including fluid and tissue composition.

Absorption. Despite reduced gastrointestinal motility, there appears to be no major defect in drug absorption except that slow gastric emptying delays the appearance in the plasma of orally administered drugs, especially during labour. Absorption from an intramuscular site is likely to be efficient because vasodilatation increases tissue perfusion.

Distribution. Total body water increases by up to 8 L, creating a larger space within which water-soluble drugs may distribute. Plasma albumin (normal 33–55 g/L) declines by some 10 g/L from haemodilution. While this gives scope for increased

---

[44]By permission from Caird F I (ed.) 1985 Drugs for the elderly. WHO (Europe), Copenhagen.

free concentration of drugs that normally bind to albumin, unbound drug is also available to distribute, be metabolised and excreted. With phenytoin, for example, the free (and pharmacologically active) concentration does not alter, despite the dilutional fall in the total plasma concentration.

Thus therapeutic drug monitoring interpreted by concentrations appropriate for non-pregnant women may mislead. A useful general guide during pregnancy is to maintain concentrations at the lower end of the recommended range. Body fat increases by about 4 kg and provides a reservoir for lipid-soluble drugs.

Hepatic metabolism increases, although not blood flow to the liver. There is increased clearance of drugs such as phenytoin and theophylline, whose elimination depends on liver enzyme activity. Drugs that are so rapidly metabolised that elimination depends on delivery to the liver, i.e. on hepatic blood flow, have unaltered clearance, e.g. pethidine.

Elimination. Renal plasma flow almost doubles and there is more rapid loss of renally excreted drugs, e.g. amoxicillin, the dose of which should be doubled for systemic infections (but not for urinary tract infections as penicillins are highly concentrated in the urine).

Placenta – see p. 83.

DISEASE

Pharmacokinetic changes

Absorption. Resection and reconstruction of the gut may lead to malabsorption, e.g. of iron, folic acid and fat-soluble vitamins after partial gastrectomy, and of vitamin B_{12} after ileal resection. Delayed gastric emptying and intestinal stasis during an attack of migraine interfere with drug absorption. Severe low-output cardiac failure or shock (with peripheral vaso-constriction) delays absorption from subcutaneous or intramuscular sites; reduced hepatic blood flow prolongs the presence in the plasma of drugs that are so rapidly extracted by the liver that removal depends on their rate of presentation to it, e.g. lidocaine.

Distribution. Hypoalbuminaemia from any cause, e.g. burns, malnutrition, sepsis, allows a higher proportion of free (unbound) drug in plasma. Although free drug is available for metabolism and excretion, there remains a risk of enhanced or adverse responses especially with initial doses of those that are highly protein bound, e.g. phenytoin.

Metabolism. Acute inflammatory disease of the liver (viral, alcoholic) and cirrhosis affect both the functioning of the hepatocytes and blood flow through the liver. Reduced extraction from the plasma of drugs that are normally highly cleared in first pass through the liver results in increased systemic availability of drugs such as metoprolol, labetalol and chlomethiazole. Many other drugs exhibit prolonged $t_{1/2}$ and reduced clearance in patients with chronic liver disease, e.g. diazepam, tolbutamide, rifampicin (see p. 90). Thyroid disease has the expected effects, i.e. drug metabolism accelerates in hyperthyroidism and decelerates in hypothyroidism.

Elimination. Renal disease has profound effects on the elimination and thence duration of action of drugs eliminated by the kidney (see p. 489).

Pharmacodynamic changes

- *Asthmatic attacks* can be precipitated by β-adrenoceptor blockers.
- *Malfunctioning of the respiratory centre* (raised intracranial pressure, severe pulmonary insufficiency) causes patients to be intolerant of opioids, and indeed any sedative may precipitate respiratory failure.
- *Myocardial infarction* predisposes to cardiac arrhythmia with digitalis glycosides or sympathomimetics.
- *Myasthenia gravis* is aggravated by quinine and quinidine, and myasthenics are intolerant of competitive neuromuscular blocking agents and aminoglycoside antibiotics.

FOOD

- The presence of food in the stomach, especially if it is fatty, delays gastric emptying and the absorption of certain drugs, e.g. ampicillin and rifampicin. More specifically, calcium, for instance in milk, interferes with absorption of tetracyclines and iron (by chelation).
- Substituting protein for fat or carbohydrate in the diet is associated with an increase in drug oxidation rates. Some specific dietary factors induce drug metabolising enzymes, e.g. alcohol, charcoal grilled (broiled) beef, cabbage and Brussels sprouts.

Protein malnutrition causes changes that are likely to influence pharmacokinetics, e.g. loss of body-weight, reduced hepatic metabolising capacity, hypoproteinaemia.

Citrus flavinoids in grapefruit (but not orange) juice decrease hepatic metabolism and may lead to toxicity from amiodarone, terfenadine (cardiac arrhythmia), benzodiazepines (increased sedation), ciclosporin, felodipine (reduced blood pressure).

DRUG INTERACTIONS

When a drug is administered, a response occurs; if a second drug is given and the response to the first drug is altered, a drug–drug interaction is said to have occurred.

Dramatic *unintended* interactions excite most notice but they should not distract attention from the many *intended* interactions that are the basis of rational polypharmacy, e.g. multi-drug treatment of tuberculosis, naloxone for morphine overdose.

For completeness, alterations in drug action caused by diet (above) are termed *drug–food* interactions, and those by herbs *drug–herb* interactions.[45]

CLINICAL IMPORTANCE OF DRUG INTERACTIONS

The quantity of drugs listed in any national formulary provides ample scope for possible alteration in the disposition or effect of one drug by another drug. But, in practice, *clinically important adverse drug–drug interactions* become likely with:

- Drugs that have a steep dose–response curve and a small therapeutic index (see p. 79) because small quantitative changes at the target site, e.g. receptor or enzyme, lead to substantial changes in effect, e.g. digoxin or lithium.
- Drugs that are known enzyme inducers or inhibitors (see pp. 97, 98).
- Drugs that exhibit saturable metabolism (zero-order kinetics), when small interference with kinetics may lead to large alteration of plasma concentration, e.g. phenytoin, theophylline.
- Drugs that are used long term, where precise plasma concentrations are required, e.g. oral

contraceptives, antiepilepsy drugs, cardiac antiarrhythmia drugs, lithium.

- Severely ill patients, for they may be receiving several drugs; signs of iatrogenic disease may be difficult to distinguish from those of existing disease and the patients' condition may be such that they cannot tolerate further adversity.
- Patients who have significantly impaired liver or kidney function, for these are the principal organs that terminate drug action.
- The elderly, for they tend to have multiple pathology, and may receive several drugs concurrently (see p. 109).

PHARMACOLOGICAL BASIS OF DRUG INTERACTIONS

Listings of recognised or possible adverse drug–drug interactions are now readily available in national formularies, on compact disk or as part of standard prescribing software. We provide here an overview of the pharmacological basis for wanted and unwanted, expected and unexpected effects when drug combinations are used.

Drug interactions are of two principal kinds:

- *Pharmacodynamic interaction*: both drugs act on the target site of clinical effect, exerting synergism (below) or antagonism. The drugs may act on the same or different receptors or processes, mediating similar biological consequences. Examples include: alcohol + benzodiazepine (to produce sedation), atropine + β-adrenoceptor blocker (to reverse β-adrenoceptor blocker overdose).
- *Pharmacokinetic interaction*: the drugs interact remotely from the target site to alter plasma (and other tissue) concentrations so that the amount of the drug at the target site of clinical effect is altered, e.g. enzyme induction by rifampicin reduces the plasma concentration of warfarin; enzyme inhibition by ciprofloxacin increases the concentration of theophylline.

Interaction may result in antagonism or synergism.

Antagonism occurs when the action of one drug opposes that of another. The two drugs simply have opposite pharmacodynamic effects, e.g. histamine and adrenaline (epinephrine) on the bronchi exhibit physiological or functional antagonism;

---

[45]Hu Z, Yang X, Ho P C et al 2005 Herb–drug interactions: a literature review. Drugs 65:1239–1282.

or they compete reversibly for the same drug receptor, e.g. flumazenil and benzodiazepines exhibit competitive antagonism.

Synergism[46] is of two sorts:

1. *Summation* or addition occurs when the effects of two drugs having the same action are additive, i.e. $2 + 2 = 4$ (a β-adrenoceptor blocker plus a thiazide diuretic have an additive antihypertensive effect).
2. *Potentiation* (to make more powerful) occurs when one drug increases the action of another, i.e. $2 + 2 = 5$. Sometimes the two drugs both have the action concerned (trimethoprim plus sulphonamide), and sometimes one drug lacks the action concerned (benserazide plus levodopa), i.e. $0 + 2 = 5$.

In broad terms, it is useful to distinguish the drug–drug interactions that occur:

- before drugs enters the body
- at important points during their disposition and metabolism
- at receptor sites.

Before administration. Intravenous fluids offer special scope for interactions (incompatibilities). Drugs commonly are weak organic acids or bases, presented as salts to improve their solubility. Plainly, the mixing of solutions of salts can result in instability, which may or may not be evident from visible change in the solution, i.e. precipitation. While specific sources of information are available in manufacturers' package inserts and formularies, issues of compatibility are complex and lie within the professional competence of the hospital pharmacy, which should prepare drug additions to infused solutions.

At the site of absorption. The complex environment of the gut provides opportunity for drugs to interfere with one another, both directly and indirectly by altering gut physiology. Usually the result is to impair absorption.

By direct chemical interaction in the gut. Antacids that contain aluminium and magnesium form insoluble complexes with tetracyclines, iron and prednisolone.

Milk contains sufficient calcium to warrant its avoidance as a major article of diet with tetracyclines. Colestyramine interferes with the absorption of levothyroxine, digoxin and some acidic drugs, e.g. warfarin. Separating the dosing of interacting drugs by at least 2 h should largely avoid the problem.

By altering gut motility. Slowing of gastric emptying, e.g. opioid analgesics, tricyclic antidepressants (antimuscarinic effect), may delay and reduce the absorption of other drugs. Purgatives reduce the time spent in the small intestine and give less opportunity for the absorption of poorly soluble substances such as adrenal corticosteroids and digoxin.

By altering gut flora. Antimicrobials potentiate oral anticoagulants by reducing bacterial synthesis of vitamin K (usually only after antimicrobials are given orally in high dose, e.g. to treat *Helicobacter pylori*).

Interactions other than in the gut. Hyaluronidase promotes dissipation of a subcutaneous injection, and vasoconstrictors, e.g. adrenaline, felypressin, delay absorption of local anaesthetics, usefully to prolong local anaesthesia.

During distribution. Carrier-mediated transporters control processes such as bioavailability, passage into the CNS, hepatic uptake and entry into bile, and renal tubular excretion (see p. 97). Inhibitors and inducers of drug transporters can profoundly influence the disposition of drugs. The transporter MDR1 controls the entry of digoxin into cells; quinidine, verapamil and ciclosporin inhibit this transporter and increase the plasma concentration of digoxin (with potentially toxic effects). Probenecid inhibits the organic anion renal transporter, which decreases the renal clearance of penicillin (usefully prolonging its effect) but also that of methotrexate (with danger of toxicity). Elucidation of the location and function of transport systems will give the explanation for, and allow the prediction of, many more drug–drug interactions.

During metabolism. Enzyme induction (see p. 97) and, even more powerfully, enzyme inhibition (see p. 98) are important sources of drug–drug interction.

At receptor sites. There are numerous examples. Beneficial interactions are sought in overdose, as with naloxone for morphine overdose (opioid receptor), atropine for anticholinesterase, i.e. insecticide poisoning (acetylcholine receptor), phentolamine for the monoamine oxidase inhibitor–sympathomimetic interaction (α-adrenoceptor). Unwanted interactions include the loss of the antihypertensive effect of β-blockers with common cold remedies containing ephedrine, phenylpropanolamine or phenylephrine, usually taken unknown to the doctor (their α-adrenoceptor agonist action is unrestrained in the β-blocked patient).

GUIDE TO FURTHER READING

Andersson T, Flockhart D A, Goldstein D B et al 2005 Drug-metabolizing enzymes: evidence for clinical utility of pharmacogenomic tests. Clinical Pharmacology and Therapeutics 78(6):559–581

Baber N S (ed.) 2005 Paediatric special issue. British Journal of Clinical Pharmacology 59(6):651–755

Cooper R S, Kaufman J S, Ward R 2003 Race and genomics. New England Journal of Medicine 348(12):1166–1170

Guttmacher A E, Collins F S 2002 Genomic medicine – a primer. New England Journal of Medicine 347(19):1512–1520

Ito S 2000 Drug therapy for breast-feeding women. New England Journal of Medicine 343(2):118–126

Kearns G L, Abdel-Rahman S M, Alander S W et al 2003 Developmental pharmacology – drug disposition, action, and therapy in infants and children. New England Journal of Medicine 349(12):1157–1167

Khoury M J, McCabe L L, McCabe E R B 2003 Population screening in the age of genomic medicine. New England Journal of Medicine 348(1):50–58

Koren G, Pastuszak A, Ito S 1998 Drugs in pregnancy. New England Journal of Medicine 338(16):1128–1137

Mallet L, Spinewine A, Huang A Prescribing in elderly people 2 The challenge of managing drug interactions in elderly people. Lancet 370:185–191

Nebert D W, Russell D W 2002 Clinical importance of the cytochromes P450. Lancet 360:1155–1162

Rehman H U, Han S 2004 Pharmacotherapy in old age. Journal of the Royal College of Physicians of Edinburgh 34:21–27

Spinewine A, Schmader K E, Barber N et al 2007 Prescribing in elderly people 1 Appropriate prescribing in elderly people: how well can it be measured and optimised? Lancet 370:173–184

Tucker G T 2000 Chiral switches. Lancet 355:1085–1087

Weinshilboum R 2003 Inheritance and drug response. New England Journal of Medicine 348(6):529–537

8

Unwanted effects and adverse drug reactions

SYNOPSIS

As drugs are intended to relieve suffering, patients find it peculiarly offensive that they can also cause disease (especially if they are not forewarned). Therefore it is important to know how much disease drugs do cause and why they cause it, so that preventive measures can be taken. The chapter will examine:

- Background
- Definitions
- Attribution and degrees of certainty
- Pharmacovigilance and pharmacoepidemiology
- Sources of adverse drug reactions
- Allergy in response to drugs
- Effects of prolonged administration: chronic organ toxicity
- Adverse effects on reproduction

BACKGROUND

Cured yesterday of my disease, I died last night of my physician.[1]

Nature is neutral, i.e. it has no 'intentions' towards humans, though it is often unfavourable to them. It is humankind, in its desire to avoid suffering and death, that decides that some of the biological effects of drugs are desirable (therapeutic) and others are undesirable (adverse). In addition to this arbitrary division, which has no fundamental biological basis, unwanted effects of drugs are promoted, or even caused, by numerous non-drug factors. Because of the variety of these factors, attempts to make a simple account of the unwanted effects of drugs must be imperfect.

There is general agreement that drugs prescribed for disease are themselves the cause of a serious amount of disease (adverse reactions), ranging from mere inconvenience to permanent disability and death.

It is not enough to measure the incidence of adverse reactions to drugs, their nature and their severity, although accurate data are obviously useful. It is necessary to take, or to try to take, into account which effects are avoidable (by skilled choice and use) and which are unavoidable (inherent in drug or patient).

As there can be no hope of eliminating all adverse effects of drugs, it is necessary to evaluate patterns of adverse reaction against one another. One drug may frequently cause minor ill-effects but pose no threat to life, though patients do not like it and may take it irregularly, to their own detriment. Another drug may be pleasant to take, so that patients take it consistently, with benefit, but it may rarely kill someone. It is not obvious which drug is to be preferred.

Some patients, e.g. those with a history of allergy or previous reactions to drugs, are up to four times more likely to have another adverse reaction, so that the incidence does not fall evenly. It is also useful to discover the causes of adverse reactions, e.g. individuals who lack certain enzymes, for such knowledge can be used to render avoidable what are at present unavoidable reactions.

Avoidable adverse effects will be reduced by more skilful prescribing and this means that doctors, amongst all the other claims on their time, must find time better to understand drugs, as well as to understand their patients and their diseases.

DEFINITIONS

Many unwanted effects of drugs are medically trivial and, in order to avoid inflating the figures of drug-induced disease, it is convenient to retain the term *side-effects* for minor reactions that occur at normal therapeutic doses, are predictable and usually dose related.

The term *adverse drug reaction* (ADR) should be confined to: harmful or seriously unpleasant effects

---

[1]From: The remedy worse than the disease. Matthew Prior (1664–1721).

occurring at doses intended for therapeutic (including prophylactic or diagnostic) effect and which call for reduction of dose or withdrawal of the drug and/or forecast hazard from future administration; it is effects of this order that are of importance in evaluating drug-induced disease in the community. The term adverse 'reaction' is almost synonymous with adverse 'effect', save that an 'effect' relates to the drug and a 'reaction' to the patient. Both terms should be distinguished from an adverse 'event', which is an adverse happening that occurs during exposure to a drug without any assumption being made about its cause (see Prescription Event Monitoring. p. 59).

Toxicity implies a direct action of the drug, often at high dose, damaging cells, e.g. liver damage from paracetamol overdose, eighth cranial nerve damage from gentamicin. All drugs, for practical purposes, are toxic in overdose[2] and overdose can be absolute or relative; in the latter case an ordinary dose may be administered but may be toxic due to an underlying abnormality in the patient, e.g. disease of the kidney. *Mutagenicity, carcinogenicity* and *teratogenicity* (see Index) are special cases of toxicity.

Secondary effects are the indirect consequences of a primary drug action. Examples are: vitamin deficiency or opportunistic infection which may occur in patients whose normal bowel flora has been altered by antimicrobials; diuretic-induced hypokalaemia causing digoxin intolerance.

Intolerance means a low threshold to the normal pharmacodynamic action of a drug. Individuals vary greatly in their susceptibility to drugs, those at one extreme of the normal distribution curve being intolerant of the drugs, those at the other, tolerant.

Idiosyncrasy (see Pharmacogenetics) implies an inherent qualitative abnormal reaction to a drug, usually due to genetic abnormality, e.g. porphyria.

---

[2]A principle appreciated by Paracelsus who stated that 'All things are poisons and there is nothing that is harmless; the dose alone decides that something is no poison.' The physician, alchemist and philosopher is regarded as the founder of chemical therapeutics; he was the first to use carefully measured doses of mercury to treat syphilis.

ATTRIBUTION AND DEGREES OF CONVICTION

When an unexpected event, for which there is no obvious cause, occurs in a patient already taking a drug, the possibility that it is drug attributable must always be considered. Distinguishing between natural progression of a disease and drug-induced deterioration is particularly challenging, e.g. sodium in antacid formulations may aggravate cardiac failure, tricyclic antidepressants may provoke epileptic seizures, and bronchospasm may be caused by aspirin in some asthmatics.

The following elements are useful in attributing the cause of an adverse event to a drug:

1. The *time sequence* in relation to taking the drug. The majority of reactions develop soon after exposure. Anaphylactic reactions (within minutes or hours) and hypersensitivity reactions (within weeks) may readily suggest an association, but delayed effects such as carcinogenesis or tardive dyskinesia (after years) present more difficulty.
2. The effects of *withdrawing* or *reintroducing* the drug. Most reactions subside when the drug is discontinued, unless an autoimmune reaction is established, when effects persist. Planned re-exposing a patient to a drug is rarely indicated unless treatment with it is essential and there is no reliable alternative.
3. The relationship to what is *already known* about the drug. This evokes questions about consistency with the established pharmacology and toxicology of the drug or related substances.

Degrees of conviction for attributing adverse reactions to drugs may be ascribed as:[3]

■ *Definite*: time sequence from taking the drug is reasonable; event corresponds to what is known of the drug and is not explicable by concurrent disease or drugs; event ceases on stopping the drug; event returns on restarting the drug (rarely advisable).
■ *Probable*: time sequence is reasonable; event corresponds to what is known of the drug; event ceases on stopping the drug; event not

---

[3]Journal of the American Medical Association (1975) 234:1236.

reasonably explained by patient's disease or other drugs.

- *Possible*: time sequence is reasonable; event corresponds to what is known of the drug; uncertain relationship to effect of stopping the drug; event could readily have been result of the patient's disease or other therapy.
- *Conditional*: time sequence is reasonable; event does not correspond to what is known of the drug; event could not reasonably be explained by the patient's disease or other drugs.
- *Doubtful*: event not meeting the above criteria.

Caution. About 80% of well people not taking any drugs admit on questioning to symptoms (often several) such as are commonly experienced as lesser adverse reactions to drugs. These symptoms are intensified (or diminished) by administration of a placebo. Thus, many (minor) symptoms may be wrongly attributed to drugs. Similarly, minor and possibly transient abnormalities in laboratory results, e.g. liver function tests, are often recorded in apparently healthy people.

PRACTICALITIES OF DETECTING RARE ADVERSE REACTIONS

For reactions with no background incidence, the number of patients required to give a good (95%) chance of detecting the effect is given in Table 8.1. Assuming that three events are required before any regulatory or other action should be taken, it shows the large number of patients that must be monitored to detect even a relatively high-incidence adverse effect. The problem can be many orders of magnitude worse if the adverse reactions closely resemble spontaneous disease with a background incidence in the population.

Table 8.1 Detecting rare adverse drug reactions[4]

Expected incidence of adverse reaction	Required number of patients for event		
	1 event	2 events	3 events
1 in 100	300	480	650
1 in 200	600	960	1300
1 in 1000	3000	4800	6500
1 in 2000	6000	9600	13 000
1 in 10 000	30 000	48 000	65 000

[4]By permission from: Dollery C D, Bankowski Z (eds) 1983 Safety requirements for the first use of new drugs and diagnostic agents in man. CIOMS (WHO), Geneva.

PHARMACOVIGILANCE AND PHARMACOEPIDEMIOLOGY

The principal methods of collecting data on ADRs (pharmacovigilance) are:

- *Experimental studies*, i.e. formal therapeutic trials of Phases 1–3. These provide reliable data on only the commoner events as they involve relatively small numbers of patients (hundreds); they detect an incidence of up to about 1 in 200.
- *Observational studies*, where the drug is observed epidemiologically under conditions of normal use in the community, i.e. pharmacoepidemiology and pharmacovigilance. Techniques used for post-marketing (Phase 4) studies include the observational cohort study and the case–control study. The surveillance systems are described on page 58.

DRUG-INDUCED ILLNESS

The discovery of drug-induced illness can be analysed thus:[5]

- A *drug commonly induces an otherwise rare illness*: this effect is likely to be discovered by clinical observation in the licensing (pre-marketing) formal therapeutic trials and the drug will almost always be abandoned; but some patients are normally excluded from such trials, e.g. pregnant women, and detection will then occur later.
- A *drug rarely or uncommonly induces an otherwise common illness*: this effect is likely to remain undiscovered. Cardiovascular risk from coxibs (e.g. rofecoxib, Vioxx) approximates as an example, but the degree of increased risk did become apparent after meta-analysis of several clinical trials and observational studies.
- A *drug rarely induces an otherwise rare illness*: this effect is likely to remain undiscovered before the drug is released for general prescribing; the effect could be detected by informal clinical observation or during any special post-registration surveillance and confirmed by a case–control study (see p. 58); aplastic

[5]After Jick H 1977 The discovery of drug-induced illness. New England Journal of Medicine 296:481–485.

anaemia with chloramphenicol[6] and the oculomucocutaneous syndrome with practolol were uncovered in this way.

■ *A drug commonly induces an otherwise common illness*: this effect will not be discovered by informal clinical observation. If very common, it may be discovered in formal therapeutic trials and in case–control studies, but if only moderately common it may require observational cohort studies, e.g. pro-arrhythmic effects of antiarrhythmic drugs.

■ *Drug adverse effects and illness incidence in an intermediate range*: both case–control and cohort studies may be needed.

Some impression of the features of drug-induced illness can be gained from the following statistics:

■ In a large UK study, the prevalence of ADRs as a cause of admission to hospital was 6.5%, with a median bed stay 8 days (4% of hospital bed capacity); most reactions were definitely or possibly avoidable; the commonest drugs were: low-dose aspirin, diuretics, warfarin, non-steroidal anti-inflammatory drugs (other than aspirin); the commonest adverse reaction was gastrointestinal bleeding.[7]

■ Overall incidence in hospital inpatients is 10–20%, with possible prolongation of hospital stay in 2–10% of patients in acute medical wards.

■ ADRs cause 2–3% of consultations in general practice.

■ A study of 661 ambulatory patients found that 25% experienced adverse events of which 13% were serious and 11% were preventable.[8]

■ Predisposing factors for ADRs are: age over 60 years or under 1 month, female sex, previous history of adverse reaction, hepatic or renal disease, number of medications taken.

■ A review of records of Coroner's Inquests for a (UK) district with a population of 1.19 million during the period 1986–1991 found that, of 3277 inquests on deaths, 10 were due to errors of prescribing and 36 were caused by adverse drug reactions.[9] Nevertheless, 17 doctors in the UK were charged with manslaughter in the 1990s, compared with two in each of the preceding decades, a reflection of 'a greater readiness to call the police or to prosecute'.[10]

It is important to avoid alarmist or defeatist extremes of attitude. Many treatments are dangerous, e.g. surgery, electroshock, drugs, and it is irrational to accept the risks of surgery for biliary stones or hernia and to refuse to accept any risk at all from drugs for conditions of comparable severity.

Many patients whose death is deemed to be partly or wholly caused by drugs are dangerously ill already; justifiable risks may be taken in the hope of helping them; ill-informed criticism in such cases can act against the interest of the sick. On the other hand there is no doubt that some of these accidents are avoidable. This is often more obvious when reviewing the conduct of treatment after the event, i.e. with the benefit of hindsight.

Sir Anthony Carlisle,[11] in the first half of the 19th century, said that 'medicine is an art founded on conjecture and improved by murder'. Although medicine has advanced rapidly, there is still a ring of truth in that statement to anyone who follows the introduction of new drugs and observes how, after the early enthusiasm, the reports of serious toxic effects appear. The challenge is to find and avoid these, and, indeed, the present systems for detecting adverse reactions came into being largely in the wake of the thalidomide, practolol and benoxaprofen disasters (see Chapter 5); they are now an increasingly sophisticated and effective part of medicines development.

> It is an absolute obligation on doctors to use only drugs about which they have troubled to inform themselves.

---

[6]Scott J L, Finegold S M, Belkin G A, Lawrence J S 1965 A controlled double-blind study of the hematologic toxicity of chloramphenicol. New England Journal of Medicine 272:1137–1142.

[7]Pirmohamed M, James S, Meakin S et al 2004 Adverse drug reactions as a cause of admission to hospital: prospective analysis of 18 820 patients. British Medical Journal 329:15–19.

[8]Gandhi T K, Weingart S N, Borus J et al 2003 Adverse events in ambulatory care. New England Journal of Medicine 348:1556–1564.

[9]Ferner R E, Whittington R M 1994 Coroner's cases of death due to errors in prescribing or giving medicines or to adverse drug reactions: Birmingham 1986–1991. Journal of the Royal Society of Medicine 87:145–148.

[10]Ferner R E 2000 Medication errors that have led to manslaughter charges. British Medical Journal 321:1212–1216.

[11]Noted for his advocacy of the use of 'the simple carpenter's saw' in surgery.

DRUGS AND SKILLED TASKS

Many medicines affect performance, and it is relevant to review here some examples with their mechanisms of action. As might be expected, centrally acting and psychotropic drugs are prominent, e.g. the sedative antidepressants, benzodiazepines, non-benzodiazepine and other hypnotics, and antipsychotics (the 'classical' type more so than the 'atypicals'; see p. 342). Many drugs possess anticholinergic activity either directly (atropine, oxybutinin) or indirectly (tricyclic antidepressants, antipsychotics), the central effects of which cause confusion and impaired ability to process information. The first-generation H_1-receptor antihistamines (chlorpheniramine, diphenhydramine) are notably sedating and impair alertness and concentration, features that are often not recognised by the recipient. Drugs may also affect performance through cerebral depression (anti-epileptics, opioids), hypoglycaemia (antidiabetics) and hypotension (antihypertensives). Alcohol and cannabis are discussed on pages 148 and 164.

Car driving is a complex multifunction task that includes: visual search and recognition, vigilance, information processing under variable demand, decision-making and risk-taking, and sensorimotor control. It is plain that prescribers have a major responsibility here, both to warn patients and, in the case of those who need to drive for their work, to choose medicines with a minimal liability to cause impairment.[12] Patients who must drive when taking a drug of known risk, e.g. benzodiazepine, should be specially warned of times of peak impairment.[13]

A patient who has an accident and was not warned of drug hazard, whether orally or by labelling, may successfully sue the doctor in law. It is also necessary that patients be advised of the additive effect of alcohol with prescribed medicines.

How the patient feels is not a reliable guide to recovery of skills, and drivers may be more than usually accident prone without any subjective feeling of sedation or dysphoria. The criteria for safety in aircrew are more stringent than those for car drivers.

Resumption of car driving or other skilled activity after anaesthesia is a special case, and an extremely variable one, but where a sedative, e.g. intravenous benzodiazepine, opioid or neuroleptic, or any general anaesthetic, has been used it seems reasonable not to drive for 24 h at least.

The emphasis on psychomotor and physical aspects (injury) should not distract from the possibility that those who live by their intellect and imagination (politicians and even journalists may be included here) may suffer cognitive disability from thoughtless prescribing.

SOURCES OF ADVERSE DRUG REACTIONS

The reasons why patients experience ADRs are varied and numerous, but reflection on the following may help a prescriber to anticipate and avoid unwelcome events:

- *The patient may be predisposed to an ADR* by age, sex, genetic constitution, known tendency to allergy, disease of drug eliminating organs (see Chapter 7), or social habits, e.g. use of tobacco, alcohol, other recreational drugs (see Chapter 10).
- *The known nature of the drug may forewarn.* Some drugs, e.g. digoxin, have steep dose–response curves and small increments of dose are more likely to induce adverse or toxic reactions (see p. 116). The capacity of the body to eliminate certain drugs, e.g. phenytoin, may saturate within the therapeutic dose range so that standard increases cause disproportionate rise in plasma concentration, risking toxic effects (see p. 80). Some drugs, e.g. antimicrobials, have a tendency to cause allergy. Anticancer agents warrant special care as they are by their nature cytotoxic (see Chapter 30). Use of these and other drugs may raise longer-term issues of mutagenicity, carcinogenicity and teratogenicity. Ingredients of a formulation, rather than the active drug may also cause adverse reactions. Examples include the high sodium content of some antacids, and colouring and flavouring agents. The latter are

---

[12]Gull D G, Langford N J 2006 Drugs and driving. Adverse Drug Reactions Bulletin 238:911–914.

[13]Nordic countries require that medicines liable to impair ability to drive or to operate machinery be labelled with a red triangle on a white background. The scheme covers antidepressants, benzodiazepines, hypnotics, drugs for motion sickness and allergy, cerebral stimulants, antiepileptics and antihypertensive agents. In the UK there are some standard labels that pharmacists are recommended to apply, e.g. 'Warning. May cause drowsiness. If affected do not drive or operate machinery. Avoid alcoholic drink'.

SECTION 2

designated in the list of contents by E numbers; tartrazine (E102) may cause allergic reactions.

■ *The prescriber* needs to be aware that adverse reactions may occur after a drug has been used for a long time, at a critical phase in pregnancy, is abruptly discontinued (see p. 104) or given with other drugs (see Drug interactions, Chapter 7).

Aspects of the above appear throughout the book as is indicated. Selected topics are now discussed.

AGE

The very old and the very young are liable to be intolerant of many drugs, largely because the mechanisms for disposing of them in the body are less efficient. The young, it has been aptly said, are not simply 'small adults' and 'respect for their pharmacokinetic variability should be added to the list of our senior citizens' rights'.[14] The old are also frequently exposed to multiple drug therapy which further predisposes to adverse effects (see Prescribing for the elderly, p. 109).

SEX

Females are more likely to experience adverse reactions to certain drugs, e.g. mefloquine (neuropsychiatric effects).

GENETIC CONSTITUTION

Inherited factors that influence response to drugs are discussed in general under Pharmacogenetics (see p. 105). It is convenient here to describe *the porphyrias*, a specific group of disorders for which careful prescribing in a subgroup, the acute porphyrias, is vital.

Healthy people need to produce *haem*, e.g. for erythrocytes and haem-dependent enzymes. Haem is synthesised by a sequence of enzymes and in non-erythroid cells (including the liver) the *rate* of the synthetic process is controlled by the first of these, D-aminolaevulinic acid (ALA) synthase, upon which haem provides a negative feedback.

The *porphyrias* comprise a number of rare, genetically determined, single-enzyme defects in haem biosynthesis and give rise to two main clinical manifestations: acute neurovisceral attacks and/or skin lesions. *Non-acute porphyrias* (porphyria cutanea tarda, erythropoietic protoporphyria and congenital erythropoietic porphyria) present with cutaneous photosensitivity that results from the overproduction of porphyrins, which are photosensitising. In porphyria cutanea tarda, a mainly acquired disorder of hepatic enzyme function, one of the main provoking agents is alcohol (and prescribed oestrogens in women).

The *acute hepatic porphyrias* (acute intermittent porphyria, variegate porphyria and hereditary co-proporphyria) are characterised by severe attacks of neurovisceral dysfunction precipitated principally by a wide variety of drugs (and also by alcohol, fasting and infection). Clinical effects arise from the accumulation of the precursors of haem synthesis, D-ALA, porphobilinogen.

The exact *precipitating mechanisms* are uncertain. Induction of the haem-containing hepatic oxidising enzymes of the cytochrome P450 group causes an increased demand for haem. Therefore drugs that induce these enzymes would be expected to precipitate acute attacks of porphyria, and they do so; tobacco smoking and alcohol excess may also act via this mechanism. Apparently unexplained attacks of porphyria should be an indication for close enquiry into all possible chemical intake, including recreational substances such as marijuana, cocaine, amfetamines and ecstasy. Patients must be educated to understand their condition, to possess a list of safe and unsafe drugs, and to protect themselves from themselves and from others, including prescribing doctors.

Great care in prescribing for these patients is required if serious illness is to be avoided and it is therefore essential that patients and their clinicians have access to information concerning the safe use of prescription medication. Drug lists should be reviewed regularly, and a recent initiative in Europe has made a consensus based list of safe drugs available at (http://www.porphyria-europe.org as well as details of common prescribing problems and a link to a searchable drug safety database (http://www.drugs-porphyria.org).

If no recognised safe option is available, use of a drug about which there is uncertainty may be justified. Dr M. Badminton[15] writes: 'Essential treatment should never be withheld, especially for a condition that is serious or life threatening. The clinician

[14]Fogel B S 1983 New England Journal of Medicine 308:1600.

[15]Department of Medical Biochemistry, University Hospital of Wales, Cardiff, UK. We are grateful to Dr Badminton for contributing the section on porphyria.

should assess the severity of the condition and the activity of the porphyria and make a risk versus benefit assessment.' In these circumstances the clinician may wish to contact an expert centre for advice (see the list at http://www.porphyria-europe.com), which is likely to recommend that the patient be monitored as follows:

1. Measure urine and porphobilinogen before starting treatment.
2. Repeat the measurement at regular intervals or if the patient has symptoms in keeping with an acute attack. If there is an increase in the precursor levels, stop the treatment and consider giving haem arginate for acute attack (see below).

In treatment of the acute attack the rationale to use means of reducing D-ALA synthase activity. *Haem arginate* (human haematin) infusion, by replenishing haem and so removing the stimulus to D-ALA synthase, is effective if given early, and may prevent chronic neuropathy. Additionally, attention to nutrition, particularly the supply of carbohydrate, relief of pain (with an opioid), and of hypertension and tachycardia (with a β-adrenoceptor blocker) are important. Hyponatraemia is a frequent complication, and plasma electrolytes should be monitored.

THE ENVIRONMENT AND SOCIAL HABITS

Drug metabolism may be increased by hepatic enzyme induction from insecticide accumulation, e.g. dicophane (DDT), and from alcohol use and the tobacco habit, e.g. smokers require a higher dose of theophylline. Antimicrobials used in feeds of animals for human consumption have given rise to concern in relation to the spread of resistant bacteria that may affect man. Penicillin in the air of hospitals or in milk (see below) may cause allergy.

ALLERGY IN RESPONSE TO DRUGS

Allergic reactions to drugs are the result of the interaction of drug or metabolite (or a non-drug element in the formulation) with patient and disease, and subsequent re-exposure.

Lack of previous exposure is not the same as lack of history of previous exposure, and 'first dose reactions' are among the most dramatic. Exposure is not necessarily medical, e.g. penicillins may occur in dairy products following treatment of mastitis in cows (despite laws to prevent this), and penicillin antibodies are commonly present in those who deny ever having received the drug. Immune responses to drugs may be harmful (allergy) or harmless; the fact that antibodies are produced does not mean a patient will necessarily respond to re-exposure with clinical manifestations; most of the UK population has antibodies to penicillins but, fortunately, comparatively few react clinically to penicillin administration.

Whilst macromolecules (proteins, peptides, dextran polysaccharides) can act as complete antigens, most drugs are simple chemicals (mol. wt. less than 1000) and act as incomplete antigens or haptens, which become complete antigens in combination with a body protein.

The chief target organs of drug allergy are the skin, respiratory tract, gastrointestinal tract, blood and blood vessels.

Allergic reactions in general may be classified according to four types of hypersensitivity, and drugs can elicit reactions of all types.

Type I reactions: immediate or anaphylactic type. The drug causes formation of tissue-sensitising immunoglobulin (Ig) E antibodies that are fixed to mast cells or leucocytes; on subsequent administration the allergen (conjugate of drug or metabolite with tissue protein) reacts with these antibodies, activating but not damaging the cell to which they are fixed and causing release of pharmacologically active substances, e.g. histamine, leukotrienes, prostaglandins, platelet activating factor, and causing effects such as urticaria, anaphylactic shock and asthma. Allergy develops within minutes and lasts for 1–2 h.

Type II reactions: antibody-dependent cytotoxic type. The drug or metabolite combines with a protein in the body so that the body no longer recognises the protein as self, treats it as a foreign protein and forms antibodies (IgG, IgM) that combine with the antigen and activate complement which damages cells, e.g. penicillin- or methyldopa-induced haemolytic anaemia.

Type III reactions: immune complex-mediated type. Antigen and antibody form large complexes and activate complement. Small blood vessels are damaged or blocked. Leucocytes attracted to the site of reaction engulf the immune complexes and release pharmacologically active substances (including lysosomal enzymes), starting an inflammatory process.

These reactions include serum sickness, glomerulo-nephritis, vasculitis and pulmonary disease.

Type IV reactions: lymphocyte-mediated type. Antigen-specific receptors develop on T lympho-cytes. Subsequent administration leads to a local or tissue allergic reaction, e.g. contact dermatitis.

Cross-allergy within a group of drugs is usual, e.g. the penicillins. When allergy to a particular drug is established, a substitute should be selected from a chemically different group. Patients with allergic diseases, e.g. eczema, are more likely to develop allergy to drugs.

The distinctive features of allergic reactions are:[16]

- Lack of correlation with known pharmacological properties of the drug.
- Lack of linear relation with drug dose (very small doses may cause very severe effects).
- Rashes, angio-oedema, serum sickness syndrome, anaphylaxis or asthma; characteristics of classic protein allergy.
- Requirement of an induction period on primary exposure, but not on re-exposure.
- Disappearance on cessation of administration and reappearance on re-exposure to a small dose.
- Occurrence in a minority of patients receiving the drug.
- Possible response to desensitisation.

PRINCIPAL CLINICAL MANIFESTATIONS AND TREATMENT

1. Urticarial rashes and angioedema (types I, III). These are probably the commonest type of drug allergy. Reactions may be generalised, but frequently are worst in and around the external area of administration of the drug. The eyelids, lips and face are usually most affected. They are usually accompanied by itching. Oedema of the larynx is rare but may be fatal. They respond to adrenaline (epinephrine), ephedrine, H_1-receptor antihistamine and adrenal steroid (see below).

2a. Nonurticarial rashes (types I, II, IV). These occur in great variety; frequently they are weeping exudative lesions. It is often difficult to be sure

when a rash is due to a drug. Apart from stopping the drug, treatment is non-specific; in severe cases an adrenal steroid should be used. Skin sensitisation to antimicrobials may be very troublesome, especially amongst those who handle them (see Chapter 16 for more detail).

2b. Diseases of the lymphoid system. Infectious mononucleosis (and lymphoma, leukaemia) is associated with an increased incidence (>40%) of a characteristic maculopapular, sometimes purpuric, rash which is probably allergic, when an aminopenicillin (ampicillin, amoxicillin) is taken; patients may not be allergic to other penicillins. Erythromycin may cause a similar reaction.

3. Anaphylactic shock (Type I) occurs with penicillin, anaesthetics (intravenous), iodine-containing radio-contrast media and a huge variety of other drugs. A severe fall in blood pressure occurs, with broncho-constriction, angio-oedema (including larynx) and sometimes death due to loss of fluid from the intra-vascular compartment. Anaphylactic shock usually occurs suddenly, in less than an hour after the drug, but within minutes if it has been given intravenously.

Treatment is urgent. The following account combines advice from the UK Resuscitation Council with comment on the action of the drugs used. Advice on the management of anaphylactic shock is altered periodically and the reader should check the relevant website (http://www.resus.org.uk) for the latest information.

- First, 500 micrograms of *adrenaline* (epinephrine) injection (0.5 mL of the 1 in 1000 solution) should be given intramuscularly to raise the blood pressure and dilate the bronchi (vasoconstriction renders the subcutaneous route less effective). If there is no clinical improvement, further intramuscular injections of adrenaline 500 micrograms should be given at 5-min intervals according to blood pressure, pulse and respiration.
- If shock is profound, cardiopulmonary resuscitation/advanced life support are necessary. Consider also giving adrenaline 1 : 10 000 by slow intravenous infusion, at a rate of 100 micrograms/min (1 mL/min of the dilute 1 in 10 000 solution over 5 min), preferably with continuous ECG monitoring, stopping when a response has been obtained. This procedure is hazardous and

---

[16]Assem E-S K 1998 Drug allergy and tests for its detection. In: Davies D M (ed.) Davies's textbook of adverse drug reactions. Chapman & Hall, London, p. 790.

should be undertaken only by an experienced practitioner who can obtain immediate intravenous access.

- The adrenaline should be accompanied by an H_1-receptor antihistamine, e.g. *chlorphenamine* 10–20 mg intramuscularly or by slow intravenous injection, and *hydrocortisone* 100–500 mg intramuscularly or by slow intravenous injection. The adrenal steroid acts by reducing vascular permeability and by suppressing further response to the antigen–antibody reaction. Benefit from an adrenal steroid is not immediate; it is unlikely to begin for 30 min and takes hours to reach its maximum.
- In severe anaphylaxis, hypotension is due to vasodilatation and loss of circulating volume through leaky capillaries. Thus, when there is no response to drug treatment, 1–2 L of plasma substitute should be infused rapidly. Crystalloid may be safer than colloid, which is associated with more allergic reactions.
- Where bronchospasm is severe and does not respond rapidly to other treatment, a β_2-adrenoceptor agonist is a useful adjunctive measure. Noradrenaline (norepinephrine) lacks any useful bronchodilator action (β effect) (see Adrenaline, Chapter 23).
- Where susceptibility to anaphylaxis is known, e.g. in patients with allergy to bee or wasp stings, preventive self-management is feasible. The patient is taught to administer adrenaline intramuscularly from a pre-filled syringe (EpiPen Auto-injector, delivering adrenaline 300 micrograms per dose).
- Half of the above doses of adrenaline may be safer for patients who are receiving amitriptyline or imipramine (increased effect; see p. 338), or a β-adrenoceptor (hypertension; see p. 433).

Any hospital ward or other place where anaphylaxis may be anticipated should have all the drugs and equipment necessary to deal with it in one convenient kit, for when they are needed there is little time to think and none to run about from place to place (see also Pseudo-allergic reactions, p. 125).

4a. Pulmonary reactions: asthma (type I). Aspirin and other non-steroidal anti-inflammatory drugs may cause an asthmatic attack. Whether this is an allergic or pseudo-allergic reaction, or a mixture of the two, is uncertain.

4b. Other types of pulmonary reaction (type III) include syndromes resembling acute and chronic lung infections, pneumonitis, fibrosis and eosinophilia.

5. The serum sickness syndrome (type III). This occurs about 1–3 weeks after administration. Treatment is by an adrenal steroid, and as above if there is urticaria.

6. Blood disorders[17]

6a. Thrombocytopenia (type II, but also pseudo-allergic) may occur after exposure to any of a large number of drugs, including: gold, quinine, quinidine, rifampicin, heparin, thionamide derivatives, thiazide diuretics, sulphonamides, oestrogens, indometacin. Adrenal steroid may help.

6b. Granulocytopenia (type II, but also pseudo-allergic), sometimes leading to agranulocytosis, is a very serious allergy which may occur with many drugs, e.g. clozapine, carbamazepine, carbimazole, chloramphenicol, sulphonamides (including diuretic and hypoglycaemic derivatives), colchicine, gold.

The value of precautionary leucocyte counts for drugs having special risk remains uncertain.[18] Weekly counts may detect presymptomatic granulocytopenia from antithyroid drugs, but onset can be sudden and an alternative view is to monitor only with drugs having special risk, e.g. clozapine. The chief clinical manifestation of agranulocytosis is sore throat or mouth ulcers, and patients should be warned to report such events immediately and to stop taking the drug, but they should not be frightened into non-compliance with essential therapy. Treatment of the agranulocytosis involves both stopping the drug responsible and giving a bactericidal drug, e.g. a penicillin, to prevent or treat infection.

---

[17]Where cells are being destroyed in the periphery and production is normal, transfusion is useless or nearly so, as the transfused cells will be destroyed, though in an emergency even a short cell life (platelets, erythrocytes) may tip the balance usefully. Where the bone marrow is depressed, transfusion is useful and the transfused cells will survive normally.

[18]In contrast to the case of a drug causing bone marrow depression as a pharmacodynamic dose-related effect, when blood counts are part of the essential routine monitoring of therapy, e.g. cytotoxics.

6c. Aplastic anaemia (type II, but not always allergic). Causal agents include chloramphenicol, sulphonamides and derivatives (diuretics, antidiabetics), gold, penicillamine, allopurinol, felbamate, phenothiazines and some insecticides, e.g. dicophane (DDT). In the case of chloramphenicol, bone marrow depression is a normal pharmacodynamic effect, although aplastic anaemia may also be due to idiosyncrasy or allergy.

Death occurs in about 50% of cases, and treatment is as for agranulocytosis, with, obviously, blood transfusion.

6d. Haemolysis of all kinds is included here for convenience. There are three principal categories:

■ *Allergy (type II)* occurs with penicillins, methyldopa, levodopa, quinine, quinidine, sulfasalazine and organic antimony. In some of these cases a drug–protein–antigen/antibody interaction may involve erythrocytes only casually, i.e. a true 'innocent bystander' phenomenon.

■ *Dose-related pharmacodynamic action on normal cells,* e.g. lead, benzene, phenylhydrazine, chlorates (weed-killer), methyl chloride (refrigerant), some snake venoms.

■ *Idiosyncrasy* (see Pharmacogenetics). Precipitation of a haemolytic crisis may also occur with the above drugs in the rare genetic haemoglobinopathies. Treatment is to withdraw the drug, and an adrenal steroid is useful in severe cases if the mechanism is immunological. Blood transfusion may be needed.

7. Fever is common; a mechanism is the release of interleukin-1 by leucocytes into the circulation which acts on receptors in the hypothalamic thermoregulatory centre, releasing prostaglandin E_1.

8. Collagen diseases (type II) and syndromes resembling them. Systemic lupus erythematosus is sometimes caused by drugs, e.g. hydralazine, procainamide, isoniazid, sulphonamides. Adrenal steroid is useful.

9. Hepatitis and cholestatic jaundice are sometimes allergic (see Drugs and the Liver, p. 584). Adrenal steroid may be useful.

10. Nephropathy of various kinds (types II, III) occurs, as does damage to other organs, e.g. myocarditis. Adrenal steroid may be useful.

DIAGNOSIS OF DRUG ALLERGY

This still depends largely on clinical criteria, history, type of reaction, response to withdrawal and systemic re-challenge (if thought safe to do so).

Simple patch skin testing is naturally most useful in diagnosing contact dermatitis, but it is unreliable for other allergies. Skin prick tests are helpful in specialist hands for diagnosing IgE-dependent drug reactions, notably due to penicillin, cephalosporins, muscle relaxants, thiopental, streptokinase, cisplatin, insulin and latex. They can cause anaphylactic shock. False-positive results occur.

Development of reliable in vitro predictive tests, e.g. employing serum or lymphocytes, is a matter of considerable importance, not merely to remove hazard but also to avoid depriving patients of a drug that may be useful. Detection of drug-specific circulating IgE antibodies by the radioallergosorbent test (RAST) is best developed for penicillins and succinyl choline.

Drug allergy, once it has occurred, is not necessarily permanent, e.g. less than 50% of patients giving a history of allergy to penicillin have a reaction if it is given again.

DESENSITISATION

Once patients become allergic to a drug, it is better that they should never again come into contact with it. Desensitisation may be considered (in hospital) where a patient has suffered an IgE-mediated reaction to penicillin and requires the drug for serious infection, e.g. meningitis or endocarditis. Such people can be desensitised by giving very small amounts of allergen, which are than gradually increased (usually every few hours) until a normal dose is tolerated.

The procedure may necessitate cover with a corticosteroid and a β-adrenoceptor agonist (both of which inhibit mediator synthesis and release), and an H_1-receptor antihistamine may be added if an adverse reaction occurs. A full kit for treating anaphylactic shock should be at hand. Desensitisation may also be carried out for other antimicrobials, e.g. antituberculous drugs.

The mechanism underlying desensitisation may involve the production by the patient of blocking antibodies that compete successfully for the allergen but whose combination with it is innocuous; or the threshold of cells to the triggering antibodies may be raised. Sometimes allergy is to an ingredient of the preparation other than the essential drug, and merely changing the preparation is sufficient. Impurities are sometimes responsible, and purified penicillins and insulins reduce the incidence of reactions.

PREVENTION OF ALLERGIC REACTIONS

Prevention is important because these reactions are unpleasant and may be fatal; it provides good reason for taking a drug history. Patients should always be told if there is reason to believe they are allergic to a drug.

When looking for an alternative drug to avoid an adverse reaction, it is important not to select one from the same chemical group, as may inadvertently occur because the proprietary name gives no indication of the nature of the drug. This is another good reason for using the non-proprietary (generic) names as a matter of course.

> If a patient claims to be allergic to a drug then that drug should not be given without careful enquiry that may include testing (above): **neglect of this has caused death.**

PSEUDO-ALLERGIC REACTIONS

These are effects that mimic allergic reactions but have no immunological basis and are largely genetically determined. They are due to release of endogenous, biologically active substances, e.g. histamine and leukotrienes, by the drug. A variety of mechanisms is probably involved, direct and indirect, including complement activation leading to formation of polypeptides that affect mast cells, as in true immunological reactions. Some drugs may produce both allergic and pseudo-allergic reactions.

Pseudo-allergic effects mimicking type I reactions (above) are called *anaphylactoid*; they occur with aspirin and other non-steroidal anti-inflammatory drugs (indirect action as above) (see also Pulmonary reactions, above); corticotropin (direct histamine release); intravenous anaesthetics and a variety of other drugs given intravenously (morphine, tubocurarine, dextran, radiographic contrast media) and inhaled (cromoglicate). Severe cases are treated as for true allergic anaphylactic shock (above), from which, at the time, they are not distinguishable.

Type II reactions are mimicked by the haemolysis induced by drugs (some antimalarials, sulphonamides and oxidising agents) and food (broad beans) in subjects with inherited abnormalities of erythrocyte enzymes or haemoglobin (see p. 107).

Type III reactions are mimicked by nitrofurantoin (pneumonitis) and penicillamine (nephropathy). Lupus erythematosus due to drugs (procainamide, isoniazid, phenytoin) may be pseudo-allergic.

MISCELLANEOUS ADVERSE REACTIONS

Transient reactions to intravenous injections are fairly common, resulting in hypotension, renal pain, fever or rigors, especially if the injection is very rapid.

EFFECTS OF PROLONGED ADMINISTRATION: CHRONIC ORGAN TOXICITY

Although the majority of adverse events occur within days or weeks after a drug is administered, some reactions develop only after months or years of exposure. In general, pharmacovigilance programmes reveal such effects; once recognised, they demand careful monitoring during chronic drug therapy for their occurrence may carry serious consequences for the patient (and the non-vigilant doctor, medicolegally). Descriptions of such reactions appear with the accounts of relevant drugs; some examples are given.

Eye. Toxic cataract can be due to chloroquine and related drugs, adrenal steroids (topical and systemic), phenothiazines and alkylating agents. Corneal opacities occur with phenothiazines and chloroquine. Retinal injury develops with thioridazine (particularly, of the antipsychotics), chloroquine and indometacin, and visual field defects with vigabatrin.

Nervous system. Tardive dyskinesias occur with neuroleptics; polyneuritis with metronidazole; optic neuritis with ethambutol.

Lung. Amiodarone may cause pulmonary fibrosis. Sulfasalazine is associated with fibrosing alveolitis.

Kidney. Gold salts may cause nephropathy; see also analgesic nephropathy (p. 257).

Liver. Methotrexate may cause liver damage and hepatic fibrosis; amiodarone may induce steatohepatitis (fatty liver) (see also alcohol, p. 152).

Carcinogenesis: see also Preclinical testing (p. 32). Mechanisms of carcinogenesis are complex; prediction from animal tests is uncertain and causal attribution in humans has finally to be based on epidemiological studies. The principal mechanisms are:

- *Alteration of DNA* (genotoxicity, mutagenicity). Many chemicals or their metabolites act by causing mutations, activating oncogenes; those substances that are used as medicines include griseofulvin and alkylating cytotoxics. Leukaemias and lymphomas are the most common malignancies.
- *Immunosuppression.* Malignancies develop in immunosuppressed patients, e.g. after organ transplantation and cancer chemotherapy. There is a high incidence of lymphoid neoplasm. Chlorambucil, melphelan and thiotepa present particular high relative risks. The use of immunosuppression in, e.g. rheumatoid arthritis, also increases the incidence of neoplasms.
- *Hormonal.* Long-term use of oestrogen replacement in postmenopausal women induces endometrial cancer. Combined oestrogen/progestogen oral contraceptives may both suppress and enhance cancers (see p. 646, 651). Diethylstilbestrol caused vaginal adenosis and cancer in the *offspring* of mothers who took it during pregnancy in the hope of preventing miscarriage. It was used for this purpose for decades after its introduction in the 1940s, on purely theoretical grounds. Controlled therapeutic trials were not done and there was no valid evidence of therapeutic efficacy. Male fetuses developed non-malignant genital abnormalities.[19]

Carcinogenesis due to medicines requires that drug exposure be prolonged,[20] i.e. months or years; the cancers develop most commonly over 3–5 years, but sometimes years after treatment has ceased. There is a higher incidence of secondary cancers in patients treated for a primary cancer.

---

[19]Herbst A L 1984 Diethylstilboestrol exposure – 1984 [effects of exposure during pregnancy on mother and daughters]. New England Journal of Medicine 311:1433–1435.
[20]Carcinogens that are effective as a single dose in animals are known, e.g. nitrosamines.

ADVERSE EFFECTS ON REPRODUCTION

The medical profession has a grave duty to refrain from all unessential prescribing for women of childbearing potential of drugs with, say, less than 10–15 years of widespread use behind them. It is not sufficient safeguard merely to ask a woman if she is or may be pregnant, for it is also necessary to consider the possibility of a woman, who is not pregnant at the time of prescribing, may become so whilst taking the drug.

Testing of new drugs on animals for their effects on reproduction has been mandatory since the thalidomide disaster, even though the extrapolation of the findings to humans is uncertain (see Preclinical testing, p. 32). The placental transfer of drugs from the mother to the fetus is considered on page 83.

Drugs may act on the embryo and fetus:

- *Directly* (thalidomide, cytotoxic drugs, antithyroid drugs, aromatic retinoids, e.g. isotretinoin): any drug affecting cell division, enzymes, protein synthesis or DNA synthesis is a potential teratogen, e.g. many antimicrobials.
- *Indirectly*:
  - on the uterus (vasoconstrictors reduce blood supply and cause fetal anoxia, misoprostol causes uterine contraction leading to abortion)
  - on the mother's hormone balance.

Early pregnancy. During the first week after fertilisation, exposure to antimetabolites, misoprostol, ergot alkaloids or diethylstilbestrol can cause abortion, which may not be recognised as such. The most vulnerable period for major anatomical abnormality is that of organogenesis which occurs during weeks 2–8 of intrauterine life (4–10 weeks after the first day of the last menstruation). After the organs are formed, abnormalities are less anatomically dramatic. Thus the activity of a teratogen (*teratos*, monster) is most devastating soon after implantation, at doses that may not harm the mother and at a time when she may not know she is pregnant.

Drugs known to be teratogenic include cytotoxics, warfarin, alcohol, lithium, methotrexate, phenytoin, sodium valproate, angiotensin-converting enzyme (ACE) inhibitors and isotretinoin. Selective interference can produce characteristic anatomical abnormalities; the phocomelia (flipper-like) limb defect was one factor that caused the effects of thalidomide to be recognised so readily (see p. 62).

Innumerable drugs have come under suspicion. Those for which evidence of safety was subsequently found include diazepam, oral contraceptives, spermicides and salicylates. Naturally the subject is a highly emotional one for prospective parents. A definitive list of unsafe drugs is not practicable. Much depends on the dose taken and at what stage of pregnancy. The topic must be followed in the current literature.

Late pregnancy. Because the important organs are already formed, drugs will not cause the gross anatomical defects that can occur following exposure in early pregnancy. Administration of hormones, androgens or progestogens, can cause fetal masculinisation; iodide and antithyroid drugs in high dose can cause fetal goitre, as can lithium; tetracyclines can interfere with tooth and bone development, ACE inhibitors are associated with renal tubular dysgenesis and a skull ossification defect. Tobacco smoking retards fetal growth; it does not cause anatomical abnormalities in humans as far as is known.

Inhibitors of prostaglandin synthesis (aspirin, indometacin) may delay onset of labour and, in the fetus, cause closure of the ductus arteriosus, patency of which is dependent on prostaglandins.

The suggestion that congenital cataract (due to denaturation of lens protein) might be due to drugs has some support in humans. Chloroquine and chlorpromazine are concentrated in the fetal eye. As both can cause retinopathy, it would seem wise to avoid them in pregnancy if possible.

For a discussion of anticoagulants in pregnancy, see page 518.

Drugs given to the mother just prior to labour can cause postnatal effects. CNS depressants may persist in and affect the baby for days after birth; vasoconstrictors can cause fetal distress by reducing uterine blood supply; β-adrenoceptor blockers may impair fetal response to hypoxia; sulphonamides displace bilirubin from plasma protein (risk of kernicterus).

Babies born to mothers dependent on opioids may show a physical withdrawal syndrome.

Drugs given during labour. Any drug that acts to depress respiration in the mother can cause respiratory depression in the newborn; opioid analgesics are notorious in this respect, but there can also be difficulty with any sedatives and general anaesthetics; they may also cause fetal distress by reducing uterine blood flow, and prolong labour by depressing uterine muscle.

Diazepam (and other depressants) in high doses may cause hypotonia in the baby and possibly interfere with suckling. There remains the possibility of later behavioural effects as a result of impaired development of the central nervous system due to psychotropic drugs used during pregnancy; such effects have been shown in animals.

Detection of teratogens. Anatomical abnormalities are the easiest to detect. Non-anatomical (functional) effects can also occur; they include effects on brain biochemistry that may have late behavioural consequences.

There is a substantial spontaneous background incidence of birth defect in the community (up to 2%), so the detection of a low-grade teratogen that increases the incidence of one of the commoner abnormalities presents an intimidating task. In addition, most teratogenic effects are probably multifactorial. In this emotionally charged area it is indeed hard for the public, and especially for parents of an affected child, to grasp that:

> The concept of absolute safety of drugs needs to be demolished ... In real life it can never be shown that a drug (or anything else) has no teratogenic activity at all, in the sense of never being a contributory factor in anybody under any circumstances. This concept can neither be tested nor proved.
>
> Let us suppose for example, that some agent doubles the incidence of a condition that has natural incidence of 1 in 10 000 births. If the hypothesis is true, then studying 20 000 pregnant women who have taken the drug and 20 000 who have not may yield respectively two cases and one case of the abnormality. It does not take a statistician to realise that this signifies nothing, and it may need ten times as many pregnant women (almost half a million) to produce a statistically significant result. This would involve such an extensive multicentre study that hundreds of doctors and hospitals have to participate. The participants then each tend to bend the protocol to fit in with their clinical customs and in the end it is difficult to assess the validity of the data.
>
> Alternatively, a limited geographical basis may be used, with the trial going on for many years. During this time other things in the environment change, so again the results would not command our confidence. If it were to be suggested that there was something slightly teratogenic in milk, the hypothesis would be virtually untestable.

In practice we have to make up our minds which drugs may reasonably be given to pregnant women. Do we start from a position of presumed guilt or from one of presumed innocence? If the former course is chosen then we cannot give any drugs to pregnant women because we can never prove that they are completely free of teratogenic influence. It therefore seems that we must start from a position of presumed innocence and then take all possible steps to find out if the presumption is correct.

Finally, we must put the matter in perspective by considering the benefit/risk ratio. The problem of prescription in pregnancy cannot be considered from the point of view of only one side of the equation. Drugs are primarily designed to do good, and if a pregnant woman is ill it is in the best interests of her baby and herself that she gets better as quickly as possible. This often means giving her drugs. We can argue about the necessity of giving drugs to prevent vomiting, but there is no argument about the need for treatment of women with meningitis, septicaemia or venereal disease.

What we must try to avoid is medication by the media or prescription by politicians. A public scare about a well-tried drug will lead to wider use of less-tried alternatives. We do not want to be forced to practise the kind of defensive medicine that is primarily designed to avoid litigation.[21]

MALE REPRODUCTIVE FUNCTION

Impotence may occur with drugs affecting autonomic sympathetic function, e.g. some antihypertensives.

Spermatogenesis is reduced by a number of drugs including sulfasalazine and mesalazine (reversible), cytotoxic anticancer drugs (reversible and irreversible) and nitrofurantoin. There has been a global decline in sperm concentration and an environmental cause, e.g. chemicals that possess oestrogenic activity, seems likely.

Causation of birth defects due to abnormal sperm remains uncertain.

GUIDE TO FURTHER READING

Aronson J K, Ferner R E 2003 Joining the DoTS: new approach to classifying adverse drug reactions. British Medical Journal 327:1222–1225

Edwards I R, Aronson J K 2000 Adverse drug reactions: definitions, diagnosis, and management. Lancet 356:1255–1259

Eigenmann P A, Haenggeli C A 2004 Food colourings and preservatives – allergy and hyperactivity. Lancet 364:823–824

Ferner R E, McDowell S E 2006 Doctors charged with manslaughter in the course of medical practice, 1795–2005: a literature review. Journal of the Royal Society of Medicine 99(6):309–314

Gray J 2007 Why can't a woman be more like a man? Clinical Pharmacology and Therapeutics 82(1):15–17

Greenhalgh T, Kostopoulou O, Harries C 2004 Making decisions about benefits and harms of medicines. British Medical Journal 329:47–50

Gruchalla R S 2000 Clinical assessment of drug-induced disease. Lancet 356:1505–1511

Kaufman D W, Shapiro S 2000 Epidemiological assessment of drug-induced disease. Lancet 356:1339–1343

Knowles S R, Uetrecht J, Shear N H 2000 Idiosyncratic drug reactions: the reactive metabolite syndromes. Lancet 356:1587–1591

Koren D, Pastuszak A, Ito S 1998 Drugs in pregnancy. New England Journal of Medicine 338(16):1128–1137 *Article lists drugs that are safe and unsafe to use in pregnancy*

Meyer U A 2000 Pharmacogenetics and adverse drug reactions. Lancet 356:1667–1671

Morrison-Griffiths S, Walley T J, Park B K, Breckenridge A M, Pirmohamed M 2003 Reporting of adverse drug reactions by nurses. Lancet 361:1347–1348

Peters T J, Sarkany R 2005 Porphyria for the general physician. Clinical Medicine 5(3):275–281

Strickler B H C, Psaty B M 2004 Detection, verification, and quantification of adverse drug reactions. British Medical Journal 329:44–47

Trontell A 2004 Expecting the unexpected – drug safety, pharmacovigilance and the prepared mind. New England Journal of Medicine 351(14):1385–1387

Woosley R L 2004 Discovering adverse reactions: Why does it take so long? Clinical Pharmacology and Therapeutics 76(4):287–289

[21]By permission from Smithells R W 1983 In: Hawkins D F (ed.) Drugs and pregnancy. Churchill Livingstone, Edinburgh.

9

Poisoning, overdose, antidotes

SYNOPSIS

Deliberate overdose with drugs is a common clinical problem. Poisoning also occurs in other ways: by accident, use of recreational substances and occupational exposure. Specific methods of counteracting acute and chronic poisons arise from an understanding of the mechanisms involved; together with general measures, these offer scope for effective management.

- Deliberate and accidental self-poisoning
- Principles of treatment
- Poison-specific measures and antidotes
- General measures
- Specific poisonings: cyanide, methanol, ethylene glycol, hydrocarbons, volatile solvents, heavy metals, herbicides and pesticides, biological substances (overdose of medicinal drugs is dealt with under individual agents)
- Incapacitating agents: drugs used for torture

SELF-POISONING

Poisoning is the means chosen in over 90% of instances of deliberate self-harm in the UK, usually by medicines taken in overdose. These amount to at least 70 000 hospital admissions per annum in England and Wales (population 51 million). Prescribed drugs are used in more than 75% of episodes, but teenagers tend to favour non-prescribed analgesics available by direct sale, e.g. paracetamol, which is important bearing in mind its potentially serious toxicity. The mortality rate of self-poisoning is very low (less than 1% of acute hospital admissions), but 'completed' suicides by poisoning still number 3500 per annum in England and Wales.

Accidental self-poisoning, causing admission to hospital, occurs predominantly amongst children under 5 years of age, usually from medicines left within their reach or with domestic chemicals, e.g. bleach, detergents.

PRINCIPLES OF TREATMENT

Successful treatment of acute poisoning depends on a combination of speed and common sense, as well as on the nature of the poison, the amount taken and the time that has since elapsed. The majority of those admitted to hospital require only observation and medical and nursing supportive measures while they metabolise and eliminate the poison. Some require a specific antidote or a specific measure to increase elimination. Only a few need intensive care facilities.

In the UK regional medicines information centres provide specialist advice and information over the telephone throughout the day and night (0870 600 6266). Additionally, TOXBASE, the primary clinical toxicology database of the UK National Poisons Information Service, is available on the internet to registered users for the routine diagnosis, treatment and management of patients exposed to drugs, household products, and industrial and agricultural chemicals at: http://www.spib.axl.co.uk.

POISON-SPECIFIC MEASURES

IDENTIFICATION OF THE POISON(S)

The key pieces of information are:

- the identity of the substance(s) taken
- the dose(s)
- the time that has since elapsed.

Adults may be sufficiently conscious to give some indication of the poison or may have referred to it in a suicide note, or there may be other circumstantial evidence. Rapid (1–2 h) biochemical 'screens' of plasma or urine are available but are best reserved for seriously ill or unconscious patients in whom the cause of coma is unknown.

Analysis of plasma for specific substances is essential in suspected cases of paracetamol or iron poisoning, to indicate which patients should receive antidotes; plasma concentration measurement is also used to quantify the risk in overdose of salicylate, lithium and some sedative drugs, e.g. trichloroethanol derivatives, phenobarbital, when particular treatments, e.g. haemodialysis, urine alkalinisation, may be indicated.

Response to a specific antidote may provide a diagnosis, e.g. dilatation of constricted pupils and increased respiratory rate after intravenous naloxone (opioid poisoning) or arousal from unconsciousness in response to intravenous flumazenil (benzodiazepine poisoning).

PREVENTION OF FURTHER ABSORPTION OF THE POISON

From the environment

When a poison has been inhaled or absorbed through the skin, the patient should be taken from the toxic environment, the contaminated clothing removed and the skin cleansed.

From the alimentary tract ('gut decontamination')[1]

Gastric lavage confers little benefit and is associated with risk (laryngospasm, hypoxia, arrhythmia, perforation). It may be considered in extraordinary circumstances for the hospitalised adult who is believed to have ingested a potentially life-threatening amount of a poison within the previous hour, and provided the airways are protected by a cuffed endotracheal tube. It is contraindicated for a corrosive substance, a hydrocarbon with high aspiration potential or if there is risk of haemorrhage from an underlying gastrointestinal condition.

Emesis, using Syrup of Ipecacuanha, is no longer practised in hospital, as there is no clinical trial evidence that the procedure improves outcome. Rarely, it may be justified out of hospital, e.g. with no alternative therapy and anticipated delay in reaching an emergency facility.

Oral adsorbents. Activated charcoal (Carbomix) consists of a very fine black powder prepared from vegetable matter, e.g. wood pulp, coconut shell, which is 'activated' by an oxidising gas flow at high temperature to create a network of small (10–20 nm) pores to create an enormous surface area in relation to weight ($1000 \, \text{m}^2/\text{g}$). This binds to, and thus inactivates, a wide variety of compounds in the gut. Indeed, activated charcoal comes nearest to fulfilling the long-sought notion of a 'universal antidote'.[2] Thus it is simpler to list the exceptions, i.e. substances that are *poorly adsorbed* by charcoal, namely:

- metal salts (iron, lithium)
- cyanide
- alcohols (ethanol, methanol, ethylene glycol)
- petroleum distillates
- clofenotane (dicophane, DDT)
- malathion
- strong acids and alkalis
- corrosive agents.

To be most effective, five to ten times as much charcoal as poison, weight for weight, is needed. In the adult an initial dose of 50 g is usual, repeated if necessary. If the patient is vomiting, give the charcoal through a nasogastric tube.

Activated charcoal is most effective when given quickly after ingestion of a potentially toxic amount of a poison and whilst a significant amount remains yet unabsorbed; administration within 1 h can be expected to prevent some 40–50% of absorption.

Charcoal in repeated doses accelerates the elimination of poison that has been absorbed (see p. 133).

Activated charcoal, although unpalatable, appears to be relatively safe but constipation or mechanical bowel obstruction may follow repeated use. In the drowsy or comatose patient there is particular risk of aspiration into the lungs causing hypoxia through obstruction and arteriovenous shunting. Note that methionine, used orally for paracetamol poisoning, is adsorbed.

---

[1] Joint position statements and guidelines agreed by the American Academy of Clinical Toxicology and the European Association of Poison Centres and Clinical Toxicologists review the therapeutic usefulness of various procedures for gut decontamination. These appear in the *Journal of Toxicology. Clinical Toxicology* from 1997 onwards.

[2] For centuries it was supposed not only that there could be, but that there actually was, a single antidote to all poisons. This was Theriaca Andromachi, a formulation of 72 (a magical number) ingredients amongst which particular importance was attached to the flesh of a snake (viper). The antidote was devised by Andromachus, whose son was physician to the Roman Emperor, Nero (AD 37–68).

Other oral adsorbents have specific uses. Fuller's earth (a natural form of aluminium silicate) binds and inactivates the herbicides paraquat (activated charcoal is superior) and diquat; colestyramine and colestipol will adsorb warfarin.

Whole-bowel irrigation[3] has been used for the removal of sustained-release or enteric-coated formulations from patients who present more than 2 h after ingestion, e.g. iron, theophylline, aspirin. Evidence of benefit is conflicting. Activated charcoal in frequent (50 g) doses is generally preferred. Sustained-release formulations are common, and patients have died from failure to recognise the danger of continued release of drug from such products. Whole-bowel irrigation is also an option for the removal of ingested packets of illicit drugs (see p. 146).

Cathartics have no routine role in gut decontamination, but a single dose of an osmotic agent (sorbitol, magnesium sulphate) may be justified on occasion.

SPECIFIC ANTIDOTES[4]

Specific antidotes reduce or abolish the effects of poisons through a variety of mechanisms, indicated in Figure 9.1. Table 9.1 illustrates these mechanisms with antidotes that are of therapeutic value.

CHELATING AGENTS

Acute or chronic exposure to heavy metals can harm the body.[5] Treatment is with chelating agents which

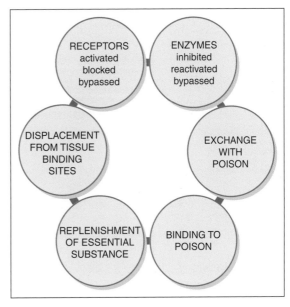

Fig. 9.1 Mechanisms by which specific antidotes reduce or abolish the effects of poisons.

incorporate the metal ions into an inner ring structure in the molecule (Greek: *chele*, claw) by means of structural groups called ligands (Latin: *ligare*, to bind). Effective agents form stable, biologically inert complexes that pass into the urine.

Dimercaprol (British Anti-Lewisite, BAL). Arsenic and other metal ions are toxic in low concentration because they combine with the SH- groups of essential enzymes, thus inactivating them. Dimercaprol provides SH- groups, which combine with the metal ions to form relatively harmless ring compounds that pass from the body, mainly in the urine. As dimercaprol itself is oxidised in the body and excreted renally, repeated administration is necessary to ensure that an excess is available to eliminate all of the metal.

---

[3]Irrigation with large volumes of a polyethylene glycol–electrolyte solution, e.g. Klean-Prep, by mouth causes minimal fluid and electrolyte disturbance (it was developed for preparation for colonoscopy). Magnesium sulphate may also be used.

[4]Mithridates the Great (?132–63 BC), king of Pontus (in Asia Minor), was noted for 'ambition, cruelty and artifice'. 'He murdered his own mother … and fortified his constitution by drinking antidotes' to the poisons with which his domestic enemies sought to kill him (Lemprière). When his son also sought to kill him, Mithridates was so disappointed that he compelled his wife to poison herself. He then tried to poison himself, but in vain; the frequent antidotes that he had taken in the early part of his life had so strengthened his constitution that he was immune. He was obliged to stab himself, but had to seek the help of a slave to complete his task. Modern physicians have to be content with less comprehensively effective antidotes, some of which are listed in Table 9.1.

[5]Sometimes in unexpected ways; an initiation custom in an artillery regiment involved pouring wine through the barrel of a gun after several shots had been fired. A healthy 19-year-old soldier drank 250 mL of the wine and within 15 min convulsed and became unconscious. His plasma, urine and the wine contained high concentrations of tungsten. He received haemodialysis and recovered. Investigation revealed that the gun barrels had recently been hardened by the addition of tungsten to the steel. Marquet P, François B, Vignon P, Lachâtre G 1996 A soldier who had seizures after drinking a quarter of a litre of wine. Lancet 348:1070.

Table 9.1 Some specific antidotes, indications and modes of action (see Index for a fuller account of individual drugs)

Antidote	Indication	Mode of action
acetylcysteine	paracetamol, chloroform, carbon tetrachloride, radiocontrast nephropathy	Replenishes depleted glutathione stores
atropine	cholinesterase inhibitors, e.g. organophosphorus insecticides	Blocks muscarinic cholinoceptors
	β-blocker poisoning	Vagal block accelerates heart rate
benzatropine	drug-induced movement disorders	Blocks muscarinic cholinoceptors
calcium gluconate	hydrofluoric acid, fluorides	Binds or precipitates fluoride ions
desferrioxamine	iron	Chelates ferrous ions
dicobalt edetate	cyanide and derivatives, e.g. acrylonitrile	Chelates to form non-toxic cobalti- and cobalto-cyanides
digoxin-specific antibody fragments (FAB)	digitalis glycosides	Binds free glycoside in plasma, complex excreted in urine
dimercaprol (BAL)	arsenic, copper, gold, lead, inorganic mercury	Chelates metal ions
ethanol (or fomepizole)	ethylene glycol, methanol	Competes for alcohol and acetaldehyde dehydrogenases, preventing formation of toxic metabolites
flumazenil	benzodiazepines	Competes for benzodiazepine receptors
folinic acid	folic acid antagonists, e.g. methotrexate, trimethoprim	Bypasses block in folate metabolism
glucagon	β-adrenoceptor antagonists	Bypasses blockade of the β-adrenoceptor; stimulates cyclic AMP formation with positive cardiac inotropic effect
isoprenaline	β-adrenoceptor antagonists	Competes for and activates β- adrenoceptors
methionine	paracetamol	Replenishes depleted glutathione stores
naloxone	opioids	Competes for opioid receptors
neostigmine	antimuscarinic drugs	Inhibits acetylcholinesterase, causing acetylcholine to accumulate at cholinoceptors
oxygen	carbon monoxide	Competitively displaces carbon monoxide from binding sites on haemoglobin
penicillamine	copper, gold, lead, elemental mercury (vapour), zinc	Chelates metal ions
phenoxybenzamine	hypertension due to α-adrenoceptor agonists, e.g. with MAOI, clonidine, ergotamine	Competes for and blocks α-adrenoceptors (long acting)
phentolamine	as above	Competes for and blocks α-adrenoceptors (short acting)
phytomenadione (vitamin K_1)	coumarin (warfarin) and indandione anticoagulants	Replenishes vitamin K
pralidoxime	cholinesterase inhibitors, e.g. organophosphorus insecticides	Competitively reactivates cholinesterase
propranolol	β-adrenoceptor agonists, ephedrine, theophylline, thyroxine	Blocks β-adrenoceptors
protamine	heparin	Binds ionically to neutralise
Prussian blue (potassium ferric hexacyanoferrate)	thallium (in rodenticides)	Potassium exchanges for thallium
sodium calciumedetate	lead	Chelates lead ions
unithiol	lead, elemental and organic mercury	Chelates metal ions

Dimercaprol may be used in cases of poisoning by antimony, arsenic, bismuth, gold and mercury (inorganic, e.g. $HgCl_2$).

Adverse effects are common, particularly with larger doses, and include nausea and vomiting, lachrymation and salivation, paraesthesiae, muscular aches and pains, urticarial rashes, tachycardia and raised blood pressure. Gross overdosage may cause over-breathing, muscular tremors, convulsions and coma.

Unithiol (dimercaptopropanesulphonate, DMPS) effectively chelates lead and mercury; it is well tolerated.

Sodium calciumedetate is the calcium chelate of the disodium salt of ethylenediaminetetra-acetic acid (calcium EDTA). It is effective in acute lead poisoning because of its capacity to exchange calcium for lead: the kidney excretes the lead chelate, leaving behind a harmless amount of calcium. Dimercaprol may usefully be combined with sodium calciumedetate when lead poisoning is severe, e.g. with encephalopathy.

Adverse effects are fairly common, and include hypotension, lachrymation, nasal stuffiness, sneezing, muscle pains and chills. Renal damage can occur.

Dicobalt edetate. Cobalt forms stable, non-toxic complexes with cyanide (see p. 136). It is toxic (especially if the wrong diagnosis is made and no cyanide is present), causing hypertension, tachycardia and chest pain; consequent cobalt poisoning is treated by giving sodium calciumedetate and intravenous glucose.

Penicillamine (dimethylcysteine) is a metabolite of penicillin that contains SH- groups; it may be used to chelate lead and copper (see Hepatolenticular degeneration, p. 386). Its principal use is for rheumatoid arthritis (see Index).

Desferrioxamine. See Iron (p. 533).

ACCELERATION OF ELIMINATION OF THE POISON

Techniques for eliminating poisons have a role that is limited, but important when applicable. Each method depends, directly or indirectly, on removing drug from the circulation and successful use requires that:

- The poison should be present in high concentration in the plasma relative to that in the rest of the body, i.e. it should have a small distribution volume.
- The poison should dissociate readily from any plasma protein binding sites.
- The effects of the poison should relate to its plasma concentration.

Methods used are:

Repeated doses of activated charcoal

Activated charcoal by mouth not only adsorbs ingested drug in the gut, preventing absorption into the body (see above), it also adsorbs drug that diffuses from the blood into the gut lumen when the concentration there is lower. As binding is irreversible, the concentration gradient is maintained and drug is continuously removed; this has been called 'intestinal dialysis'. Charcoal may also adsorb drugs that secrete into the bile, i.e. by interrupting an enterohepatic cycle.

The procedure is effective for overdose of *carbamazepine, dapsone, phenobarbital, quinine, salicylate* and *theophylline*. Repeated-dose activated charcoal is increasingly preferred to alkalinisation of urine (below) for phenobarbital and salicylate poisoning.

In adults, activated charcoal 50 g is given initially, then 50 g every 4 h. Vomiting should be treated with an antiemetic drug because it reduces the efficacy of charcoal treatment. Where there is intolerance, the dose may be reduced and the frequency increased, e.g. 25 g every 2 h *or* 12.5 g every hour, but efficacy may be compromised.

Alteration of urine pH and diuresis

It is useful to alter the pH of the glomerular filtrate such that a drug that is a weak electrolyte will ionise, become less lipid soluble, remain in the renal tubular fluid, and leave the body in the urine (see p. 82).

Maintenance of a good urine flow (e.g. 100 mL/h) helps this process, but the alteration of tubular fluid pH is the important determinant. The practice of forcing diuresis with furosemide and large volumes of intravenous fluid does not add significantly to drug clearance but may cause fluid overload; it is obsolete.

Alkalinisation[6] may be used for salicylate (>500 mg/L + metabolic acidosis, or in any case >750 mg/L), phenobarbital (75–150 mg/L) or phenoxy herbicides, e.g. 2,4-D, mecoprop, dichlorprop.

The objective is to maintain a urine pH of 7.5–8.5 by an intravenous infusion of sodium bicarbonate. Available preparations of sodium bicarbonate vary between 1.2 and 8.4% (1 mL of the 8.4% preparation contains 1 mmol sodium bicarbonate) and the concentration given will depend on the patient's fluid needs.

Acidification may be used for severe, acute amfetamine, dexfenfluramine or phencyclidine poisoning. The objective is to maintain a urine pH of 5.5–6.5 by giving an intravenous infusion of arginine hydrochloride (10 g) over 30 min, followed by ammonium chloride (4 g) every 2 h by mouth. It is rarely necessary. Hypertension due to amfetamine-like drugs, for example, will respond to phenoxybenzamine (by α-adrenoceptor block).

Haemodialysis

The system requires a temporary extracorporeal circulation, e.g. from an artery to a vein in the arm. A semipermeable membrane separates blood from dialysis fluid; the poison passes passively from the blood, where it is present in high concentration to enter the dialysis fluid, which is flowing and thus constantly replaced.

Haemodialysis significantly increases the elimination of: salicylate (>750 mg/L + renal failure, or in any case >900 mg/L), isopropanol (present in aftershave lotions and window-cleaning solutions), lithium and methanol, ethylene glycol, ethanol.

Haemofiltration

An extracorporeal circulation brings blood into contact with a highly permeable membrane. Water is lost by ultrafiltration (the rate being dependent on the hydrostatic pressure gradient across membrane) and solutes by convection; the main change in plasma concentrations results from replacement of ultrafiltrate with an appropriate solution.

Haemofiltration is effective for: phenobarbital (>100–150 mg/L, but repeat-dose activated charcoal by mouth appears to be as effective; see above)

---

[6]Proudfoot A T, Krenzelok E P, Vale J A 2004 Position paper on urine alkalinization. Journal of Toxicology Clinical Toxicology 42:1–26.

and other barbiturates, ethchlorvynol, glutethimide, meprobamate, methaqualone, theophylline, trichloroethanol derivatives.

Peritoneal dialysis

This involves instilling appropriate fluid into the peritoneal cavity. Poison in the blood diffuses down the concentration gradient into the dialysis fluid, which undergoes repeated drainage and replacement. The technique requires little equipment; it may be worth using for lithium and methanol poisoning.

Haemofiltration and peritoneal dialysis are more readily available but are less efficient (one-half to one-third) than haemodialysis.

Haemodialysis and haemoperfusion are invasive, demand skill and experience on the part of the operator and are costly in terms of staffing. Their use should be confined to cases of severe, prolonged or progressive clinical intoxication, when high plasma concentration indicates a dangerous degree of poisoning, and their effect constitutes a significant addition to natural methods of elimination.

GENERAL MEASURES

INITIAL ASSESSMENT AND RESUSCITATION

The initial clinical review should include a search for known toxic syndromes (see below).

Maintenance of an adequate oxygen supply is the first priority and the airway must be sucked clear of oropharyngeal secretions or regurgitated matter.

Shock in acute poisoning is usually due to expansion of the venous capacitance bed and placing the patient in the head-down position to encourage venous return to the heart, or a colloid plasma expander such as gelatin or etherified starch administered intravenously restores blood pressure.

External cardiac compression may be necessary and should be continued until the cardiac output is self-sustaining, which may be a long time when the patient is hypothermic or poisoned with a cardiodepressant drug, e.g. tricyclic antidepressant, β-adrenoceptor blocker.

Investigations include biochemical screening of plasma for commonly used agents, e.g. paracetamol (which initially produces no characteristic signs), and measurement of plasma electrolytes. Hypokalaemia (e.g. due to β$_2$-agonist, theophylline, chloroquine, alkalosis or gastrointestinal loss) is commoner than hyperkalaemia (e.g. due to acidosis or rhabdomyolysis). Respiratory insufficiency or hyperventilation calls for blood gas analysis.

SUPPORTIVE TREATMENT

The salient fact is the most efficient eliminating mechanisms are the patient's own, which, given time, will inactivate and eliminate all the poison. Most patients recover from acute poisonings provided they are adequately oxygenated, hydrated and perfused. Special problems introduced by poisoning are:

Airway maintenance is essential; some patients require a cuffed endotracheal tube but seldom for more than 24 h.

Ventilation. A mixed respiratory and metabolic acidosis is common. Supplementing the inspired air with oxygen corrects hypoxia and mechanical ventilation is necessary if the $Paco_2$ exceeds 6.5 kPa.

Hypotension is common and, in addition to the resuscitative measures indicated above, infusion of a combination of dopamine and dobutamine in low dose may be required to maintain renal perfusion.

Convulsions should be treated if they are persistent or protracted. Intravenous diazepam is the first choice.

Cardiac arrhythmia frequently accompanies poisoning, e.g. with tricyclic antidepressants, theophylline, β-adrenoceptor blockers. Acidosis, hypoxia and electrolyte disturbance are often important contributory factors and it is preferable to observe the effect of correcting these before considering resort to an antiarrhythmic drug. If arrhythmia does lead to persistent peripheral circulatory failure, an appropriate drug may be justifed, e.g. a β-adrenoceptor blocker for poisoning with a sympathomimetic drug.

Hypothermia may occur if CNS depression impairs temperature regulation. A low-reading rectal thermometer is used to monitor core temperature, while the patient is nursed in a heat-retaining 'space blanket'.

Immobility may lead to pressure lesions of peripheral nerves, cutaneous blisters and necrosis over bony prominences.

Rhabdomyolysis may result from prolonged pressure on muscles, from agents that cause muscle spasm or convulsions (phencyclidine, theophylline) or be aggravated by hyperthermia due to muscle contraction, e.g. with MDMA ('ecstasy'). Aggressive volume repletion and correction of acid–base abnormality are needed, and urine alkalinisation may prevent acute tubular necrosis.

PSYCHIATRIC AND SOCIAL ASSESSMENT

Interpersonal or social problems precipitate most cases of self-poisoning and require attention. Treat major psychiatric illness, when it is identified.

> There are said to be occasions when a wise man chooses suicide – but generally speaking it is not in an excess of reasonableness that people kill themselves.[7]

SOME POISONINGS

CHARACTERISTIC TOXIC SYNDROMES ('TOXIDROMES')[8]

Many substances used in accidental or self-poisoning produce recognisable symptoms and signs. Some arise from dysfunction of the central or autonomic nervous systems; other agents produce individual effects. They can be useful diagnostically.

Antimuscarinic syndromes consist of tachycardia, dilated pupils, dry, flushed skin, urinary retention, decreased bowel sounds, mild increase in body temperature, confusion, cardiac arrhythmias and seizures. Antipsychotics, tricyclic antidepressants, antihistamines, antispasmodics and many plants (see p. 138) are causal.

Cholinergic (muscarinic) syndromes comprise salivation, lachrymation, abdominal cramps, urinary and faecal incontinence, vomiting, sweating, miosis, muscle fasciculation and weakness, bradycardia, pulmonary oedema, confusion, CNS depression and fitting. Common causes include organophosphorus and carbamate insecticides, neostigmine

---

[7]Voltaire (pseudonym of Francois-Marie Arouet, French writer, 1694–1778).
[8]Based on Kulig K 1992 Initial management of ingestions of toxic substances. New England Journal of Medicine 326:1677–1681.

and other anticholinesterase drugs, and some fungi (mushrooms).

Sympathomimetic syndromes include tachycardia, hypertension, hyperthermia, sweating, mydriasis, hyperreflexia, agitation, delusions, paranoia, seizures and cardiac arrhythmias. Amphetamine and its derivatives, cocaine, ecstasy, proprietary decongestants, e.g. ephedrine, and theophylline (in the latter case, excluding psychiatric effects), are common causes.

Sedatives, opioids and ethanol cause signs that may include respiratory depression, miosis, hyporeflexia, coma, hypotension and hypothermia.

Other drugs and non-drug chemicals that produce characteristic effects include: salicylates, methanol and ethylene glycol, iron, selective serotonin reuptake inhibitors (see Index).

Effects of overdose with other individual drugs or drug groups appear in the relevant accounts throughout the book.

POISONINGS BY (NON-DRUG) CHEMICALS

Cyanide causes tissue anoxia by chelating the ferric part of the intracellular respiratory enzyme, cytochrome oxidase. Poisoning may occur as a result of self-administration of hydrocyanic (prussic) acid, by accidental exposure in industry, through inhaling smoke from burning polyurethane foams in furniture, through ingesting amygdalin which is present in the kernels of several fruits including apricots, almonds and peaches (constituents of the unlicensed anticancer agent, laetrile), or from excessive use of sodium nitroprusside for severe hypertension.[9]

The symptoms of acute poisoning are due to tissue anoxia, with dizziness, palpitations, a feeling of chest constriction and anxiety; characteristically the breath smells of bitter almonds. In more severe cases there is acidosis and coma. Inhaled hydrogen cyanide may lead to death within minutes, but with the ingested salt several hours may elapse before the patient is seriously ill.

The principles of specific therapy are as follows:

- *Dicobalt edetate* to chelate the cyanide is the treatment of choice when the diagnosis is certain (see p. 133). The dose is 300 mg given intravenously over 1 min (5 min if condition is less serious), followed immediately by a 50-mL intravenous infusion of 50% glucose; a further 300 mg dicobalt edetate should be given if recovery is not evident within 1 min.
- Alternatively, a two-stage procedure may be followed by intravenous administration of:
  1. *Sodium nitrite*, which rapidly converts haemoglobin to methaemoglobin, the ferric ion of which takes up cyanide as cyanmethaemoglobin (up to 40% methaemoglobin can be tolerated).
  2. *Sodium thiosulphate*, which more slowly detoxifies the cyanide by permitting the formation of thiocyanate. When the diagnosis is uncertain, administration of thiosulphate plus oxygen is a safe course.

Hydroxocobalamin (5 g for an adult) is a newer antidote that appears to be effective and well tolerated.

There is evidence that oxygen, especially if at high pressure (hyperbaric), overcomes the cellular anoxia in cyanide poisoning; the mechanism is uncertain, but it is reasonable to administer high-flow oxygen.

Carbon monoxide (CO) forms when substances containing carbon and hydrogen are incompletely combusted; poisoning results from inhalation. The concentration of CO in the blood may confirm exposure (cigarette smoking alone may account for up to 10%) but is no guide to the severity of poisoning. Myocardial and neurological injury result from impaired oxygen transport to cells; delayed (2–4 weeks) neurological sequelae include parkinsonism and cerebellar signs. Administer oxygen through a tight-fitting mask and continue for at least 12 h. Evidence for the efficacy of hyperbaric oxygen is conflicting and transport to hyperbaric chambers may present logistic problems, but it is advocated when the blood carboxyhaemoglobin concentration

---

[9]Or in other more bizarre ways. 'A 23-year-old medical student saw his dog (a puppy) suddenly collapse. He started external cardiac massage and a mouth-to-nose ventilation effort. Moments later the dog died, and the student felt nauseated, vomited and lost consciousness. On the victim's arrival at hospital, an alert medical officer detected a bitter almonds odour on his breath and administered the accepted treatment for cyanide poisoning after which he recovered. It turned out that the dog had accidentally swallowed cyanide, and the poison eliminated through the lungs had been inhaled by the master during the mouth-to-nose resuscitation.' Journal of the American Medical Association (1983) 249:353.

exceeds 40%, there is unconsciousness, neurological defect, ischaemic change on the ECG, or pregnancy.

Lead poisoning arises from a variety of occupational (house renovation and stripping old paint), and recreational sources. Environmental exposure has been a matter of great concern, as witnessed by the protective legislation introduced by many countries to reduce pollution, e.g. by removing lead from petrol.

Lead in the body comprises a rapidly exchangeable component in blood (2%, biological $t_{1/2}$ 35 days) and a stable pool in dentine and the skeleton (95%, biological $t_{1/2}$ 25 years).

In severe lead poisoning *sodium calciumedetate* is commonly used to initiate lead excretion. It chelates lead from bone and the extracellular space, and urinary lead excretion diminishes over 5 days thereafter as the extracellular store is exhausted. Redistribution of lead from bone to brain may account for subsequent worsening of symptoms (colic and encephalopathy). *Dimercaprol* is more effective than sodium calciumedetate at chelating lead from the soft tissues such as brain, which is the rationale for combined therapy with sodium calciumedetate.

More recently *succimer* (2,3-dimercaptosuccinic acid, DMSA), a water-soluble analogue of dimercaprol, has been increasingly preferred. Succimer has a high affinity for lead, is suitable for administration by mouth and is better tolerated (has a wider therapeutic index) than dimercaprol. It is licensed for such use in the USA but not in the UK.

Methanol is widely available as a solvent and in paints and antifreezes, and constitutes a cheap substitute for ethanol. As little as 10 mL may cause permanent blindness and 30 mL may kill, through its toxic metabolites. Methanol, like ethanol, is metabolised by zero-order processes that involve the hepatic alcohol and aldehyde dehydrogenases, but, whereas ethanol forms acetaldehyde and acetic acid (partly responsible for the unpleasant effects of 'hangover'), methanol forms formaldehyde and formic acid. Blindness may occur because aldehyde dehydrogenase present in the retina (for the interconversion of retinol and retinene) allows the local formation of formaldehyde. Acidosis is due to the formic acid, which itself enhances pH-dependent hepatic lactate production, adding the problems of lactic acidosis.

The clinical features include severe malaise, vomiting, abdominal pain and tachypnoea (due to the acidosis). Loss of visual acuity and scotomata indicate ocular damage and, if the pupils are dilated and non-reactive, permanent loss of sight is probable. Coma and circulatory collapse may follow.

Therapy is directed at:

- *Correcting the acidosis.* Achieving this largely determines the outcome; sodium bicarbonate is given intravenously in doses up to 2 mol in a few hours, carrying an excess of sodium which must be managed. Methanol is metabolised slowly and relapse may accompany too early discontinuation of bicarbonate.
- *Inhibiting methanol metabolism.* Ethanol, which occupies the dehydrogenase enzymes in preference to methanol, competitively prevents metabolism of methanol to its toxic products. A single oral dose of ethanol 1 mL/kg (as a 50% solution or as the equivalent in gin or whisky) is followed by 0.25 mL/kg/h orally or intravenously, aiming to maintain the blood ethanol at about 100 mg/100 mL until no methanol is detectable in the blood. Fomepizole (4-methylpyrazole), another competitive inhibitor of alcohol dehydrogenase, is effective in severe methanol poisoning and is less likely to cause cerebral depression (it is available in the UK on a named-patient basis).
- *Eliminating methanol* and its metabolites by dialysis. Haemodialysis is two to three times more effective than is peritoneal dialysis. Folinic acid 30 mg intravenously 6-hourly may protect against retinal damage by enhancing formate metabolism.

Ethylene glycol is readily accessible as a constituent of antifreezes for car radiators. Its use to give 'body' and sweetness to white table wines was criminal. Metabolism to glycolate and oxalate causes acidosis and renal damage, a situation that is further complicated by lactic acidosis. In the first 12 h after ingestion the patient appears as though intoxicated with alcohol but without the characteristic odour; subsequently there is increasing acidosis, pulmonary oedema and cardiac failure, and in 2–3 days renal pain and tubular necrosis develop because calcium oxalate crystals form in the urine. Intravenous sodium bicarbonate corrects the acidosis, and with calcium gluconate, the hypocalcaemia. As with methanol (above), ethanol or fomepizole competitively inhibit the metabolism of ethylene glycol and haemodialysis eliminates the poison.

Hydrocarbons e.g. paraffin oil (kerosene), petrol (gasoline), benzene, chiefly cause CNS depression and pulmonary damage from inhalation. It is vital to avoid aspiration into the lungs with spontaneous vomiting.

Volatile solvent abuse or 'glue sniffing' is common among teenagers, especially males. The success of the modern chemical industry provides easy access to these substances as adhesives, dry cleaners, air fresheners, deodorants, aerosols and other products. Viscous products are taken from a plastic bag, liquids from a handkerchief or plastic bottle.

The immediate euphoriant and excitatory effects give way to confusion, hallucinations and delusions as the dose is increased. Chronic abusers, notably of toluene, develop peripheral neuropathy, cerebellar disease and dementia; damage to the kidney, liver, heart and lungs also occurs with solvents. Over 50% of deaths from the practice follow cardiac arrhythmia, probably caused by sensitisation of the myocardium to catecholamines and by vagal inhibition from laryngeal stimulation due to aerosol propellants sprayed into the throat.

Acute solvent poisoning requires immediate cardiorespiratory resuscitation and antiarrhythmia treatment. Toxicity from carbon tetrachloride and chloroform involves the generation of phosgene, a 1914–1918 war gas, which is inactivated by cysteine and by glutathione, formed from cysteine. Recommended treatment is *N*-acetylcysteine, as for poisoning with paracetamol.

POISONING BY HERBICIDES AND PESTICIDES

Organophosphorus pesticides are anticholinesterases; an account of poisoning and its management appears on page 395. Organic carbamates are similar.

Dinitro-compounds. Dinitro-orthocresol (DNOC) and dinitrobutylphenol (DNBP) are selective weed-killers and insecticides, and cases of poisoning occur accidentally, e.g. by ignoring safety precautions. These substances can be absorbed through the skin and the hands, resulting in yellow staining of face or hair. Symptoms and signs indicate a very high metabolic rate (due to uncoupling of oxidative phosphorylation); copious sweating and thirst proceed to dehydration and vomiting, weakness, restlessness, tachycardia and deep, rapid breathing, convulsions and coma. Treatment is urgent and consists of cooling the patient and attention to fluid and electrolyte balance. It is essential to differentiate this type of poisoning from that due to anticholinesterases, because atropine given to patients poisoned with dinitro-compound will stop sweating and may cause death from hyperthermia.

Phenoxy herbicides (2,4-D, mecoprop, dichlorprop) are used to control broad-leaved weeds. Ingestion causes nausea, vomiting, pyrexia (due to uncoupling of oxidative phosphorylation), hyperventilation, hypoxia and coma. Urine alkalinisation accelerates elimination. Organochlorine pesticides, e.g. dicophane (DDT), may cause convulsions in acute overdose. Treat as for status epilepticus.

Rodenticides include warfarin and thallium (see Table 9.1); for strychnine, which causes convulsions, give diazepam.

Paraquat is a widely used herbicide that is extremely toxic if ingested; a mouthful of the commercial solution taken and spat out may be sufficient to kill. A common sequence is: ulceration and sloughing of the oral and oesophageal mucosa, renal tubular necrosis (5–10 days later), pulmonary oedema and pulmonary fibrosis. Whether the patient lives or dies depends largely on the condition of the lung. Treatment is urgent and includes activated charcoal or aluminium silicate (Fuller's earth) by mouth as adsorbents. Haemodialysis may have a role in the first 24 h, the rationale being to reduce the plasma concentration and protect the kidney, failure of which allows the slow but relentless accumulation of paraquat in the lung.

Diquat is similar to paraquat but the late pulmonary changes may not occur.

POISONING BY BIOLOGICAL SUBSTANCES

Many plants form substances that are important for their survival either by enticing animals, which disperse their spores, or by repelling potential predators. Poisoning occurs when children eat berries or chew flowers, attracted by their colour; adults may mistake non-edible for edible varieties of salad plants and fungi (mushrooms) for they may resemble one another closely and some are greatly prized by epicures. Some biologicals, e.g. yellow oleander seeds, are a common means of suicide.[10]

The range of toxic substances that these plants produce is exhibited in a diversity of symptoms that may be grouped broadly thus:

- *Atropinic*, e.g. from deadly nightshade (*Atropa belladonna*) and thorn apple (*Datura*), causing dilated pupils, blurred vision, dry mouth, flushed skin, confusion and delirium.
- *Nicotinic*, e.g. from hemlock (*Conium*) and *Laburnum*, causing salivation, dilated pupils, vomiting, convulsions and respiratory paralysis.
- *Muscarinic*, e.g. from *Inocybe* and *Clitocybe* fungi (mushrooms), causing salivation, lachrymation, miosis, perspiration, bradycardia and bronchoconstriction, also hallucinations.
- *Hallucinogenic*, e.g. from psilocybin-containing mushrooms (liberty cap), which may be taken specifically for this effect ('magic mushrooms').
- *Cardiovascular*, e.g. from foxglove (*Digitalis*), mistletoe (*Viscum album*), lily-of-the-valley (*Convallaria*) and yellow oleander (*Thevetia peruviana*), which contain cardiac glycosides that cause vomiting, diarrhoea and cardiac arrhythmia.
- *Hepatotoxic*, e.g. from *Amanita phalloides* (death cap mushroom), *Senecio* (ragwort) and *Crotalatia*, and 'bush teas' prepared from these plants in the Caribbean. Aflatoxin, from *Aspergillus flavus*, a fungus that contaminates foods, is probably a cause of primary liver cancer.
- *Convulsant*, e.g. from water dropwort (*Oenanthe*) and cowbane (*Cicuta*), which contain the related and very dangerous substances, oenanthotoxin and cicutoxin.
- *Cutaneous irritation*, e.g. directly with nettle (*Urtica*), or dermatitis following sensitisation with *Primula*.
- *Gastrointestinal* symptoms, nausea, vomiting, diarrhoea and abdominal pain occur with numerous plants.

Treatment of plant poisonings consists mainly of *activated charcoal* to adsorb toxin in the gastrointestinal tract. Control convulsions with diazepam. In 'death cap' mushroom poisoning, penicillin may be used to displace toxin from plasma albumin, provided haemodialysis is being used, which latter may also benefit the renal failure; intensive fluid and supportive therapy and restitution of altered coagulation factors are also required.

BIOLOGICAL AGENTS AS WEAPONS

Many natural agents can cause life-threatening infections but their recruitment as biological weapons against communities of people requires particular qualities of infectivity, pathogenicity, stability and ease of production. Among the pathogens that may be considered candidates for this horrific purpose are *Bacillus anthracis* (the causal agent of anthrax), *Brucella* (brucellosis), *Clostridium botulinum* (botulism), *Francisella tularensis* (tularaemia), *Yersinia pestis* (plague), influenza and variola virus (smallpox). Drugs used for the treatment and prophylaxis of some of the bacterial infections appear in Table 11.1 (p. 184). Special centres retain vaccines to immunise against anthrax, plague and smallpox, and an antitoxin for botulism. Even this short account on the subject of bioterrorism is surely a sad commentary on the times in which we live.

INCAPACITATING AGENTS

(harassing, disabling, anti-riot agents)

> Harassing agents may be defined as chemical substances that are capable when used in field conditions, of rapidly causing a temporary disablement that lasts for little longer than the period of exposure.[11]

The pharmacological requirements for a safe and effective harassing agent must be stringent (it is hardly appropriate to refer to benefit versus risk). As well as potency and rapid onset and offset of effect in open areas under any atmospheric condition, it must be safe in confined spaces where concentration may be very high and may affect an innocent, bedridden invalid should a projectile enter a window.

CS (chlorobenzylidene malononitrile, a tear 'gas') is a favoured substance at present. This is a solid that is disseminated as an aerosol (particles of 1 micron in diameter) by including it in a pyrotechnic mixture. Television renders familiar the spectacle of its dissemination. It is an aerosol or smoke, not a gas.

[10]Eddleston M, Rezvi Sheriff MH, Hawton K 1998 Deliberate self-harm in Sri Lanka: an overlooked tragedy in the developing world. British Medical Journal 317:133–135.

[11]World Health Organization 1970 Health aspects of chemical and biological weapons. WHO, Geneva.

The particles aggregate and settle to the ground in minutes, so that the risk of prolonged exposure out of doors is not great.

> According to the concentration of CS to which a person is exposed, the effects vary from a slight pricking or peppery sensation in the eyes and nasal passages up to the maximal symptoms of streaming from the eyes and nose, spasm of the eyelids, profuse lachrymation and salivation, retching and sometimes vomiting, burning of the mouth and throat, cough and gripping pain in the chest.[12]

The onset of symptoms occurs immediately on exposure (an important factor from the point of view of the user) and they disappear dramatically:

> At one moment the exposed person is in their grip. Then he either stumbles away, or the smoke plume veers or the discharge from the grenade stops, and, immediately, the symptoms begin to roll away. Within a minute or two, the pain in the chest has gone and his eyes, although still streaming, are open. Five or so minutes later, the excessive salivation and pouring tears stop and a quarter of an hour after exposure, the subject is essentially back to normal.[11]

Exposed subjects absorb small amounts only, and the plasma $t_{1/2}$ is about 5 s.

Investigations of the effects of CS are difficult in 'field use', but some have been done and at present there is no evidence that even the most persistent rioter will suffer any permanent effect. The hazard to the infirm or sick seems to be low, but, plainly, it would be prudent to assume that patients with asthma or chronic bronchitis could suffer an exacerbation from high concentrations, although bronchospasm does not occur in healthy people. Vomiting seems to be due to swallowing contaminated saliva. Transient looseness of the bowels may follow exposure. Hazard from CS is probably confined to situations where the missiles enter enclosed spaces.

CN (chloroacetophenone, a tear gas) is generally used as a solid aerosol or smoke; solutions (Mace) are used at close quarters.

CR (dibenzoxazepine) entered production in 1973 after testing on army volunteers. In addition to the usual properties (above) it may induce a transient rise in intraocular pressure. Its solubility allows use in water 'cannons'.

'Authority' is reticent about the properties of all these substances and no further important information is readily available.

This brief account has been included, because, in addition to helping victims, even the most well conducted and tractable students and doctors may find themselves exposed to CS smoke in our troubled world, and some may even feel it their duty to incur exposure. The following points are worth making:

- Wear disposable plastic gloves, for the object of treating the sufferer is frustrated if the physician becomes affected.
- Contaminated clothing should be placed in plastic bags and skin washed with soap and water. Showering or bathing may cause symptoms to return by releasing the agent from contaminated hair. Cutaneous erythema is usual and blistering may occur with high concentrations of CS and CN in warm, moist conditions.
- The eyes will irrigate themselves. Dry air blown directly on the eye with an electric fan, if available, helps dissolved CS gas to vaporise. Raised intraocular pressure may cause acute glaucoma in those aged over 40 years.

DRUGS USED FOR TORTURE, INTERROGATION AND JUDICIAL EXECUTION

Regrettably, drugs have been and are used for torture, sometimes disguised as 'interrogation' or 'aversion therapy'. Facts are, not surprisingly, hard to obtain, but it seems that suxamethonium, hallucinogens, thiopental, neuroleptics, amfetamines, apomorphine and cyclophosphamide have been engaged to hurt, frighten, confuse or debilitate in such ways as callous ingenuity can devise. When the definition of criminal activity becomes distorted to include activities in defence of human liberty, the employment of drugs offers inducement to inhuman behaviour. Such use, and any doctors or others who engage in it, or who misguidedly allow themselves to believe that it can be in the interest of victims to monitor the activity by others, must surely be outlawed.

It might be urged that it is justifiable to use drugs to protect society by uncovering serious crimes such as murder. There is no such thing as a 'truth drug'

---

[12]Home Office Report (1971) of the enquiry into the medical and toxicological aspects of CS. Part II. HMSO, London: Cmnd 4775.

in the sense that it guarantees the truth of what the subject says. There always must be uncertainty of the truth of evidence obtained with drugs, e.g. thiopental, without independent confirmation. But accused people, convinced of their own innocence, sometimes volunteer to undergo such tests. The problem of discerning truth from falsehood remains.

In some countries drugs are used for judicial execution, e.g. combinations of thiopental, pancuronium and potassium chloride, given intravenously and sequentially. There is concern that the degree of anaesthesia achieved is inadequate. In 43 of 49 executed prisoners in the USA, blood concentrations of thiopental were lower than are required for surgery, and 21 had concentrations consistent with awareness. Constraints of ethics prohibit many doctors from participating in the design of the protocol or the execution itself.[13]

GUIDE TO FURTHER READING

Beeching N J, Dance D A B, Miller A R O, Spencer R C 2002 Biological warfare and bioterrorism. British Medical Journal 324:336–339

Camidge R, Bateman D N 2003 Self-poisoning in the UK: epidemiology and toxidromes. Clinical Medicine 3(2):111–114

Chyka P A, Erdman A R, Christianson G et al 2007 Salicylate poisoning: An evidence-based consensus guideline for out-of-hospital management. Clinical Toxicology 45:95–131

Dawson A H, Whyte I M 1999 Therapeutic drug monitoring in drug overdose. British Journal of Clinical Pharmacology 48(3):278–283

Evison D, Hinsley D, Rice P 2002 Chemical weapons. British Medical Journal 324:332–335

Gawande A 2006 When law and ethics collide – why physicians participate in executions. New England Journal of Medicine 354(12):1221–1229

Hawton K, Simkin S, Deeks J J et al 1999 Effects of a drug overdose in a television drama on presentation to hospital for self poisoning: time series and questionnaire study. British Medical Journal 318:972–977

Kales S N, Christiani D C 2004 Acute chemical emergencies. New England Journal of Medicine 350(8):800–808

Kerins M, Dargan P I, Jones A L 2003 Pitfalls in the management of the poisoned patient. Journal of the Royal College of Physicians of Edinburgh 33:90–103

Reisman R E 1994 Insect stings. New England Journal of Medicine 331(8):523–527

Ruben Thanacoody H K, Thomas S H L 2003 Antidepressant poisoning. Clinical Medicine 3(2):114–118

Skegg K 2005 Self-harm. Lancet 366:1471–1483

Tibbles P M, Edelsberg J S 1996 Hyperbaric-oxygen therapy. New England Journal of Medicine 334(25):1642–1648

Volans G, Hartley V, McCrea S, Monaghan J 2003 Non-opioid analgesic poisoning. Clinical Medicine 3(2):119–123

Woolf A D, Erdman A R, Nelson L S et al 2007 Tricyclic antidepressant poisoning: An evidence-based consensus guideline for out-of-hospital management. Clinical Toxicology 45:203–233

Yawar A 2004 Healing in survivors of torture. Journal of the Royal Society of Medicine 97(8):366–370

[13]Koniaris L G, Zimmers T A, Lubarsky D A, Sheldon J P 2005 Inadequate anaesthesia in lethal injection for execution. Lancet 365:1412–1414.

10

Drug abuse

SYNOPSIS

Drugs used for non-medical purposes (abused, mis-used, used for recreational purposes) present a range of social problems, all of which have important phar-macological dimensions. General topics include:

- Social aspects
- Terms used
- Rewards for the individual
- Drug dependence and its management
- Drugs and sport

Individual substances are discussed:
- Opioids (see pp. 297–306)
- Ethyl alcohol and other cerebral depressants (benzodiazepines, GHB)
- Tobacco
- Psychodysleptics (LSD, mescaline, tenamfetamine, phencyclidine, cannabis)
- Psychostimulants (cocaine, amfetamines, methylxanthines, ginseng, khat)
- Volatile substances
- Drugs as adjuvants to crime

SOCIAL ASPECTS

The enormous social importance of this subject warrants comment here.

> All the naturally occurring sedatives, narcotics, euphoriants, hallucinogens and excitants were discovered thousands of years ago, before the dawn of civilisation … By the late Stone Age man was systematically poisoning himself. The presence of poppy heads in the kitchen middens of the Swiss Lake Dwellers shows how early in his history man discovered the techniques of self-transcendence through drugs. There were dope addicts long before there were farmers.[1]

The drives that induce a more or less mentally healthy person to resort to drugs to obtain chemical vacations from intolerable self-hood will be briefly considered here, as well as some account of the phar-macological aspects of drug dependence.

The dividing line between legitimate use of drugs for social purposes and their abuse is indistinct, for it is not only a matter of which drug, but of the amount of drug and of whether the effect is anti-social or not. In the UK and elsewhere, the classifi-cation of drugs of abuse continues to be subject to controversy.[2]

'Normal' people seem to be able to use alcohol for their occasional purposes without harm but, given the appropriate personality and/or environ-mental adversity, many may turn to it for relief and become dependent on it, both psychologically and physically. But drug abuse is not primarily a phar-macological problem; it is a social problem with important pharmacological aspects.

A further issue is whether a boundary can be drawn between the therapeutic and non-therapeutic use of a therapeutic drug and, some would argue, if it can be drawn, should it be? The matter has been highlighted by the use of selective serotonin-reuptake inhibitor antidepressants, e.g. fluoxetine (Prozac), not to treat depression but to elevate mood – make a person feel 'better than well' – and of sildenafil to heighten sexual experience rather than to correct erectile dysfunction.

Abuse of drugs to improve performance in sport stems from a distinct and different motivation, the obtaining of advantage in competition, but the prac-tice yet has major implications for the health of the individual and for the participating and spectating sporting community.

---

[1]Huxley A 1957 The history of tension. Annals of the New York Academy of Sciences 67:675–684.

[2]MacDonald R, Das A 2006 UK classification of drugs of abuse: an un-evidence-based mess. Lancet 368:559–561.

SOME TERMS USED

Drug abuse is defined as 'persistent or sporadic excessive drug use inconsistent with or unrelated to acceptable medical practice. Thus, the intentional use of excessive doses, or the intentional use of thera-peutic doses for purposes other than the indication for which the drug was prescribed, is drug abuse. *Misuse* and *non-medical* use are synonyms of drug abuse.'[3] (There is here a clear conceptual distinction from inappropriate prescribing or medication errors, which constitute drug *maladministration*.) This defi-nition recognises the need to continue treatment with a dependence-producing drug even after the patient has become dependent on it, e.g. opioids in palliative care. Such drug dependence is unwanted but it is not drug abuse.

Individuals abuse drugs either from their own 'free' choice or under feelings of compulsion, to achieve their own well-being, or what they conceive as their own well-being (see motives below). Abused drugs are often divided into two groups, hard and soft.

Hard drugs are those that are liable seriously to disable the individual as a functioning member of society by inducing severe psychological and, in the case of cerebral depressants, physical, dependence. The group includes heroin and cocaine.

Soft drugs are less dependence producing. There may be psychological dependence, but there is lit-tle or no physical dependence except with heavy doses of depressants (alcohol). The group includes sedatives and tranquillisers, amfetamines, cannabis, hallucinogens, alcohol, tobacco and caffeine.

This classification fails to recognise individual variation in drug use. Alcohol can be used in heavy doses that are gravely disabling and induce severe physical dependence with convulsions on sudden withdrawal; i.e. for the individual the drug is 'hard'. But there are many people mildly psychologically dependent on it who retain their position in home and society.

Hard-use, where the drug is central in the user's life, and soft-use, where it is merely incidental, are terms of assistance in making this distinction, i.e.

what is classified is not the drug but the effect it has on, or the way it is used by, the individual. The term '*recreational*' is often applied to such use, conferring an apparent sanction that relates more to the latter category.

Abuse liability of a drug is related to its capacity to produce immediate gratification, which may be a feature of the drug itself (amfetamine and heroin give rapid effect whereas tricyclic antidepressants do not) and its route of administration in descend-ing order: inhalation/intravenous, intramuscular/subcutaneous, oral. Abuse liability is the central issue and is usefully distinguished from dependence liability, for not all dependence-producing drugs are abused: caffeine, for example, is dependence producing but seldom abused.

Drug dependence (see p. 144) now replaces terms such as drug *addiction* and drug *habituation*. Nevertheless, the terms 'addict' or 'addiction' have not been completely abandoned in this book because they remain convenient. Addiction refers to the most severe forms of *dependence* where compul-sive craving dominates the subject's daily life. Such cases pose problems as grave as dependence on tea drinking is trivial. But the use of the term drug dependence is welcome, because it renders irrelevant arguments about whether some drugs are addictive or merely habit forming.

Drug abuse use has two principal forms:

- *Continuous use*, when there is a true dependence, e.g. opioids, alcohol, benzodiazepines.
- *Intermittent or occasional use* to obtain a recreational experience, e.g. 'ecstasy' (tenamfetamine), LSD, cocaine, cannabis, solvents, or to relieve stress, e.g. alcohol.

Some drugs, e.g. alcohol, are used in both ways, but others, e.g. 'ecstasy', LSD, cannabis, are virtually con-fined to the second use.

Drives to drug abuse are:

- Relief of anxiety, tension and depression; escape from personal psychological problems; detachment from harsh reality; ease of social intercourse.
- Search for self-knowledge and for meaning in life, including religion. The cult of 'experience' including aestheticism and artistic creation,

---

[3]WHO Expert Committee on Drug Dependence 2003 33rd Report. WHO, Geneva. Other aspects of the report are referred to in this chapter.

sex and 'genuine', 'sincere' interpersonal relationships, to obtain a sense of 'belonging'.

- Rebellion against or despair about orthodox social values and the environment. Fear of missing something, and conformity with own social subgroup (the young, especially).
- Fun, amusement, recreation, excitement, curiosity (the young, especially).
- Improvement of performance in competitive sport (a distinct motivation, see below).

REWARDS FOR THE INDIVIDUAL

It is inherently unlikely that mind-affecting chemicals could be central to a constructive culture, and no convincing support for the assertion has yet been produced. (That chemicals might be central to a destructive culture is another matter.) Certainly, like-minded people practising what are often illegal activities will gather into closely knit subgroups for mutual support, and will feel a sense of community, but that is hardly a 'culture'. Even when drug-using subgroups are accepted as representing a subculture, it may be doubted whether drugs are sufficiently central to their ideology to justify using 'drug' in the title. But claims for value to the individual and to society of drug experience must surely be tested by the criterion of fruitfulness for both, and the judgement of the individual concerned alone is insufficient; it must be agreed by others. The results of both legal and illegal drug use do not give encouragement to press for a large-scale experiment in this field.

It is claimed that drugs provide mystical experience and that this has valid religious content. Mystical experience may be defined as a combination of feelings of unity (oneness with nature and/or God), ineffability (experience beyond the subject's power to express), joy (peace, sacredness), knowledge (insight into truths of life and values, illuminations) and transcendence (of space and time).

When such states do occur there remains the question of whether they tell us something about a reality outside the individual or merely something about the mind of the person having the experience. Mystical experience is not a normal dose-related pharmacodynamic effect of any drug; its occurrence depends on many factors such as the subject's personality, mood, environment, conditioning. The drug facilitates rather than induces the experience, and drugs can facilitate unpleasant as well as pleasant experiences. It is not surprising that mystical experience can occur with a wide range of drugs that alter consciousness:

> … I seemed at first in a state of utter blankness … with a keen vision of what was going on in the room around me, but no sensation of touch. I thought that I was near death; when, suddenly, my soul became aware of God, who was manifestly dealing with me, handling me, so to speak, in an intense personal, present reality … I cannot describe the ecstasy I felt.[4]

This experience occurred in the 19th century with chloroform, a general anaesthetic now obsolete because of cardiac depression and hepatotoxicity.

There is no good evidence that drugs can produce experience that passes the test of results, i.e. fruitfulness to the individual and to society. Plainly there is a risk of the experience becoming an end in itself rather than a means of development.

GENERAL PATTERN OF USE

Divisions are not rigid and they change with fashion. The general picture in the UK is:

- *Any age*: alcohol, tobacco, mild dependence on hypnotics and tranquillisers, occasional use of LSD and cannabis.
- *Age 16–35 years*: hard-use drugs, chiefly heroin, cocaine and amfetamines (including 'ecstasy'). Surviving users tend to reduce or relinquish heavy use as they enter middle age.
- *Aged 14–16*: cannabis, ecstasy, cocaine.
- *Under 14 years*: volatile inhalants, e.g. solvents of glues, aerosol sprays, vaporised (by heat) paints, 'solvent or substance' abuse, 'glue sniffing'.
- *Miscellaneous*: any drug or combination of drugs reputed to alter consciousness may have a local vogue, however brief, e.g. drugs used in parkinsonism and metered aerosols for asthma.

Ketamine (see p. 319) is increasingly popular.

DEPENDENCE

Drug dependence is a state arising from repeated administration of a drug that results in harm to the individual and sometimes to society. The features

---

[4]Quoted in James W 1902 Varieties of religious experience. Longmans, Harlow, and many subsequent editions of this classic. See also Leary T 1970 The politics of ecstasy. MacGibbon and Kee, London. Other editions, USA.

common to experience with such drugs are: an initial pleasurable or euphoric sensation ('kick'), tolerance with repeated use so that the subject feels a desire, need or compulsion to continue using the drug and feels ill if abruptly deprived of it (abstinence or withdrawal syndrome). Subsequently there is difficulty in controlling use of the drug which leads to impairment of important social activities.

Dependence may be regarded as possessing both physical (physiological) and psychological elements. The distinction is criticised as being difficult to make in practice and inconsistent with the modern view that all drug effects are potentially understandable in biological terms, but it has sufficient usefulness to be retained here.

PSYCHOLOGICAL DEPENDENCE

This is the first to appear and there is emotional distress if the drug is withdrawn. It may occur with any drug that alters consciousness, however bizarre, e.g. muscarine (see p. 394), and with some that, in ordinary doses, do not, e.g. non-narcotic analgesics, purgatives, diuretics; these latter provide problems of psychopathology rather than of psychopharmacology.

Psychological dependence can occur merely to a tablet or injection, regardless of its content, as well as to drug substances. Mild dependence does not require that a drug should have important psychic effects; the subject's beliefs as to what it does are as important, e.g. purgative and diuretic dependence in people obsessed with dread of obesity. We are all physically dependent on food, and some develop a strong emotional dependence and eat too much (or the reverse); sexual activity, with its unique mix of arousal and relaxation, can for some become compulsive or addictive.

There is danger in personal experimentation; as an American addict has succinctly put it, 'They all think they can take just one joy-pop but it's the first one that hooks you'.[5] Unfortunately, subjects cannot decide for themselves that their dependence will remain mild.

PHYSICAL (PHYSIOLOGICAL) DEPENDENCE

Physical (physiological) dependence implies that continued exposure to a drug induces adaptive

changes in body tissues so that *tolerance* occurs, and that abrupt withdrawal of the drug leaves these changes unopposed, resulting generally in a *discontinuation (withdrawal) syndrome*, usually of rebound over-activity.

Tolerance follows the operation of homeostatic adaptation, e.g. to continued high occupancy of opioid receptors. Changes of similar type may occur with γ-aminobutyric acid (GABA) transmission, involving benzodiazepines. It also results from metabolic changes (enzyme induction) and physiological or behavioural adaptation to drug effects, e.g. opioids. Physiological adaptation develops to a substantial degree with cerebral depressants, but is minor or absent with excitant drugs. There is commonly cross-tolerance between drugs of similar, and sometimes even of dissimilar, chemical groups, e.g. alcohol and benzodiazepines. A general account of tolerance appears on page 80.

A discontinuation (withdrawal) syndrome occurs, for example, when administration of an opioid is suddenly stopped. Morphine-like substances (endomorphins, dynorphins) act as CNS neurotransmitters, and exogenously administered opioid suppresses their endogenous production by a feedback mechanism. Abrupt discontinuation results in an immediate deficiency of endogenous opioid, which thus causes the withdrawal syndrome. A general discussion of abrupt withdrawal of drug therapy appears on page 104.

SITES AND MECHANISMS OF ACTION

Drugs of abuse are extremely diverse in their chemical structures, mechanisms of action and anatomical and cellular targets. Nevertheless, there is an emerging consensus that addictive drugs possess a parallel ability to affect glutaminergic and dopaminergic transmission in the ventral striatum of the basal forebrain and in the extended nucleus amygdala. It seems that drugs of abuse can converge on common neural mechanisms in these areas to produce acute reward and chronic alterations in reward systems that lead to addiction.

ROUTE OF ADMINISTRATION AND EFFECT

With the intravenous route or inhalation, much higher peak plasma concentrations can be reached

[5]Maurer D W, Vogel V H 1962 Narcotica and narcotic addiction. Thomas, Springfield.

than with oral administration. This accounts for the 'kick' or 'flash' that abusers report and which many seek, likening it to sexual orgasm or better. As an addict said, 'The ultimate high is death', and it has been reported that, when hearing of someone dying from an overdose, some addicts will seek out the vendor as it is evident he is selling 'really good stuff.[6] Addicts who rely on illegal sources are inevitably exposed to being supplied diluted or even inert preparations at high prices. North American addicts who have come to the UK believing themselves to be accustomed to high doses of heroin have suffered acute poisoning when given, probably for the first time, pure heroin at an official UK drug dependence clinic.

PRESCRIBING FOR DRUG DEPENDENCE

In the UK, supply of certain drugs for the purpose of sustaining addiction or managing withdrawal is permitted under strict legal limitations, usually by designated doctors. Guidance about the responsibilities and management of addiction is available.[7] By such procedures it is hoped to limit the expansion of the illicit market, and its accompanying crime and dangers to health, e.g. from infected needles and syringes. The object is to sustain young (usually) addicts, who cannot be weaned from drug use, in reasonable health until they relinquish their dependence (often over about 10 years).

When injectable drugs are prescribed there is currently no way of assessing the truth of an addict's statement that he or she needs x mg of heroin (or other drug), and the dose has to be assessed intuitively by the doctor. This has resulted in addicts obtaining more than they need and selling it, sometimes to initiate new users. The use of oral methadone or other opioid for maintenance by prescription is devised to mitigate this problem.

TREATMENT OF DEPENDENCE

Withdrawal of the drug. Whilst obviously important, this is only a step on what can be a long and

often disappointing journey to psychological and social rehabilitation, e.g. in 'therapeutic communities'. A heroin addict may be given methadone as part of a gradual withdrawal programme (see p. 302) for this drug has a long duration of action and blocks access of injected opioid to the opioid receptor so that if, in a moment of weakness, the subject takes heroin, the 'kick' is reduced. More acutely, the physical features associated with discontinuing high alcohol use may be alleviated by chlordiazepoxide given in decreasing doses for 7–14 days. Sympathetic autonomic overactivity can be treated with a β-adrenoceptor blocker.

Maintenance and relapse. Relapsed addicts who live a fairly normal life are sometimes best treated by supplying drugs under supervision. There is no legal objection to doing this in the UK (see above), but naturally this course, which abandons unrealistic hope of cure, should not be adopted until it is certain that cure is virtually impossible. A less harmful drug by a less harmful route may be substituted, e.g. oral methadone for intravenous heroin. Addicts are often particularly reluctant to abandon the intravenous route, which provides the 'immediate high' that they find, or originally found, so desirable.

Severe pain in an opioid addict presents a special problem. High-efficacy opioid may be ineffective (tolerance) or overdose may result; low-efficacy opioids will not only be ineffective but may induce withdrawal symptoms, especially if they have some antagonist effect, e.g. pentazocine. This leaves as drugs of choice non-steroidal anti-inflammatory drugs (NSAIDs), e.g. indometacin, and nefopam (which is neither opioid nor a NSAID).

MORTALITY

Young illicit users by intravenous injection (heroin, benzodiazepines, amfetamine) have a high mortality rate. Death either follows overdose, or the occurrence of septicaemia, endocarditis, hepatitis, AIDS, gas gangrene, tetanus or pulmonary embolism from the contaminated materials used without aseptic precautions (schemes to provide clean equipment mitigate this). Smugglers of illicit cocaine or heroin sometimes carry the drug in plastic bags concealed by swallowing or in the rectum ('body packing').

---

[6]Bourne P 1976 Acute drug abuse emergencies. Academic Press, New York.

[7]See Department of Health 1999 Drug misuse and dependence – guidelines on clinical management. The Stationery Office, London (3rd impression 2005).

Leakage of the packages, not surprisingly, may have a fatal result.[8]

ESCALATION

A variable proportion of subjects who start with cannabis eventually take heroin. This disposition to progress from occasional to frequent soft use of drugs through to hard drug use, when it occurs, is less likely to be due to pharmacological actions, than to psychosocial factors, although increased suggestibility induced by cannabis may contribute.

De-escalation also occurs as users become disillusioned with drugs over about 10 years.

'DESIGNER DRUGS'

This unhappily chosen term means molecular modifications produced in secret for profit by skilled and criminally minded chemists. Manipulation of fentanyl has resulted in compounds of extraordinary potency.

In 1976 a too-clever 23-year-old addict seeking to manufacture his own pethidine took a synthetic shortcut and injected himself with what later, with his help, proved to be two closely related byproducts; one was MPTP (methylphenyltetrahydropyridine).[9,10] Three days later he developed a severe parkinsonian syndrome that responded to levodopa. MPTP selectively destroys melanin-containing cells in the substantia nigra. Further such cases have occurred from use of supposed synthetic heroin. MPTP has since been used in experimental research on parkinson-

ism. What the future holds for individuals and for society in this area can only be imagined.

DRUGS AND SPORT

The rewards of competitive sport, both financial and in personal and national prestige, are the cause of determination to win at (almost) any cost. Drugs are used to enhance performance, although efficacy is largely undocumented. Detection can be difficult when the drugs or metabolites are closely related to or identical with endogenous substances, and when the drug can be stopped well before the event without apparent loss of efficacy, e.g. anabolic steroids (but suppression of endogenous trophic hormones can be measured, and can assist).

PERFORMANCE ENHANCEMENT

There follow illustrations of the mechanisms by which drugs can enhance performance in various sports; naturally, these are proscribed by the authorities (International Olympic Committee [IOC] Medical Commission, and the governing bodies of individual sports).

For *'strength sports'* in which body-weight and brute strength are the principal determinants (weight lifting, rowing, wrestling): anabolic agents, e.g. clenbuterol (β-adrenoceptor agonist), androstenedione, methandienone, nandrolone, stanozolol, testosterone. Taken together with a high-protein diet and exercise, these increase lean body-weight (muscle) but not necessarily strength. It is claimed they allow more intensive training regimens (limiting cell injury in muscles). Rarely, there may be episodes of violent behaviour, known amongst athletes as 'roid [steroid] rage'.

High doses are used, with risk of liver damage (cholestatic, tumours) especially if the drug is taken long term, which is certainly insufficient to deter 'sportsmen'. They may be more inclined to take more seriously the fact that anabolic steroids suppress pituitary gonadotrophin, and so testosterone production.

Growth hormone (somatrem, somatropin) and corticotropin use may be combined with that of anabolic steroids. Chorionic gonadotrophin may be taken to stimulate testosterone production (and prevent testicular atrophy). Similarly, tamoxifen (antioestrogen) may be used to attenuate some of the effects of anabolic steroids.

---

[8]A 49-year-old man became ill after an international flight. An abdominal radiograph showed a large number of spherical packages in his gastrointestinal tract, and body-packing was suspected. As he had not defaecated, he was given liquid paraffin. He developed ventricular fibrillation and died. Post-mortem examination showed that he had ingested more than 150 latex packets, each containing 5 g cocaine, making a total of almost 1 kg (lethal oral dose 1–3 g). The liquid paraffin may have contributed to his death as the mineral oil dissolves latex. Sorbitol or lactulose with activated charcoal should be used to remove ingested packages, or surgery if there are signs of intoxication. (Visser L, Stricker B, Hoogendoorn M, Vinks A 1998 Do not give paraffin to packers. Lancet 352:1352.)
[9]Williams A 1984 MPTP parkinsonism. British Medical Journal 289:1401–1402.
[10]Davis G C, Williams A C, Markey S P et al 1979 Chronic parkinsonism secondary to intravenous injection of meperidine analogues. Psychiatry Research 1:249–254.

For events in which *output of energy* is explosive (100-m sprint): stimulants, e.g. amfetamine, bromantan, carphendon, cocaine, ephedrine and caffeine (>12 mg/L in urine). Death has occurred in bicycle racing (continuous hard exercise with short periods of sprint), probably due to hyperthermia and cardiac arrhythmia in metabolically stimulated and vasoconstricted subjects exercising maximally under a hot sun.

For *endurance sports* to enhance the oxygen-carrying capacity of the blood (bicycling, marathon running): *erythropoietin*, also *'blood doping'* (the athlete has blood withdrawn and stored, then transfused once the deficit had been made up naturally, so raising the plasma haemoglobin level above normal).

For events in which *steadiness of hand* is essential (pistol, rifle shooting): *β-adrenoceptor blockers*. Tremor is reduced by the β_2-adrenoceptor blocking effect, as are somatic symptoms of anxiety.

For events in which *body pliancy* is a major factor (gymnastics): delaying puberty in child gymnasts by endocrine techniques.

For *weight reduction*, e.g. boxers, jockeys: diuretics. These are also used to flush out other drugs in the hope of escaping detection; severe volume depletion can cause venous thrombosis and pulmonary embolism.

Generally, owing to recognition of natural biological differences, most competitive events are sex segregated. In many events men have a natural physical biological advantage and the (inevitable) consequence has been that women have been deliberately virilised (by administration of androgens) so that they may outperform their sisters.

It seems safe to assume that anything that can be thought up to gain advantage will be tried by competitors eager for immediate fame. Reliable data are difficult to obtain in these areas. No doubt placebo effects are important, i.e. beliefs as to what has been taken and what effects ought to follow.

The dividing line between what is and what is not acceptable practice is hard to draw. Caffeine can improve physical performance and illustrates the difficulty of deciding what is 'permissible' or 'impermissible'. A cup of coffee is part of a normal diet, but some consider taking the same amount of caffeine in a tablet, injection or suppository to be 'doping'. The fact that success and failure can be separated by mere factions of a second only compounds the problem.

For any minor injuries sustained during athletic training, NSAIDs and corticosteroids (topical, intra-articular) suppress symptoms and allow the training to proceed maximally. Their use is allowed subject to restrictions about route of administration, but strong opioids are disallowed. Similarly, the IOC Medical Code defines acceptable and unacceptable treatments for relief of cough, hay fever, diarrhoea, vomiting, pain and asthma. Doctors should remember that they may get their athlete patients into trouble with sports authorities by inadvertent prescribing of banned substances. The *British National Formulary* provides general advice for UK prescriber. Further information and advice, including the status of specific drugs in sport, can be obtained at http://www.uksport.gov.uk.

Some of the issues seem to be ethical rather than medical, as witnessed by the reported competition success of a swimmer who, it is alleged, had been persuaded under hypnosis into the belief that he was being pursued by a shark, or the instructors at a swimming club in Darwin, Australia, who made their students swim faster by having a (muzzled) crocodile chase them during speed trials.[11]

TYPES OF DRUG DEPENDENCE

The World Health Organization recommends that drug dependence be specified by type for purposes of detailed discussion. The subject can be treated according to the following principal types:

- Opioids (see pp. 304–306).
- Alcohol and other cerebral depressants (benzodiazepines, GHB).
- Tobacco.
- Psychodysleptics (LSD, mescaline, tenamfetamine, phencyclidine, cannabis).
- Psychostimulants (cocaine, amfetamines, methylxanthines, khat).
- Volatile substances.

ETHYL ALCOHOL (ETHANOL)

According to legend, Jamsheed, King of Persia in about 5000 BC kept grapes in containers for use throughout the year. Inevitably, some fermented

---

[11]*The Times* 12 October 2004.

and he concluded that the liquid was poisonous; the containers were appropriately labelled. A member of his harem suffered from severe headaches and drank the liquid, preferring death to the constant pain. She fell asleep and awoke with her headache relieved, whereupon Jamsheed ordered that (the wine) be made regularly available to him. Legend aside, the history of alcohol is part of the history of civilisation 'ever since Noah made his epoch-making discovery'.[12]

Alcohol is important in medicine chiefly because of the consequences of its misuse/abuse. Its misuse is a social problem with pharmacological aspects, which latter are discussed here.

PHARMACOKINETICS

Gastrointestinal absorption of alcohol taken orally is rapid, for it is highly lipid soluble and diffusible. Solutions above 20% are absorbed more slowly because high concentrations of alcohol inhibit gastric peristalsis, thus delaying the arrival of the alcohol in the small intestine which is the major site of absorption.

Absorption is delayed by food, especially milk, the effect of which is probably due to the fat it contains. Carbohydrate also delays absorption of alcohol.

Distribution of alcohol is rapid and throughout the body water (dist. vol. 0.7 L/kg men; 0.6 L/kg women); it is not selectively stored in any tissue.

Maximum blood concentrations after oral alcohol therefore depend on numerous factors including the total dose, sex, the strength of the solution, the time over which it is taken, the presence or absence of food, the time relations of taking food and alcohol, and the kind of food eaten, as well as on the speed of metabolism and excretion. Alcoholic drinks taken on an empty stomach will probably produce maximal blood concentration at 30–90 min and will not all be disposed of for 6–8 h or even more (Fig. 10.1). There are very great individual variations.

Metabolism. About 95% of absorbed alcohol is metabolised, the remainder being excreted in the breath, urine and sweat; convenient methods of estimation of alcohol in all these are available.

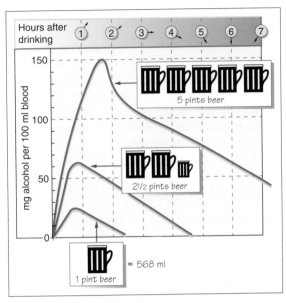

Fig. 10.1 Approximate blood concentrations after three doses of alcohol.

Alcohol in the systemic circulation is oxidised in the liver, principally (90%) by alcohol dehydrogenase to acetaldehyde and then by aldehyde dehydrogenase to products that enter the citric acid cycle or are utilised in various anabolic reactions. Other alcohol-metabolising enzymes are microsomal cytochrome P4502E1 (which alcohol also induces) and catalase.

Alcohol metabolism by alcohol dehydrogenase follows first-order kinetics after the smallest doses. Once the blood concentration exceeds about 10 mg/100 mL the enzymatic processes are saturated and elimination rate no longer increases with increasing concentration but becomes steady at 10–15 mL/h in occasional drinkers. Thus alcohol is subject to dose-dependent kinetics, i.e. saturation or zero-order kinetics, with potentially major consequences for the individual.

Induction of hepatic drug-metabolising enzymes occurs with repeated exposure to alcohol and this contributes to tolerance in habitual users, and to toxicity. Increased formation of metabolites causes organ damage in chronic over-consumption (acetaldehyde in the liver and probably fatty ethyl esters in other organs) and increases susceptibility to liver injury when heavy drinkers are exposed to anaesthetics, industrial solvents and drugs. But chronic use of large amounts reduces hepatic metabolic capacity by causing cellular damage. An acute substantial dose

---

[12]See *Genesis* 9:21; Huxley A 1957 The history of tension. Annals of the New York Academy of Sciences 67:675–684.

of alcohol (binge drinking) inhibits hepatic drug metabolism.

Inter-ethnic variation is recognised in the ability to metabolise alcohol (see p. 152).

The blood concentration of alcohol (see Fig. 10.1) has great medicolegal importance. Alcohol in alveolar air is in equilibrium with that in pulmonary capillary blood, and reliable, easily handled, measurement devices (breathalyser) are used by police at the roadside on both drivers and pedestrians.[13]

PHARMACODYNAMICS

Alcohol exerts on cells in the CNS a generally depressant effect that is probably mediated through particular membrane ion channels and receptors. It seems likely that acetaldehyde acts synergistically with alcohol to determine the range of neurochemical and behavioural effects of alcohol consumption. Alcohol enhances (inhibitory) $GABA_A$-stimulated flux of chloride through receptor-gated membrane ion channels, a receptor subtype effect that may be involved in the motor impairment caused by alcohol (see pp. 151, 152). Other possible modes of action include inhibition of the (excitatory) *N*-methyl-D-aspartate (NMDA) receptor and inhibition of calcium entry via voltage-gated (L type) calcium channels.

Alcohol is not a stimulant; hyperactivity, when it occurs, is due to removal of inhibitory effects. Alcohol in ordinary doses may act chiefly on the arousal mechanisms of the brainstem reticular formation, inhibiting polysynaptic function and enhancing presynaptic inhibition. Direct cortical depression probably occurs only with large amounts. With increasing doses the subject passes through all the stages of general anaesthesia and may die from respiratory depression. Loss of consciousness occurs at blood concentrations around 300 mg/100 mL; death at about 400 mg/100 mL. But the usual cause of death in acute alcohol poisoning is inhalation of vomit.

Psychic effects are the most important socially, and it is to obtain these that the drug is habitually used in so many societies, to make social intercourse not merely easy but even pleasant. They were admirably described by Sollmann half a century ago:

> The first functions to be lost are the finer grades of judgement, reflection, observation and attention – the faculties largely acquired through education, which constitute the elements of the restraint and prudence that man usually imposes on his actions. The orator allows himself to be carried by the impulse of the moment, without reflecting on ultimate consequences, and as his expressions become freer, they acquire an appearance of warmth, of feeling, of inspiration. Not a little of this inspiration is contributed by the audience if they are in a similar condition of increased appreciation … Another characteristic feature, evidently resulting from paralysis of the higher functions, is the loss of power to control moods.[14]

Environment, personality, mood and dose of alcohol are all relevant to the final effect on the individual. These and other effects that are characteristic of alcohol, have been celebrated in the following couplets:[15]

> You may drunk I am think, but I tell you I'm not,
> I'm as sound as a fiddle and fit as a bell,
> And stable quite ill to see what's what …
> And I've swallowed, I grant, a beer of lot –
> But I'm not so think as you drunk I am …
> I shall stralk quite weight and not yutter an ell,
> My feech will not spalter the least little jot:
> If you knownly had own! – well, I gave him a dot,
> And I said to him, 'Sergeant, I'll come like a lamb –
> The floor it seems like a storm in a yacht,
> But I'm not so think as you drunk I am.
> I'm sorry, I just chair over a fell –
> A trifle – this chap, on a very day hot –
> If I hadn't consumed that last whisky of tot!
> As I said now, this fellow, called Abraham –
> Ah? One more? Since it's you! just a do me will spot –
> But I'm not so think as you drunk I am.

---

[13]An arrested man was told, in a police station by a doctor, that he was drunk. The man asked, 'Doctor, could a drunk man stand up in the middle of this room, jump into the air, turn a complete somersault, and land down on his feet?' The doctor was injudicious enough to say, 'Certainly not' – and was then and there proved wrong (Worthing C L 1957 British Medical Journal i:643). The introduction of the breathalyser, which has a statutory role only in road traffic situations, has largely eliminated such professional humiliations.

---

[14]Sollmann T 1957 Manual of pharmacology, 8th edn. Saunders, Philadelphia.

[15]By Sir J C Squire (1884–1958). Quoted by permission of R H A Squire.

Innumerable tests of physical and mental performance have been used to demonstrate the effects of alcohol. Results show that alcohol reduces visual acuity and delays recovery from visual dazzle; it impairs taste, smell and hearing, muscular coordination and steadiness, and prolongs reaction time. It also causes nystagmus and vertigo. At the same time, subjects commonly have an increased confidence in their ability to perform well when tested and underestimate their errors, even after quite low doses. There is a decline in attentiveness and ability to assimilate, sort and take quick decisions on continuously changing information input. This results particularly in inattentiveness to the periphery of the visual field, which is important in motoring. All of these are evidently highly undesirable effects when a person is in a position where failure to perform well may be dangerous.

OTHER EFFECTS OF ALCOHOL CONSUMPTION

Vomiting. This common accompaniment of acute alcoholism seems to be partly a central effect, for the incidence of vomiting at equivalent blood alcohol concentrations is similar following oral or intravenous administration. This is not to deny that very strong solutions and dietary indiscretions accompanying acute and chronic alcoholism can cause vomiting by local gastric effects. When death occurs, it is commonly due to suffocation from inhaled vomit.

Diuretic effect. Alcohol acts by inhibiting secretion of antidiuretic hormone by the posterior pituitary gland. The reason it is useless as a diuretic in heart failure is that the diuresis is of water, not of salt.

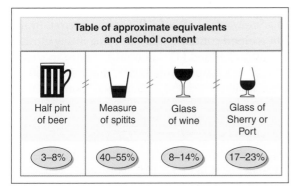

Fig. 10.2 Four standard units of drink (in which social consumption is measured). A unit contains approximately 10 mL (8 g) alcohol. Knowledge of blood alcohol concentration does not allow a reliable estimate of how much has been consumed.

Gastric mucosa. Injury occurs because alcohol allows back diffusion of acid from the gastric lumen into the mucosa. After an acute binge the mucosa shows erosions and also petechial haemorrhages (recovery may take 3 weeks) and up to 60% of chronic alcoholics have chronic gastritis.

Glucose tolerance. Alcohol initially increases the blood glucose level, due to reduced uptake by the tissues. This leads to increased glucose metabolism. But alcohol also inhibits gluconeogenesis and a person whose hepatic glycogen is already low, e.g. a person who is getting most of their calories from alcohol or who has not eaten adequately for 3 days, can experience *hypoglycaemia* that can be severe enough to cause irreversible brain damage. Hypoglycaemia can be difficult to recognise clinically in a person who has been drunk, and this adds to the risk.

Hyperuricaemia occurs (with precipitation of gout) due to accelerated degradation of adenine nucleotides resulting in increased production of uric acid and its precursors. Only at high alcohol concentrations does alcohol-induced high blood lactate compete for renal tubular elimination and so diminish excretion of urate.

Effects on sexual function. Nothing really new has been said since William Shakespeare wrote that alcohol 'provokes the desire, but it takes away the performance'. Performance in other forms of athletics is also impaired. Prolonged substantial consumption lowers plasma testosterone concentration at least partly as a result of hepatic enzyme induction; feminisation may be seen and men have been threatened with genital shrinkage.

Source of energy. Alcohol may be useful as an energy source (rather than a food) in debilitated patients. It is rapidly absorbed from the alimentary tract without requiring digestion and it supplies 7 calories per gram, compared with 9 from fat and 4 from carbohydrate and protein. Heavy doses cause hyperlipidaemia in some people (see p. 152).

Tolerance to alcohol can be acquired and the point has been made that it costs the regular heavy drinker 2.5 times as much to get visibly drunk as it would cost the average abstainer. This is probably due both to enzyme induction and to adaptation of the CNS.

Intolerance. Inter-ethnic variation in tolerance to alcohol is well recognised, for Asian persons, particularly Japanese, develop flushing, headache and nausea after what are, by caucasian standards, small amounts of the substance. Slow metabolism of (toxic) acetaldehyde by variant forms of alcohol dehydrogenase may explain these features. (see p. 149).

Acute alcohol poisoning is a sufficiently familiar condition not to require detailed description. It is notorious that the characteristic behaviour changes, excitement, mental confusion (including 'blackouts'), incoordination and even coma, can be due to numerous other conditions and diagnosis can be difficult if a sick or injured patient happens to have taken alcohol as well. Alcohol can cause severe hypoglycaemia (see above). Measurement of blood alcohol may clarify the situation.

If sedation is essential, diazepam in low dose is least hazardous. Alcohol dialyses well, but dialysis is used only in extreme cases.

Acute hepatitis, which may be extremely severe, can occur with extraordinarily heavy acute drinking bouts. The single case report that, after a binge, the cerebrospinal fluid tasted of gin remains unconfirmed.

CHRONIC CONSUMPTION

Chronic heavy alcohol use is associated with organ damage including: hepatic cirrhosis; deteriorating brain function (psychotic states, dementia, seizures, Wernicke's encephalopathy, episodes of loss of memory); peripheral neuropathy and, separately, myopathy (including cardiomyopathy); cancer of the upper alimentary and respiratory tracts (many alcoholics also smoke heavily, and this contributes); and chronic pancreatitis.

Malnutrition. With heavy continuous drinking, subjects take all the calories they need from alcohol, cease to eat adequately and develop deficiency of B-group vitamins in particular, including megaloblastosis (due to the alcohol and to alcohol-induced folate deficiency).

Hypertension. Heavy chronic use of alcohol is an important cause of hypertension and this should always be considered in both diagnosis and management. Cessation of use may be sufficient to eliminate or reduce the need for drug therapy. But even social drinking can raise blood pressure, and hypertensives should be told this.

Blood lipoproteins. Moderate intake of alcoholic drinks may increase high-density lipoprotein (HDL) and diminish low-density lipoprotein (LDL) concentrations, which may account for the observed protective effect against ischaemic heart disease (see below).

Reversal of all or most of the above effects is usual in early cases if alcohol is abandoned. In more advanced cases the disease may be halted (except cancer), but in severe cases it may continue to progress. When wine rationing was introduced in Paris, France, in the 1939–1945 war, deaths from hepatic cirrhosis dropped to about one-sixth of the previous level; 5 years after the war they had regained their former level.

CAR DRIVING AND ALCOHOL

The effects of alcohol and psychotropic drugs on motor driving (Fig. 10.3) have been the subject of well deserved attention, and many countries have made laws designed to prevent motor accidents caused by alcohol. The problem has nowhere been solved. In general it can be said that the weight of evidence points to a steady deterioration of driving skill and an increased liability to accidents beginning with the entry of alcohol into the blood and steadily increasing with blood concentration.

Alcohol plays a huge part in causing motor accidents, being a factor in as many as 50%. For this reason, the compulsory use of a roadside breath test is acknowledged to be in the public interest. In the UK a blood concentration exceeding 80 mg alcohol per 100 mL blood (17.4 mmol/L)[16] whilst in charge of a car is a statutory offence. At this concentration, the liability to accident is about twice normal. Other

---

[16]Approximately equivalent to 35 micrograms alcohol in 100 mL expired air (or 107 mg in 100 mL urine). In practice, prosecutions are undertaken only when the concentration is significantly higher to avoid arguments about biological variability and instrumental error. Urine concentrations are little used as the urine is accumulated over time and does not provide the immediacy of blood and breath.

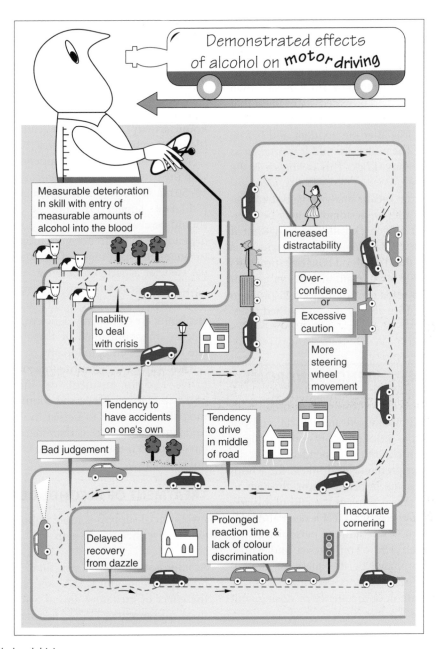

Fig. 10.3 Alcohol and driving.

countries set lower limits, e.g. Nordic countries,[17] some states of the USA, Australia, Greece.

So clearly is it in the public interest that drunken driving be reduced and that the privileges normally attaching to freedom of conscience as well as to personal eccentricity must take second place. In one instance, an ingenious driver, having provided a positive breath test, offered a blood sample on the condition it should be taken from his penis; the physician refused to take it; the police demanded a urine sample; the subject refused on the ground that he had offered blood and that his offer had been refused. He was acquitted, but a

[17]In 1990 Sweden lowered the limit to 20 mg/100 mL, which has been approached by ingestion of glucose which becomes fermented by gut flora in some people – the 'autobrewery' syndrome.

Court has since decided that the choice of site for blood-taking is for the physician, not for the subject, and that such transparent attempts to evade justice should be treated as unreasonable refusal to supply a specimen under the law. The subject is then treated as though he had provided a specimen that was above the statutory limit. Yet another trick is to take a dose of spirits after the accident and before the police arrive. The police are told it was taken as a remedy for nervous shock. This is known is the 'hip flask' defence.

Where blood or breath analysis is not immediately available after an accident, it may be measured hours later and 'back calculated' to what it would have been at the time of the accident. It is usual to assume that the blood concentration falls at about 15 mg/100 mL/h. Naturally, the validity of such calculations leads to acrimonious disputes in the courts of law. (See also: Drugs and skilled tasks, p. 369.)

ALCOHOL DEPENDENCE SYNDROME

Alcohol dependence is a complex disorder with environmental, drug-induced and genetic components with multiple genes probably contributing to vulnerability to the condition. Dependence (chronic alcoholism) varies from social drinkers for whom companionship is the principal factor, through to individuals who take a drink at the end of a working (or indeed any) day, who feel a need and who would be reluctant to give it up, to persons who are overcome by need, who cannot resist and whose whole life is dominated by the quest for alcohol (Fig. 10.4). The major factors determining physical dependence are dose, frequency of dosing, and duration of abuse.

The development involves alterations in CNS neurotransmission. The *acute* effect of alcohol appears to be the blockade of NMDA receptors for which the normal agonist is glutamate, the main excitatory transmitter in the brain. *Chronic* exposure increases the number of (excitatory) NMDA receptors and also 'L type' calcium channels, while the action of the (inhibitory) $GABA_A$ neurotransmitter is reduced. The resulting excitatory effects may explain the anxiety, insomnia and craving that accompanies sudden withdrawal of alcohol (and may explain why resumption of drinking brings about relief, perpetuating dependence).

WITHDRAWAL OF ALCOHOL

Abrupt withdrawal of alcohol from a person who has developed physical dependence, such as may occur when an ill or injured alcoholic is admitted to hospital, can precipitate withdrawal syndrome (agitation, anxiety and excess sympathetic autonomic activity) in 6 h and an acute psychotic attack (delirium tremens) and seizures (by 72 h).

Withdrawal should be supervised in hospital with the patient receiving *chlordiazepoxide* by mouth, 10–50 mg four times daily, gradually reducing over 7–14 days. Longer exposure to chlordiazepoxide should be avoided as it has the potential to induce dependence. A β-adrenoceptor blocker may be given to attenuate symptoms of sympathetic overactivity. General aspects of care, e.g. attention to fluid and electrolyte balance, are important. It is usual to administer vitamins, especially thiamine, in which alcoholics are commonly deficient, and intravenous glucose unaccompanied by thiamine may precipitate Wernicke's encephalopathy.

Clomethiazole (chlormethiazole) is an alternative, also for inpatient use, but carries significant risk of dependence and should not be given if the patient is likely to persist in drinking alcohol. Anticonvulsants, e.g. carbamazepine, topiramate, have also been used to alleviate symptoms of alcohol withdrawal.

TREATMENT OF ALCOHOL DEPENDENCE

Psychosocial support is more important than drugs, which nevertheless may help.

Acamprosate bears a structural resemblance to both glutamate and $GABA_A$ and appears to reduce the effect of excitatory amino acids such as glutamate, and modifies $GABA_A$ neurotransmission during withdrawal. Taken for 1 year (accompanied by counselling and psychosocial support), acamprosate increases the number of alcohol-free days and also the chance of subsequent complete abstinence. The benefit may last for 1 year after stopping treatment. Acamprosate may cause diarrhoea, and cutaneous eruptions.

Disulfiram (Antabuse). In alcoholics who are well and motivated, an attempt may be made to discourage drinking by inducing immediate unpleasantness. Disulfiram inhibits the enzyme aldehyde dehydrogenase so that acetaldehyde (toxic metabolite of

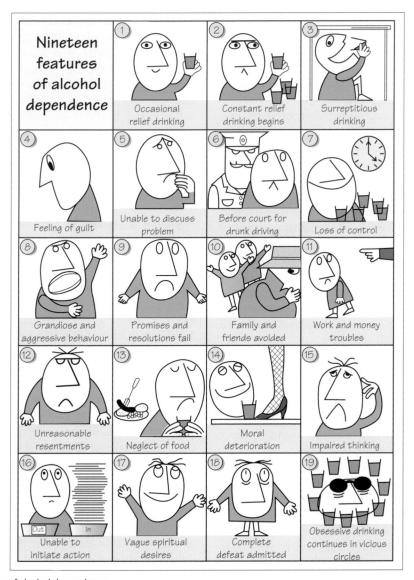

Fig. 10.4 Features of alcohol dependence.

alcohol) accumulates. The objective of administering disulfiram is that patients will find the experience so unpleasant that they will avoid alcohol. It should be administered only under specialist supervision.

A typical reaction of medium severity comes on about 5 min after taking alcohol and consists of generalised vasodilatation and fall in blood pressure, sweating, dyspnoea, headache, chest pain, nausea and vomiting. It may result from even small amounts of alcohol (such as may be present in some oral medicines or mouthwashes). Severe reactions include convulsions and circulatory collapse; they may last several hours. Some advocate the use of a

test dose of alcohol under supervision (after the fifth day of taking), so that patients can be taught what to expect and also to induce an aversion from alcohol.

SAFE LIMITS FOR CHRONIC CONSUMPTION

These cannot be defined accurately. But both patients and non-patients justifiably expect some guidance, and doctors and government departments will wish to be helpful. They may reasonably advise as a 'safe' or prudent maximum (there being no particular individual contraindication): for men not more than

21 units per week (and not more than 4 units in any 1 day), and for women 14 units per week (and not more than 3 units in any 1 day).[18] Consistent drinking of more than these amounts carries a progressive risk to health. In other societies recommended maxima are higher or lower.

Alcoholics with established cirrhosis have usually consumed about 23 units (230 mL; 184 g) daily for 10 years. It has long been thought that total consumption accumulated over time was the crucial factor for cirrhosis. Heavy drinkers may develop hepatic cirrhosis at a rate of about 2% per annum. The type of drink (beer, wine, spirits) is not particularly relevant to the adverse health consequences. A standard bottle of spirits (750 mL) contains 300 mL (240 g) of alcohol (i.e. 40% by volume). A standard human cannot metabolise more than about 170 g/day. People whose intake is concentrated at the weekend allow their livers time for repair and have a lower risk of liver injury than do those who consume the same total on an even daily basis.

Regular low alcohol consumption may even confer benefit: up to one drink per day appears not to impair cognitive function in women and may actually decrease the risk of cognitive decline[19], and light-to-moderate alcohol consumption may reduced risk of dementia in people aged 55 years or more.[20]

The curve that relates mortality (vertical axis) to alcoholic drink consumption (horizontal axis) is J-shaped; i.e. as consumption rises above zero the all-cause mortality declines, then levels off, and then progressively rises. The benefit is largely a reduction of deaths due to cardiovascular and cerebrovascular disease for regular drinkers of 1–2 units per day for men aged over 40 years and postmenopausal women.

Consuming more than 2 units a day does not provide any major additional health benefit. The mechanism may be an improvement in lipoprotein (HDL/LDL) profiles and changes in haemostatic factors.[21] The effect appears to be due mainly to ethanol itself, but non-ethanol ingredients (antioxidants, phenols, flavinoids) may contribute. The rising (adverse) arm of the curve is associated with known harmful effects of alcohol (already described), but also, for example, with pneumonia (which may be secondary to direct alcohol effects, or with the increased smoking of alcohol users).

PREGNANCY, THE FETUS AND LACTATION

Pregnancy is unlikely to occur in severely alcoholic women (who have amenorrhoea secondary to liver injury). The spontaneous miscarriage rate in the second trimester is doubled by consumption of 1–2 units/day.

Fetal injury can occur in early pregnancy (fetal alcohol syndrome). It may be due to the metabolite, acetaldehyde, and so acute (binge) consumption is more hazardous than similar total intake on a daily basis. The vulnerable period of pregnancy is at 4–10 weeks. Because of this, prevention cannot be reliably achieved after diagnosis of pregnancy (usually 3–8 weeks).

There is no level of maternal consumption that can be guaranteed safe for the fetus. But it is plainly unrealistic to leave the matter there, and it has been suggested that if the ideal of total abstinence is unachievable then women who are pregnant or are thinking of becoming pregnant should not drink more than 1–2 units of alcohol per week and should avoid periods of intoxication.[22]

In addition to the fetal alcohol syndrome there is general fetal/embryonic growth retardation (1% for every 10 g alcohol per day) and this is not 'caught up' later.

Fetal alcohol syndrome is a term that covers a spectrum of disorders[23]; it includes the following characteristics: microcephaly, mental retardation with irritability in infancy, low body-weight and

[18]Report of an Inter-Departmental Working Group 1995 Sensible drinking. Department of Health, London.

[19]Stampfer M J, Kang J H, Chen J, Cherry R, Grodstein F 2005 Effects of moderate alcohol consumption on cognitive function in women. New England Journal of Medicine 352:245–253.

[20]Ruitenberg A, van Swieten J C, Witteman J C M et al 2002 Alcohol consumption and the risk of dementia: the Rotterdam study. Lancet 359:281–286.

[21]Rimm E B, Williams P, Fosher K, Criqui M, Stampfer M J 1999 Moderate alcohol intake and lower risk of coronary heart disease: meta-analysis of effects on lipids and haemostatic factors. British Medical Journal 319:1523–1528.

[22]Report of an Inter-Departmental Working Group 1995 Sensible drinking. Department of Health, London.

[23]Mukherjee R A S, Hollins A, Turk J 2006 Fetal alcohol spectrum disorder: an overview. Journal of the Royal Society of Medicine 99:298–302.

length, poor coordination, hypotonia, small eyeballs and short palpebral fissures, lack of nasal bridge.[24]

Children of about 10% of alcohol abusers may show the syndrome. In women consuming 12 units of alcohol per day the incidence may be as high as 30%.

Lactation. Even small amounts of alcohol taken by the mother delay motor development in the child; an effect on mental development is uncertain.

ALCOHOL AND OTHER DRUGS

All cerebral depressants (hypnotics, tranquillisers, antiepileptics, antihistamines) can either potentiate or synergise with alcohol, and this can be important at ordinary doses in relation to car driving. But, when supplies of hypnotics or tranquillisers are given to patients known to drink heavily, they should be warned to omit the drugs when they have been drinking. Deaths have occurred from these combinations.

Alcohol-dependent people with a physical tolerance are relatively tolerant of some other cerebral depressant drugs (hydrocarbon anaesthetics), but the synergism with these drugs still occurs. There is no significant acquired cross-tolerance with opioids.

A *disulfiram-like reaction* occurs with metronidazole, griseofulvin, cefamandole, chlorpropamide, procarbazine and (possibly) tinidazine.

Oral anticoagulants. Control may be disturbed by alcohol inhibiting hepatic metabolism acutely, or enhancing it by enzyme induction; moderate drinking is unlikely to cause trouble.

Anti-epilepsy drugs can be metabolised faster due to enzyme induction by alcohol, and this contributes to its well known adverse effect on epilepsy.

Monoamine oxidase inhibitors (MAOIs). Some alcoholic (and de-alcoholised) drinks contain tyramine, sufficient to cause a hypertensive crisis in a patient taking a MAOI.

Miscellaneous uses of alcohol

Alcohol precipitates protein and is used to harden the skin in bedridden patients. Local application also reduces sweating and may allay itching. As a skin antiseptic, 70% by weight (76% by volume) is most effective. Stronger solutions are less effective. Alcohol injections are sometimes used to destroy nervous tissue in cases of intractable pain (trigeminal neuralgia, carcinoma involving nerves).

OTHER CEREBRAL DEPRESSANTS

Alcohol, benzodiazepines, clomethiazole and barbiturates broadly possess the common action of influencing GABA neurotransmission through the $GABA_A$–benzodiazepine receptor complex (see p. 358 and Fig. 19.6) and all readily induce tolerance and dependence.

γ-Hydroxybutyrate (GHB) is a metabolite of GABA, the major inhibitory transmitter in the CNS. It acts by binding to GABA receptors but additionally affects dopamine, serotonin and endogenous systems. GHB has euphoric and sedative effects and is popular at dance parties where it has achieved notoriety as a 'date-rape drug'. It is highly addictive and frequent ingestion may induce dependency and a severe withdrawal state.

Benzodiazepine dependence is discussed on page 362.

Clomethiazole and barbiturate use, and accordingly opportunity for abuse, is now very limited. Barbiturate use is confined to severe intractable insomnia only in patients already taking barbiturates. Clomethiazole is given short term for severe intractable insomnia, restlessness and agitation in the elderly.

TOBACCO

In 1492, Columbus observed Native Americans using the dried leaves of the tobacco plant (later named *Nicotiana*[25]) for pleasure and also to treat ailments.

---

[24]For pictures see Streissguth A P, Clarren S K, Jones K L 1985 Natural history of the fetal alcohol syndrome: a 10-year follow-up of eleven patients. Lancet ii:85–91.

[25]After the French diplomat, Jean Nicot de Villemain, who introduced tobacco to Europe.

Following its introduction to Europe in the 16th century, tobacco enjoyed popularity to the extent of a panacea, being called 'holy herb' and 'God's remedy'.[26] Later, in a bizarre use, tobacco smoke was administered by bellows as an enema to revive victims of drowning, and special tobacco resuscitation kits were stationed for this purpose at various points along the River Thames in England.[27] Only relatively recently have the harmful effects of tobacco come to light, notably from mortality studies among British doctors.[28] Current estimates hold that there are more than a billion smokers worldwide. In 1990 there were 3 million smoking-related deaths per year, projected to reach 10 million by 2030.[29]

COMPOSITION

The principal components are tar and nicotine, the amounts of which can vary greatly depending on the country in which cigarettes are sold. Regulation and voluntary agreement by manufacturers aspires to achieve a 'global cigarette' containing at most 12 mg tar and 1 mg nicotine.

The composition of tobacco smoke is complex (over 4000 compounds have been identified) and varies with the type of tobacco and the way it is smoked. The chief pharmacologically active ingredients are nicotine (acute effects) and tars (chronic effects).

Smoke of cigars and pipes is alkaline (pH 8.5) and nicotine is relatively un-ionised and lipid soluble, so it is readily absorbed in the mouth. Cigar and pipe smokers thus obtain nicotine without inhaling (they also have a lower death rate from lung cancer; which is caused by non-nicotine constituents).

The smoke of cigarettes is acidic (pH 5.3) and nicotine is relatively ionised and insoluble in lipids. Desired amounts are absorbed only if nicotine is taken into the lungs, where the enormous surface area for absorption compensates for the lower lipid solubility. Cigarette smokers therefore inhale (and have a high rate of death from tar-induced lung cancer). The amount of nicotine absorbed from tobacco smoke varies from 90% in those who inhale to 10% in those who do not.

Smoke drawn through the tobacco and taken in by the smoker is known as main-stream smoke. Smoke that arises from smouldering tobacco and passes directly into the surrounding air, whence it may be inhaled by smokers and non-smokers alike, is known as side-stream smoke. Main-stream and side-stream smoke differ in composition, partly because of the different temperatures at which they are produced.

Side-stream smoke constitutes about 85% of smoke generated in an average room during cigarette smoking. Environmental tobacco smoke has been classified as a known human carcinogen in the USA since 1992.[30] Although the risks of passive smoking are naturally smaller, the number of people affected is large. One study estimated that breathing other people's smoke increases a person's risk of ischaemic heart disease by a quarter.[31]

Tobacco smoke contains 1–5% carbon monoxide and habitual smokers have 3–7% (heavy smokers as much as 15%) of their haemoglobin as carboxyhaemoglobin, which cannot carry oxygen. This is sufficient to reduce exercise capacity in patients with angina pectoris. Chronic carboxyhaemoglobinaemia causes polycythaemia (which increases the viscosity of the blood).

Substances carcinogenic to animals (polycyclic hydrocarbons and nicotine-derived N-nitrosamines) have been identified in tobacco smoke condensates from cigarettes, cigars and pipes. Polycyclic hydrocarbons are responsible for the hepatic enzyme induction that occurs in smokers.

TOBACCO DEPENDENCE

Psychoanalysts have made a characteristic contribution to the problem. 'Getting something orally', one asserted …, 'is the first great libidinous experience in life; first the breast, then the bottle, then the comforter, then food and finally the cigarette.'[32]

[26]Dickson S A 1954 Panacea or precious bane. Tobacco in 16th century literature. New York Public Library, New York. Quoted in Charlton A 2004 Medicinal uses of tobacco in history. Journal of the Royal Society of Medicine 97:292–296.

[27]Lawrence G 2002 Tobacco smoke enemas. British Medical Journal 359:1442.

[28]Doll R, Hill A B 1954 The mortality of doctors in relation to their smoking habits. British Medical Journal i:1451–1455.

[29]Peto R, Lopez A D, Boreham A et al 1996 Mortality from smoking worldwide. British Medical Bulletin 52:12–21.

[30]Environmental Protection Agency (EPA 1992A/600/6–90/006F).

[31]Law M R, Morris J K, Wald N J 1997 Environmental tobacco smoke exposure and ischaemic heart disease: an evaluation of the evidence. British Medical Journal 315:973–988.

[32]Scott R B 1957 British Medical Journal i:671.

Sigmund Freud, inventor of psychoanalysis, was a lifelong tobacco addict. He suggested that some children may be victims of a 'constitutional intensification of the erotogenic significance of the labial region', which, if it persists, will provide a powerful motive for smoking.[33]

The immediate satisfaction of smoking is due to nicotine and also to tars, which provide flavour. Initially the factors are psychosocial; pharmacodynamic effects are unpleasant. But under the psychosocial pressures the subject continues, learns to limit and adjust nicotine intake, so that the pleasant pharmacological effects of nicotine develop and tolerance to the adverse effects occurs. Thus to the psychosocial pressure is now added pharmacological pleasure.

Nicotine possesses all the characteristics of a drug of dependence. It modulates dopamine activity in the midbrain, particularly in the mesolimbic system, which promotes the development and maintenance of reward behaviour. Nicotine inhaled in cigarette smoke reaches the brain in 10–19 s and its short elimination $t_{1/2}$ requires regular smoking to maintain the effect. Inhaling cigarette smoke is thus an ideal drug delivery system to institute behavioural reinforcement and then dependence. A report on the subject concludes that most smokers do not do so from choice but because they are addicted to nicotine.[34]

Tolerance and some physical dependence occur. Transient withdrawal effects include EEG and sleep changes, impaired performance in some psychomotor tests, disturbance of mood and increased appetite (with weight gain), though it is difficult to disentangle psychological from physical effects in these last.

ACUTE EFFECTS OF SMOKING TOBACCO

- *Increased airways resistance* occurs due to the non-specific effects of submicronic particles, e.g. carbon particles less than 1 micrometre across. The effect is reflex: even inert particles of this size cause bronchial narrowing sufficient to double airways resistance; this is insufficient to cause dyspnoea, though it might affect athletic performance. Pure nicotine inhalations of concentration comparable to that reached in smoking do not increase airways resistance.

- *Ciliary activity*, after transient stimulation, is depressed, and particles are removed from the lungs more slowly.

- *Carbon monoxide absorption* may be clinically important in the presence of coronary heart disease (see above), although it is physiologically insignificant in healthy young adults.

NICOTINE PHARMACOLOGY

Pharmacokinetics

Nicotine is absorbed through mucous membranes in a highly pH-dependent fashion. The $t_{1/2}$ is 2 h. It is metabolised largely by P450 (CYP) 2A6 to inert substances, e.g. cotinine, although some is excreted unchanged in the urine (pH dependent, it is un-ionised at acid pH). Cotinine is used as a marker for nicotine intake in smoking surveys because of its conveniently long $t_{1/2}$ (20 h).

Pharmacodynamics

Large doses[35] Nicotine is an agonist to receptors at the ends of peripheral cholinergic nerves whose cell bodies lie in the CNS, i.e. it acts at autonomic ganglia and at the voluntary neuromuscular junction (see Fig. 21.1). This is what is meant by the term 'nicotine-like' or 'nicotinic' effect. Higher doses paralyse at the same points. The CNS is stimulated, including

---

[33]Quoted in Royal Collage of Physicians 1977 Smoking or health. Pitman, London. In 1929 Freud posed for a photograph holding a large cigar prominently. 'He was always a heavy smoker – twenty cigars a day were his usual allowance and he tolerated abstinence from it with the greatest difficulty'. Jones E 1953 Sigmund Freud: life and work. Hogarth Press, London.

[34]Tobacco Advisory Group, Royal College of Physicians 2000 Nicotine addiction in Britain. RCP, London.

[35]Fatal nicotine poisoning has been reported from smoking, from swallowing tobacco, from tobacco enemas, from topical application to the skin and from accidental drinking of nicotine insecticide preparations. In 1932 a florist sat down on a chair, on the seat of which a 40% free nicotine insecticide solution had been spilled. Fifteen minutes later he felt ill (vomiting, sweating, faintness and respiratory difficulty, followed by loss of consciousness and cardiac irregularity). He recovered in hospital over about 24 h. On the fourth day he was deemed well enough to leave hospital and was given his clothes, which had been kept in a paper bag. He noticed the trousers were still damp. Within 1 h of leaving hospital he had to be readmitted, suffering again from poisoning due to nicotine absorbed transdermally from his still contaminated trousers. He recovered over 3 weeks, apart from persistent ventricular extrasystoles (Faulkner J M 1933 Journal of the American Medical Association 100:1663).

the vomiting centre, both directly and via chemo-receptors in the carotid body; tremors and convulsions may occur. As with the peripheral actions, depression follows stimulation.

Doses from/with smoking. Nicotine causes release of catecholamines in the CNS, also serotonin, antidiuretic hormone, corticotropin and growth hormone. The effects of nicotine on viscera are probably largely reflex, from stimulation of sensory receptors (chemoreceptors) in the carotid and aortic bodies, pulmonary circulation and left ventricle. Some of the results are mutually antagonistic.

The following account tells what generally happens after one cigarette, from which about 1 mg of nicotine is absorbed, although much depends on the amount and depth of inhalation and on the duration of end-inspiratory breath-holding.

On the *cardiovascular system* the effects are those of sympathetic autonomic stimulation. There is vasoconstriction in the skin and vasodilatation in the muscles, tachycardia and a rise in blood pressure of about 15 mmHg systolic and 10 mmHg diastolic, and increased plasma noradrenaline (norepinephrine). Ventricular extrasystoles may occur. Cardiac output, work and oxygen consumption rise. Nicotine increases platelet adhesiveness, an effect that may be clinically significant in the development of atheroma and thrombosis.

Metabolic rate. Nicotine increases the metabolic rate, only slightly at rest,[36] but approximately doubles it during light exercise (occupational tasks, housework). This may be due to increase in autonomic sympathetic activity. The effect declines over 24 h on stopping smoking and accounts for the characteristic weight gain that is so disliked and which is sometimes given as a reason for continuing or resuming smoking. Smokers weigh 2–4 kg less than non-smokers (not enough to be a health issue).

Tolerance develops to some of the effects of nicotine, taken repeatedly over a few hours; a first experience commonly causes nausea and vomiting, which quickly ceases with repetition of smoking. Tolerance is usually rapidly lost; the first cigarette of the day

has a greater effect on the cardiovascular system than do subsequent cigarettes.

Conclusion. The pleasurable effects of smoking are derived from a complex mixture of multiple pharmacological and non-pharmacological factors.

In this account nicotine is represented as being the major (but not the sole) determinant of tobacco dependence after the smoker has adapted to the usual initial unpleasant effects. But there remains some uncertainty as to its role, e.g. intravenous nicotine fails adequately to substitute the effects of smoking. An understanding of the full function of nicotine is important if less harmful alternatives to smoking, such as nicotine chewing gum, are to be exploited.

EFFECTS OF CHRONIC SMOKING

Bronchogenic carcinoma. Between 1920 and 1950 an epidemic of bronchogenic carcinoma occurred (the rate in men increased 20-fold) that can be attributed to cigarette smoking; lesser causes include exposure to a variety of industrial chemicals and atmospheric pollution. The most persuasive evidence came from a cohort study of 34 439 British doctors. When follow-up ceased in 2004 some 6000 non-smokers were alive whereas all of the smokers were dead.[37] The risk of death from lung cancer is related to the number of cigarettes smoked and the age of starting. It is similar between smokers of medium (15–21 mg), low (8–14 mg) and very low (> mg) tar cigarettes. Giving up smoking reduces the risk of death progressively from the time of cessation.[38]

Other cancers. The risk of smokers developing cancer of the mouth, throat and oesophagus is five to ten times greater than that of non-smokers. It is as great for pipe and cigar smokers as it is for cigarette smokers. Cancer of the pancreas, kidney and urinary tract is also commoner in smokers.

---

[36]The metabolic rate at rest accounts for about 70% of daily energy expenditure.

[37]Doll R, Peto R, Boreham J, Sutherland I 2004 Mortality in relation to smoking: 50 years' observations of male British doctors. British Medical Journal 328:1519.

[38]Peto R, Darby S, Deo H et al 2000 Smoking, smoking cessation and lung cancer in the UK since 1950: combination of national statistics with two case–control studies. British Medical Journal 321:323–329.

Coronary heart disease (CHD). In the UK about 30% of CHD deaths can be attributed to smoking. Sudden death may be the first manifestation of CHD and, especially in young men, is related to cigarette smoking. Smoking is especially dangerous for people in whom other risk factors (raised blood cholesterol, high blood pressure) are present.

Atherosclerotic narrowing of the smallest coronary arteries is enormously increased in heavy and even in moderate smokers; the increased platelet adhesiveness caused by smoking increases the readiness with which thrombi form.

Stopping smoking reduces the excess risk of CHD in people under the age of 65 years, and after about 4 years of abstinence the risk approximates to that of non-smokers.

Chronic lung disease. The adverse effects of cigarette smoke on the lungs may be separated into two distinct conditions:

- *Chronic mucus hypersecretion*, which causes persistent cough with sputum and fits with the original definition of simple chronic bronchitis. This condition arises chiefly in the large airways, usually clears up when the subject stops smoking and does not on its own carry any substantial risk of death.
- *Chronic obstructive lung disease*, which causes difficulty in breathing chiefly due to narrowing of the small airways, includes a variable element of destruction of peripheral lung units (emphysema), is progressive and largely irreversible and may ultimately lead to disability and death.

Both conditions can coexist in one person and they predispose to recurrent acute infective illnesses.

The *obstructive syndrome* is as specifically related to smoking as is lung cancer. Despite this, in discussing the health effects of tobacco, there has generally been far more emphasis on lung cancer than on this more disabling, but equally fatal disorder.

Other effects. About 120 000 men in the UK aged 30–50 years are impotent because of smoking.[39]

Interactions with drug therapy. Induction of hepatic drug metabolising enzymes by non-nicotine constituents of smoke causes increased metabolism of a range of drugs, including oestrogens, theophylline and warfarin.

WOMEN AND SMOKING

Fertility. Women who smoke are more likely to be infertile or take longer to conceive than women who do not smoke. In addition, smokers are more liable to have an earlier menopause than are non-smokers. Increased metabolism of oestrogens may not be the whole explanation.

Complications of pregnancy. The risks of spontaneous abortion, stillbirth and neonatal death are approximately doubled. The placenta is heavier in smoking than non-smoking women and its diameter larger, possibly from adaptations to lack of oxygen due to smoking, secondary to raised concentrations of circulating carboxyhaemoglobin.

The child. The babies of women who smoke are approximately 200 g lighter than those of women who do not smoke. They have an increased risk of death in the perinatal period which is independent of other variables such as social class, level of education, age of mother, race or extent of antenatal care. The increased risk rises two-fold or more in heavy smokers and appears to be accounted for entirely by the placental abnormalities and the consequences of low birth-weight. Ex-smokers and women who give up smoking in the first 20 weeks of pregnancy have offspring whose birth-weight is similar to that of the children of women who have never smoked.

STARTING AND STOPPING USE

Contrary to popular belief it is not generally difficult to stop, only 14% finding it 'very difficult'. But ex-smoker status is unstable and the long-term success rate of a smoking withdrawal clinic is rarely above 30%. The situation is summed up by the witticism, 'Giving up smoking is easy, I've done it many times'.

Though they are as aware of the risks of smoking as men, women find it harder to stop; they have consistently lower success rates. This trend crosses every age group and occupation. Women particularly dislike the weight gain.

---

[39]*Smoking and Reproductive Life: The Impact of Smoking on Sexual, Reproductive and Child Health.* Available at: http://www.bma.org.uk.

Aids to giving up

For those smoking more than 10 cigarettes per day, nicotine replacement and bupropion (amfebutamone) can provide effective therapy, particularly if supported by access to a smoking cessation clinic for behavioural support. Ideally, smoking should stop completely before embarking on a cessation regimen.

Nicotine, being principally responsible for the addictive effects of tobacco smoking, is a logical pharmacological aid to quitting. It is available in a number of formulations, including chewing gum, transdermal patch, oral and nasal spray. When used casually without special attention to technique, nicotine formulations have proved no better than other aids but, if used carefully and withdrawn as recommended, the accumulated results are almost two times better than in smokers who try to stop without this assistance.[40] Restlessness during terminal illness may be due to nicotine withdrawal and go unrecognised; a nicotine patch may benefit a (deprived) heavy smoker. Nicotine transdermal patches may cause nightmares and abnormal dreaming, and skin reactions (rash, pruritus and 'burning' at the application site). Immunotherapy, using a vaccine of antibodies specific for nicotine, holds promises to prevent relapse in abstinent smokers or for adolescents to avoid initiation.[41]

Bupropion may provide an alternative, or addition, to nicotine. When the drug was being investigated as an antidepressant, researchers noticed that patients gave up smoking, and it was developed as an aid to smoking cessation. Bupropion selectively inhibits neuronal uptake of noradrenaline (norepinephrine) and dopamine, and may reduce nicotine craving by an action on the mesolimbic system. Evidence suggests that bupropion may be at least as effective as the nicotine patch with which it may usefully be combined.

Bupropion may cause dry mouth and insomnia. It is contraindicated in patients with a history of eating disorder or epilepsy or who are experiencing acute symptoms of alcohol or benzodiazepine

withdrawal; where potential for seizure exist, e.g. use of drugs that lower the seizure threshold, this hazard must be weighed against the possible benefits of smoking cessation.

If the patient is heavily tobacco-dependent and severe anxiety, irritability, headache, insomnia and weight gain (about 3 kg) and tension are concomitants of attempts to stop smoking, an anxiolytic sedative (or β-adrenoceptor blocker) may be useful for a short time, but it is important to avoid substituting one drug dependence for another.

There is ample evidence to warrant strong advice against starting to smoke but over-hasty and unreasonable prohibitions on patients' longstanding pleasures (or vices) do no good. The pliable patient is made wretched, but most are merely alienated.

> My doctor's issued his decree
> That too much wine is killing me,
> And furthermore his ban he hurls
> Against my touching naked girls.
> How then? Must I no longer share
> Good wine or beauties, dark and fair?
> Doctor, goodbye, my sail's unfurled,
> I'm off to try the other world.
>
> D G Rossetti, poet (1828–1882)

PSYCHODYSLEPTICS OR HALLUCINOGENS

These substances produce mental changes that resemble those of some psychotic states in which the subject experiences hallucinations or illusions, i.e. disturbance of perception with the apparent awareness of sights, sounds and smells that are not actually present. They are used by people seeking a new experience or escape.

Experiences with these drugs vary greatly with the subject's expectations, existing frame of mind and personality and environment. Subjects can be prepared so that they are more likely to have a good 'trip' than a bad one.

EXPERIENCES WITH PSYCHODYSLEPTICS

The following brief account of experiences with LSD (lysergic acid diethylamide, lysergide) in normal subjects will serve as a model. Experiences with mescaline and psilocybin are similar:

[40]Lancaster T, Stead L, Silagy C, Sowden A 2000 Effectiveness of interventions to help people to stop smoking: findings from the Cochrane Library. British Medical Journal 321:355–358.

[41]Le Houezec J 2005 Why a nicotine vaccine? Clinical Pharmacology and Therapeutics 78:453–455.

- Vision may become blurred and there may be hallucinations; these generally do not occur in the blind and are fewer if the subject is blindfolded. Objects appear distorted, and trivial things, e.g. a mark on a wall, may change shape and acquire special significance.
- Auditory acuity increases, but hallucinations are uncommon. Subjects who do not ordinarily appreciate music may suddenly come to do so.
- Foods may feel coarse and gritty in the mouth.
- Limbs may be left in uncomfortable positions.
- Time may seem to stop or to pass slowly, but usually it gets faster and thousands of years may seem suddenly to go by.
- The subject may feel relaxed and supremely happy, or may become fearful or depressed. Feelings of depersonalisation and dreamy states occur.

The experience lasts for a few hours, depending on the dose; intervals of normality then occur and become progressively longer.

Somatic symptoms and signs include nausea, dizziness, paraesthesiae, weakness, drowsiness, tremors, dilated pupils, ataxia. Effects on the cardiovascular system and respiration vary and probably reflect fluctuating anxiety.

There is no shortage of sensational accounts of experience with psychodysleptics, because there has been a vogue amongst intellectuals, begun by Mr Aldous Huxley,[42] for publishing their experiences. Subsequent accounts are tedious to most except their authors and to those who would do the same; they have little pharmacological importance and reveal more about the author's egocentricity than about pharmacology. The same applies to published accounts of what it is like to be a drug addict.

LYSERGIDE (LSD)

Lysergic acid provides the nucleus of the ergot alkaloids and it was during a study of derivatives of this in a search for an analeptic that in 1943 a Swiss worker investigating LSD felt peculiar and had visual hallucinations. This led him to take a dose of the substance and so to discover its remarkable potency, an effective oral dose being about 30 microgams.

The $t_{1/2}$ is 3 h. (See description of experience, above.) Mechanisms of action are complex and include agonist effect at pre-synaptic 5-HT receptors in the CNS.

Tachyphylaxis (acute tolerance) occurs to LSD. Psychological dependence may occur; physical dependence does not.

Serious adverse effects include psychotic reactions (which can be delayed in onset) with suicide.

LSD has curious effects in animals: green sunfish become aggressive, Siamese fighting fish float nose up, tail down, and goats walk in unaccustomed stereotyped patterns. The elephant exhibits episodically a form of sexual or delinquent behaviour known as 'musth'.

Mescaline is an alkaloid from the Mexican peyote cactus (derived from the Indian word peyotl, meaning 'divine messenger'), the top of which is cut off and dried and used as 'mescal buttons' in religious ceremonies. Mescaline does not induce serious dependence and the drug has little importance except to members of some North and Central American societies and to psychiatrists and biochemists who are interested in the mechanism of induced psychotic states.

Psilocybin is derived from varieties of the fungus Psilocybe ('magic mushrooms') that grow in many countries. It is related to LSD.

Tenamfetamine ('ecstasy', MDMA: methylenedioxymethamfetamine) is structurally related to mescaline as well as to amfetamine. It was originally patented in 1914 as an appetite suppressant and has recently achieved widespread popularity as a dance drug at 'rave' parties (where it is deemed necessary to keep pace with the beat and duration of the music). An estimated 5% of the American adult population have used tenamfetamine at least once.[43] Popular names reflect the appearance of the tablets and capsules and include White Dove, White Burger, Red and Black, Denis the Menace.

Tenamfetamine stimulates central and peripheral α- and β-adrenoceptors; thus the pharmacological effects are compounded by those of physical

---

[42]Huxley A 1964 The doors of perception. Chatto & Windus, London.

[43]Roehr B 2005 Half a million Americans use methamfetamine every week. British Medical Journal 332:476.

exertion, dehydration and heat. In susceptible individuals (poor metabolisers who exhibit the CYP450 2D6 polymorphism) a severe and fatal idiosyncratic reaction may occur with fulminant hyperthermia, convulsions, disseminated intravascular coagulation, rhabdomyolysis, and acute renal and hepatic failure. Treatment includes: activated charcoal, diazepam for convulsions, β-blockade (atenolol) for tachycardia, α-blockade (phentolamine) for hypertension, and dantrolene if the rectal temperature exceeds 39°C.

In chronic users, positive emission tomographic (PET) brain scans show selective dysfunction of serotonergic neurones, raising concerns that neurodegenerative changes accompany long-term use of MDMA.[44]

Phencyclidine ('angel dust') was made in a search for a better intravenous anaesthetic. It is structurally related to pethidine. Phencyclidine was found to induce analgesia without unconsciousness, but with amnesia, in humans (dissociative anaesthesia, see p. 314). Ketamine originated from this work. The postoperative course, however, was complicated by psychiatric disturbance. As the interest of anaesthetists waned, so that of psychiatrists grew and the drug has been used in experimental therapy. Phencyclidine acts as an antagonist at NMDA glutamate receptors.

Overdose can cause agitation, abreactions, hallucinations and psychosis, and if severe can result in seizures, coma, hyperthermia, muscular rigidity, and rhabdomyolysis.

CANNABIS

Cannabis is obtained from the annual plant *Cannabis sativa* (hemp) and its varieties *Cannabis indica* and *Cannabis americana*. The preparations that are smoked are called marijuana (also grass, pot, weed) and consist of crushed leaves and flowers. There is a wide variety of regional names, e.g. ganja (India, Caribbean), kif (Morocco), dagga (Africa). The resin scraped off the plant is known as hashish (hash). The term cannabis is used to include all the above preparations. As most preparations are illegally prepared it is not surprising that they are impure and of variable potency. The plant grows wild in the Americas,[45] Africa and Asia. It can also be grown successfully in the open in the warmer southern areas of Britain. Some 27% of the adult UK population report having used cannabis in their lifetime.

PHARMACOKINETICS

Of the scores of chemical compounds that the resin contains, the most important are the oily cannabinoids, including tetrahydrocannabinol (THC), which is the main psychoactive ingredient. Samples of resin vary greatly in the amounts and proportions of these cannabinoids according to their country of origin; as the sample ages, its THC content declines. As a result, the THC content of samples can vary from 8% to almost zero.

Smoke from a cannabis cigarette (the usual mode of use is to inhale and hold the breath to allow maximum absorption) delivers 25–50% of the THC content to the respiratory tract.

THC ($t_{1/2}$ 4 days) and other cannabinoids undergo extensive biotransformation in the body, yielding scores of metabolites, several of which are themselves psychoactive. They are extremely lipid soluble and are stored in body fat from which they are slowly released.[46] Hepatic drug-metabolising enzymes are inhibited acutely but may also be induced by chronic use of crude preparations.

PHARMACODYNAMICS

Cannabinoid CB_1-receptors (expressed by hypothalamic and peripheral neurones, e.g. sensory terminals in the gastrointestinal tract, and by adipocytes) and CB_2-receptors (expressed only in the periphery

---

[44]In an extreme usage, a man was estimated to have taken about 40 000 tablets of ecstasy between the ages of 21 and 30 years. At maximum he took 25 pills per day for 4 years. At age 37 years, and after 7 years off the drug, he was experiencing paranoia, hallucinations, depression, severe short-term memory loss, and painful muscle rigidity around the neck and jaw. Several of these features were thought to be permanent. (Kouimtsidis C 2006 Neurological and psychopathological sequelae associated with a lifetime intake of 40 000 ecstasy tablets. Psychosomatics 47:86–87.)

[45]The commonest pollen in the air of San Francisco, California is said to be that of the cannabis plant, illegally cultivated.

[46]When a chronic user discontinues, cannabinoids remain detectable in the urine for an average of 4 weeks and it can be as long as 11 weeks before ten consecutive daily tests are negative (Ellis G M et al 1986 Clinical Pharmacology and Therapeutics 38:572).

by immune cells) together with their endogenous ligands (called endocannabinoids) are components of the *endocannabinoid neuromodulatory system* which has a role in many physiological processes including food intake and energy homeostasis. Cannabinoids act as agonists at CB_1-receptors (mediating addictive effects) and CB_2-receptors. Understanding this system offers scope for developing novel drug therapies (see below).

Psychological reactions are very varied, being much influenced by the behaviour of the group. They commence within minutes of starting to smoke and last for 2–3 h. Euphoria is common and is believed to follow stimulation of the limbic system reward pathways causing release of dopamine from the nucleus accumbens, i.e. the same effect that provides the 'kick' with other addictive drugs. There may be giggling or laughter which can seem pointless to an observer. Sensations become more vivid, especially visual, and contrast and intensity of colour can increase, although no change in acuity occurs. Size of objects and distance are distorted. Sense of time can disappear altogether, leaving a sometimes distressing sense of timelessness. Recent memory and selective attention are impaired; the beginning of a sentence may be forgotten before it is finished, and the subject is very suggestible and easily distracted. Psychological tests such as mental arithmetic, digit-symbol substitution and pursuit meter tests show impairment. These effects may be accompanied by feelings of deep insight and truth. Memory defect may persist for weeks after abstinence.

Once memory is impaired, concentration becomes less effective, because the object of attention is less well remembered. With this may go an insensitivity to danger or the consequences of actions.

A striking phenomenon is the intermittent wave-like nature of these effects which affects mood, visual impressions, time sense, spatial sense, and other functions.

The desired effects of cannabinoids, as of other psychodysleptics, depend not only on the expectation of the user and the dose, but also on the environmental situation and personality. Genial or revelatory experiences may indeed occur, e.g. 'Haschich Fudge'.[47]

(which anyone can whip up on a rainy day). This is the food of Paradise … euphoria and brilliant storms of laughter, ecstatic reveries and extension of one's personality on several simultaneous planes are to be complacently expected. Almost anything St Teresa[48] did, you can do better …

But this cannot be relied upon.

Cannabinoids and skilled tasks, e.g. car driving. General performance in both motor and psychological tests deteriorates, more in naive than in experienced subjects. Effects may be similar to alcohol, but experiments in which the subjects are unaware that they are being tested (and so do not compensate voluntarily) are difficult to do, as with alcohol. Some scientists claim the effects are negligible but this view has been 'put in proper perspective' by a commentator[49] who asked how these scientists 'would feel if told that the pilot of their international jet taking them to a psychologists' conference, was just having a reefer or two before opening up the controls'. He had a point: in a placebo-controlled trial of airline pilots in a flight simulator, performance was impaired for up to 50 h after the pilots smoked a joint containing THC 20 mg (a relatively low dose by current standards).[50]

USES

A therapeutic role has been suggested for cannabinoids in a variety of conditions including chronic pain, migraine headaches, muscle spasticity in multiple sclerosis or spinal cord injury, movement disorders, appetite stimulation in patients with AIDS, and nausea and vomiting. Use of specific cannabinoids rather than the resin allows a clearer picture to emerge.

THC is currently available as *dronabinol*, a synthetic form and as *nabilone*, a synthetic analogue, and both are approved to alleviate:

- chemotherapy-induced vomiting in patients who have shown inadequate response to conventional antiemetics
- AIDS-related wasting syndrome.

---

[47]From Toklas A B 1954 The Alice B Toklas cook book. Michael Joseph, London. The author was companion to Gertrude ('rose is a rose is a rose') Stein (1874–1946).

[48]St Teresa of Avila (1515–1582) was noted for her power of levitation.
[49]Dr G Milner.
[50]Yesavage J A, Leirer V O, Denari M, Hollister L E 1985 'Hangover' effects of marijuana intoxication in airline pilots. American Journal of Psychiatry 142:1325–1328.

Issues of cannabis and cannabis-based medicines were the subject of a working party report[51] whose main conclusions were:

- Inhibition of cannabinoid action can be used to help obese patients to *lose weight*. The first of a new class of CB_1-receptor antagonists, rimonabant, reduced body-weight and improved cardiovascular risk factors (HDL-cholesterol, triglycerides, insulin resistance) in obese patients over 1 year.[52] It may cause nausea and depression and is contraindicated in pregnancy.
- In *neuropathic pain*, i.e. due to damaged neural tissue, data from well controlled but limited duration trials suggest that THC is similar to codeine in potency, is safe and is not associated with tolerance or dependence.
- Cannabinoids regulate bone mass, and cannabinoid receptor antagonists may have a role in the treatment of osteoporosis.
- Data on the value of cannabis preparations for multiple sclerosis are not conclusive, although there is some support for a therapeutic effect.

ADVERSE EFFECTS

The *psychological* effects can be unpleasant, especially in inexperienced subjects, particularly timelessness and the feeling of loss of control of mental processes. Feelings of unease, sometimes amounting to anguish and acute panic, occur as well as 'flashbacks' of previously experienced hallucinations, e.g. on LSD. The effect of an acute dose usually ends in drowsiness and sleep. It is claimed that death has not occurred.

There is also, especially in the habitual user, a tendency to paranoid thinking. Cognitive defect occurs and persists in relation to the duration of cannabis use. High or habitual use can be followed by a psychotic state; this is usually reversible, quickly with brief periods of cannabis use, but more slowly after sustained exposures. Evidence indicates that chronic use may precipitate psychosis in vulnera-

ble individuals.[53] Increase in appetite is commonly experienced.

Tolerance, with continued heavy use, and a *withdrawal* syndrome occur (depression, anxiety, sleep disturbance, tremor and other symptoms). Abandoning cannabis is difficult for many users. In studies of self-administration by monkeys, spontaneous use did not occur but, once use was initiated, drug-seeking behaviour developed. Subjects who have become tolerant to LSD or opioids as a result of repeated dosage respond normally to cannabis but there appears to be cross-tolerance between cannabinoids and alcohol.

The term '*amotivational syndrome*' dignifies an imprecisely characterised state, with features ranging from a feeling of unease and sense of not being fully effective, up to a gross lethargy, with social passivity and deterioration. It is difficult to assess, when personal traits and intellectual rejection of technological civilisation are also taken into account. Yet the reversibility of the state, its association with cannabinoid use, and its recognition by cannabis users make it impossible to ignore. (See Escalation theory, p. 147.)

The smoke produces the usual smoker's cough and delivers much more tar than tobacco cigarettes. In terms of damage to the bronchial epithelium, e.g. squamous metaplasia, (a pre-cancerous change), three or four cannabis cigarettes are the equivalent of 20 tobacco cigarettes.

Cannabinoids are teratogenic in animals, but effect in humans is unproved, although there is impaired fetal growth with repeated use.

MANAGEMENT OF ADVERSE REACTIONS TO PSYCHODYSLEPTICS

Mild and sometimes even severe episodes ('bad trips') can be managed by reassurance including talk, 'talking the patient down' and physical contact, e.g. hand-holding (LSD and mescaline). The objective is to help patients relate their experience to reality and to appreciate that the mental experiences are drug induced and will abate. Because short-term memory is disrupted the treatment can be very time

[51]Working Party Report 2005 Cannabis and cannabis-based medicines. Potential benefits and risks to health. Royal College of Physicians, London.

[52]Van Gaal L F, Rissanen A M, Scheen A J et al 2005 Effects of the cannabinoid-1 receptor blocker rimonabant on weight reduction and cardiovascular risk factors in overweight patients: 1-year experience from the RIO-Europe study. Lancet 365:1389–1397.

[53]Henquet C, Murray R, Linszen D, van Os J 2005 Prospective cohort study of cannabis use, predisposition for psychosis, and psychotic symptoms in young people. British Medical Journal 330:11–14.

consuming, as therapists cannot absent themselves without risking relapse. But with phencyclidine such intervention may have the opposite effect, i.e. over-stimulation. It is therefore appropriate to sedate all anxious or excited subjects with diazepam (or haloperidol). With sedation the 'premorbid ego' may be rapidly re-established.

If the user's 'bad trip' is due to overdose of an antimuscarinic drug, natural or synthetic, then diazepam is specially preferred, or a neuroleptic with no or minimal antimuscarinic effects, e.g. haloperidol. A dose of an anticholinesterase that penetrates the CNS (physostigmine, tacrine) is effective in severe reaction to an antimuscarinic.

PSYCHOSTIMULANTS

COCAINE

Cocaine is found in the leaves of the coca plant (*Erythroxylum coca*), a bush commonly found growing wild in Peru, Ecuador and Bolivia, and cultivated in many other countries. A widespread and ancient practice amongst South American peasants is to chew coca leaves with lime to release the alkaloid which gives relief from fatigue and hunger, and from altitude sickness in the Andes, experienced even by natives of the area when journeying; it also induces a pleasant introverted mental state. The physical constraints of leaf chewing act as a protection against the type of acute toxicity seen with abuse. But what may have been (or even still may be) an acceptable feature of these ancient stable societies has now developed into a massive, criminal business, not for leaf chewing, but for the manufacture and export of purified cocaine to supply an eager and lucrative demand from unhappy but economically richer societies where its use constitutes an intractable social problem. An estimated 344 000 people abused cocaine in the UK in 2003–2004.

Cocaine hydrochloride, extracted from the coca leaves, is a fine white powder (called 'snow' but it has innumerable popular names, including 'dandruff of the Andes'). The powder is used as snuff (snorting), swallowed, smoked (below) or injected intravenously. It is taken to obtain the immediate characteristic intense euphoria which is often followed in a few minutes by dysphoria. This leads to repeated use (10–45 min) during 'runs' of usually about 12 h. After the 'run' there follows the 'crash' (dysphoria, irritability, hypersomnia), lasting for hours to days. After the 'crash' there may be depression ('cocaine blues') and decreased capacity to experience pleasure (anhedonia) for days to weeks.

Mode of action. Cocaine binds to and blocks the dopamine reuptake transporter which plays a key role in controlling entry of dopamine into central nerve terminals after release. Dopamine then accumulates in the synapse and acts on adjacent neurones to produce the characteristic 'high'.

The psychotropic effects of cocaine are similar to those of amfetamine (euphoria and excitement) but briefer. Psychological dependence with intense compulsive drug-seeking behaviour is characteristic of even short-term use, but physical dependence is arguably slight or absent. Tachyphylaxis, acute tolerance, occurs.

Cocaine is metabolised by plasma esterases; the $t_{1/2}$ is 50 min.

Modes of use. Intranasal use causes mucosal vasoconstriction, anosmia and eventually necrosis and perforation of the nasal septum.

Smoking involves converting the non-volatile cocaine HCl into the volatile 'free base' or 'crack' (by extracting the HCl with alkali); for use it is vaporised by heat (it pops or cracks) in a special glass 'pipe'; or mixed with tobacco in a cigarette. Inhalation with breath-holding allows pulmonary absorption that is about as rapid as an intravenous injection. It induces an intense euphoric state. The mouth and pharynx become anaesthetised. (See Local anaesthetic action of cocaine, p. 323.)

Intravenous use gives the expected rapid effect (kick, flash, rush). Cocaine may be mixed with heroin (as 'speedball').

Overdose is common amongst users (up to 22% of heavy users report losing consciousness). The desired euphoria and excitement turns to acute fear, with psychotic symptoms, convulsions, hypertension, haemorrhagic stroke, tachycardia, arrhythmias, hyperthermia; coronary artery vasospasm (sufficient to present as the acute coronary syndrome with chest pain and myocardial infarction) may occur, and acute left ventricular dysfunction.

Treatment is chosen according to the clinical picture (and the known mode of action), from amongst, e.g. haloperidol (rather than chlorpromazine) for mental disturbance; diazepam for convulsions; a vasodilator, e.g. a calcium channel blocker, for hypertension; glyceryl trinitrate for myocardial ischaemia (but not a β-blocker which aggravates cocaine-induced coronary vasospasm).

Fetal growth is retarded by maternal use, but teratogenicity is uncertain.

AMFETAMINES

Amfetamine has had multifarious uses. It is now obsolete for depression and as an appetite suppressant, and its use in sport is abuse (see before). An easily prepared crystalline form of methylamfetamine (known as 'crystal meth' or 'ice') is in widespread illicit use as a psychostimulant. Amfetamine is a racemic compound: the *laevo* form is relatively inactive but dexamfetamine (the *dextro* isomer) finds use in medicine. Amfetamine will be described, and structurally related drugs only in the ways in which they differ.

Mode of action. Amfetamine acts centrally by releasing dopamine stored in nerve endings and peripherally by α- and β-adrenoceptor actions common to indirectly acting sympathomimetics. As with all drugs acting on the CNS, the psychological effects vary with mood, personality and environment, as well as with dose.

Subjects become euphoric and fatigue is postponed. Although physical and mental performance may improve, this cannot be relied on; subjects may be more confident and show more initiative, and be better satisfied with a more speedy performance that has deteriorated in accuracy. On the other hand there may be anxiety and a feeling of nervous and physical tension, especially with large doses, and subjects develop tremors and confusion, and feel dizzy. Time seems to pass with greater rapidity. The sympathomimetic effect on the heart, causing palpitations, may intensify discomfort or alarm. Amfetamine increases the peripheral oxygen consumption and this, together with vasoconstriction and restlessness, leads to hyperthermia in overdose, especially if the subject exercises.

Dependence on amfetamine and similar sympathomimetics occurs; it is chiefly psychological, but there is a withdrawal syndrome, suggesting physical dependence; tolerance occurs.

Mild dependence on (formerly) prescribed amfetamines became common, particularly amongst people with unstable personalities, depressives and tired, lonely people. Unfortunately, drugs provide only the temporary solution of avoidance and postponement of such challenges, retarding rather than assisting progress to maturity.

As well as oral use, intravenous administration (with the pleasurable 'flash' as with opioids) is employed. Severe dependence induces behaviour disorders, hallucinations and even florid psychosis, which can be controlled by haloperidol. Withdrawal is accompanied by lethargy, sleep, desire for food and sometimes severe depression, which leads to an urge to resume the drug.

Pharmacokinetics. Amfetamine ($t_{1/2}$ 12 h) is readily absorbed by any usual route and is largely eliminated unchanged in the urine. Urinary excretion is pH dependent; being a basic substance, elimination will be greater in an acid urine.

Interactions are as expected from mode of action, e.g. antagonism of antihypertensives; severe hypertension with MAOIs and β-adrenoceptor blocking drugs.

Acute poisoning is manifested by excitement and peripheral sympathomimetic effects; convulsions may occur; also, in acute or chronic overuse, a state resembling hyperactive paranoid schizophrenia with hallucinations develops. Hyperthermia occurs with cardiac arrhythmias, vascular collapse, intracranial haermorrhage and death. Treatment is chlorpromazine with added antihypertensive, e.g. labetalol, if necessary; these provide sedation and β-adrenoceptor blockade (but not a β-blocker alone, see p. 433), rendering unnecessary the optional enhancement of elimination by urinary acidification.

Chronic overdose can cause a psychotic state mimicking schizophrenia. A vasculitis of the cerebral and/ or renal vessels can occur, possibly due to release of vasoconstrictor amines from both platelets and nerve endings. Severe hypertension can result from the renal vasculitis.

Structurally related drugs include dexamfetamine, used for narcolepsy and in attention deficit hyperactivity disorder (ADHD) (see p. 368), methylphenidate (used for ADHD), tenamfetamine (Ecstasy, see p. 163), phentermine, diethylpropion and pemoline.

METHYLXANTHINES (XANTHINES)

The three xanthines, *caffeine, theophylline* and *theobromine*, occur in plants. They are qualitatively similar but differ markedly in potency:

- Tea contains caffeine and theophylline.
- Coffee contains caffeine.
- Cocoa and chocolate contain caffeine and theobromine.
- The cola nut ('cola' drinks) contains caffeine.

Theobromine is weak and of no clinical importance.

Mode of action. Caffeine and theophylline have complex and incompletely elucidated actions, which include inhibition of phosphodiesterase (the enzyme that breaks down cyclic AMP, see pp. 493, 526), effects on intracellular calcium distribution, and noradrenergic function. When theophylline (as aminophylline) is used alongside salbutamol in asthma, its action adds up to increased benefit to the bronchi, but increased risk to the heart.

Pharmacokinetics. Absorption of xanthines after oral or rectal administration varies with the preparation used. It is generally extensive (>95%). Caffeine metabolism varies much between individuals ($t_{1/2}$ 2–12 h). Xanthines are metabolised (>90%) by numerous mixed function oxidase enzymes, and xanthine oxidase. (For further details on theophylline, see Asthma.)

Actions on mental performance. Caffeine is more potent than theophylline, but both drugs stimulate mental activity where it is below normal. They do not raise it above normal; thought is more rapid and fatigue is removed or its onset delayed. The effects on mental and physical performance vary according to the mental state and personality of the subject. Reaction time is decreased. Performance that is inferior because of excessive anxiety may become worse. Caffeine can also improve physical performance, both in tasks requiring more physical effort than skill (athletics) and in tasks requiring more skill than physical effort (monitoring instruments and taking corrective action in an aircraft flight simulator). It is uncertain whether the improvement consists only of restoring to normal performance that is impaired by fatigue or boredom, or whether caffeine can also enable subjects to improve their normal maximum performance. The drugs may produce their effects by altering both physical capacity and mental attitude.

There is insufficient information on the effects on learning to be able to give any useful advice to students preparing for examination other than that intellectual performance may be assisted when it has been reduced by fatigue or boredom. Effects on mood vary greatly amongst individuals and according to the environment and the task in hand. In general, caffeine induces feelings of alertness and well-being, euphoria or exhilaration. Onset of boredom, fatigue, inattentiveness and sleepiness is postponed.

Overdose will certainly reduce performance (see Chronic overdose, below). Acute overdose, e.g. intravenous aminophylline (see p. 467), can cause convulsions, hypotension, cardiac arrhythmia and sudden death.

Other effects

Respiratory stimulation occurs with substantial doses.

Sleep. Caffeine affects sleep of older people more than it does that of younger people; this may be related to the fact that older people show greater catecholamine turnover in the CNS than do the young. Onset of sleep (sleep latency) is delayed, bodily movements are increased, total sleep time is reduced and there are increased awakenings. Tolerance to this effect does not occur, as is shown by the provision of decaffeinated coffee.[54]

Skeletal muscle. Metabolism is increased, and this may play a part in the enhanced athletic performance mentioned above. There is significant improvement of diaphragmatic function in chronic obstructive pulmonary disease.

Cardiovascular system. Both caffeine and theophylline directly stimulate the myocardium and cause increased cardiac output, tachycardia, and sometimes ectopic beats and palpitations. This effect occurs almost at once after intravenous injection and lasts for half an hour. Theophylline contributes

---

[54]The European Union regulations define 'decaffeinated' as coffee (bean) containing 0.3% or less of caffeine (normal content 1–3%).

usefully to the relief of acute left ventricular failure. There is peripheral (but not cerebral) vasodilatation due to a direct action of the drugs on the blood vessels, but stimulation of the vasomotor centre tends to counter this.

Changes in the blood pressure are therefore somewhat unpredictable, but caffeine 250 mg (single dose) usually causes a transient rise of blood pressure of about 14/10 mmHg in occasional coffee drinkers (but has no additional effect in habitual drinkers); this effect can be used advantageously in patients with autonomic nervous system failure who experience postprandial hypotension (two cups of coffee with breakfast may suffice for the day). In occasional coffee drinkers two cups of coffee (about 160 mg caffeine) per day raise blood pressure by 5/4 mmHg. Increased coronary artery blood flow may occur but increased cardiac work counterbalances this in angina pectoris.

When theophylline (aminophylline) is given intravenously, slow injection is essential in order to avoid transient peak concentrations which are equivalent to administering an overdose (below).

Smooth muscle (other than vascular muscle, which is discussed above) is relaxed. The only important clinical use for this action is in reversible airways obstruction (asthma), when the action of theophylline can be a very valuable addition to therapy.

Kidney. Diuresis occurs in normal people chiefly due to reduced tubular reabsorption of sodium, similar to thiazide action, but weaker.

Preparations and uses of caffeine and theophylline

Aminophylline. The most generally useful preparation is aminophylline, which is a soluble, irritant salt of theophylline with ethylenediamine (see Asthma).

Attempts to make non-irritant, orally reliable, preparations of theophylline have resulted in choline theophyllinate and numerous variants. Sustained-release formulations are convenient for asthmatics, but they cannot be assumed to be bio-equivalent and repeat prescriptions should adhere to the formulation of a particular manufacturer. Suppositories are available. Aminophylline is used in:

- Asthma. In severe asthma (given intravenously) when β-adrenoceptor agonists fail to give adequate response; and for chronic asthma (orally) to provide a background bronchodilator effect.
- Acute left ventricular failure (see p. 467).
- Neonatal apnoea; caffeine is also effective.

Caffeine is used as an additional ingredient in analgesic tablets; about 60 mg potentiates the effects of NSAIDs; also as an aid in hypotension of autonomic failure (above) and to enhance oral ergotamine absorption in migraine.

XANTHINE-CONTAINING DRINKS (SEE ALSO ABOVE)

Coffee, tea and cola drinks in excess can make people tense and anxious. Small children are not usually given tea and coffee because they are thought to be less tolerant of the CNS stimulant effect, but cola drinks irrationally escape this prohibition. It is possible to make an imposing list of diseases that may be caused or made worse by caffeine-containing drinks, but there is no conclusive evidence to warrant any general constraints. High doses of caffeine in animals damage chromosomes and cause fetal abnormalities; but studies in humans suggest that normal consumption poses no risk.

Epidemiological studies are not conclusive but indicate either no, or only slight, increased risk (2–3-fold) of coronary heart disease in heavy (including decaffeinated) coffee consumers (more than four cups daily) (see Lipids, below).

Tolerance and dependence. The regular, frequent use of caffeine-containing drinks is part of normal social life, and mild overdose is common. Slight tolerance to the effects of caffeine (on all systems) occurs. Withdrawal symptoms, attributable to psychological and perhaps mild physical dependence occur in habitual coffee drinkers (five or more cups/day) 12–16 h after the last cup; they include headache (lasting up to 6 days), irritability and jitteriness; they may occur with transient changes in intake, e.g. high at work, lower at the weekend. Habitual tea and coffee drinkers are seldom willing to recognise that they have a mild drug dependence.

Chronic overdose. Excessive prolonged consumption of caffeine causes anxiety, restlessness, tremors, insomnia, headache, cardiac extrasystoles and confusion. The cause can easily be overlooked if specific enquiry into habits is not made, including children regarding cola drinks. Of coffee drinkers, up to 25% who complain of anxiety may benefit from reduction of caffeine intake. An adult heavy user may be defined as one who takes more than 300 mg caffeine per day, i.e. four cups of 150 mL of brewed coffee, each containing 80 ± 20 mg caffeine per cup or five cups (60 ± 20 mg) of instant coffee. The equivalent for tea would be 10 cups at approximately 30 mg caffeine per cup; and of cola drinks about 2.0 L. Plainly, caffeine drinks brewed to personal taste of consumer or vendor must have an extremely variable concentration according to source of coffee or tea, amount used, method and duration of brewing. There is also great individual variation in the effect of coffee both between individuals and sometimes in the same individual at different times of life (see Sleep, above).

Decaffeinated coffee contains about 3 mg per cup; cola drinks contain 8–13 mg caffeine per 100 mL; cocoa as a drink, 4 mg per cup; chocolate (solid) 6–20 mg/30 g.

In *young people* high caffeine intake has been linked to behaviour disorders and a limit of 125 mg/L has been proposed for cola drinks.

Blood lipids. Drinking five cups of boiled coffee per day increases plasma total cholesterol by up to 10%; this does not occur with coffee made by simple filtration. Cessation of coffee drinking can reduce plasma cholesterol concentration in hypercholesterolaemic men.

Breast-fed infants may become sleepless and irritable if there is high maternal intake. Fetal cardiac arrhythmias have been reported with exceptionally high maternal caffeine intake, e.g. 1.5 L cola drinks per day.

GINSENG

Ginseng is the root of two plants of the same family (oriental, *Panax ginseng*; Siberian, *Eleutherococcus senticosis*) and contains a range of biologically active substances (ginsenosides).

It has been used as a tonic or stimulant for thousands of years. In animal studies ginseng doubles the time that mice placed in water can swim before becoming exhausted; it appears to have anti-fatigue effects in various other tests in mice (climbing up a rope that is moving downwards) and it increases sexual activity. In humans, ginseng has been claimed to benefit the performance of athletes and astronauts (fewer fatigue-caused errors), and to reduce absenteeism due to respiratory illness in mining and steel workers and truck drivers. Oriental soldiers at war have used ginseng. Despite accumulating evidence and wide use by the public, the medical profession in Western countries remains sceptical of the value of this tonic. A range of adverse effects is reported, including oedema, hypertension, rashes, diarrhoea, sleeplessness and oestrogen-like effects.

KHAT

The leaves of the khat shrub (*Catha edulis*) contain alkaloids (cathinine, cathine, cathidine) that are structurally like amfetamine and produce similar effects. They are chewed fresh (for maximal alkaloid content), so that the habit was confined to geographical areas favourable to the shrub (Arabia, East Africa) until modern transportation allowed wider distribution. Khat chewers (mostly male) became euphoric, loquacious, excited, hyperactive and even manic. As with some other drug dependencies, subjects may give priority to their drug needs above personal, family, and other social and economic responsibilities. Cultivation takes up serious amounts of scarce arable land and irrigation water.

VOLATILE SUBSTANCE ABUSE

Seekers of the 'self-gratifying high' also inhale any volatile substance that may affect the CNS. These include: adhesives ('glue sniffing'), lacquer-paint solvents, petrol, nail varnish, any pressurised aerosol and butane liquid gas (which latter especially may 'freeze' the larynx, allowing fatal inhalation of food, drink, gastric contents, or even the liquid itself to flood the lungs). Even solids, e.g. paint scrapings, solid shoe polish, may be volatilised over a fire.

These substances are particularly abused by the young (13–15 years), no doubt largely because they are accessible at home and in ordinary shops, and these children cannot easily buy alcohol or 'street' drugs (although this latter may be changing as dealers target the youngest). CNS effects include confusion and hallucinations, ataxia, dysarthria, coma, convulsions and respiratory failure. Liver, kidney, lung and heart damage occur. Sudden cardiac death may be due to sensitisation of the heart to endogenous catecholamines. If the substance is put in a plastic bag from which the user takes deep inhalations, or is sprayed in a confined space, e.g. cupboard, there is particularly high risk.

A 17-year-old boy was offered the use of a plastic bag and a can of hair spray at a beach party. The hair spray was released into the plastic bag and the teenager put his mouth to the open end of the bag and inhaled … he exclaimed, 'God, this stuff hits ya fast!' He got up, ran 100 yards; and died.[55]

Signs of frequent volatile substance abuse include perioral eczema and inflammation of the upper respiratory tract.

DRUGS AS ADJUVANTS TO CRIME

Since time immemorial drugs have been used to facilitate sexual excess and robbery, e.g. opium and plants containing antimuscarinics, e.g. hyoscine. All such acts constitute a criminal offence. The advent of synthetic drugs widened the scope and ease of administration.

In 19th-century Chicago (USA) the proprietor of the Lone Palm Saloon, Michael J Finn, employed girls to ensure his customers consumed drinks to which he had added chloral hydrate –the 'Mickey Finn' – they were robbed when unconscious. In our present times, the benzodiazepine flunitrazepam (Rohypnol), has become known as a 'date rape' drug, being used by sexual predators chemically to incapacitate their victims. In addition to its intoxicant and relaxant effects, it frequently causes retrograde amnesia. (See also γ-hydroxybutyrate, GHB, p. 157).

GUIDE TO FURTHER READING

Clark S 2005 Personal account: on giving up smoking. Lancet 365:1855

Doll R 1997 One for the heart. British Medical Journal 315:1664–1668

Edwards R 2004 The problem of tobacco smoking. British Medical Journal 328:217–219 (and subsequent articles in this series on the 'ABC of Smoking Cessation')

Fergusson D M, Poulton R, Smith P F, Boden J M 2006 Cannabis and psychosis. British Medical Journal 322:172–176

Flower R 2004 Lifestyle drugs: pharmacology and the social agenda. Trends in Pharmacological Sciences 25(4):182–185

Gerada C 2005 Drug misuse: a review of treatments. Clinical Medicine 5(1):69–73

Gordon R J, Lowy F D 2005 Bacterial infections in drug users. New England Journal of Medicine 353(18):1945–1954

Jamrozik K 2005 Estimate of deaths attributable to passive smoking among UK adults: database analysis. British Medical Journal 330:812–815

Karch S B 1999 Cocaine: history, use, abuse. Journal of the Royal Society of Medicine 92(8):393–397

Kosten T R, O'Connor P G 2003 Management of drug and alcohol withdrawal. New England Journal of Medicine 348(18):1786–1795

Lange R A, Hillis L D 2001 Cardiovascular complications of cocaine use. New England Journal of Medicine 345(5):351–358

Malaiyandi V, Sellers E M, Tyndale R F 2005 Implications of CYP2A6 genetic variation for smoking behaviours and nicotine dependence. Clinical Pharmacology and Therapeutics 77(3):145–158

Nutt D, King L A, Saulsbury W, Blakemore C 2007 Development of a rational scale to assess the harm of drugs of potential misuse. Lancet 369:1047–1053

Ricaurte G A, McCann U D 2005 Recognition and management of complications of new recreational drug use. Lancet 365:2137–2145 (see also page 2146, the anonymous Personal Account: GHB – sense and sociability)

Room R, Babor T, Rehm J 2005 Alcohol and public health. Lancet 365:519–530

Snead O C, Gibson K M 2005 γ-hydroxybutyric acid. New England Journal of Medicine 352(26):2721–2732

[55]Bass M 1970 Sudden sniffing death. Journal of the American Medical Association 212:2075.

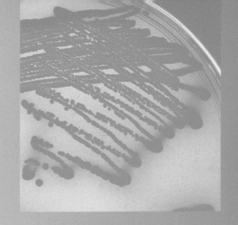

Section 3

INFECTION AND INFLAMMATION

11

Chemotherapy of infections

SYNOPSIS

Infection is a major category of human disease and skilled management of antimicrobial drugs is of the first importance. The term *chemotherapy* is used for the drug treatment of infections in which the infecting agents (viruses, bacteria, protozoa, fungi, worms) are destroyed or removed without injuring the host. The use of the term to cover all drug or synthetic drug therapy needlessly removes a distinction that is convenient to the clinician and has the sanction of long usage. By convention the term is also used to include therapy of cancer.

- Classification of antimicrobial drugs
- How antimicrobials act
- Principles of optimal antimicrobial therapy
- Use of antimicrobial drugs: choice, combinations, chemoprophylaxis and pre-emptive suppressive therapy
- Problems with antimicrobial drugs: resistance, opportunistic infection, masking of infections
- Antimicrobial drugs of choice (Reference table)

HISTORY

Many substances that we now know to possess therapeutic efficacy were first used in the distant past. The Ancient Greeks used male fern, and the Aztecs chenopodium, as intestinal anthelminthics. The Ancient Hindus treated leprosy with chaulmoogra. For hundreds of years, moulds, some no doubt containing penicillin (see below), were applied to wounds. Despite the introduction of mercury as a treatment for syphilis (16th century), and the use of cinchona bark against malaria (17th century), the history of modern rational chemotherapy did not begin until Ehrlich[1] developed

the idea from his observation that aniline dyes selectively stained bacteria in tissue microscopic preparations and could selectively kill them. He invented the word 'chemotherapy' and in 1906 he wrote:

> In order to use chemotherapy successfully, we must search for substances which have an affinity for the cells of the parasites and a power of killing them greater than the damage such substances cause to the organism itself … This means … we must learn to aim, learn to aim with chemical substances.

The antimalarials, pamaquin and mepacrine, came from dyes and in 1935 the first sulphonamide, linked with a dye (Prontosil) was introduced following systematic studies by Domagk.[2] The results obtained with sulphonamides in puerperal sepsis, pneumonia and meningitis were dramatic and caused a revolution in scientific and medical thinking.

In 1928, Fleming[3] accidentally rediscovered the long-known ability of *Penicillium* fungi to suppress the growth of bacterial cultures, but put the finding aside as a curiosity.

In 1939, principally as an academic exercise, Florey[4] and Chain[5] undertook an investigation of antibiotics, i.e. substances produced by microorganisms that are antagonistic to the growth

---

[1] Paul Ehrlich (1854–1915), the German scientist who was the pioneer of chemotherapy and discovered the first cure for syphilis (Salvarsan).

[2] Gerhard Domagk (1895–1964), bacteriologist and pathologist, who made his discovery while working in Germany. Awarded the 1939 Nobel prize for Physiology or Medicine, he had to wait until 1947 to receive the gold medal because of Nazi policy at the time.
[3] Alexander Fleming (1881–1955). He researched for years on antibacterial substances that would not be harmful to humans. His findings on penicillin were made at St Mary's Hospital, London.
[4] Howard Walter Florey (1898–1969), Professor of Pathology at Oxford University.
[5] Ernest Boris Chain (1906–1979), biochemist. Fleming, Florey and Chain shared the 1945 Nobel prize for Physiology or Medicine.

or life of other microorganisms.[6] They prepared penicillin and confirmed its remarkable lack of toxicity.[7]

When the preparation was administered to a police officer with combined staphylococcal and streptococcal septicaemia, there was dramatic improvement; unfortunately the manufacture of penicillin in the local pathology laboratory could not keep pace with the requirements (it was also extracted from the patient's urine and re-injected); it ran out and the patient later succumbed to infection. Subsequent development amply demonstrated the remarkable therapeutic efficacy of penicillin.

The 'bullets' have lost some of their magic with the rise of resistant organisms, and there is an urgent need for new antibiotics. Fewer pharmaceutical companies are involved in antibiotic production: 'The high cost of development, the prolonged safety evaluation, and the probable short duration of field use and the present tendency for any new compound to induce resistance all militate against major investment in new compounds.'[8]

---

[6]Strictly, the definition should refer to substances that are antagonistic in dilute solution because it is necessary to exclude various common metabolic products such as alcohols and hydrogen peroxide. The term antibiotic is now commonly used for antimicrobial drugs in general, and it would be pedantic to object to this. Today, many commonly used antibiotics are either fully synthetic or produced by major chemical modification of naturally produced molecules; hence, 'antimicrobial agent' is perhaps a more accurate term, although 'antibiotic' is much the commoner usage.

[7]The importance of this discovery for a nation at war was obvious to these workers, but the time, July 1940, was unpropitious, for invasion was feared. The mood of the time is shown by the decision to ensure that, by the time invaders reached Oxford, the essential records and apparatus for making penicillin would have been deliberately destroyed; the productive strain of *Penicillium* mould was to be secretly preserved by several of the principal workers smearing the spores of the mould into the linings of their ordinary clothes where it could remain dormant but alive for years; any member of the team who escaped (wearing the right clothes) could use it to start the work again (Macfarlane G 1979 Howard Florey, the making of a great scientist. Oxford University Press, Oxford).

[8]Lord Soulsby of Swaffham Prior 2005 Resistance to antimicrobials in humans and animals. British Medical Journal 331:1219.

CLASSIFICATION OF ANTIMICROBIAL DRUGS

Antimicrobial agents may be classified according to the type of organism against which they are active and in this book follow the sequence:

- Antibacterial drugs.
- Antiviral drugs.
- Antifungal drugs.
- Antiprotozoal drugs.
- Anthelminthic drugs.

A few antimicrobials have useful activity across several of these groups. For example, metronidazole inhibits obligate anaerobic bacteria as well as some protozoa that rely on anaerobic metabolic pathways (such as *Trichomonas vaginalis*).

Antimicrobial drugs have also been classified broadly into:

- *Bacteriostatic*, i.e. those that act primarily by arresting bacterial multiplication, such as sulphonamides, tetracyclines and chloramphenicol.
- *Bactericidal*, i.e. those that act primarily by killing bacteria, such as penicillins, aminoglycosides and rifampicin.

The classification is in part arbitrary because most bacteriostatic drugs are bactericidal at high concentrations, under certain incubation conditions in vitro, and against some bacteria. There is clinical evidence to support use of conventionally bactericidal drugs even for infective endocarditis and meningitis.

Bactericidal drugs act most effectively on rapidly dividing organisms. Thus a bacteriostatic drug, by reducing multiplication, may protect the organism from the killing effect of a bactericidal drug. Such mutual antagonism of antimicrobials may be clinically important, but the matter is complex because of the multiple and changing factors that determine therapeutic efficacy at the site of infection. In vitro tests of antibacterial synergy and antagonism may replicate these conditions only distantly. Probably more important is whether its antimicrobial effect is *concentration* dependent or *time* dependent.

Examples of the former include the quinolones and aminoglycosides in which the outcome relates to the peak antibiotic concentration achieved at the site of infection in relation to the minimum concentration necessary to inhibit multiplication of the organism (the 'minimum inhibitory concentration', or MIC). These antimicrobials produce a prolonged inhibitory effect on bacterial multiplication (the post-antibiotic effect, or PAE), suppressing growth until the next dose is given. In contrast, the β-lactams and macrolides have PAEs that are more modest and exhibit time-dependent killing; for optimal efficacy, their concentrations should be kept above the MIC for a high proportion of the time between each dose.

Figure 11.1 shows the results of an experiment in which a culture broth initially containing 10^6 bacteria per millilitre responds to various concentrations of two antibiotics, one of which exhibits concentration-dependent and the other time-dependent killing. The 'control' series contains no antibiotic, and the other series contain progressively higher antibiotic concentrations ranging from 0.5 to 64 times the MIC. Over 6h of incubation, the time-dependent antibiotic exhibits killing, but there is no difference between the 1× and 64× MIC. The additional cidal effect of rising

concentrations of the antibiotic that has concentration-dependent killing can be clearly seen.

HOW ANTIMICROBIALS ACT – SITES OF ACTION

Drugs are seldom the sole instruments of cure but act together with the natural defences of the body. Antimicrobials act at different sites in the target organism as follows.

The cell wall gives the bacterium its characteristic shape and provides protection against the lower osmotic pressure of the environment. Bacterial multiplication involves breakdown and extension of the wall; interference with these processes prevents the organism from resisting osmotic pressures, so that it bursts. As the cells of higher, e.g. human, organisms do not possess this type of wall, drugs that act here may be especially selective; obviously, the drugs are effective only against growing cells. They include penicillins, cephalosporins, vancomycin, bacitracin, cycloserine.

The cytoplasmic membrane inside the cell wall is the site of much of biochemical activity. Drugs that interfere with its structure include polyenes (nystatin, amphotericin), azoles (fluconazole, itraconazole), polymyxins (colistin, polymixin B) and daptomycin.

Protein synthesis. Drugs that interfere at various points with the build-up of peptide chains on the ribosomes of the organism include: chloramphenicol, erythromycin, fusidic acid, tetracyclines, aminoglycosides, quinupristin/dalfopristin, linezolid.

Nucleic acid metabolism. Drugs may interfere:

- directly with microbial DNA or its replication or repair, e.g. quinolones, metronidazole, or with RNA, e.g. rifampicin
- indirectly on nucleic acid synthesis, e.g. sulphonamides, trimethoprim.

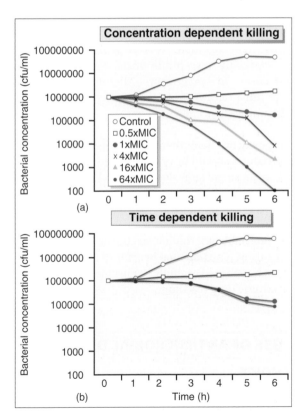

Fig. 11.1 Efficacy of antimicrobials: examples of concentration-dependent and time-dependent killing (see text). cfu, Colony-forming units; MIC, minimum inhibitory concentration.

PRINCIPLES OF ANTIMICROBIAL CHEMOTHERAPY

The following principles, many of which apply to drug therapy in general, are a guide to good practice with antimicrobial agents.

Make a diagnosis as precisely as is possible and define the site of infection, the organism(s) responsible and their sensitivity to drugs. This objective will be more readily achieved if all relevant samples for laboratory culture are taken before treatment is begun. Once antimicrobials have been administered, isolation of the underlying organism may be inhibited and its place in diagnostic samples may be taken by resistant, colonising bacteria, thereby obscuring the true causative pathogen.

Remove barriers to cure, e.g. lack of free drainage of abscesses, obstruction in the urinary or respiratory tracts, infected intravenous catheters.

Decide whether chemotherapy is really necessary. As a general rule, acute infections require chemotherapy whereas other measures may be more important for resolution of chronic infections. For example, chronic abscess or empyema respond poorly to antibiotics alone and require surgical drainage, although chemotherapeutic cover may be essential during surgery to avoid dissemination of infection. Symptomatic management may be preferred to antimicrobials for some acute infections; the risks of adverse drug reactions for previously healthy individuals may outweigh the modest clinical benefits that follow antibiotic therapy of salmonella gastroenteritis and streptococcal sore throat.

Select the best drug. This involves consideration of:

- *Specificity.* Ideally the antimicrobial activity of the drug should match that of the infecting organisms. Indiscriminate use of broad-spectrum drugs promotes antimicrobial resistance and encourages opportunistic infections (see p. 183). At the beginning of treatment, empirical 'best guess' chemotherapy of reasonably broad spectrum must often be given because the precise identification of the responsible microbe is usually uncertain. This problem eases when the causative organisms are known.
- *Pharmacokinetic factors* – to ensure that the chosen drug is capable of reaching the site of infection in adequate amounts, e.g. by crossing the blood–brain barrier.
- *The patient,* who may previously have exhibited allergy to antimicrobials or whose routes of elimination may be impaired, e.g. by renal disease.

Administer the drug in optimal dosage and frequency, and by the most appropriate route(s). Inadequate dose may encourage the development of microbial resistance. In general, on grounds of practicability, intermittent dosing is preferred to continuous infusion. Plasma concentration monitoring can be performed to optimise therapy and reduce adverse drug reactions (e.g. aminoglycosides, vancomycin, 5-flucytosine).

Continue therapy until apparent cure has been achieved; most acute infections are treated for 5–10 days. There are many exceptions to this, such as typhoid fever, tuberculosis and infective endocarditis, in which relapse is possible long after apparent clinical cure and so the drugs are continued for a longer period determined by comparative or observational trials. Otherwise, prolonged therapy is to be avoided because it risks adverse drug reactions and increases costs.

Test for cure. In some infections, microbiological proof of cure is desirable because disappearance of symptoms and signs occurs before the organisms are eradicated. This is generally restricted to especially susceptible hosts, e.g. urinary tract infection in pregnancy. Microbiological culture must be done, of course, after withdrawal of chemotherapy.

Prophylactic chemotherapy for surgical and dental procedures should be of very limited duration, often to only a single large dose (see p. 543).

Carriers of pathogenic or resistant organisms. Allowing normal flora to re-establish naturally may be preferable to routine treatment to remove the organisms. The potential benefits of clearing carriage must be weighed carefully against the inevitable risks of adverse drug reactions.

USE OF ANTIMICROBIAL DRUGS

CHOICE

The general rule is that selection of antimicrobials should be based on identification of the microbe and susceptibility tests. All appropriate specimens (blood, pus, urine, sputum, etc.) must be cultured before administering an antimicrobial.

This process inevitably takes time, and therapy, at least of the more serious infections, must usually be started on the basis of the 'best guess' (i.e. 'empirical' therapy). Especially in critically ill patients, choosing initial therapy to which the infecting microbes are susceptible improves the outcome, and with the worldwide rise in prevalence of multiply resistant bacteria knowledge of the local antimicrobial resistance pattern is essential. Publication of these resistance rates (and corresponding guidelines for choice of empirical therapy for common infections) is now an important role for clinical diagnostic microbiology laboratories. Regular guideline review is necessary to keep pace with changing resistance patterns.

When considering 'best guess' therapy, infections are those in which:

1. Choice of antimicrobial follows automatically from the clinical diagnosis because the causative organism is always the same, and is virtually always sensitive to the same drug, e.g. meningococcal septicaemia (benzylpenicillin), some haemolytic streptococcal infections, e.g. scarlet fever, erysipelas (benzylpenicillin), typhus (tetracycline), leprosy (dapsone with rifampicin).
2. The clinical diagnosis identifies the infecting organism, but without safe assumption as to its sensitivity to any one antimicrobial, e.g. tuberculosis.
3. The infecting organism is not identified by the clinical diagnosis, e.g. in urinary tract infection or abdominal surgical wound infection.

In the second and third categories, particularly, choice of an antimicrobial may be guided by:

Knowledge of the likely pathogens (and their current local susceptibilities to antimicrobials). Cefalexin may be a reasonable first choice for lower urinary tract infection (coliform organisms – depending on the prevalence of resistance locally), and benzylpenicillin for meningitis in the adult (meningococcal or pneumococcal).

Rapid diagnostic tests. There is a revolution in affordable, sensitive and specific nucleic acid detection assays (especially those based on the polymerase chain reaction, PCR). Classically, antimicrobial choice followed direct microscopy of smears of body secretions or tissues, e.g. Ziehl–Neelsen staining for acid-fast tubercle bacilli. Light microscopy will remain useful, but PCR detection of DNA sequences specific for individual microbial species or resistance mechanisms speeds the institution of definitive, reliable therapy, e.g. for meningitis due to *Neisseria meningitidis*, *Streptococcus pneumoniae* and *Haemophilus influenzae*, tuberculosis (including detection of rifampicin resistance) and many viral infections. Quantitative PCR allows monitoring of response to therapy, e.g. copy numbers of circulating cytomegalovirus DNA in a transplant recipient receiving ganciclovir.

Modification of treatment can be made later if necessary, in the light of culture and susceptibility tests. Treatment otherwise should be changed only after adequate trial, usually 2–3 days, for over-hasty alterations cause confusion and encourage the emergence of resistant organisms.

Route of administration. Parenteral therapy (intramuscular or intravenous) is preferred for serious infections because high therapeutic concentrations are reliably and rapidly obtained. Initial parenteral therapy should change to oral whenever possible once the patient has improved clinically and is able to absorb the drug, i.e. without vomiting, ileus or diarrhoea. Many antibiotics are well absorbed orally, and the long-held assumption that prolonged parenteral therapy is necessary for adequate therapy of serious infections, e.g. osteomyelitis, lacks support from clinical trials. Although intravenous therapy is usually restricted to hospital patients, continuation parenteral therapy of certain infections, e.g. cellulitis, is sometimes appropriately performed in the community by specially trained nurses.[9]

Oral therapy of infections is usually cheaper and avoids the risks of maintaining intravenous access, but the gastrointestinal tract experiences higher local concentrations of antibiotic and chance of antibiotic-associated diarrhoea. Some antimicrobials are available only for topical use to skin, anterior nares, eye or mouth; this usage may predispose to the selection of resistant strains and is generally unsuitable with antibiotics that are also used for systemic therapy. Topical therapy to the conjunctival sac is appropriate for therapy of infections of the conjunctiva and the anterior chamber of the eye.

[9]Corwin P, Toop L, McGeoch G, Than M, Wynn-Thomas S 2005 Randomised controlled trial of intravenous antibiotic treatment for cellulitis at home compared with hospital. British Medical Journal 330:129–132.

Other routes used for antibiotics on occasion include inhalational, rectal (as suppositories), intraophthalmic, intrathecal (to the cerebrospinal fluid), and by direct injection or infusion to infected tissues.

COMBINATIONS

Treatment with a single antimicrobial is sufficient for most infections. The indications for use of two or more antimicrobials are to:

- avoid the development of drug resistance, especially in chronic infections where many bacteria are present (encouraging the emergence of a resistant mutant), e.g. tuberculosis;
- broaden the spectrum of antibacterial activity: (1) in a known mixed infection, e.g. peritonitis following gut perforation or (2) where the infecting organism is unpredictable but treatment is essential before a diagnosis has been reached, e.g. septicaemia complicating neutropenia or severe community-acquired pneumonia; full doses of each drug are needed;
- obtain potentiation (or 'synergy'), i.e. an effect unobtainable with either drug alone, e.g. penicillin plus gentamicin for enterococcal endocarditis, and ceftazidime plus gentamicin for serious *Pseudomonas aeruginosa* infections;
- enable reduction of the dose of one component and hence reduce the risks of adverse drug reactions, e.g. flucytosine plus amphotericin B for *Cryptococcus neoformans* meningitis.

Selection of agents. A bacteriostatic drug, by reducing multiplication, may protect the organism from a bactericidal drug (see above, Antagonism). When a combination must be used blind, it is theoretically preferable to use two bacteriostatic or two bactericidal drugs, lest there be antagonism.

CHEMOPROPHYLAXIS AND PRE-EMPTIVE SUPPRESSIVE THERAPY

It is sometimes assumed that what a drug can cure it will also prevent, but this is not necessarily so. The basis of effective, true, chemoprophylaxis is the use of a drug in a healthy person to prevent infection by one organism of virtually uniform susceptibility, e.g. benzylpenicillin against a group A streptococcus. But the term chemoprophylaxis is commonly extended to include suppression of existing infection. To

design effective chemoprophylaxis it is essential to know the organisms causing infection and their local resistance patterns, and the period of time for which the patient is at risk. A narrow-spectrum antibiotic regimen should be administered only during this period – ideally for a few minutes before until a few hours after the risk period. It is much easier to define chemotherapeutic regimens for short-term exposures, e.g. surgical operations, than it is for longer-term and less well defined risks. The main categories of chemoprophylaxis are:

- *True prevention of primary infection*: rheumatic fever,[10] recurrent urinary tract infection.
- *Prevention of opportunistic infections*, e.g. due to commensals getting into the wrong place (bacterial endocarditis after dentistry and peritonitis after bowel surgery). Note that these are both high-risk situations of short duration; prolonged administration of drugs before surgery would result in the areas concerned (mouth and bowel) being colonised by drug-resistant organisms with potentially disastrous results (see below). Immunocompromised patients can benefit from chemoprophylaxis, e.g. of Gram-negative septicaemia complicating neutropenia with an oral quinolone or of *Pneumocystis carinii* pneumonia with co-trimoxazole.
- *Suppression of existing infection* before it causes overt disease, e.g. tuberculosis, malaria, animal bites, trauma.
- *Prevention of acute exacerbations of a chronic infection*, e.g. bronchitis, cystic fibrosis.
- *Prevention of spread amongst contacts* (in epidemics and/or sporadic cases). Spread of influenza A can be partially prevented by amantadine; rifampicin may be used when there is a case of meningococcal meningitis in a family; very young and fragile non-immune child contacts of pertussis might benefit from erythromycin.

---

[10]Rheumatic fever is caused by a large number of types of Group A streptococci and immunity is type specific. Recurrent attacks are commonly due to infection with different strains of these, all of which are sensitive to penicillin and so chemoprophylaxis is effective. Acute glomerulonephritis is also due to Group A streptococci, but only a few types cause it, so that natural immunity is more likely to protect and, in fact, second attacks are rare. Therefore, chemoprophylaxis is not used (see also p. 178).

Long-term prophylaxis of bacterial infection can be achieved often by doses that are inadequate for therapy once the acute infection has been fully treated. Details of the practice of chemoprophylaxis are given in the appropriate sections.

Attempts to use drugs routinely to prevent infection by a range of organisms, e.g. pneumonia in the unconscious or in patients with heart failure, in the newborn after prolonged labour, and in patients with long-term urinary catheters, have not only failed but have sometimes encouraged infections with less susceptible organisms. Attempts routinely to prevent bacterial infection secondary to virus infections, e.g. in respiratory tract infections and measles, have not been sufficiently successful to outweigh the disadvantages of drug allergy and infection with drug-resistant bacteria. In these situations it is generally better to be alert for complications and then to treat them vigorously rather than to try to prevent them.

CHEMOPROPHYLAXIS IN SURGERY

The principles governing use of antimicrobials in this context are as follows.

Chemoprophylaxis is justified when:

- the risk of infection is high because of the presence of large numbers of bacteria at the operative site, e.g. the large bowel
- the risk of infection is low but the consequences of infection would be disastrous, e.g. infection of prosthetic joints or prosthetic heart valves, or of abnormal heart valves following the transient bacteraemia of dentistry
- risks of infection are low but randomised controlled trials in large numbers of patients have shown the benefits of prophylaxis to outweigh the risks, e.g. single-dose antistaphylococcal prophylaxis for uncomplicated hernia and breast surgery. This indication remains controversial.

Antimicrobials should be selected in the light of knowledge of the likely pathogens at the sites of surgery and their prevailing antimicrobial susceptibility.

Antimicrobials should be given intravenously, intramuscularly or occasionally rectally at the beginning of anaesthesia and for no more than 48 h. A single preoperative dose, given at the time of induc-

tion of anaesthesia, has been shown to give optimal cover for many different operations. Vancomycin is often included in prophylactic regimens when the patient is known to be a carrier of meticillin-resistant *Staphylococcus aureus* (MRSA) or its local prevalence is high (ask microbiological advice). Specific instances are:

1. *Colorectal surgery*, because there is a high risk of infection with *Escherichia coli*, *Clostridium* spp., streptococci and *Bacteroides* spp. which inhabit the gut (a cephalosporin plus metronidazole, or benzylpenicillin plus gentamicin plus metronidazole are commonly used).
2. *Gastroduodenal surgery*, because colonisation of the stomach with gut organisms occurs especially when acid secretion is low, e.g. in gastric malignancy, following use of a histamine H_2-receptor antagonist or following previous gastric surgery (usually a cephalosporin will be adequate).
3. *Gynaecological surgery*, because the vagina contains *Bacteroides* spp. and other anaerobes, streptococci and coliforms (metronidazole and a cephalosporin are often used).
4. *Leg amputation*, because there is a risk of gas gangrene in an ischaemic limb and the mortality rate is high (benzylpenicillin, or metronidazole for the patient with allergy to penicillin).
5. *Insertion of prosthetic joints*: chemoprophylaxis is justified because infection (*S. aureus*, coagulase-negative staphylococci and coliforms are commonest) often means that the artificial joint, valve or vessel must be replaced (various regimens are used). Single perioperative doses of appropriate antibiotics with plasma elimination $t_{1/2}$ of several hours (e.g. cefotaxime) are adequate, but if short $t_{1/2}$ agents are used (e.g. flucloxacillin) several doses should be given during the first 24 h.

PROBLEMS WITH ANTIMICROBIAL DRUGS

RESISTANCE

Microbial resistance to antimicrobials is a matter of great importance; if sensitive strains are supplanted by resistant ones, then a valuable drug may become useless. Just as:

Some are born great, some achieve greatness, and some have greatness thrust upon them.[11]

so microorganisms may be naturally ('born') resistant, 'achieve' resistance by mutation, or have resistance 'thrust upon them' by transfer of plasmids and other mobile genetic elements.

Resistance may become more prevalent by spread of microorganisms containing resistance genes, and also by dissemination of the resistance genes among different microbial species. Because resistant strains are encouraged (selected) at the population level by use of antimicrobial agents, antibiotics are the only group of therapeutic agents that can alter the actual diseases suffered by untreated individuals. About half of the use of antimicrobials is in human medicine (the other half is in animals) and 80% of human use occurs in domiciliary practice, out of hospitals.

Problems of antimicrobial resistance have burgeoned during the past few decades in most countries of the world, both in and out of hospital. Some resistant microbes are currently restricted mainly to patients in, or recently in, hospital, e.g. MRSA, vancomycin-resistant enterococci (VRE). Others more commonly infect patients in the community, e.g. penicillin- and macrolide-resistant *Streptococcus pneumoniae* and multiply resistant *Mycobacterium tuberculosis*, whereas some, such as coliforms that produce 'extended spectrum β-lactamases' (ESBLs), are commoner in hospital but occur also quite often in those who have never been inpatients. The outcomes of infections with antibiotic-resistant bacteria are generally poorer, and the costs of therapy and associated length of hospital stay are greater, than those with susceptible strains.

Mechanisms of resistance act as follows:

- *Naturally resistant strains*. Some bacteria are innately resistant to certain classes of antimicrobial agent, e.g. coliforms and many other Gram-negative bacteria possess outer cell membranes that protect their cell walls from the action of certain penicillins and cephalosporins. Facultatively anaerobic bacteria (such as *E. coli*) lack the ability to reduce the nitro group of metronidazole, which therefore remains in an

inactive form. In the course of therapy, naturally sensitive organisms are eliminated and those naturally resistant proliferate and occupy the biological space newly created by the drug.

- *Spontaneous mutation* brings about organisms with novel antibiotic resistance mechanisms. If these cells are viable in the presence of the antimicrobial agent, selective multiplication of the resistant strain occurs so that it eventually dominates as above.

- *Transmission of genes from other organisms* is the commonest and most important mechanism. Genetic material may be transferred, e.g. in the form of *plasmids* which are circular strands of DNA that lie outwith the chromosomes and contain genes capable of controlling various metabolic processes including formation of β-lactamases (which destroy some penicillins and cephalosporins) and enzymes that inactivate aminoglycosides. Alternatively, genetic transfer may occur through *bacteriophages* (viruses that infect bacteria), particularly in the case of staphylococci.

Resistance is mediated most commonly by the production of enzymes that modify the drug, e.g. aminoglycosides are phosphorylated, β-lactamases hydrolyse penicillins. Other mechanisms include decreasing the passage into or increasing the efflux of drug from the bacterial cell (e.g. imipenem resistance in *Pseudomonas aeruginosa*), modification of the target site so that the antimicrobial binds less effectively (e.g. meticillin resistance in staphylococci), and bypassing of inhibited metabolic pathways (e.g. resistance to trimethoprim in many bacteria). The complex molecular systems that control expression of antimicrobial resistance are the subject of a review.[12]

Limiting resistance to antimicrobials involves issues of 'antibiotic stewardship', as follows:

- Avoid indiscriminate use by ensuring that the indication for, and the dose and duration of treatment are appropriate; up to 35% antimicrobial courses administered in the UK (in both hospital and domiciliary practice) may be too long or not indicated at all.

[11]Malvolio in Twelfth Night, Act 2 Scene 5, by William Shakespeare (1564–1616).

[12]Stix G 2006 An antibiotic resistance fighter. Scientific American 294(4):80–83.

- Restrict use of antimicrobial combinations to appropriate circumstances, e.g. tuberculosis.
- Constantly monitor resistance patterns in a hospital or community and change recommended antibiotics used for empirical treatment when the prevalence of resistance becomes high; good infection control in hospitals, such as the isolation of carriers, hand hygiene practices for ward staff, prevent the spread of resistant bacteria.
- Restrict drug use, e.g. limit the use of the newest member of a group of antimicrobials so long as the current drugs are effective; avoid a drug that promotes the proliferation of resistant strains.

The fundamental principle of therapeutics is 'first, do no harm', 'yet, in the case of antibiotics, harm is inevitable, for use (even appropriate usage) selects for resistance, complicating the treatment of future patients'.[13]

Certain policies and practices address the problem. 'Antibiotic cycling', where first-choice antibiotics for commonly treated infections in a hospital or ward are formally rotated over several months or years, does not appear to reduce overall resistance rates or total antibiotic usage. The issuing of 'delayed prescriptions' (used only if symptoms fail to improve in 24–48 h) seems to reduce antibiotic usage without impairing outcomes in upper and lower respiratory tract infection in community practice.

Measures of routine practice can be effective, such as avoiding transmission of resistant bacteria among patients and staff in hospital by performing careful hand hygiene between each patient contact, and through identification and isolation of carriers. Evidence is accumulating that resistance rates do not rise inevitably and irreversibly. In both hospital and domiciliary practice, reductions in antibiotic usage are often followed by reductions in the prevalence of microbial resistance, although there can be a 'lag' of months or years.

SUPERINFECTION

When any antimicrobial drug is used, there is usually suppression of part of the normal bacterial flora of the patient that is susceptible to the drug. Often, this causes no ill effects, but sometimes a drug-resistant organism, freed from competition, proliferates to an extent that allows an infection to be established. The principal organisms responsible are *Candida albicans* and pseudomonads. Careful clinical assessment of the patient is essential, as the mere presence of such organisms in diagnostic specimens taken from a site in which they may be present as commensals does not necessarily mean they are causing disease.

Antibiotic-associated (Clostridium difficile-associated) colitis is an example of a superinfection. It follows alteration of the normal bowel flora by antimicrobials, allowing multiplication of *C. difficile*, which releases several toxins that damage the mucosa of the bowel and promote excretion of fluid. Almost any antimicrobial may initiate this condition, but the drugs most commonly reported today are injectable cephalosporins and amoxicillin/ampicillin. An acute colitis results (pseudomembranous colitis), with diarrhoeal stools containing blood or mucus, abdominal pain, leucocytosis and dehydration. A history of antibiotic use in the previous 3 weeks, even if the drug therapy has been stopped, should alert the physician to the diagnosis, which is confirmed by detection of *C. difficile* toxin in the stools. Mild cases usually respond to discontinuing the offending antimicrobial, and allowing the patient's normal bowel flora to re-establish. More severe cases merit oral metronidazole. Symptomatic patients should be isolated. *C. difficile* may spread among hospitalised patients on the unwashed hands of health-care workers, and it survives well in the environment.

Opportunistic infection arises in patients with compromised immune systems or reduced phagocytic cellular defences, by disease (AIDS, hypogammaglobulinaemia, leukaemia) or drugs (cytotoxics, adrenal steroids). Infections involve organisms that rarely or never cause clinical disease in normal hosts.

Treatment should be prompt, initiated before the results of bacteriological tests are known, and usually involves combinations of bactericidal drugs administered parenterally. Infections of this type include *Pneumocystis carinii* pneumonia and 'primary' septicaemia with gut organisms such as *E. coli* and *Klebsiella*, which cross the mucosa of the gut and invade the bloodstream directly. Compromised local defences may allow

[13]Livermore D M 2005 Minimising antibiotic resistance. Lancet Infectious Diseases 5:450–459.

opportunistic infection with lowly pathogens even in otherwise healthy hosts; the best example is *Staphylococcus epidermidis* infection of intravenous catheters.

MASKING OF INFECTIONS

Masking of infections by chemotherapy is an important possibility. Recognising the possibility, combined with intelligent use of antimicrobials, can minimise the risk. A course of penicillin, adequate to cure gonorrhoea, may prevent simultaneously contracted syphilis from showing primary and secondary stages without effecting a cure; a serological test for syphilis should be done 3 months after treatment for gonorrhoea.

DRUGS OF CHOICE

Table 11.1 is provided for reference. It is a summary of the choice of antimicrobial drugs and owes its form and much of its contents to Medical Letter on Drugs and Therapeutics (USA). The authors are grateful to the Chairman of the Editorial Board for permission to use this material, which has been modified for predominantly UK usage.

The table supplements the general text. Some differences will be noted between text and table, for there may be no single correct procedure for each infection. Suggested alternatives do not necessarily comprise all options.

Tables on drugs for viruses, fungi, protozoa and helminths appear in Chapter 14.

Table 11.1 Reference data on antimicrobial drugs of choice

Infecting organism	Drug(s) of first choice	Alternative drugs
Gram-positive cocci		
Enterococcus		
endocarditis or other severe infection	benzylpenicillin or amoxicillin + gentamicin or streptomycin	vancomycin + gentamicin or streptomycin, or linezolid
uncomplicated urinary tract infection	amoxicillin	a quinolone
Staphylococcus aureus or *epidermidis*		
non-penicillinase-producing	benzylpenicillin or phenoxymethylpenicillin	a cephalosporin or vancomycin or meropenem or erythromycin
penicillinase-producing	flucloxacillin	a cephalosporin or vancomycin or co-amoxiclav or meropenem or erythromycin
meticillin-resistant	vancomycin ± gentamicin ± rifampicin	co-trimoxazole or a tetracycline or linezolid or quinupristin–dalfopristin or sodium fusidate + rifampicin
Streptococcus pyogenes (Group A) and Groups C and G	benzylpenicillin or phenoxymethylpenicillin or amoxicillin	erythromycin or a cephalosporin or vancomycin or clindamycin (the latter for necrotising fasciitis)
Group B	benzylpenicillin or amoxicillin	a cephalosporin or vancomycin or erythromycin
Streptococcus, viridans group (endocarditis)	benzylpenicillin ± gentamicin	vancomycin or a cephalosporin
Streptococcus, anaerobic	benzylpenicillin	metronidazole or a cephalosporin or clindamycin or vancomycin
Streptococcus pneumoniae (pneumococcus)	benzylpenicillin or phenoxymethylpenicillin or amoxicillin	erythromycin or vancomycin or a cephalosporin or rifampicin or a quinolone (or chloramphenicol for meningitis)
Gram-negative cocci		
Moraxella (Branhamella) catarrhalis	co-amoxiclav	erythromycin or a tetracycline
Neisseria gonorrhoeae (gonococcus)	amoxicillin (+ probenecid) or ceftriaxone	spectinomycin or cefixime or cefotaxime
Neisseria meningitidis (meningococcus)	benzylpenicillin	cefotaxime or chloramphenicol

Table 11.1   Reference data on antimicrobial drugs of choice—*Cont'd*

Infecting organism	Drug(s) of first choice	Alternative drugs
Gram-positive bacilli		
Bacillus anthracis (anthrax)	benzylpenicillin or ciprofloxacin	erythromycin or a tetracycline; prophylaxis, ciprofloxacin orally for 60 days (inhalational form) or 7 days (cutaneous form)
Clostridium difficile (pseudomembranous colitis)	metronidazole (oral)	vancomycin (oral)
Clostridium perfringens (gas gangrene)	benzylpenicillin	metronidazole or clindamycin
Clostridium tetani (tetanus)	benzylpenicillin	a tetracycline
Corynebacterium diphtheriae (diphtheria)	erythromycin	benzylpenicillin
Listeria monocytogenes (listeriosis)	amoxicillin ± gentamicin	trimethoprim–sulfamethoxazole
Enteric Gram-negative bacilli		
*Bacteroides		
oropharyngeal strains	benzylpenicillin	metronidazole or clindamycin
gastrointestinal strains	metronidazole	co-amoxiclav or clindamycin or meropenem
*Campylobacter jejuni	erythromycin or a quinolone	tetracycline
*Enterobacteriaceae, e.g.		
*Escherichia coli		
*Klebsiella pneumoniae		
*Proteus spp.		
*Enterobacter aerogenes		
lower urinary tract septicaemia	a quinolone or an oral cephalosporin; gentamicin or cefuroxime or cefotaxime	amoxicillin or trimethoprim or meropenem
*Helicobacter pylori	amoxicillin + clarithromycin + metronidazole (with omeprazole)	amoxicillin + metronidazole + bismuth chelate or tetracycline + clarithromycin + bismuth chelate
*Salmonella typhi (typhoid fever)	a quinolone	chloramphenicol or co-trimoxazole or amoxicillin or ceftriaxone or cefixime or azithromycin
*other Salmonella	a quinolone	amoxicillin or co-trimoxazole or chloramphenicol or ceftriaxone
*Shigella	a quinolone	trimethoprim or ampicillin
*Yersinia enterocolitica (yersiniosis)	co-trimoxazole	a quinolone or gentamicin or tetracycline
Yersinia pestis (plague)	streptomycin or gentamicin	tetracycline; for prophylaxis, ciprofloxacin
Other Gram-negative bacilli		
*Bordetella pertussis (whooping cough)	erythromycin	ampicillin
*Brucella (brucellosis)	doxycycline + streptomycin	co-trimoxazole or rifampicin + doxycycline; for prophylaxis, ciprofloxacin
Calymmatobacterium granulomatis (granuloma inguinale)	a tetracycline	streptomycin or gentamicin or co-trimoxazole
Francisella tularensis (tularaemia)	streptomycin or gentamicin	for prophylaxis, ciprofloxacin
*Fusobacterium	benzylpenicillin	metronidazole or clindamycin or co-amoxiclav
Gardnerella vaginalis (bacterial vaginosis)	oral metronidazole	topical clindamycin or metronidazole, or oral clindamycin or amoxicillin
*Haemophilus ducreyi (chancroid)	erythromycin	a quinolone

(Continued)

Table 11.1 Reference data on antimicrobial drugs of choice—*Cont'd*

Infecting organism	Drug(s) of first choice	Alternative drugs
*Haemophilus influenzae		
meningitis, epiglottitis, arthritis or other serious infections	cefotaxime or ceftriaxone or amoxicillin	cefuroxime (but not for meningitis) or chloramphenicol
upper respiratory infections and bronchitis	amoxicillin	co-amoxiclav or cefuroxime
Legionella pneumophila (legionnaires' disease)	erythromycin ± rifampicin	a quinolone ± rifampicin
Pasteurella multocida (from animal bites)	benzylpenicillin	co-amoxiclav or a cephalosporin
*Pseudomonas aeruginosa		
urinary tract infection	a quinolone	ticarcillin or piperacillin or mezlocillin
other infections	ticarcillin or mezlocillin, or piperacillin or gentamicin or amikacin	ceftazidime or meropenem
Vibrio cholerae (cholera)	tetracycline	a quinolone
Acid-fast bacilli		
*Mycobacterium tuberculosis	isoniazid + rifampicin + pyrazinamide + ethambutol or streptomycin	a quinolone or cycloserine or capreomycin or para-aminosalicylic acid or ethionamide
Mycobacterium leprae (leprosy)	dapsone + rifampicin ± clofazimine	ethionamide or cycloserine
Actinomycetes		
Actinomyces israelii (actinomycosis)	benzylpenicillin	a tetracycline
Nocardia	co-trimoxazole	amikacin or minocycline or meropenem
Chlamydiae		
Chlamydia psittaci (psittacosis, ornithosis)	tetracycline	a macrolide or chloramphenicol
Chlamydia trachomatis		
trachoma	azithromycin	tetracycline (topical plus oral) or a sulphonamide (topical plus oral)
inclusion conjunctivitis	erythromycin (oral or intravenous)	a sulphonamide
pneumonia	erythromycin	a sulphonamide
urethritis, cervicitis	azithromycin or doxycycline	erythromycin or ofloxacin
lymphogranuloma venereum	tetracycline	erythromycin
Chlamydia pneumoniae (TWAR strain)	tetracycline	a macrolide
Ehrlichia		
Ehrlichia chaffeensis	doxycycline	
Mycoplasma		
Mycoplasma pneumoniae	erythromycin or tetracycline or clarithromycin or azithromycin	a quinolone
Ureaplasma urealyticum	erythromycin	tetracycline or clarithromycin
Rickettsia		
Q fever, typhus	doxycycline	chloramphenicol or a quinolone
Spirochaetes		
Borrelia burgdorferi (Lyme disease)	doxycycline or amoxicillin or cefuroxime	cefuroxime or ceftriaxone or cefotaxime or benzylpenicillin
Borrelia recurrentis (relapsing fever)	a tetracycline	benzylpenicillin
Leptospira (leptospirosis)	benzylpenicillin	a tetracycline
Treponema pallidum (syphilis)	benzylpenicillin	a tetracycline or ceftriaxone
Treponema pertenue (yaws)	benzylpenicillin	a tetracycline

*Resistance may be a problem; sensitivity tests should be performed.

GUIDE TO FURTHER READING

Resources on the World Wide Web

The 'Antimicrobial Resistance' section of the website of the UK Health Protection Agency (http://www.hpa.org.uk/infections/topics_az/antimicrobial_resistance/menu.htm) is a valuable resource of contemporary background information on the prevalence and epidemiology of infectious diseases and antimicrobial resistance in the UK.

Global Antimicrobial Resistance Alerts and Implications: the report of the Global Advisory on Antibiotic Resistance Data (GAARD, 2005). Available: http://www.journals.uchicago.edu/CID/journal/contents/v41nS4.html

The Path of Least Resistance: the Report of the Standing Medical Advisory Committee of the UK Department of Health, September 1998. Available: http://www.dh.gov.uk/PublicationsAndStatistics/Publications/PublicationsPolicyAndGuidance/PublicationsPolicyAndGuidanceArticle/fs/en?CONTENT_ID=4009357&chk=87ei43

Recommendations for antimicrobial prophylaxis of infective endocarditis in the UK, 2006. Available: http://jac.oxfordjournals.org/cgi/content/abstract/dkl121v1

Printed resources

Amyes S 2005 Treatment of staphylococcal infection. British Medical Journal 330:976–977

Colebrook L, Kenny M 1936 Treatment with prontosil for puerperal infections: due to haemolytic streptococci. Lancet ii:1319–1322 (a classic paper)

Dancer S J 2004 How antibiotics can make us sick: the less obvious adverse effects of antimicrobial chemotherapy. Lancet Infectious Diseases 4(10):611–619

Fletcher C 1984 First clinical use of penicillin. British Medical Journal 289:1721–1723 (a classic paper)

Jacoby G A, Munoz-Price L S 2005 The new β-lactamases. New England Journal of Medicine 352:380–391

Kwiatkowski D 2000 Science, medicine and the future: susceptibility to infection. British Medical Journal 321:1061–1065

Leibovici L, Shraga I, Andreassen S 1999 How do you choose antibiotic treatment? British Medical Journal 318:1614–1618

Levy S B, Marshall B 2004 Antibacterial resistance worldwide: causes, challenges and responses. Nature Medicine 10(suppl):S122–S129

Livermore D M 2005 Minimising antibiotic resistance. Lancet Infectious Diseases 5:450–459

Loudon I 1987 Puerperal fever, the streptococcus, and the sulphonamides, 1911–1945. British Medical Journal 295:485–490

Lowy F D 1998 Staphylococcus aureus infections. New England Journal of Medicine 339:520–532

Mackowiak P A 1982 The normal microbial flora. New England Journal of Medicine 307:83–93

Russell J A 2006 Management of sepsis. New England Journal of Medicine 355:16

Ryan E T, Wilson M E, Kain K C 2002 Illness after international travel. New England Journal of Medicine 347(7):505–516

Safdar N, Handelsman J, Maki D G 2004 Does combination antimicrobial therapy reduce mortality in Gram-negative bacteraemia? A meta-analysis. Lancet Infectious Diseases 4(8):519–527

12

Antibacterial drugs

SYNOPSIS

The range of antibacterial drugs is wide and affords the clinician scope to select with knowledge of the likely or proved pathogen(s) and of factors relevant to the patient, e.g. allergy, renal disease. Antibacterial drugs are here discussed in groups primarily by their site of antibacterial action and secondly by molecular structure, because members of each structural group are usually handled by the body in a similar way and have the same range of adverse effects.

Table 11.1 (p. 184) is a general reference for this chapter.

Glossary

ESBL	extended-spectrum β-lactamase-producing
GISA	glycopeptide-resistant *Staphylococcus aureus*
MRSA	meticillin-resistant *Staphylococcus aureus*
VISA	vancomycin-intermediate resistant *Staphylococcus aureus*
VRE/GRE	vancomycin-resistant/glycopeptide-resistant enterococci
VMRSA	vancomycin–meticillin-resistant *Staphylococcus aureus*

CLASSIFICATION

INHIBITION OF CELL WALL SYNTHESIS

β-Lactams the structure of which contains a β-lactam ring. The major subdivisions are:

- *Penicillins*, whose official names usually include or end in 'cillin'.
- *Cephalosporins and cephamycins*, which are recognised by the inclusion of 'cef' or 'ceph' in their official names. In the UK recently all these names have been standardised to begin with 'cef'.

Other subcategories of β-lactams include:

- carbapenems, e.g. meropenem
- monobactams, e.g. aztreonam
- β-lactamase inhibitors, e.g. clavulanic acid.

Other inhibitors of cell wall synthesis include vancomycin and teicoplanin.

INHIBITION OF PROTEIN SYNTHESIS

Aminoglycosides. The names of aminoglycosides that derived from streptomyces end in 'mycin', e.g. tobramycin. Others include gentamicin (from *Micromonospora purpurea*, which is not a fungus – hence the spelling as 'micin') and semi-synthetic drugs, e.g. amikacin.

Tetracyclines, as the name suggests, are four-ringed structures and their names end in '-cycline'.

Macrolides, e.g. erythromycin. Clindamycin, structurally a lincosamide, has a similar action and overlapping antibacterial activity.

Other drugs that act by inhibiting protein synthesis include quinupristin–dalfopristin, linezolid, chloramphenicol and sodium fusidate.

INHIBITION OF NUCLEIC ACID SYNTHESIS

Sulphonamides. Usually their names contain 'sulpha' or 'sulfa'. These drugs, sometimes in combination with trimethoprim, inhibit synthesis of nucleic acid precursors.

Quinolones are structurally related to nalidixic acid; the names of the most recently introduced members of the group end in '-oxacin', e.g. ciprofloxacin. They act by preventing DNA replication.

Azoles all contain an azole ring and the names end in '-azole', e.g. metronidazole. They act by the production of short-lived intermediate compounds, which are toxic to DNA of sensitive organisms. Rifampicin inhibits bacterial DNA-dependent RNA polymerase.

Antimicrobials that are restricted to certain specific uses, e.g. tuberculosis or urinary tract infections, appear with the treatment of these conditions in Chapter 13.

INHIBITION OF CELL WALL SYNTHESIS

β-LACTAMS

PENICILLINS

Benzylpenicillin (1942) is produced by growing one of the penicillium moulds in deep tanks. Following synthesis of the penicillin nucleus (6-amino-penicillanic acid) in 1957, it became possible to add side-chains and so to make semi-synthetic penicillins with different properties. Penicillins differ widely in antibacterial spectrum.

A general account of the penicillins (Table 12.1) follows and then of the individual drugs in so far as they differ.

Mode of action. Penicillins act by inhibiting the enzymes (penicillin binding proteins, PBPs) involved in the cross-linking of the peptidoglycan layer of the cell wall, which protects the bacterium from its environment; incapable of withstanding the osmotic gradient between its interior and its environment, the cell swells and ruptures. Penicillins are thus bactericidal and are effective only against multiplying organisms because resting organisms are not making new cell wall.

The main defence of bacteria against penicillins is to produce enzymes, β-lactamases, which open the β-lactam ring and terminate antimicrobial activity. Other possible mechanisms include modifications to PBPs to render them unable to bind β-lactams, reduced permeability of the outer cell membrane of Gram-negative bacteria, and possession of pumps in the outer membrane, which remove β-lactam molecules that manage to enter. Some particularly resistant bacteria may possess several mechanisms that act in concert. The remarkable safety and high therapeutic index of the penicillins is because human cells, although bounded by a cell membrane, lack a cell wall. They exhibit time-dependent bacterial killing (see p. 105).

Pharmacokinetics. Gastric acid destroys benzylpenicillin, which is therefore unsuitable for oral use. Others, e.g. phenoxymethylpenicillin, resist acid and are absorbed in the upper small bowel. The plasma $t_{1/2}$ of penicillins is usually less than 2 h. Penicillins distribute mainly in the body water and enter well into the cerebrospinal fluid (CSF) if the meninges are inflamed. Penicillins are organic acids and their rapidly clearance from plasma is due to tubular secretion by the renal anion transporter. Renal clearance therefore greatly exceeds the glomerular filtration rate (127 mL/min). Concurrent probenecid usefully delays excretion of penicillin by competing successfully for the transport mechanism. Patients with severely impaired renal function require a reduced dose.

Adverse effects. The main hazard with the penicillins is *allergic reactions*. These include itching, rashes (eczematous or urticarial), fever and angio-oedema. Rarely (about 1 in 10 000) there is anaphylactic shock,

Table 12.1 Penicillins	
Group	**Examples**
Narrow spectrum (natural penicillins)	benzylpenicillin, phenoxymethylpenicillin
Antistaphylococcal penicillins (β-lactamase resistant)	cloxacillin, flucloxacillin
Broad spectrum	ampicillin, amoxicillin, bacampicillin
Mecillinam	pivmecillinam
Monobactam (active only against Gram-negative bacteria)	aztreonam[1]
Anti-pseudomonal	
Carboxypenicillin	ticarcillin
Ureidopenicillin	piperacillin
Penicillin–β-lactamase inhibitor combinations	co-amoxiclav, piperacillin–tazobactam, ticarcillin–clavulanate
Carbapenems	meropenem, imipenem–cilastatin

[1]While not strictly a penicillin, aztreonam has a similar spectrum of action including some antipseudomonal activity.

which can be fatal (about 1 in 50 000–100 000 treatment courses). Allergies are least likely with oral penicillins and most likely with local application. Metabolic opening of the β-lactam ring creates a highly reactive penicilloyl group, which polymerises and binds with tissue proteins to form the major antigenic determinant. The anaphylactic reaction involves specific immunoglobulin (Ig) E antibodies, detectable in the plasma of susceptible persons.

There is *cross-allergy* between all the various forms of penicillin, probably due in part to their common structure, and in part to the degradation products common to them all. Partial cross-allergy exists between penicillins and cephalosporins (a maximum of 10%); this is of particular concern when the reaction to either group of antimicrobials has been angio-oedema or anaphylactic shock. Carbapenems (meropenem and imipenem–cilastatin) and the monobactam aztreonam apparently have a much lower risk of cross-reactivity.

When attempting to predict whether a patient will have an allergic reaction, a reliable history of a previous adverse response to penicillin is valuable. Immediate-type reactions such as urticaria, angio-oedema and anaphylactic shock are indicative of allergy, but interpretation of maculopapular rashes is more difficult. As an alternative drug can usually be found, a penicillin is best avoided if there is suspicion of allergy, although the condition is undoubtedly over-diagnosed and may be transient (see below).

When the history of allergy is not clear-cut and a penicillin is necessary, the presence of IgE antibodies in serum is a useful indicator of reactions mediated by these antibodies, i.e. immediate (type 1) reactions. Additionally, an intradermal test for allergy may be performed using standard amounts of a mixture of a major determinant (metabolite) (benzylpenicilloyl polylysine) and minor determinants (such as benzylpenicillin) of the allergic reaction; appearance of a flare and weal reaction indicates a positive response. The fact that only about 10% of patients with a history of 'penicillin allergy' respond suggests that many who are so labelled are not, or are no longer, allergic to penicillin.

Other (non-allergic) adverse effects include diarrhoea due to alteration in normal intestinal flora, which may progress to *Clostridium difficile*-associated diarrhoea. Neutropenia is a risk of high-dose penicillins (or other β-lactam antibiotics), usually for a period of longer than 10 days. Rarely the penicillins cause anaemia, sometimes haemolytic, and thrombocytopenia or interstitial nephritis. Penicillins come as their sodium or potassium salts, and patients inevitably experience significant amounts when the antimicrobial dose is high. Physicians should be aware of this unexpected source of sodium or potassium, especially in patients with renal or cardiac disease. Extremely high plasma penicillin concentrations cause convulsions. Co-amoxiclav and flucloxacillin given in high doses for prolonged periods in the elderly may cause hepatic toxicity.

NARROW-SPECTRUM PENICILLINS

Benzylpenicillin (penicillin G)

Benzylpenicillin ($t_{1/2}$ 0.5 h) is used when high plasma concentrations are required. The short $t_{1/2}$ means that reasonably spaced doses have to be large to maintain a therapeutic concentration. Fortunately, the unusually large therapeutic ratio of penicillin allows the resulting fluctuations to be tolerable.[2] The kidney eliminates benzylpenicillin, some 80% by active secretion by the renal tubule, which probenecid usefully blocks in single-dose therapy for gonorrhoea.

Uses (see Table 11.1, p. 184). Benzylpenicillin is highly active against *Streptococcus pneumoniae* and the Lancefield group A, β-haemolytic streptococcus (*Streptococcus pyogenes*). Viridans streptococci are usually sensitive unless the patient has recently received penicillin. *Enterococcus faecalis* is less susceptible and, especially for endocarditis, penicillin is combined with an aminoglycoside, usually gentamicin. This combination is synergistic unless the enterococcus is highly resistant to the aminoglycoside; such strains are becoming more frequent in hospital patients and present major difficulties in therapy. Benzylpenicillin was active against most strains of *Staphylococcus aureus*, but now more than 90% are resistant in hospital and domiciliary practice. Benzylpenicillin is the drug of choice for infections due to *Neisseria meningitidis* (meningococcal meningitis and septicaemia), *Bacillus anthracis* (anthrax), *Clostridium perfringens*

---

[2]Is it surprise at the answer that reduces most classes of students to silence when asked the trough : peak ratio for a drug given 6-hourly with a $t_{1/2}$ of 0.5 h? (answer: $2^{12} = 4096$).

(gas gangrene) and *tetani* (tetanus), *Corynebacterium diphtheriae* (diphtheria), *Treponema pallidum* (syphilis), *Leptospira* spp. (leptospirosis) and *Actinomyces israelii* (actinomycosis). It is also the drug of choice for *Borrelia burgdorferi* (Lyme disease) in children. Penicillin resistance in *Neisseria gonorrhoeae* is rising in many parts of the world.

Adverse effects are in general uncommon, apart from allergy (above). It is salutary to reflect that the first clinically useful true antibiotic (1942) is still in use and is amongst the least toxic.

Preparations and dosage for injection. Benzylpenicillin is given intramuscularly or intravenously (by bolus injection or by continuous infusion). For a sensitive infection, benzylpenicillin[3] 600 mg 6-hourly is sufficient. In domiciliary practice, a mixture of benzylpenicillin and one of its long-acting variants may be preferred (see below).

Where sensitive organisms sequester within avascular tissue, e.g. infective endocarditis, give 7.2 g daily i.v. in divided doses. When an infection is controlled, change to the oral route with phenoxymethylpenicillin, or amoxicillin, which is more reliably absorbed in adults.

Procaine benzylpenicillin, given i.m. only, is a stable salt and liberates benzylpenicillin over 12–24 h, according to the dose administered. There is no general agreement on its place in therapy, and it is no longer available in a number of countries. Benzylpenicillin is preferred in most severe infections, especially at the outset, as procaine penicillin will not give therapeutic blood concentrations for some hours after injection and peak concentrations are much lower.

Preparations and dosage for oral use. Phenoxymethylpenicillin (penicillin V) resists gastric acid and so reaches the small intestine intact where it is moderately well absorbed, but sometimes erratically in adults. It is less active than benzylpenicillin against *Neisseria gonorrhoeae* and *meningitidis*, and so is unsuitable for use in gonorrhoea and meningococcal meningitis. It is a satisfactory substitute for benzylpenicillin against *Staphylococcus pneumoniae* and *Staphylococcus pyogenes*, especially after intra-

venous therapy has controlled the acute infection. The dose is 500 mg 6-hourly. Give all oral penicillins on an empty stomach to avoid the absorption delay caused by food.

Antistaphylococcal penicillins

Certain bacteria produce β-lactamases, which open the β-lactam ring that is common to all penicillins, and thus terminate the antibacterial activity. β-Lactamases vary in their activity against different β-lactam antibiotics because stearic hindrance from added side-chains limits access of the drug to the enzymes' active site. Drugs that resist the action of staphylococcal β-lactamase do so by possession of an acyl side-chain. The drugs do have activity against other bacteria for which penicillin is indicated, but benzylpenicillin is substantially more active against these organisms – up to 20 times more so in the cases of pneumococci, β-haemolytic streptococci and *Neisseria*. Hence, when infection is mixed, it may be preferable to give benzylpenicillin as well as a β-lactamase-resistant drug in severe cases.

Examples include:

- *Flucloxacillin* ($t_{1/2}$ 1 h), which is better absorbed and so gives higher blood concentrations than cloxacillin. It may cause cholestatic jaundice, particularly when used for more than 2 weeks or to patients aged more than 55 years.
- *Cloxacillin* ($t_{1/2}$ 0.5 h), which resists degradation by gastric acid and is absorbed from the gut, but food markedly interferes with its absorption (it has been withdrawn from the market in some countries, including the UK).
- *Meticillin* and *oxacillin* are now used only for laboratory sensitivity tests. *Staphylococcus aureus* resistance to meticillin (MRSA) indicates resistance to all β-lactam antibiotics (and often to other antibacterial drugs), and evokes the institution of special infection control measures.

BROAD-SPECTRUM PENICILLINS

The activity of these semi-synthetic penicillins extends beyond the Gram-positive and Gram-negative cocci, which are susceptible to benzylpenicillin, and includes many Gram-negative bacilli. They do not resist β-lactamases, and their usefulness has reduced markedly because of the increased prevalence of organisms that produce these enzymes.

---

[3]600 mg = 1 000 000 units, 1 mega-unit.

In general, these agents are less active than benzylpenicillin against Gram-positive cocci, but more active than the β-lactamase-resistant penicillins (above). They have useful activity against *Enterococcus faecalis* and many strains of *Haemophilus influenzae*. *Enterobacteriaceae* are variably susceptible. The differences between the members of this group are pharmacological rather than bacteriological.

Amoxicillin ($t_{1/2}$ 1 h; previously known as amoxycillin) is a structural analogue of ampicillin (below) and is better absorbed from the gut (especially after food), achieving for the same dose approximately double the plasma concentration. Diarrhoea is less frequent with amoxicillin than with ampicillin. The oral dose is 250 mg 8-hourly, and this drug is preferred to ampicillin because of its greater bioavailability and fewer adverse effects; the parenteral form offers no advantage over ampicillin.

Co-amoxiclav (Augmentin). Clavulanic acid ($t_{1/2}$ 1 h) is a β-lactam molecule with little intrinsic antibacterial activity, which binds irreversibly to β-lactamases. It competitively protects the penicillin, so potentiating its effect against bacteria that are resistant by producing β-lactamases, i.e. clavulanic acid acts as a 'suicide' inhibitor. It is formulated in tablets as its potassium salt (equivalent to 125 mg clavulanic acid) in combination with amoxicillin (250 or 500 mg), as co-amoxiclav. It is a satisfactory oral treatment for infections due to β-lactamase-producing organisms, notably in the respiratory or urogenital tracts, i.e. when β-lactamase-producing amoxicillin-resistant organisms are either suspected or proven by culture. These include many strains of *Staphyloccocus aureus*, many strains of *Escherichia coli* and an increasing number of strains of *Haemophilus influenzae*. It also has useful activity against β-lactamase-producing *Bacteroides* spp. The dose one tablet 8-hourly.

Ampicillin ($t_{1/2}$ 1 h) is acid stable and is moderately well absorbed when swallowed. The oral dose is 250 mg to 1 g 6–8-hourly; or i.m. or i.v. 500 mg 4–6-hourly. Approximately one-third of a dose appears unchanged in the urine. The drug is concentrated in the bile.

Adverse effects. Ampicillin may cause diarrhoea but the incidence (12%) is less with amoxicillin. Ampicillin and amoxicillin are the commonest antibiotics to be associated with *Clostridium difficile* diarrhoea, although this relates to their frequency of use rather than to innate risk of causing the disease. Ampicillin and its analogues have a peculiar capacity to cause a macular rash resembling measles or rubella, usually unaccompanied by other signs of allergy. Rashes are very common in patients with disease of the lymphoid system, notably infectious mononucleosis and lymphoid leukaemia. A macular rash is not necessarily indicative of allergy to other penicillins, which tend to cause a true urticarial reaction. Patients with renal failure and those taking allopurinol for hyperuricaemia also seem more prone to ampicillin rashes. Cholestatic jaundice has been associated with use of co-amoxiclav even up to 6 weeks after cessation of the drug; the clavulanic acid may be responsible.

MECILLINAM

Pivmecillinam ($t_{1/2}$ 1 h) is an oral agent closely related to the broad-spectrum penicillins but with differing antibacterial activity. It is active against Gram-negative organisms including many extended-spectrum β-lactamase-producing (ESBL) *Enterobacteriaceae*, but is inactive against *Pseudomonas aeruginosa* and its relatives, and against Gram-positive organisms. Pivmecillinam is hydrolysed in vivo to the active form mecillinam (which is poorly absorbed by mouth). It can be used to treat urinary tract infection.

MONOBACTAM

Aztreonam ($t_{1/2}$ 2 h) is the first member of this class of β-lactam antibiotics. It is active against Gram-negative organisms including *Pseudomonas aeruginosa*, *Haemophilus influenzae*, and *Neisseria meningitidis* and *gonorrhoeae*. Aztreonam is effective in septicaemia and complicated urinary tract infections, Gram-negative lower urinary tract infections and gonorrhoea.

Adverse effects include reactions at the site of infusion, rashes, gastrointestinal upset, hepatitis, thrombocytopenia and neutropenia. Aztreonam appears to carry a remarkably low risk of β-lactam allergy, and may be an option for some penicillin-allergic patients.

ANTIPSEUDOMONAL PENICILLINS

Carboxypenicillins

In general these have the same antibacterial spectrum as ampicillin (being susceptible to β-lactamases), but have the additional capacity to destroy *Pseudomonas aeruginosa* and indole-positive *Proteus* spp.

Ticarcillin ($t_{1/2}$ 1 h) is presented in combination with clavulanic acid (as Timentin), so to provide greater activity against β-lactamase-producing organisms, and is given by i.m. or slow i.v. injection or by rapid i.v. infusion. Note that ticarcillin comes as its disodium salt and each 1 g delivers about 5.4 mmol sodium; this should be borne in mind when treating patients with impaired cardiac or renal function.

Ureidopenicillins

These are adapted from the ampicillin molecule, with a side-chain derived from urea. Their major advantages over the carboxypenicillins are higher efficacy against *Pseudomonas aeruginosa* and that as monosodium salts they are safer in respect of sodium overload. They are susceptible to many β-lactamases. Ureidopenicillins are administered parenterally.

Elimination is mainly by the kidney, but accumulation with renal impairment is less than with other penicillins as the bile excretes 25%. An unusual feature of their kinetics is that the plasma concentration rises disproportionately with dose, i.e. they exhibit saturation (zero order) kinetics.

For pseudomonas septicaemia, a ureidopenicillin plus an aminoglycoside provides a synergistic effect, but the co-administration in the same fluid results in inactivation of the aminoglycoside (as with carboxypenicillins, above).

Piperacillin ($t_{1/2}$ 1 h) has the same or slightly greater activity as azlocillin against *Pseudomonas aeruginosa* but is more effective against the common Gram-negative organisms. It is also available as a combination with the β-lactamase inhibitor tazobactam (as Tazocin).

CEPHALOSPORINS

Cephalosporins were discovered in a filamentous fungus, *Cephalosporium*, cultured from the sea near a Sardinian sewage outfall in 1945; their molecular structure is closely related to that of penicillin, and many semi-synthetic forms have been introduced. They now comprise a group of antibiotics having a wide range of activity and low toxicity. 'Cephalosporins' is used here as a general term, recognising that some are strictly cephamycins, e.g. cefoxitin and cefotetan.

Mode of action is that of the β-lactams, i.e. cephalosporins impair bacterial cell wall synthesis and hence are bactericidal. They exhibit time-dependent bacterial killing (see p. 189).

Addition of various side-chains on the cephalosporin molecule confers variety in pharmacokinetic and antibacterial activities because the β-lactam ring is protected. The result is a range of compounds with improved activity against Gram-negative organisms, but having less anti-Gram-positive activity. The cephalosporins resist attack by β-lactamases, but bacteria develop resistance to them by other means.

Pharmacokinetics. Most cephalosporins enter the urine unchanged, but some, including cefotaxime, form a desacetyl metabolite, which retains some antibacterial activity. Many undergo active secretion by the renal tubule, a process that probenecid can block. As a rule, patients with poor renal function require reduced dose. Cephalosporins in general have a $t_{1/2}$ of 1–4 h, but with exceptions, e.g. ceftriaxone $t_{1/2}$ 8 h. Wide distribution in the body allows treatment of infection at most sites, including bone, soft tissue, muscle and (in some cases) CSF. Data on individual cephalosporins appear in Table 12.2.

Classification and uses. The cephalosporins conventionally separate into 'generations' of broadly similar antibacterial and pharmacokinetic properties; newer agents have rendered this classification less precise but it retains sufficient usefulness to be presented in Table 12.2.

Adverse effects. Cephalosporins are well tolerated. The most usual unwanted effects are allergic reactions of the penicillin type. There is cross-allergy between penicillins and cephalosporins involving up to 10% patients; if a patient has had a severe or immediate allergic reaction or if serum or skin testing for penicillin allergy is positive (see p. 189), then a cephalosporin should not be used. Sites of i.v. or i.m. injection may be painful. Cephalosporins continued for more than 2 weeks may cause reversible thrombocytopenia, haemolytic anaemia, neutropenia, interstitial nephritis or abnormal liver function test results, especially at high dosage. The broad spectrum of activity of the third-generation cephalosporins may predispose to opportunist infection with resistant bacteria or *Candida albicans* and to *Clostridium difficile* diarrhoea. Ceftriaxone achieves high concentrations in bile and, as the

Table 12.2 The cephalosporins

Drug	$t_{\frac{1}{2}}$ (h)	Excretion in urine (%)	Comment
First generation			
Parenteral			
cefazolin	2	90	May be used for staphylococcal infections but generally have been replaced by the newer cephalosporins
cefradine (also oral)	1	86	
Oral			
cefaclor	1	86	All very similar. Effective against the common respiratory pathogens *Streptococcus pneumoniae* and *Moraxella catarrhalis* but (excepting cefaclor) have poor activity against *Haemophilus influenzae*. Also active against *Escherichia coli* which, increasingly, is demonstrating resistance to amoxicillin and trimethoprim. May be used for uncomplicated upper and lower respiratory tract, urinary tract and soft tissue infections, and also as follow-on treatment once parenteral drugs have brought an infection under control
cefadroxil	2	88	
cefalexin	1	88	
Second generation			
Parenteral			
cefoxitin (a cephamycin) (cefotetan is similar)	1	90	More resistant to β-lactamases than the first-generation drugs and active against *Staphylococcus aureus*, *Streptococcus pyogenes*, *Streptococcus pneumoniae*, *Neisseria* spp., *Haemophilus influenzae* and many Enterobacteriaceae. Cefoxitin also kills *Bacteroides fragilis* and is effective in abdominal and pelvic infections. Cefuroxime may be given for community-acquired pneumonia, commonly due to *Streptococcus pneumoniae* (not when causal organism is *Mycoplasma pneumoniae*, *Legionella* or *Chlamydia*). The oral form, cefuroxime axetil, is also used for the range of infections listed for the first-generation oral cephalosporins (above)
cefuroxime (also oral)	1	80	
Third generation			
Parenteral			
cefpirome	2.3	75	More effective than the second-generation drugs against Gram-negative organisms whilst retaining useful activity against Gram-postive bacteria. Cefotaxime, ceftizoxime and ceftriaxone are used for serious infections such as septicaemia, pneumonia and meningitis. Ceftriaxone is also used for gonorrhoea and Lyme disease; also once-daily outpatient intravenous therapy
cefotaxime	1	60	
ceftazidime	2	88	
ceftriaxone	8	56 (44 bile)	
Oral			
cefixime	4	23 (77 bile)	Active against a range of Gram-positive and Gram-negative organisms including *Staphylococcus aureus* (excepting cefixime), *Streptococcus pyogenes*, *Streptococcus pneumoniae*, *Neisseria* spp., *Haemophilus influenzae* and (excepting cefpodoxime) many Enterobacteriaceae. Used to treat urinary, upper and lower respiratory tract infections
cefprozil	2	40	
cefpodoxime proxetil	2	80	

calcium salt, may precipitate to cause symptoms resembling cholelithiasis (biliary pseudolithiasis). Cefamandole may cause prothrombin deficiency and a disulfiram-like reaction after ingestion of alcohol.

OTHER β-LACTAM ANTIBACTERIALS

CARBAPENEMS

Members of this group have the widest spectrum of all currently available antimicrobials, being bactericidal against most Gram-positive and Gram-negative aerobic and anaerobic pathogenic bacteria. They resist hydrolysis by most β-lactamases, including ESBLs. Only occasional pseudomonas relatives are naturally resistant, and acquired resistance is uncommon in all species.

IMIPENEM

Imipenem ($t_{1/2}$ 1 h) is inactivated by metabolism in the kidney to products that are potentially toxic to renal tubules; combining imipenem with cilastatin (as Primaxin), a specific inhibitor of dihydropeptidase (the enzyme responsible for its renal metabolism), prevents both inactivation and toxicity.

Imipenem finds use in septicaemia, intra-abdominal infection and nosocomial pneumonia. In terms of imipenem, the dose is 1–2 g daily by i.v. infusion in three to four doses, reduced when renal function is impaired.

Adverse effects include gastrointestinal upset including nausea, blood disorders, allergic reactions, confusion and convulsions.

Meropenem ($t_{1/2}$ 1 h) is similar to imipenem, but is stable to renal dihydropeptidase and can therefore be given without cilastatin. It penetrates into the CSF and is not associated with nausea or convulsions.

Ertapenem ($t_{1/2}$ 4 h) is given as a single daily i.v. injection and has found a niche indication for parenteral therapy of multiply resistant Gram-negative bacteria, such as ESBL-producing coliforms, outside hospital. It is much less active against *Pseudomonas aeruginosa*, *Acinetobacter* and their relatives than are the other carbapenems.

OTHER INHIBITORS OF CELL WALL SYNTHESIS AND MEMBRANE FUNCTION

Vancomycin

Vancomycin ($t_{1/2}$ 8 h), a 'glycopeptide' or 'peptolide', acts on multiplying organisms by inhibiting cell wall formation at a site different from that of the β-lactam antibacterials. It is bactericidal against most strains of clostridia (including *Clostridium difficile*), almost all strains of *Staphylococcus aureus* (including those that produce β-lactamase and meticillin-resistant strains), coagulase-negative staphylococci, viridans group streptococci and enterococci.

Vancomycin is poorly absorbed from the gut and the i.v. route is necessary for systemic infections, there being no satisfactory i.m. preparation. It distributes effectively into body tissues and is excreted in urine.

Uses. Vancomycin is effective for antibiotic-associated pseudomembranous colitis (caused by *Clostridium difficile* or, less commonly, staphylococci) in a dose of 125 mg 6-hourly by mouth (although oral metronidazole is preferred, being as effective and less costly). It is combined with an aminoglycoside for treating streptococcal endocarditis in patients who are allergic to benzylpenicillin, and for serious infection with multiply resistant staphylococci. It is not as effective as flucloxacillin for serious infections caused by meticillin-susceptible *Staphylococcus aureus*. Dosing is guided by plasma concentration with the aim of achieving trough concentrations between 5 and 15 mg/L, or 10–15 mg/L in patients being treated for infective endocarditis.

Adverse effects. Tinnitus and deafness may arise, but may improve on stopping the drug. Nephrotoxicity and allergic reactions also occur. Rapid i.v. infusion may cause a maculopapular rash possibly due to histamine release (the 'red person' syndrome).

Teicoplanin

Teicoplanin, structurally related to vancomycin, is active against Gram-positive bacteria. The $t_{1/2}$ of 50 h allows once-daily i.v. or i.m. administration. It is less likely than vancomycin to cause ototoxicity or nephrotoxicity, but plasma monitoring is required to assure adequate concentrations for severely ill patients and those with changing renal function.

A serious concern is the emergence of vanco-mycin-resistant/glycopeptide-resistant enterococci (VRE/GRE), and vancomycin-intermediate resistant *Staphylococcus aureus* (VISA or GISA), and the very rare vancomycin–meticillin-resistant *Staphylococcus aureus* (VMRSA). VISA and VMRSA occur in patients treated for long periods with vancomycin or teicoplanin.

Daptomycin

Daptomycin ($t_{1/2}$ 9 h) is a lipopeptide antibiotic, naturally produced by *Streptomyces roseosporus*, with activity against virtually all Gram-positive bacteria, including penicillin-resistant *Streptococcus pneumoniae* and MRSA, regardless of vancomycin resistance phenotype. Daptomycin demonstrates concentration-dependent bactericidal activity, including against most enterococci (for which van-comycin is generally bacteriostatic). Emergence of resistance (or reduction in susceptibility) during clinical use has rarely been reported to date.

Excretion is predominantly renal, with some 60% of a dose appearing unchanged from the urine; patients with renal impairment require reduced dose. Administration is by single daily i.v. injection.

Uses. Daptomycin is currently approved in the UK for complicated skin and skin structure infections caused by Gram-positive bacteria, but wider applications appear likely.

Adverse reactions. Muscle pain and weakness, with rise in plasma levels of creatinine phosphokinase (CPK), may be due to effects on the myocyte cell membrane, and appear to be dose related. They are fully reversible but CPK monitoring is desirable.

Cycloserine

See Drug-resistant tuberculosis (p. 220).

INHIBITION OF PROTEIN SYNTHESIS

AMINOGLYCOSIDES

The purposeful search that followed the discovery of penicillin uncovered streptomycin from *Streptomyces griseus* in 1943, cultured from a heavily manured field and also from a chicken's throat. The scientist who made the discovery was Albert Schatz but credit went to the head of the laboratory, Selman Waksman, a injustice that has belatedly been acknowledged. Aminoglycosides resemble one another in their mode of action, and in their pharmacokinetic, therapeutic and toxic properties. The main differences in usage reflect variation in their range of antibacterial activity; cross-resistance is variable.

Mode of action. Aminoglycosides act inside the cell by binding to the ribosomes in such a way that incorrect amino acid sequences enter into peptide chains. The resulting abnormal proteins are fatal to the microbe, i.e. aminoglycosides are bactericidal and exhibit concentration-dependent bacterial killing (see p. 179).

Pharmacokinetics. Aminoglycosides are water soluble and do not readily cross cell membranes. Poor absorption from the intestine necessitates their administration i.v. or i.m. for systemic use, and they distribute mainly to the extracellular fluid; transfer into the CSF is poor, even with inflamed meninges. Their $t_{1/2}$ ranges from 2 to 5 h.

Aminoglycosides are eliminated unchanged mainly by glomerular filtration, and attain high concentration in the urine. Significant accumulation occurs in the renal cortex. Plasma concentration should be measured frequently in renally impaired patients, and it is prudent to monitor approximately twice weekly even when renal function is normal. Reduced dosing is necessary to compensate for varying degrees of renal impairment, including that of normal aging. With prolonged therapy, e.g. endocarditis (gentamicin), monitoring must be meticulous. Algorithms are available to guide dosing according to patients' weight and renal function, and assay of trough concentrations.

Current practice is moving towards administration of aminoglycosides as a single daily dose, which is probably less ototoxic and nephrotoxic than divided dose regimens, and appears to be as effective. The immediate high plasma concentrations that result from single daily dosing are advantageous, e.g. for acutely ill septicaemic patients, as aminoglycosides exhibit concentration-dependent killing (see p. 179).

Antibacterial avctivity. Aminoglycosides are in general active against staphylococci and aerobic Gram-negative organisms including almost all of the *Enterobacteriaceae*. Bacterial resistance to aminoglyco-sides is an increasing but variable problem, notably by acquisition of plasmids that carry genes coding for the formation of drug-destroying enzymes. Gentamicin resistance is rare in community-acquired pathogens in many hospitals in the UK.

Uses include:

- *Gram-negative bacillary infection*, particularly septicaemia, renal, pelvic and abdominal sepsis. Gentamicin remains the drug of choice, but tobramycin may be preferred for *Pseudomonas aeruginosa*. Amikacin has the widest antibacterial spectrum of the aminoglycosides but is best reserved for infection caused by gentamicin-resistant organisms. If local resistance rates are low, an aminoglycoside may be included in the initial best-guess regimen for treatment of serious septicaemia. A potentially less toxic antibiotic may be substituted when culture results are known (48–72 h), and toxicity is very rare after such short use.
- *Bacterial endocarditis*. An aminoglycoside, usually gentamicin, should comprise part of the antimicrobial combination for enterococcal, streptococcal or staphylococcal infection of the heart valves, and for the therapy of clinical endocarditis that fails to yield a positive blood culture.
- *Other infections*: tuberculosis, tularaemia, plague, brucellosis.
- *Topical uses*. Neomycin and framycetin, too toxic for systemic use, are effective for topical treatment of infections of the conjunctiva or external ear. Tobramycin is given by inhalation for therapy of infective exacerbations of cystic fibrosis; sufficient systemic absorption may occur to recommend assay of serum concentrations in such patients.

Adverse effects. Aminoglycoside toxicity is a risk when the dose is high or of long duration; the risk is higher when renal clearance is inefficient (because of disease or age), other potentially nephrotoxic drugs are co-administered (e.g. loop diuretics, amphotericin B) or the patient is dehydrated. It may take the following forms:

- *Ototoxicity*. Both vestibular and auditory damage[4] may occur, causing hearing loss, vertigo and tinnitus, which may be permanent (see above). Tinnitus may give warning of auditory nerve damage. Early signs of vestibular toxicity include motion-related headache, dizziness or nausea. Serious ototoxicity can occur with topical application, including ear-drops.
- *Nephrotoxicity*. Dose-related changes, which are usually reversible, occur in renal tubular cells, where aminoglycosides accumulate. Low blood pressure, loop diuretics and advanced age are recognised as added risk factors.
- *Neuromuscular blockade*. Aminoglycosides may impair neuromuscular transmission and aggravate (or reveal) myasthenia gravis, or cause a transient myasthenic syndrome in patients whose neuromuscular transmission is normal.
- *Other reactions* include rashes and haematological abnormalities, including marrow depression, haemolytic anaemia and bleeding due to antagonism of factor V.

INDIVIDUAL AMINOGLYCOSIDES

Gentamicin is active against aerobic Gram-negative bacilli including *Escherichia coli*, *Enterobacter*, *Klebsiella*, *Proteus* and *Pseudomonas*. In streptococcal and enterococcal endocarditis, gentamicin is combined with benzylpenicillin; in staphylococcal endocarditis with an antistaphylococcal penicillin; and in enterococcal endocarditis with ampicillin (true synergy is seen provided the enterococcus is not highly resistant to gentamicin).

Dosage is 3–5 mg/kg body-weight per day (the highest dose for more serious infections) as a single dose, or 8-hourly in equally divided doses. The rationale behind single-dose administration is to achieve high peak plasma concentrations (10–14 mg/L, which correlate with therapeutic efficacy) and more time at lower trough concentrations (16 h at less than 1 mg/L, which are associated with reduced risk of toxicity). Therapy should rarely exceed 7 days. Patients with cystic fibrosis eliminate gentamicin rapidly and require higher doses. Gentamicin applied to the eye gives effective corneal and aqueous humour concentrations.

Tobramycin is similar to gentamicin; it is more active against most strains of *Pseudomonas aeruginosa* and may be less nephrotoxic.

---

[4]Aspirin 3 g daily may reduce the incidence of hearing loss by the antioxidant effect of salicylate. Sha S 2006 Aspirin to prevent gentamicin-induced hearing loss. New England Journal of Medicine 354:1856–1857.

Amikacin is expensive and is of value mainly because it is more resistant to aminoglycoside-inactivating bacterial enzymes than gentamicin. Peak plasma concentrations of 20–30 mg/L and trough concentrations below 10 mg/L are desirable.

Netilmicin is active against some strains of bacteria that resist gentamicin and tobramycin; it may be less ototoxic and nephrotoxic.

Neomycin principally finds use topically for skin, eye and ear infections. Sufficient absorption can occur from both oral and topical use to cause eighth cranial nerve damage, especially if there is renal impairment.

Framycetin is similar to neomycin in use and in toxicity.

Streptomycin, superseded as a first-line choice for tuberculosis, may be used to kill resistant strains of the organism. The first effective antituberculosis drug, streptomycin was discovered by Albert Schatz in 1943 although the credit (and Nobel Prize) went to Edwin Waksman, head of the laboratory.

Spectinomycin is active against Gram-negative organisms but its use is limited to gonorrhoea in patients allergic to penicillin, or for infection with gonococci that are β-lactam drug resistant. The steady growth of resistant gonococci, particularly β-lactamase-producing strains, suggests that spectinomycin will continue to have a significant role in this disease.

TETRACYCLINES

Tetracyclines have a broad range of antimicrobial activity. New tetracyclines and relatives have a wider spectrum of activity that includes bacteria with acquired resistance to other classes of antibiotic.

Mode of action. Tetracyclines interfere with protein synthesis by binding to bacterial ribosomes, and their selective action is due to higher uptake by bacterial than by human cells. They are bacteriostatic.

Pharmacokinetics. Most tetracyclines are absorbed only partially from the alimentary tract, enough remaining in the intestine to alter the flora and cause diarrhoea. They distribute throughout the body and cross the placenta. Tetracyclines pass mainly unchanged into the urine and should be avoided when renal function is severely impaired. Exceptionally, doxycycline and minocycline depend on non-renal elimination routes and are preferred when kidney function is impaired.

Uses. Tetracyclines are active against nearly all Gram-positive and Gram-negative pathogenic bacteria, but increasing bacterial resistance and low innate activity limit their clinical use. The 4-quinolone drugs are preferred, especially in the developed world, but tetracyclines remain drugs of first choice for infection with chlamydiae (psittacosis, trachoma, pelvic inflammatory disease, lymphogranuloma venereum), mycoplasma (pneumonia), rickettsiae (Q fever, typhus), *Bartonella* spp., and borreliae (Lyme disease, relapsing fever) (for use in acne, see p. 287). Doxycycline has a place in therapeutic and prophylactic regimens for malaria (see p. 238), and is active against amoebae and a variety of other protozoa. The most common other uses of tetracyclines are as second-line therapy of minor skin and soft tissue infections, especially in β-lactam-allergic patients; surprisingly, many MRSA strains currently remain susceptible to tetracyclines in the UK.

An unexpected use for a tetracycline is in the treatment of chronic hyponatraemia due to the syndrome of inappropriate antidiuretic hormone secretion (SIADH) when water restriction has failed. *Demeclocycline* produces a state of unresponsiveness to ADH, probably by inhibiting the formation and action of cyclic AMP in the renal tubule. It is effective and convenient to use in SIADH because this action is both dose dependent and reversible.

Adverse reactions. Heartburn, nausea and vomiting due to gastric irritation are common, and attempts to reduce this with milk or antacids impair the absorption of tetracyclines (see below). Diarrhoea and opportunistic infection (antibiotic associated or pseudomembranous colitis) may supervene. Disorders of epithelial surfaces, perhaps due partly to vitamin B complex deficiency and partly to mild opportunistic infection with yeasts and moulds, lead to sore mouth and throat, black hairy tongue, dysphagia and perianal soreness. Vitamin B preparations may prevent or arrest alimentary tract symptoms.

Tetracyclines selectively enter the teeth and growing bones of the fetus and of children, owing to their chelating properties with calcium phosphate. This causes hypoplasia of dental enamel with pitting, cusp malformation, yellow or brown pigmentation, and increased susceptibility to caries. After the 14th week of pregnancy and in the first few months of life, even short courses can be damaging. Prevention of discoloration of the permanent front teeth requires that tetracyclines be avoided from the last 2 months of pregnancy to the age of 4 years, and of other teeth to 8 years of age (or 12 years if the third molars are valued). Prolonged tetracycline therapy can also stain the fingernails at all ages.

Effects on bone formation in the fetus are of less clinical importance because pigmentation has no cosmetic disadvantage and a short exposure to tetracycline is unlikely to delay growth significantly.

As tetracyclines act by inhibiting bacterial protein synthesis, the same effect occurring in humans causes blood urea levels to rise (the antianabolic effect). The increased nitrogen load can be clinically important in renal failure and in the elderly.

Tetracyclines induce photosensitisation and other rashes. Liver and pancreatic damage can occur, especially in pregnancy and with renal disease, with i.v. administration. Tetracyclines can cause benign intracranial hypertension, dizziness and other neurological reactions, after tetracyclines have been taken for 2 weeks or a year.[5] Any patient who develops headaches or visual disturbance requires assessment of visual function and ocular fundi.

Interactions. Dairy products reduce absorption to a degree, but antacids and iron preparations do so much more, by chelation to calcium, aluminium and iron.

INDIVIDUAL TETRACYCLINES

Tetracycline may be taken as representative of most tetracyclines. Because of incomplete absorption from the gut, i.v. doses need be less than half of the oral dose to be similarly effective. Tetracycline is eliminated by the kidney and in the bile ($t_{1/2}$ 6 h).

Doxycycline is well absorbed from the gut, even after food, and is cleared intact from the body by biliary and renal mechanisms ($t_{1/2}$ 16 h). Biliary and faecal excretion compensate effectively when renal function is impaired and no reduction of dose is necessary; 200 mg on the first day, then 100 mg daily.

Minocycline differs from other tetracyclines by having activity against *Neisseria meningitidis*, and finds use in prophylaxis of meningococcal meningitis. It is well absorbed from the gut, even after a meal, partly metabolised in the liver and excreted in the bile and urine ($t_{1/2}$ 15 h). Dose reduction is not necessary when renal function is impaired; 200 mg initially is followed by 100 mg 12-hourly. Minocycline, but not other tetracyclines, may cause a reversible vestibular disturbance with dizziness, tinnitus and impaired balance, especially in women.

Other tetracyclines include demeclocycline (see above), lymecycline and oxytetracycline.

Tigecycline

Tigecycline ($t_{1/2}$ 42 h) is the first of the *glycylcyclines* to be licensed. Structurally similar to minocycline, it binds to the 30S bacterial ribosomal subunit, preventing amino acid chain elongation. Probably because of stearic hindrance from its 9-glycylamide structure and avid ribosomal binding, tigecycline is unaffected by the two commonest tetracycline resistance mechanisms – ribosomal alteration and efflux pumps.

Tigecycline has useful bacteriostatic activity against a wide range of pathogens including streptococci and staphylococci (also VRE and MRSA), coliforms (but not *Proteus* spp.) and anaerobes. Body distribution is widespread; some 60% of a dose appears in the bile and faeces, and 33% in the urine (22% unchanged). It is available only for parenteral use. Dose reduction is required in severe hepatic failure but not when renal function is impaired.

Tigecycline is effective for skin, soft tissue and intra-abdominal infections, with clinical trial outcomes equivalent to carbapenems and similar agents.

Adverse effects. The drug is generally well tolerated; reported unwanted effects are similar to those of the tetracyclines.

MACROLIDES

Erythromycin

Erythromycin ($t_{1/2}$ 2–4 h) binds to bacterial ribosomes and interferes with protein synthesis; it is bacteriostatic and exhibits time-dependent bacterial killing (see p. 181). Erythromycin is effective against Gram-positive organisms because these accumulate the drug more efficiently than Gram-negative organisms, and its antibacterial spectrum is similar to that of penicillin.

---

[5]Lochead J, Elston J S 2003 Doxycycline induced intracranial hypertension. British Medical Journal 326:641–642.

Absorption after oral administration is best with erythromycin estolate, even when there is food in the stomach. Hydrolysis of the estolate releases the active erythromycin, which diffuses readily into most tissues. It is metabolised in the liver by P450 3A; the $t_{1/2}$ is dose dependent, and elimination is almost exclusively in the bile and faeces.

Uses. Erythromycin is the drug of choice for:

- *Mycoplasma pneumoniae* in children, although in adults a tetracycline may be preferred.
- *Legionella* spp. (including legionnaires' disease), with or without rifampicin.
- Diphtheria (including carriers), pertussis, and some chlamydial infections.

In gastroenteritis caused by *Campylobacter jejuni*, erythromycin effectively eliminates the organism from the faeces, but does not reduce the duration of the symptoms unless given very early in the course of the illness.

Erythromycin is an effective alternative for penicillin-allergic patients infected with *Staphylococcus aureus*, *Streptococcus pyogenes*, *Streptococcus pneumoniae* or *Treponema pallidum*.

Use in acne: see page 287.

Dose is 250 mg 6-hourly, or twice this in serious infection and four times this for legionnaires' disease. The ethylsuccinate and stearate esters of erythromycin produce lower plasma concentrations of the active drug than does the same dose of the estolate.

Adverse reactions. Erythromycin is remarkably non-toxic, but the estolate can cause cholestatic hepatitis, probably as a result of allergy; recovery is usual but patients with liver disease should not receive the estolate. Other allergies are rare. Gastrointestinal disturbances occur frequently (up to 28%), particularly diarrhoea and nausea, but opportunistic infection is uncommon.

Interactions. Erythromycin and the other macrolides interfere with the metabolic inactivation of some drugs, notably those also metabolised by P450 3A. The effects of co-administered warfarin, carbamazepine, theophylline and disopyramide are increased. Reduced inactivation of terfenadine may lead to serious cardiac arrhythmias, and that of ergot alkaloids may cause ergotism.

Clarithromycin

Clarithromycin acts like erythromycin and has a similar spectrum of antibacterial activity, i.e. mainly against Gram-positive organisms, although it is usefully more active against *Haemophilus influenzae*. It is rapidly and completely absorbed from the gastrointestinal tract; 60% of a dose is inactivated by metabolism that is saturable ($t_{1/2}$ 3 h after 250 mg, 9 h after 1200 mg), and the remainder is eliminated in the urine. Clarithromycin is effective for respiratory tract infections including atypical pneumonias and soft tissue infections. It is concentrated intracellularly, allowing effective combination therapy for mycobacterial infections such as *Mycobacterium avium-intracellulare* in patients with AIDS. Gastrointestinal tract adverse effects are uncommon (7%). For interactions, see erythromycin (above).

Azithromycin

Azithromycin is usefully active against a number of important Gram-negative organisms including *Haemophilus influenzae* and *Neisseria gonorrhoeae*, and against *Chlamydiae*, but is a little less effective than erythromycin against Gram-positive organisms.

Azithromycin achieves high concentrations in tissues relative to those in plasma. It remains largely unmetabolised, passing into the bile and faeces ($t_{1/2}$ 50 h). Azithromycin is effective for respiratory tract and soft tissue infections and sexually transmitted diseases, especially genital chlamydia infections, and for travellers' diarrhoea. Gastrointestinal effects (9%) are less than with erythromycin, but diarrhoea, nausea and abdominal pain occur. In view of its high hepatic excretion, its use should be avoided in patients with liver disease. For interactions, see erythromycin (above).

Telithromycin

Telithromycin ($t_{1/2}$ 10 h) is the first of the ketolides, which are semi-synthetic relatives of the macrolides that bind to the 50S bacterial ribosomal subunit, preventing translation and ribosome assembly. It exhibits greater acid stability, less susceptibility to bacterial export pumps and increased ribosomal binding compared with erythromycin. The antibacterial spectrum of telithromycin is similar to that of the macrolides, but includes most erythromycin-resistant strains of *Streptococcus pneumoniae*. It is not active against erythromycin-resistant staphylococci, including most MRSA.

Telithromycin is effective as once-daily oral therapy for upper and lower respiratory tract infections. Dose adjustment is not required in hepatic disease, but it is prudent to half the dose in severe renal impairment.

The drug causes diarrhoea more commonly than the macrolides and some patients experience transient visual disturbance (blurred or double vision).

Interaction with itraconazole, rifampicin, midazolam and atorvastatin increases their effects, by interference with metabolic inactivation (see Erythromycin, above).

Clindamycin

Clindamycin, structurally a lincosamide rather than a macrolide, binds to bacterial ribosomes to inhibit protein synthesis. Its antibacterial spectrum is similar to that of erythromycin (with which there is partial cross-resistance) and benzylpenicillin (but includes penicillin-resistant staphylococci); it has the useful additional property of efficacy against anaerobes such as *Bacteroides fragilis* that are involved in gut-associated sepsis. Clindamycin is well absorbed from the gut and distributes to most body tissues including bone. The drug is metabolised by the liver and enterohepatic cycling occurs with bile concentrations two to five times those of plasma ($t_{1/2}$ 3 h). Significant excretion of metabolites occurs by the gut.

Clindamycin is used for staphylococcal bone and joint infections, dental infections and serious intra-abdominal sepsis (in the latter case, it is usually combined with an agent active against Gram-negative pathogens such as gentamicin). It is also a second choice in combination for some *Toxoplasma* infections. Topical preparations serve for therapy of severe acne and non-sexually transmitted infection of the genital tract in women. It is the antibiotic of choice for serious invasive *Streptococcus pyogenes* infections, although surgical resection of affected tissue plays a prime role.

The most serious *adverse effect* is antibiotic-associated (pseudomembranous) colitis (see p. 183), usually due to opportunistic infection of the bowel with *Clostridium difficile*; discontinue clindamycin should diarrhoea occur.

OTHER INHIBITORS OF PROTEIN SYNTHESIS

Chloramphenicol

Chloramphenicol has a broad spectrum of activity and is primarily bacteriostatic, but may be bactericidal against *Haemophilus influenzae, Neisseria meningitidis* and *Streptococcus pneumoniae.*

Pharmacokinetics. Chloramphenicol succinate is hydrolysed to the active chloramphenicol and there is much individual variation in the capacity to perform this reaction. Chloramphenicol is inactivated by conjugation with glucuronic acid in the liver ($t_{1/2}$ 5 h in adults). In the neonate (especially in the premature), this process of glucuronidation is slow and plasma concentrations are variable (see below). Monitoring of plasma concentration is therefore essential, as it is in the adult with serious infection. Chloramphenicol penetrates well into all tissues, including the CSF and brain, even in the absence of meningeal inflammation.

Uses. Rare but serious toxic effects influence the decision to use chloramphenicol for systemic infection (see below). Broad-spectrum cephalosporins, e.g. cefotaxime and ceftriaxone, are now preferred in meningitis and brain abscess, but chloramphenicol is a second-line agent for these indications and for haemophilus epiglottitis in children. Chloramphenicol is an option for salmonella infections (typhoid fever, salmonella septicaemia) but ciprofloxacin is preferred. Topical administration is effective for bacterial conjunctivitis.

Adverse effects. Systemic use of chloramphenicol is dominated by rare (1 in 18 000–100 000 courses), though serious, bone marrow toxicity. This may be a *dose-dependent* reversible depression of erythrocyte, platelet and leucocyte formation that occurs early in treatment, or an *idiosyncratic* (probably genetically determined), non-dose-related and usually fatal aplastic anaemia which may develop during, or even weeks after, prolonged treatment, and sometimes on re-exposure to the drug. Marrow depression is detectable at an early and recoverable stage by frequent checking of the full blood count. Optic and peripheral neuritis occur with prolonged use (avoid if possible) but are uncommon.

The 'grey baby' syndrome occurs in neonates as circulatory collapse, in which the skin develops a cyanotic grey colour. It is due to failure of the liver to conjugate, and of the kidney to excrete the drug.

Sodium fusidate

Sodium fusidate is a steroid antimicrobial that finds use almost exclusively against β-lactamase-producing staphylococci. Because staphylococci may rapidly become resistant by a one-step genetic mutation, the drug is combined with another antistaphylococcal agent, e.g. flucloxacillin. Sodium fusidate is readily absorbed from the gut and distributes widely in body tissues including bone. It is metabolised and very little is excreted unchanged in the urine; the $t_{1/2}$ is 5 h.

Uses. Sodium fusidate is valuable for treating severe staphylococcal infections, including osteomyelitis, and is available as i.v. and oral preparations. In an ointment or gel, sodium fusidate is effective for staphylococcal skin infection, and as a cream to eradicate the staphylococcal nasal carrier state. Another gel preparation serves for application to the eye; it contains such a high fusidic acid concentration that it possesses useful activity against most bacteria that cause conjunctivitis.

Adverse effects. Mild gastrointestinal upset is frequent. Jaundice may develop, particularly with high doses given intravenously (monitor of liver function).

RESISTANCE TO ANTIMICROBIALS: QUINUPRISTIN–DALFOPRISTIN AND LINEZOLID

These novel antibiotics emerged in response to the challenge of multiply resistant Gram-positive pathogens during the 1990s. Both have useful activity against MRSA (including vancomycin-intermediate and -resistant strains), vancomycin-resistant enterococci and penicillin-resistant *Streptococcus pneumoniae*, but are inactive against most Gram-negative bacteria. They are currently reserved for treatment of infections caused by such bacteria and for patients who are allergic to more established antibiotics. Difficult decisions arise about the use of novel but expensive antimicrobial agents:

> No antibiotic should be used recklessly, however difficult it appears to be to select for resistance in vitro. On the other hand, the attitude that 'All new antibiotics should be locked away' risks stifling innovation whilst denying life-saving treatments ... Debates on the use of new anti-Gram-positive agents are sure to intensify ... and it is vital that they take place on a basis of science not knee-jerk restrictions or over-zealous marketing.[6]

[6]Livermore D M 2000 Quinupristin/dalfopristin and linezolid: where, when, which and whether to use? Journal of Antimicrobial Chemotherapy 46:347–350.

Quinupristin–dalfopristin is a 30:70% combination of two streptogramin molecules; the dalfopristin component binds first to the 50S bacterial ribosome, inducing a conformational change that allows the additional binding of quinupristin. The combination results in premature release of polypeptide chains from the ribosome; the summative effect is bactericidal.

Acquired resistance is currently rare. Most strains of *Enterococcus faecalis* are naturally resistant, but *Enterococcus faecium* is sensitive. Most Gram-negative bacteria have impermeable membranes and hence are resistant, but the respiratory pathogens *Legionella pneumophila*, *Moraxella catarrhalis* and *Mycoplasma pneumoniae* are susceptible. The $t_{1/2}$ is 1.5 h.

The UK licence covers *Enterococcus faecium* infections, skin and soft tissue infection, and hospital-acquired pneumonia.

Injection to peripheral veins frequently causes phlebitis, so a central line is required. Arthralgia and myalgia occur in some 10% patients. The dose is reduced in moderate hepatic disease and the drug should generally be avoided if impairment is severe.

Linezolid, a synthetic oxazolinidone, is the first member of this new class of antibacterial agent that provides effective therapy for MRSA, and the oral therapy against VRE. Its unique mode of action involves binding to domain V of the 23S component of the 50S ribosomal subunit and inhibiting formation of the initiation complex between transfer RNA, messenger RNA and the ribosomal subunits at the first stage of protein synthesis.

Linezolid is bacteriostatic against most Gram-positive bacteria, including staphylococci, streptococci and enterococci resistant to other antimicrobial agents, but is bactericidal against pneumococci.

Resistance has occurred in a few *Enterococcus* and *Staphylococcus aureus* isolates from immunocompromised patients and others with chronic infections treated with linezolid for long periods.

Cross-resistance to other antibiotics has yet to appear. Most Gram-negative bacteria are resistant by virtue of possessing membrane efflux pumps, but many obligate anaerobes are susceptible.

Linezolid is eliminated via both renal and hepatic routes ($t_{1/2}$ 6 h), 30–55% in the urine as the active drug. Absorption after oral administration is rapid, almost complete and little affected by food.

Linezolid has a UK licence for skin, soft tissue and respiratory tract infections, but use is restricted on grounds of cost to those caused by multiply resistant pathogens. The oral formulation provides useful continuation therapy for severe and chronic infections caused by bacteria resistant to other agents, e.g. MRSA osteomyelitis.

Adverse effects include nausea, vomiting and headache. Reversible optic and irreversible peripheral neuropathy occur and, importantly, marrow suppression, especially with pre-existing renal disease (blood counts and neurological assessments should be performed weekly in patients exposed to linezolid for longer than 2 weeks). Potentiation of pressor effect of monoamine oxidase inhibitors (see p. 331) may occur.

INHIBITION OF NUCLEIC ACID SYNTHESIS

SULPHONAMIDES AND SULPHONAMIDE COMBINATIONS

Sulphonamides, amongst the first successful chemotherapeutic agents, now find use mainly in combination with trimethoprim. Because of risks of adverse drug reactions, their use is generally restricted to specific indications where other therapeutic agents have clearly inferior efficacy. Their individual names are standardised in the UK to begin with 'sulfa-'.

The enzyme dihydrofolic acid (DHF) synthase converts *p*-aminobenzoic acid (PABA) to DHF, which subsequently metabolises to tetrahydrofolic acid (THF), purines and DNA. The sulphonamides are structurally similar to PABA, compete with it successfully for DHF synthase and thus ultimately impair DNA formation. Susceptible bacteria cannot use preformed folate, but humans derive DHF from dietary folate, which protects their cells from the metabolic effect of sulphonamides. Trimethoprim acts at the subsequent step by inhibiting DHF reductase, which converts DHF to THF. The drug is relatively safe because bacterial DHF reductase is much more sensitive to trimethoprim than is the human form. Both sulphonamides and trimethoprim are bacteriostatic.

Pharmacokinetics. Sulphonamides for systemic use are absorbed rapidly from the gut. The princi-

pal metabolic path is acetylation and the capacity to acetylate is genetically determined in a bimodal form, i.e. there are slow and fast acetylators (see Pharmacogenetics) but the differences are of limited practical importance in therapy. The kidney is the principal route of excretion of drug and acetylate.

CLASSIFICATION AND USES

Sulphonamides may be classified as follows:

Systemic use

Sulphonamide–trimethoprim combination. *Co-trimoxazole* (sulfamethoxazole plus trimethoprim). The optimum synergistic in vitro effect against most susceptible bacteria is achieved with a 5:1 ratio of sulfamethoxazole to trimethoprim, although concentrations achieved in the tissues vary considerably. Each drug is well absorbed from the gut, has a $t_{1/2}$ of 10 h and is 80% excreted by the kidney; impaired renal function necessitates reduction in dose.

Trimethoprim on its own finds use in many conditions for what were originally indications for the combination, and it may cause fewer adverse reactions (see below). Co-trimoxazole is retained for:

■ Prevention and treatment of pneumonia due to *Pneumocystis carinii*, a life-threatening infection in immunosuppressed patients.
■ Prevention and treatment of toxoplasmosis, and treatment of nocardiasis.

Sulfadiazine ($t_{1/2}$ 10 h), sulfametopyrazine ($t_{1/2}$ 38 h) and sulfadimidine (sulfamethazine) ($t_{1/2}$ approx. 6 h, dose dependent) are available in some countries for urinary tract infections, meningococcal meningitis and other indications, but are not drugs of first choice (resistance rates are high).

Topical application

Silver sulfadiazine finds use for prophylaxis and treatment of infected burns, leg ulcers and pressure sores because of its wide antibacterial spectrum (which includes pseudomonads).

Miscellaneous

Sulfasalazine (salicylazosulfapyridine) is used in inflammatory bowel disease (see p. 580); in effect, the sulfapyridine component acts as a carrier to release the active 5-aminosalicylic acid in the colon (see also rheumatoid arthritis, p. 269).

Adverse effects of sulphonamides include malaise, diarrhoea and, rarely, cyanosis (due to methaemoglobinaemia). These may all be transient and are not necessarily indications for stopping the drug. Crystalluria may rarely occur.

Allergic reactions include rash, fever, hepatitis, agranulocytosis, purpura, aplastic anaemia, peripheral neuritis and polyarteritis nodosa. Rarely, severe skin reactions including erythema multiforme bullosa (Stevens–Johnson syndrome) and toxic epidermal necrolysis (Lyell's syndrome) occur.

Haemolysis may occur in glucose-6-phosphate dehydrogenase-deficient subjects. Patients with AIDS have a high rate of allergic systemic reactions (fever, rash) to co-trimoxazole used for treatment of *Pneumocystis carinii* pneumonia.

Trimethoprim

Following its extensive use in combination with sulphonamides, trimethoprim ($t_{1/2}$ 10 h) has emerged as a useful broad-spectrum antimicrobial on its own. It is active against many Gram-positive and Gram-negative aerobic organisms, excepting the enterococci and *Pseudomonas aeruginosa*; resistant organisms are becoming a problem. Absorption from the gastrointestinal tract is rapid and complete, and the drug passes largely unchanged into the urine. Trimethoprim is effective as sole therapy in treating urinary and respiratory tract infections, and for prophylaxis of urinary tract infections.

Adverse effects are fewer than with co-trimoxazole; they include skin rash, anorexia, nausea, vomiting, abdominal pain and diarrhoea.

QUINOLONES

(4-quinolones, fluoroquinolones)

The first widely used quinolone, nalidixic acid, emerged serendipitously as a byproduct of chloroquine synthesis. Being concentrated in urine, it is effective for urinary tract infections, but has little systemic activity. Fluorination of the quinolone structure produced compounds that were up to 60 times more active than nalidixic acid and killed a wider range of organisms.

These newer '4-quinolones' act principally by inhibiting bacterial (but not human) DNA gyrase (topoisomerase II and IV), thus preventing the supercoiling of DNA, a process that is necessary for compacting chromosomes into the bacterial cell; they are bactericidal and exhibit concentration-dependent bacterial killing. In general, quinolones are extremely active against Gram-negative organisms and most have useful activity against *Pseudomonas aeruginosa*, mycobacteria and *Legionella pneumophila*. Most are less active against Gram-positive organisms (resistance commonly emerges) and are not effective against anaerobes.

Resistance typically arises by mutation of the target enzymes that are coded on mobile plasmids (in 'quinolone resistance-determining regions'); efflux pumps may also contribute. Quinolone resistance rates for a wide range of Gram-negative bacteria have risen alarmingly across the world in the past 10 years, and cross-resistance across all members of the group is common.

Pharmacokinetics. Quinolones are well absorbed from the gut and widely distributed in body tissue. Mechanisms of inactivation (hepatic metabolism, renal and biliary excretion) for individual members appear below. There is substantial excretion and re-absorption by colonic mucosa, and patients with renal failure or intestinal malfunction, e.g. ileus, are prone to accumulate quinolones.

Uses vary between individual drugs (see below).

Adverse effects include gastrointestinal upset and allergic reactions (rash, pruritus, arthralgia, photosensitivity and anaphylaxis). CNS effects may develop with dizziness, headache and confusion, and are sufficient to require cautioning the patient against driving a motor vehicle. Convulsions have occurred during treatment (avoid or use with caution where there is a history of epilepsy or concurrent use of non-steroidal anti-inflammatory drugs, which potentiate this effect).

Reversible arthropathy has developed in weight-bearing joints in immature animals exposed to quinolones. Quinolone use is restricted to serious infections, and then with caution, in children and adolescents; ciprofloxacin is licensed for *Pseudomonas aeruginosa* lung infection in children over 5 years of age with cystic fibrosis. Rupture of tendons, notably the Achilles tendon, occurs, more commonly in the elderly and those concurrently taking corticosteroids.

Some of the quinolones are potent liver enzyme inhibitors and impair the metabolic inactivation of other drugs including warfarin, theophylline and sulphonylureas, increasing their effect. Magnesium- and aluminium-containing antacids impair the absorption of quinolones from the gastrointestinal tract, probably by forming a chelate complex; ferrous sulphate and sucralfate also reduce quinolone absorption.

Individual members of the group include the following:

Ciprofloxacin $(t_{1/2}$ 3 h) is effective against a range of bacteria but particularly the Gram-negative organisms (see above); it has less activity against Grampositive bacteria. Chlamydia and mycoplasma are susceptible. Ciprofloxacin finds use in infections of the urinary, gastrointestinal and respiratory tracts, tissue infections, gonorrhoea and septicaemia. It has proven especially useful for oral therapy of chronic Gram-negative infections such as osteomyelitis, and for acute exacerbations of *Pseudomonas* infection in cystic fibrosis. Uses include the prophylaxis and therapy of anthrax, including instances resulting from bioterrorism. The dose of 250–750 mg 12-hourly by mouth, 200–400 mg 12-hourly i.v., should be halved when the glomerular filtration rate is less than 20 mL/min. Ciprofloxacin impairs the metabolism of theophylline and of warfarin, both of which should be monitored when co-administered.

Norfloxacin $(t_{1/2}$ 3 h) is used for acute or chronic recurrent urinary tract infections.

Ofloxacin $(t_{1/2}$ 4 h) has modestly greater Gram-positive activity, but less Gram-negative activity than ciprofloxacin. It is used for urinary and respiratory tract infections, gonorrhoea and topically for eye infection.

Nalidixic acid $(t_{1/2}$ 6 h) is now used principally for the prevention of urinary tract infection. It may cause haemolysis in glucose-6-phosphate dehydrogenase-deficient subjects.

Others *Levofloxacin* $(t_{1/2}$ 7 h) has greater activity against *Streptococcus pneumoniae* than ciprofloxacin, and is used for respiratory and urinary tract infection. *Moxifloxacin* $(t_{1/2}$ 10 h) has strong anti-Gram-positive activity and is also effective against many anaerobes, but only weakly active against *Pseudomonas*. It is a second-line agent for upper and lower respiratory tract infections including those caused by 'atypical' pathogens and penicillin-resistant *Streptococcus pneumoniae*. Moxifloxacin prolongs the QTc interval and is contraindicated in patients with cardiac failure or rhythm disorders. Newer 4-quinolones available in various parts of the world include *gemifloxacin* and *gatifloxacin*.

AZOLES

This group includes:

- metronidazole and tinidazole (antibacterial and antiprotozoal), described here
- fluconazole, itraconazole, clotrimazole, econazole, ketoconazole, isoconazole and miconazole described under Antifungal drugs (see p. 233)
- albendazole, mebendazole and thiabendazole, described under Anthelminthic drugs (see p. 247).

Metronidazole

In obligate anaerobic microorganisms (but not in aerobic microorganisms, which it also enters) metronidazole is converted into an active form by reduction of its nitro group; this binds to DNA and prevents nucleic acid formation. It is bacteriostatic.

Pharmacokinetics. Metronidazole is well absorbed after oral or rectal administration and distributed to achieve sufficient concentration to eradicate infection in liver, gut wall and pelvic tissues. It is eliminated in the urine, partly unchanged and partly as metabolites. The $t_{1/2}$ is 8 h.

Uses. Metronidazole is active against a wide range of anaerobic bacteria, and protozoa. Its clinical indications are:

- Treatment of sepsis to which anaerobic organisms, e.g. *Bacteroides* spp. and anaerobic cocci, are contributing, including post-surgical infection, intra-abdominal infection and septicaemia, osteomyelitis and abscesses of brain or lung.
- Antibiotic-associated pseudomembraneous colitis (caused by *Clostridium difficile*).
- Trichomoniasis of the urogenital tract in both sexes.

- Amoebiasis (*Entamoeba histolytica*), including both intestinal and extra-intestinal infection.
- Giardiasis (*Giardia lamblia*).
- Acute ulcerative gingivitis and dental infections (*Fusobacterium* spp. and other oral anaerobic flora).
- Anaerobic vaginosis (*Gardnerella vaginalis* and vaginal anaerobes).

Dose. Established anaerobic infection is treated with metronidazole by mouth 400 mg 8-hourly; by rectum 1 g 8-hourly for 3 days followed by 1 g 12-hourly; or by i.v. infusion of 500 mg 8-hourly. A topical gel preparation is useful for reducing the odour associated with anaerobic infection of fungating tumours.

Adverse effects include nausea, vomiting, diarrhoea, furred tongue and an unpleasant metallic taste in the mouth; also headache, dizziness and ataxia. Rashes, urticaria and angio-oedema occur. Peripheral neuropathy occurs when treatment is prolonged, and epileptiform seizures when the dose is high. Large doses of metronidazole are carcinogenic in rodents and the drug is mutagenic in bacteria; long-term studies have failed to discover oncogenic effects in humans.

A disulfiram-like effect (see p. 154) occurs with alcohol because metronidazole inhibits alcohol and aldehyde dehydrogenase; warn the patient.

Tinidazole is similar to metronidazole but has a longer $t_{1/2}$ (13 h). It is excreted mainly unchanged in the urine. The indications for use and adverse effects are essentially those of metronidazole. The longer duration of action of tinidazole may be an advantage, e.g. in giardiasis, trichomoniasis and acute ulcerative gingivitis, in which tinidazole 2 g by mouth in a single dose is as effective as a course of metronidazole.

MINOR ANTIMICROBIALS

These are effective topically (except colistin) without serious risk of allergy, but toxicity or chemical instability limits or precludes their systemic use.

Mupirocin is primarily active against Gram-positive organisms including those commonly associated with skin infections. It is available as an ointment for use, e.g. in folliculitis and impetigo, and to eradicate nasal staphylococci, e.g. in carriers of resistant staphylococci. It is rapidly hydrolysed in the tissues.

POLYPEPTIDE ANTIBIOTICS

Colistin ($t_{1/2}$ 6 h) is effective against Gram-negative organisms. It finds use for bowel decontamination in neutropenic patients, for inhalational use in patients with cystic fibrosis infected with *Pseudomonas aeruginosa*, and is applied to skin, including external ear infections. Colistin is currently undergoing a renaissance, being given systemically for severe infections with multiply resistant Gram-negative pathogens such as pseudomonads and *Acinetobacter* when no alternative agents are available. Adverse effects of systemic administration include nephrotoxicity, neurological symptoms and neuromuscular blockade; renal function should be monitored daily and the dose reduced in patients with a creatinine clearance rate of less than 10–20 mL/min.

Polymyxin B is also active against Gram-negative organisms, particularly *Pseudomonas aeruginosa*. Its principal use now is topical application for skin, eye and external ear infections.

Gramicidin is used in various topical applications as eye and ear drops, combined with neomycin and framycetin.

GUIDE TO FURTHER READING

Alvarez-Elcoro S, Enzler M J 1999 The macrolides: erythromycin, clarithromycin, and azithromycin. Mayo Clinic Proceedings 74(6):613–634

Andriole V T 2005 The quinolones: past present and future. Clinical Infectious Diseases 41(suppl 2):S113–S119

Anonymous 1996 Penicillin allergy. Drug and Therapeutics Bulletin 34:87–88

Chambers H F 1997 Methicillin resistance in staphylococci: molecular and biochemical basis and clinical implications. Clinical Microbiology Reviews 10(4):781–791

Diekema D J, Jones R N 2001 Oxazolidinone antibiotics. Lancet 358:1975–1982

Farr B M 2002 Mupirocin to prevent *S. aureus* infections. New England Journal of Medicine 346:1905–1906

Fisman D N, Kaye K M 2000 Once-daily dosing of aminoglycoside antibiotics. Infectious Disease Clinics of North America 14:475–488

Hancock R E W 1997 Peptide antibiotics. Lancet 349:418–422

Jacoby G A, Munoz-Price L S 2005 The new β-lactamases. New England Journal of Medicine 352:380–391

Kelkar P S, Li J T-C 2001 Cephalosporin allergy. New England Journal of Medicine 345:804–809

Moellering R C 1998 Vancomycin-resistant enterococci. Clinical Infectious Diseases 26(5):1196–1199

Zopf D, Roth S 1996 Oligosaccharide anti-infective agents. Lancet 347:1017–1021

13

Chemotherapy of bacterial infections

SYNOPSIS

We live in a world heavily populated by microorganisms of astonishing diversity. This chapter considers the bacteria that cause disease in individual body systems, the drugs that combat them, and how they are best used. The chapter discusses infection of:

- Blood
- Paranasal sinuses and ears
- Throat
- Bronchi, lungs and pleura
- Endocardium
- Meninges
- Intestines
- Urinary tract
- Genital tract
- Bones and joints
- Eye
- Also mycobacteria, that infect many sites.

Table 11.1 (see p. 186) is a general reference for this chapter.

INFECTION OF THE BLOOD

Septicaemia is a medical emergency. Usually, the infecting organism(s) is not known at the time of presentation and treatment must be instituted on the basis of a 'best guess'. The clinical circumstances and knowledge of local resistance patterns may provide some clues. Patients who have been in hospital for some time before presenting with septicaemia need antibiotic regimens that provide more reliable cover for multiply resistant pathogens, and examples of suitable choices are given in the list below in square brackets.

- When septicaemia follows gastrointestinal or genital tract surgery, *Escherichia coli* (or other Gram-negative bacteria), anaerobic bacteria, e.g. *Bacteroides*, streptococci or enterococci are likely pathogens and the following combinations are effective: cefuroxime plus metronidazole or gentamicin plus benzylpenicillin plus metronidazole [meropenem plus vancomycin].
- Septicaemia related to urinary tract infection usually involves *Escherichia coli* (or other Gram-negative bacteria), enterococci: gentamicin plus benzylpenicillin or cefotaxime alone [meropenem plus vancomycin].
- Neonatal septicaemia is usually due to streptococci or coliforms: benzylpenicillin plus gentamicin.
- Staphylococcal septicaemia may be suspected where there is an abscess, e.g. of bone or lung, or with acute infective endocarditis or infection of intravenous catheters: high-dose flucloxacillin is indicated [vancomycin].
- Toxic shock syndrome occurs in circumstances that include healthy women using vaginal tampons, abortion or childbirth, and occasionally with skin and soft tissue infection. The clinical problem is due to systemic effects of toxins produced by staphylococci; although this is not strictly an infection of the blood, flucloxacillin is used. Elimination of the source by removal of the tampon and drainage of abscesses is also important.

Antimicrobials are given i.v. initially, and their combination with optimal circulatory and respiratory support and glycaemic control, and administration of hydrocortisone and recombinant human activated protein C, provides the best outcome.

Patients who have had a splenectomy are at risk of fulminant septicaemia especially from capsulate bacteria, e.g. *Streptococcus pneumoniae, Neisseria meningitidis*. The risk is greatest in the first 2 years after splenectomy (but is lifelong), in children, and in those with splenectomy for haematological malignancy. Patients must be immunised against appropriate pathogens and receive continuous low-dose oral prophylaxis with penicillin V, or erythromycin in those allergic to penicillin.

INFECTION OF PARANASAL SINUSES AND EARS

SINUSITIS

As oedema of the mucous membrane hinders the drainage of pus, a logical first step is to open the obstructed passage with a sympathomimetic vaso-constrictor, e.g. ephedrine nasal drops. Antibiotic therapy produces limited additional clinical benefit, but the common infecting organism(s) – *Streptococcus pneumoniae*, *Haemophilus influenzae*, *Streptococcus pyogenes*, *Moraxella (Branhamella) catarrhalis* – usually respond to oral amoxicillin (with or without clavulanic acid) or doxycycline, if the case is serious enough to warrant antibiotic therapy.

In chronic sinusitis, correction of the anatomical abnormalities (polypi, nasal septum deviation) is often important. Very diverse organisms, many of them normal inhabitants of the upper respiratory tract, may be cultured, e.g. anaerobic streptococci, *Bacteroides* spp., and a judgement is required as to whether any particular organism is acting as a pathogen. Choice of antibiotic should be guided by culture and sensitivity testing; therapy may need to be prolonged.

OTITIS MEDIA

Mild cases are normally viral and often resolve spontaneously, needing only analgesia and observation. A bulging, inflamed eardrum indicates bacterial otitis media usually due to *Streptococcus pneumoniae*, *Haemophilus influenzae*, *Moraxella (Branhamella) catarrhalis*, *Streptococcus pyogenes* (Group A) or *Staphylococcus aureus*. Amoxicillin or co-amoxiclav is satisfactory, but the clinical benefit of antibiotic therapy is very small when tested in controlled trials. Chemotherapy has not removed the need for myringotomy when pain is very severe, and also for later cases, as sterilised pus may not be completely absorbed and may leave adhesions that impair hearing. Chronic infection presents a similar problem to that of chronic sinus infection, above. Pneumococcal vaccination is modestly effective at reducing recurrences in children who are prone to them.

INFECTION OF THE THROAT

Pharyngitis is usually viral but the more serious cases may be due to *Streptococcus pyogenes* (Group A) (always sensitive to benzylpenicillin), which cannot be differentiated from virus infection with any certainty. Prevention of complications is more important than relief of the symptoms, which seldom last long.

There is no general agreement as to whether chemotherapy should be employed in mild sporadic sore throat, and expert reviews reflect this diversity of opinion.[1,2,3] The disease usually subsides in a few days, septic complications are uncommon and rheumatic fever rarely follows. It is reasonable to withhold penicillin unless streptococci are cultured or the patient develops a high fever. Severe sporadic or epidemic sore throat is likely to be streptococcal and the risk of these complications is limited by phenoxymethylpenicillin by mouth (erythromycin/clarithromycin or an oral cephalosporin in the penicillin allergic), given, ideally, for 10 days, although compliance is bad once the symptoms have subsided and 5 days should be the minimum objective. Do not use amoxicillin if the circumstances suggest pharyngitis due to infectious mononucleosis, as the patient is very likely to develop a rash (see p. 192). In a closed community, chemoprophylaxis of unaffected people to stop an epidemic may be considered, for instance with oral phenoxymethylpenicillin 125 mg 12-hourly, for a period depending on the course of the epidemic.

In scarlet fever and erysipelas, the infection is invariably streptococcal (Group A), and benzylpenicillin should be used even in mild cases, to prevent rheumatic fever and nephritis.

CHEMOPROPHYLAXIS

Chemoprophylaxis of streptococcal (Group A) infection with phenoxymethylpenicillin is necessary for

[1]Cooper R J, Hoffman J R, Bartlett J G et al 2001 Principles of appropriate antibiotic use for acute pharyngitis in adults: background. Annals of Internal Medicine 134:506.
[2]Del Mar C B, Glasziou P P, Spinks A B 2001 Antibiotics for sore throat (Cochrane review). The Cochrane Library 2. Update Software, Oxford.
[3]Thomas M, Del Mar C, Glasziou P 2000 How effective are treatments other than antibiotics for acute sore throat? British Journal of General Practice 50:817.

patients who have had one attack of rheumatic fever. Continue for at least 5 years, or until aged 20 years, whichever is the longer period (although some hold that it should continue for life, for histological study of atrial biopsies shows that the cardiac lesions may progress despite absence of clinical activity). Chemoprophylaxis should be continued for life after a second attack of rheumatic fever. A single attack of acute nephritis is not an indication for chemoprophylaxis, but, in the rare cases of nephritis in which recurrent haematuria occurs after sore throats, chemoprophylaxis should be used. Ideally, chemoprophylaxis should continue throughout the year but, if the patient is unwilling to submit to this, cover at least the colder months (see also p. 178).

Adverse effects are uncommon. Patients taking penicillin prophylaxis are liable to have penicillin-resistant viridans type streptococci in the mouth, so that during even minor dentistry, e.g. scaling, there is a risk of bacteraemia and thus of infective endocarditis with a penicillin-resistant organism in those with any residual rheumatic heart lesion. The same risk applies to urinary, abdominal and chest surgery, and patients need special chemoprophylaxis (see Endocarditis). Patients taking penicillins are also liable to be carrying resistant staphylococci and pneumococci.

OTHER CAUSES OF PHARYNGITIS

Vincent's infection (microbiologically complex, includes anaerobes, spirochaetes) responds readily to benzylpenicillin; a single i.m. dose of 600 mg is often enough except in a mouth needing dental treatment, when relapse may follow. Metronidazole 200 mg 8-hourly by mouth for 3 days is also effective.

Diphtheria (*Corynebacterium diphtheriae*). Antitoxin 10 000–100 000 units i.v. in two divided doses 0.5–2 h apart is given to neutralise toxin already formed according to the severity of the disease. Erythromycin or benzylpenicillin is also used, to prevent the production of more toxin.

Whooping cough (*Bordetella pertussis*). Chemotherapy is needed in children who are weak, have damaged lungs or are less than 3 years old. Erythromycin is usually recommended at the catarrhal stage and

should be continued for 14 days (also as prophylaxis in cases of special need). It may curtail an attack if given early enough (before paroxysms have begun) but is not dramatically effective; it also reduces infectivity to others. A corticosteroid, salbutamol and physiotherapy may be helpful for relief of symptoms, but reliable evidence of efficacy is lacking.

INFECTION OF THE BRONCHI, LUNGS AND PLEURA

BRONCHITIS

Most cases of acute bronchitis are viral; where bacteria are responsible, the usual pathogens are *Streptococcus pneumoniae* and/or *Haemophilus influenzae*. It is questionable whether there is role for antimicrobials in uncomplicated acute bronchitis, but amoxicillin, a tetracycline or trimethoprim is appropriate if treatment is considered necessary. Whether newer antimicrobials, e.g. moxifloxacin, confer significant outcome advantages to justify their expense is a matter of debate.

In chronic bronchitis, suppressive chemotherapy, generally needed only during the colder months (in temperate, colder regions), may be considered for patients with symptoms of pulmonary insufficiency, recurrent acute exacerbations or permanently purulent sputum. Amoxicillin or trimethoprim is suitable.

For intermittent therapy, the patient is given a supply of the drug and told to take it in full dose at the first sign of a 'chest' cold, e.g. purulent sputum, and to stop the drug after 3 days if there is rapid improvement. Otherwise, the patient should continue the drug until recovery takes place. If the exacerbation lasts for more than 10 days, there is a need for clinical reassessment.

PNEUMONIAS

The clinical setting is a useful guide to the causal organism and hence to the 'best guess' early choice of antimicrobial. It is not possible reliably to differentiate between pneumonias caused by 'typical' and 'atypical' pathogens on clinical grounds alone and most experts advise initial cover for both types of pathogen in seriously ill patients.

Pneumonia in previously healthy people (community acquired)

Disease that is segmental or lobar in its distribution is usually due to *Streptococcus pneumoniae* (pneumococcus). *Haemophilus influenzae* is a rare cause in this group, although it more often leads to exacerbations of chronic bronchitis and does cause pneumonia in patients infected with HIV infection. Benzylpenicillin i.v. or amoxicillin p.o. are the treatments of choice if pneumococcal pneumonia is very likely; use erythromycin/clarithromycin in a penicillin-allergic patient. Seriously ill patients should receive benzylpenicillin (to cover the pneumococcus) plus ciprofloxacin (to cover *Haemophilus* and 'atypical' pathogens). Where penicillin-resistant pneumococci are prevalent, i.v. cefotaxime is a reasonable 'best guess' choice.

Pneumonia following influenza is more often caused by *Staphylococcus aureus*, and 'best guess' therapy usually involves adding flucloxacillin to one of the regimens above. When staphylococcal pneumonia is proven, sodium fusidate p.o. plus flucloxacillin i.v. should be used in combination.

'Atypical' cases of pneumonia may be caused by *Mycoplasma pneumoniae*, which may be epidemic, or more rarely *Chlamydia pneumoniae* or *psittaci* (psittacosis/ornithosis), *Legionella pneumophila* or *Coxiella burnetii* (Q fever), and a tetracycline or erythromycin/clarithromycin should be given by mouth. Treatment of ornithosis should continue for 10 days after the fever has settled, and that of mycoplasma pneumonia and Q fever for 3 weeks to prevent relapse.

At an early stage, once there is clinical improvement, i.v. administration should change to oral.

Pneumonia acquired in hospital

Pneumonia is usually defined as being nosocomial (Greek: *nosokomeian*, hospital) if it presents after at least 2 days in hospital. It occurs primarily among patients admitted with medical problems or recovering from abdominal or thoracic surgery or on mechanical ventilators. The common pathogens are *Staphylococcus aureus*, Enterobacteriaceae, *Streptococcus pneumoniae*, *Pseudomonas aeruginosa* and *Haemophilus influenzae*. It is reasonable to initiate therapy with ciprofloxacin, meropenem or ceftazidime (plus vancomycin if the local prevalence of MRSA is high) pending the results of sputum culture and antimicrobial susceptibility tests.

Pneumonia in people with chronic lung disease

Normal commensals of the upper respiratory tract proliferate in damaged lungs especially following virus infections, pulmonary congestion or pulmonary infarction. Mixed infection is therefore common, and as *Haemophilus influenzae* and *Streptococcus pneumoniae* are often the pathogens, amoxicillin or trimethoprim is a reasonable choice in domiciliary practice; if response is inadequate, co-amoxiclav or a quinolone should be substituted.

Klebsiella pneumoniae is a rare cause of lung infection ('Friedlander's pneumonia') in the alcoholic and debilitated elderly. Abscesses form, particularly in the upper lobes; cefotaxime possibly with an aminoglycoside is recommended.

Moraxella (previously *Branhamella*) *catarrhalis*, a commensal of the oropharynx, may be a pathogen in patients with chronic bronchitis; because many strains produce β-lactamase, co-amoxiclav or erythromycin/clarithromycin is used.

Pneumonia in immunocompromised patients

Pneumonia is common, e.g. in acquired immune deficiency syndrome (AIDS) or in those who are receiving immunosuppressive drugs.

Common pathogenic bacteria may be responsible (*Staphylococcus aureus*, *Streptococcus pneumoniae*) but often organisms of lower natural virulence (Enterobacteriaceae, viruses, fungi) are causal and necessitate strenuous efforts to identify the microbe including, if feasible, bronchial washings or lung biopsy.

- Until the pathogen is known the patient should receive broad-spectrum antimicrobial treatment, such as an aminoglycoside plus ceftazidime.
- Aerobic Gram-negative bacilli, e.g. Enterobacteriaceae, *Klebsiella* spp., are pathogens in half of the cases, especially in neutropenic patients, and respond to cefotaxime or ceftazidime. *Pseudomonas aeruginosa* may also cause pneumonia in these patients; for treatment see Table 11.1.
- The fungus *Pneumocystis carinii* is an important respiratory pathogen in patients with deficient

cell-mediated immunity; treat with co-trimoxazole 120 mg/kg daily by mouth or i.v. in two to four divided doses for 14 days, or with pentamidine (see p. 247).

Legionnaires' disease

Legionella pneumophila responds to erythromycin 4 g/day i.v. in divided doses, with the addition of rifampicin in more severe infections. Ciprofloxacin is emerging as possibly more effective.

Pneumonia due to anaerobic microorganisms

Pneumonia often follows aspiration of material from the oropharynx, or accompanies other lung pathology such as pulmonary infarction or bronchogenic carcinoma. In addition to conventional microbial causes, pathogens include anaerobic and aerobic streptococci, *Bacteroides* spp. and *Fusobacterium*. Cefuroxime plus metronidazole may be needed for several weeks to prevent relapse.

Pulmonary abscess: treat the identified organism and with surgery if necessary.

Empyema: aspiration or drainage is essential followed by treatment of the isolated organism.

ENDOCARDITIS

When there is suspicion, two or three blood cultures should be taken over a few hours and antimicrobial treatment commenced, to be adjusted later in the light of the results. Delay in treating only exposes the patient to the risk of grave cardiac damage or systemic embolism. Streptococci, enterococci and staphylococci are causal in 80% of cases, with viridans group streptococci the most common pathogens. In intravenous drug users, *Staphylococcus aureus* is most likely. Culture-negative endocarditis (up to 20% of cases) is usually due to previous antimicrobial therapy or to special culture requirements of the microbe; it is best regarded as being due to streptococci and treated accordingly.

PRINCIPLES FOR TREATMENT

- Use high doses of bactericidal drugs because the organisms are difficult to access in avascular vegetations on valves.
- Give drugs parenterally, at least initially, and preferably by i.v. bolus injection to achieve the necessary high peak concentration to penetrate the vegetations.

- Examine the infusion site daily and change it regularly to prevent opportunistic infection, which is usually with coagulase-negative staphylococci or fungi. Alternatively, use a central subclavian venous catheter.
- Continue therapy, usually for 2–4 weeks, and, in the case of infected prosthetic valves, 6 weeks. Valve replacement may be needed at any time during and after antibiotic therapy if cardiovascular function deteriorates or the infection proves impossible to control.
- Adjust the dose according to the sensitivity of the infecting organism. Use the minimum inhibitory concentration test (see p. 177), rather than testing dilutions of the patient's serum against the organism (the serum cactericidal titre), which has not proved useful.

DOSE REGIMENS

The following regimens are commonly recommended:

1. Initial ('best guess') treatment should comprise benzylpenicillin 7.2 g i.v. daily in six divided doses), plus gentamicin (1 mg/kg bodyweight 8-hourly – synergy allows this dose of gentamicin and minimises risk of adverse effects). Regular serum gentamicin assay is vital: trough concentrations should be below 1 mg/L and peak concentrations about 3 mg/L; if *Staphylococcus aureus* is suspected, high-dose flucloxacillin plus rifampicin should be used. Patients allergic to penicillin and those with intracardiac prostheses or suspected MRSA infection should receive vancomycin plus rifampicin plus gentamicin. Patients presenting acutely (suggesting infection with *Staphylococcus aureus*) should receive flucloxacillin (8–12 g/day in four to six divided doses) plus gentamicin.

2. When an organism is identified and its sensitivity determined:

- *Viridans group streptococci*: the susceptibility of the organism determines the antimicrobial(s) and its duration use, e.g. benzylpenicillin plus gentamicin for 2 weeks, to vancomycin plus gentamicin for 4–6 weeks. Some patients with uncomplicated endocarditis caused by very sensitive strains may be managed as outpatients; for these patients ceftriaxone for 4 weeks may be suitable, its prolonged $t_{1/2}$ allowing convenient once-daily administration.

- *Enterococcus faecalis* (Group D): ampicillin 2 g 4-hourly plus gentamicin 1 mg/kg 8–12-hourly i.v. for 4–6 weeks. The prolonged gentamicin administration carries a significant risk of adverse drug reactions, but is essential to assure eradication of the infection.
- *Staphylococcus aureus*: flucloxacillin 2 g 4–6-hourly i.v. for at least 4 weeks. In the presence of intracardiac prostheses, flucloxacillin is combined with rifampicin orally (or fusidic acid) for at least the first 2 weeks. MRSA may be treated with vancomycin plus rifampicin plus fusidic acid (or gentamicin) for 4–6 weeks.
- *Staphylococcus epidermidis* and other coagulase-negative staphylococci infecting native heart valves are managed as for *Staphylococcus aureus* if the organism is sensitive.
- *Coxiella* or *Chlamydia*: Give doxycycline 100 mg once daily orally, plus ciprofloxacin 500 mg 8-hourly for at least 3 years. Valve replacement is advised in many cases, but some may continue indefinitely on tetracycline.
- *Fungal endocarditis*: amphotericin plus flucytosine are used. Valve replacement is usually essential.
- *Culture-negative endocarditis*: benzylpenicillin plus gentamicin i.v. are given for 4–6 weeks.

PROPHYLAXIS

Transient bacteraemia is provoked by dental procedures that induce gum bleeding, surgical incision of the skin, instrumentation of the urinary tract, parturition and even seemingly innocent activities such as brushing the teeth or chewing toffee. Bacteraemia may lead to infection of acquired or congenital heart defects, and antimicrobials are used prophylactically (although the evidence base for their efficacy is lacking). The drugs are given as a short course in high dose at the time of the procedure to coincide with the bacteraemia and avoid emergence of resistant organisms. The following recommendations on antimicrobial prophylaxis are based on those published in 2006 by the British Society for Antimicrobial Chemotherapy (see Guide for further reading); they are abbreviated and not every contingency is covered. The guidelines are based on a careful assessment of the risks of bacteraemia and reported cases of endocarditis after each procedure. Other national working parties may recommend different measures, and the physician should consult special sources, their local microbiologist and exercise a clinical judgement that relates to individual circumstances. All oral drugs should be taken under supervision.

Dental procedures

Adults who are not allergic to penicillins and who have not taken penicillin more than once in the previous month (including those with a prosthetic valve) require amoxicillin 3 g by mouth 1 h before the procedure.

Patients allergic to penicillins or who have taken penicillin more than once in the previous month should receive clindamycin 600 mg by mouth 1 h before the procedure. Azithromycin 500 mg is an alternative, which is available as a suspension for those unable to swallow capsules. If parenteral prophylaxis is required, use amoxicillin 1 g i.v. or clindamycin 300 mg i.v.

Patients having a series of separate procedures all requiring prophylaxis should receive amoxicillin or clindamycin alternately. Where practicable, a preoperative mouthwash of the antiseptic chlorhexidine gluconate (0.2%) should be used to reduce oral bacterial numbers.

Consult the guideline publication (above) for prophylactic regimens for children and other procedures, including instrumentation of the urogenital or gastrointestinal tracts, which are now recognised to carry a greater risk of endocarditis than dental procedures.

MENINGITIS

Speed of initiating treatment and accurate bacteriological diagnosis are the major factors determining the fate of the patient. With suspected meningococcal disease (and unless the patient has a history of penicillin anaphylaxis) benzylpenicillin should be started by the general practitioner before transfer to hospital; the benefit of rapid treatment outweighs the reduced chance of identifying the causative organism. Newly introduced diagnostic methods such as the polymerase chain reaction (PCR) for bacterial DNA in CSF or blood enable accurate and rapid diagnosis even when the causative organisms have been destroyed by antibiotics.

Drugs must be given i.v. in high dose. The regimens below provide the recommended therapy, with alternatives for patients allergic to first choices, and septic shock requires appropriate management (see p. 412). Intrathecal therapy is now considered unnecessary and can be dangerous, e.g. encephalopathy with penicillin.

INITIAL THERAPY

Initial therapy should be sufficient to kill all pathogens, which are likely to be:

All ages over 5 years

For *Neisseria meningitidis* and *Streptococcus pneumoniae*, give benzylpenicillin 2–4 g 4–6-hourly followed, in the case of *Neisseria meningitidis*, by rifampicin for 2 days prior to discharge from hospital (to eradicate persisting organisms). Some prefer cefotaxime 2–3 g 6–8-hourly in all cases pending the results of susceptibility tests, and this may be generally preferred with the rising prevalence of penicillin resistance to pneumococci and meningococci. Optimal therapy for known penicillin-resistant pneumococcal meningitis may comprise cefotaxime 2–3 g 6–8-hourly plus vancomycin 1 g 12-hourly plus rifampicin 600 g 12-hourly.

Children under 5 years

Neisseria meningitidis is now commonest and *Haemophilus influenzae*, formerly a frequent pathogen, is much less often isolated (following immunisation programmes). *Streptococcus pneumoniae* is also less common than in older patients. Give a cephalosporin, e.g. cefotaxime.

Neonates

For *Escherichia coli*, give cefotaxime or ceftazidime perhaps with gentamicin. For Group B streptococci, give benzylpenicillin plus gentamicin. Consult a specialist text for details of doses. Add ampicillin if *Listeria monocytogenes* is suspected.

Dexamethasone given i.v. and early appears to reduce long-term neurological sequelae, especially sensorineural deafness, in infants and children. There is no general agreement about the value of dexamethasone for meningitis in adults.

Chloramphenicol remains a good alternative for 'blind' therapy in patients giving a history of β-lactam anaphylaxis.

SUBSEQUENT THERAPY

Specific therapy follows identification of the infecting organism, as below. Necessarily, i.v. administration should continue until the patient can take drugs by mouth, but whether or when continuation therapy should be oral or i.v. is a matter of debate. Antimicrobials (except aminoglycosides) enter well into the CSF when the meninges are inflamed; relapse may be due to restoration of the blood–CSF barrier as inflammation reduces. The following are recommended (adult doses).

Neisseria meningitidis. Give benzylpenicillin 2.4 g 4–6-hourly or cefotaxime 2–3 g 6–8-hourly for a minimum of 5 days.

Streptococcus pneumoniae. Give cefotaxime 2–3 g 6–8-hourly or benzylpenicillin 2.4 g 4–6-hourly if the organism is penicillin-sensitive and continue for 10 days after the patient has become afebrile.

Haemophilus influenzae. Give cefotaxime 2–3 g 6–8-hourly or chloramphenicol 100 mg/kg daily for 10 days after the temperature has settled. Subdural empyema, often presenting as persistent fever, is relatively common after haemophilus meningitis and may require surgical drainage.

Chemoprophylaxis

The three common pathogens (below) are spread by respiratory secretions. Asymptomatic nasopharyngeal carriers seldom develop meningitis but may transmit the pathogens to close personal contacts. Rifampicin by mouth is effective at reducing carriage rates.

Meningococcal meningitis often occurs in epidemics in closed communities, but also in isolated cases. Patients and close personal contacts should receive rifampicin 600 mg 12-hourly by mouth for 2 days. Single doses of ciprofloxacin (500 mg by mouth) or ceftriaxone (2 g i.m.) are alternatives, the latter of particular value for pregnant women.

Haemophilus influenzae type b has an infectivity similar to that of the meningococcus; give rifampicin 600 mg by mouth daily for 4 days.

Pneumococcal meningitis tends to occur in isolated cases and contacts do not need chemoprophylaxis.

INFECTION OF THE INTESTINES

(For *Helicobacter pylori*, see p. 565)

Both wit and truth are contained in the aphorism that 'travel broadens the mind but opens the bowels'.

Antimicrobial therapy should be reserved for specific conditions with identified pathogens where benefit has been shown; acute diarrhoea can be caused by bacterial toxins in food, dietary indiscretions, anxiety and by drugs as well as by infection. Even if diarrhoea is infective, it may be due to viruses; or, if bacterial, antimicrobial agents may not reduce the duration of symptoms and may aggravate the condition by permitting opportunistic infection and encouraging *Clostridium difficile*-associated diarrhoea. Maintaining water and electrolyte balance either orally or by i.v. infusion with a glucose–electrolyte solution, and administration of an antimotility drug (except in small children), are the mainstays of therapy in such cases (see Oral rehydration therapy, p. 575). Some specific intestinal infections do benefit from chemotherapy:

Campylobacter jejuni. Erythromycin or ciprofloxacin by mouth will eliminate the organism from the stools and a 5-day course is worth giving early in the illness if it is severe.

Shigella. Mild disease requires no specific antimicrobial therapy but toxic shigellosis with high fever should be treated with ciprofloxacin or amoxicillin by mouth.

Salmonella. Give an antimicrobial for severe salmonella gastroenteritis, or for bacteraemia or salmonella enteritis in an immunocompromised patient. The choice lies between ciprofloxacin, amoxicillin or a parenteral cephalosporin, according to the sensitivity of the pathogen.

Typhoid fever is a generalised infection and requires treatment with ciprofloxacin. Chloramphenicol, amoxicillin or co-trimoxazole are less effective alternatives. The i.v. route is used at least initially, followed by oral administration. A longer period of treatment may be required for those who develop complications such as osteomyelitis or abscess.

A carrier state develops in a few individuals who have no symptoms of disease but who can infect others.[4] Organisms reside in the biliary or urinary

---

[4]The most famous carrier was Mary Mallon ('Typhoid Mary') who worked as a cook in New York City, USA, using various assumed names and moving through several different households. She caused at least 10 outbreaks with 51 cases of typhoid fever and 3 deaths. To protect the public, she was kept in detention for 23 years.

tracts. Ciprofloxacin in high dose by mouth for 3–6 months may be successful for what can be a very difficult problem, requiring investigation for urinary tract abnormalities or even cholecystectomy.

Escherichia coli is a normal inhabitant of the bowel but some enterotoxigenic strains are pathogenic and are frequently a cause of travellers' diarrhoea. A quinolone, e.g. ciprofloxacin, is the drug of choice for a severe attack, and azithromycin or the non-absorbable rifampicin-relative rifaximin are alternatives (see Travellers' diarrhoea, p. 576). Prophylactic use of an antimicrobial is not usual but, should it be deemed necessary, a quinolone is best.

Verotoxic *Escherichia coli* (VTEC; O157) may cause severe bloody diarrhoea and systemic effects such as the haemolytic uraemic syndrome (HUS); antibiotic therapy has been shown in some trials to worsen the prognosis, perhaps by releasing more toxin from dying bacteria. In general, avoid using an antibiotic for bloody diarrhoea unless VTEC has been excluded bacteriologically.

Vibrio cholerae. Death in cholera is due to electrolyte and fluid loss in the stools, and this may exceed 1 L/h. Prompt replacement and maintenance of water and electrolyte balance with i.v. and oral electrolyte solutions are vital. Doxycycline, given early, significantly reduces the amount and duration of diarrhoea and eliminates the organism from the faeces (thus lessening the contamination of the environment). Carriers may be treated by doxycycline by mouth in high dose for 3 days. Ciprofloxacin may be given for resistant organisms.

Suppression of bowel flora has been shown to be useful in hepatic encephalopathy. Here, absorption of products of bacterial breakdown of protein (ammonium, amines) in the intestine lead to cerebral symptoms and even to coma. In acute coma, neomycin 6 g daily should be given by gastric tube; as prophylaxis, 1–4 g/day may be given to patients with protein intolerance who fail to respond to dietary protein restriction (see also Lactulose, p. 573).

Selective decontamination of the gut may reduce the risk of nosocomial infection from gut organisms (including fungi) in patients who are immunocompromised or receiving intensive care (notably mechanical ventilation). The commonest regimen involves combinations of nonabsorbable (framycetin, colistin, nystatin and amphotericin) and i.v. (cefotaxime) antimicrobials to reduce the number of Gram-negative bacilli and yeasts while maintaining a normal anaerobic flora. An alternative is to administer oral ciprofloxacin alone.

Peritonitis is usually a mixed infection and antimicrobial choice must take account of coliforms, anaerobes and streptococci; a combination of gentamicin, benzylpenicillin plus metronidazole, or of cefuroxime plus metronidazole, or meropenem alone is usually appropriate. Surgical drainage of peritoneal collections and abscesses is usually required as well.

Chemoprophylaxis in surgery. See page 181.

Antibiotic-associated colitis. See page 183.

INFECTION OF THE URINARY TRACT

(excluding sexually transmitted infections)

Common pathogens include *Escherichia coli* (commonest in all patient groups), *Proteus* spp., *Klebsiella* spp., other Enterobacteriaceae, *Pseudomonas aeruginosa*, *Enterococcus* spp. and *Staphylococcus saprophyticus*.

Patients with abnormal urinary tracts, e.g. renal stones, prostatic hypertrophy, indwelling urinary catheters, are likely to be infected with a more varied and antimicrobial-resistant microbial flora. Identification of the causative organism and of its sensitivity to drugs are important because of the range of organisms and the prevalence of resistant strains.

For infection of the lower urinary tract a low dose may be effective, as many antimicrobials are concentrated in the urine. Infections of the substance of the kidney require the doses needed for any systemic infection. A large urine volume (over 1.5 L/day) and frequent micturition hasten elimination of infection.

Drug treatment of urinary tract infection falls into several categories:

Lower urinary tract infection

Initial treatment with an oral cephalosporin (e.g. cefalexin), trimethoprim, amoxicillin or co-amoxiclav is usually satisfactory, although current resistance rates of 20–50% among common pathogens for trimethoprim and amoxicillin threaten their value for empirical therapy. Therapy should normally last for 3 days and may need to be altered once the results of bacterial sensitivity are known.

Upper urinary tract infection

Acute pyelonephritis may be accompanied by septicaemia and it is advisable to start with gentamicin plus amoxicillin i.v. or alternatively cefotaxime i.v. alone. If oral therapy is considered suitable, ciprofloxacin is recommended for 2 weeks. This is an infection of the kidney substance and so needs adequate blood as well as urine concentrations.

Recurrent urinary tract infection

Attacks following rapidly with the same organism may be relapses and indicate a failure to eliminate the original infection. Attacks with a longer interval between them and produced by differing bacterial types may be regarded as due to reinfection, most often by ascending infection from the perineal skin. Repeated short courses of antimicrobials should overcome most recurrent infections but, if these fail, 7–14 days of high-dose treatment may be given, following which continuous low-dose prophylaxis may be needed.

Asymptomatic infection ('asymptomatic bacteriuria')

This may be found by routine urine testing of pregnant women or patients with known structural abnormalities of the urinary tract. Such infection may explain micturition frequency or incontinence in the elderly. Appropriate antimicrobial therapy should be given, chosen on the basis of susceptibility tests, and normally for 7–10 days. Amoxicillin or a cephalosporin is preferred in pregnancy, although nitrofurantoin may be used if imminent delivery is not likely (see below).

Prostatitis

The commonest pathogens here are Gram-negative aerobic bacilli, although chlamydia may also be involved. A quinolone such as ciprofloxacin is commonly used, although trimethoprim or erythromycin is also effective. Being lipid soluble, these drugs penetrate the prostate in adequate concentration; they may usefully be combined. Response to a single, short course is often good, but recurrence is common and a patient can be regarded as cured only if he has been symptom-free without resort to antimicrobials for a year. Four weeks of oral therapy is often given for recurrent attacks.

Chemoprophylaxis

Chemoprophylaxis is sometimes undertaken in patients liable to recurrent attacks or acute exacerbations of ineradicable infection. It may prevent progressive renal damage in children who are found to have asymptomatic bacteriuria on routine screening. Nitrofurantoin (50–100 mg/day), nalidixic acid (0.5–1.0 g/day) or trimethoprim (100 mg/day) is satisfactory. The drugs are best given as a single oral dose at night.

Tuberculosis of the genitourinary tract is treated on the principles described for pulmonary infection (see p. 219).

SPECIAL DRUGS FOR URINARY TRACT INFECTIONS

General antimicrobials used for urinary tract infections are described elsewhere. A few agents find use solely for infection of the urinary tract:

Nitrofurantoin, a synthetic antimicrobial, is active against the majority of urinary pathogens except pseudomonads. It is well absorbed from the gastrointestinal tract and is concentrated in the urine ($t_{1/2}$ 1 h), but plasma concentrations are too low to treat infection of kidney tissue. Excretion is reduced when there is renal insufficiency, rendering the drug both more toxic and less effective. Adverse effects include nausea and vomiting (much reduced with the macrocrystalline preparation) and diarrhoea. Peripheral neuropathy occurs especially in patients with significant renal impairment, in whom the drug is contraindicated. Allergic reactions include rashes, generalised urticaria and pulmonary infiltration with lung consolidation or pleural effusion. Nitrofurantoin is safe in pregnancy, except near to term (because it may cause neonatal haemolysis), and it must be avoided in patients with glucose-6-phosphate dehydrogenase deficiency (see p. 107).

Nalidixic acid. See page 204.

GENITAL TRACT INFECTIONS

A general account of orthodox literature is given below, but treatment is increasingly the prerogative of specialists, who, as is so often the case, get the best results. Interested readers are referred to specialist texts. Sexually transmitted infections are commonly multiple. Screening of contacts plays a vital part in controlling spread and reducing reinfection.

GONORRHOEA

The problems of β-lactam and quinolone resistance in *Neisseria gonorrhoeae* infection are increasing (ciprofloxacin resistance rates rose from 2.1% in 2000 to 9.8% in 2002 in England and Wales), and selection of a particular drug will depend on sensitivity testing and a knowledge of resistance patterns in different geographical locations. Effective treatment requires exposure of the organism briefly to a high concentration of the drug. Single-dose regimens are practicable as well as being obviously desirable for social reasons, including compliance. The following schedules are effective:

Uncomplicated anogenital infections. Amoxicillin with probenecid (in areas where the local penicillin resistance rate is less than 5%), or high-dose cefixime (3 g) by mouth; spectinomycin i.v., or ceftriaxone i.m. UK resistance rates for oral ciprofloxacin are now considered too high for recommendation unless the isolate is known to be susceptible.

Pharyngeal gonorrhoea responds less reliably, and i.m. ceftriaxone is recommended.

Coexistent infection. *Chlamydia trachomatis* is frequently present with *Neisseria gonorrhoeae*; tetracycline by mouth for 7 days or a single oral dose of azithromycin 1 g will treat the chlamydial urethritis.

NON-GONOCOCCAL URETHRITIS

The vast majority of cases of urethritis with pus in which gonococci cannot be identified are due to sexually transmitted organisms, usually *Chlamydia trachomatis* and sometimes *Ureaplasma urealyticum*. Tetracycline or azithromycin by mouth is effective.

PELVIC INFLAMMATORY DISEASE

Several pathogens are involved including *Chlamydia trachomatis*, *Neisseria gonorrhoeae* and *Mycoplasma hominis*, and there may be superinfection with bowel and other urogenital tract bacteria. A combination of antimicrobials is usually required, e.g. metronidazole plus doxycycline by mouth.

SYPHILIS

Treponema pallidum is invariably sensitive to penicillin.

Primary and secondary syphilis are effectively treated by benzylpenicillin or procaine penicillin i.m. daily for 10–21 days. Tetracycline or erythromycin orally may be used for penicillin-allergic patients, and a single dose of azithromycin appears to have equivalent efficacy, but macrolide resistance to *Treponema pallidum* has been reported uncommonly but worldwide.

Tertiary syphilis should have the same treatment, ensuring that it continues for 3 weeks.

Congenital syphilis in the newborn should be treated with benzylpenicillin for 10 days at least. Some advocate that a pregnant woman with syphilis should be treated as for primary syphilis, in each pregnancy, in order to avoid all danger to children. Therapy is best given between the third and sixth month, as there may be a risk of abortion if it is given earlier.

Results of treatment of syphilis with penicillin are excellent. Follow-up of all cases is essential, for 5 years if possible.

The *Herxheimer* (or Jarisch–Herxheimer) reaction is probably caused by cytokine (mainly tumour necrosis factor) release following massive slaughter of spirochaetes. Presenting as pyrexia, it is common during the few hours after the first penicillin injection; other features include tachycardia, headache, myalgia and malaise, which last for up to a day. It cannot be avoided by giving graduated doses of penicillin. Prednisolone may prevent it and should probably be given if a reaction is specially to be feared, e.g. in a patient with syphilitic aortitis.

CHANCROID

The causal agent, *Haemophilus ducreyi*, normally responds to erythromycin for 7 days or a single dose of ceftriaxone or azithromycin.

GRANULOMA INGUINALE

Calymmatobacterium granulomatis infection responds to co-trimoxazole or doxycycline for 2 weeks or a single dose of azithromycin weekly for 4 weeks.

BACTERIAL VAGINOSIS (BACTERIAL VAGINITIS, ANAEROBIC VAGINOSIS)

Bacterial vaginosis is a common form of vaginal discharge in which neither *Trichomonas vaginalis* nor *Candida albicans* can be isolated and inflammatory cells are not present. The condition is associated with overgrowth of several normal commensals of the vagina including *Gardnerella vaginalis*, Gram-negative curved bacilli and anaerobic organisms, especially of the *Bacteroides* genus, the latter being responsible for the characteristic fishy odour of the vaginal discharge. The condition responds well to a single dose of metronidazole 2 g by mouth, with topical clindamycin offering an alternative.

Candida vaginitis. See page 183.

Trichomonas vaginitis. See page 234.

INFECTION OF BONES AND JOINTS

Osteomyelitis may be acute or chronic and the causative bacteria arrive in the bloodstream or are implanted directly (through a compound fracture, chronic local infection of local tissue, or surgical operation). *Staphylococcus aureus* is the commonest isolate in all patient groups, but *Haemophilus influenzae* is frequently seen in children (now much reduced by the Hib vaccine), and salmonella species in the tropics. Chronic osteomyelitis of the lower limbs (especially when underlying chronic skin infection in the elderly) frequently involves obligate anaerobes (such as *Bacteroides* spp.) and coliforms.

Strenuous efforts should be made to obtain bone for culture because superficial and sinus cultures are poorly predictive of the underlying flora, and prolonged therapy is required for chronic osteomyelitis (usually 6–8 weeks, sometimes longer). Surgical removal of dead bone improves the outcome of chronic osteomyelitis.

Definitive therapy is guided by the results of culture but commonly used regimens include flucloxacillin with or without fusidic acid (for *Staphylococcus aureus*), cefotaxime or co-amoxiclav (in children), and ciprofloxacin (for coliforms). Short courses of therapy (3 weeks) may suffice for acute osteomyelitis.

Septic arthritis is a medical emergency if good joint function is to be retained. *Staphylococcus aureus* is the commonest pathogen, but a very wide range of bacteria may be involved including streptococci coliforms and *Neisseria*. Aspiration of the joint allows specific microbiological diagnosis, differentiation from non-infectious causes such as crystal synovitis, and has therapeutic benefit, e.g. for the hip joint where formal drainage is recommended. Initial therapy is as for chronic osteomyelitis.

EYE INFECTIONS

Superficial infections, caused by a variety of organisms, are treated by chloramphenicol, fusidic acid, framycetin, gentamicin, ciprofloxacin, ofloxacin or neomycin in drops or ointments. Ciprofloxacin, ofloxacin, gentamicin or tobramycin is used for *Pseudomonas aeruginosa*, and fusidic acid principally for *Staphylococcus aureus*. Preparations often contain hydrocortisone or prednisolone, but the steroid masks the progress of the infection, and should it be applied with an antimicrobial to which the organism is resistant (bacterium or virus) it may aggravate the disease by suppressing protective inflammation. Local chemoprophylaxis without corticosteroid is used to prevent secondary bacterial infection in viral conjunctivitis. A variety of antibiotics may be given by direct injection to the chambers of the eye for treatment of bacterial endophthalmitis.

Chlamydial conjunctivitis. In the developed world, the genital (D–K) serotypes of the organism are responsible, and the reservoir and transmission is maintained by sexual contact. Endemic trachoma in developing countries is usually caused by serotypes A, B and C. In either case, oral tetracycline is effective. Pregnant or lactating women may receive systemic erythromycin. Neonatal ophthalmia responds to systemic erythromycin and topical tetracycline.

Herpes keratitis (see p. 219). A corticosteroid should never be put on the eye; the disease is exacerbated and permanent blindness can result.

MYCOBACTERIAL INFECTIONS

PULMONARY TUBERCULOSIS

Nearly one-third of the world's population is infected with *Mycobacterium tuberculosis*, and it is the second leading cause of death due to an identified pathogen, after HIV infection. Drug therapy has transformed tuberculosis from a disabling and often fatal disease into one in which almost 100% cure is obtainable, although the recent emergence of multi-

ply drug-resistant strains of *Mycobacterium tuberculosis* (MDR-TB) and its interaction with HIV infection has disturbed this optimistic view. Chemotherapy was formerly protracted, but a better understanding of the mode of action of antituberculous drugs and of effective immune reconstitution in HIV infection has allowed the development of shorter-course regimens.

Principles of antituberculous therapy

- Kill a large number of actively multiplying bacilli: *isoniazid* achieves this.
- Treat persisters, i.e. semidormant bacilli that metabolise slowly or intermittently: *rifampicin* and *pyrazinamide* are the most efficacious.
- Prevent the emergence of drug resistance by multiple therapy to suppress single-drug-resistant mutants that may exist de novo or emerge during therapy: *isoniazid* and *rifampicin* are best.
- Combined formulations are used to ensure that poor compliance does not result in monotherapy with consequent drug resistance.

Most contemporary regimens employ an *initial* phase with at least three drugs to reduce the bacterial load as rapidly as possible (usually for 2 months), followed by a *continuation* phase with usually two drugs given for 4 months.

All short-course regimens include isoniazid, pyrazinamide and rifampicin. After extensive clinical trials, the following three have been found satisfactory:

1. An *unsupervised* regimen of daily dosing comprising isoniazid and rifampicin for 6 months, plus pyrazinamide for the first 2 months.
2. A *supervised* (directly observed therapy, DOT) regimen for patients who cannot be relied upon to comply with treatment, comprising thrice-weekly dosing with isoniazid and rifampicin for 6 months, plus pyrazinamide for the first 2 months (isoniazid and pyrazinamide are given in higher dose than in the unsupervised regimen). With both of the above regimens, ethambutol by mouth or streptomycin i.m. should be added for the first 2 months if there is a likelihood of drug-resistant organisms, or if the patient is severely ill with extensive active lesions.
3. A *less costly*, yet still effective, regimen favoured by some countries comprises supervised

daily administration of isoniazid, rifampicin, pyrazinamide and either ethambutol or streptomycin for 2 months followed by 6 months of unsupervised daily isoniazid and thiacetazone.

All of the regimens are highly effective, with relapse rates of 1–2% in those who continue for 6 months; even if patients default after, say, 4 months, tuberculosis can be expected to recur in only 10–15%. Drug resistance seldom develops with any of these regimens.

Compliance is often a concern with multiple drug therapy given for long periods, especially in the developing world, and (surprisingly) DOT did improve relapse rates in many trials. Combination therapy is assumed to improve compliance; some commonly used combinations include Rifater (rifampicin, isoniazid plus pyrazinamide), and Rifinah or Rimactazid (rifampicin plus isoniazid). In all cases, effective control of tuberculosis in a population requires optimal therapy of index cases combined with careful screening and case finding among their contacts.

Special problems

Resistant organisms. Initial resistance occurs in about 4% of isolates in the UK, usually to isoniazid. Patients with multiply drug-resistant tuberculosis, i.e. resistant to rifampicin and isoniazid at least, should be treated with three or four drugs to which the organisms are sensitive, and treatment should extend for 12–24 months after cultures become negative. Treatment of such cases requires expert management.

Atypical mycobacteria are often resistant to standard drugs; their virulence is low but they can produce serious infection in immunocompromised patients which may respond, e.g. to clarithromycin or a quinolone, often in combination.

Chemoprophylaxis may be either:

- *primary*, i.e. the giving of antituberculous drugs to uninfected but exposed individuals, which is seldom justified; or
- *secondary*, which is the treatment of infected but symptom-free individuals, e.g. those known to be in contact with the disease and who develop a positive tuberculin reaction. Secondary chemoprophylaxis may be justified in children

under the age of 3 years because they have a high risk of disseminated disease; isoniazid alone for 6–9 months may be used as there is little risk of resistant organisms emerging because the organism load is low.

Pregnancy. Drug treatment should never be interrupted or postponed during pregnancy. On the general principle of limiting exposure of the fetus, the standard three-drug, 6-month course (no. 1 above) is best. Exclude streptomycin from any regimen (danger of fetal eighth cranial nerve damage).

Non-respiratory tuberculosis. The principles of treatment, i.e. multiple therapy and prolonged follow-up, are the same as for respiratory tuberculosis. Many chronic tuberculous lesions may be relatively inaccessible to drugs as a result of avascularity of surrounding tissues, so treatment frequently has to be prolonged and dosage high, especially if damaged tissue cannot be removed by surgery, e.g. tuberculosis of bones.

Meningeal tuberculosis. It is essential to use isoniazid and pyrazinamide, which penetrate well into the CSF. Rifampicin enters inflamed meninges well, but non-inflamed meninges less so. An effective regimen is isoniazid, rifampicin, pyrazinamide and streptomycin. Treatment may need to continue for much longer than modern short-course chemotherapy for pulmonary tuberculosis.

Adrenal steroid and tuberculosis. In pulmonary tuberculosis a corticosteroid may be given to severely ill patients, and increases survival in tuberculous meningitis. Corticosteroids reduce the injurious reaction of the body to tuberculoprotein and buy time for the chemotherapy to take effect. The patient also feels better much more quickly. In the absence of effective chemotherapy, an adrenal steroid will cause tuberculosis to extend and should never be used alone, e.g. for another disease, if tuberculosis is suspected.

Tuberculosis in the immunocompromised. Such patients require special measures because they may be infected more readily when exposed; their infections usually involve large numbers of tubercle bacilli (multibacillary disease), and patients with AIDS are more likely to be infected with multiply antibiotic-resistant strains. Usually at least four drugs are started, and patients are isolated until bacteriological results have been obtained and they have shown clinical improvement. If infections are proved to involve antibiotic-susceptible mycobacteria, therapy can continue with a conventional 6-month regimen with careful follow-up. Particular problems may occur with multiple drug interactions during antituberculous treatment of patients receiving antiretroviral therapy.

ANTITUBERCULOSIS DRUGS

Isoniazid

Isoniazid (INH, INAH, isonicotinic acid hydrazide) is selectively effective against *Mycobacterium tuberculosis* because it prevents the synthesis of components that are unique to mycobacterial cell walls. Hence it is bactericidal against actively multiplying bacilli (whether within macrophages or at extracellular sites) but is bacteriostatic against non-dividing bacilli; it has little or no activity against other bacteria. Isoniazid is well absorbed from the alimentary tract and is distributed throughout the body water, readily crossing tissue barriers and entering cells and CSF. It should always be given in cases where there is special risk of meningitis (miliary tuberculosis and primary infection). Isoniazid is inactivated by conjugation with an acetyl group and the rate of the reaction is bimodally distributed (see Pharmacogenetics, p. 105). The $t_{1/2}$ is 1 h in fast and 4 h in slow acetylators; fast acetylators achieve less than half the steady-state plasma concentration of slow acetylators but standard oral doses (300 mg/day) on daily regimens give adequate tuberculocidal concentrations in both groups.

Adverse effects. Isoniazid is in general well tolerated. The most severe adverse effect is liver damage, which may range from a moderate rise in the level of hepatic enzymes to severe hepatitis and death. It is probably caused by a chemically reactive metabolite(s), e.g. acetylhydrazine. Most cases are in patients aged over 35 years, and develop within the first 8 weeks of therapy; liver function should be monitored monthly during this period at least.

Isoniazid is a structural analogue of pyridoxine and accelerates its excretion, the principal result of which is peripheral neuropathy with numbness and tingling of the feet, motor involvement being less common. Neuropathy is more frequent in slow acetylators, malnourished people, the elderly and those with HIV infection, liver disease and alcohol-

ism. Such patients should receive pyridoxine 10 mg/day by mouth, which prevents neuropathy and does not interfere with the therapeutic effect; some prefer simply to give pyridoxine to all patients. Other adverse effects include mental disturbances, incoordination, optic neuritis and convulsions.

Isoniazid inhibits the metabolism of phenytoin, carbamazepine and ethosuximide, increasing their effect.

Rifampicin

Rifampicin has bactericidal activity against the tubercle bacillus, comparable to that of isoniazid. It is also used in leprosy.

It acts by inhibiting RNA synthesis, bacteria being sensitive to this effect at much lower concentrations than mammalian cells; it is particularly effective against mycobacteria that lie semi-dormant within cells. Rifampicin has a wide range of antimicrobial activity. Other uses include leprosy, severe legionnaires' disease (with erythromycin or ciprofloxacin), the chemoprophylaxis of meningococcal meningitis, and severe staphylococcal infection (with flucloxacillin or vancomycin).

Rifampicin is well absorbed from the gastrointestinal tract. It penetrates into most tissues. Entry into the CSF when meninges are inflamed is sufficient to maintain therapeutic concentrations at normal oral doses but transfer is reduced as inflammation subsides in 1–2 months.

Enterohepatic recycling takes place, and eventually about 60% of a single dose is eliminated in the faeces; urinary excretion of unchanged drug also occurs. The $t_{1/2}$ is 4 h after initial doses, but shortens on repeated dosing because rifampicin is a very effective enzyme inducer and increases its own metabolism (as well as that of several other drugs, see below).

Adverse reactions. Rifampicin rarely causes any serious toxicity. Adverse reactions include flushing and itching with or without a rash, and thrombocytopenia. Rises in plasma levels of bilirubin and hepatic enzymes may occur when treatment starts, but are often transient and are not necessarily an indication for stopping the drug; fatal hepatitis, however, has occurred. Hepatic function should be checked before starting treatment and at least for the first few months of therapy. Intermittent dosing, i.e. less than twice weekly, either as part of a regimen or through poor compliance, promotes an influenza-like syndrome (malaise, headache and fever, shortness of breath and wheezing), acute haemolytic anaemia and thrombocytopenia, and acute renal failure sometimes with haemolysis. These may have an immunological basis. Red discoloration of urine, tears and sputum is a useful indication that the patient is taking the drug. Rifampicin also causes an orange discoloration of soft contact lenses.

Interactions. Rifampicin is a powerful enzyme inducer and speeds the metabolism of numerous drugs, including warfarin, steroid contraceptives, narcotic analgesics, oral antidiabetic agents, phenytoin and dapsone. Appropriate increase in dosage, and alternative methods of contraception, are required to compensate for increased drug metabolism (see also Paracetamol overdose, p. 259).

Rifabutin ($t_{1/2}$ 36 h) has similar activity and adverse reactions, and is used for prophylaxis of *Mycobacterium avium* infection in patients with AIDS, and for treatment of tuberculous and non-tuberculous mycobacterial infection in combination with other drugs.

Rifaximin is a semi-synthetic rifamycin that is not absorbed from the gastrointestinal tract (less than 0.4%). Because of the very high faecal concentrations achieved after a 400-mg oral dose (about 8000 micrograms/g faeces), it has broad activity against the common bacterial causes of travellers' diarrhoea and has proved as effective as an oral quinolone or azithromycin (see p. 200), and adverse effects are rare.

Pyrazinamide

Pyrazinamide is a derivative of nicotinamide and is included in first-choice combination regimens because of its particular ability to kill intracellular persisters, i.e. mycobacteria that are dividing or semi-dormant, often within cells. Its action is dependent on the activity of intrabacterial pyrazinamidase, which converts pyrazinamide to the active pyrazinoic acid; this enzyme is most effective in an acidic environment such as the interior of cells. It is inactive against *Mycobacterium bovis*. Pyrazinamide is well absorbed from the gastrointestinal tract and metabolised in the liver, very little unchanged drug appearing in the urine ($t_{1/2}$ 9 h). CSF concentrations are almost identical to those in the blood. Pyrazinamide is safe to use in pregnancy.

Adverse effects include hyperuricaemia and arthralgia, which is relatively frequent with daily but less so with intermittent dosing and, unlike gout, affects both large and small joints. Pyrazinoic acid, the principal metabolite of pyrazinamide, inhibits renal tubular secretion of urate. Symptomatic treatment with a non-steroidal anti-inflammatory drug is usually sufficient and it is rarely necessary to discontinue pyrazinamide because of arthralgia. Hepatitis, which was particularly associated with high doses, is not a problem with modern short-course schedules. Sideroblastic anaemia and urticaria also occur.

Ethambutol

Ethambutol, being bacteriostatic, is used in conjunction with other antituberculous drugs to delay or prevent the emergence of resistant bacilli. It is well absorbed from the gastrointestinal tract and effective concentrations occur in most body tissues including the lung; in tuberculous meningitis, sufficient may reach the CSF to inhibit mycobacterial growth but insignificant amounts cross into the CSF if the meninges are not inflamed. Excretion is mainly by the kidney, by tubular secretion as well as by glomerular filtration ($t_{1/2}$ 4 h); the dose should be reduced when renal function is impaired.

Adverse effects. In recommended oral doses (15 mg/kg/day), with dose adjustment for reduced renal function, ethambutol is relatively non-toxic. The main problem is rare *optic neuritis* (unilateral or bilateral) causing loss of visual acuity, central scotomata, occasionally also peripheral vision loss and red–green colour blindness. The changes reverse if treatment is stopped promptly; if not, the patient may go blind. It is prudent to note any history of eye disease and to get baseline tests of vision before starting treatment with ethambutol. The drug should not be given to a patient whose vision is much reduced and who may not notice further minor deterioration. Patients should be told to make a point of reading small print in newspapers (with each eye separately) and, if there is any deterioration, to stop the drug immediately and seek advice. Patients who cannot understand and comply (especially children) should be given alternative therapy if possible. The need for repeated specialist ophthalmological monitoring is controversial. Peripheral neuritis occurs but is rare.

Streptomycin

See page 196.

Thiacetazone

Thiacetazone is tuberculostatic and is used with isoniazid to inhibit the emergence of resistance to the latter drug. It is absorbed from the gastrointestinal tract, partly metabolised and partly excreted in the urine ($t_{1/2}$ 13 h).

Adverse reactions include gastrointestinal symptoms, conjunctivitis and vertigo. More serious effects are erythema multiforme, haemolytic anaemia, agranulocytosis, cerebral oedema and hepatitis.

Alternative or reserve drugs are used where there are problems of drug intolerance and bacterial resistance. They are in this class because of either greater toxicity or of lesser efficacy, and include ethionamide (gastrointestinal irritation, allergic reactions), capreomycin (nephrotoxic) and cycloserine (effective but neurotoxic). Quinolone antibiotics such as ciprofloxacin and moxifloxacin, linezolid, and the more recently introduced macrolides such as clarithromycin and azithromycin also have useful activity against mycobacteria.

LEPROSY

Effective treatment of leprosy is complex and requires much experience to obtain the best results. Problems of resistant leprosy now require that multiple drug therapy be used and involve:

- For *paucibacillary disease*: dapsone and rifampicin for 6 months.
- For *multibacillary disease*: dapsone, rifampicin and clofazimine for 2 years. Follow-up for 4–8 years may be necessary.

Dapsone is a bacteriostatic sulphone related to sulphonamides (and acts by the same mechanism; see p. 107). It has long been the standard drug for all forms of leprosy. Irregular and inadequate duration of treatment with a single drug have allowed the emergence of resistance, both primary and secondary, to become a major problem. Dapsone is also used to treat dermatitis herpetiformis and *Pneumocystis carinii* pneumonia, and (with pyrimethamine) for malaria prophylaxis. The $t_{1/2}$ is 27 h. Adverse effects range from gastrointestinal symptoms to agranulocytosis, haemolytic anaemia and generalised allergic reactions that include exfoliative dermatitis.

Rifampicin (see above) is bactericidal, and is safe and effective when given once monthly. This long interval renders feasible the directly observed administration of rifampicin which the above regimens require.

Clofazimine has a leprostatic action and an anti-inflammatory effect which prevents erythema nodosum leprosum. It causes gastrointestinal symptoms. Reddish discoloration of the skin and other cutaneous lesions also occur, and may persist for months after the drug has been stopped. The $t_{1/2}$ is 70 days.

Other antileprotics include ethionamide and prothionamide. Thalidomide (see Index), despite its notorious past, still finds a use with corticosteroid in the control of allergic lepromatous reactions.

OTHER BACTERIAL INFECTIONS

Burns. Infection may be reduced by application of silver sulfadiazine cream. Substantial absorption can occur from any raw surface and use of aminoglycoside, e.g. neomycin, preparations can cause ototoxicity.

Gas gangrene. The skin between the waist and the knees is normally contaminated with anaerobic faecal organisms. However assiduous the skin preparation for orthopaedic operations or thigh amputations, this will not kill or remove all the spores. Surgery done for vascular insufficiency where tissue oxygenation may be poor is likely to be followed by infection. Gas gangrene (*Clostridium perfringens*) may occur; prophylaxis with benzylpenicillin or metronidazole is used.

Wounds. Systemic chemoprophylaxis is necessary for several days at least in dirty wounds where sutures have to be left below the skin, and in penetrating wounds of body cavities. Flucloxacillin is probably best, but in the case of penetrating abdominal wounds metronidazole should be added and consideration given to adding an agent active against aerobic Gram-negative bacteria, e.g. gentamicin (see also Tetanus).

Bites from humans and other mammals are common and involve the inoculation of the rich bacterial flora of the mouth deep in the tissues; secondary infection is frequent. Appropriate management beyond direct care of the wound includes prevention of tetanus, wound infection and transmission of viruses such as hepatitis B and C, and

HIV. Antibiotic prophylaxis appears to reduce wound infection risks only in bites of the hand and those made by humans or cats, and co-amoxiclav is considered the best choice; microbiological advice should be sought for patients allergic to penicillin.

Abscesses and infections in serous cavities are treated according to the antimicrobial sensitivity of the organism concerned but require high doses because of poor penetration. Local instillation of the drug may be needed.

Actinomycosis. The anaerobe *Actinomyces israelii* is sensitive to several drugs, but not to metronidazole, and access is poor because of granulomatous fibrosis. High doses of benzylpenicillin or amoxicillin are given for several weeks; the infections are often mixed with other anaerobic bacteria, so metronidazole is often given in addition to ensure activity against all components of the mixture. Co-amoxiclav may be a convenient alternative. Surgery is likely to be needed.

Leptospirosis. To be maximally effective against *Leptospira*, start chemotherapy within 4 days of the onset of symptoms. Benzylpenicillin is recommended; a Herxheimer reaction may be induced (see Syphilis). General supportive management is important, including attention to fluid balance and observation for signs of hepatic, renal or cardiac failure.

Lyme disease. Keeping the skin covered and use of insect repellants are effective to prevent tick bites; tick removal shortly after attachment (within 24 h) will prevent infection. A single dose of doxycycline 200 mg is effective as prophylaxis after tick removal, but should be used only in high-risk areas (expert advice should be sought). In most manifestations of the established disease, *Borrelia burgdorferi* responds to amoxicillin or doxycycline orally for up to 21 days but invasion of the CNS calls for large doses of cefotaxime i.v. for 14 days.

GUIDE TO FURTHER READING

Resources on the world wide web

Algorithm for the early management of suspected bacterial meningitis and meningococcal septicaemia in immunocompetent adults. Available: http://www.britishinfectionsociety.org/adult_men_early_poster%202004.pdf

British Thoracic Society guidelines on management of community-acquired pneumonia in adults updated 2004. Available: http://www.brit-thoracic.org.uk/iqs/dlsfa.view/dldbitemid.311/dlcpti.175/page269.html

British Society for Antimicrobial Chemotherapy recommendations for treatment of infective endocarditis in the UK, 2006. Available: http://jac.oxfordjournals.org/cgi/content/short/dkh474v1

Printed resources

Annane D, Bellissant E, Cavaillon J M 2005 Septic shock. Lancet 365:63–76

Anonymous 2004 Managing bites from humans and other mammals. Drugs and Therapeutics Bulletin 42:67–71

Bhan M K, Bahl R, Bhatnagar S 2005 Typhoid and paratyphoid fever. Lancet 366:749–762

Bharti A R, Nally J E, Ricaldi J N et al 2003 Leptospirosis: a zoonotic disease of global importance. Lancet Infectious Diseases 3(12):757–771

Campion E W 1999 Liberty and the control of tuberculosis. New England Journal of Medicine 340(5):385–386

Donovan B 2004 Sexually transmissible infections other than HIV. Lancet 363:545–556

Dye C 2006 Global epidemiology of tuberculosis. Lancet 367:938–940

Gould F K, Elliott T S, Foweraker J et al 2006 Guidelines for the prevention of endocarditis: report of the Working Party of the British Society for Antimicrobial Chemotherapy. Journal of Antimicrobial Chemotherapy 57(6):1035–1042

Hasham S, Matteucci P, Stanley P R W, Hart N B 2005 Necrotising fasciitis. British Medical Journal 330:830–833

Lever A (ed.) 2004 Infection. Clinical Medicine 4(6):494–523 (a series of articles on the management of various types of infection)

Lew D P, Waldvogel F A 2004 Osteomyelitis. Lancet 364:369–379

Newland A, Provan D, Myint S 2005 Preventing severe infection after splenectomy. British Medical Journal 331:417–418

Quagliarello V 2004 Adjunctive steroids for tuberculous meningitis – more evidence, more questions. New England Journal of Medicine 351(17):1792–1794

Ryan E T, Wilson M E, Kain K C 2002 Illness after international travel. New England Journal of Medicine 347(7):505–516

Sack D A, Sack R B, Nair G B, Siddique A K 2004 Cholera. Lancet 363:223–233

Swartz M N 2004 Bacterial meningitis – a view of the past 90 years. New England Journal of Medicine 351(18):1826–1828

Thomas C F, Limper A H 2004 *Pneumocystis* pneumonia. New England Journal of Medicine 350(24):2487–2498

Whitty C J M 1999 Erasmus, syphilis, and the abuse of stigma. Lancet 354:2147–2148

Wormser G P 2006 Early Lyme disease. New England Journal of Medicine 354(26):2794–2801

14

Viral, fungal, protozoal and helminthic infections

SYNOPSIS

- **Viruses** present a more difficult problem of chemotherapy than do higher organisms, e.g. bacteria, for they are intracellular parasites that use the metabolism of host cells.[1] Highly selective toxicity is, therefore, harder to achieve. In the past 15 years, identification of the molecular differences between viral and human metabolism has led to the development of many effective antiviral agents; four were available in 1990, now there are over 40.
- **Fungal infections** range from inconvenient skin conditions to life-threatening systemic diseases; the latter have become more frequent as opportunistic infections in patients immunocompromised by drugs or AIDS, or receiving intensive medical and surgical interventions in intensive care units.
- **Protozoal infections**. Malaria is the major transmissible parasitic disease in the world. Drug resistance is an increasing problem and differs with geographical location, and species of plasmodium.
- **Helminthic infestations** cause considerable morbidity. The drugs that are effective against these organisms are summarised.

---

[1]The large-scale screening for natural compounds able to kill bacteria in vitro, which was the basis for the boom of antibiotics in the 1950s, was not successful for antivirals … The driving force for the boom of antivirals in this period has been the pressure to contain the HIV pandemic, combined with the increased understanding of the molecular mechanisms … which has allowed the identification of new targets for therapeutic intervention.' (Rappuoli R 2004 From Pasteur to genomics: progress and challenges in infectious diseases. Nature Medicine 10:1177–1185.)

VIRAL INFECTIONS

Antiviral agents are most active when viruses are replicating. The earlier that treatment is given, therefore, the better the result. Apart from primary infection, viral illness is often the consequence of reactivation of latent virus in the body. Patients whose immune systems are compromised may suffer particularly severe illness. Viruses are capable of developing resistance to antimicrobial drugs, with similar implications for the individual patient, for the community and for drug development. An overview of drugs that have proved effective against virus diseases appears in Table 14.1.

HERPES SIMPLEX AND VARICELLA-ZOSTER

ACICLOVIR

Aciclovir ($t_{1/2}$ 3 h) inhibits viral DNA synthesis only after phosphorylation by virus-specific *thymidine kinase* this accounts for its high therapeutic index. Phosphorylated aciclovir inhibits DNA polymerase and so prevents viral DNA being formed. It is effective against susceptible herpes viruses if started early in the course of infection, but it does not eradicate persistent infection because viral DNA is integrated in the host genome. About 20% is absorbed from the gut, but this is sufficient for oral systemic treatment of some infections. It distributes widely in the body; the concentration in CSF is approximately half that of plasma, and the brain concentration may be even lower. These differences are taken into account in dosing for viral encephalitis (for which aciclovir must be given i.v.). The drug is excreted in the urine. For oral and topical use the drug is given five times daily.

Table 14.1 Drugs of choice for virus infections

Organism	Drug of choice	Alternative
Varicella-zoster		
chickenpox	aciclovir	valaciclovir or famciclovir
zoster	aciclovir or famciclovir	valaciclovir
Herpes simplex		
keratitis	aciclovir (topical)	
labial	aciclovir (topical and/or oral)	valaciclovir or famciclovir
genital	aciclovir (topical and/or oral)	valaciclovir
	famciclovir (oral)	penciclovir
encephalitis	aciclovir	
disseminated	aciclovir	foscarnet
Human immunodeficiency virus (HIV)	zidovudine	zalcitabine
	tenofovir	didanosine
	ritonavir	lamivudine
	emtricitabine	indinavir
	atazanavir	abacavir
	nelfinavir	enfuvirtide
	efavirenz	
	saquinavir	
	nevirapine	
	fosamprenavir	
	lopinavir	
Hepatitis B, C or D	pegylated interferon α-2a and interferon 2b	lamivudine, ribavirin, adefovir
Influenza A	zanamivir, oseltamivir	amantadine
Cytomegalovirus (CMV)	valganciclovir, ganciclovir	foscarnet (for retinitis in patients with HIV) oidofovir
Respiratory syncytial virus	ribavirin	palivizumab
Papillomavirus (genital warts)	imiquimod	
Molluscum contagiosum	cidofovir	

Indications for aciclovir include:

Herpes simplex virus:

- skin infections, including initial and recurrent labial and genital herpes (as a cream), most effectively when new lesions are forming; skin and mucous membrane infections (as tablets or oral suspension)
- ocular keratitis (as an ointment)
- prophylaxis and treatment in the immunocompromised (oral, as tablets or suspension)
- encephalitis, disseminated disease (i.v.).

Aciclovir-resistant herpes simplex virus has been reported in patients with AIDS; foscarnet (p. 232) and cidofovir (p. 232) have been used in these cases.

Varicella-zoster virus:

- chickenpox, particularly in the immuno-compromised (i.v.) or in the immunocompetent with pneumonitis or hepatitis (i.v.)

- shingles in immunocompetent persons (as tablets or suspension, and best started within 48 h of the appearance of the rash). Immunocompromised persons will often have more severe symptoms and require i.v. administration.

Adverse reactions are remarkably few. The ophthalmic ointment causes a mild transient stinging sensation and a diffuse superficial punctate keratopathy which clears when the drug is stopped. Oral or i.v. use may cause gastrointestinal symptoms, headache and neuropsychiatric reactions. Extravasation with i.v. use causes severe local inflammation.

Valaciclovir is a pro-drug (ester) of aciclovir, i.e. after oral administration the parent aciclovir is released. The higher bioavailability of valaciclovir (about 60%) allows dosing only 8-hourly. It is used for treating herpes zoster infections and herpes simplex infections of the skin and mucous membranes.

Famciclovir ($t_{1/2}$ 2 h) is a pro-drug of *penciclovir*, which is similar to aciclovir; it is used for herpes zoster and genital herpes simplex infections, and a single dose is effective at reducing the time to healing of labial herpes simplex. It need be given only 8-hourly. Penciclovir is also available as a cream for treatment of labial herpes simplex.

Idoxuridine was the first widely used antiviral drug; it is variably effective topically for ocular and cutaneous herpes simplex, with few adverse reactions. It has been superseded by aciclovir.

HUMAN IMMUNODEFICIENCY VIRUS (HIV)

According to World Health Organization data, more than 40 million people worldwide were infected with human immunodeficiency virus (HIV) in 2004, 95% in the developing world; 6 million needed antiretroviral therapy but fewer than 8% of these were receiving it.

GENERAL COMMENTS

- The aims of antiretroviral therapy are to delay disease progression and prolong survival by suppressing the replication of the virus. Optimal suppression also prevents the emergence of drug resistance and reduces the risks of onward transmission to sexual partners and the unborn children of HIV-infected mothers. Virological failure is defined as the inability to reduce plasma HIV viral load to fewer than 400 copies per microlitre after 24 weeks, or fewer than 50 copies by 48 weeks.
- No current antiviral agents or combinations eliminate HIV infection, but the most effective combinations (so-called 'highly active antiretroviral therapy', HAART) produce profound suppression of viral replication in many patients and allow useful reconstitution of the immune system, measured by a fall in the plasma viral load and an increase in the numbers of cytotoxic T cells (CD4 count). Rates of opportunistic infections such as *Pneumocystis carinii* pneumonia and cytomegalovirus (CMV) retinitis are reduced when CD4 counts are restored, and life expectancy is markedly increased. Efficacy of viral suppression comes at the cost of unwanted effects from the multiple drugs used.

- Combination therapy reduces the risks of emergence of resistance to antiretroviral drugs, which is increasing in incidence even in patients newly diagnosed with HIV. Mutations in the viral genome either prevent binding of the drug to the active site of the protease or reverse transcriptase enzymes, or lead to removal of the drug from the reverse transcriptase active site. The potential for rapid development of resistance is immense because untreated HIV replicates rapidly (50% of circulating virus is replaced daily), the spontaneous mutation rate is high, the genome is small, the virus will develop single mutations at every codon every day, and for many antiretroviral agents a single mutation will render the virus fully resistant.
- Currently two types of antiretroviral combination are generally recommended for initial HIV therapy:
  1. A ritonavir-boosted protease inhibitor plus two nucleoside analogue reverse transcriptase inhibitors.
  2. A non-nucleoside reverse transcriptase inhibitor plus two nucleoside analogue reverse transcriptase inhibitors.
- The decision to begin antiretroviral therapy is based on:
  1. the CD4 cell count (most current recommendations are to start in patients with counts below 200 cells per microlitre, and to consider treating those with counts below 350 cells per microlitre and those with rapidly falling counts)
  2. the plasma viral load (especially if over 100 000 viral genome copies per mL)
  3. in pregnancy (to reduce the risk of vertical transmission).
- Alternative combinations are used if these variables deteriorate or unwanted drug effects occur. Antiretroviral resistance testing, both genetic (by searching viral RNA for sequences coding for resistance) and phenotypic (by testing antiretroviral agents against the patient's virus in cell culture), also guide the choice of drug regimen, especially after virological failure.
- There are currently more than 20 antiretroviral agents in four classes approved in most countries, plus five combinations. The choice for the individual patient is best made after reference to contemporary, expert advice (see the websites listed at the end of this chapter).

- Pregnancy and breast-feeding pose special problems. The objectives of therapy are to minimise drug toxicity to the fetus while reducing the maternal viral load and the catastrophic results of HIV transmission to the neonate. Prevention of maternal–fetal and maternal–infant spread is the most cost-effective way of using antiretroviral drugs in less developed countries, and available regimens reduce transmission to less than 10% of the untreated rate.

- Combination antiretroviral therapy, especially the thymidine nucleoside analogue reverse transcriptase inhibitors zidovudine and stavudine, cause redistribution of body fat in some patients, the 'lipodystrophy syndrome'. Protease inhibitors can disturb lipid and glucose metabolism to a degree that warrants a change to drugs with limited effects on lipid metabolism, e.g. ritonavir-boosted atazanavir, and the introduction of lipid-lowering agents.

- Impaired cell-mediated immunity leaves the host prey to opportunistic infections including: candidiasis, coccidioidomycosis, cryptosporidiosis, CMV disease, herpes simplex, histoplasmosis, *Pneumocystis carinii* pneumonia, toxoplasmosis and tuberculosis (often with multiply resistant organisms). Treatment of these conditions is referred to elsewhere in this text.[2]

- Improvement in immune function as a result of antiretroviral treatment may provoke an inflammatory reaction against residual opportunistic organisms.

- Antiretroviral drugs may also be used in combination to reduce the risks of infection with HIV from injuries, e.g. from HIV-contaminated needles. The decision to offer such post-exposure prophylaxis (PEP), and the optimal combination of drugs used, is a matter for experts; administration must begin within a few hours of the injury.

- Some drugs described here have found additional indications, or are used only, for therapy of non-HIV infections, e.g. lamivudine and adefovir, for chronic hepatitis B infection.

[2]For a comprehensive review, see Kovacs J A, Masur H 2000 Prophylaxis against opportunistic infections in patients with human immunodeficiency virus infection. New England Journal of Medicine 342:1416–1429.

NUCLEOSIDE REVERSE TRANSCRIPTASE INHIBITORS

Zidovudine (AZT, Retrovir)

The HIV replicates by converting its single-stranded RNA into double-stranded DNA, which is incorporated into host DNA; this crucial conversion, the reverse of the normal cellular transcription of nucleic acids, is accomplished by the enzyme *reverse transcriptase*. Zidovudine has a high affinity for reverse transcriptase and is integrated by it into the viral DNA chain, causing premature chain termination. The drug must be present continuously to prevent viral integration to the host DNA, which is permanent once it occurs.

Pharmacokinetics. Zidovudine is well absorbed from the gastrointestinal tract (it is available as capsules and syrup) and is rapidly cleared from the plasma ($t_{1/2}$ 1 h); concentrations in cerebrospinal fluid (CSF) are approximately half of those in plasma. Zidovudine is also available i.v. for patients temporarily unable to take oral medications. The drug is inactivated mainly by metabolism, but 20% is excreted unchanged by the kidney.

Uses. Zidovudine is indicated for serious manifestations of HIV infection in patients with acquired immunodeficiency syndrome (AIDS) or AIDS-related complex, i.e. those with opportunistic infection, constitutional or neurological symptoms, or with low CD4 counts; treatment reduces the frequency of opportunistic infections and prolongs survival when used in effective combinations.

Adverse reactions early in treatment may include anorexia, nausea, vomiting, headache, dizziness, malaise and myalgia, but tolerance develops to these and usually the dose does not need to be altered. More serious are anaemia and neutropenia, which develop more commonly when the dose is high, with advanced disease, and in combination with ganciclovir, interferon-α and other marrow suppressive agents. A toxic myopathy (not easily distinguishable from HIV-associated myopathy) may develop with long-term use. Rarely, a syndrome of hepatic necrosis with lactic acidosis may occur with zidovudine (and with other reverse transcriptase inhibitors).

Didanosine

Didanosine (ddI) has a short plasma half-life ($t_{1/2}$ 1 h) but a much longer intracellular duration than zidovudine, and thus prolonged antiretroviral activity. Didanosine is rapidly but incompletely absorbed from the gastrointestinal tract and is widely distributed in body water; 30–65% is recovered unchanged in the urine. Didanosine may cause pancreatitis with an incidence of 7% at a dose of 500 mg/day; a reduced dose may be tolerated after symptoms have resolved. Other adverse effects include peripheral neuropathy, hyperuricaemia and diarrhoea, any of which may give reason to reduce the dose or discontinue the drug. Didanosine is administered with a buffer that reduces gastric acidity, and this impairs absorption of a number of drugs frequently used in patients with AIDS including dapsone, ketoconazole, quinolones and indinavir.

Zalcitabine

Zalcitabine (ddC) ($t_{1/2}$ 1 h) is similar. Adverse effects include peripheral neuropathy, hepatitis and pancreatitis which are reason to discontinue the drug. Oral ulceration, gastrointestinal symptoms and bone marrow suppression are reported.

Lamivudine

Lamivudine (3TC) is a reverse transcriptase inhibitor with a relatively long intracellular half-life (14 h; plasma $t_{1/2}$ 6 h). In combination with zidovudine, lamivudine appears to reduce viral load effectively and to be well tolerated, although bone marrow suppression may be produced. Rarely, pancreatitis may occur. The drug is excreted mainly by the kidney, and dose modification is necessary in renal impairment. Lamivudine was the first nucleoside analogue to be licensed for therapy of chronic hepatitis B infection, for which it is sometimes used in combination with interferon (see p. 233) Emergence of resistant mutants of hepatitis B is troublesome (due to mutations of the viral reverse transcriptase/DNA polymerase), occurring in up to about 30% patients after 1 year and 70% after 5 years of therapy.

Emtricitabine has a similar structure, tolerability, efficacy and resistance profile.

Abacavir

Abacavir ($t_{1/2}$ 2 h) has high therapeutic efficacy; it is usually well tolerated, but adverse effects include hypersensitivity reactions especially during the first 6 weeks of therapy, affecting about 5% of patients; the drug must be stopped immediately and avoided in future if hypersensitivity is suspected.

Tenofovir

Tenofovir ($t_{1/2}$ 17 h), admnistered orally as the pro-drug tenofovir disoproxil fumarate, is hydrolysed to tenofovir, which is activated by phosphorylation. It is also effective against hepatitis B virus. Some 80% is excreted by renally and dose adjustment is recommended in patients with a creatinine clearance rate of less than 50 mL/min.

Tenofovir competes with didanosine for renal tubular excretion, raising didanosine plasma concentrations with associated risk of pancreatitis, peripheral neuropathy and lactic acidosis. It lowers plasma concentrations of atazanavir (the mechanism is unclear), which must therefore be given at higher dose.

Stavudine

Stavudine (d4T) inhibits reverse transcriptase by competing with the natural substrate deoxythymidine triphosphate, and additionally is incorporated into viral DNA causing termination of chain elongation ($t_{1/2}$ 1.5 h). Troublesome lipoatrophy has limited its use by most authorities outside the developing world. Hepatic toxicity and pancreatitis are reported, and a dose-related peripheral neuropathy may occur, all probably related to mitochondrial toxicity.

Adefovir

Adefovir dipivoxil is a nucleoside analogue used for chronic hepatitis B infection, including against lamivudine-resistant strains. It is administered as the oral pro-drug (plasma $t_{1/2}$ 8 h, intracellular $t_{1/2}$ of active metabolite 17 h). Adverse effects are uncommon, but include headache, abdominal pain and diarrhoea. Resistance emerges over time, but much less commonly than with lamivudine therapy, possibly due to the flexibility of the adefovir molecule, which allows it to conform to mutated binding sites.

PROTEASE INHIBITORS

In its process of replication, HIV produces protein and also a *protease*, which cleaves the protein into component parts that are subsequently reassembled into virus particles; protease inhibitors disrupt this essential process.

Protease inhibitors reduce viral RNA concentration ('viral load'), increase the CD4 count and improve survival when used in combination with other agents. They are metabolised extensively by isoenzymes of the cytochrome P450 system, notably by

CYP 3A4, and most protease inhibitors inhibit these enzymes. They have a plasma $t_{1/2}$ of 2–4 h, except for fosamprenavir (8 h) and atazanavir (7 h with food). The drugs have broadly similar therapeutic effects. Members of the group include:

- amprenavir, atazanavir, fosamprenavir (a pro-drug of amprenavir), indinavir, lopinavir, nelfinavir, ritonavir, saquinavir and tipranavir.

Adverse effects include gastrointestinal disturbance, headache, dizziness, sleep disturbance, raised liver enzymes, neutropenia, pancreatitis and rashes.

Interactions. Involvement with the cytochrome P450 system provides scope for numerous drug–drug interactions. Agents that induce P450 enzymes, e.g. rifampicin, St John's Wort, accelerate their metabolism, reducing plasma concentration and therapeutic efficacy; enzyme inhibitors, e.g. ketoconazole, cimetidine, raise their plasma concentration with risk of toxicity.

The powerful inhibiting effect of ritonavir on CYP 3A4 and CYP 2D6 is harnessed usefully by its combination in low (subtherapeutic) dose with *lopinavir*; the result is to decrease the metabolism and increase the therapeutic efficacy of the latter (called ritonavir 'boosting' or 'potentiation'), i.e. a *beneficial* drug–drug interaction. The effect appears more advantageous in patients infected with low-level resistant virus. Ritonavir also inhibits the metabolism and increases the persistence in plasma of amprenavir, atazanavir, indinavir, lopinavir, saquinavir and tipranavir.

NON-NUCLEOSIDE REVERSE TRANSCRIPTASE INHIBITORS

This group is structurally different from the reverse transcriptase inhibitors; members are active against the subtype HIV-1 but not HIV-2, a subtype encountered mainly in Africa. Non-nucleoside reverse transcriptase inhibitors tend to be inducers of CYP 450 enzymes.

Efavirenz is taken once per day ($t_{1/2}$ 52 h). Rash is relatively common during the first 2 weeks of therapy, but resolution usually occurs within a further 2 weeks; the drug should be stopped if the rash is severe or if there is blistering, desquamation, mucosal involvement or fever. Neurological adverse reactions occur in about 50% patients and may be reduced by taking the drug before retiring at night; gastrointestinal side-effects, and occasional hepatitis and pancreatitis, have also been reported. Efavirenz is teratogenic, so should be avoided in pregnancy.

Nevirapine is used in combination with at least two other antiretroviral drugs, usually for progressive or advanced HIV infection, although it also appears to be effective and relatively safe in pregnancy. It penetrates the CSF well, and undergoes hepatic metabolism ($t_{1/2}$ 28 h); it induces its own metabolism and the dose should be increased gradually. Nevirapine is taken once daily, increasing to twice daily if rash is not seen. Rash (including Stevens–Johnson syndrome) and occasionally fatal hepatitis are the commonest unwanted effects.

Delavirdine ($t_{1/2}$ 6 h) is administered thrice daily; rash is the commonest adverse effect, generally appearing within the first month of therapy and disappearing over a 2-week period, during which the drug usually does not need to be discontinued.

ENTRY INHIBITOR

Enfuvirtide is the first antiretroviral agent to target the host cell attachment/entry stage in the HIV replication cycle; the linear 36-amino acid synthetic peptide inhibits fusion of the cellular and viral membranes. It is given by s.c. injection ($t_{1/2}$ 4 h). The drug seems most effective when combined with several antiretroviral agents to which the virus is susceptible, and in patients whose CD4 counts are above 100 cells per microlitre.

Adverse effects are usually limited to mild injection-site reactions, although hypersensitivity, peripheral neuropathy and other adverse reactions are reported rarely. HIV isolates with decreased susceptibility have been recovered from enfuvirtide-treated patients; these exhibit mutations in the gp41 outer envelope glycoprotein of the virus (which plays a key role in infection of CD4 cells by fusing the HIV envelope with the host cell membrane).

Fixed-dose combinations of antiretroviral drugs include Combivir (zidovudine plus lamivudine), Truvada (tenofovir plus emtricitabine), Epzicom (abacavir plus lamivudine), Trizivir (zidovudine plus lamivudine plus abacavir) and Kaletra (lopinavir plus ritonavir). Although these are convenient, the components of the combination may differ in their dependence on metabolic inactivation or renal excretion; particular attention to these is necessary when use in patients with renal or hepatic impairment is proposed.

INFLUENZA A

Neuraminidase inhibitors are highlighted by the emergence of avian influenza viruses with the potential for mutation to cause pandemic spread in the human population, although their clinical effectiveness is not high. There is little scientific evidence to recommend any of these agents for public health control of seasonal influenza, and amantadine is not recommended for therapy or prophylaxis of avian influenza.

Amantadine

Amantadine is effective only against influenza A; it acts by interfering with the uncoating and release of viral genome into the host cell. It is well absorbed from the gastrointestinal tract and is eliminated in the urine ($t_{1/2}$ 3 h). Amantadine may be used orally for the prevention and treatment of infection with influenza A virus: if commenced within 48 h of the onset of symptoms, it reduces the duration of symptoms by an average of 1 day. Those most likely to benefit include the debilitated, persons with respiratory disability or those living in crowded conditions, especially during an influenza epidemic. Amantadine reduces the risk of acquiring influenza A by 70–90% if started before exposure. Natural resistance is very rare, but may emerge on treatment, and the resistant virus is fully pathogenic and transmissible; it remains susceptible to oseltamivir and zanamivir.

Adverse reactions include dizziness, nervousness, lightheadedness and insomnia. Drowsiness, hallucinations, delirium and coma may occur in patients with impaired renal function. Convulsions may be induced, and amantadine should be avoided in epileptic patients.

Amantadine for Parkinson's disease: see page 384.

Zanamivir (Relenza)

Zanamivir is a viral neuraminidase inhibitor that blocks both entry of influenza A and B viruses to target cells and the release of their progeny. It is administered as a dry powder twice daily in a 5-day course by a special inhaler. The duration of symptoms is reduced from about 6 to 5 days, with a smaller reduction in the mean time taken to return to normal activities. In high-risk groups the reduction in duration of symptoms is a little greater, and fewer patients need antibiotics. It is also effective for prophylaxis given as a once-daily inhalation.

The UK National Institute for Health and Clinical Excellence (NICE) recommends that zanamivir be reserved for:

- at-risk patients (those with chronic respiratory or cardiovascular disease, immunosuppression or diabetes mellitus, or over the age of 65 years)
- when virological surveillance in the community indicates that influenza virus is circulating
- only those presenting within 48 h of the onset of influenza-like symptoms.

Zanamivir retains activity against amantadine- and some oseltamivir-resistant strains.

Unwanted effects are uncommon, but bronchospasm may be precipitated in asthmatics, and gastrointestinal disturbance and rash are occasionally seen.

Oseltamivir (Tamiflu)

Oseltamivir is an oral pro-drug of a viral neuraminidase inhibitor. It reduces the severity and duration of symptoms caused by influenza A or B in adults and children if commenced within 36 h of the onset of symptoms. More specifically, the risk of respiratory complications such as secondary pneumonia, antibiotic use and hospital admission are reduced. It is effective for prophylaxis when given daily for 10 days, a usage that might be appropriate for healthcare workers and those especially likely to suffer serious complications from pre-existing illness. Prophylaxis may be given for 2 weeks after influenza immunisation while protective antibodies are being produced.

Oseltamivir is one option for treatment and prophylaxis of avian H5N1 influenza. In the event of a pandemic, treatment for 5 days and prophylactic use for up to 6 weeks (or until 48 h after last exposure) are suggested.

Unwanted effects are uncommon; some people experience gastrointestinal symptoms that are reduced by taking the drug with food. No naturally occurring oseltamivir resistance has yet been detected, but resistant virus can be found in 1% of immunocompetent adults and 9% of children during treatment, owing to mutations in viral neuraminidase. Mutated isolates appear less virulent and transmissible than native strains, and human-to-human transmission has not yet been detected.

CYTOMEGALOVIRUS

Ganciclovir

Ganciclovir resembles aciclovir in its mode of action, but is much more toxic. It is given orally or i.v. and is eliminated in the urine, mainly unchanged ($t_{1/2}$ 4 h). Ganciclovir is active against several types of virus but toxicity limits its i.v. use to life- or sight-threatening CMV infection in immunocompromised patients. A ganciclovir-releasing intraocular implant is more effective than i.v. ganciclovir for CMV retinitis and avoids systemic toxicity. It is given by mouth for maintenance suppressive treatment of retinitis in patients with AIDS, and to prevent CMV disease in patients receiving immunosuppressive therapy following organ transplantation (especially liver transplants).

Ganciclovir-resistant CMV isolates have been reported, and require treatment with foscarnet or cidofovir.

Adverse reactions include neutropenia and thrombocytopenia, which are usually but not always reversible. Concomitant use of potential marrow-depressant drugs, e.g. co-trimoxazole, amphotericin B, azathioprine, zidovudine, should be avoided, and co-administration of granulocyte colony-stimulating factor may ameliorate the myelosuppressive effects. Other reactions are fever, rash, gastrointestinal symptoms, confusion and seizure (the last especially when imipenem is co-administered).

Valganciclovir is an oral pro-drug of ganciclovir that provides systemic concentrations almost as high as those following i.v. therapy.

Foscarnet

Foscarnet finds use i.v. for CMV retinitis in patients with HIV infection when ganciclovir is contraindicated, and for aciclovir-resistant herpes simplex virus infection (see p. 225). It is generally less well tolerated than ganciclovir; adverse effects include renal toxicity (usually reversible), nausea and vomiting, neurological reactions and marrow suppression.

Hypocalcaemia is seen especially when foscarnet is given with pentamidine, e.g. during treatment of multiple infections in patients with AIDS.

Cidofovir

Cidofovir is given by i.v. infusion (usually every 1–2 weeks) for CMV retinitis in patients with AIDS when other drugs are unsuitable or resistance is a problem. It has also been used i.v. and topically to produce resolution of molluscum contagiosum skin lesions in immunosuppressed patients, and it may be effective in other poxvirus infections. Nephrotoxicity is common with i.v. use, but is reduced by hydration with i.v. fluids before each dose and co-administration with probenecid. Other unwanted effects include bone marrow suppression, nausea and vomiting, and iritis and uveitis, and cause about 25% patients to discontinue therapy.

Fomivirsen

Fomivirsen, an antisense oligonucleotide, is available in some countries as an intravitreal injection for CMV retinitis in HIV-infected patients who cannot tolerate or who have failed treatment with other drugs.

RESPIRATORY SYNCYTIAL VIRUS (RSV)

Ribavirin (Tribavirin) is a synthetic nucleoside used for RSV bronchiolitis in infants and children, inhaled by a special ventilator. As therapeutic efficacy for this indication is controversial, it is usually reserved for the most severe cases and those with co-existing illnesses, such as immunosuppression. Systemic absorption by the inhalational route is negligible.

Ribavirin is effective by mouth ($t_{1/2}$ 45 h) for reducing mortality from Lassa fever and hantavirus infection (possibly also other viral haemorrhagic fevers and West Nile virus) and, when combined with interferon α-2b or peg-interferon, for chronic hepatitis C infection (see below). It does not cross the blood–brain barrier, so is unlikely to be effective in viral encephalitides. Systemic ribavirin is an important teratogen, and it may cause cardiac, haematological, gastrointestinal and neurological adverse effects.

Palivizumab is a humanised monoclonal antibody that is given by monthly i.m. injection in the winter and early spring to infants at high risk of RSV infection. Transient fever and local injection site reactions are seen and rarely, gastrointestinal disturbance, rash, leucopenia or disturbed liver function occur.

DRUGS THAT MODULATE THE HOST IMMUNE SYSTEM

Interferons

Virus infection stimulates the production of protective glycoproteins (*interferons*) which act:

- *directly* on uninfected cells to induce enzymes that degrade viral RNA
- *indirectly* by stimulating the immune system
- to modify cell regulatory mechanisms and inhibit neoplastic growth.

Interferons are classified as α, β or γ according to their antigenic and physical properties. α-Interferons (subclassified -2a, -2b and -N1) are effective against conditions that include hairy cell leukaemia, chronic myelogenous leukaemia, recurrent or metastatic renal cell carcinoma, Kaposi's sarcoma in patients with AIDS (an effect that may be due partly to its activity against HIV) and condylomata acuminata (genital warts).

Interferon α-2a and -2b also improve the manifestations of viral hepatitis, but responses differ according to the infecting agent (see p. 539). Therapy with interferon α-2b leads in about a third of patients with chronic hepatitis B to loss of circulating 'e' antigen, a return to normal liver enzyme levels, histological improvement in liver architecture, and a lowered rate of progression of liver disease. Pegylated (bound to polyethylene glycol) interferon α-2a may be more effective.

Over 50% patients with hepatitis C respond to the combination of pegylated interferon plus ribavirin, and 30–40% to peg-interferon alone. Successful treatment results in the serum concentration of viral RNA becoming undetectable by polymerase chain reaction (PCR). Hepatitis D (δ agent co-infection with hepatitis B) requires a much larger dose of interferon to obtain a response, and relapse may yet occur when the drug is withdrawn. Interferon α-2b may be effective in West Nile Virus encephalitis.

See also page 229 for lamivudine, and page 229 for adefovir, use in chronic hepatitis B infection.

Adverse reactions are common and include an influenza-like syndrome (naturally produced interferon may be responsible for symptoms in natural influenza infection), fatigue and depression, which respond to lowering the dose but tend to improve after the first week. Other effects are anorexia (sufficient to induce weight loss), alopecia, convulsions, hypotension, hypertension, cardiac arrhythmias and bone marrow depression (which may respond to granulocyte colony-stimulating factors and erythropoietin). Interferons inhibit the metabolism of theophylline, increasing its effect, and autoimmune diseases such as thyroiditis may be induced or exacerbated.

Imiquimod is used topically for genital warts (caused by papillomaviruses). Treatment for 2–3 months results in gradual clearance of warts in about 50% patients, and recurrence is less common than after physical removal, e.g. with liquid nitrogen.

Inosine pranobex is reported to stimulate the host immune response to virus infection and has been used for mucocutaneous herpes simplex and genital warts. It is administered by mouth and metabolised to uric acid, so should be used with caution in patients with hyperuricaemia or gout.

FUNGAL INFECTIONS

Widespread use of immunosuppressive chemotherapy and the emergence of AIDS have contributed to a rise in the incidence of opportunistic infection ranging from comparatively trivial cutaneous infections to systemic disease that demands prolonged treatment with potentially toxic agents.

SUPERFICIAL MYCOSES

DERMATOPHYTE INFECTIONS (RINGWORM, TINEA)

Longstanding remedies such as Compound Benzoic Acid Ointment (Whitfield's ointment) are still acceptable for mild infections, but a topical imidazole (clotrimazole, econazole, miconazole, sulconazole), which is also effective against candida, is now usually preferred. Tioconazole is effective topically for nail infections. When multiple areas are affected, especially if the scalp or nails are included, and when topical therapy fails, oral itraconazole or terbinafine are used.

CANDIDA INFECTIONS

Cutaneous infection is generally treated with topical amphotericin, clotrimazole, econazole, miconazole or nystatin. Local hygiene is also important. An underlying explanation should be sought when a patient fails to respond to these measures, e.g. diabetes, the use of a broad-spectrum antibiotic or of immunosuppressive drugs.

Candidiasis of the alimentary tract mucosa responds to amphotericin, fluconazole, ketoconazole, miconazole or nystatin as lozenges (to suck, for oral infection), gel (held in the mouth before swallowing), suspension or tablets.

Vaginal candidiasis is treated by clotrimazole, econazole, isoconazole, ketoconazole, miconazole or nystatin as pessaries or vaginal tablets or cream inserted once or twice a day with cream or ointment on surrounding skin. Failure may be due to a concurrent intestinal infection causing re-infection, and nystatin tablets may be given by mouth 8-hourly with the local treatment. Alternatively, oral fluconazole may be used, now available without prescription ('over the counter') in the UK. The male sexual partner may use a similar antifungal ointment for his benefit and for the patient's (reinfection).

Fluconazole is often given orally or i.v. to heavily immunocompromised patients, e.g. during periods of profound granulocytopenia, and to severely ill patients on intensive care units to reduce the incidence of systemic candidiasis. *Candida albicans* is rarely (1% of clinical isolates) resistant to fluconazole, but other *Candida* species may be, more commonly in hospitals where prophylactic fluconazole use is extensive.

Isolation of candida from the bloodstream or intravenous catheter tips of patients with predisposing factors for systemic candidasis, e.g. prolonged intravenous access, neutropenia, is associated with a significant risk of serious sequelae, e.g. retinal or renal deposits, and should be treated with oral fluconazole for at least 3 weeks.

SYSTEMIC MYCOSES

The principal treatment options are summarised in Table 14.2.

Table 14.2 Drugs of choice for some fungal infections

Infection	Drug of first choice	Alternative
Aspergillosis	amphotericin or voriconazole	caspofungin or itraconazole
Blastomycosis[a]	itraconazole or amphotericin	fluconazole
Candidiasis		
mucosal	fluconazole or amphotericin	caspofungin, voriconazole or fluconazole
systemic	fluconazole or amphotericin ± flucytosine	
Coccidioidomycosis[a]	fluconazole, amphotericin or itraconazole	
Cryptococcosis	amphotericin + flucytosine (followed by fluconazole)	fluconazole
chronic suppression	fluconazole or itraconazole	amphotericin (weekly)
Fusariosis	amphotericin or voriconazole	
Histoplasmosis	itraconazole or amphotericin	fluconazole
chronic suppression[b]	itraconazole	amphotericin
Mucormycosis	amphotericin	posaconazole
Paracoccidioidomycosis	itraconazole or amphotericin	ketoconazole[c]
Pseudallescheriasis	voriconazole, ketoconazole or itraconazole	
Sporotrichosis		
cutaneous	itraconazole	potassium iodide
deep	amphotericin	itraconazole or fluconazole
Tinea pedis	terbinafine cream or topical azole (miconazole, clotrimazole, econazole)	fluconazole

[a]Patients with severe illness, meningitis, AIDS or some other causes of immunosuppression should receive amphotericin.
[b]For patients with AIDS.
[c]Continue treatment for 6–12 months.
This table was drawn substantially from The Medical Letter on Drugs and Therapeutics (2005, USA).
The authors are grateful to the Chairman of the Editorial Board for permission to publish the material.

Pneumocystosis, caused by *Pneumocystis carinii*, is an important cause of potentially fatal pneumonia in the immunosuppressed, especially HIV-positive patients. It is treated with co-trimoxazole in high dose: 120 mg/kg daily in two to four divided doses for 14 days by mouth or i.v. infusion; monitoring of plasma concentrations is recommended. Although co-trimoxazole resistance has not yet been reported, patients who fail to respond or are intolerant may benefit from pentamidine or primaquine plus clindamycin. Other options include atovaquone and trimetrexate (given with calcium folinate). Co-trimoxazole, dapsone (alone or with pyrimethamine) or atovaquone by mouth, or intermittent inhaled pentamidine, are used for primary and secondary prophylaxis in patients with AIDS.

Classification of antifungal agents
- Drugs that disrupt the fungal cell membrane:
  - *polyenes*, e.g. amphotericin
  - *azoles*: imidazoles, e.g. ketoconazole, triazoles, e.g. fluconazole
  - *allylamine*: terbinafine.
- Drugs that inhibit mitosis: griseofulvin.
- Drugs that inhibit DNA synthesis: flucytosine.

DRUGS THAT DISRUPT THE FUNGAL CELL MEMBRANE

POLYENE ANTIBIOTICS

These act by binding tightly to sterols present in cell membranes. The resulting deformity of the membrane allows leakage of intracellular ions and enzymes, causing cell death. Those polyenes that have useful antifungal activity bind selectively to *ergosterol*, the most important sterol in fungal (but not mammalian) cell walls.

Amphotericin (amphotericin B)

Amphotericin is absorbed negligibly from the gut and must be given by i.v. infusion for systemic infection; about 10% remains in the blood and the fate of the remainder is not known but is probably bound to tissues. The $t_{1/2}$ is 15 days and, after stopping treatment, drug persists in the body for several weeks.

Amphotericin is at present the drug of choice for most systemic fungal infections (but see Table 14.2). The diagnosis of systemic infection should, when-

ever possible, be firmly established; tissue biopsy and culture may be necessary, and methods using the PCR to detect aspergillus DNA may revolutionise management of invasive infection.

A conventional course of treatment for filamentous fungal infection lasts 6–12 weeks, during which at least 2 g amphotericin is given (usually 1 mg/kg daily, and up to 10 mg/kg daily of lipid-associated formulations for the most severe, invasive infections), but lower total and daily doses (e.g. 0.6 mg/kg daily) are used for candida infections, with correspondingly better tolerance. Antifungal drugs may be combined with immune-stimulating agents, e.g. granulocyte colony-stimulating factor, and clinical response in neutropenic episodes is closely related to return of normal neutrophil counts.

Lipid-associated formulations of amphotericin offer the prospect of reduced risk of toxicity while retaining therapeutic efficacy. In an aqueous medium, a lipid with hydrophilic and hydrophobic properties will form vesicles (liposomes) comprising an outer lipid bilayer surrounding an aqueous centre. The AmBisome formulation incorporates amphotericin in a lipid bilayer (55–75 nm diameter) from which the drug is released. Other lipid-associated complexes include Abelcet ('amphotericin B lipid complex') and Amphocil ('amphotericin B colloidal dispersion'). AmBisome may be more effective for some indications because higher doses (3 mg/kg daily) may be given rapidly and safely. It is the first choice when renal function is impaired. Treatment often begins with the conventional formulation in those with normal kidneys, resorting to AmBisome if the patient's renal function deteriorates.

Adverse reactions. Gradual escalation of the dose limits toxic effects, which may be deemed justifiable in life-threatening infection if conventional amphotericin is used. A strategy of continuous i.v. infusion appears to combine therapeutic efficacy with tolerability. Renal impairment is invariable, although reduced by adequate hydration; nephrotoxicity is reversible, at least in its early stages. Hypokalaemia (due to distal renal tubular acidosis) may necessitate replacement therapy. Other adverse effects include anorexia, nausea, vomiting, malaise, abdominal, muscle and joint pains, loss of weight, anaemia, hypomagnesaemia and fever. Aspirin, an antihistamine (H_1-receptor) or an antiemetic may alleviate symptoms. Severe febrile reactions are mitigated by hydrocortisone 25–50 mg before each infusion. Lipid-formulated preparations are associated with adverse reactions much less often, but fever, chills, nausea, vomiting, nephrotoxicity, electrolyte disturbance and occasional nephrotoxicity and hepatotoxicity are reported.

Nystatin

(named after New York State Health Laboratory)

Nystatin is too toxic for systemic use. It is not absorbed from the alimentary canal and is used to prevent or treat superficial candidiasis of the mouth, oesophagus or intestinal tract (as suspension, tablets or pastilles), for vaginal candidiasis (pessaries) and cutaneous infection (cream, ointment or powder).

AZOLES

The antibacterial, antiprotozoal and anthelminthic members of this group are described in the appropriate sections. Antifungal azoles comprise the following:

- *Imidazoles* (ketoconazole, miconazole, fenticonazole, clotrimazole, isoconazole, tioconazole) interfere with fungal oxidative enzymes to cause lethal accumulation of *hydrogen peroxide*; they also reduce the formation of *ergosterol*, an important constituent of the fungal cell wall which thus becomes permeable to intracellular constituents. Lack of selectivity in these actions results in important adverse effects.
- *Triazoles* (fluconazole, itraconazole, voriconazole, posaconazole) damage the fungal cell membrane by inhibiting *lanosterol 14-α-demethylase*, an enzyme crucial to ergosterol synthesis, resulting in accumulation of toxic sterol precursors. Triazoles have greater selectivity against fungi, better penetration of the CNS, resistance to degradation and cause less endocrine disturbance than do the imidazoles.

Ketoconazole

Ketoconazole is well absorbed from the gut (poorly where there is gastric hypoacidity; see below); it is widely distributed in tissues but concentrations in CSF and urine are low; its action is terminated by metabolism by cytochrome P450 3A ($t_{1/2}$ 8 h). For systemic mycoses, ketoconazole (see Table 14.2) has been superseded by fluconazole and itraconazole on grounds of improved pharmacokinetics, tolerability and efficacy. Impairment of steroid synthesis by ketoconazole has been put to other uses, e.g. inhibition of testosterone synthesis lessens bone pain in patients with advanced androgen-dependent prostatic cancer.

Adverse reactions include nausea, giddiness, headache, pruritus and photophobia. Impairment of testosterone synthesis may cause gynaecomastia and decreased libido in men. Of particular concern is impairment of liver function, ranging from a transient increase in levels of hepatic transaminases and alkaline phosphatase to severe injury and death.

Interactions. Drugs that lower gastric acidity, e.g. antacids, histamine H_2-receptor antagonists, impair the absorption of ketoconazole from the gastrointestinal tract. Like all imidazoles, ketoconazole binds strongly to several cytochrome P450 isoenzymes, inhibiting their action and thereby increasing effects of oral anticoagulants, phenytoin and ciclosporin, and increasing the risk of cardiac arrhythmias with terfenadine. A disulfiram-like reaction occurs with alcohol. Concurrent use of rifampicin, by enzyme induction of CYP 3A, markedly reduces the plasma concentration of ketoconazole.

Other azole drugs. *Miconazole* is an alternative. *Clotrimazole* is an effective topical agent for dermatophyte, yeast and other fungal infections (intertrigo, athlete's foot, ringworm, pityriasis versicolor, fungal nappy rash). *Econazole* and *sulconazole* are similar. *Tioconazole* is used for fungal nail infections, and *isoconazole* and *fenticonazole* for vaginal candidiasis.

Fluconazole

Fluconazole is absorbed from the gastrointestinal tract and is excreted largely unchanged by the kidney ($t_{1/2}$ 30 h). It is effective by mouth for oropharyngeal and oesophageal candidiasis, and i.v. for systemic candidiasis and cryptococcosis (including cryptococcal meningitis; it penetrates the CSF well). It is used prophylactically in a variety of conditions predisposing to systemic candida infections, including at times of profound neutropenia after bone marrow transplantation, and in patients in intensive care units who have intravenous lines in situ, are receiving antibiotic therapy and have undergone bowel surgery. It may cause gastrointestinal discomfort, headaches, reversible alopecia, increased levels of liver enzymes and allergic rash, but is generally well tolerated. Animal studies demonstrate embryotoxicity, and fluconazole ought not to be given to pregnant women. High doses increase the effects of phenytoin, ciclosporin, zidovudine and warfarin.

Itraconazole

Itraconazole is available for oral and i.v. administration ($t_{1/2}$ 25 h, increasing to 40 h with continuous treatment). Absorption from the gut is about 55%, but variable. It is improved by ingestion with food, but decreased by fatty meals and therapies that reduce gastric acidity, and is often reduced in patients with AIDS; plasma concentrations should be monitored during prolonged use for critical indications. The oral suspension formulation is much less affected by gastric hypoacidity. Itraconazole is heavily protein bound and virtually none is found within the CSF. It is almost completely oxidised in the liver (by CYP 3A) and excreted in the bile; little unchanged drug enters the urine.

Itraconazole is used for a variety of superficial mycoses, as a prophylactic agent for aspergillosis and candidiasis in the immunocompromised, and i.v. for treatment of histoplasmosis. It is licensed in the UK as a second-line agent for *Candida*, *Aspergillus* and *Cryptococcus* infections, and it may be convenient as 'follow on' therapy after systemic aspergillosis has been brought under control by an amphotericin preparation. It appears to be an effective adjunct treatment for allergic bronchopulmonary aspergillosis.

Adverse effects are uncommon, but include transient hepatitis and hypokalaemia. Prolonged use may lead to cardiac failure, especially in those with pre-existing cardiac disease. Co-administration of a calcium channel blocker adds to the risk. Cyclodextrin (used as a vehicle for the i.v. formulation) accumulates and causes sodium overload in renally impaired patients, but the oral formulation avoids this problem.

Interactions. Enzyme induction of CYP 3A, e.g. by rifampicin, reduces the plasma concentration of itraconazole. Additionally, its affinity for several P450 isoforms, notably CYP 3A4, causes it to inhibit the oxidation of a number of drugs, including phenytoin, warfarin, ciclosporin, tacrolimus, midazolam, triazolam, cisapride and terfenidine (see above), increasing their intensity and/or duration of effect.

Voriconazole

Voriconazole ($t_{1/2}$ 7 h) is more active in vitro than itraconazole against *Aspergillus* because of more avid binding of the sterol synthetic enzymes of filamentous fungi; it also appears to have synergistic activity against *Aspergillus* in combination with amphotericin. It is as active as the other triazoles against yeasts and is more reliably and rapidly absorbed than itraconazole by mouth, but cross-resistance between these agents is usual. It is more effective than conventional amphotericin in invasive aspergillosis, and probably equivalent to lipid-associated formulations. Oral absorption is not significantly reduced by gastric hypoacidity. CSF and brain tissue concentrations are at least 50% of those in the plasma, and are sufficient for effective therapy of fungal infections of the eye and CNS.

Adverse effects. Administration i.v. gives rise rapidly to transient visual disturbance in 30% of patients (blurring, alerted visual perception such as reversal of light and dark, visual hallucinations and photophobia). These often resolve after the first week of therapy, and almost all of those affected are able to continue with the course of treatment.

Accumulation of the cyclodextrin vehicle (see above) may cause sodium retention in renally impaired patients with i.v. use. Patients with hepatic cirrhosis should receive a standard loading, but only half of the daily maintenance dose. Transiently raised liver enzyme levels are seen in up to 20% patients, but serious liver impairment is rare. Rashes and photosensitivity appear to be more common than with the other triazoles.

Extensive metabolism of voriconazole by the cytochrome P450 system (predominantly CYP 2C19) may lead to unwanted interaction with in patients receiving, e.g. rifampicin, ciclosporin or tacrolimus.

Posaconazole

Posaconazole ($t_{1/2}$ 20 h) is structurally related to itraconazole and has similar in vitro antifungal activity to voriconazole. It is fungistatic against *Candida* spp. but fungicidal against *Aspergillus* spp., and is also active against a range of other filamentous fungi. Absorption is less reliable by mouth but is increased by food, especially a fatty meal. More than 75% of a dose is excreted in the faeces.

Adverse effects are uncommon, but include gastrointestinal disturbance, dizziness and fatigue, neutropenia (7% patients) and transient disturbance of liver function. Dose adjustment is not required for renal or hepatic impairment.

ECHINOCANDINS

The echinocandins are large lipopeptide molecules that inhibit synthesis of β-(1,3)-D-glucan, a vital component of the cell walls of many fungi (excepting *Cryptococcus neoformans*, against which they have no useful activity). In vitro and in vivo, the echinocandins are rapidly fungicidal against most *Candida* spp. and fungistatic against *Aspergillus* spp.

Caspofungin ($t_{1/2}$ 10 h) is the first member of this group. It is licensed for i.v. treatment of invasive candidiasis, suspected fungal infections in febrile granulocytopenic patients, and *Aspergillus* infections in patients who have not responded to amphotericin or itraconazole. Caspofungin retains activity against most triazole- and polyene-resistant yeasts, and is also active against *Pneumocystis carinii*. It is widely distributed through body tissues and highly protein bound. It penetrates to the CSF poorly, but clinical responses in fungal CNS infection have been reported.

Caspofungin is generally well tolerated, but headache, fever, raised liver function tests and hypokalaemia occur. Patients with significant liver impairment should receive a reduced dose.

ALLYLAMINE

Terbinafine

Terbinafine interferes with *ergosterol* biosynthesis, and thereby with the formation of the fungal cell membrane. It is absorbed from the gastrointestinal tract and undergoes extensive metabolism in the liver ($t_{1/2}$ 14 h). Terbinafine is used topically for dermatophyte infections of the skin and orally for infections of hair and nails where the site, e.g. hair, severity or extent of the infection renders topical use inappropriate (see p. 277). Treatment may need to continue for several weeks. Terbinafine may cause nausea, diarrhoea, dyspepsia, abdominal pain, headaches and cutaneous reactions.

OTHER ANTIFUNGAL DRUGS

Griseofulvin

Griseofulvin prevents fungal growth by inhibiting mitosis. The therapeutic efficacy of griseofulvin depends on its capacity to bind to *keratin* as it is being formed in the cells of the nail bed, hair follicles and skin, for dermatophytes specifically infect keratinous tissues. Griseofulvin does not kill fungus already established; it merely prevents infection of new keratin so that the duration of treatment is governed by the time that it takes for infected keratin to be shed. On average, hair and skin infection should be treated for 4–6 weeks, although toenails may need a year or more. Treatment must continue for a few weeks after both visual and microscopic evidence has disappeared. Fat in a meal enhances absorption of griseofulvin; it is metabolised in the liver and induces hepatic enzymes ($t_{1/2}$ 15 h).

Griseofulvin is effective against all superficial ringworm (dermatophyte) infections, but ineffective against pityriasis versicolor, superficial candidiasis and all systemic mycoses.

Adverse reactions include gastrointestinal upset, rashes, photosensitivity, headache and various CNS disturbances.

Flucytosine

Flucytosine (5-fluorocytosine) is metabolised in the fungal cell to 5-fluorouracil, which inhibits nucleic acid synthesis. It is well absorbed from the gut, penetrates effectively into tissues, and almost all is excreted unchanged in the urine ($t_{1/2}$ 4 h). The dose should be reduced for patients with impaired renal function, and the plasma concentration monitored. The drug is well tolerated when renal function is normal. *Candida albicans* rapidly becomes resistant to flucytosine, which ought not to be used alone; it may be combined with amphotericin (see Table 14.2), but this increases the risk of adverse effects (leucopenia, thrombocytopenia, enterocolitis) and is reserved for serious infections where the risk:benefit balance is favourable, e.g. *Cryptococcus neoformans* meningitis.

PROTOZOAL INFECTIONS

MALARIA

Over 90 million cases of malaria occur each year (although recent estimates have been as high as 500 million) and these result in more than 1 million deaths, mainly in sub-Saharan African children.

In terms of socio-economic impact, malaria is the most important of the transmissible parasitic diseases.

Quinine as cinchona bark was introduced into Europe from South America in 1633. It was used for all fevers, amongst them malaria, the occurrence of which was associated with damp places with bad air ('mal aria').

LIFE CYCLE OF THE MALARIA PARASITE AND SITES OF DRUG ACTION

The incubation period of malaria is 10–35 days. The principal features of the life cycle (Fig. 14.1) of the malaria parasite must be known in order to understand its therapy.

Female anopheles mosquitoes require a blood meal for egg production, and in the process of feeding they inject salivary fluid containing *sporozoites* into humans. As no drugs are effective against sporozoites, infection with the malaria parasite cannot be prevented.

Hepatic cycle (site 1 in Fig. 14.1)

Sporozoites enter liver cells where they develop into *schizonts*, which form large numbers of *merozoites* which, after 5–16 days, but sometimes after months or years, are released into the circulation. *Plasmodium falciparum* differs in that it has no persistent hepatic cycle.

Primaquine, proguanil and tetracyclines (*tissue schizontocides*) act at this site and are used for:

- *Radical cure*, i.e. an attack on persisting hepatic forms (*hypnozoites*, i.e. sleeping) once the parasite has been cleared from the blood; this is most effectively accomplished with primaquine; proguanil is only weakly effective.
- *Preventing the initial hepatic cycle*. This is also called *causal prophylaxis*. Primaquine was long regarded as too toxic for prolonged use but evidence now suggests it may be used safely, and it is inexpensive; proguanil is weakly effective. Doxycycline may be used short term.

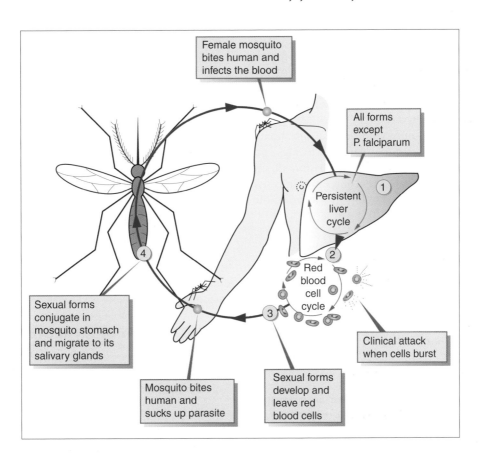

Fig. 14.1 Life cycle of the malaria parasite. The numbers are referred to in the text.

Vaccine development against both falciparum and vivax malaria concentrates mostly on antigens involved in the pre-erythrocytic stages, before invasion of liver cells (stage 1).

Erythrocyte cycle (site 2 in Fig. 14.1)

Merozoites enter red cells, where they develop into *schizonts*, which form more merozoites that are released when the cells burst, giving rise to the features of the clinical attack. The merozoites re-enter red cells and the cycle is repeated.

Chloroquine, quinine, mefloquine, halofantrine, proguanil, pyrimethamine and tetracyclines (blood schizontocides) kill these asexual forms. Drugs that act at this stage in the cycle of the parasite may be used for:

- *Treatment* of acute attacks of malaria.
- *Prevention* of attacks by early destruction of the erythrocytic forms. This is called *suppressive prophylaxis* as it does not cure the hepatic cycle (above).

Sexual forms (site 3 in Fig. 14.1)

Some merozoites differentiate into male and female gametocytes in the erythrocytes and can develop further only if they are ingested by a mosquito where they form *sporozoites* (site 4 in Fig. 14.1) and complete the transmission cycle.

Quinine, mefloquine, chloroquine, artesunate, artemether and primaquine (gametocytocides) act on sexual forms and prevent transmission of the infection because the patient becomes non-infective and the parasite fails to develop in the mosquito (site 4).

In summary, drugs may be selected for:

- treatment of clinical attacks
- prevention of clinical attacks
- radical cure.

Drugs used for malaria, and their principal actions, are classified in Table 14.3.

DRUG-RESISTANT MALARIA

Drug-resistant parasites constitute a persistent problem. *Plasmodium falciparum* is now resistant to chloroquine in many parts of the world and the picture changes monthly. Areas of high risk for resistant parasites include sub-Saharan Africa, Latin America, Oceania (Papua New Guinea,

Table 14.3 Antimalarial drugs and their sites of action

Drug	Biological activity	
	Blood schizontocide	Tissue schizontocide
4-Aminoquinolone		
chloroquine	++	0
Arylaminoalcohols		
quinine	++	0
mefloquine	++	0
Phenanthrene methanol		
halofantrine	++	0
lumefantrine	++	0
Antimetabolites		
proguanil	+	+
pyrimethamine	+	0
sulfadoxine	+	0
dapsone	+	0
Antibiotics		
tetracycline	+	+
doxycycline	+	+
minocycline	+	+
8-Aminoquinolone		
primaquine	0	+
Sesquiterpenes		
artesunate	+	0
artemether	+	0

Solomon Islands, Vanuatu) and some parts of South-East Asia. Chloroquine-resistant *Plasmodium vivax* is also reported. Any physician who is unfamiliar with the resistance pattern in the locality from which patients have come, or to which they are going, is well advised to check the current position. Because prevalence and resistance rates are so variable, advice on therapy and prophylaxis in this section is given for general guidance only and readers are referred to specialist sources for up-to-date information.

CHEMOTHERAPY OF AN ACUTE ATTACK OF MALARIA[3]

Successful management demands attention to the following points of principle:

---

[3]Treatment regimens vary in detail; those quoted here accord with the recommendations in the *British National Formulary* 2005; the BNF is a good source of contact numbers, addresses and websites to obtain expert advice on therapy and prophylaxis of malaria.

- Whenever possible, the diagnosis should be confirmed before treatment by examination of blood smears; this is not often possible in the developing world, where clinically diagnosed illnesses may receive unnecessary courses of antimalarials, thus increasing the risks of plasmodial resistance.
- When the infecting organism is not known or infection is mixed, treatment should begin as for *Plasmodium falciparum* (below).
- Drugs used to treat *Plasmodium falciparum* malaria must always be selected with regard to the prevalence of local patterns of drug resistance.
- Patients not at risk of reinfection should be re-examined several weeks after treatment for signs of recrudescence, which may result from inadequate chemotherapy or survival of persistent hepatic forms.

Falciparum ('malignant') malaria

Falciparum malaria in the non-immune is a medical emergency, and malaria of unknown infecting species should be treated as though it were falciparum. The regimen depends on the condition of the patient; the doses quoted are for adults. Chloroquine resistance is now usual. The optimal use of the newly available antimalarial drugs alone and in combination is yet to be established.

If the patient can swallow and there are no serious complications such as impairment of consciousness, treatment options are as follows:

- A quinine salt:[4] 600 mg 8-hourly by mouth for 5–7 days, followed by doxycycline 200 mg daily for at least 7 days. This additional therapy is necessary as quinine alone tends to be associated with a higher rate of relapse. Alternatively, clindamycin 300 mg may be given four times daily for 5 days or, if the parasite is likely to be sensitive, Fansidar (pyrimethamine plus sulfadoxine) 3 tablets as a single dose.
- Malarone (atovaquone and proguanil hydrochloride): 4 tablets once-daily for 3 days.
- Riamet (artemether plus lumefantrine): 4 tablets initially, followed by five further doses of 4 tablets given at 8, 24, 36, 48 and 60 h.

- Mefloquine is also effective, but resistance has been reported in several regions, including South-East Asia. It is not necessary to use follow-on therapy after Riamet, mefloquine or Malarone.

Seriously ill patients should be treated with:

- A quinine salt:[4] 20 mg/kg as a loading dose[5] (maximum 1.4 g) infused i.v. over 4 h, followed 8 h later by a maintenance infusion of 10 mg/kg (maximum 700 mg) infused over 4 h, repeated every 8 h[6] until the patient can swallow tablets to complete the 7-day course.
- Fansidar or doxycycline should be given subsequently, as above (mefloquine is an alternative, but this must begin at least 12 h after parenteral quinine has ceased).

Treatment in pregnancy should always be based on expert advice.

Non-falciparum ('benign') malarias

These are usually due to *Plasmodium vivax* or less commonly to *Plasmodium ovale* or *Plasmodium malariae*.

The drug of choice is *chloroquine*, which should be given by mouth as follows:

- Initial dose: 600 mg (base),[7] then 300 mg as a single dose 6–8 h later.
- Second day: 300 mg as a single dose.
- Third day: 300 mg as a single dose.

The total dose of chloroquine base over 3 days should be approximately 25 mg/kg base. This is sufficient for *Plasmodium malariae* infection, but for *Plasmodium vivax* and *Plasmodium ovale* eradication of the hepatic parasites is necessary to prevent relapse, by giving:

---

[5]The loading dose should not be given if the patient has received quinine, quinidine or mefloquine in the previous 24 h; see also warnings about halofantrine (below).
[6]Reduced to 5–7 mg/kg if the infusion lasts for more than 72 h.
[7]The active component of many drugs, whether acid or base, is relatively insoluble and may present a problem in formulation. This is overcome by adding an acid to a base or vice versa; the weight of the salt differs according to the acid or base component, i.e. chloroquine base 150 mg = chloroquine sulfate 200 mg = chloroquine phosphate 250 mg (approximately). Where there may be variation, therefore, the amount of drug prescribed is expressed as the weight of the active component, in the case of chloroquine, the base.

---

[4]Acceptable as quinine hydrochloride, dihydrochloride or sulfate, but not quinine bisulfate, which contains less quinine.

■ Primaquine, 15 mg/day for 14 days started after the chloroquine course has been completed (30 mg once-weekly for 8 weeks will suffice without undue risk of haemolysis). *Plasmodium vivax* infections require 30 mg/day for 14 days.

CHEMOPROPHYLAXIS OF MALARIA

Geographically variable plasmodial drug resistance has become a major factor. The World Health Organization gives advice in its annually revised booklet, *Vaccination Certificate Requirements and Health Advice for International Travel*, and national bodies publish recommendations, e.g. *British National Formulary*, that apply particularly to their own residents.

General principles

■ Chemoprophylaxis aims to prevent deaths from falciparum malaria, but only ever gives relative protection; travellers should guard against bites by using mosquito nets and repellents, and wearing well-covering clothing especially during high-risk times of day (after dusk).

■ Mefloquine, chloroquine, proguanil and Maloprim (pyrimethamine plus dapsone), alone or in combination, are most commonly advised for prophylaxis regimens, and doxycycline for special cases (drug resistance or intolerance); primaquine is being re-evaluated.

■ Effective chemoprophylaxis requires that there be a plasmodicidal concentration of drug in the blood when the first infected mosquito bites, and that it be sustained safely for long periods.

■ The progressive rise in plasma concentration to *steady state* (after $t_{1/2} \times 5$), sometimes attained only after weeks (consider mefloquine $t_{1/2}$ 21 days, chloroquine $t_{1/2}$ 50 days), allows that unwanted effects (which can impair compliance or be unsafe) may occur after a subject has entered a malarial area. Thus, it is advised that prophylaxis begin long enough before travel to reveal acute intolerance and to impress on the subject the importance of compliance (to relate drug-taking to a specific daily or weekly event).

■ Prompt achievement of efficacy and safety, i.e. *plasmodicidal concentrations*, by one (or two) doses is plainly important for travellers who cannot wait on dosage schedules to deliver both only when steady-state blood

concentrations are attained; the schedules must reflect this need.

■ Prophylaxis should continue for at least 4 weeks after leaving an endemic area to kill parasites that are acquired about the time of departure, are still incubating in the liver and will develop into the erythrocyte phase. The traveller should be aware that any illness occurring within a year, and especially within 3 months, of return may be malaria.

■ Chloroquine and proguanil may be used for periods of up to 5 years, and mefloquine for up to 1–2 years; expert advice should be taken by long-term travellers, especially those going to areas for which other prophylactic drugs are recommended.

■ *Naturally acquired immunity* offers the most reliable protection for people living permanently in endemic areas (below). Repeated attacks of malaria confer partial immunity and the disease often becomes no more than an occasional inconvenience. Vaccines to confer active immunity are under development.

■ As a rule, the *partially immune* should not take a prophylactic. The reasoning is that immunity is sustained by the red cell cycle, loss of which through prophylaxis diminishes their resistance and leaves them highly vulnerable to the disease. There are, however, exceptions to this general advice, and the partially immune may or should use a prophylactic:

 – if it is virtually certain that they will never abandon its use
 – if they go to another malarial area where the strains of parasite may differ
 – during the last few months of pregnancy in areas where *Plasmodium falciparum* is prevalent (to avert the risk of miscarriage).

Examples of standard prophylactic regimens

■ Chloroquine: 300 mg (base) once weekly (start 1 week before travel).
■ Proguanil: 200 mg once-daily (start 1 week before travel).
■ Chloroquine plus proguanil in the above doses.
■ Malarone: 1 tablet daily (start 1–2 days before travel).
■ Mefloquine: 250 mg once-weekly (start 1 week, preferably 2–3 weeks, before travel).
■ Doxycycline: 100 mg once-daily (start 1 week before travel).

For 'last minute' travellers. The standard regimens normally provide immediate protection but for special assurance a priming/loading dose may be considered, e.g. the standard prophylactic dose daily for 2–3 days (this has been suggested for mefloquine).

Drug interactions. Where subjects are already taking other drugs, e.g. antiepileptics, some cardiovascular drugs, it is desirable to start prophylaxis as much as 2–3 weeks in advance to establish safety.

Antimalarial drugs and pregnancy

Women living in endemic areas in which *Plasmodium falciparum* remains sensitive to chloroquine should take chloroquine prophylactically throughout pregnancy. Proguanil (an 'antifol', see below) may be taken for prophylaxis provided it is accompanied by folic acid 5 mg/day. Chloroquine may be used in full dose to treat chloroquine-sensitive infections. Quinine is the only widely available drug that is acceptable as suitable for treating chloroquine-resistant infections during pregnancy. Mefloquine is teratogenic in animals and a woman should avoid pregnancy whilst taking it, and for 3 months afterwards (although evidence is accruing that it may be safe for use in chloroquine-resistant areas). Maloprim (pyrimethamine plus dapsone) should not be given in the first trimester, but may be given in the second and third trimesters with a folate supplement. Doxycycline is contraindicated throughout pregnancy, and Malarone (proguanil plus atovaquone) should be avoided unless there is no suitable alternative.

INDIVIDUAL ANTIMALARIAL DRUGS

Chloroquine

Chloroquine ($t_{1/2}$ 50 days) is concentrated within parasitised red cells and forms complexes with plasmodial DNA. It is active against the blood forms and also the gametocytes (formed in the mosquito) of *Plasmodium vivax*, *Plasmodium ovale* and *Plasmodium malariae*; it is ineffective against many strains of *Plasmodium falciparum* and also its immature gametocytes. Chloroquine is readily absorbed from the gastrointestinal tract and is concentrated several-fold in various tissues, e.g. erythrocytes, liver, spleen, heart, kidney, cornea and retina; the long $t_{1/2}$ reflects slow release from these sites. A priming dose is used in order to achieve adequate free plasma concentration (see acute attack, above). Chloroquine is partly

inactivated by metabolism and the remainder is excreted unchanged in the urine.

Adverse effects are infrequent at doses normally used for malaria prophylaxis and treatment, but are more common with the higher or prolonged doses given for resistant malaria or for rheumatoid arthritis or lupus erythematosus (see p. 266).

Corneal deposits of chloroquine may be asymptomatic or may cause halos around lights or photophobia. These are not a threat to vision and reverse when the drug is stopped. Retinal toxicity is more serious, and may be irreversible. In the early stage it takes the form of visual field defects; late retinopathy classically gives the picture of macular pigmentation surrounded by a ring of pigment (the 'bull's-eye' macula). The functional defect can take the form of scotomas, photophobia, defective colour vision and decreased visual acuity resulting, in the extreme case, in blindness.

Other reactions include pruritus, which may be intolerable and is common in Africans, headaches, gastrointestinal disturbance, precipitation of acute intermittent porphyria in susceptible individuals, mental disturbances and interference with cardiac rhythm, the latter especially if the drug is given i.v. in high dose (it has a quinidine-like action). Long-term use is associated with reversible bleaching of the hair and pigmentation of the hard palate.

Acute overdose may be rapidly fatal without treatment, and indeed has even been described as a means of suicide.[8] (Chloroquine may now be bought from pharmacies in the UK without a prescription.) Pulmonary oedema is followed by convulsions, cardiac arrhythmias and coma; as little as 50 mg/kg can be fatal. These effects are principally due to the profound negative inotropic action of chloroquine. Diazepam was found fortuitously to protect the heart and adrenaline (epinephrine) reduces intraventricular conduction time; this combination of drugs, given by separate i.v. infusions, improves survival.

Halofantrine

Halofantrine ($t_{1/2}$ 2.5 days) is active against the erythrocytic forms of all four *Plasmodium* species, especially *Plasmodium falciparum* and *Plasmodium*

---

[8]Report 1993 Chloroquine poisoning. Lancet 307:49.

vivax, and at the schizont stage. Its mechanism of action is not fully understood. Absorption of halofantrine from the gastrointestinal tract is variable, incomplete and substantially increased (6–10-fold) by taking the drug with food (see below). It is metabolised to an active metabolite and no unchanged drug is recovered in the urine. Halofantrine is used for the treatment of uncomplicated chloroquine-resistant *Plasmodium falciparum* and *Plasmodium vivax malaria*. It should not be given for prophylaxis.

Adverse effects. Halofantrine may cause gastrointestinal symptoms; pruritus occurs but to a lesser extent than with chloroquine, which may be reason to prefer it. It prolongs the cardiac QTc interval and may predispose to hazardous arrhythmia. The drug should *not be taken*:

- with food
- with other potentially arrhythmic drugs, e.g. antimalarials, tricyclic antidepressants, antipsychotics, astemizole, terfenadine
- with drugs causing electrolyte disturbance
- by patients with cardiac disease associated with prolonged QTc interval.

Mefloquine

Mefloquine ($t_{1/2}$ 21 days) is similar in several respects to quinine although it does not intercalate with plasmodial DNA. It is used for malaria chemoprophylaxis, and occasionally to treat uncomplicated *Plasmodium falciparum* (both chloroquine sensitive and chloroquine resistant) and chloroquine-resistant *Plasmodium vivax* malaria. Mefloquine is rapidly absorbed from the gastrointestinal tract and its action is terminated by metabolism. When used for prophylaxis, 250 mg (base)/week should be taken, commencing 1–3 weeks before entering and continued for 4 weeks after leaving a malarious area. It should not be given to patients with hepatic or renal impairment.

Adverse effects include nausea, dizziness, disturbance of balance, vomiting, abdominal pain, diarrhoea and loss of appetite. More rarely, hallucinations, seizures and psychoses occur. Mefloquine should be avoided in patients taking β-adrenoceptor and calcium channel antagonists, because it causes sinus bradycardia; quinine can potentiate these and other dose-related effects of mefloquine.

Neuropsychiatric events, including seizures and psychoses, occur after high-dose therapy in about 1 in 10 000 of those using the drug for prophylaxis. Less severe reactions including headache, dizziness, depression and insomnia have been reported but there is uncertainty as to whether these can be ascribed to mefloquine. The drug should not be used in travellers with a history of neuropsychiatric disease including convulsions and depression, and in those whose activities require fine coordination or spatial performance, e.g. airline flight-deck crews.

Primaquine

Primaquine ($t_{1/2}$ 6 h) acts at several stages in the development of the plasmodial parasite, possibly by interfering with its mitochondrial function. Its unique effect is to eliminate the hepatic forms of *Plasmodium vivax* and *Plasmodium ovale* after standard chloroquine therapy, but only when the risk of re-infection is absent or slight. Primaquine is well absorbed from the gastrointestinal tract, is only moderately concentrated in the tissues and is rapidly metabolised.

Adverse effects include anorexia, nausea, abdominal cramps, methaemoglobinaemia and haemolytic anaemia, especially in patients with genetic deficiency of erythrocyte glucose-6-phosphate dehydrogenase (G6PD). Subjects should be tested for G6PD and, in those who are deficient, the risk of haemolytic anaemia is greatly reduced by giving primaquine in reduced dose.

Proguanil (chloroguanide)

Proguanil ($t_{1/2}$ 17 h) inhibits dihydrofolate reductase, which converts folic to folinic acid, deficiency of which inhibits plasmodial cell division. Plasmodia, like most bacteria but unlike humans, cannot make use of preformed folic acid. Pyrimethamine and trimethoprim, which share this mode of action, are collectively known as the 'antifols'. Their plasmodicidal action is markedly enhanced by combination with sulphonamides or sulphones because there is inhibition of sequential steps in folate synthesis. It is used alone (usually with chloroquine) for malaria prophylaxis, and is also available with atovaquone (as Malarone: proguanil hydrochloride 100 mg plus atovaquone 250 mg) for prophylaxis and treatment.

Proguanil is moderately well absorbed from the gut and is excreted in the urine either unchanged or as an active metabolite. Being little stored in the tissues, proguanil must be used daily when given for prophylaxis, which is its main use, particularly in pregnant women (with folic acid 5 mg/day, which does not antagonise therapeutic efficacy) and non-immune individuals.

Adverse effects. In prophylactic doses proguanil is well tolerated. Mouth ulcers and stomatitis have been reported. The drug should be avoided or used in reduced dose for patients with impaired renal function.

Pyrimethamine

Pyrimethamine ($t_{1/2}$ 4 days) inhibits plasmodial dihydrofolate reductase, for which it has a high affinity. It is well absorbed from the gastrointestinal tract and is extensively metabolised. It is seldom used alone (see below). Pregnant women should receive supplementary folic acid when taking pyrimethamine.

Adverse effects reported include anorexia, abdominal cramps, vomiting, ataxia, tremor, seizures and megaloblastic anaemia.

Pyrimethamine with sulfadoxine

Pyrimethamine acts synergistically with sulfadoxine (as Fansidar) to inhibit folic acid metabolism (see 'antifols', above); sulfadoxine is excreted in the urine. The combination is now used with quinine to treat acute attacks of malaria caused by susceptible strains of *Plasmodium falciparum*; a single dose of pyrimethamine 75 mg plus sulfadoxine 1.5 g (3 tablets) usually suffices.

Adverse effects. Any sulphonamide-induced allergic reactions can be severe, e.g. erythema multiforme, Stevens–Johnson syndrome and toxic epidermal necrolysis. Because of its 'antifol' action the combination should not be used by pregnant women unless they take a folate supplement.

Pyrimethamine with dapsone

Pyrimethamine is combined with dapsone (Maloprim) (see p. 107) for prophylaxis of *Plasmodium falciparum* malaria.

Quinine

Quinine ($t_{1/2}$ 9 h; 18 h in severe malaria) is obtained from the bark of the South American cinchona tree. It binds to plasmodial DNA to prevent protein synthesis but its exact mode of action remains uncertain. It is used to treat *Plasmodium falciparum* malaria in areas of multiple drug resistance. Apart from its antiplasmodial effect, quinine is used for myotonia and muscle cramps because it prolongs the muscle refractory period. Quinine is included in dilute concentration in tonics and aperitifs for its desired bitter taste.

Quinine is well absorbed from the gastrointestinal tract and is almost completely metabolised in the liver.

Adverse effects include tinnitus, diminished auditory acuity, headache, blurred vision, nausea and diarrhoea (common to quinine, quinidine, salicylates and called 'cinchonism'). Idiosyncratic reactions include pruritus, urticaria and rashes. Hypoglycaemia may be significant when quinine is given by i.v. infusion, and supplementary glucose may be required.

When large amounts are taken, e.g. (unreliably) to induce abortion or in attempted suicide, ocular disturbances, notably constriction of the visual fields, may occur and even complete blindness, the onset of which may be very sudden. Vomiting, abdominal pain and diarrhoea result from local irritation of the gastrointestinal tract. Quinidine-like effects include hypotension, disturbance of atrioventricular conduction and cardiac arrest. Activated charcoal should be given. Supportive measures are employed thereafter as no specific therapy has proven benefit.

Quinidine, the dextrorotatory isomer of quinine, has antimalarial activity, but is used mainly as a cardiac antiarrhythmic (see p. 450).

Artesunate and artemether are soluble derivatives of artemisinin, which is isolated from the leaves of the Chinese herb qinghao (*Artemisia annua*); they act against the blood, including sexual, forms of plasmodia and may also reduce transmissibility. Artesunate (i.v.) and artemether (i.m.) are rapidly effective in severe and multidrug-resistant malaria. They are well tolerated but should be used with caution in patients with chronic cardiac disorders as they prolong the PR and QTc interval in some experimental animals.

Riamet, a combination of artemether 20 mg and lumefantrine 120 mg, is licensed for acute uncomplicated falciparum malaria. Lumefantrine is structurally related to halofantrine and shares its enhanced absorption with food, but not its cardiotoxicity. The combination must be given in a complex 3-day regimen and may be inferior to artesunate plus mefloquine. Adverse effects are uncommon but irreversible hearing loss is reported.

AMOEBIASIS

Infection occurs when mature cysts are ingested and pass into the colon where they divide into trophozoites; these forms either enter the tissues or reform cysts. Amoebiasis occurs in two forms, both of which need treatment:

- *Bowel lumen amoebiasis* is asymptomatic, and trophozoites (noninfective) and cysts (infective) are passed into the faeces. Treatment is directed at eradicating cysts with a luminal amoebicide; *diloxanide furoate* is the drug of choice; *iodoquinol* or *paromomycin* are alternatives.
- *Tissue-invading amoebiasis* gives rise to dysentery, hepatic amoebiasis and liver abscess. A systemically active drug (tissue amoebicide) effective against trophozoites must be used, e.g. *metronidazole, tinidazole.* Parenteral forms of these are available for patients too ill to take drugs by mouth. In severe cases of amoebic dysentery, *tetracycline* lessens the risk of opportunistic infection, perforation and peritonitis when it is given in addition to the systemic amoebicide.

Treatment with tissue amoebicides should always be followed by a course of a luminal amoebicide to eradicate the source of the infection.

Dehydroemetine (from ipecacuanha), less toxic than the parent emetine, is claimed by some authorities to be the most effective tissue amoebicide. It is reserved for dangerously ill patients, but these are more likely to be vulnerable to its cardiotoxic effects. When dehydroemetine is used to treat amoebic liver abscess, chloroquine should also be given.

The drug treatment of other protozoal infections is summarised in Table 14.4.

NOTES ON DRUGS FOR PROTOZOAL INFECTIONS

Atovaquone is a quinone; it may cause gastrointestinal and mild neurological side-effects, and rare hepatotoxicity and blood dyscrasias.

Table 14.4 Drugs for some protozoal infections

Infection	Drug and comment
Giardiasis	Metronidazole, tinidazole or mepacrine
Leishmaniasis	
visceral	Sodium stibogluconate or meglumine antimoniate; resistant cases may benefit from combining antimonials with allopurinol, pentamidine, paromomycin or amphotericin (including AmBisome)
cutaneous	Mild lesions heal spontaneously, fluconazole; antimonials may be injected intralesionally
Toxoplasmosis	Most infections are self-limiting in the immunologically normal patient. Pyrimethamine with sulfadiazine for chorioretinitis, and active toxoplasmosis in immunodeficient patients; folinic acid is used to counteract the inevitable megaloblastic anaemia. Alternatives include pyrimethamine with clindamycin or clarithromycin or azithromycin or atovaquone. Spiramycin for primary toxoplasmosis in pregnant women. Expert advice is essential
Trichomoniasis	Metronidazole or tinidazole is effective
Trypanosomiasis	
African (sleeping sickness)	Suramin or pentamidine is effective during the early stages but not for the later neurological manifestations for which melarsoprol should be used. Eflornithine is effective for both early and late stages. Expert advice is recommended
American (Chagas' disease)	Prolonged (1–3 months) treatment with benznidazole or nifurtimox may be effective

Benznidazole is a nitroimidazole that may occasionally cause peripheral neuritis but is generally well tolerated, including by infants.

Dehydroemetine inhibits protein synthesis; it may cause pain at the site of injection, weakness and muscular pain, hypotension, precordial pain and cardiac arrhythmias.

Diloxanide furoate may cause troublesome flatulence, and pruritus and urticaria may occur.

Eflornithine inhibits protozoal DNA synthesis; it may cause anaemia, leucopenia and thrombocytopenia, and seizures.

Iodoquinol may cause abdominal cramps, nausea and diarrhoea. Skin eruptions, pruritus ani and thyroid gland enlargement have been attributed to its iodine content. The recognition of severe neurotoxicity with the related drug, clioquinol, in Japan in the 1960s, must give cause for caution in its use.

Meglumine antimonate is a pentavalent antimony compound, similar to sodium stibogluconate (below).

Melarsoprol, a trivalent organic arsenical, acts through its high affinity for sulphydryl groups of enzymes. Adverse effects include encephalopathy, myocardial damage, proteinuria and hypertension.

Mepacrine (quinacrine) was formerly used as an antimalarial but is now an alternative to metronidazole or tinidazole for giardiasis. It may cause gastrointestinal upset, occasional acute toxic psychosis, hepatitis and aplastic anaemia.

Nifurtimox is a nitrofuran derivative. Adverse effects include anorexia, nausea, vomiting, gastric pain, insomnia, headache, vertigo, excitability, myalgia, arthralgia and convulsions. Peripheral neuropathy may necessitate stopping treatment.

Paromomycin, an aminoglycoside, is not absorbed from the gut; it is similar to neomycin.

Pentamidine is a synthetic aromatic amidine; it must be administered parenterally or by inhalation as it is absorbed unreliably from the gastrointestinal tract; it does not enter the CSF. Given systemically it frequently causes nephrotoxicity, which is reversible; acute hypotension and syncope are common especially after rapid i.v. injection. Pancreatic damage may cause hypoglycaemia due to insulin release.

Sodium stibogluconate (Pentostam) is an organic pentavalent antimony compound; it may cause anorexia, vomiting, coughing and substernal pain. Used in mucocutaneous leishmaniasis, it may lead to severe inflammation around pharyngeal or tracheal lesions which may require control with corticosteroid. *Meglumine antimoniate* is similar.

Suramin forms stable complexes with plasma protein and is detectable in urine for up to 3 months after the last injection; it does not cross the blood–brain barrier. It may cause tiredness, anorexia, malaise, polyuria, thirst, and tenderness of the palms and soles.

HELMINTHIC INFECTIONS

Helminths have complex life cycles, special knowledge of which is required by those who treat infections. Table 14.5 will suffice here. Drug resistance has not so far proved to be a clinical problem, though it has occurred in animals on continuous chemoprophylaxis.

DRUGS FOR HELMINTHIC INFECTIONS

Albendazole is similar to mebendazole (below).

Diethylcarbamazine kills both microfilariae and adult worms. Fever, headache, anorexia, malaise, urticaria, vomiting and asthmatic attacks following the first dose are due to products of destruction of the parasite, and reactions are minimised by slow increase in dosage over the first 3 days.

Ivermectin may cause immediate reactions due to the death of the microfilaria (see diethylcarbamazine). It can be effective in a single dose, but is best repeated at intervals of 6–12 months.

Levamisole paralyses the musculature of sensitive nematodes which, unable to maintain their anchorage, are expelled by normal peristalsis. It is well tolerated, but may cause abdominal pain, nausea, vomiting, headache and dizziness.

Mebendazole blocks glucose uptake by nematodes. Mild gastrointestinal discomfort may be caused, and it should not be used in pregnancy or in children under the age of 2 years.

Metriphonate is an organophosphorus anticholinesterase compound that was originally used as an insecticide. Adverse effects include abdominal pain, nausea, vomiting, diarrhoea, headache and vertigo.

Niclosamide blocks glucose uptake by intestinal tapeworms. It may cause some mild gastrointestinal symptoms.

Piperazine may cause hypersensitivity reactions, neurological symptoms (including 'worm wobble') and may precipitate epilepsy.

Praziquantel paralyses both adult worms and larvae. It is metabolised extensively. Praziquantel may cause nausea, headache, dizziness and drowsiness; it cures with a single dose (or divided doses in 1 day).

Pyrantel depolarises neuromuscular junctions of susceptible nematodes, which are expelled in the faeces. It cures with a single dose. It may induce gastrointestinal disturbance, headache, dizziness, drowsiness and insomnia.

Table 14.5   Drugs for helminthic infections

Infection	Drug	Comment
Cestodes (tapeworms)		
Beef tapeworm *Taenia saginata*	niclosamide or praziquantel	Praziquantel cures with single dose
Pork tapeworm *Taenia solium*	niclosamide or praziquantel	Praziquantel cures with single dose
Cysticercosis *Taenia solium*	albendazole or praziquantel	Treat in hospital as dying and disintegrating cysts may cause cerebral oedema
Fish tapeworm *Diphyllobothrium latum*	niclosamide or praziquantel	
Hydatid disease *Echinococcus granulosus*	albendazole	Surgery for operable cyst disease
Nematodes (intestinal)		
Ascariasis *Ascaris lumbricoides*	levamisole, mebendazole, pyrantel, piperazine or albendazole	
Hookworm *Ancylostoma duodenale; Necator americanus*	mebendazole, pyrantel, or albendazole	Anaemic patients require iron
Strongyloidiasis *Strongyloides stercoralis*	tiabendazole or ivermectin	Alternatively, albendazole is better tolerated
Threadworm (pinworm) *Enterobius vermicularis*	pyrantel, mebendazole, albendazole or piperazine salts	
Whipworm *Trichuris trichiuria*	mebendazole or albendazole	
Nematodes (tissue)		
Cutaneous larva migrans *Ancylostoma braziliense; Ancylostoma caninum*	tiabendazole (topical for single tracks); ivermectin, albendazole or oral tiabendazole (for multiple tracks)	Calamine lotion for symptom relief
Guinea worm *Dracunculus medinensis*	metronidazole, mebendazole	Rapid symptom relief
Trichinellosis *Trichinella spiralis*	mebendazole	Prednisolone may be needed to suppress allergic and inflammatory symptoms
Visceral larva migrans *Toxocara canis; Toxocara cati*	diethylcarbamazine, albendazole or mebendazole	Progressive escalation of dose lessens allergic reactions to dying larvae; prednisolone suppresses inflammatory response in ophthalmic disease
Lymphatic filariasis *Wuchereria bancrofti; Brugia malayi; Brugia timori*	diethylcarbamazine	Destruction of microfilia may cause an immunological reaction (see below)
Onchocerciasis (river blindness) *Onchocerca volvulus*	ivermectin	Cures with single dose. Suppressive treatment; a single annual dose prevents significant complications
Schistosomiasis (intestinal)		
Schistosoma mansoni; Schistosoma japonicum	praziquantel	Oxamniquine only for *Schistosoma mansoni*
Schistosomiasis (urinary)		
Schistosoma haematobium	praziquantel	Metriphonate only for *Schistosoma haematobium*
Flukes (intestinal, lung, liver)	praziquantel	Alternatives: niclosamide for intestinal fluke, bithionol for lung fluke

Tiabendazole (formerly known as thiabendazole) inhibits cellular enzymes of susceptible helminths. Gastrointestinal, neurological and hypersensitivity reactions, liver damage and crystalluria may be induced.

GUIDE TO FURTHER READING

World wide web resources

The American Centers for Disease Control and Prevention (CDC-P) website includes a comprehensive travel section (http://www.cdc.gov/travel/) that contains high-quality and up-to-date information about prophylaxis, avoidance, diagnosis and treatment of infectious diseases of travel. Another useful contemporary source is 'Fit for travel', the NHS public access website providing travel health information for people travelling abroad from the UK (http://www.fitfortravel.scot.nhs.uk/).

Anonymous 2005 Antifungal drugs. Treatment guidelines from The Medical Letter 3(30):7–14 Available:http://medicalletter.org

World Health Organization data on HIV infection Available: http://www.who.int/topics/hiv_infections/en/

US Department of Health and Human Services guidelines on use of antiretroviral agents in adults and adolescents, and children, which are updated several times per year. Available:http://www.aidsinfo.nih.gov

University of Liverpool interactive charts on antiretroviral drug interactions, information about advances in therapeutic drug monitoring and other resources. Available:http://www.hiv-druginteractions.org

Printed resources

Baird J K 2005 Effectiveness of antimalarial drugs. New England Journal of Medicine 352(15):1565–1577

Beigel J H, Farrar J, Han A M et al of the Writing Committee of WHO Consultation on Human Influenza A/H5 2005 Avian influenza A (H5N1) infection in humans. New England Journal of Medicine 353(13):1374–1385

Bethony J, Brooker S, Albonico M et al 2006 Soil-transmitted helminth infections: ascariasis, trichuriasis, and hookworm. Lancet 367:1521–1532

Bruce-Chwatt L J 1988 Three hundred and fifty years of the Peruvian fever bark. British Medical Journal 296:1486–1487

Deeks S G 2006 Antiretroviral treatment of HIV infected adults. British Medical Journal 332:1489–1493

Edwards G, Biagini G A 2006 Resisting resistance: dealing with the irrepressible problem of malaria. British Journal of Clinical Pharmacology 61(6):690–693

Esté J A, Telenti A 2007 HIV entry inhibitors. Lancet 370:81–88

Franco-Paredes C, Santos-Preciado J I 2006 Problem pathogens: prevention of malaria in travellers. Lancet Infectious Diseases 6(3):139–149

Geisbert T W, Jahrling P B 2004 Exotic emerging viral diseases: progress and challenges. Nature Medicine (supplement review) 10(12):S110–S121

Greenwood B M, Bojang K, Whitty C J, Targett G A 2005 Malaria. Lancet 365:1487–1498

Gryseels B, Polman K, Clerinx J, Kestens L 2006 Human schistosomiasis. Lancet 368:1106–1118

Jefferson T, Demicheli V, Rivetti D et al 2006 Antivirals for influenza in healthy adults: systematic review. Lancet 367:303–313

Kremsner P G, Krishna S 2004 Antimalarial combinations. Lancet 364:285–294

McManus D P, Zhang W, Li J, Bartley P B 2003 Echinococcosis. Lancet 362:1295–1304

Merson M H 2006 The HIV-AIDS pandemic at 25 – the global response. New England Journal of Medicine 354(23):2414–2417

Montoya J G, Liesenfeld O 2004 Toxoplasmosis. Lancet 363:1965–1976

Moscona A 2005 Neuraminidase inhibitors for influenza. New England Journal of Medicine 353(13):1361–1373

Murray H W, Berman J D, Davies C R, Saravia N G 2005 Advances in leishmaniasis. Lancet 366:1561–1577

Patterson T F 2005 Advances and challenges in management of invasive mycoses. Lancet 366:1013–1025

Sepkowitz K A 2006 One disease, two epidemics – AIDS at 25. New England Journal of Medicine 354(23):2411–2414

Drugs for inflammation and rheumatological disease

SYNOPSIS

Musculoskeletal diseases are the most widespread cause of chronic illness and sickness absence from work in the UK. Common to many of these conditions are abnormalities of the inflammatory process. This chapter reviews the complex mechanisms of inflammation, and the agents that are now available to modify it.

- Inflammation, acute and chronic
- Pharmacological manipulation of inflammatory mediators
- Corticosteroids
- Manipulation of eicosanoid and platelet-activating factor
- Aspirin and NSAIDs
- Mast cell stabilisers and inhibitors of chemotaxis
- Immunomodulatory drugs
  - Inhibition of lymphocyte activation
  - Manipulation of cytokine activity
- Management of diseases affecting the joints

Abbreviation	
ANCA	antinuclear cytoplasmic antibody
COX	cyclo-oxygenase
DMARD	disease-modifying antirheumatic drug
IL	interleukin
LT	leukotriene
PAF	platelet-activating factor
PG	prostaglandin
TNF	tumour necrosis factor
TX	thromboxane

INFLAMMATION

The immune system is vital to our survival, for it acts to eradicate or contain invading substances, microorganisms, and aberrant native cells, and to repair and remodel tissues. It comprises a complex of interrelated genetic, molecular and cellular components that provide a defence system known as the *immune response*, often manifest as the process of *inflammation*.

The *innate* immune response comprises, firstly, the detection of an injurious stimulus by cells resident in tissue and, secondly, the orchestrated deployment of a variety of rapidly available *effectors* (a general term for molecules, proteins or cells that cause an effect). In many cases of microbial infection, an *adaptive* immune response, is also initiated. This is integrated with the innate system but employs additional effectors that recognise the invading agent with high specificity and contribute the important phenomenon of *immunological memory*.

The processes of acute and chronic inflammation result in the familiar features of pain, swelling and heat at the site of damage or infection. But the immune and inflammatory responses rely also on recruitment of effectors from distant sites. Thus the systemic nature of the response is often reflected by constitutional clinical features, such as fever, fatigue, malaise and, in some cases, weight loss.

The immune and inflammatory responses operate in answer to a variety of stimuli including physical damage (thermal, crush injury), microbial infection, allergy of all types (hay fever, anaphylactic shock, ABO incompatibility, post-streptococcal arthritis, contact hypersensitivity), autoimmunity (e.g. rheumatoid arthritis, systemic lupus erythematosus [SLE]), malignancy and organ transplantation.

The ideal immune/inflammatory response rapidly neutralises invading microbes, with minimal intercurrent tissue damage, and is followed by complete resolution. Unfortunately, inflammation may also occur *inappropriately*, e.g. during allergy or autoimmune disease. In addition, if microbes are not rapidly eradicated, an initially normal reaction to microbial challenge evolves into a chronic response.

The sequelae of immune/inflammation responses that require pharmacological intervention are:

- management of local pain and swelling
- management of systemic features of inflammation
- minimisation of tissue dysfunction during inflammation
- minimisation of permanent tissue damage.

ACUTE AND CHRONIC INFLAMMATION

Acute inflammation describes the rapid response of innate immune components to a challenge. The inflammatory *effectors* are numerous and varied. They include cells (leucocytes of all types, mast cells, macrophages, natural killer cells and endothelial cells), soluble plasma proteins (of the complement, coagulation, fibrinolytic and kinin systems) and soluble mediators synthesised by innate cellular components (histamine, eicosanoids, cytokines, chemokines, nitric oxide, heat shock proteins). These components interact in the following ways.

White blood cells in tissue detect microbes by pattern recognition receptors that identify molecules produced by microbes but not by host cells, e.g. components of bacterial cell walls. *Mast cells* in tissues contain granules with preformed *histamine* and *tumour necrosis factor-α* (*TNFα*, a pro-inflammatory cytokine), which are released within seconds of a stimulus and act on tissue microcirculation. Histamine (see also p. 499) causes vasodilatation and increased vascular permeability, thereby augmenting tissue blood supply and the delivery of *soluble inflammatory effectors* to the tissue, including fibrinogen and components of the complement cascade. TNFα and histamine also cause the vascular endothelium to express *adhesion molecules*, which facilitate the recruitment of leucocytes to the tissue. The local production of *chemokines*, e.g. interleukin (IL)-8, synthesised by activated endothelium, causes leucocytes to migrate to inflammatory sites (*chemotaxis*).

Neutrophils, recruited rapidly to a site of pyogenic bacterial infection, ingest particles, including bacteria, aided by a coating (opsonisation) of the bacteria by soluble effector molecules, including C-reactive protein and components of the complement cascade. Neutrophils have potent microbicial capabilities, including the respiratory burst, which generates toxic free radicals, in the compartment containing the ingested bacterium. Several leucocytes, including mast cells and macrophages, as well as endothelial cells, synthesise pro-inflammatory eicosanoids (Fig. 15.1).

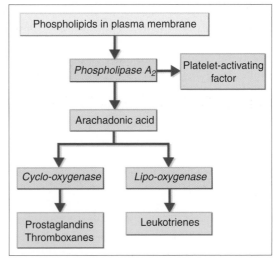

Fig. 15.1 Synthesis of eicosanoids and platelet-activating factor. The enzymes *phospholipase A₂, cyclo-oxygenase* and *lipo-oxygenase* are involved in the synthesis of eicosanoids (20-carbon unsaturated fatty acids) and platelet-activating factor, all of which are derived from phospholipid substrates in plasma membranes.

Resident tissue *macrophages* can ingest (phagocytose) bacteria and also express pattern recognition receptors, which signal the microbial presence and initiate pro-inflammatory responses in the macrophage. This includes the release of more TNFα (and the *cytokine* IL-1. As well as having local pro-inflammatory effects, IL-1 is a pyrogen and contributes to the fever that often accompanies acute inflammation.

The enzymes *phospholipase A₂, cyclo-oxygenase (COX)* and *lipo-oxygenase* are involved in the synthesis of eicosanoids (20-carbon unsaturated fatty acids) and platelet-activating factor (PAF), all of which are derived from phospholipid substrates in plasma membranes. Corticosteroids act by inducing the synthesis of lipocortin-1, a polypeptide that inhibits phospholipase A₂, and thereby exert a broad anti-inflammatory effect. Non-steroidal anti-inflammatory drugs (NSAIDs), including aspirin, inhibit COX and hence prostaglandin and thromboxane synthesis.

Chronic inflammation may arise because of (a) susceptibility in the individual to perpetuate inflammatory responses, (b) failure to eradicate the agent or factors triggering inflammation, e.g. a foreign body embedded in injured tissue, (c) persistent microbial infection, e.g. tuberculosis, hepatitis B or C virus, chronic parasitic infestation, or (d) continuing tissue damage and pro-inflammatory stimuli, such as those encountered in the atherosclerotic plaque.

Chronic inflammatory conditions include rheumatoid arthritis, SLE, inflammatory bowel disease, multiple sclerosis, glomerulonephritis, sarcoidosis and psoriasis. Although the nature of the inflammatory pathogenesis differs between these diseases, all involve interaction between *innate* and *adaptive* immune responses and probably derive from aberrant regulation of immune effectors. In many cases, microbial trigger(s) are implicated. There is also a known genetic predisposition to autoinflammatory and autoimmune disease, involving polymorphisms in genes encoding human leucocyte antigen (HLA) molecules, pattern recognition receptors and cytokines.

THE ADAPTIVE IMMUNE RESPONSE

The adaptive immune response utilises cellular and soluble effectors to provide a high degree of specificity for a given challenge, usually a microbial infection. The system is mediated by antigen receptors on T cells and B cells, and the end result is the secretion of soluble antibodies (Fig. 15.2). Each T or B cell is clonal, i.e. it specifically encodes a single T-cell or B-cell receptor. Although the B-cell receptor and antibody recognise antigen in its native form, the T-cell receptor recognises antigen only in the form of linear peptide, which is presented in a groove of a major histocompatibility (MHC) molecule. Thus complex protein antigens must be processed to allow recognition by T cells.

A primary adaptive immune response is initiated when a T cell recognises a peptide antigen presented on the surface of an antigen-presenting cell (macrophage). The activated T cell is then able to 'help' the activation of other types of T cell, as well as B

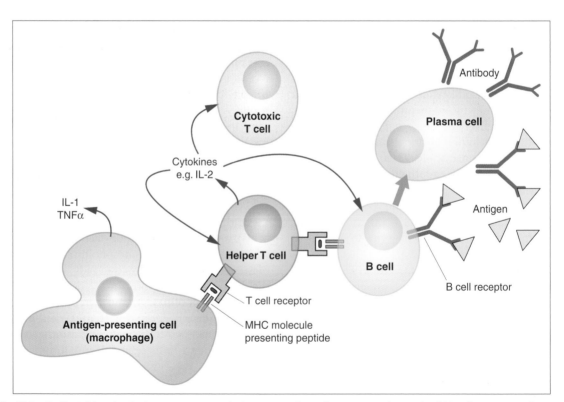

Fig. 15.2 Outline of the adaptive immune response. Antigen-presenting cells, e.g. macrophages, dendritic cells, process and present antigen to T cells. The activated T cells provide 'help' for B cells and cytotoxic T cells, which develop their respective effector functions. Some B cells differentiate into plasma cells, which secrete antibody. IL, interleukin; MHC, major histocompatibility complex; TNF, tumour necrosis factor.

cells and macrophages. This results in proliferation of adaptive cellular effectors and the production of a range of cytokines by the participating leucocytes. In chronic inflammatory disease, these amplification loops may become self-perpetuating.

EICOSANOIDS AND PLATELET-ACTIVATING FACTOR

Eicosanoids form a group of 20-carbon unsaturated fatty acids that are derived principally from phospholipids, via arachadonic acid, in plasma membranes. The group includes prostaglandins, thromboxanes and leukotrienes. Platelet-activating factor (PAF) is a phospholipid that is also derived from the phospholipid substrates in the plasma membrane. These lipid-derived autocoids are synthesised in virtually all tissues and have diverse physiological roles, including:

- protection of the gastrointestinal mucosa – prostaglindin (PG)E_2 and PGI_2
- regulation of renal perfusion and tubular function – PGE_2 and PGI_2
- regulation of vascular tone and permeability – leukotriene (LT), PGI_2 and thromoxane (TX)A_2
- regulation of coagulation/fibrinolysis – PAF, PGI_2 and TXA_2
- regulation of bronchodilatation and constriction
- regulation of pain threshold
- uterine function, embryo implantation and labour – PGF_2
- regulation of the sleep–wake cycle – PGD_2
- temperature homeostasis – PGE_2.

Orally active leukotriene *receptor antagonists*, *montelukast* and *zafirlukast*, cause bronchodilatation and are licensed for use in asthma (see p. 499). Synthetic *analogues* of eicosanoids have a variety of clinical uses including:

Misoprostol is a PGE_1 analogue that suppresses the production of gastric acid. It is used as a gastroprotective agent together with a NSAID, i.e. combined with diclofenac (as Arthrotec) or with naproxen (as Napratec). Misoprostol prevents the development of peptic ulcers during long-term NSAID use, with a therapeutic efficacy comparable to that of proton pump inhibitors. It is less effective in the context of ulcer healing.

Alprostadil is a PGE_1 analogue that is administered intravenously to maintain the patency of the ductus arteriosus in neonates with congenital heart defects. Injection of alprostadil into the corpus cavernosum of the penis is a treatment for erectile dysfunction (see p. 128). A PGE_2 analogue, *dinoprostone*, serves as a cervical and vaginal gel to induce labour and for late therapeutic abortion.

Epoprostenol is a PGI_2 (prostacyclin) analogue that has vasodilator with antithrombotic properties. It is used as a continuous intravenous infusion in severe pulmonary hypertension, and as intermittent infusions for patients with digitial ischaemia in the context of systemic sclerosis and other connective tissue diseases.

Gemeprost is a PGE_1 analogue that is the preferred prostaglandin for the medical induction of late therapeutic abortion.

Carboprost is a $PGF2\alpha$ analogue given for postpartum haemorrhage due to uterine atony in patients unresponsive to ergometrine and oxytocin.

PHARMACOLOGICAL MANIPULATION OF INFLAMMATORY MEDIATORS

CORTICOSTEROIDS

Corticosteroids exert a variety of effects on carbohydrate, protein and lipid metabolism; these and other aspects of these agents are described in Chapter 34 (and have been reviewed[1]).The powerful *anti-inflammatory* effects of corticosteroids rest on their capacity to suppress the action of many pro-inflammatory mediators.

1. Corticosteroids bind to a corticosteroid receptor (CR) and the complex translocates to the nucleus where it binds to a glucocorticoid response element (GRE). This complex *increases* the transcription of a number of *anti-inflammatory* genes, including the gene that encodes inhibitory (I)- κB, which inhibits the activation of nuclear factor (NF)- κB, genes encoding cytokines IL-4, IL-10, IL-13 and

[1]Chikanza I C, Kozaci D, Chernajovsky Y 2003 The molecular and cellular basis of corticosteroid resistance. Journal of Endocrinology 179:301–310.

transforming growth factor (TGF)β , which have T helper cell type 2 and/or suppressive activity (Fig. 15.3).

2. The corticosteroid–CR complex also interferes with the binding of transcription factors activating protein (AP)-1η and NF-κB to their response elements. This action *inhibits* the production of a range of *pro-inflammatory* mediators including IL-1β and TNFα, which are synthesised predominantly by activated macrophages, IL-2, which is pivotal for T-cell proliferation, a range of chemokines and adhesion molecules, which serve to recruit leucocytes to inflamed tissue, metalloproteinases, COX-1 and inducible nitric oxide synthase (see Fig. 15.3).

3. Corticosteroids also increase synthesis of the polypeptide lipocortin-1, which inhibits *phospholipase A$_2$* and thereby the synthesis of eicosanoids and PAF (see Fig. 15.1).

At the cellular level, corticosteroids reduce the numbers of circulating neutrophils, eosinophils, monocytes and lymphocytes. This is maximal approximately 6 h after administration and is achieved by a combination of induction of apoptosis and inhibition of proliferation of leucocytes. In contrast, chronic administration of corticosteroid is associated with a neutrophilia, owing to release of neutrophils from the bone marrow.

In inflammatory disease, the choice of corticosteroid preparation will reflect the site and the extent of inflamed tissue, e.g. oral or parenteral for systemic disease, inhaled in asthma, topical in cutaneous, ocular, oral or rectal disease. Different corticosteroid preparations, their modes of delivery and adverse effects of long-term use are discussed in Chapter 34.

NON-STEROIDAL ANTI-INFLAMMATORY DRUGS

Mode of action

The NSAIDs are chemically diverse, most being organic acids. Despite their structural heterogeneity, NSAIDs possess *a single common mode of action*, which is to block prostaglandin synthesis largely though their inhibition of the enzyme cyclo-oxygenase (COX), which catalyses the synthesis of prostaglandins and thromboxane from arachadonic acid (see Fig. 15.1). There are two isoforms of COX:

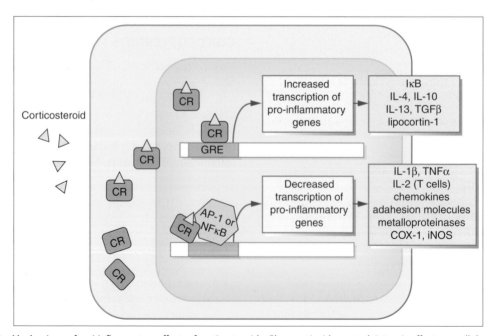

Fig. 15.3 Mechanisms of anti-inflammatory effects of corticosteroids. Glucocorticoids exert pleiotropic effects on cellular metabolism. The anti-inflammatory efficacy results from increased transcription of a number of genes encoding anti-inflammatory proteins and from decreased transcription of pro-inflammatory genes. AP, activating protein; COX, cyclo-oxygenase; CR, corticosteroid receptor; GRE, glucocorticoid response element; IL, interleukin; iNOS, inducible nitric oxide synthase; NF, nuclear factor; TGF, transforming growth factor.

- COX-1 is *constitutively* (constantly) expressed in most cell types and has a maintenance role in the body, being concerned with tissue homeostasis.
- COX-2 is *induced* (increased in amount or activity) when inflammatory cells are activated (particularly by cytokines including IL-1 and TNF α) and it produces the prostaglandin mediators of inflammation.

The significance of the two isoforms is that the useful *anti-inflammatory* action of NSAIDs is owed to their inhibition of COX-2, whereas many *adverse* effects, notably on the gastrointestinal tract, rest on inhibition of COX-1, notably with loss of cytoprotective mucosal prostaglandins PGI_2 and PGE_2. Once this had been recognised, the development of selective COX inhibitors assumed importance, and NSAIDs may now be categorised according to their COX specificity as:

- *COX-2-selective* compounds, which inhibit COX-2 with at least five times greater potency than COX-1. The group includes the coxibs (e.g. celecoxib), meloxicam, etodolac and nabumetone.
- *Non-COX-2-selective* compounds, which comprise all other NSAIDs. These drugs inhibit COX-1 as much as, or even more than, COX-2.

Various NSAIDs have other actions that may contribute to differences between the drugs, including: the inhibition of lipo-oxygenases (diclofenac, indometacin); superoxide radical production and superoxide scavenging; effects on neutrophil aggregation and adhesion, cytokine production and modification of cartilage metabolism. Nevertheless, their key action of inhibiting prostaglandin formation is reflected in the range of effects, beneficial and adverse, that the members exhibit.

Pharmacokinetics

In general, NSAIDs are absorbed almost completely from the gastrointestinal tract, tend not to undergo first-pass (presystemic) elimination, are highly bound to plasma albumin and have small volumes of distribution. Their $t_{1/2}$ values in plasma tend to group into those that are short (1–5 h) or long (10–60 h). Differences in $t_{1/2}$ are not necessarily reflected proportionately in duration of effect, as peak and trough drug concentrations at their intended site of action in synovial (joint) fluid at steady-state dosing are much less than those in plasma. The vast majority of NSAIDs are weakly acidic drugs that localise preferentially in the synovial tissue of inflamed joints (see pH partition hypothesis, p. 82).

Uses

Analgesia. All non-selective and COX-2-selective NSAIDs are analgesics. They are particularly effective for disorders that have an inflammatory component, as the analgesic action of most NSAIDs is a composite of COX inhibition, both in the brain and at the inflammatory site(s). NSAIDs are also particularly effective in conditions where local release of prostaglandins is a major contributor to the pain, e.g. dysmenorrhoea, bone malignancy. The non-selective and COX-2-selective agents have generally comparable analgesic efficacies.

Anti-inflammatory action. The majority of NSAIDs are anti-inflammatory. An important exception is acetaminophen (paracetamol), which inhibits cyclo-oxygenase in the brain but not in the periphery. Curiously, although other NSAIDs reduce eicosanoid synthesis at inflammatory sites, there is little evidence to suggest that they are effective disease-modifying agents. Their widespread use in inflammatory arthritis reflects their considerable symptomatic efficacy. The anti-inflammatory effects of NSAIDs are also employed in patients with systemic mastocytosis, in order to reduce episodes of vasodilatation and hypotension.

Antipyretic action. Both non-selective NSAIDs and coxibs reduce cytokine-induced prostaglandin synthesis in the hypothalamus, and are effective antipyretics.

Antiplatelet action. Aspirin exerts its antiplatelet effects by *irreversibly* acetylating a serine residue in COX-1, expressed in platelets. The production of thromboxane A_2 (which promotes coagulation and vasoconstriction) is thus inhibited for the life of the exposed platelet. This effect is exploited to reduce the incidence of cardiovascular events in at-risk individuals, to decrease mortality following acute myocardial infarction, and to reduce the risk of thromboembolic disease in predisposed patients, e.g. with antiphospholipid antibody syndrome. Although aspirin protects women against stroke and transient ischaemic attacks, the benefit to them may not extend to myocardial infarction.[2]

In contrast to aspirin, other non-selective NSAIDs bind *reversibly* to COX-1 and produce a variable anti-platelet action. Indeed, evidence suggests that ibuprofen may block access of aspirin to the active site on platelets and interfere with its cardioprotective effect when taken regularly (but not intermittently, and aspirin taken 2 h before ibuprofen may avoid the problem). Diclofenac and other NSAIDs appear not to exhibit this interaction.

Selective inhibition has further important consequences. Coxibs inhibit COX-2-derived synthesis of endothelial *prostacyclin* (which acts to prevent platelet aggregation and causes vasodilatation), but allow the continued production of COX-1-derived *thromboxane* (which promotes platelet aggregation and coagulation, and causes vessels to constrict). The selective inhibition of COX-2 would thus be expected to alter the balance in favour of *thromboxane,* and increase the risk of cardiovascular events. Indeed, this theoretical (but predictable) possibility found expression in adverse events following the use of the coxib, rofecoxib (see below).

Prolongation of gestation. Prostaglandins in the E and F series are potent uterotropic agents, and indometacin is used to inhibit labour.

Closure of patent ductus arteriosus. Indometacin is used to achieve closure of a patent ductus arteriosus in neonates. However, prescription of NSAIDs should generally be avoided in pregnant women, particularly in the third trimester, owing to the risk of *premature* closure of the ductus arteriosus.

Bartter's syndrome. This is characterised by hypokalaemia, hyperreninaemia, hyperaldosteronism, normotension and resistance to pressor effects of angiotensin II. Excessive production of prostaglandin has been implicated in the pathogenesis. NSAIDs (usually indometacin) may improve the metabolic abnormalities by inhibiting prostaglandin production and by promoting renal reabsorption of potassium.

Colonic cancer. Chronic administration of NSAID reduces the incidence of colonic cancer by approximately 50%. This appears to be related to the inhibition of COX-2, which is up-regulated in colonic tumours.

Adverse effects of aspirin and other NSAIDs

Gastrointestinal effects. The most common unwanted effect is dyspepsia. The propensity to alimentary, especially gastric, ulceration may also result in occult or overt blood loss. Use of NSAIDs is associated with an approximately four-fold increased incidence of severe gastrointestinal haemorrhage, and such complications account for between 700 and 2000 deaths in the UK each year. In addition, ulceration and stricture of the small intestine can result in anaemia, diarrhoea and malabsorption, which may be clinically indistinguishable from Crohn's disease.

The risk of NSAID-associated gastrointestinal disease is particularly associated with a high dose and prolonged use, age over 65 years, a previous history of peptic ulcer, concomitant use of corticosteroid, anticoagulant or other NSAID, heavy smoking and alcohol use, and the presence of *Helicobacter pylori* infection. Serious co-morbidity, e.g. cardiovascular disease, renal or hepatic impairment, is also a factor.

These adverse effects appear to result mainly from the inhibition of COX–1-mediated production of cytoprotective mucosal prostaglandins, especially PGI_2 and PGE_2, which inhibit acid secretion in the stomach, promote mucus production and enhance mucosal perfusion. Several large randomised controlled trials have compared the incidence of gastrointestinal adverse effects in traditional NSAIDs compared with coxibs. The VIGOR study (rofecoxib versus naproxen), the CLASS (celecoxib versus ibuprofen and diclofenac) and the TARGET (lumiracoxib versus ibuprofen and naproxen) all indicate that coxib use leads to an appoximately 50% reduction of upper gastrointestinal adverse events.[3]

[3]Borer J S, Simon L S 2005 Cardiovascular and gastrointestinal effects of COX-2 inhibitors and NSAIDs: achieving a balance. Arthritis Research and Therapy 7 (Suppl 4):S14–S22. VIGOR, Vioxx Gastrointestinal Outcomes Research; TARGET, Therapeutic Arthritis Research and Gastrointestinal Event Trial; CLASS, Colecoxib Long-term Arthritis Safety Study.

[2]Ridker P M, Cook N R, Lee I M, Gordon D, Gaziano J M 2005 A randomised trial of low-dose aspirin in the primary prevention of cardiovascular disease in women. New England Journal of Medicine 352:1293–1204.

The gastrointestinal toxicity of NSAIDs may be reduced by co-prescription of a proton pump inhibitor, e.g. omeprazole or lansoprazole, an H_2-receptor blocker, e.g. ranitidine, or the prostaglandin analogue misoprostol. Proton pump inhibitors are more effective than the other classes of gastroprotective agent and should be considered in all patients with at least one of the above risk factors. This strategy is often overlooked, and approximately 16% of patients at risk receive an appropriate gastroprotective strategy.[4] The risk of recurrent ulcer bleeding appears to be equal between patients who receive a coxib or a non-selective NSAID plus a proton pump inhibitor.

Cardiovascular effects. The theoretical possibility of increased cardiovascular risk (see above) with a coxib was supported by the VIGOR trial, which reported a four-fold higher incidence of non-fatal myocardial infarction in patients who received rofecoxib (Vioxx) compared with naproxen.[5] The effect was initially ascribed to a cardioprotective effect of naproxen rather than to cardiotoxicity of rofecoxib, but analysis of 18 subsequent randomised clinical trials and 11 observational studies confirmed a two-fold increased relative risk with the coxib.[6] The data from epidemiological studies on other coxibs indicate a cardiovascular risk somewhere between equivalence and a three-fold greater risk of cardiovascular events, compared with non-selective NSAIDs. A reasonable conclusion is that increased cardiovascular risk with coxibs is indeed a class effect; variation between individual drugs may reflect their differential affinity for COX-1 and COX-2, and the resulting balance between prostacyclin and thromboxane production. Because of these concerns, patients with ischaemic heart or cerebrovascular disease should not receive a coxib unless there is a specific indication, i.e. patients who are at a particularly high risk of developing gastroduodenal ulcer, perforation or bleeding.[7]

Non-selective NSAIDs are also associated with increased risk of cardiovascular events. This finding may be explained by a mean 5.0 mmHg increase in systolic blood pressure, compared with that in non-users of NSAIDs, possibly due to retention of sodium and water.

Renal effects. NSAIDs decrease renal perfusion in individuals with congestive cardiac failure, chronic renal disease, cirrhosis with ascites and hypovolaemia; these are all states in which renal perfusion is dependent upon prostaglandin-mediated vasodilatation. NSAIDs may also promote sodium and water retention, causing oedema and hypertension in some individuals. Papillary necrosis and interstitial nephritis are rare complications, often in the context of chronic and excessive NSAID usage, and with chronic use of analgesic mixtures.

Intolerance. NSAID intolerance probably reflects the diversion of arachidonic acid metabolism towards excessive products of the lipo-oxygenase pathway. It is not immune mediated, but clinically may resemble hypersensitivity, with manifestations including vasomotor rhinitis, urticaria, bronchoconstriction, flushing, hypotension and shock.

Other unwanted effects. include headache, photosensitivity, erythema multiforme, toxic epidermal necrolysis, cholestasis, hepatocellular toxicity, cytopaenia, haemolytic anaemia and inhibition of ovulation.

Principal interactions

NSAIDs offer scope for interaction with other drugs by differing pharmacokinetic and pharmacodynamic mechanisms with:

- Angiotensin-converting enzyme (ACE) inhibitors and angiotensin receptor blockers: there is a risk of renal impairment and hyperkalaemia.
- Quinolone antimicrobials: convulsions may occur if NSAIDs are co-administered.

[4]Scheiman J M 2005 Practical approaches to minimizing gastrointestinal and cardiovascular safety concerns with COX-2 inhibitors and NSAIDs. Arthritis Research and Therapy 7(Suppl 4):S23–S29.

[5]Bombardier C, Laine L, Reicin A et al 2000 Comparison of upper gastrointestinal toxicity of rofecoxib and naproxen in patients with rheumatoid arthritis. New England Journal of Medicine 343:1520–1528.

[6]Jüni P, Nartey L, Reichenbach S et al 2004 Risk of cardiovascular events and rofecoxib: cumulative meta-analysis. Lancet 364:2021–2029.

[7]Delay in recognising the cardiovascular toxicity of coxibs was acknowledged by the drug regulatory agency involved (the US Food and Drug Administration) as a failure of post-marketing surveillance and evoked a major reorganisation of the process.

- Anticoagulant (warfarin) and antiplatelet agents (ticlopidine, clopidogrel): increased risk of alimentary bleeding with NSAIDs (notably with azapropazone). Phenylbutazone, and probably azapropazone, inhibit the metabolism of warfarin, increasing its effect.
- Oral hypoglycaemics: azapropazone and phenylbutazone inhibit the metabolism of sulphonylurea hypoglycaemics, increasing their intensity and duration of action.
- Antiepileptics: azapropazone and phenylbutazone inhibit the metabolism of phenytoin and sodium valproate, increasing their risk of toxicity.
- Antihypertensives: their effect is lessened due to sodium retention by inhibition of renal prostaglandin formation.
- Antivirals: ritonavir may raise plasma concentrations of piroxicam; NSAIDs may increase haematological toxicity from zidovudine.
- Ciclosporin and tacrolimus: nephrotoxic effect is exacerbated by NSAIDs.
- Cytotoxics: renal tubular excretion of methotrexate is reduced by competition with NSAIDs, with risk of methotrexate toxicity (low-dose methotrexate given weekly avoids this hazard).
- Diuretics: NSAIDs cause sodium retention and reduce diuretic and antihypertensive efficacy; risk of hyperkalaemia with potassium-sparing diuretics; increased nephrotoxicity risk (with indometacin, ketorolac).
- Lithium: NSAIDs delay the excretion of lithium by the kidney and may cause lithium toxicity.

Different classes of NSAID and their key distinguishing features are summarised in Table 15.1. Paracetamol and aspirin are discussed in more detail below.

PARACETAMOL (ACETAMINOPHEN) (PANADOL)

Mode of action. Paracetamol inhibits prostaglandin synthesis in the brain but hardly at all in the periphery, and it does not affect platelet function. Paracetamol has analgesic efficacy equivalent to aspirin, but in therapeutic doses it has only weak anti-inflammatory effects, a functional separation that reflects its differential inhibition of enzymes

Table 15.1 Classes of non-steroidal anti-inflammatory drug (NSAID)

Class	Representatives	Comment
Para-amino phenol	paracetamol	Analgesic effect but weak anti-inflammatory activity due to predominantly central COX inhibition
Salicylic acids	aspirin	Irreversibly inhits COX-2 – hence predictable anti-platelet effect
Acetic acids	indometacin, diclofenac, etodolac, sulindac,	Indometacin and diclofenac have potent analgesic, antipyretic and anti-inflammatory activities; indometacin has adverse effects in 35–50%, diclofenac in about 20%
	ketorolac	Etodolac is relatively COX-2 selective and is uricosuric. Ketorolac has analgesic but not anti-inflammatory activity
Fenamic acid	mefenamic acid	Used mainly for inflammatory arthritis and dysmenorrhea; may cause non-oliguric renal failure in the elderly
Propionic acids	ibuprofen, naproxen, fenbufen, fenoprofen, flurbiprofen, ketoprofen, tiaprofenic acid	Lower incidence of gastrointestinal side-effects than salicylic or acetic acids
Enolic acids	piroxicam, meloxicam, azapropazone, phenylbutazone, tenoxicam	The generally long half-life of drugs in this group enables once-daily dosing Azapropazone has high toxicity; use only in rheumatoid arthritis, ankylosing spondylitis and acute gout, when other drugs have failed. Uricosuric action useful in gout Phenylbutazone toxicity restricts use to ankylosing spondylitis under specialist supervision
Non-acidic NSAIDs	celecoxib, etoricoxib	Lower incidence of gastrointestinal adverse effects, but probable increased cardiovascular risk

responsible for prostaglandin synthesis.[8] For this reason, some would not class paracetamol as an NSAID. (See also p. 251.)

Uses. Paracetamol is effective in mild to moderate pain such as that of headache or dysmenorrhoea, and it is also useful in patients who should avoid aspirin because of gastric intolerance, a bleeding tendency or allergy, or because they are aged less than 12 years.

Pharmacokinetics. Paracetamol ($t_{\frac{1}{2}}$ 2 h) is well absorbed from the alimentary tract and is inactivated in the liver, principally by conjugation as glucuronide and sulphate. Minor metabolites of paracetamol are also formed, of which one oxidation product, N-acetyl-p-benzoquinoneimine (NABQI), is highly reactive chemically. This substance is normally rendered harmless by conjugation with glutathione. However, the supply of hepatic glutathione is limited and, if the amount of NABQI formed is greater than the amount of glutathione available, the excess metabolite oxidises thiol (SH-) groups of key enzymes, causing cell death. This explains why a normally safe drug can, in overdose, give rise to hepatic and renal tubular necrosis (the kidneys also contain drug-oxidising enzymes).

Dose. The oral dose is 0.5–1 g every 4–6 h; maximum daily dose 4 g.

Adverse effects. Paracetamol is usually well tolerated by the stomach because inhibition of prostaglandin synthesis in the periphery is weak; allergic reactions and skin rash sometimes occur. Heavy, long-term, daily use may predispose to chronic renal disease.

Acute overdose. Severe hepatocellular damage and renal tubular necrosis can result from taking 150 mg/kg body-weight (about 10 or 20 tablets) in one dose. Patients at particular risk include:

- those whose enzymes are induced as a result of taking drugs or alcohol; their livers and kidneys form more NABQI

- those who are malnourished (chronic alcohol abuse, eating disorder, HIV infection) to the extent that their livers and kidneys are depleted of glutathione to conjugate with NABQI.

The international normalised ratio (INR: ratio of prothrombin time to normal prothrombin time) is used to monitor liver damage, and renal impairment is assessed by measurement of plasma creatinine level, rather than urea (which is metabolised by the liver). The clinical signs (jaundice, abdominal pain, hepatic tenderness) do not become apparent for 24–48 h, and liver failure, when it occurs, does so between 2 and 7 days after the overdose. The plasma concentration of paracetamol is of predictive value; if it lies above a semilogarithmic graph joining points between 200 mg/L (1.32 mmol/L) at 4 h after ingestion to 50 mg/L (0.33 mmol/L) at 12 h, then serious hepatic damage is likely. Patients who are enzyme induced or malnourished are regarded as being at risk at 50% of these plasma concentrations (plasma concentrations measured earlier than 4 h are unreliable because of incomplete absorption).

The general principles for limiting drug absorption apply (see Chapter 9) if the patient is seen within 4 h. Activated charcoal by mouth is effective and should be considered if paracetamol in excess of 150 mg/kg body-weight or 12 g, whichever is the smaller, is thought to have been ingested within the previous hour. The decision to use activated charcoal must take into account its capacity to bind an oral antidote (methionine).

Specific therapy is directed at replenishing the store of liver glutathione, which conjugates with and so diminishes the amount of toxic metabolite available to do harm. Glutathione itself cannot be used as it penetrates cells poorly, but N-acetylcysteine (NAC) (Parvolex) and methionine are effective as they are precursors for the synthesis of glutathione. NAC is more effective because its conversion into glutathione requires fewer enzymes; also, it is administered by intravenous infusion – an advantage if the patient is vomiting. Methionine alone may be used to initiate treatment when facilities for infusing NAC are not immediately available.

The earlier such therapy is instituted the better and it should be started if:

- a patient is estimated to have taken more than 150 mg/kg body-weight, without waiting for the measurement of the plasma concentration

[8]Aronoff D M, Oates J A, Boutaud O et al 2006 New insights into the mechanism of action of acetaminophen: its clinical pharmacological characteristics reflect inhibition of the two prostaglandin H₂ synthases. Clinical Pharmacology and Therapeutics 79:9–19.

■ plasma concentration indicates the likelihood of liver damage (above), or

■ there is uncertainty about the amount taken or its timing.

NAC is administered by intravenous infusion, 150 mg/kg in dextrose 5% (200 mL) over 15 min; then 50 mg/kg in dextrose 5% (500 mL) over 4 h; then 100 mg/kg in dextrose 5% (1000 mL) over 16 h, to a total of about 300 mg/kg in 20 h. While it is most effective if administered within 8 h of the overdose, evidence shows that treatment continuing for up to 72 h still provides benefit.

The INR and serum creatinine levels should be measured daily. If the INR exceeds 2 there is risk of infection and gastric bleeding, and an antimicrobial plus either sucralfate or a histamine H_2-receptor antagonist is given prophylactically. The patient is kept well hydrated and in fluid balance; falling urine output, indicative of acute renal tubular necrosis, will necessitate measures to improve urine flow (see Chapter 23).

ASPIRIN (ACETYLSALICYLIC ACID)

In the 18th century, the Reverend Edmund Stone, an English clergyman, wrote about the value of an extract of bark from the willow tree (of the family *Salix*) for alleviating pain and fever. The active principle was salicin, which is metabolised to salicylic acid in vivo. In due course, sodium salicylate manufactured from salicin proved highly successful in the treatment of rheumatic fever and gout, but it was a gastric irritant. In 1897, Felix Hoffman, a chemist at the Bayer Company whose father experienced pain from taking sodium salicylate, succeeded in producing acetylsalicylic acid in a form that was chemically stable. The new preparation proved acceptable to his father and paved the way for the production of aspirin.

Mode of action. The anti-inflammatory, analgesic and antipyretic actions of aspirin are those of NSAIDs in general (see above). The following additional actions are relevant:

■ The antiplatelet effect is due to permanent inactivation, by acetylation, of COX in platelets, preventing synthesis of thromboxane. Being non-nucleated, platelets cannnot regenerate the enzyme as can nucleated cells, and the resumption of thromboxane production is dependent on the entry of new platelets into the circulation (platelet lifespan is 8 days). Thus continuous antiplatelet effect is readily achieved with low doses.

■ Respiratory stimulation is a characteristic of aspirin intoxication and occurs both directly by stimulation of the respiratory centre and indirectly through increased carbon dioxide production.

■ Metabolic effects, including increased oxygen consumption and carbon dioxide production, are relevant when aspirin is taken in overdose.

■ Aspirin in high dose reduces renal tubular *reabsorption* of uric acid, increasing its elimination (both substances are transported by the same mechanism), but other treatments for hyperuricaemia are preferred. Indeed aspirin should be *avoided in gout* as low doses (less than 2 g/day) inhibit uric acid *secretion*, causing uric acid retention, and on balance its effects on uric acid elimination are adverse.

Pharmacokinetics. Aspirin ($t_{1/2}$ 15 min) is well absorbed from the stomach and upper intestinal tract. Hydrolysis removes the acetyl group, and the resulting salicylate ion is inactivated largely by conjugation with glycine. At low therapeutic doses this reaction proceeds by first-order kinetics with a $t_{1/2}$ of about 4 h, but at higher therapeutic doses and in overdose the process becomes saturated, i.e. kinetics become zero order, and most of the drug in the body is present as the salicylate. The problem in overdose is to remove salicylate.

A reasonably steady plasma concentration can be maintained if aspirin is given 6-hourly by mouth, but if a high dose is given repeatedly there is risk of accumulation to toxic amounts; tinnitus is a useful warning sign. Salicylate is an organic anion and, in addition to undergoing glomerular filtration, is secreted by the proximal renal tubule.

Doses of 75–150 mg/day are used to prevent thrombotic vascular occlusion; 300 mg as immediate treatment for myocardial infarction; 300–900 mg every 4–6 h for analgesia.

Adverse effects. Gastrointestinal effects are those of NSAIDs in general. Effects particularly associated with aspirin are:

■ *Salicylism* (the symptoms of an excessive dose) is expressed as tinnitus and hearing difficulty, dizziness, headache and confusion.

- *Allergy*. Aspirin is a common cause of allergic or pseudoallergic symptoms and signs. Patients exhibit severe rhinitis, urticaria, angio-oedema, asthma or shock. Those who already suffer from recurrent urticaria, nasal polyps or asthma are more susceptible.
- *Reye's syndrome*. Epidemiological evidence relates aspirin use to the development of the rare Reye's syndrome (encephalopathy, liver injury) in children recovering from febrile viral infections. Acknowledging this, aspirin should not be given to children aged under 12 years and should be avoided in those up to and including age 15 years (paracetamol is preferred).

Overdose. A moderate overdose (plasma salicylate 500–750 mg/L) will cause nausea, vomiting, epigastric discomfort, tinnitus, deafness, sweating, pyrexia, restlessness, tachypnoea and hypokalaemia. A large overdose (plasma salicylate level above 750 mg/L) may result in pulmonary oedema, convulsions and coma, with severe dehydration and ketosis. Bleeding is unusual, despite the antiplatelet effect of aspirin.

Adults who have taken a single large quantity usually develop a respiratory alkalosis. Metabolic acidosis suggests severe poisoning. Often, a mixed picture is seen. In children aged less than 4 years, severe metabolic acidosis is more likely than respiratory alkalosis, especially if the drug has been ingested over many hours (mistaken for sweets).

Treatment. Serial measurements of plasma salicylate are necessary to monitor the course of the overdose, for the concentration may rise over the early hours after ingestion. The general management described in Chapter 9 applies, but the following are relevant for salicylate overdose.

- *Activated charcoal* 50 g p.o. adsorbs salicylate and prevents its absorption from the alimentary tract; gastric lavage or the use of an emetic is no longer recommended.
- *Correction of dehydration*. Dextrose 5% i.v. with additional potassium is often indicated.
- *Acid–base disturbance*. Alkalosis or mixed alkalosis/acidosis need no specific treatment. Metabolic acidosis is treated with sodium bicarbonate, which alkalinises the urine and accelerates the removal of salicylate in the urine (see p. 133).
- *Haemodialysis* may be necessary, if either renal failure develops or the plasma salicylate concentration exceeds 900 mg/L.

OTHER NSAID PREPARATIONS

Several NSAIDs can be administered topically, e.g. ibuprofen (Ibugel), diclofenac (Voltarol emulgel), piroxicam (Feldene gel) and ketoprofen (Oruvail gel). Their objective is to deliver high local concentrations without undesirable effects. These drugs should not be used on broken or inflamed skin, or on mucous membranes; they may cause photosensitivity and local skin reactions. NSAIDs are also available as suppositories, which some patients prefer. Both local and systemic side-effects may occur.

MAST CELL STABILISERS AND INHIBITORS OF CHEMOTAXIS

Cromolyn sodium and nedocromil inhibit the release of mediators from mast cells and also inhibit leucocyte trafficking. They are used as an adjunct inhaled therapy in asthma (see p. 501) and are administered orally in patients with systemic mastocytosis with gastrointestinal involvement.

Colchicine is derived from the autumn crocus *Colchicum autumnale*. It was regarded as a poisonous plant from ancient times, but Alexander of Tralles recommended colchicum for gout in the 6th century AD.

Colchicine is an effective anti-inflammatory agent in gout and is also used for some features of the multi-system inflammatory Behçet's disease, including oral and genital ulceration. It does not have broad efficacy as an anti-inflammatory agent and its selective effects in gout and Behçet's disease probably relate to the prominent role played by neutrophil infiltration and activation in both conditions. Colchicine inhibits the assembly of microtubules and thereby interferes with the mitotic spindle and with cell migration. It also decreases release of histamine from mast cells, probably again by inhibition of microtuble assembly.

In an acute attack of gout, colchicine is taken orally with 1 mg initially, followed by 500 micrograms every 2–3 h until either pain relief is achieved or further doses are precluded by gastrointestinal effects or until a total dose of 6 mg is reached. The course must not be repeated within 3 days. For prophylaxis of gout, during institution of allopurinol, colchicine 500 micrograms b.d. or t.d.s. may be used.

Adverse effects. The most common is diarrhoea, from effects of colchicine on the rapidly proliferating gastrointestinal epithelial cells; the problem usually responds to reduction of the dose. Agranulocytosis and aplastic anaemia may complicate chronic use of colchicine.

IMMUNOMODULATOR DRUGS

Immunomodulator drugs are used both to control symptoms and to retard or arrest progression of chronic inflammatory diseases. The latter constitutes an important distinction from NSAIDs, which have no significant impact on accumulation of tissue damage.

The terminology surrounding immunomodulator drugs has evolved separately in different specialties, although the underlying management principles are similar. The concept in rheumatoid disease has been used to establish the role of disease-modifying antirhheumatic drugs (DMARDs) as agents that reduce disease activity and prevent radiologically determined 'disease progression'. DMARDs are often described as 'steroid-sparing' agents, particularly in older literature. In contrast, the terminology of the management of life-threatening inflammatory disease, epitomised by lupus nephritis or antineutrophil cytoplasmic antibody (ANCA)-positive nephritis, is drawn from oncological practice, and describes regimes for 'inducing remission' or for 'maintenance'. Disease progression is measured in terms of tissue 'damage', using a variety of indices.

The choice and combination of immunomodulator agent in an individual patient depends on the following considerations:

- Severity of disease: this determines the risk : benefit ratio.
- Adverse-effect profile: both the probability and severity of potential adverse effects need to be considered.
- Organ involvement: e.g. cerebral or renal lupus is more hazardous than rash or arthritis.
- Evidence base for the drug: this may reflect greater efficacy or greater number/quality of studies in one disease compared with another.
- Age: the risk of future malignancy less significant in elderly patient.
- Co-morbidity: e.g. agents causing hypertension or adverse lipid profile in patients with high cardiovascular risk.
- Pregnancy/breast-feeding: an absolute contraindication for many immunomodulators.

- Importance of future fertility: e.g. cyclophosphamide likely to decrease fertility; leflunomide requires long washout period prior to pregnancy.

Most conventional immunomodulator agents fall into the broad categories of those that inhibit *lymphocyte activation* and those that interfere with *cytokine expression* or *signalling*. Figure 15.4 presents an overview of these drugs and their mechanisms of action that are relevant to the following discussion.

Several immunomodulators, including many *conventional DMARDs*, are antimetabolites with a predilection for proliferating lymphocytes. This is due to the dependence of proliferating (but not resting) lymphocytes on *de novo* synthesis of both purine and pyrimidines. The *calcineurin antagonists* and *sirolimus* exhibit selective inhibition of activated T cells, owing to their effects on IL-2 expression and signalling, respectively. *Other conventional immunomodulators* also influence the expression of a range of pro-inflammatory cytokines. *Cyclophosphamide* is cytotoxic to dividing cells and, in an autoimmune response, is particularly toxic to rapidly proliferating lymphocytes. The *biological immunomodulators* introduce new mechanisms of action, including cytokine blockade, depletion of specific leucocyte populations or interference with co-stimulation.

Immunomodulators have well recognised *toxicity profiles* but adverse effects occur in only a proportion of patients and/or are reversible on cessation of drug, or have less impact on quality of life than the inevitable effect of chronic high-dose corticosteroid. *Drug interactions* are given where these are relevant for individual agents. *A general caveat applies to the use of live vaccines* with any potent immunomodulator, as this creates a real hazard of disseminated infection.

The complexity of the prescribing of most immunomodulator drugs demands collaboration between specialists, general practitioners and the well informed patient. *All call for close monitoring*, e.g. of bone marrow, liver, kidney or other functions, as known toxicity dictates.

INHIBITION OF LYMPHOCYTE ACTIVATION

Corticosteroid

Adrenal corticosteroids may be considered DMARDs, because they reduce disease severity and associated damage and, unlike most other immunomodulators,

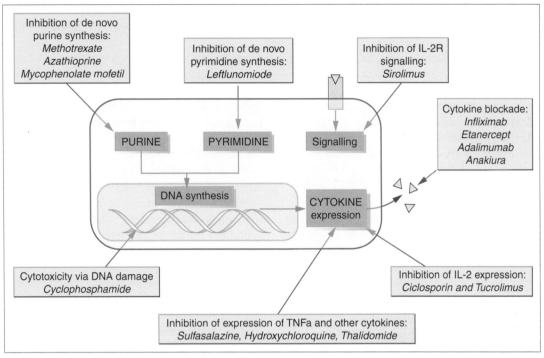

Fig. 15.4 Overview of action of immunomodulatory drugs. Many conventional immunomodulatory drugs used in rheumatology practice are *antimetabolites*, inhibiting de novo synthesis of either purines or pyrimidines, pathways on which activated lymphocytes are particularly dependent. The mechanisms of action of *sulfasalazine* and *hydroxychloroquine* are less clear but appear to involve inhibition of expression of pro-inflammatory cytokines; thalidomide is also used occasionally for this purpose. The *calcineurin* inhibitors and *sirolimus* interfere with either the expression of IL-2 or signalling downstream of the IL-2 receptor; these effects target activated T cells. *Cyclophosphamide* is a cytotoxic agent that indiscriminately targets proliferating cells. Several *biological agents* block specific pro-inflammatory cytokines; the most important currently is TNFα. IL, interleukin; TNF, tumour necrosis factor.

their clinical effects are usually noticeable within 24 h. The catalogue of adverse effects associated with chronic corticosteroid use highlight the importance of controlling disease activity and progression with less toxic agents (see above and Chapter 34).

Methotrexate

This drug inhibits dihydrofolate reductase; its antimetabolic effects arise from the importance of tetrahydrofolate as a co-factor in the de novo purine synthetic pathway to form DNA. The immunomodulatory effects of methotrexate, used at rheumatological rather than (higher) oncological doses, may depend partly on the anti-inflammatory activity of increased plasma concentrations of adenosine.

Methotrexate is used as first-line treatment in rheumatoid arthritis and psoriatic arthritis and, less commonly, in connective tissue diseases or vasculitides. It is usually prescribed orally, starting at 7.5–10 mg once-weekly and increasing as bone marrow and liver function allows. Baseline chest radiography and, in some centres, lung function tests are performed. Folic acid is usually prescribed (variably 5 mg weekly, three times weekly or on all days apart from on the methotrexate dosing day), in order to mitigate some of the adverse effects. This appears to have little effect on the blockade of de novo purine synthesis, unlike folinic acid (tetrahydrofolic acid) (see folinic acid rescue, p. 132).

Adverse effects. The most important are bone marrow toxicity, hepatic toxicity and pulmonitis; regular (at least monthly) monitoring of full blood count and liver function testing are required. Methotrexate is also embryotoxic and must not be prescribed for women who are or may become pregnant. Mouth ulcers and other gastrointestinal symptoms occur commonly but may be improved by co-prescription of folic acid.

Interactions. Methotrexate used with trimethoprim, co-trimoxazole or sulphonamides creates a risk of megaloblastic anaemia and pancytopenia due to the additive antifolate effect. Leucovorin (folinic acid) rescue may be effective should this occur.

Contraindications include moderate to severe renal impairment, liver disease, pregnancy (both male and female patients should avoid conception for at least 6 months after cessation of methotrexate), breast-feeding and active infection.

Azathioprine

Azathioprine undergoes reduction in the presence of glutathione to 6-mercaptopurine and subsequently to a variety of methylated metabolites. It appears to act by both triggering apoptosis and inhibiting de novo purine synthesis, which particularly targets proliferating lymphocytes. Azathioprine and mercaptopurine are metabolised predominantly by methylation and oxidation in the liver and/or erythrocytes.

Azathioprine is used, in daily doses of 1.5–2.5 mg/kg, to treat SLE, other connective tissue diseases and vasculitides, and, occasionally, in rheumatoid arthritis that is refractory to other DMARDs.

Adverse effects. The major serious reactions are leukopenia (common), anaemia and thrombocytopenia, hepatotoxicity, increased susceptibility to infection and increased risk of neoplasia. Other side-effects include nausea (common), alopecia and, rarely, allergy.

Polymorphisms in the gene encoding the enzyme *thiomethylpurine transferase* (TMPT) are associated with variable catabolism and hence toxicity of azathioprine and, in some centres either the genotype or phenotype of TMPT is assessed prior to prescribing azathioprine.

Interactions. *Sulfasalazine* and *NSAIDs* inhibit TMPT and thereby the metabolism of azathioprine, increasing the risk of myelotoxicity. Xanthine oxidase is also important in the catabolism of azathioprine and is inhibited by *allopurinol*. Azathioprine must be decreased to 25–33% of the usual dose if it becomes necessary to use the drugs in combination. Co-prescription of *angiotensin-converting enzyme inhibitors* and azathioprine increases the risk of myelosuppression; the mechanism is incompletely understood but has assumed greater importance with the recent appreciation that patients with rheumatoid arthritis, SLE and probably other chronic inflammatory disorders, have an increased risk of cardiovascular diseases.

Contraindications. Although immunomodulators are contraindicated in pregnancy, experience with azathioprine in pregnant women with renal transplants indicates that it is relatively safe. It is absolutely contraindicated during breast-feeding.

Mycophenolate mofetil

This drug is metabolised to mycophenolic acid, which inhibits inosine monophosphate dehydrogenase. This enzyme forms part of the de novo pathway of guanine nucleotide synthesis. Mycophenolate mofetil is licensed for the prophylaxis of acute rejection following renal or cardiac transplantation. It is also used (unlicensed in the UK) under specialist supervision for lupus nephritis and primary systemic vasculitides.

Adverse reactions include gastrointestinal disturbances, leucopenia, anaemia, thrombocytopenia, abnormal liver function test results, hepatitis, electrolyte disturbances, adverse lipid profile, increased risk of malignancy and pancreatitis.

Leflunomide

Leflunomide[9] inhibits dihydro-orotate dehydrogenase, a mitochondrial enzyme required for the de novo synthesis of pyrimidines. It arrests the proliferation of activated T cells and is licensed for the treatment of rheumatoid arthritis.

Adverse effects. Diarrhoea is reported in more than 40% of patients; other gastrointestinal disturbances, allergic responses, alopecia, hypertension, leucopenia and abnormal liver function test results also occur. In the event of a serious adverse event, the elimination of leflunomide can be accelerated by cholestyramine (8 g t.i.d.) or activated charcoal (50 g q.i.d.).

Contraindications include renal impairment, liver disease, severe hypoproteinaemia (e.g. nephrotic syndrome), immunodeficiency, serious infection, cytopenia, pregnancy, breast-feeding or possibility of future pregnancy; a gap of at least 2 years is recommended between cessation of leflunomide treatment and conception.

---

[9]Drug and Therapeutics Bulletin 2000 Leflunomide for rheumatoid arthritis. 38:52–54.

Calcineurin inhibitors and sirolimus

The calcineurin inhibitors (*ciclosporin* and *tacrolimus*) and *sirolimus* (rapamycin) inhibit the proliferation of activated T cells by interfering with synthesis of IL-2 and signalling via the IL-2 receptor.

Calcineurin inhibitors and rapamycin are used to prevent rejection after solid organ transplantation and (under specialist supervision) in autoinflammatory disorders, including psoriasis, Behçet's ocular disease, primary systemic vasculitis and, occasionally, rheumatoid arthritis.

Biological agent that inhibits lymphocyte activation

Efalizumab is a humanised monoclonal anti-CD11a (leucocyte functional antigen [LFA]-1α chain) antibody. It inhibits activation of T cells by blocking CD11a-mediated co-stimulation. It is used in moderate to severe plaque psoriasis.

OTHER CONVENTIONAL DISEASE-MODIFYING ANTIRHEUMATIC DRUGS (DMARDs)

Sulfasalazine

Sulfasalazine is a conjugate of mesalamine (5-aminosalicylic acid) coupled to sulfapyridine. It is poorly absorbed from the gut but is cleaved by bacterial azoreductases in the colon to release mesalazine and sulfapyridine (Fig. 15.5). Mesalamine is retained mostly in the colon and excreted in faeces, but some 25% is absorbed.

Anti-inflammatory effects of mesalamine, both in the colonic epithelial cell and in peripheral blood mononuclear cells, include inhibition of cyclo-oxygenase and lipo-oxygenase, scavenging of free radicals, and inhibition of the production of pro-inflammatory cytokines and immunoglobulins. In the treatment of inflammatory bowel disease (see p. 580), preparations containing the mesalamine component alone have efficacy comparable to that of sulfasalazine, but with fewer unwanted effects. In contrast, the sulfapyridine component is more effective than mesalamine in rheumatoid arthritis, possibly due to effects of sulfapyridine on IL-8 production and angiogenesis. Sulfasalazine has recently also been reported to inhibit folate uptake by cells.

Sulfasalazine is used to treat rheumatoid arthritis, particularly in seronegative patients (i.e. lacking rheumatoid factor), and peripheral (but not spinal) joint involvement in the spondyloarthropathies, including ankylosing spondylitis and enteropathic arthritides.

Sulfasalazine is associated with a number of adverse effects, many of which appear to be caused by the sulfapyridine moiety (see p. 577). A lupus-like

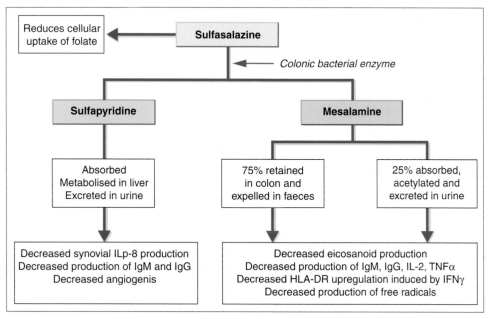

Fig. 15.5 Metabolism and activity of sulfasalazine. Sulfasalazine is reduced to sulfapyridine and mesalamine in the colon. Each component has distinct anti-inflammatory activities. HLA, human leucocyte antigen; IFN, interferon; Ig, immunoglobulin; IL, interleukin; TNF, tumour necrosis factor.

syndrome, including several of these allergic manifestations, may occur; the risk of these adverse effects is higher in rheumatoid patients who are antinuclear antibody positive.

Gold

The main preparations are *auranofin* (administered orally) and *sodium aurothiomalate* (given by intramuscular injection); the latter is more effective for rheumatoid arthritis. The use of all gold compounds has decreased as a result of increased use of methotrexate and, more recently, anti-TNFα biological agents.

The mechanism of action is uncertain but gold is sequestered in phagocytic cells, including type A synoviocytes. Gold decreases chemotaxis and phagocytic activity of macrophages, which may affect antigen presentation and therefore reduce T-cell activation.

Adverse effects include mouth ulcers, rashes, skin pigmentation, proteinuria, thrombocytopenia and other blood dyscrasias, hepatitis, peripheral neuropathy and pulmonary infiltrates. Auranofin is generally associated with fewer unwanted effects than sodium aurothiomalate, but it does causes gastrointestinal disturbances.

Contraindications to gold therapy include hepatic or renal disease, pregnancy or breast-feeding and colitis.

D-Penicillamine

This drug has disease-modifying activity in rheumatoid arthritis but is poorly tolerated and thus used infrequently. Its mechanism of action is unknown. Adverse effects include blood dyscrasias, rashes, nausea, proteinuria, Goodpasture's syndrome, myasthenia gravis-like syndrome, inflammatory myositis, loss of taste, lupus-like syndrome and breast enlargement.

Hydroxychloroquine

Hydroxychloroquine is used commonly for mild manifestations of SLE and other connective tissue diseases, particularly those with rashes and arthralgia. In rheumatoid arthritis, it is used as an adjunct to other disease-modifying agents.

The mechanism of action is unclear, but in vitro studies suggest that chloroquine and hydroxychloroquine can reduce the production of pro-inflammatory cytokines including TNFα, interferon (IFN) γ and IL-6. Both drugs inhibit the acidification of lysosomes; this could impair antigen processing and presentation in phagocytes, leading to decreased T-cell activation.

Adverse effects of hydroxychloroquine include nausea and other gastrointestinal disturbances, headache, rashes, discoloration of skin and mucous membranes, alopecia and, rarely, blood dyscrasias. Retinal toxicity occurs with hydroxychloroquine; it is rare, but measurement of visual acuity initially and at annual intervals is advisable.[10]

Hydroxychloroquine should be used with caution in the presence of hepatic or renal impairment, in neurological disorders, in glucose 6-phosphate dehydrogenase deficiency and porphyria. Although the manufacturer's instructions advise against use in pregnancy and breast-feeding, data on over 250 pregnancies in women with connective tissue disease, who were taking hydroxychloroquine, have provided preliminary evidence that the treatment is safe in pregnancy, and probably also during breast-feeding.[11]

ALKYLATING AGENT

Cyclophosphamide an alkylating agent, is cytotoxic largely by damaging DNA in dividing cells; this eventually triggers apoptosis in affected cells. In an autoimmune response it is particularly toxic to rapidly proliferating lymphocytes.

Cyclophosphamide is used to induce remission in renal lupus, ANCA-positive vasculitides (especially with renal involvement), rheumatoid vasculitis and other severe vasculitic complications. It is given only under specialist supervision; use in oncology is described in Chapter 30.

In rheumatological practice, cyclophosphamide most commonly given as an intravenous pulse, repeated at 3–4-week intervals, for six pulses. A serious consequence is haemorrhagic cystitis, due to the action of acrolein (a drug metabolite) on the epithelium of the urinary tract. This is prevented or

[10]Fielder A, Graham E, Jones S, Silman A, Tullo A 1998 Royal College of Ophthalmologists guidelines: ocular toxicity and hydroxychloroquine. Eye 12:907–909.

[11]Costedoat-Chalumeau N, Amoura Z, du Huong L T et al 2005 Safety of hydroxychloroquine in pregnant patients with connective tissue diseases. Review of the literature. Autoimmunity Reviews 4:111–115.

minimised by adequate prior intravenous hydration and oral administration of *mesna*, which reacts with and inactivates the metabolite in the urinary tract.

Other adverse effects are highly significant and include marrow toxicity, infertility, teratogenicity, nausea and increased incidence of malignancy including that of the bladder. In male patients, sperm may be stored prior to cyclophosphamide treatment.

INTERFERENCE WITH CYTOKINE EXPRESSION OR SIGNALLING

Corticosteroid (see above)

Anti-TNFα agents. The pro-inflammatory cytokine, TNFα, is produced predominantly by macrophages, but also by T helper 1 CD4+ cells. It plays an important role in macrophage activation and the eradication of intracellular bacterial and fungal infections. TNFα is also prominent in the pathogenesis of granulomatous conditions, such as rheumatoid arthritis and Crohn's disease. TNFα blockade by biological agents has proved highly effective for many (although not all) chronic inflammatory diseases and this has ushered in a new era of disease-modifying therapy particularly for inflammatory arthritis and in Crohn's disease (see p. 578).

Infliximab is a humanised monoclonal IgG1 antibody (Fig. 15.6). In rheumatoid arthritis it is generally given, with methotrexate, by intravenous infusion at doses of 3 mg/kg, repeated 2 and 6 weeks after the initial infusion and then at 8-week intervals. In ankylosing spondylitis, psoriatic arthritis and psoriasis, it is used at doses of 5 mg/kg. In Crohn's disease, it is also used at 5 mg/kg, but usually without methotrexate.

Adalimumab, in contrast with infliximab, is a fully human monoclonal IgG1 (see Fig. 15.6). The recommended dose is 40 mg s.c., on alternate weeks, usually in combination with methotrexate. It is licensed for use in rheumatoid arthritis, including aggressive early disease (less than 3 years from diagnosis) and psoriatic arthritis.

Etanercept is a recombinant molecule, consisting of two human p75 TNFα receptors coupled to an Fc component of a human IgG1 (see Fig. 15.6). It is licensed for twice-weekly subcutaneous injection in adult patients with rheumatoid arthritis (25 mg),

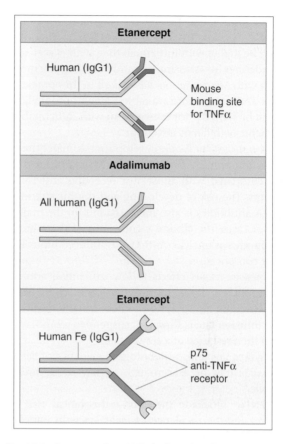

Fig. 15.6 Structure of anti-TNFα biologicals. Infliximab and adalimumab are monoclonal antibodies. Etanercept is a fusion molecule, including the p75 anti-TNFα receptor coupled to a human immunoglobulin Fc component. Ig, immunoglobulin; TNF, tumour necrosis factor.

for children over 4 years with polyarticular juvenile idiopathic arthritis (400 micrograms/kg; maximum dose 25 mg), psoriatic arthritis, psoriasis and ankylosing spondylitis.

The mechanism of action of etanercept differs from that of the monoclonal IgG antibodies in that it:

- does not fix complement and will therefore not cause lysis of cells that express TNFα on their surface
- binds trimeric (active) TNFα, in contrast with infliximab, which binds both monomeric (inactive) and trimeric (active) TNFα
- also binds lymphotoxin (TNFβ).

Adverse effects. There is increased susceptibility to reactivation of *tuberculosis* and to infection with other intracellular pathogens, leading to histoplasmosis, coccidiomycosis or nocardiosis. The risks may be higher with infliximab than with etanercept. Guidelines for assessing risk and for managing infection with *Mycobacterium tuberculosis* in the context of anti-TNFα agents are available.[12] Chemoprophylaxis must be started prior to treatment with infliximab in patients with latent infection.

Antinuclear antibodies develop approximately twice as commonly in patients with rheumatoid arthritis compared with those not receiving anti-TNFα agents. The risk of developing anti-double-stranded DNA antibodies is also increased but, in the majority of cases, the clinical significance of these autoantibodies is unclear. Anti-TNFα -induced lupus is a rare complication.

Infusion-related effects follow infliximab administration, e.g. fever, pruritus, urticaria, chest pain, hypotension and dyspnoea. These usually resolve if the infusion rate is slowed or suspended temporarily and then restarted at a slower rate.

Symptoms and/or radiological evidence of *demyelination* may be exacerbated, as may *severe cardiac failure*.

TNFα blockade presents a theoretical risk of increasing the incidence of *malignancy*. In patients with rheumatoid arthritis, current data do not suggest an overall augmented tumour risk but the chance of developing *lymphoma* may be increased.

Thalidomide has a notorious past for its teratogenic effects (see p. 62). Surprisingly, it is re-emerging as effective treatment of certain inflammatory dermatoses, including discoid lupus erythematosus, cutaneous manifestations of Behçet's disease, erythema nodosum leprosum, aphthous stomatitis and graft-versus-host disease (see also Chapter 30). These effects may relate to its antiangiogenic and anti-TNFα actions. Apart from its known teratogenicity, the use of thalidomide is limited by cumulative peripheral nerve damage, and nerve conduction should be monitored.

Anti-IL-1 agents. *Anakinra* is a monoclonal anti-IL-1 antibody licensed for use in rheumatoid arthritis,

but anti-TNFα agents are currently preferred for their greater therapeutic efficacy.

Other anticytokine agents. Other anticytokine biologicals under development or undergoing clinical trial include antibodies that block IL-4, IL-5, IL-6, IL-8, IL-12 and TGFβ.

Recombinant cytokines. *Aldesleukin* (recombinant IL-2) is licensed for use in metastatic renal cell carcinoma. Interferon-α is used in certain lymphomas and solid tumours and in chronic hepatitis B or C, ideally in combination with ribavirin. Pegylated IFNα is licensed for chronic hepatitis C.

LEUCOCYTE DEPLETION

Rituximab is a humanised monoclonal IgG1 specific for CD20, which is expressed on B cells but not plasma cells. Initially used for B-cell lymphomas, it is now prescribed for a variety of autoimmune disorders, including rheumatoid arthritis and SLE.[13]

MANAGEMENT OF DISEASES AFFECTING THE JOINTS

OSTEOARTHRITIS

Osteoarthritis (OA) is the most common disease of synovial joints. It reflects a dynamic bone and cartilage response to joint trauma and aging. OA is a common cause of disability, particularly in the elderly, and is the major indication for joint replacement. In the UK, OA of the hips affects 10–20% of people over the age of 65 years, and the knees in approximately 15% people aged more than 55 years.

The aims of management of OA are to control pain, reduce progression of joint damage, and minimise functional impairment and disability. In addition to pharmacological management of pain, physical measures, such as addressing obesity and maintaining muscle strength, are important. Patient education in pain management is pivotal to minimising the adverse affects associated with analgesics. NSAIDs have been shown to be only marginally

[12]British Thoracic Society Standards of Care Committee 2005 BTS recommendations for assessing risk and for managing *Mycobacterium tuberculosis* infection and disease in patients due to start anti-TNF-α treatment. Thorax 60:800–805.

[13]Silverman G J, Weisman S 2003 Rituximab therapy and autoimmune disorders: prospects for anti-B cell therapy. Arthritis and Rheumatism 48:1484–1492.

more effective but are associated with more adverse effects than simple analgesics such as paracetamol or ibuprofen.[14,15] Use of regular paracetamol and/or co-dyramol should therefore be tried before introducing a NSAID. A topical NSAID gel can provide modest improvement in symptoms but further evidence from long-term use is required adequately to clarify efficacy. For patients with large-joint OA, occasional intra-articular injection of corticosteroid and local anaesthetic (e.g. for a knee joint injection: triamcinolone 80 mg with 2 mL 1% lidocaine) can provide some respite for up to 6 weeks.

RHEUMATOID ARTHRITIS

The symptoms of rheumatoid arthritis (RA) are predominantly those of pain and stiffness in synovial joints, but RA is a systemic autoinflammatory disorder, with frequent extra-articular manifestations affecting blood vessels, bone marrow, gut, skin, lungs and eyes. Co-morbidity and/or complications of RA reflect the interaction of the disease process with adverse effects of medication. The increased risks from cardiovascular disease, osteoporosis and gastrointestinal haemorrhage are particularly important. Mortality in patients with RA is increased up to three-fold compared with that in the general population; most of the excess is cardiovascular.

Management of the patient who presents with recent-onset inflammatory polyarthritis should aim to reduce systemic symptoms with the joint pain and stiffness (and damage) whilst the diagnosis is clarified (Fig. 15.7).[16] This may be achieved initially by a pulse of depomedrone 80–120 mg i.m., combined with paracetamol 1 g q.i.d. (or co-dydramol 1–2 tablets q.i.d.) with a COX non-selective NSAID (e.g. diclofenac 50 mg t.i.d., meloxicam 7.5 mg o.d. or etodolac 600 mg o.d.).

A definitive diagnosis of RA requires the use of one or more DMARDs. As these agents reduce the progression of joint damage, it is imperative to start treatment in *early disease;* it is no longer acceptable to attempt to treat patients with early RA solely symptomatically. *Methotrexate* is the most common first-line DMARD used in RA. Careful education and counselling of the patient is important to ensure regular monitoring (of bone marrow, liver and lung function) and early detection of adverse effects. Folic acid 5 mg (once weekly or up to 6 days weekly) is co-prescribed with methotrexate to reduce unwanted effects, such as mouth ulcers.

Hydroxychloroquine is often used as an adjunct DMARD with methotrexate. Where methotrexate is contraindicated, ineffective or toxic, azathioprine, sulfasalazine, leflunomide or gold is an alternative. When at least two DMRDs have failed, current UK recommendations are to use biological agents, including infliximab, etanercept or adalimumab.

The pathogenesis of RA and of vascular disease is closely related, and this underlies the importance of cardiovascular risk reduction. Aggressive management of RA with DMARDs appears to reduce cardiovascular disease, and the cholesterol-reducing drug atorvastatin has been reported to have some DMARD activity.[17,18]

Osteoprotection is particularly important for patients who receive long-term adrenal corticosteroids. Corticosteroid is sometimes used as an adjunct DMARD, or even as the primary DMARD, if other agents are ineffective or not tolerated. The UK guideline[19] for the prevention and treatment of glucocorticoid-induced osteoporosis is summarised in Figure 15.8. Bone loss is most rapid in the first few months of treatment and even prednisolone less than 7.5 mg daily increases fracture risk. Osteoprotection must therefore be considered

[14]Bradley J D, Brandt K D, Katz B P et al 1991 Comparison of an antiinflammatory dose of ibuprofen, an analgesic dose of ibuprofen, and acetaminophen in the treatment of patients with osteoarthritis of the knee. New England Journal of Medicine 325:87–91.

[15]Pincus T, Koch G G, Sokka T et al 2001 A randomized, double-blind, crossover clinical trial of diclofenac plus misoprostol versus acetaminophen in patients with osteoarthritis of the hip or knee. Arthritis and Rheumatism 44:1587–1598.

[16]Kennedy T, McCabe C, Struthers G et al 2005 BSR guidelines on standards of care for persons with rheumatoid arthritis. Rheumatology (Oxford) 44:553–556.

[17]McCarey D W, McInnes I B, Madhok R et al 2004 Trial of atorvastatin in rheumatoid arthritis (TARA): double-blind, randomised placebo-controlled trial. Lancet 363:2015–2021.

[18]Kitas G D, Sattar N 2005 Potential role of statins in the treatment of rheumatoid arthritis. Journal of the Royal College of Physicians of Edinburgh 35:309–316.

[19]Bone and Tooth Society, National Osteoporosis Society and Royal College of Physicians. Glucocorticoid-induced osteoporosis – guidelines for prevention and treatment. 2002. Available: http://www.nos.org.uk/about/corticosteroid-induced-osteoporosis.htm

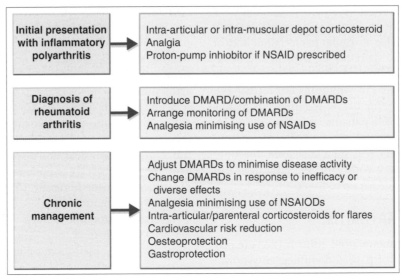

Fig. 15.7 Pharmacotherapy of rheumatoid arthritis. The cornerstone of management of rheumatoid arthritis is effective disease modification from the time of presentation. Attention to cardiovascular, gastrointestinal and skeletal co-morbidity is also important. DMARD, disease-modifying antirheumatic drug; NSAID, non-steroidal anti-inflammatory drug.

at the onset of treatment, whenever the intention is to continue for more than 3 months, at any dose. This includes minimising the dose of corticosteroid, prescribing calcium 1 g daily, in conjunction with vitamin D by mouth, and giving advice on smoking, alcohol excess, nutrition and exercise. Activated vitamin D (alfacalcidol or calcitriol) is more effective than vitamin D in maintaining bone mineral density and reducing fractures in patients treated with corticosteroid.[20] Emerging evidence suggests that this may be of particular significance in chronic inflammatory conditions. The role of activated vitamin D in combination with bisphosphonates requires clarification, and patients receiving this combination should have careful monitoring of blood calcium levels.

Bisphosphonates should be provided for all patients aged over 65 years, or who have a history of a fragility fracture. Other patients should undergo bone densitometry and should be prescribed a bisphosphonate if the T score is −1.5 or less[21] at either spine or hip.

Patients with RA have a five-fold increased risk of gastrointestinal haemorrhage compared with the general population, mainly, it appears, from the risks associated with NSAIDs, alone or in combination with corticosteroids. Therefore, any patient with RA taking regular NSAIDs should be given a *gastroprotective* agent, usually a proton pump inhibitor.

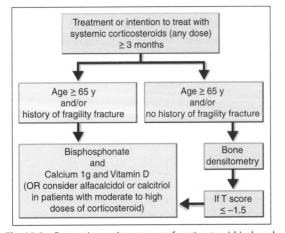

Fig. 15.8 Prevention and treatment of corticosteroid-induced osteoporosis. UK guidelines for osteoprotection in patients treated with corticosteroids.

[20]Ringe J D, Faber H, Fahramand P, Schacht E 2005 Alfacalcidol versus plain vitamin D in the treatment of glucocorticoid/inflammation-induced osteoporosis. Journal of Rheumatology. Supplement 76:33–40.

[21]The T score is the number of standard deviations above or below the mean bone mineral density of a 25-year-old (sex-matched) individual. A T score below −2.5 indicates osteoporosis.

PSORIATIC ARTHRITIS

Psoriatic arthritis affects some 0.5% of the population and 10% of people with psoriasis. The objectives of management are to relieve symptoms and prevent joint damage.

As there is greater likelihood of spontaneous remission and of mild disease, compared with that in RA, initial treatment with a NSAID alone or in combination with intra-articular corticosteroid to large joints may be justified.

When DMARDs are required, methotrexate is most commonly used. Sulfasalazine, ciclosporin, leflunomide and gold tend to have a lower therapeutic efficacy and are more toxic. Anti-TNFα biologicals are reported to be effective in psoriatic arthritis and in severe psoriasis.[22] It remains to be established which of these agents has greatest efficacy and whether DMARDs should be used in combination.

SPONDYLOARTHRITIS

The traditional objectives in the management of spondyloarthritis, epitomised by anklyosing spondylitis (AS), are to relieve pain and stiffness and to maintain mobility through a combination of regular NSAIDs and physiotherapy. NSAIDs provide symptomatic relief in the majority of patients with AS but are not disease modifying. Sulfasalazine is used for peripheral arthritis in AS but appears to have no value in spinal disease.

The anti-TNFα agents infliximab and etanercept are now also licensed for use in AS in the UK.[23] They are symptomatically effective for spondyloarthritis, and preliminary evidence from serial magnetic resonance imaging indicates that bone oedema regresses following TNFα blockade. There are as yet insufficient data to comment on the true disease-modifying effect of these agents. It is as yet unclear whether TNFα blockade should be used for peripheral arthritis.

GOUT

Patients with gout but no visible tophi have a uric acid pool that is two to three times normal and, as this exceeds the amount that can be carried in solution in the extracellular fluid, microcrystalline deposits form in tissues, including the joints, and cause pain; patients with tophi have a uric acid pool that may be 15 to 26 times normal.

Hyperuricaemia and gout from whatever cause, e.g. metabolic, renal disease, neoplasia, depends essentially on over-production and under-excretion of uric acid. Both mechanisms may operate in the same patient, but decreased renal clearance contributes to hyperuricaemia in most patients. Drugs may influence these processes as follows:

- *Overproduction* of uric acid, with excessive cell destruction releasing nucleic acids, occurs when myeloproliferative or lymphoproliferative disorders are treated by drugs.
- *Under-excretion* of uric acid is caused by all diuretics (except spironolactone), aspirin in low as opposed to high dose (see p. 260) (warn the patient), ethambutol, pyrazinamide, nicotinic acid, ciclosporin and alcohol (which increases uric acid synthesis and also causes a rise in blood lactic acid that inhibits tubular secretion of uric acid).[24]

The priority in an *acute attack* is to relieve the intense pain. NSAIDs are most commonly prescribed; indometacin, diclofenac, ketoprofen, naproxen, piroxicam, sulindac and etoricoxib are used, and azapropazone only for patients who have not responded. When NSAIDs are contraindicated, colchicine (see p. 261) is an alternative, with 1 mg taken orally followed by 500 micrograms every 2 h until the patient responds or develops adverse effects. A short course of oral prednisolone or intra-articular corticosteroid is also effective, except that the severity of joint pain may preclude intra-articular injection during an acute attack.

[22]Kyle S, Chandler D, Griffiths C E M et al 2005 Guideline for anti-TNF-alpha therapy in psoriatic arthritis. Rheumatology (Oxford) 44:390–397.

[23]Keat A, Barkham N, Bhalla A, Gaffney K, Marzo-Ortega H 2005 BSR guidelines for prescribing TNF-α blockers in adults with ankylosing spondylitis. Report of a working party of the British Society for Rheumatology. Rheumatology (Oxford) 44:939–947.

[24]Knowledge that alcohol induces acute gout is of long standing, and has been celebrated in verse:
A taste for drink, combined with gout,
Had doubled him up for ever.
Of that there is no matter of doubt—
No probable, possible shadow of doubt—
No possible doubt whatever.
(Don Alhambra's song in Act 1 of the Savoy opera, The Gondoliers or the King of Barataria. W S Gilbert [1836–1911].) But the author did not know the mechanisms.

Management of *chronic gout* should include a review of modifiable risk factors for hyperuricaemia, including obesity, hypertension, excessive alcohol intake, high dietary intake of purines (red meat, game, seafood, legumes), severe psoriasis and drugs (see above). Attention to these may be sufficient to prevent further attacks. Alternatively, or in addition, plasma uric acid levels may be reduced by allopurinol (see below) or a uricosuric agent such as sulfinpyrazone (see below) or probenecid (see p. 113). Rapid lowering of plasma uric acid by any means may actually precipitate acute gout, probably by causing the dissolution of tophi. Thus a NSAID or colchicine must be prescribed concomitantly for the first 3 months with uric acid-reducing medication. It can create an unfavourable impression if the patient, who has been told only that the drug will prevent gout, promptly has a severe attack.

Allopurinol inhibits xanthine oxidase, the enzyme that converts xanthine and hypoxanthine to uric acid. Patients taking allopurinol excrete less uric acid and more xanthine and hypoxanthine in the urine. These compounds are more soluble than uric acid (renal stones are rarely xanthine) and are more readily excreted in renal failure.

Allopurinol ($t_{1/2}$ 2 h) is readily absorbed from the gut, metabolised in the liver to alloxanthine ($t_{1/2}$ 25 h), which is also a xanthine oxidase inhibitor, and excreted unchanged by the kidney.

Allopurinol is indicated in recurrent gout (above), in blood diseases where there is spontaneous hyperuricaemia, and during treatment of myeloproliferative disorders where cell destruction creates a high uric acid load. Allopurinol prevents the hyperuricaemia due to diuretics and may be combined with a uricosuric agent.

Adverse effects include precipitation of an acute attack of gout (see above) and allergic reactions, which are uncommon but may be severe, e.g. exfoliative rash, arthralgia, fever, lymphadenopathy, vasculitis and hepatitis. Deaths have been reported. For this reason, allopurinol should not be commenced unless the diagnosis is certain, and attacks of gout are frequent despite lifestyle changes (see below). Allergy to allopurinol can be managed by desensitisation, using very small doses of the drug initially, and continuing over a long period.

Allopurinol prevents the oxidation of azathioprine, causing dangerous potentiation (see p. 113).

Sulfinpyrazone competitively inhibits the active transport of organic anions across the kidney tubule, both from the plasma to the tubular fluid and vice versa. The effect is dose dependent: at low dose sulfinpyrazone prevents secretion of uric acid into tubular fluid, and at high dose, and more powerfully, it prevents reabsorption, increasing its excretion in the urine. A net beneficial uricosuric action is obtained with an initial dose of 100–200 mg/day by mouth with food, increasing over 2–3 weeks to 600 mg/day, which should be continued until the plasma uric acid level is normal. The dose may then be reduced for maintenance, to as little as 200 mg daily. During initial therapy ensure that fluid intake is at least 2 L/day to prevent uric acid crystalluria. Other adverse effects are mainly gastrointestinal; sulfinpyrazone is contraindicated in peptic ulcer.

SYSTEMIC LUPUS ERYTHEMATOSUS

Management depends on the nature and severity of the disease, which range from mild rashes and polyarthralgia to life-threatening renal or cerebral vasculitis.

Mild lupus may be treated with hydroxychloroquine and lifestyle advice, such as avoidance of sun exposure or extreme stress. Most patients with SLE require a more potent immunomodulator, such as azathioprine, methotrexate or mycophenolate mofetil. Flares may be controlled by pulses of corticosteroid i.v. or i.m., or a progressively reduced oral course. Topical or intra-articular steroids are used, where appropriate. Severe manifestations, e.g. lupus nephritis, are generally managed with i.v. pulses of methylprednisolone and cyclophosphamide, often given as six pulses at 3–4-week intervals. The B cell-depleting therapy with rituximab is being used increasingly in moderate or severe SLE, particularly in young patients or to preserve child-bearing potential.

Co-morbidity is an important feature; in addition to excess cardiovascular mortality there is risk of osteoporosis (for protective measures, see RA, above), infection, malignancy and other autoimmune diseases. Patients with SLE should be screened for antiphospholipid antibodies, and antiplatelet therapy should be considered in those who are positive.

GIANT CELL ARTERITIS

The spectrum of giant cell arteritis (GCA) ranges from polymyalgia rheumatica to large arterial vasculitis, and includes temporal arteritis. Any form of the disease, but particularly temporal arteritis, may be complicated by visual loss; control of disease activity is therefore a medical emergency. Temporal arteritis necessitates corticosteroid in high oral dose, e.g. prednisolone 60 mg o.d. Polymyalgia rheumatica may be contolled with lower doses, e.g. prednisolone 30 mg o.d.

Other immunomodulators, e.g. azathioprine, methotrexate, anti-TNFα agents, do not have proven efficacy. As adrenal corticosteroids must usually be continued for at least 2 years, osteoprotection and gastroprotection (see above) assume importance.

OSTEOPOROSIS

See p. 664.

GUIDE TO FURTHER READING

Borer J S, Simon L S 2005 Cardiovascular and gastro-intestinal effects of COX-2 inhibitors and NSAIDs: achieving a balance. Arthritis Research and Therapy 7(Suppl 4):S14–S22

Choy E H S, Panayi G S 2001 Mechanisms of disease: cytokine pathways and joint inflammation in rheumatoid arthritis. New England Journal of Medicine 344(12):907–916

D'Cruz D P, Khamashta M A, Hughes G R V 2007 Systemic lupus erythematosus. Lancet 369:587–596

Emery P 2006 Treatment of rheumatoid arthritis. British Medical Journal 332:152–155

Hall F C, Dalbeth N 2005 Disease modification and cardiovascular risk reduction: two sides of the same coin? Rheumatology 44:1473–1482

Halushka M K, Halushka P V 2006 Towards individualized analgesic therapy: functional cyclooxygenase 1 and 2 haplotypes. Clinical Pharmacology and Therapeutics 79(5):404–406

Hunter D J, Felson D T 2006 Osteoarthritis. British Medical Journal 332:639–642

Littlejohn G O 2005 Musculoskeletal pain. Journal of the Royal College of Physicians of Edinburgh 35(4):340–344

Neame R, Doherty M 2005 Osteoarthritis update. Clinical Medicine 5(3):207–210

O'Dell J R 2004 Therapeutic strategies for rheumatoid arthritis. New England Journal of Medicine 350(25):2591–2602

Olsen N J, Stein C M 2004 New drugs for rheumatoid arthritis. New England Journal of Medicine 350(21):2167–2179

Rhen T, Cidlowski J A 2005 Antiinflammatory action of glucocorticoids: new mechanisms for old drugs. New England Journal of Medicine 353(16):1711–1723

Simpson C, Franks C, Morrison C, Lempp H 2005 The patient's journey: rheumatoid arthritis. British Medical Journal 331:887–889

Underwood M 2006 Diagnosis and management of gout. British Medical Journal 332:1315–1319

16

Drugs and the skin

SYNOPSIS

This account is confined to therapy directed primarily at the skin.

- Dermal pharmacokinetics
  –Vehicles for presenting drugs to the skin
- Selected topical preparations
  –Emollients and barrier preparations
  –Topical analgesics
  –Antipruritics
  –Analgesics
  –Adrenal corticosteroids
  –Sunscreens
- Cutaneous adverse drug reactions
  –Drug-specific rashes
- Approaches to some skin disorders
  –Psoriasis
  –Acne
  –Urticaria
  –Atopic dermatitis

DERMAL PHARMACOKINETICS

Human skin is a highly efficient self-repairing barrier that permits terrestrial life by regulating heat and water loss whilst preventing the ingress of noxious chemicals and microorganisms. A drug applied to the skin may diffuse from the stratum corneum into the epidermis and then into the dermis, to enter the capillary microcirculation and thus the systemic circulation (Fig. 16.1). The features of components of the skin in relation to drug therapy, whether for local or systemic effect, are worthy of examination.

The principal barrier to penetration resides in the multiple-layered lipid-rich stratum corneum. The passage of a drug through this layer is influenced by its:

- *Physicochemical features*: lipophilic drugs can utilise the *intra*cellular route because they readily cross cell walls, whereas hydrophilic drugs

principally take the *inter*cellular route, diffusing in fluid-filled spaces between cells.
- *Molecular size*: most therapeutic agents suitable for topical delivery measure 100–500 Da.

Drugs are presented in vehicles (bases[1]), designed to vary in the extent to which they increase hydration of the stratum corneum; e.g. oil-in-water creams promote hydration (see below). Increasing the water content of the stratum corneum via occlusion or hydration generally increases the penetration of both lipophilic and hydrophilic materials. This may be due to an increased fluid content of the lipid bilayers. The stratum corneum and stratum granulosum layers become more similar with hydration and occlusion, thus lowering the partition coefficient of the molecule passing through the interface. Some vehicles also contain substances intended to enhance penetration by reducing the barrier properties of the stratum corneum, e.g. fatty acids, terpenes, surfactants. Encapsulation of drugs into vesicular liposomes may enhance drug delivery to specific compartments of the skin, e.g. hair follicles.

Absorption through normal skin varies with site. From the sole of the foot and the palm of the hand it is relatively low; it increases progressively on the forearm, trunk, head and neck; and on the scrotum and vulva absorption is very high. Where the skin is damaged by inflammation, burn or exfoliation, barrier function is reduced and absorption is further increased.

If an occlusive dressing (impermeable plastic membrane) is used, absorption increases by as much as 10-fold (plastic pants for babies are occlusive, and some ointments are partially occlusive). Systemic toxicity can result from use of occlusive dressing over large areas.

Transdermal delivery systems are now used to administer drugs via the skin for systemic effect; the

---

[1]The chief ingredient of a mixture.

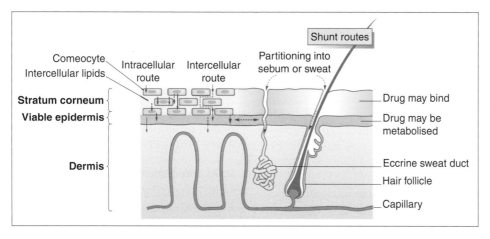

Fig. 16.1 Principal pathways opeating during topical drug delivery.

advantages and disadvantages of this route are discussed on p. 92.

VEHICLES FOR PRESENTING DRUGS TO THE SKIN

Dermatological formulations tend to be classified by their physical properties. The formulations below are described in order of decreasing water content. All water-based formulations must contain preservatives, e.g. chlorocresol, but these rarely cause allergic contact dermatitis.

Liquid formulations

Water or a solvent is the most important component. The preparation can be a soak, a bath or a paint. Wet dressings are generally used to cleanse, cool and relieve pruritus in acutely inflamed lesions, especially where there is much exudation, e.g. atopic eczema. The frequent reapplication and the cooling effect of evaporation of the water reduce the inflammatory response by inducing superficial vasoconstriction (an effect enhanced when alcohol is present in the formulation). Sodium chloride solution 0.9%, stringent substances, e.g. aluminium acetate lotion, or potassium permanganate soaks or compresses of approximately 0.01–0.05% can be used. The use of *lotions* (wet dressings) over very large areas can reduce body temperature dangerously in the old or the very ill.

Two-phase or multiple liquid shake lotions, e.g. calamine lotion, are essentially a convenient way of applying a powder to the skin with additional cooling due to evaporation of the water. They are contraindicated when there is much exudate, because crusts form. Lotions, after evaporation, sometimes produce excessive drying of the skin, but this can be reduced if oils are included, as in oily calamine lotion.

Creams

These are emulsions of either oil in water (washable; cosmetic 'vanishing' creams) or water in oil. The water content allows the cream to rub in well. A cooling effect (cold creams) is obtained with both groups as the water evaporates.

Oil-in-water creams, e.g. aqueous cream (see emulsifying ointment, below), mix with serous discharges and are especially useful as vehicles for water-soluble drugs. They may contain a wetting (surface tension-reducing) agent (cetomacrogol). Various other ingredients, e.g. calamine, zinc, may be added to it.

Water-in-oil creams, e.g. oily cream, zinc cream, behave like oils in that they do not mix with serous discharges, but their chief advantage over ointments (below) is that the water content makes them easier to spread and they give a better cosmetic effect. They act as lubricants and emollients, and can be used on hairy parts. Water-in-oil creams can be used as vehicles for lipid-soluble substances.

Creams, being less occlusive and effective at hydrating the stratum corneum, are not as effective for drug delivery as ointments.

Ointments

Ointments are greasy and thicker than creams. Some are both lipophilic and hydrophilic, i.e. by occlusion they promote dermal hydration, but are also water miscible. Other ointment bases are composed largely of lipid; by preventing water loss they have a hydrating effect on skin and are used in chronic dry conditions. Ointments contain fewer preservatives and are less likely to sensitise. There are two main kinds:

Water-soluble ointments include mixtures of macrogols and polyethylene glycols; their consistency can be varied readily. They are easily washed off and are used in burn dressings, as lubricants and as vehicles that readily allow passage of drugs into the skin, e.g. hydrocortisone.

Emulsifying ointment is made from emulsifying wax (cetostearyl alcohol and sodium lauryl sulphate) and paraffins. Aqueous cream is an oil-in-water emulsion of emulsifying ointment.

Non-emulsifying ointments do not mix with water. They adhere to the skin to prevent evaporation and heat loss, i.e. they can be considered a form of occlusive dressing (with increased systemic absorption of active ingredients); skin maceration may occur. Non-emulsifying ointments are helpful in chronic dry and scaly conditions, such as atopic eczema, and as vehicles; they are not appropriate where there is significant exudation. They are difficult to remove except with oil or detergents, and are messy and inconvenient, especially on hairy skin. Paraffin ointment contains beeswax, paraffins and cetostearyl alcohol.

Collodions and gels

Collodions are preparations of a thickening agent, e.g. cellulose nitrate (pyroxylin) dissolved in an organic solvent. The solvent evaporates rapidly and the resultant flexible film is used to hold a medicament, e.g. salicylic acid, in contact with the skin. They are irritant and inflammable, and are used to treat only small areas of skin.

Gels or *jellies* are semi-solid colloidal solutions or suspensions used as lubricants and as vehicles for drugs. They are sometimes useful for treating the scalp.

Pastes

Pastes, e.g. zinc compound paste, are stiff, semi-occlusive ointments containing insoluble powders. They are very adhesive and are valuable for treating highly circumscribed lesions whilst preventing spread of active ingredients on to surrounding skin. Their powder content enables them to absorb a moderate amount of discharge. They can be used as vehicles, e.g. coal tar paste, which is zinc compound paste with 7.5% coal tar. Lassar's paste is used as a vehicle for dithranol in the treatment of well circumscibed plaque psoriasis.

Solid preparations

Solid preparations such as dusting powders, e.g. zinc starch and talc,[2] may cool by increasing the effective surface area of the skin and they reduce friction between skin surfaces by their lubricating action. Although usefully absorbent, they cause crusting if applied to exudative lesions. They may be used alone or as specialised vehicles for, e.g., fungicides.

EMOLLIENTS AND BARRIER PREPARATIONS

Emollients hydrate the skin, and soothe and smooth dry scaly conditions. They need to be applied frequently as their effects are short lived. There is a variety of preparations but aqueous cream, in addition to its use as a vehicle (above), is effective when used as a soap substitute. Various other ingredients may be added to emollients, e.g. menthol, camphor or phenol for its mild antipruritic effect, and zinc and titanium dioxide as astringents.[3]

Barrier preparations. Many different kinds have been devised for use in medicine, in industry and in the home to reduce dermatitis. They rely on water-repellent substances, e.g. silicones (dimethicone cream), and on soaps, as well as on substances that form an impermeable deposit (titanium, zinc, calamine). The barrier preparations are useful in protecting skin from discharges and secretions (colostomies, nappy rash), but are ineffective when used under industrial working conditions. Indeed, the irritant properties of some barrier creams can enhance the percutane-

---

[2]Talc is magnesium silicate. It must not be used for dusting surgical gloves as it causes granulomas if it gets into mounds or body cavities.

[3]Astringents are weak protein precipitants, e.g. tannins, salts of aluminium and zinc.

ous penetration of noxious substances. A simple after-work emollient is more effective.

Silicone sprays and *occlusives*, e.g. hydrocolloid dressings, may be effective in preventing and treating pressure sores. Masking creams (camouflaging preparations) for obscuring unpleasant blemishes from view are greatly valued by patients.[4] They may consist of titanium oxide in an ointment base with colouring appropriate to the site and the patient.

TOPICAL ANALGESICS

Counterirritants and rubefacients are irritants that stimulate nerve endings in intact skin to relieve pain in skin (e.g. post-herpetic), viscera or muscle supplied by the same nerve root. All produce inflammation of the skin, which becomes flushed – hence the term 'rubefacients'. The best counterirritants are physical agents, especially heat. Many compounds have been used for this purpose and suitable preparations contain salicylates, nicotinates, menthol, camphor and capsaicin. Specific transient receptor potential (TRP) cation channels involved in sensory perception in skin can be stimulated by these drugs. The moderate heat receptor TRPV1 is sensitive to capsaicin as well as moderate heat (42–52°C), whereas TRPM8 is stimulated specifically by temperatures below 26°C and by menthol.

Topical non-steroidal anti-inflammatory drugs (NSAIDs) can be used to relieve musculoskeletal pain.

Local anaesthetics. Lidocaine and prilocaine are available as gels, ointments and sprays to provide reversible block of conduction along cutaneous nerves. Benzocaine and amethocaine (tetracaine) carry a high risk of sensitisation.

Volatile aerosol sprays, beloved by sportspeople, produce analgesia by cooling and by placebo effect.

ANTIPRURITICS

Mechanisms of itch are both peripheral and central. Itch (at least histamine-induced itch) is not a minor or low-intensity form of pain. Cutaneous histamine injection stimulates a specific group of C fibres with very low conduction speeds and large fields, distinct from those that signal pain. Second-order neurones then ascend via the spinothalamic tract to the thalamus. In the central nervous sytem, endogenous opioid peptides are released (the opioid antagonist naloxone can relieve some cases of intractable itch). Itch signalling appears to be under tonic inhibition by pain. If pain after histamine injection is reduced by opioid then itch results and, if pain is ablated by lidocaine, itch sensation increases. Prolonged inflammation in the skin may lead to peripheral and central sensitisation, thus leading non-itchy stimuli to be reinterpreted as itch.

Liberation of histamine and other autacoids in the skin also contributes and may be responsible for much of the itch of urticarial allergic reactions. Histamine release by bile salts may explain some, but not all, of the itch of obstructive jaundice. It is likely that other chemical mediators, e.g. serotonin and prostaglandins, are involved.

Generalised pruritus

In the absence of a primary dermatosis it is important to search for an underlying cause, e.g. iron deficiency, liver or renal failure, and lymphoma, but there remain patients in whom the cause either cannot be removed or is not known. Antihistamines (H_1-receptor), especially chlorphenamine and hydroxyzine orally, are used for their sedative or anxiolytic effect (except in urticaria); they should not be applied topically over a prolonged period because of risk of allergy. In severe pruritus, a sedative antidepressant may also help.

The itching of obstructive jaundice may be relieved by colestyramine and phototherapy with ultraviolet B light can be tried. Naltrexone offers short-term relief of the pruritus associated with haemodialysis.

Localised pruritus

Scratching or rubbing seems to give relief by converting the intolerable persistent itch into a more bearable pain. A vicious cycle can be set up in which itching provokes scratching, and scratching leads to infected skin lesions that itch, as in prurigo nodularis. Covering the lesion or enclosing it in a medicated bandage so as to prevent any further scratching or rubbing may help.

Topical corticosteroid preparations are used to treat the underlying inflammatory cause of pruritus, e.g. in eczema. A cooling application such as 0.5–2% menthol in aqueous cream is temporarily antipruritic.

---

[4]In the UK, the Red Cross offers a free cosmetic camouflage service through hospital dermatology departments.

Calamine and *astringents* (aluminium acetate, tannic acid) may help. Local anaesthetics do not offer any long-term solution and, as they are liable to sensitise the skin, they are best avoided. Topical doxepin can be helpful in localised pruritus but extensive use induces sedation and may cause allergic contact dermatitis.

Pruritus ani is managed by attention to any underlying disease, e.g. haemorrhoids, parasites, and hygiene. Emollients, e.g. washing with aqueous cream and a weak corticosteroid with antiseptic/anticandida application, may be used briefly to settle any acute eczema or superinfection. Some cases are a form of neurodermatitis, and an antihistamine with antianxiolytic properties, e.g. hydroxyzine, or a low-dose sedative antidepressant, e.g. doxepin, may be helpful. Secondary contact sensitivity, e.g. to local anaesthetics, must be considered.

ADRENOCORTICAL STEROIDS

Actions. Adrenal steroids possess a range of actions, of which the following are relevant to topical use:

- Inflammation is suppressed, particularly when there is an allergic factor, and immune responses are reduced.
- Antimitotic activity suppresses proliferation of keratinocytes, fibroblasts and lymphocytes (useful in psoriasis, but also causes skin thinning).
- Vasoconstriction reduces ingress of inflammatory cells and humoral factors to the inflamed area; this action (blanching effect on human skin) has been used to measure the potency of individual topical corticosteroids (see below).

Penetration into the skin is governed by the factors outlined at the beginning of the chapter. The vehicle should be appropriate to the condition being treated: an ointment for dry, scaly conditions; a water-based cream for weeping eczema.

Uses. Adrenal corticosteroids should be considered a symptomatic and sometimes curative, but not preventive, treatment. Ideally a potent steroid (see below) should be given only as a short course and reduced as soon as the response allows. Corticosteroids are most useful for eczematous disorders (atopic, discoid, contact), whereas dilute corticosteroids are especially useful for flexural psoriasis (where other therapies are highly irritant). Adrenal corticosteroids of highest potency are reserved for recalcitrant der-

matoses, e.g. lichen simplex, lichen planus, nodular prurigo and discoid lupus erythematosus.

Topical corticosteroids should be applied sparingly. The 'fingertip unit'[5] is a useful guide in educating patients (Table 16.1). The difficulties and dangers of systemic adrenal steroid therapy are sufficient to restrict such use to serious conditions (such as pemphigus and generalised exfoliative dermatitis) not responsive to other forms of therapy.

> **Guidelines for the use of topical corticosteroids**
>
> - Use for symptom relief and not prophylactically.
> - Choose the appropriate therapeutic potency (Table 16.2), e.g. mild for the face. In cases likely to be resistant, use a very potent preparation, e.g. for 3 weeks, to gain control, after which change to a less potent preparation.
> - Choose the appropriate vehicle, e.g. a water-based cream for weeping eczema, an ointment for dry scaly conditions.
> - Prescribe in small but adequate amounts so that serious overuse is unlikely to occur without the doctor knowing, e.g. weekly quantity by group (see Table 16.2): very potent 15 g; potent 30 g; other 50 g.
> - Occlusive dressing should be used only briefly. Note that babies' plastic pants are an occlusive dressing as well as being a social amenity.
> - If it's wet, dry it; if it's dry, wet it. The traditional advice contains enough truth to be worth repeating.
> - One or two applications a day are all that is usually necessary.

Choice. Topical corticosteroids are classified according to both drug and potency, i.e. therapeutic efficacy in relation to weight (see Table 16.2). Their potency is determined by the amount of vasoconstriction a topical corticosteroid produces (MacKenzie skin blanching test) and the degree to which it inhibits inflammation. Choice of preparation relates both to the disease and the site of intended use. High-potency preparations are commonly needed for lichen planus and discoid lupus erythematosus; weaker preparations (hydrocortisone 0.5–2.5%) are usually adequate for eczema, for use on the face and in childhood.

---

[5]The distance from the tip of the index finger to the first skin crease.

Table 16.1 Fingertip unit dosimetry for topical corticosteroids (distance from the tip of the adult index finger to the first crease)

Age	Face/neck	Arm/hand	Leg/foot	Trunk (front)	Trunk (back, including buttocks)
3–6 months	1	1	1.5	1	1.5
1–2 years	1.5	1.5	2	2	3
3–5 years	1.5	2	3	3	3.5
6–10 years	2	2.5	4.5	3.5	5
Adult	2.5	Arm: 3 Hand: 1	Leg: 6 Foot: 2	7	7

Table 16.2 Topical corticosteroid formulations conventionally ranked according to therapeutic potency

Potency	Formulations
Very potent	Clobetasol (0.05%); also formulations of diflucortolone (0.3%), halcinonide
Potent	Beclometasone (0.025%); also formulations of betamethasone, budesonide, desoximetasone, diflucortolone (0.1%), fluclorolone, fluocinolone (0.025%), fluocinonide, fluticasone, hydrocortisone butyrate, mometasone (once daily), triamcinolone
Moderately potent	Clobetasone (0.05%); also formulations of alclometasone, clobetasone, desoximetasone, fluocinolone (0.00625%), fluocortolone, fluandrenolone
Mildly potent	Hydrocortisone (0.1–1.0%); also formulations of alclomethasone, fluocinolone (0.0025%), methylprednisolone

Important note: the ranking is based on agent and its concentration; the same drug appears in more than one rank.

When a skin disorder requiring a corticosteroid is already infected, a preparation containing an antimicrobial is added, e.g. fusidic acid or clotrimazole. When the infection has been eliminated, the corticosteroid may be continued alone. Intralesional injections are used occasionally to provide high local concentrations without systemic effects in chronic dermatoses, e.g. hypertrophic lichen planus and discoid lupus erythematosus.

Adverse effects. Used with restraint, topical corticosteroids are effective and safe. Adverse effects are more likely with formulations ranked therapeutically as very potent or potent in Table 16.2.

Short-term use. Infection may spread.

Long-term use. Skin atrophy can occur within 4 weeks and may or may not be fully reversible. It reflects loss of connective tissue, which also causes striae (irreversible) and generally occurs at sites where dermal penetration is high (face, groins, axillae).

Other effects include: local hirsutism; perioral dermatitis (especially in young women), which responds to steroid withdrawal and may be mitigated by tetracycline by mouth for 4–6 weeks; depigmentation (local); monomorphous acne (local). Potent corticosteroids should not be used on the face unless this is unavoidable. Systemic absorption can lead to all the adverse effects of systemic corticosteroid use. Fluticasone propionate and mometasone furoate are rapidly metabolised following cutaneous absorption, which may reduce the risk of systemic toxicity. Suppression of the hypothalamic–pituitary axis occurs readily with overuse of the very potent agents, and when 20% of the body is under an occlusive dressing with mildly potent agents.

Other complications of occlusive dressings include infections (bacterial, candidal) and even heat stroke when large areas are occluded. Antifungal cream containing hydrocortisone and used for vaginal candidiasis may contaminate the urine and misleadingly suggest Cushing's syndrome.[6]

Applications to the eyelids may get into the eye and cause glaucoma.

[6]Kelly C J G, Ogilvie A, Evans J R et al 2001 Raised cortisol excretion rate in urine and contamination by topical steroids. British Medical Journal 322:594.

Rebound exacerbation of the disease can occur after abrupt cessation of therapy. This can lead the patient to reapply the steroid and so create a vicious cycle.

Allergy. Corticosteroids, particularly hydrocortisone and budesonide, or other ingredients in the formulation, may cause allergic contact dermatitis. The possibility of this should be considered when expected benefit fails to occur, e.g. varicose eczema.

SUNSCREENS (SUNBURN AND PHOTOSENSITIVITY)

Ultraviolet (UV) solar radiation (Fig. 16.2) is defined as:

- UVA (320–400 nm), which damages collagen, contributes to skin cancer and drug photosensitivity.
- UVB (280–320 nm), which is 1000 times more active than UVA, acutely causes sunburn and chronically skin cancer and skin aging.
- UVC (200–280 nm), which is prevented, at present, from reaching the earth at sea level by the stratospheric ozone layer, although it can cause skin injury at high altitude.

Protection of the skin

Protection from UV radiation is effected by:

Absorbent sunscreens. These organic chemicals absorb UVB and UVA at the surface of the skin (generally more effective for UVB).

UVB protection is provided by aminobenzoic acid and aminobenzoates (padimate-0), cinnamates, salicylates, camphors.

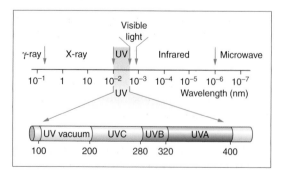

Fig. 16.2 The ultraviolet component of the electromagnetic spectrum.

UVA protection is provided by benzophenones (mexenone, oxybenzone), dibenzoylmethanes.

Reflectant sunscreens. Opaque inorganic minerals such as titanium dioxide, zinc oxide and calamine act as a physical barrier to UVB and UVA (especially zinc oxide); they are cosmetically unattractive; but the newer micronised preparations are more acceptable. Because they are able to protect against visible light; they are especially useful in photosensitivity disorders, e.g. porphyria.

The performance of a sunscreen is expressed as the sun protective factor (SPF), which refers to UVB (UVA is more troublesome to measure and the protection is indicated by a star rating system, with four stars providing the greatest). A SPF of 10 means that the dose of UVB required to cause erythema must be 10 times greater on protected than on unprotected skin. The SPF should be interpreted only as a rough guide; consumer use is more haphazard, and less liberal amounts are applied to the skin in practice.

Sunscreens should protect against both UVB and UVA. Absorbent and reflectant components are combined in some preparations. The washability of the preparation (including removal by sweat and swimming) is also relevant to efficacy and frequency of application; some penetrate the stratum corneum (padimate-0) and are more persistent than others.

Uses. Sunscreens are no substitute for light-impermeable clothing and sun avoidance (especially during peak hours of UV light). Daily application of sunscreen appears to protect more against UV-induced skin changes than intermittent use of the product. Methodical use has been demonstrated to reduce the incidence of cutaneous squamous cell carcinoma. Sunscreens are especially beneficial in protecting those who are photosensitive due to drugs (below) or disease, i.e. for photodermatoses such as photosensitivity dermatitis, polymorphic light eruption, cutaneous porphyrias and lupus erythematosus.

Treatment of mild sunburn is usually with a lotion such as oily calamine lotion. Severe cases are helped by topical corticosteroids. NSAIDs, e.g. indometacin, can help if given early, by preventing the formation of prostaglandins.

Drug photosensitivity

Drug photosensitivity means that an adverse effect occurs as a result of drug plus light, usually UVA;

sometimes even the amount of UV radiation from fluorescent light tubes is sufficient.

Systemically taken drugs that can induce photosensitivity are many, the most common being:[7]

- antimitotics: dacarbazine, vinblastine
- antimicrobials: demeclocycline, doxycycline, nalidixic acid, sulphonamides
- antipsychotics: chlorpromazine, prochlorperazine
- cardiac arrhythmic: amiodarone
- diuretics: furosemide, chlorothiazide, hydrochlorothiazide
- fibric acid derivatives, e.g. fenofibrate
- hypoglycaemics: tolbutamide
- NSAIDs: piroxicam
- psoralens (see below).

Topically applied substances that can produce photosensitivity include:

- para-aminobenzoic acid and its esters (used as sunscreens)
- coal tar derivatives
- psoralens from juices of various plants, e.g. bergamot oil
- 6-methylcoumarin (used in perfumes, shaving lotions, sunscreens).

There are two forms of photosensitivity:

Phototoxicity, like drug toxicity, is a normal effect of too high a dose of UV light in a subject who has been exposed to the drug. The reaction is like severe sunburn. The threshold returns to normal when the drug is withdrawn. Some drugs, notably NSAIDs, induce a 'pseudoporphyria', clinically resembling porphyria cutanea tarda and presenting with skin fragility, blisters and milia on sun-exposed areas, notably the backs of the hands.

Photoallergy, like drug allergy, is a cell-mediated immunological effect that occurs only in some people, and which may be severe with a small dose. Photoallergy due to drugs is the result of a photochemical reaction caused by UVA in which the drug combines with tissue protein to form an antigen. Reactions may persist for years after the drug is withdrawn; they are usually eczematous.

Systemic protection, as opposed to application of drug to exposed areas, should be considered when the topical measures fail.

Antimalarials such as hydroxychloroquine may be effective for short periods in polymorphic light eruption and in cutaneous lupus erythematosus.

Psoralens (obtained from citrus fruits and other plants), e.g. methoxsalen, are used to induce photochemical reactions in the skin. After topical or systemic administration of the psoralen and subsequent exposure to UVA there is an erythematous reaction that goes deeper than ordinary sunburn and may reach its maximum only after 48 h (sunburn maximum is 12–24 h). Melanocytes are activated and pigmentation occurs over the following week. This action is used to repigment areas of disfiguring depigmentation, e.g. vitiligo in blackskinned persons.

In the presence of UVA the psoralen interacts with DNA, forms thymine dimers and inhibits DNA synthesis. Psoralen plus UVA (PUVA) treatment is used chiefly in severe psoriasis (a disease characterised by increased epidermal proliferation) and cutaneous T-cell lymphoma.

Severe *adverse reactions* can occur with psoralens and UV radiation, including sunburn, increased risk of skin cancer (due to mutagenicity inherent in their action), cancer of the male genitalia, cataracts and accelerated skin aging; the treatment is used only by specialists.

Chronic exposure to sunlight induces wrinkling and yellowing due to the changes in the dermal connective tissue. Topical retinoids are used widely in an attempt to reverse some of these tissue changes.

MISCELLANEOUS COMPOUNDS

Keratolytics are used to destroy unwanted tissue, including warts and corns. Great care is obviously necessary to avoid ulceration. They include trichloracetic acid, salicylic acid and many others. Resorcinol and sulphur are mild keratolytics used in acne. Salicylic acid may enhance the efficacy of a topical steroid in hyperkeratotic disorders.

Tars are mildly antiseptic, antipruritic and inhibit keratinisation in an ill-understood way. They are safe in low concentrations and are used in psoriasis. Photosensitivity occurs and tar–UVB regimens

---

[7]Data from The Medical Letter 1995; 37:35.

are highly effective therapies for extensive psoriasis. There are very many preparations, which usually contain other substances, e.g. coal tar and salicylic acid ointment.

Ichthammol is a sulphurous, tarry, distillation product of fossilised fish (obtained in the Austrian Tyrol); it has a weaker effect than coal tar.

Zinc oxide provides mild astringent, barrier and occlusive actions. Calamine is basic zinc carbonate that owes its pink colour to added ferric oxide. It has a mild astringent action, and is used as a dusting powder and in shake and oily lotions.

Urea is used topically to assist skin hydration, e.g. in ichthyosis.

Insect repellents, e.g. against mosquitoes, ticks, fleas, such as deet (diethyl toluamide), dimethyl phthalate. These are applied to the skin and repel insects principally by vaporisation. They must be applied to all exposed skin, and sometimes also to clothes if their objective is to be achieved (some damage plastic fabrics and spectacle frames). Their duration of effect is limited by the rate at which they vaporise (dependent on skin and ambient temperature), by washing off (sweat, rain, immersion) and by mechanical factors causing rubbing (physical activity). They can cause allergic and toxic effects, especially with prolonged use.

Benzyl benzoate may be used on clothes; it resists one or two washings.

CUTANEOUS DRUG REACTIONS

Drugs applied locally or taken systemically often cause rashes. These take many different forms and the same drug may produce different rashes in different people. Types of drug rash include:

- Exanthems.
- Acute generalised exanthematous pustulosis.
- Fixed drug rash.
- Stevens–Johnson syndrome/erythema multiforme/toxic epidermal necrolysis.
- DRESS (drug rash with eosinophilia and systemic symptoms), e.g. hepatitis. The

> **Box 16.1   Mechanisms of cutaneous drug reactions**
>
> Immunological mechanisms
> - IgE dependent
> - Cytotoxic
> - Immune complex mediated
> - Cell mediated
>
> **Non-immunological mechanisms**
> - Overdosage
> - Cumulative toxicity
> - Delayed toxicity
> - Drug–drug–food interactions
> - Excacerbation of disease
>
> **Idiosyncratic**
> - Drug rash with eosinophilia and systemic symptoms (DRESS)
> - Toxic epidermal necrolysis/Stevens–Johnson syndrome
> - Drug reactions in setting of HIV
> - Drug-induced lupus

pathogenesis of DRESS is likely to be mulitfactorial. The factors include deficient detoxification of a drug metabolite in patients who are genetically susceptible, drug interactions, and direct effects of drug-specific T cells. Recent reports of co-infection with human herpesvirus (HHV)-6 or HHV-7 and a transient hypogammaglobulinaemia may prove important in anticonvulsant hypersensitivity.

Some of the mechanisms involved in drug-induced cutaneous reactions are described in Box 16.1.

Although drugs may change, the clinical problems remain depressingly the same: a patient develops a rash; he or she is taking many different tablets; which, if any, of these caused the eruption, and what should be done about it? It is no answer simply to stop all drugs, although the fact that this can often be done casts some doubt on the patient's need for them in the first place. All too often, potentially valuable drugs are excluded from further use on totally inadequate grounds. Clearly some guidelines are useful, but no simple set of rules exists that can cover this complex subject:[8]

[8]Hardie R A, Savin J A 1979 Drug-induced skin diseases. British Medical Journal 1:935 (to whom we are grateful for the quotation and classification).

1. *Can other skin diseases be excluded and are the skin changes compatible with a drug cause?* Clinical features that indicate a drug cause include the type of primary lesion (blisters, pustules), distribution of lesions (acral lesions in erythema multiforme), mucosal involvement and evidence of systemic involvement (fever, lymphadenopathy, visceral involvement).

2. *Which drug is most likely to be responsible?* Document all of the drugs the patient has been exposed to and the date of introduction of each drug. Determine the interval between commencement date and the date of the skin eruption. Chronology is important, with most reactions occurring about 10–12 days after starting a new drug or within 2–3 days in previously exposed patients. A search of standard literature sources of adverse reactions, including the pharmaceutical company data, can be helpful in identifying suspect drugs.

3. *Are any further tests worthwhile?* Excluding infectious causes of skin eruptions is important, e.g. viral exanthems, mycoplasma. A skin biopsy in cases of non-specific dermatitis is helpful as a predominance of eosinophils would support a drug precipitant.

4. *Is any treatment needed?* Supporting the ill patient and stopping the causative drug is crucial.

DRUG-SPECIFIC RASHES

Despite great variability, some hints at drug-specific or characteristic rashes from drugs taken systemically can be discerned; some examples are as follows:

- *Acne and pustular*: corticosteroids, androgens, ciclosporin, penicillins.
- *Allergic vasculitis*: sulphonamides, NSAIDs, thiazides, chlorpropamide, phenytoin, penicillin, retinoids.
- *Anaphylaxis*: X-ray contrast media, penicillins, angiotensin-converting enzyme (ACE) inhibitors.
- *Bullous pemphigoid*: furosemide (and other sulphonamide-related drugs), ACE inhibitors, penicillamine, penicillin, PUVA therapy.
- *Eczema*: penicillins, phenothiazines.
- *Exanthematic/maculopapular* reactions are the most frequent; unlike a viral exanthem, the eruption typically starts on the trunk; the face is relatively spared. Causes include antimicrobials, especially ampicillin, sulphonamides and derivatives (sulphonylureas, furosemide and thiazide diuretics).

- *Morbilliform* (measles-like) eruptions typically recur on rechallenge.
- *Erythema multiforme*: NSAIDs, sulphonamides, barbiturates, phenytoin.
- *Erythema nodosum*: dermatitis and sulphonamides, oral contraceptives, prazosin.
- *Exfoliative erythroderma*: gold, phenytoin, carbamazepine, allopurinol, penicillins, neuroleptics, isoniazid.
- *Fixed eruptions* are eruptions that recur at the same site, often circumoral, with each administration of the drug: phenolphthalein (laxative self-medication), sulphonamides, quinine (in tonic water), tetracycline, barbiturates, naproxen, nifedipine.
- *Hair loss*: cytotoxic anticancer drugs, acitretin, oral contraceptives, heparin, androgenic steroids (women), sodium valproate, gold.
- *Hypertrichosis*: corticosteroids, ciclosporin, doxasosin, minoxidil.
- *Lichenoid eruption*: β-adrenoceptor blockers, chloroquine, thiazides, furosemide, captopril, gold, phenothiazines.
- *Lupus erythematosus*: hydralazine, isoniazid, procainamide, phenytoin, oral contraceptives, sulfazaline.
- *Purpura*: thiazides, sulphonamides, sulphonylureas, phenylbutazone, quinine. Aspirin induces a capillaritis (pigmented purpuric dermatitis).
- *Photosensitivity*: see above.
- *Pemphigus*: penicillamine, captopril, piroxicam, penicillin, rifampicin.
- *Pruritus* unassociated with rash: oral contraceptives, phenothiazines, rifampicin (cholestatic reaction).
- *Pigmentation*: oral contraceptives (chloasma in photosensitive distribution), phenothiazines, heavy metals, amiodarone, chloroquine (pigmentation of nails and palate, depigmentation of the hair), minocycline.
- *Psoriasis* may be aggravated by β-blockers, lithium and antimalarials.
- *Scleroderma-like*: bleomycin, sodium valproate, tryptophan contaminants (eosinophila–myalgia syndrome).
- *Serum sickness*: immunoglobulins and other immunomodulatory blood products.
- *Stevens–Johnson syndrome and toxic epidermal necrolysis* (TENS): e.g. anticonvulsants, sulphonamides, aminopenicillins, NSAIDs, allopurinol, chlormezanone, corticosteroids.

- *Urticaria and angio-oedema*: penicillins, ACE inhibitors, gold, NSAIDs, e.g. aspirin, codeine.

Patients with the acquired immunodeficiency syndrome (AIDS) have an increased risk of adverse reactions, which are often severe. Recovery after withdrawal of the causative drug generally begins within a few days, but lichenoid reactions may not improve for weeks.

Diagnosis

The patient's drug history may give clues. Reactions are commoner during early therapy (days) than after the drug has been given for months. Diagnosis by purposeful readministration of the drug (challenge) is not recommended, especially in patients suffering a generalised effect or with mucosal involvement as it may precipitate toxic epidermal necrolysis.

Patch and photopatch tests are useful in contact dermatitis as they reproduce the causative process, but should be performed only by those with special experience. Fixed drug eruptions can sometimes be reproduced by patch testing with the drug over the previously affected site.

Intradermal tests introduce all the problems of allergy to drugs, e.g. metabolism, combination with protein, fatal anaphylaxis.

Treatment

Treatment involves supportive care and removal of the causative drug. Use cooling applications and antipruritics; use a histamine H_1-receptor blocker systemically for acute urticaria. The use of adrenal corticosteroids is controversial. It may be useful for severe exanthems if the incriminated drug is crucial for other concurrent disease, and is useful for internal organ disease involvement in DRESS. The use of human-derived immunoglobulin infusions is increasingly advocated in the treatment of toxic epidermal necrolysis.

SAFETY MONITORING

Several drugs commonly used in dermatology should be monitored regularly for (principally systemic) adverse effects. These include:

- *aciclovir* (plasma creatinine)
- *azathioprine* (blood count and liver function)
- *colchicine* (blood count, plasma creatinine)
- *ciclosporin* (plasma creatinine)
- *dapsone* (liver function, blood count including reticulocytes)

- *methotrexate* (blood count, liver function)
- *PUVA* (liver function, antinuclear antibodies)
- *aromatic retinoids* (liver function, plasma lipids).

INDIVIDUAL DISORDERS

Table 16.3 is not intended to give the complete treatment of even the commoner skin conditions but merely to indicate a reasonable approach. Secondary infections of ordinarily uninfected lesions may require added topical or systemic antimicrobials. Analgesics, sedatives or tranquillisers may be needed in painful or uncomfortable conditions, or where the disease is intensified by emotion or anxiety.

PSORIASIS

In psoriasis there is increased epidermal undifferentiated cell proliferation and inflammation of the epidermis and dermis. The consequence of increased numbers of immature horn cells containing abnormal keratin is that an abnormal stratum corneum is formed. Drugs are used to:

- dissolve keratin (keratolysis)
- inhibit cell division.

An emollient such as aqueous cream will reduce the inflammation. The proliferated cells may be eliminated by a *dithranol* (antimitotic) preparation applied accurately to the lesions (but not on the face or scalp) for 1 h and then removed as it is irritant to normal skin and stains skin, blond hair and fabrics. A suitable regimen may begin with 0.1% dithranol, increasing to 1%. Dithranol is available in cream bases or in Lassar's paste (the preparations are not interchangeable). It is used daily until the lesions have disappeared and may produce prolonged remissions of psoriasis. Tar (antimitotic) preparations are used in a similar way, are less irritating to normal skin and are commonly used for psoriasis of the scalp.[9]

[9]But are not without risk. A 46-year-old man whose psoriasis was treated with topical corticosteroids, UV light and tar was seen in the hospital courtyard bursting into flames. A small ring of fire began several centimetres above the sternal notch and encircled his neck. The patient promptly put out the fire. He admitted to lighting a cigarette just before the fire, the path of which corresponded to the distribution of the tar on his body (Fader D J, Metzman M S 1994 Smoking, tar, and psoriasis: a dangerous combination. New England Journal of Medicine 330:1541).

Table 16.3 Summary of treatment for selected skin disorders

Condition	Treatment	Remarks
Androgenic alopecia	Topical 2% or 5% minoxidil is worth trying. Finasteride can stop hair loss and increase hair density in 50% of men.	The response occurs in 4–12 months; hair loss resumes when therapy is stopped.
Alopecia areata	Potent topical or intralesional corticosteroids may be useful in the short term.	Although distressing, the condition is often self-limiting. A few individuals have responded to PUVA or contact sensitisation induced by diphencyprone.
Dermatitis herpetiformis	Dapsone is typically effective in 24 h, or sulfapyridine. Long-term gluten-free diet.	Methaemoglobinaemia may complicate dapsone therapy.
Hirsutism in women	Combined oestrogen–progestogen contraceptive pill: cyproterone plus ethinylestradiol (Dianette). Spironolactone, cimetidine have been used.	Local cosmetic approaches: epilation by wax or electrolysis; depilation (chemical), e.g. thioglycollic acid, barium sulfide. Laser epilation is expensive and the results are transient.
Hyperhidrosis	Astringents reduce sweat production, especially aluminium chloride hexahydrate. Antimuscarinics, e.g. glycoppyrolate (topical or systemic), may help and may be used with iontophoresis. Botulinum toxin can be used to provide temporary remission (3–4 months) and is most useful for the axilla. Sympathectomy is used occasionally but may be complicated by compensatory hyperhidrosis.	The characteristic smell is produced by bacterial action, so cosmetic deodorants contain antibacterials rather than substances that reduce sweat.
Impetigo	Topical antibiotics, e.g. mupirocin, fusidic acid.	In severe cases (resistant organisms) sytemic macrolide, cephalosporin antibiotics.
Intertrigo	Cleansing lotions, powders to cleanse, lubricate and reduce friction. A dilute corticosteroid with anticandidal cream is often helpful.	No evidence that new azoles are superior to nystatin.
Larva migrans	Cryotherapy. Albendazole (single dose) or topical thiabendazole.	
Lichen planus	Antipruritics (menthol); potent topical corticosteroid.	PUVA or retinoids in severe cases.
Lichen simplex (neurodermatitis)	Antipruritics (menthol); topical corticosteroid; sedating antihistamines.	Occluding the lesion so as to prevent scratch–itch cycle to patient.
Lupus erythematosus	Photoprotection (including against UVA) is essential. Potent adrenal corticosteroid topically or intralesionally. Hydroxychloroquine or mepacrine. Monitor for retinal toxicity when treatment is long term. Other agents include acetretin and auranofin.	
Malignancies	Actinic keratoses and Bowen's disease can be treated with topical 5-fluorouracil (skin irritation is to be expected) or cryotherapy. Imiquimod is a possible topical alternative. Extensive lesions may respond to photodynamic therapy: the skin is sensitised using a topical haematoporphyrin derivative, e.g. aminolaevulinic acid, and irradiated with a visible light or laser source. Cutaneous T-cell lymphoma in its early stages is best treated conservatively; PUVA will often clear lesions for several months or years; alternatives include topical nitrogen mustard, e.g. carmustine.	
Nappy rash	Prevention: rid re-usable nappies of soaps, detergents and ammonia by rinsing. Change frequently and use an emollient cream, e.g. aqueous cream, to protect skin. Costly disposable nappies are useful but must also be changed regularly. Cure: zinc cream or calamine lotion plus above measures.	

(Continued)

Table 16.3 Summary of treatment for selected skin disorders—Cont'd

Condition	Treatment	Remarks
Onychomycosis	Confirm dermatophyte infection with microscopy and culture. Terbinafine, two pulses of itraconazole or 6–9 months of once-weekly fluconazole is used for fingernail onychomycosis. For toenail disease, terbinafine is used for 12–16 weeks; 3–4 pulses of itraconazole or fluconazole once per week for 9–15 months can be used.	The newer oral antifungals have not been approved for use in children.
Pediculosis (lice)	Permethrin, phenothrin, carbaryl or malathion (anticholinesterases, with safety depending on more rapid metabolism in humanas than in insects, and on low absorption).	Usually two applications 7 days apart to kill lice from eggs that survive the first dose. Physical measures including regular combing and keeping hair short are important.
Pemphigus and pemphigoid	Milder cases can be treated with topical corticosteroids and tetracyclines. Systemic steroids and immunosuppressants (azathioprine, mycophenylate) are useful for severe disease. Plasmapheresis and IVIg may also be useful.	
Pityriasis rosea	Antipruritics and emollients as appropriate; UVB phototherapy.	The disease is self-limiting.
Pyoderma gangrenosum	Topical therapies may include corticosteroids, tacrolimus. Systemic corticosteroids are usually effective. Immunosuppressives, e.g. ciclosporin, may be used for steroid-sparing effect. Some patients respond to dapsone, minocycline or clofazamine.	
Rosacea	Topical metronidazole and systemic tetracycline. Retinoids are useful for severe cases.	Control pustulation in order to prevent secondary scarring and rhinophyma.
Scabies (*Sarcoptes scabiei*)	Permethrin dermal cream. Alternatives include benzyl benzoate or ivermectin (single dose), especially for outbreaks in closed communities. Crotamiton or calamine for residual itch. Topical corticosteroid to settle persistent hypersensitivity.	Apply to all members of the household, immediate family or partner. Change underclothes and bedclothes after application.
Seborrhoeic dermatitis: dandruff (*Pityriasis capitis*)	A proprietary shampoo with pyrithione, selenium sulfide or coal tar; ketoconazole shampoo in more severe cases. Occasionally a corticosteroid lotion may be necessary.	
Tinea capitis	In children griseofulvin for 6–8 weeks is effective and safe. Terbinafine for 4 weeks is effective against *Trichophyton* spp. Microsporum will respond to 6 weeks' therapy with terbinafine.	Antifungal shampoos can reduce active shedding in patients treated with oral antifungals.
Tinea pedis	Most cases will respond to tolnaftate or undecenoic acid creams. Allylamine (terbinafine) creams are possibly more effective than azoles in resistant cases.	
Venous leg ulcers	Limb compression is the mainstay of therapy. Other agents including pentoxifylline and skin grafts are useful adjuncts to compression therapy.	
Viral warts	All treatments are destructive and should be applied with precision. Salicylic acid in collodion daily. Many other caustic (keratolytic) preparations exist, e.g. salicylic and lactic acid paint or gel. For plantar warts, formaldehyde or glutaraldehyde; for plantar or anogenital warts, podophyllin (antimitotic). Follow the manufacturer's instructions meticulously. If one topical therapy fails it is worth trying a different type. Topical imiquimod is an alternative for genital warts; it is irritant. Careful cryotherapy (liquid nitrogen).	Warts often disappear spontaneously. Cryotherapy can cause ulceration, damage the nail matrix and leave permanent scars.

Topical adrenal corticosteroids act principally by reducing inflammation. Application, especially under occlusive dressings, can be very effective at suppressing the disease, but increased doses (concentrations) become necessary and rebound, which may be severe, follows withdrawal. For this reason potent corticosteroids should never be used except for lesions on the scalp, palms and soles. Corticosteroids of mild potency may be used for flexural psoriasis where other drugs are too irritating.

Systemic corticosteroid administration should be avoided, for high doses are needed to suppress the disease, which is liable to recur in a more unstable form when treatment is withdrawn, as it must be if complications of long-term steroid therapy are to be avoided.

Calcipotriol and tacalcitol are analogues of calcitriol, the most active natural form of vitamin D (see p. 588). They inhibit cell proliferation and encourage cell differentiation. Although they have less effect on calcium metabolism than does calcitriol, excessive use (more than 100 g/week) can raise the plasma calcium concentration.

Vitamin A (retinols) plays a role in epithelial function, and the retinoic acid derivative *acitretin* (orally) inhibits psoriatic hyperkeratosis over 4–6 weeks. Acitretin should be used in courses (6–9 months) with intervals (3–4 months). It is teratogenic, like the other vitamin A derivatives. It is not recommended for use in women of childbearing potential because the drug is stored in the liver and in fat, and active metabolites are released many months after cessation of therapy.

UVB light is effective in guttate psoriasis and potentiates the effects of topical agents such as calcipotriol (act by reducing cell division), antimitotic agents like tar (Goeckerman's regimen) and dithranol (Ingram's regimen). Oral psoralen followed by UVA light (PUVA) may be used to clear severe cases of psoriasis, with remissions of more than a year being achievable. Long-term PUVA therapy is associated with an increased risk of cutaneous squamous cell carcinoma and melanoma development (especially in those given maintenance treatment).

Ciclosporin, the systemic calcineurin inhibitor (see p. 556), has been instrumental in shifting the focus of psoriasis research from keratinocyte abnormalities to immune perturbations. It has a rapid onset of action and is useful in achieving remissions in all forms of psoriasis. Monitoring of blood pressure and renal function is mandatory. Severe adverse effects, including renal toxicity, preclude its being used as long-term suppressive therapy.

Since the introduction of ciclosporin for psoriasis, much research has focused on new ways of disrupting T lymphocytes and the cytokines involved in the induction and maintenance of psoriasis. These drugs target specific cellular events, e.g. induction of T-lymphocytic apoptosis, inhibition of tumour necrosis factor. The exact role of these promising therapies is still evolving.

Folic acid antagonists, e.g. methotrexate, can also suppress epidermal activity and inhibit T and B lymphocytes, and are especially useful when psoriasis is severe and remits rapidly with other treatments. Methotrexate is particularly of use if there is associated disabling arthritis. Platelet count, renal and liver function must be monitored regularly. When 1.5 g of the total dose has been taken, liver biopsy should be considered, especially in those with predisposing hepatic steatosis.

It is plain from this brief outline that treatment of psoriasis requires considerable judgement and choice will depend on the patient's sex, age and the severity of the condition. Topical therapies such as calcipotriol, tar or dithranol-containing compounds should be the mainstay of limited mild psoriasis. Topical corticosteroids can be used for psoriasis inversus under close supervision, as over-use can lead to cutaneous atrophy. Phototherapy is useful for widespread psoriasis where compliance with topical treatments is difficult. Resistant disease is best managed by the specialist who may utilise a rotation of treatments, including retinoids, methotrexate, ciclosporin, UVB plus dithranol and PUVA + acitretin, to reduce the unwanted effects of any single therapy. Fumaric acid compounds, hydroxyurea and specific biological agents are useful for severe cases.

ACNE

Acne vulgaris results from disordered function of the pilosebaceous follicle whereby abnormal keratin and sebum (the production of which is androgen driven) form debris that plugs the mouth of the follicle. *Propionibacterium acnes* colonises the debris.

287

Bacterial action releases inflammatory fatty acids from the sebum, resulting in inflammation. Acne is a chronic disorder and if uncontrolled can lead to irreversible scarring.

The following measures are used progressively and selectively as the disease becomes more severe; they may need to be applied for up to 3–6 months:

- *Mild keratolytic* (exfoliating, peeling) formulations unblock pilosebaceous ducts, e.g. benzoyl peroxide, sulphur, salicylic acid, azelaic acid.
- *Systemic or topical antimicrobial therapy* (tetracycline, erythromycin, lymecycline) is used over months (expect 30% improvement after 3 months). Bacterial resistance is not a problem; benefit is due to suppression of bacterial lipolysis of sebum, which generates inflammatory fatty acids. (Avoid minocycline because of adverse effects, including raised intracranial pressure and drug-induced lupus.)
- *Vitamin A (retinoic acid) derivatives* reduce sebum production and keratinisation. Vitamin A is a teratogen. *Tretinoin* (Retin-A) is applied topically (but not in combination with other keratolytics). Tretinoin should be avoided in sunny weather and in pregnancy. Benefit is seen in about 10 weeks. *Adapalene*, a synthetic retinoid, may be better tolerated as it is less irritant. *Isotretinoin* (Roaccutane) orally is highly effective (a single course of treatment to a cumulative dose of 100 mg/kg is curative in 94% of patients), but is known to be a *serious teratogen*; its use should generally be confined to the more severe cystic and conglobate cases, where other measures have failed. Fasting blood lipids should be measured before and during therapy (levels of cholesterol and triglycerides may rise). Women of childbearing potential should be fully informed of this risk, pregnancy-tested before commencement and use contraception for 4 weeks before, during and for 4 weeks after cessation.[10] Other adverse effects are described, including mood change and severe depression.

- *Hormone therapy*. The objective is to reduce androgen production or effect by using (1) oestrogen, to suppress hypothalamic–pituitary gonadotrophin production, or (2) an antiandrogen (cyproterone). An oestrogen alone as initial therapy to get the acne under control or, in women, the cyclical use of an oral contraceptive containing 50 micrograms of oestrogen diminishes sebum secretion by 40%. A combination of ethinylestradiol and cyproterone (Dianette) orally is also effective in women (it has a contraceptive effect, which is desirable as the cyproterone may feminise a male fetus).

URTICARIA

Acute urticaria (named after its similarity to the sting of a nettle, *Urtica*) and *angio-oedema* usually respond well to H_1-receptor antihistamines, although severe cases are relieved more quickly with use of adrenaline (epinephrine) (adrenaline injection 1 mg/mL: 0.1–0.3 mL s.c.). A systemic corticosteroid may be needed in severe cases, e.g. urticarial vasculitis.

In some individuals, urticarial weals are provoked by physical stimuli, e.g. friction (dermographism), heat or cold. Exercise may induce weals, particularly on the upper trunk (cholinergic urticaria). Physical urticarias are particularly challenging to treat.

Chronic urticaria usually responds to an H_1-receptor antihistamine with low sedating properties, e.g. cetirizine or loratidine. Terfenadine is also effective, but may cause dangerous cardiac arrhythmias if the recommended dose is exceeded or if it is administered with drugs (or grapefruit juice) that inhibit its metabolism. But lack of sleep increases the intensity of itch (similar to pain), and a sedating antihistamine may be useful at night. H_2-receptor antihistamines may be added for particularly resistant cases. In some patients with antibodies against the Fc receptor on mast cells, immunosuppressive therapies (e.g. ciclosporin, methotrexate or intravenous immunoglobulin) may be required.

Hereditary angio-oedema, with deficiency of C_1-esterase inhibitor (a complement inhibitor), may not respond to antihistamines or corticosteroid but only to fresh frozen plasma or, preferably, C_1-inhibitor concentrate. Delay in initiating the treatment may lead to death from laryngeal oedema (try adrenaline (epinephrine) i.m. in severe cases). For long-term prophylaxis an androgen (stanozolol,

---

[10]The risk of birth defect in a child of a woman who has taken isotretinoin when pregnant is estimated at 25%. Thousands of abortions have been performed in such women in the USA. It is probable that hundreds of damaged children have been born. There can be no doubt that there has been irresponsible prescribing of this drug, e.g. in less severe cases. The fact that a drug with such a grave effect is still permitted to be available is attributed to its high efficacy.

danazol) can be effective. Hereditary angio-oedema is a very rare cause of simple urticaria.

ATOPIC DERMATITIS

Atopic dermatitis is a chronic condition, and treatment must be individualised and centred around preventive measures. Successful management includes the elimination of precipitating and exacerbating factors, and maintaining the skin barrier function by use of topical or systemic agents.

Immunological triggers of atopic dermatitis vary and can include aeroallergens, detergents (including soaps), irritants, climate and microorganisms. Identification and modification of these factors is useful.

Antiseptic containing soap substitutes are useful in reducing pro-inflammatory *Staphylococcus aureus* colonies.

In *acute* weeping dermatitis, lotions, wet dressing or soaks (sodium chloride, potassium permanganate) are used.

In *subacute* and *chronic* disease, skin care with occlusive emollients helps to offset the xerosis (dryness) that creates microfissures in the skin and disturbs its normal barrier function. Topical corticosteroids form the cornerstone of pharmacological therapy. In general, the lowest-potency topical steroid should be used initially and higher-potency agents considered only if these fail, the aim being to switch to intermittent steroid-use protocols once the disease has been controlled. Higher-potency agents are usually inappropriate for young children and highly permeable areas. Very potent steroids should not be used for longer than two consecutive weeks to minimise the likelihood of unwanted effects.

The calcineurin inhibitors, tacrolimus and pimecrolimus, are effective topically. Local irritation may result but they do not cause skin atrophy and so are especially useful on the face. Long-term safety data are still lacking.

Sedating H_1-receptor antihistamines with anxiolytic properties may assist with sleep and nocturnal itch. A 2-week course of systemic corticosteroid is useful, especially in cases of acute allergic contact dermatitis. Long-term oral immunosuppression with ciclosporin, mycophenylate or azathioprine should be undertaken only in specialist centres. Although there is minimal objective improvement in atopic dermatitis with UVB phototherapy, patients have consistently reported subjective improvement in itch.

SKIN INFECTIONS

Superficial bacterial infections, e.g. impetigo, eczema, are commonly staphylococcal or streptococcal. They are treated with a topical antimicrobial for less than 2 weeks, applied twice daily after removal of crusts that prevent access of the drug, e.g. with a povidone–iodine preparation. Very extensive cases need systemic treatment.

Topical *sodium fusidate* and *mupirocin* are preferred (as they are not used ordinarily for systemic infections and therefore development of drug-resistant strains is less likely to have any serious consequences). Framycetin and polymyxins are also used. Absorption of neomycin from all topical preparations can cause serious injury to the eighth cranial nerve. It is also a contact sensitiser.

When prolonged treatment is required, topical antiseptics (e.g. chlorhexidine) are preferred and bacterial resistance is less of a problem.

Combination of an antimicrobial drug with a corticosteroid (to suppress inflammation) can be useful for secondarily infected eczema.

The *disadvantages* of antimicrobials are contact allergy and developments of resistant organisms (which may cause systemic, as well as local, infection). Failure to respond may be due to the development of a contact allergy (which may be masked by corticosteroid).

Infected leg ulcers generally do not benefit from long-term antimicrobials, although topical metronidazole is useful when the ulcer is malodorous due to colonisation with Gram-negative organisms. An antiseptic (plus a protective dressing with compression) is preferred if antimicrobial therapy is needed.

Nasal carriers of staphylococci may be cured (often temporarily) by topical mupirocin or neomycin plus chlorhexidine.

Deep bacterial infections, e.g. boils, generally do not require antimicrobial therapy, but if they do it should be systemic. Cellulitis requires systemic chemotherapy initially with benzylpenicillin and flucloxacillin.

Infected burns are treated with a variety of antimicrobials, including silver sulfadiazine and mupirocin.

Fungal infections. Superficial dermatophyte or *Candida* infections purely involving the skin can be treated with a topical imidazole, e.g. clotrimazole, miconazole. Pityriasis versicolor, a yeast infection, primarily involves the trunk in young adults. It responds to topical antifungals or selenium sulfide preparations; severe infection may require systemic itraconazole. It tends to recur and regular treatments are frequently necessary. Invasion of hair or nails by a dermatophyte or a deep mycosis requires systemic therapy; terbinafine is the most effective drug. Terbinafine and griseofulvin are ineffective against yeasts, for which itraconazole is an alternative. Itraconazole can be used in weekly pulses each month for 3–4 months; it is less effective against dermatophytes than terbinafine.

Viral infections. Topical antivirals, e.g. aciclovir, penetrate the stratum corneum poorly. Aciclovir is used systemically for severe infections, e.g. eczema herpeticum.

Parasitic infection. Topical parasiticides (see Table 16.3 for details).

Disinfection and cleansing of the skin. Numerous substances are used according to circumstances:

- for skin preparation prior to injection: ethanol or isopropyl alcohol
- for disinfection: chlorhexidine salts, cationic surfactant (cetrimide), soft soap, povidone–iodine (iodine complexed with polyvinylpyrrollidone), phenol derivatives (hexachlorophene, triclosan) and hydrogen peroxide.

GUIDE TO FURTHER READING

Bystryn J-C, Rudolph J 2005 Pemphigus. Lancet 366:61–73

Griffiths C E M, Barker J N W N 2007 Psoriasis 1 Pathogenesis and clinical features of psoriasis. Lancet 370:263–271

Heukelbach J, Feldmeier H 2006 Scabies. Lancet 367:1767–1774

James W D 2005 Acne. New England Journal of Medicine 352(14):1463–1472

Kaplan K P 2002 Chronic urticaria and angioedema. New England Journal of Medicine 346(3):175–179

Kullavanijaya P, Lim H W 2005 Photoprotection. Journal of the American Academy of Dermatology 52(6):937–958

Lebwohl M 2005 A clinician's paradigm in the treatment of psoriasis. Journal of the American Academy of Dermatology 53(Suppl 1):S59–S69

Menter A, Griffiths C E M 2007 Psoriasis 2 Current and future management of psoriasis. Lancet 370:272–284

Powell F C 2005 Rosacea. New England Journal of Medicine 352(8):793–803

Rosenfield R L 2005 Hirsutism. New England Journal of Medicine 353(24):2578–2588

Schwartz R A 2004 Superficial fungal infections. Lancet 364:1173–1182.

Smith C H, Barker J N W N 2006 Psoriasis and its management. British Medical Journal 333:380–384

Stern R S 2004 Treatment of photoaging. New England Journal of Medicine 350:1526–1534

Thompson J F, Scolyer R, Kefford R 2005 Cutaneous melanoma. Lancet 365:687–701

Williams H C 2005 Atopic dermatitis. New England Journal of Medicine 352(22):2314–2324

Yosipovitch G, Greaves M, Schmelz M 2003 Itch. Lancet 361:690–694

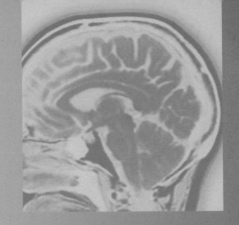

Section 4

NERVOUS SYSTEM

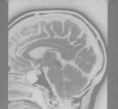

17

Pain and analgesics

SYNOPSIS

One of the greatest services doctors can do their patients is to acquire skill in the management of pain. This chapter describes the following:

- The phenomenon of pain: definition of pain; physiology of nociception; classification of pain; clinical evaluation of pain
- Pharmacotherapy: classification of analgesics; principles of analgesic pharmacotherapy
- Non-opioid analgesics: non-steroidal anti-inflammatory drugs; paracetamol (Acetaminophen); nefopam
- Opioid analgesics: mechanism of action; classification of opioid analgesics; pharmacodynamics of opioids; adverse effects and their management
- Opioid agonist drugs: mixed agonist–antagonist drugs; partial agonist drugs; antagonist drugs; tolerance, dependence and addiction
- Co-analgesic agents: multipurpose adjuvant analgesics; drugs used in neuropathic pain; adjuvants used for bone pain
- Drug treatment of migraine: pharmacotherapy of acute migraine; drugs used in migraine prophylaxis

PAIN AND ANALGESICS

The work that you are accomplishing is immensely important for the good of humanity, as you seek the ever more effective control of physical pain and of the oppression of mind and spirit that physical pain so often brings with it.[1]

[1]Pope John Paul II (26 July 1987). Letter handed to John Bonica on the occasion of the Fifth World Congress on Pain. In: Benedetti C, Chapman C R, Giron G (eds) 1990 Opioid analgesia: recent advances in systemic administration (Advances in Pain Research and Therapy, vol. 14). Raven Press, New York.

DEFINITION OF PAIN

The International Association for the Study of Pain defines pain as 'an unpleasant sensory and emotional experience associated with actual or potential tissue damage, or described in terms of such damage'. This implies that the degree of pain experienced by the patient may be unrelated to the extent or presence of underlying tissue damage, and that emotional or spiritual distress can add to the patient's experience of pain (Fig. 17.1).

This chapter is about the use of drugs for relieving pain and describes analgesics that are encountered in clinical practice. Clinicians should recognise

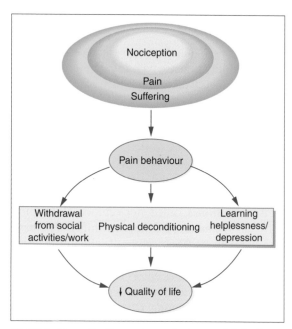

Fig. 17.1 The patient's experience of pain: a model of pain perception. Modified with permission from Carr D B, Loese J L, Morris D (eds) 2005 Narrative, pain, and suffering. The challenge of narrative to pain. Progress in Pain Research and Management series, vol. 34. IASP Press, Seattle.

that the patient's experience of pain is influenced by physical, emotional and psychological factors. Drug therapy is often an expedient (and familiar) form of treatment. But the successful management of pain in patients may require a more holistic approach that addresses all the components of pain, as the following account illustrates:

> Another event at Elsterhorst had a marked effect on me. The Germans dumped a young Soviet prisoner in my ward late one night. The ward was full, so I put him in my room as he was moribund and screaming and I did not want to wake the ward. I examined him. He had obvious gross bilateral cavitation and a severe pleural rub. I thought the latter was the cause of the pain and the screaming. I had no morphia, just aspirin, which had no effect. I felt desperate. I knew very little Russian then and there was no one in the ward who did. I finally instinctively sat down on the bed and took him in my arms, and the screaming stopped almost at once. He died peacefully in my arms a few hours later. It was not the pleurisy that caused the screaming but loneliness. It was a wonderful education about the care of the dying. I was ashamed of my misdiagnosis and kept the story secret.[2]

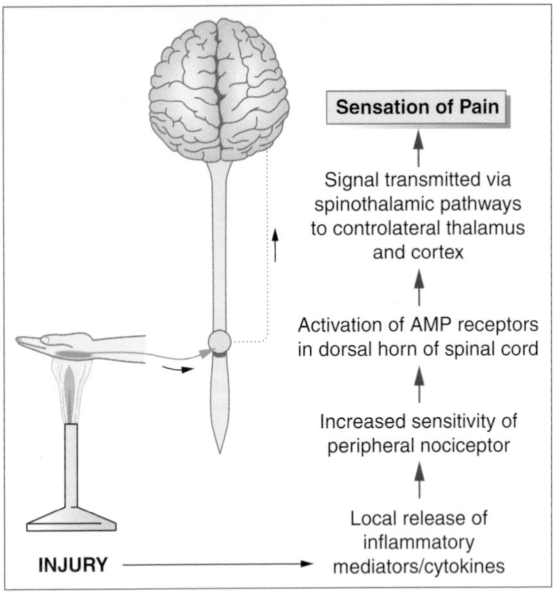

NOCICEPTION

Pain alerts us to ongoing or potential tissue damage, and the ability to sense pain is vital to our survival. The physiological process by which pain is perceived is known as *nociception* (Fig. 17.2). Although the neurobiology of nociception is complex, its appreciation provides a useful framework for understanding the way analgesics work.

Our nervous system is alerted to actual or potential tissue injury by the activation of the peripheral terminals of highly specialised primary sensory neurones called nociceptors. Nociceptors have *unmyelinated* (C-fibre) or thinly *myelinated* (Aδ-fibre) axons. Their cell bodies lie in the dorsal root ganglia of the spinal cord or in the trigeminal ganglia. Different nociceptors encode discrete intensities and modalities of pain, depending upon their expression of ion channel receptors. These receptors are transducers. They convert noxious stimuli into

Fig. 17.2 Schematic representation of nociceptive pathways. In acute pain, tissue damage causes the release of inflammatory mediators that activate and increase the sensitivity of peripheral nociceptors. The release of neurotransmitters such as glutamate at the dorsal horn of the spinal cord causes activation, via AMP (α-amino-3-hydroxy-5-methylisoxazole-4-propionate) and other receptors, of second-order neurones leading to the thalamus and, eventually, the cortex. This cortical activation produces the sensation of pain. In chronic pain, changes to receptor expression, neurotransmitters, and the balance of inhibition and excitation can cause activation of the nociceptive pathways without the need for any ongoing peripheral injury process.

action potentials. Some of these transducers have been identified, including those that respond to heat (>46°C), cold (<10°C) and direct chemical irritants such as capsaicin.

Action potentials that result from the transduction of noxious stimuli are conducted along the axon of the sensory neurone into the spinal cord. Conduction of the action potentials in sensory neurones depends on voltage-gated sodium channels, including two that are unique to nociceptors: Nav1.8 and Nav1.9.

The central terminal of the nociceptor makes synaptic contact with dorsal horn neurones within the spinal cord. *Glutamate*, an amino acid, is the main excitatory neurotransmitter released at these synapses. Its release can be inhibited by ligands that act to activate receptors found on the central terminal of the nociceptors (presynaptic inhibition).

---

[2]Cochrane A L (with M Blythe) 1989 One man's medicine: an autobiography of Professor Archie Cochrane. British Medical Journal, London, p. 82.

These include the *opioids, cannabinoids, γ-aminobutyric acid* (GABA) receptor ligands and the anticonvulsant *gabapentin*, which acts on the $\alpha_2\delta$ subunit of voltage-gated calcium channels. Opioids and GABA also influence the action of glutamate on the dorsal horn neurones. They act on postsynaptic receptors to produce hyperpolarising inhibitory potentials by the opening of potassium or chloride channels.

Other neurotransmitters may also be released by the central terminal of the nociceptors. For example, *substance P* is released during high-intensity and repetitive noxious stimulation. It mediates slow excitatory postsynaptic potentials and results in a localised depolarisation that facilitates the activation of N-*methyl-D-aspartate* (NMDA) receptors by glutamate. The end result is a progressive increase in the output from dorsal horn neurones. This amplified output is thought to be responsible for the escalation of pain when the skin is repeatedly stimulated by noxious heat – a phenomenon known as 'wind-up'.

Nociceptive output from the spinal cord is further modulated by descending inhibitory neurones that originate from supraspinal sites, such as the periaqueductal grey or the rostroventromedulla, and terminate on nociceptive neurones in the spinal cord as well as on spinal inhibitory interneurones that store and release opioids. Stimulation of these brain regions, either electrically or chemically, e.g. with opioids, produces analgesia in humans. Transmission through these inhibitory pathways is facilitated by monoamine neurotransmitters such as *noradrenaline (norepinephrine)* and *serotonin*.

Finally, dorsal horn neurones send projections to supraspinal areas in the brainstem, hypothalamus and thalamus, and then, through relay neurones, to the cortex where the sensation of pain is perceived. The mechanism by which the cortex produces the conscious appreciation of pain is poorly understood and remains the focus of much research.

CLASSIFICATION OF CLINICAL PAIN

Rational pharmacological treatment of clinical pain considers a number of factors that include the underlying cause and duration of pain, the patient's general medical condition and prognosis. Clinical pain is generally divided into three broad categories: acute, chronic and cancer related.

Acute pain, such as that experienced after trauma or surgery, typically resolves with healing of the injured tissue, and can usually be managed effectively with the appropriate use of pharmacotherapy. Poorly controlled postsurgical pain is associated with complications such as pneumonia, myocardial ischaemia, paralytic ileus and thromboembolism, as well as an increased risk of the patient developing chronic pain. Effective analgesia in this setting not only reduces patient anxiety and provides subjective comfort, but also helps to blunt autonomic and somatic reflex responses. Early mobilisation and improved food intake resulting from effective analgesia can improve postoperative outcome. Moreover, research suggests that analgesia given before surgical incision may reduce subsequent postoperative pain. Clinicians have attempted to exploit the concept of pre-emptive analgesia with varying success.

Chronic pain is commonly defined as pain that persists beyond the period expected for healing, or pain that is associated with progressive or persistent non-malignant disease. Chronic pain may be due to the continuing stimulation of nociceptors in areas of ongoing tissue damage (e.g. chronic pain due to rheumatoid arthritis). Chronic pain can persist long after the healing of damaged tissue. In some patients, chronic pain presents without any identified ongoing tissue damage or antecedent injury.

Neuropathic pain is defined as a chronic pain resulting from damage to the nervous system. Neuropathic pain can result from damage to the peripheral nervous system, such as in patients with diabetic or AIDS polyneuropathy, post-herpetic neuralgia or lumbar radiculopathy; or to the central nervous system (CNS), such as patients with spinal cord injury, multiple sclerosis or stroke. The mechanisms of neuropathic pain remain the subject of much research.

Cancer-related pain refers to pain that is the result of primary tumour growth, metastatic disease, or the toxic effects of chemotherapy and radiation, such as neuropathies due to neurotoxic antineoplastic drugs.

EVALUATION OF PAIN

Optimal pharmacological management of the patient's pain depends on the type and cause of pain, as well as the psychological and physical condition of the patient. A comprehensive evaluation of the pain is therefore essential to treat the patient successfully and safely. Underlying organic pathology must be excluded unless an obvious cause of pain is apparent, e.g. after recent surgery or trauma. The presence of organic pathology should also be suspected if the patient's pain presents in an unusual way, or is of a much greater magnitude than would normally be expected from the assumed pathology.

Once an organic explanation has been eliminated, additional tests are useless. The illusory sense of progress such tests provide for both physician and patient may perpetuate maladaptive behaviour and impede the return to more normal function.

The evaluation of persistent pain should include pain location, quality, severity, duration, course, timing (including frequency of remissions and degree of fluctuation), exacerbating and relieving factors, and co-morbidities associated with the pain (with emphasis on psychological issues, depression and anxiety). The efficacy and adverse effects of currently or previously used drugs and other treatments should also be determined.

If appropriate, the patient should be asked whether litigation is in progress or whether financial compensation for injury will be sought. A personal or family history of chronic pain can often give insight into the current problem. The patient's level of function should be assessed in detail, focusing on family relationships (including sexual), social network, and employment or vocation. The interviewer should elicit how the patient's pain affects the activities of normal living.

It is also important to determine what pain means to the patient. In some patients, reporting pain may be more socially acceptable than reporting feelings of depression or anxiety. Pain and suffering should also be distinguished. In cancer patients, suffering may be due as much to the loss of function and fear of impending death as to the experience of pain. The patient's expression of pain represents more than the pathology intrinsic to the disease.

Thorough physical examination is essential, and can often help to identify underlying causes and to evaluate further the degree of functional impairment. A basic neurological examination may identify features associated with neuropathic pain including:

- *Allodynia* – pain caused by a stimulus that would not normally provoke pain, e.g. light touch.
- *Hyperalgesia* – an increased response to a stimulus that would normally be painful.
- *Paraesthesia* – abnormal sensation, e.g. 'pins and needles'.

- *Dysaesthesia* – a painful paraesthesia, e.g. burning foot pain in diabetic neuropathy.

PHARMACOTHERAPY

An *analgesic* is defined as a drug that relieves pain. Analgesics are classified as opioids and non-opioids, e.g. non-steroidal anti-inflammatory drugs (NSAIDs). *Co-analgesics* or *adjuvants* are drugs that have a primary indication other than pain but are analgesic in some conditions. For example, antidepressants and anticonvulsants also act to reduce nociceptive processing in neuropathic pain.

The therapeutic efficacy of any given analgesic varies widely between individuals. Analgesics also have a relatively narrow therapeutic window, and drug dosages may be limited by the onset of adverse effects. For these reasons, the dose of analgesic drugs should be titrated for individual patients until an acceptable balance is achieved between subjective pain relief and adverse drug effects.

NON-OPIOID ANALGESICS

NON-STEROIDAL ANTI-INFLAMMATORY DRUGS

The account below should be read in conjunction with the description of NSAIDs in Chapter 15 (pp. 254–61).

Mechanism of analgesia. Endothelial damage produces an inflammatory response in tissues. Damaged cells release intracellular contents, such as adenosine triphosphate, hydrogen and potassium ions. Inflammatory cells recruited to the site of damage produce cytokines, chemokines and growth factors. A profound change to the chemical environment of the peripheral terminal of nociceptors occurs. Some factors act directly on the nociceptor terminal to activate it and produce pain, whereas others sensitise the terminal to subsequent stimuli. This process is known as 'peripheral sensitisation'.

Prostanoids (a term that encompasses the prostaglandins and thromboxanes) are major sensitisers that are produced at the site of tissue injury. NSAIDs act by inhibiting cyclo-oxygenase (COX), an enzyme involved in the production of prostanoids, and other prostaglandins. The enzyme has a number of isoforms, the most studied being COX-1 and COX-2. Their actions are inhibited by NSAIDs. Increased COX-2 production is induced by tissue injury and accounts for the efficacy of COX-2-specific inhibitor drugs (COXIBs).

Clinical use. NSAIDs are among the most commonly prescribed analgesics and, unless contraindicated, are effective and appropriate analgesics for use in acute inflammatory pain. There is much evidence to suggest that NSAIDs are effective in cancer-related pain. The benefit of NSAIDs in chronic non-cancer-related pain is less certain, with efficacy proven only in chronic inflammatory musculoskeletal pain, mainly from studies in rheumatoid arthritis. NSAIDs are generally ineffective in neuropathic pain conditions, and a careful risk:benefit assessment should be made prior to use in view of the side-effects associated with long-term use.

Choice of NSAID and route of administration. There is little difference in the clinical benefit conferred by any particular NSAID, but differences in pharmacokinetic properties and profiles of unwanted effects should be taken into account when choosing an agent for long-term use. For example, the oxicams, e.g. piroxicam, tenoxicam, are metabolised slowly and have a high degree of enteropathic circulation. These NSAIDs have long plasma half-lives but also higher incidences of unwanted gastrointestinal and renal effects.

NSAIDs are generally given orally. Topical application of NSAIDs for musculoskeletal pain is an exception as it is effective and associated with a lower incidence of unwanted effects.

Adverse effects. See Chapter 15.

PARACETAMOL (ACETAMINOPHEN)

The major advantage of paracetamol over the NSAIDs is its relative lack of unwanted effects; this justifies its use as a first-line analgesic. It can be used on its own, or synergistically with non-steroidal drugs or opioids. Paracetamol is also an antipyretic with very weak anti-inflammatory properties. There is considerable evidence that part of its analgesic effect is central and results from the activation of descending serotonergic pain-inhibiting pathways. Its primary mode of action, however, is inhibition of prostagladin synthesis (by inhibition of a recently discovered isoform, COX-3).

NEFOPAM

Nefopam is chemically distinct and pharmacologically unrelated to any presently known analgesic. It is a racemic mixture of two enantiomers. Although its mechanism of action is unclear, nefopam is thought to increase the inhibiting tone of serotonergic and noradrenergic (norepinephrinergic) descending pathways by inhibiting the synaptic uptake of dopamine, noradrenaline (norepinephrine) and serotonin. Compared with NSAIDs and opioids, nefopam has the advantage of minimally affecting platelet aggregation and having no CNS depressive effect.

Minor unwanted effects include nausea, dizziness and sweating, and are observed in 15–30% of patients. Rare fatal overdoses with the oral form of the drug were characterised by convulsions and cardiac arrhythmia. Nefopam is contraindicated in patients with limited coronary reserve, prostatitis and glaucoma because of its sympathomimetic action. Nefopam has been used as a drug of abuse, primarily because of its psychostimulant effects. These may be linked to its dopamine-reuptake inhibiting properties.

OPIOID ANALGESICS

Opium, the dried juice of the seed-head of the opium poppy (of the family Papaveraceae), was used in prehistoric times. Modern medical practice still benefits from the use of its alkaloids, employing them as analgesics, tranquillisers, antitussives and in the treatment of diarrhoea. Friedrich Sertürner crystallised an extract of opium and obtained morphine in 1801. On testing the pure morphine on himself and three young men, he observed that the drug caused cerebral depression and relieved toothache, and named it after Morpheus, the Greek god of dreams.[3] Opium contains many alkaloids, but the

---

[3]In classical mythology Morpheus was the son of Somnus, the infernal deity who presided over sleep. He was generally represented as a corpulent, winged boy holding opium poppies in his hand. His principal function seems to have been to stand by his sleeping father's black-curtained bed of feathers, on watch to prevent his being awakened by noise.

only important opiates (drugs derived from opium) are morphine (10%) and codeine. Papaverine is occasionally used as a vasodilator.

Opioid is a generic term for natural or synthetic substances that bind to specific opioid receptors in the CNS, producing an agonist action.

Mechanism of action. Opioids act to reduce the intensity and unpleasantness of pain. They produce their effects by activating specific G-protein-coupled receptors in the brain, spinal cord and peripheral nervous system. There are three major classes of opioid receptor: δ-opioid (*OPRD1*), κ-opioid (*OPRK1*) and μ-opioid (*OPRM1*)[4], which correspond respectively to their endogenous ligands, *dynorphin, enkephalin* and *β-endorphin*. Although studies suggest the existence of subtypes of all three major opioid receptor classes, the evidence is controversial and the subclassification is of little practical value except, perhaps, to explain the change in toxicity profile often seen during opioid rotation in long-term opioid use or cancer-related pain.

Agonist activity at opioid receptors acts to open potassium channels and prevent the opening of voltage-gated calcium channels. This reduces neuronal excitability and inhibits the release of pain neurotransmitters.

Classification. Opioids have been traditionally classified as strong, intermediate and weak, according to their perceived analgesic properties and propensity for addiction (Table 17.1). This approach can be misleading, as it implies that weak opioids such as codeine are less effective but safe. Codeine may be less potent than morphine but can cause respiratory depression if given in sufficient quantities. Codeine-like drugs are also frequently abused. Opioids may also be classified according to their structure. As described below, the properties of opioids may be predicted on the basis of activity on opioid and other receptor systems. The functional classification is probably of most clinical use.

Adverse effects. The common unwanted effects of opioids are due to their action on different opioid receptors. They include sedation, euphoria, dysphoria, respiratory depression, constipation, pruritus,

and nausea and vomiting. It is important to note that many of these effects tend to diminish as tolerance develops. Constipation and dry mouth (leading to increased risk of dental caries) are more resistant to tolerance and remain problems with long-term use. Impairment of hypothalamic function also occurs with long-term use and may lead to loss of libido and impotence, and to infertility.

Unwanted effects associated with opioid use in acute pain (and occasionally in chronic non-malignant pain) can often be managed simply by reducing the dose or switching to a different opioid. In palliative medicine, adverse effects related to long-term opioid use are often treated proactively: laxatives are given for constipation, and methylphenidate or dextroamfetamine for excessive sedation in cancer patients.

SYSTEMIC EFFECTS OF OPIOID ANALGESICS

Central nervous system

Patients taking opioid analgesics often report less distress, even when they can still perceive pain. *Sedation* often occurs, particularly in the early stages of treatment, but can remain a problem, especially at higher doses, and is a common cause of drug discontinuation in the chronic pain population.

The sensitivity of the *respiratory centre* to hypercarbia and hypoxaemia is reduced by opioids. Hypoventilation, due to a reduction in respiratory rate and tidal volume, ensues. Prolonged apnoea and respiratory obstruction can occur during sleep. These effects are more pronounced when the respiratory drive is impaired by disease, for example in chronic obstructive lung disease, obstructive sleep apnoea and raised intracranial pressure.

Opioid-related respiratory depression is more common in patients being treated for acute pain than in patients established on long-term opioids, and is a consequence of high plasma opioid concentrations. This may follow an inappropriately large dose that fails to account for differences in patient physiology, e.g. after hypovolaemic trauma or in the elderly patient, or because the patient is unable to excrete the drug efficiently, e.g. in renal impairment. Respiratory depression is unusual in patients established on long-term opioids due to tolerance, but abrupt changes in the physiological state, e.g. acute renal failure, may increase plasma opioid concentrations and precipitate toxic effects.

---

[4]The gene associated with the receptor is indicated within the parenthesis. For example, the gene for μ-opioid receptor is termed *OPRM1*, short for OPioid Receptor Mu 1.

Cough is inhibited by a central action. *Nausea* and *vomiting* are common with opioids used for acute pain relief, probably following activation of opioid receptors within the chemoreceptor trigger zone within the medulla, but opioid effects on the gastrointestinal tract and vestibular function probably play a role. Antiemetics are often prescribed for the prophylaxis or treatment of nausea.

Miosis occurs due to an excitatory effect on the parasympathetic nerve innervating the pupil. Pinpoint pupils are characteristic of acute poisoning; at therapeutic doses the pupils are merely smaller than normal.

Cardiovascular system

Opioids cause *peripheral vasodilatation* and impair sympathetic vascular reflexes. *Hypotension* may occur on rising from the supine position, but this is seldom troublesome in the reasonably fit patient and is rare with long-term use. Intravenous administration of opioids to patients who are hypovolaemic or have poor cardiac reserve can cause marked hypotension but intravenous morphine incremented carefully may benefit patients with acute myocardial infarction and left ventricular failure as the drug reduces sympathetic drive (from pain and anxiety) and preload (by venodilatation), thereby reducing the work of the heart.

Gastrointestinal tract

Opioids increase smooth muscle tone along the gastrointestinal tract. Reduced peristalsis (propulsion) and delayed gastric emptying cause *constipation*. Delayed passage of the intestinal contents allows for greater absorption of water, increasing the viscosity of faeces and aggravating the constipation (but the effect is useful in the treatment of diarrhoea). Opioid-induced constipation commonly occurs in palliative care and can be managed by increasing the fibre content of the diet to more than 10 g/day (unless bowel obstruction exists) and prescribing a stool softener, e.g. docusate sodium 100 mg b.d. or t.i.d., usually along with a stimulant laxative, e.g. senna or bisacodyl. Stimulant laxatives should be started in low dose, e.g. senna 15 mg o.d. and increased as necessary. Persisting constipation can be managed with an osmotic laxative, e.g. magnesium citrate given for 2–3 days or with lactulose 15 mL b.d.

Opioids contract the sphincter of Oddi and thereby increase pressure within the biliary tree. Some patients experience colicky pain after receiving morphine, owing to biliary spasm. This can be relieved by giving a small dose of the opioid antagonist, naxolone. It is a commonly held belief that pethidine (meperidine) produces less spasm in the sphincter of Oddi than do other opioids (due to its atropine-like effects) and that it should be the opioid of choice for treatment of biliary tree and pancreatic pain. At higher equi-analgesic doses, however, the effect on the sphincter is similar to that of other opioids, and pethidine confers no advantage.

Urogenital tract

Increased contraction of the ureters is probably clinically unimportant. Raised tone in the detrusor muscle and contraction of the external sphincter, together with inhibition of the voiding reflexes, may cause urinary retention.

Others

Opioid administration is often associated with cutaneous vasodilatation that results in the flushing of the face, neck and thorax. This may, in part, be due to histamine release. Pruritus is common with epidural or intrathecal administration of opioids and appears to be mediated by opioid receptor activation, as it is reversed by naxolone.

Pharmacokinetics

Systemic availability after oral administration varies from 30% with morphine, diamorphine and pethidine (meperidine) to 60% with codeine and oxycodone, and 80% with tramadol and methadone. The differences in therapeutic effect between oral and intravenous dosing are generally less than these percentages would suggest, because opioids tend to produce active metabolites.

Most opioids have a large volume of distribution and many have similar elimination $t_{1/2}$. A notable exception is remifentanil, which has a relatively short $t_{1/2}$ (8–20 min) that does not vary significantly with prolonged administration, owing to metabolism by plasma esterases. Methadone has a low body clearance and a large volume of distribution; consequently both the $t_{1/2}$ after a single dose (7.3 h, but varies greatly) and time to reach steady state, i.e. $5 \times t_{1/2}$, are long.

Controlled-release opioids typically require days to approach steady-state plasma concentrations.

The duration of analgesia usually correlates with $t_{1/2}$ unless the parent drug produces active metabolites (morphine) or has high affinity for opioid receptors (buprenophine), when the effect is prolonged.

Inter-individual variation

Individuals vary in their responses, and the neonate and elderly exhibit particular sensitivity to opioids. The inconsistency of response and the narrow therapeutic index of opioids require that the dose be individually titrated and its effects monitored for each patient. For opioid-naive patients with acute pain, frequent monitoring of pain relief, sedation, respiratory rate and blood pressure is necessary to guide dosage adjustment.

Route of administration

The *oral route* is generally satisfactory for the relief of pain that is not acute. Administration by mouth is obviously unsuitable for patients with emesis, dysphagia, gastrointestinal obstruction or in acute trauma where the patient may have delayed gastric emptying.

The *intravenous route* provides rapid and effective relief for acute pain and is more appropriate than (the more painful) intramuscular injection when repeated administration is necessary. Additionally, intramuscular and subcutaneous routes should not be used if the patient is peripherally vasoconstricted (e.g. following acute trauma), as the re-establishment of normal peripheral blood flow, subsequent to resuscitation, may result in too sudden redistribution of drug to the central circulation with danger of toxicity.

Continuous intravenous or subcutaneous infusion should be considered if repeated parenteral doses produce a prominent bolus effect, i.e. toxicity, at peak concentrations early in the dosing interval or breakthrough pain at trough levels. Patient-controlled analgesia (PCA) systems (in which the patient can trigger additional drug delivery) can be added to an infusion to provide supplementary doses. These systems are safe for both home and hospitalised patients, but are contraindicated for sedated and confused patients.

Epidural and intrathecal administration of opioids requires special expertise. The dorsal horn of the spinal cord is rich in opioid receptors, and analgesia can be provided using low-dose opioids, resulting in fewer unwanted systemic effects. Rostral (towards the head) spread of the drug can result in delayed toxicity, e.g. respiratory depression, during acute administration, and the cost of infusion systems, staffing

and monitoring must also be taken into account. The use of *intraventricular* morphine appears to be beneficial in treating recalcitrant pain due to head and neck malignancies and tumours (e.g. superior sulcus tumours, breast carcinoma) that affect the brachial plexus.

PHARMACOLOGY OF INDIVIDUAL OPIOIDS

OPIOID AGONISTS

Morphine

Morphine remains the most widely used opioid analgesic for the treatment of severe pain and is the 'gold standard' against which other opioids are compared. Commonly given intramuscularly, intravenously or orally; it can also be administered per rectum and into the epidural space or cerebrospinal fluid. Unlike most opioids, it is relatively water soluble. It is metabolised by conjugation in the liver and its $t_{1/2}$ is 3 h. The duration of useful analgesia provided by morphine is 3–6 h, but varies greatly with different preparations and routes of administration.

Morphine-6-glucuronide (M6G), one of its major metabolites, is an agonist at the μ receptor and also at the distinct M6G receptor. It is more potent than the parent morphine. As it is excreted in the urine, M6G accumulates when renal function is impaired, and may cause toxic effects with repeated doses of morphine.[5]

Diamorphine (heroin)

Diamorphine (3,6-diacetyl morphine), or heroin, is a semi-synthetic drug that was first made from morphine at St Mary's Hospital, London, in 1874. In almost every country the manufacture of diamorphine, even for use in medicine, is now illegal. The USA, not yet discouraged by the experience of alcohol prohibition (1919–1933), was the first to prohibit diamorphine manufacture in 1924 as a remedy for widespread drug addiction. An effort was made in 1953 to achieve a worldwide ban on diamorphine in medicine (so that any diamorphine, wherever it was found, must be illegal) and many countries agreed. The UK did not agree because legitimate

---

[5]Conway B R, Fogarty D G, Nelson W E, Doherty C C 2006 Opiate toxicity in patients with renal failure. British Medical Journal 332:345–346.

supplies for medicine were not then getting into illicit channels. A ban now would be pointless, as illegal diamorphine is readily available worldwide. As such, diamorphine has remained available for medicinal use within the UK.

Diamorphine has no direct activity at the μ receptor. It is converted within minutes to morphine and 6-monoacetylmorphine, a metabolite of both drugs. The effects of diamorphine are principally due to the actions of morphine and 6-monoacetylmorphine on μ receptors and, to a lesser extent, on the κ receptors.

Diamorphine given parenterally as a single bolus has a $t_{1/2}$ of 3 min. By the oral route, it is subject to complete presystemic or 'first-pass' metabolism, and only morphine and other metabolites reach the systemic circulation. Thus oral diamorphine is essentially a pro-drug. It is likely that there are no significant differences in the pharmacodynamics of diamorphine when compared with morphine when used for acute pain, despite the common belief that diamorphine is associated with more euphoria and less nausea and vomiting. Its greater potency (greater efficacy in relation to weight, and therefore requiring a smaller volume) and lipid solubility make diamorphine suitable for delivery by subcutaneous infusion through a syringe driver when continuous pain control is required in palliative care that can no longer be achieved by the enteral route (oral, buccal, rectal).

Codeine

Codeine is obtained naturally or by methylation of morphine. It has a low affinity for opioid receptors and most of its analgesic effects results from its metabolism (about 10%) to morphine. The polymorphic CYP2D6 enzyme is responsible for this transformation and is absent in some individuals, e.g. 7% of Caucasians, suggesting that these patients will derive little benefit from codeine.

Its principal uses are for mild and moderate pain, treatment of persistent cough and for the short-term symptomatic control of mild acute diarrhoea. Long-term use is often associated with chronic constipation, especially at higher doses (more than 30 mg q.i.d.). Numerous formulations exist, for cough, e.g. Codeine Linctus, and for pain commonly combined with paracetamol and/or aspirin.

Dihydrocodeine

Dihydrocodeine (DF118) is a low-efficacy opioid with an analgesic potency similar to that of codeine.

It is used to relieve moderate acute and chronic pain on its own or as a compound tablet (co-dydramol; dihydrocodeine 10 mg plus paracetamol 500 mg). Although active metabolites (dihydromorphine and dihydromorphine-6-O-glucuronide) account for some of its pharmacological effects, dihydrocodeine itself is active and may be a more reliable analgesic than codeine.

Oxycodone

Oxycodone is a semi-synthetic opioid that has been in clinical use since 1917. Its potency is approximately twice that of morphine. Oxycodone is currently used as a controlled-release preparation for cancer and chronic non-malignant pain. An immediate-release solution and tablets are available for acute or breakthrough pain. Parental oxycodone is an alternative when opioids cannot be given orally. Oxycodone provides as effective analgesia as morphine in acute and chronic pain but its higher systemic availability after oral administration confers the advantage of reduced inter-individual variation in plasma concentrations. It has a similar adverse effect profile to morphine, with a slightly reduced incidence of psychotropic effects.

Hydromorphone

Hydromorphone is a semi-synthetic opioid used primarily for the treatment of cancer-related pain. It can be administered intravenously, orally and rectally. Hydromorphone is five times as potent as morphine when given by the oral route and eight to nine times as potent when given intravenously, with a similar duration of action. The liver is its principal site of metabolism. In contrast to morphine, the 6-glucuronide metabolite is not produced in any significant amount, the main metabolite being hydromorphone-3-glucuronide. Some metabolites are active but they are present in such small amounts that they are unlikely to have a significant effect, except perhaps when renal function is significantly impaired.

Methadone

Methadone is a synthetic opioid used commonly as a maintenance drug in opioid addicts and increasingly used in cancer and chronic non-malignant pain. It is rapidly absorbed after oral administration and is metabolised extensively to products that are excreted in the urine. The principal feature of methadone is its long duration of action, due to high protein binding and slow liver metabolism. The elimination $t_{1/2}$ is 7 h after a single intramuscular dose, 15 h after an oral dose, but 25 h after repeated dosing. The latter reflects redistribution from the tissue reservoir, and makes the drug compatible with use in long-term therapy but less appropriate for use in acute pain. On average, steady-state plasma concentration is reached after approximately 36 h with regular administration (but can take several days), and dosages must be titrated carefully.

When used in cancer-related pain or chronic non-malignant pain, an opioid of short half-life should be provided for breakthrough pain, rather than an extra dose of methadone. The long duration of action also favours its use for the treatment of opioid withdrawal.

Because of its long duration of action, methadone has been used to cover opioid withdrawal in addicted patients. Methadone occupies opioid receptors, thus reducing the desire to take other opioids and the intensity of euphoria, should any be taken. The slow offset also diminishes the severity of the withdrawal. Addicts who are cooperative enough to take oral methadone experience reduced craving and less 'kick/buzz/rush' from intravenous heroin or morphine, because their opioid receptors are already occupied by methadone and the intravenous drug must compete. Recent evidence, however, indicates that methadone lengthens the cardiac QTc interval in direct proportion to the dose given. Although higher doses of methadone can reduce illicit heroin abuse, it may also predispose to cardiac arrhythmia. ECG screening of patients seems prudent in at-risk patients prior to prescribing methadone. The partial agonist buprenorphine, which has less capacity to lengthen the QTc interval, may be a satisfactory alternative.[6]

Fentanyl

Fentanyl is one of the first short-acting opioids developed for use in anaesthesia. It is approximately 100 times more potent than morphine; hepatic metabolism produces inactive metabolites. At low doses, fentanyl has a short duration of action due to rapid initial distribution of drug in the body. Its terminal $t_{1/2}$ is 1–6 h, depending on dose and, at higher doses, when tissue sites are saturated, its duration of action

is much longer. The long terminal $t_{1/2}$ and high lipid solubility render fentanyl ideal for use as a transdermal patch. These preparations are used commonly in cancer-related pain and chronic non-malignant pain. Fentanyl mixed with heroin and cocaine, and marketed illicitly as the 'ultimate high', has caused many deaths.

Alfentanil

Alfentanil is less potent and has a shorter $t_{1/2}$ (80 min) than fentanyl. Despite its lower lipid solubility, it has a more rapid onset of action. This is because the lower pK_a of alfentanil compared with fentanyl results in a much greater concentration of the un-ionised form of the drug, which is then able to diffuse freely across the blood–brain barrier. The plasma $t_{1/2}$ of alfentanil reaches its maximum after 90 min of continuous administration; this favours its use over fentanyl as a short-term intravenous opioid infusion in anaesthesia and intensive care.

Remifentanil

Remifentanil is a μ-opioid receptor agonist with an analgesic potency similar to that of fentanyl and a speed of onset similar to that of alfentanil. It is metabolised by blood and tissue esterases, and has a predictable $t_{1/2}$ (8–20 min) that is not affected by renal or hepatic function or plasma cholinesterase deficiency.

Its main metabolite is a carboxylic acid derivative that is excreted in urine. Although this accumulates in renal failure, significant pharmacological effects are unlikely as its potency relative to that of remifentanil is only 0.1–0.3%.

Remifentanil is unique in that its plasma $t_{1/2}$ remains constant even after prolonged infusion. This property favours its use during anaesthesia, when a rapid wake-up time is desirable, e.g. after neurosurgery.

Papaveretum

Papaveretum is a mixture of opium alkaloids, the principal constituents being morphine (50%), codeine, papaverine and noscapine. Noscapine may be teratogenic, and is no longer a component of commercially available papaveretum in UK.

PARTIAL AGONIST OPIOID ANALGESICS

Buprenorphine

Buprenorphine is a partial agonist at the μ receptor. It has less liability to induce dependence and

[6]Krantz M J, Mehler P S 2006 QTc prolongation: methadone's efficacy–safety paradox. Lancet 368:556–557.

respiratory depression than pure agonists. It is 30 times more potent than morphine and dissociates very slowly from the receptor. The therapeutic effect of parenteral buprenorphine reaches a peak up to 3 h after administration, and may last for 10 h. Its high receptor affinity (tenacity of binding) may explain why respiratory depression is only partially reversed by naloxone, and a respiratory stimulant (doxapram) or mechanical ventilation may be necessary in overdose.

Because of extensive first-pass metabolism by the oral route, buprenorphine is normally given by the buccal (sublingual) route or by intramuscular or slow intravenous injection. It is a useful analgesic in acute pain because administration by injection can be avoided (for children, or for patients with a bleeding disorder or needle phobia). The low incidence of drug dependency has led to its increased use in withdrawing opioid addicts and in chronic non-malignant pain. The relatively long $t_{1/2}$ and high lipid solubility make buprenorphine suitable for use as a transdermal patch preparation.

Meptazinol

Meptazinol is a high-efficacy partial agonist opioid with central cholinergic activity that may add to its analgesic effect. It is used to relieve acute or chronic pain of moderate intensity. It appears to have a low incidence of confusion and a low potential for abuse. Its poor systemic availability by mouth and partial agonist activity makes it less useful in severe pain.

MIXED AGONIST–ANTAGONIST OPIOID ANALGESICS

Drugs in this class include *pentazocine*, *butorphanol* and *nalbuphine*. They act as partial agonists at the κ receptor and as weak antagonists at the µ receptor. Consequently, they may cause withdrawal symptoms in patients dependent on other opioids. As analgesics, mixed agonist–antagonist opioids are not as efficacious as pure µ agonists. Compared with morphine, they produce less dependence (although this definitely occurs), more psychotomimetic effects (κ receptor), and less sedation and respiratory depression (naloxone can reverse the respiratory depression in overdose). They are given to relieve moderate to severe pain, but dysphoric adverse effects often limit their usefulness.

Pentazocine is one-sixth as potent as morphine; nalbuphine is slightly less potent than morphine; and butorphanol is five to nine times as potent.

Adverse effects include nausea, vomiting, dizziness, sweating, hypertension, palpitations, tachycardia and CNS disturbance (euphoria, dysphoria, psychotomimesis). Pentazocine has effects on the cardiovascular system, raising systolic blood pressure and pulmonary artery pressure, and should be avoided in myocardial infarction.

OPIOIDS WITH ACTIONS ON OTHER SYSTEMS

Pethidine (meperidine)

Pethidine was discovered in 1939 during a search for atropine-like compounds. Its use as a treatment for asthma was abandoned when its opioid agonist properties were appreciated.

Pethidine is primarily a µ agonist. Despite its structural dissimilarity to morphine, pethidine shares many similar properties, including antagonism by naloxone. In general, a 75–100 mg dose given parenterally is approximately equivalent to 10 mg morphine. Pethidine is metabolised extensively in the liver, and the parent drug and metabolites are excreted in the urine ($t_{1/2}$ 5 h). Norpethidine, a pharmacologically active metabolite, can cause central excitation and, eventually, convulsions, if it accumulates after prolonged intravenous administration or in renal impairment.

Pethidine has atropine-like effects, including dry mouth and blurred vision (cycloplegia and sometimes mydriasis, though usually miosis). It can produce euphoria and is associated with a high incidence of dependence. Its use for analgesia in obstetric practice was based on early clinical research which showed that, unlike morphine, pethidine did not appear to delay labour. The doses of pethidine used in these studies were low, and it is now established that pethidine confers no advantage over other opioids at higher equi-analgesic doses.

Tramadol

Tramadol is a centrally acting analgesic with relatively weak µ-opioid receptor activity. It also inhibits neuronal reuptake of noradrenaline (norepinephrine) and enhances serotonin release; these actions may account for some of the analgesic action.

Tramadol is rapidly absorbed from the gastrointestinal tract. Some 20% of an oral dose undergoes first-pass metabolism, and less than 30% of a dose is excreted unchanged in the urine ($t_{1/2}$ 6 h). Production of the O-desmethyl-tramadol metabolite is dependent on the cytochrome CYP 2D6 enzyme. This metabolite is an active μ agonist with a greater receptor affinity than tramadol. Tramadol is approximately as effective as pethidine for postoperative pain.

Tramadol is less likely to depress respiration and has a lower incidence of constipation compared with opioids, but has a high incidence of nausea and dizziness. Rarely, it can cause seizures, a fact that ought to be taken into account in susceptible patients.

OPIOID ANTAGONISTS

Naloxone

Naloxone is a competitive antagonist at μ-, δ-, κ- and σ-opioid receptors, and can reverse the effects of most opioid analgesics. It acts within minutes when given intravenously, and slightly less rapidly intramuscularly. As the duration of antagonism (approximately 20 min) is usually shorter than that of opioid-induced respiratory depression, close monitoring of the patient and repeated doses of naloxone may be necessary.

A common starting dosage in an opioid-naive patient with acute opioid overdose is 0.4 mg i.v. every 2–3 min until the desired effect is obtained. For patients receiving long-term opioid therapy, naloxone should be used only to reverse respiratory depression, with care taken to avoid precipitating withdrawal or severe pain. A reasonable starting dose is 0.04 mg (dilute a 0.4-mg ampoule in 10 mL isotonic saline) i.v. every 2–3 min until the respiratory rate improves.

Naltrexone ($t_{1/2}$ 4 h; active metabolite 13 h) is similar to naloxone but longer acting, with an effect that lasts for 1–3 days according to dose. It can be used orally to assist in the rehabilitation of ex-opioid abusers who are fully withdrawn (otherwise it will induce an acute withdrawal syndrome). A patient who then takes an opioid fails to experience the 'kick' or euphoria, although naltrexone does not reduce craving as does the agonist methadone. This use of naltrexone requires careful selection and supervision of subjects.

CHOICE OF OPIOID ANALGESIC

An opioid may be preferred because of favourable experience, route of administration or duration of

action. Opioids with a short $t_{1/2}$ (morphine and diamorphine) should be used as first-line agents for acute pain, but may be replaced with longer-acting drugs if pain persists.

Knowledge of equi-analgesic doses of opioids is essential when changing drugs or routes of administration (Tables 17.2 & 17.3).

Cross-tolerance between drugs is incomplete, so when one drug is substituted for another the equi-analgesic dose should be reduced by 50%. The only exception is methadone, which should be reduced by 75–90%. Opioid rotation is commonly used in cancer-related and chronic non-malignant pain as a means of reducing unwanted effects and limiting the development of tolerance.

OPIOID TOLERANCE, DEPENDENCE AND ADDICTION

(For general discussions, see also the relevant sections of Chapter 7 and 10.)

Although the use of strong opioid analgesics in cancer-related pain is well established, physicians are often reluctant to prescribe opioids in acute, and especially in chronic, non-malignant pain. Patients (and their families, friends and employers) are, likewise, wary about the long-term use of opioids. The reasons for this reluctance may stem from previous

Table 17.1 Classification of opioids

Type	Examples
Traditional	
Strong	morphine, diamorphine, fentanyl
Intermediate	partial agonists, mixed agonist–antagonists (see below)
Weak	codeine
Structural	
Morphinans	morphine, codeine
Phenylperidines	meriperidine, fentanyl
Diphenylprophylamines	methadone, dextropropoxyphene
Esters	remifentanil
Functional	
Pure agonists	morphine, codeine
Partial agonists	buprenorphine
Mixed action	pentazocine, nalbupine, butorphanol
Antagonists	naxolone

Table 17.2 Relative potency of opioids, i.e. therapeutic efficacy in relation to weight

Drug	Mode of action	Potency relative to oral morphine (24 h)
Codeine/dihydrocodeine	Weak μ-receptor agonist. Metabolised to morphine	0.1
Tramadol[a]	μ-receptor agonist. 5-HT/NA reuptake inhibition	0.2
Morphine	μ-receptor agonist	1
Oxycodone	μ-receptor agonist	2
Methadone[b]	μ-receptor agonist. NMDA receptor antagonist	≈10
Buprenorphine (transdermal)	μ-receptor partial agonist	60
Fentanyl (transdermal)	μ-receptor agonist	150

[a]Normal maintenance dose 100 mg q.i.d.
[b]Conversion to methadone is complex and requires specialist expertise.
5-HT, serotonin; NA, noradrenaline (norepinephrine); NMDA, *N*-methyl-D-aspartate.

experiences of the genuine problems associated with long-term opioid use in patients or, more often, due to the perception of opioids as dangerous and addictive drugs. Patients and physicians also frequently confuse tolerance and dependence with drug addiction.

Tolerance (see p. 80 and p. 145) indicates the need to increase the dose of a drug with time to achieve the same analgesic effect. It is due to physiological adaptation to the drug and can be managed by increasing the dose of the opioid over time. Tolerance to the adverse effects of opioids, e.g. constipation, is often less predictable, and the development of unwanted effects may prevent further escalation of the drug.

It is important to distinguish a gradual reduction in efficacy of an analgesic that is due to acquiring tolerance, from the onset of pain due to progression of the underlying disease process or new pathology.

Dependence (see p. 144) is the physical manifestation of tolerance and its effects are observed soon after abrupt withdrawal of a long-term opioid (the *discontinuation* or *withdrawal syndrome*). The severity of withdrawal symptoms varies depending on the patient, the drug and the length of treatment, and includes symptoms such as coryza, tremor, sweating, abdominal cramps, myalgia, vomiting and diarrhoea. Acute withdrawal can usually be avoided by reducing the drug dose gradually at the end of treatment by about 50% every 2 days (but may require a slower rate of withdrawal in some long-term users). Patients on long-term opioid therapy should not be given mixed agonist–antagonist drugs, which can precipitate a withdrawal state.

Addiction (see p. 143) is a behavioural problem characterised by drug-seeking activity in the individual in order to experience a drug's psychotropic effects. This behaviour may persist in despite of the knowledge that continued use of the drug will result in considerable physical, emotional, social or economic harm. The incidence of addiction in patients taking opioid medications for acute pain is negligible, and is low even in patients on long-term opioids for chronic non-malignant pain (<10%). The risk of iatrogenic addiction in patients prescribed opioids for cancer-related pain is extremely low.

PAIN RELIEF IN OPIOID ADDICTS

Physicians, particularly hospitals, are often guilty of withholding or under-prescribing opioids for drug-addicted patients in acute pain. This stems from unfounded fears of 'worsening' the addiction, distrust of the patient's motives or misguided attempts to 'cure' the patient of his or her addiction.

Before treating opioid addicts with acute pain, physicians should attempt to establish the patient's

Table 17.3 Opioid oral analgesic equivalents

Analgesic	Single dose	Equi-analgesic dose of oral morphine
Codeine	60 mg	5 mg
Dihydrocodeine	60 mg	8 mg
Tramadol	50 mg	10 mg
Meptazinol	200 mg	8 mg
Buprenorphine sublingual	200 micrograms	10 mg
Hydromorphone	1.3 mg	10 mg
Methadone	1 mg	10 mg
Oxycodone	5 mg	10 mg

daily opioid intake prior to hospital admission. The patient should then continue with an equivalent daily dose of opioid throughout their admission. Physicians should be aware that the strength of illicitly acquired 'street' drugs is highly variable. The addicted patient may also have an acute medical condition that alters opioid pharmacokinetics unpredictably. It is safer, therefore, first to prescribe an appropriate dose of an opioid with a short duration of action on an 'as required' basis, in order to assess opioid needs, before conversion to longer-acting opioids for maintenance.

The opioid-addicted patient with acute pain will require appropriate analgesia in addition to the calculated maintenance dose. This may involve NDAIDs, e.g. indometacin, or nefopam (which is neither opioid nor a NSAID). Non-opioid analgesics are useful adjuncts, but should not be used as a substitute for opioid analgesia.

Importantly, the use of opioid agonist–antagonist compounds in known or suspected active opioid addicts is absolutely contraindicated as these drugs may precipitate the withdrawal syndrome.

CO-ANALGESICS

Co-analgesics (adjuvant analgesics) are important for the treatment of cancer-related and chronic non-malignant pain. These agents provide an 'opioid-sparing' effect and are effective for the treatment of neuropathic pain associated with many cancers. In chronic non-malignant pain, co-analgesics are frequently used as 'first-line' drugs, and form the mainstay of treatment for chronic neuropathic pain. The general aspects of co-analgesics, e.g. as anticonvulsants or antidepressants, appear in the relevant chapters. The present account covers co-analgesics in the context of pain management.

MULTIPURPOSE ADJUVANT ANALGESICS

Corticosteroids

Corticosteroids are amongst the most widely used adjuvant analgesics in palliative care. They improve quality of life in cancer patients by virtue of their analgesic effects and other beneficial effects on appetite, nausea, mood and malaise. Corticosteroids may also reduce oedema around metastases or damaged nerve plexuses. Patients with advanced cancer who experience pain and other symptoms often respond favourably to a relatively small dose of corticosteroid, e.g. dexamethasone 1–2 mg twice daily by mouth.

Neuroleptics

Levomepromazine (*Methotrimeprazine*) has proven very useful in bedridden patients with advanced cancer who experience pain associated with anxiety, restlessness or nausea. In this setting, the sedative, anxiolytic and antiemetic effects of this drug can be useful, and unwanted effects, such as orthostatic hypotension, are less significant. Treatment can be started at 12.5–50 mg/day by mouth in three divided doses at mealtimes and increased until optimum effect is reached. Alternatively, as a sedative, a single night-time dose of 10–25 mg can be given.

Benzodiazepines

Benzodiazepines have limited analgesic effects but are often used as a short-term treatment for painful muscle spasm. Their use, however, must be balanced by the potential for unwanted effects, including sedation and confusion. With the important exception of clonazepam, which is widely accepted for use in the management of neuropathic pain, these drugs are generally prescribed only if another indication exists, such as anxiety or insomnia.

ADJUVANT ANALGESICS USED FOR NEUROPATHIC PAIN

Antidepressants

At present, the evidence for analgesic efficacy is greatest for the tertiary amine tricyclic drugs, such as *amitriptyline*, *doxepin* and *imipramine*. The secondary amine tricyclic antidepressants (such as *desipramine* and *nortriptyline*) have fewer adverse effects and are preferred when there are serious concerns about sedation, antimuscarinic effects or cardiovascular toxicity. Dual-reuptake inhibitors (*venlafaxine*, *duloxetine*) may be beneficial for patients who obtain relief from tricyclics but find the adverse effects a problem. The selective serotonin-reuptake inhibitors (SSRIs) appear to be less efficacious in neuropathic pain than other antidepressant drugs.

In contrast to their effect on depression, the analgesic effect of the above drugs is achieved at a smaller dose and within a shorter time from onset (1–2 weeks). The drugs should be started at a low dose to minimise initial unwanted effects, e.g. amitriptyline 10 mg o.d. in the elderly and 10–25 mg o.d. in younger patients. Education of patients is essential. It is common for patients to report taking the medication intermittently as a supplement to simple analgesics 'when the pain is bad'. Patients need to be told that the analgesic effect of the antidepressant medication can take days or weeks to develop, and that the drug must be taken regularly. Patient compliance is often improved when physicians emphasise that the drugs are being prescribed for their analgesic effects and not for their antidepressant properties.

Abrupt withdrawal of the antidepressant drugs should be avoided as unpleasant symptoms may result, possibly related to rebound cholinergic activity, including vivid dreams, restlessness and gastrointestinal hyperactivity. These can be minimised by gradual reduction of the dose, e.g. at intervals of 5–10 days.

Anticonvulsants

In 1853, Alfred Trousseau, then director of the medical clinic at Hotel Dieu (hospital) in Paris, suggested that painful paroxysms seen in trigeminal neuralgia were due to discharges in the trigeminal system that were similar to the neuronal discharges seen in epilepsy. Trousseau's hypothesis was tested by Bergouigan, who successfully used phenytoin to treat trigeminal neuralgia. Carbamazepine was studied in the same condition by a placebo-controlled double-blind design that was among the first of its kind in pain medicine. Since then, anticonvulsants have been extensively used in a wide variety of neuropathic pain syndromes.

Carbamazepine, phenytoin and sodium valproate have been used for many years to treat neuropathic pain. Carbamazepine remains the only anticonvulsant licensed in the UK for the treatment of trigeminal neuralgia. All anticonvulsants produce unwanted effects such as dizziness and drowsiness. Carbamazepine, in particular, may suppress bone marrow function and cause hyponatraemia. Its use requires regular plasma concentration monitoring.

Gabapentin and Pregabalin are more recently introduced anticonvulsant agents that show good efficacy in clinical trials of neuropathic pain. They appear to have a central site of action and may act by binding to the $\alpha 2 \delta$ subunit of voltage-dependent calcium channels, modulating the influx of calcium ions into the neuronal cell. Gabapentin is generally better tolerated than the older anticonvulsants and is licensed in the UK for neuropathic pain. It is excreted unchanged in the urine ($t_{1/2}$ 6h). It should be started at a dose of 300mg at night (100mg in the elderly) and increased as tolerated or to a dose of 600mg t.i.d. (although higher doses are frequently used).

Local anaesthetics

The use of local anaesthetics in neuropathic pain was popularised by studies that showed effectiveness in painful diabetic neuropathy. Parenteral administration is clearly impractical for long-term treatment, but infusions of lidocaine can identify the subgroup of patients with neuropathic pain who respond to sodium channel blockade; a trial of mexiletine, the oral analogue of lidocaine, is then worth considering.

An adhesive topical dressing infused with a preparation containing 5% lidocaine (Lidoderm) has proven effectiveness in post-herpetic neuralgia and other neuropathic pain disorders.

Capsaicin

Capsaicin (derived from chili peppers) activates specific vanilloid receptors found in C-nociceptors. Initial topical application causes a transient burning sensation. With repeated applications, desensitisation of the nociceptors occurs and is the basis for its use in chronic pain conditions.

Capsaicin cream 0.075% (applied four times daily) may benefit some patients with diabetic neuropathy and post-herpetic neuralgia, but the intense burning sensation during initial treatment and the need for repeated applications for several weeks may limit use.

Clonidine

Clonidine has agonist activity at adrenergic α_2 and imidazoline receptors, and is an effective analgesic when given intravenously or by the epidural or intrathecal route. Oral preparations also exist. Its greater potency, when given centrally, means that analgesic efficacy can be obtained with smaller doses and a reduced incidence of unwanted effects. Clonidine augments the analgesic effectiveness of epidural local anaesthetic agents and opioids, and has proven efficacy in chronic pain disorders, including cancer pain. The major adverse effects are sedation and hypotension. The latter is caused primarily by central sympatholysis, and may be compounded by concomitant bradycardia. Abrupt withdrawal after long-term administration leads to a risk of rebound hypertension (see p. 439).

Ketamine

Ketamine (see also p. 319) is a non-competitive NMDA antagonist that acts at the phencyclidine (PCP) binding site in the NMDA receptor. Controlled studies show good analgesic efficacy in peripheral and central neuropathic pain, fibromyalgia and chronic ischaemic pain. Ketamine may have a synergistic effect when combined with opioids. The drug can be given by various routes, but mostly as intravenous boluses of 100–450 micrograms/kg, followed sometimes by infusions of 10–45 micrograms/kg/min adjusted according to response.

Oral administration is generally unsatisfactory because systemic availability is low and the taste is unpleasant. Other adverse effects include unpleasant dreams, hallucinations, and visual and auditory disturbances, and the drug is best avoided in those prone to these symptoms.

ADJUVANTS USED FOR BONE PAIN

Bisphosphonates

Bisphosphonates (see p. 666) are analogues of inorganic pyrophosphate that inhibit osteoclast activity and, consequently, reduce bone resorption in a variety of illnesses. This effect, presumably, underlines the use of these compounds for metastatic bone pain that persists despite the use of other analgesic measures. Current evidence for analgesic effects is best for *pamidronate*, particularly for bone pain related to breast cancer or myeloma. Neither dose-dependent effects nor long-term risks or benefits in cancer patients are yet established. The use of any bisphosphonate requires monitoring of plasma calcium, phosphate, magnesium and potassium levels.

ASPECTS OF PALLIATIVE CARE

Analgesia in palliative care is referred to at various points in this chapter. The pharmacotherapy of other aspects of this important subject is described briefly below. It is important to note that in palliative care 'up to a quarter of all prescriptions are for licensed drugs given for unlicensed indication or via an unlicensed route'.[7]

The cause of any distressing symptom must be identified and corrected whenever possible. Non-pharmacological approaches to symptomatic relief are vital in palliative care.

Alimentary symptoms include the following:

- *Anorexia* is common in patients with widespread cancer. Appetite stimulants, however, are indicated in only a minority of patients. Prednisolone (15–30 mg daily) or megesterol (160–800 mg o.m.) may prove beneficial in some patients. The use of these drugs must be monitored carefully and stopped if no perceived benefit occurs after 1–2 weeks.

- A *mouth that is dry* and painful may be due to candidiasis (treat with nystatin), or to dehydration (rehydrate the patient judiciously where this can be done orally). In drug-related dry mouth caused by antimuscarinic drugs, including some antidepressants, withdraw the drug or adjust its dose.

- *Constipation* is common in dying patients, and may be due to a combination of opioid analgesics, inadequate intake of food and fluid, and physical inactivity. It can be exceedingly troublesome, and management should begin early to forestall the need for the use of enemas or of manual removal of faeces. Dietary measures should be used where practicable. A stimulant laxative and faecal softener (danthron plus poloxamer: co-danthramer) is commonly effective. Suppositories, e.g. glycerol or bisacodyl, should be used if the bowels have not been opened for 3 days and the rectum is found to be loaded.

- *Nausea* and *vomiting* can be caused by the underlying disease process, but is commonly related to drug therapy, especially opioid analgesics. These symptoms often cause great distress and can be more difficult to manage than pain. Two drugs acting by different mechanisms may be needed when a single agent fails, e.g. metoclopramide (dopamine D_2-receptor antagonist) or ondansetron (5-hydroxytryptamine$_3$ [HT$_3$]-receptor antagonist) or hyoscine (antimuscarinic). The phenothiazine, levomepromazine, has been shown to be particularly effective in nausea secondary to drug therapy or radiotherapy. For vomiting related to hypercalcaemia, use an antiemetic and treat the cause (see p. 568).

[7]Twycross R, Wilcock A, Charlesworth S, Dickman A 2002 Pallative care formulary, 2nd edn. Radcliffe Medical Press, Oxon, UK.

Respiratory symptoms include:

- *Dyspnoea*. Chronic dyspnoea (not due to respiratory failure) may be relieved by judicious use of opioids (by causing respiratory centre depression and reducing its sensitivity to chemical stimuli). When there is respiratory failure due to pulmonary disease, however, any drug-induced sedation may be life threatening. Oxygen is used as appropriate. A benzodiazepine can reduce the anxiety associated with dyspnoea. Dexamethasone reduces inflammation around obstructive tumours that cause dyspnoea.
- *'Death rattle'* is a symptom that results from accumulation of mucus when the patient is too weak to expectorate. This terminal event (often more distressing to others than to the patient) may be resolved by drying up secretions with an antimuscarinic drug (hyoscine or atropine 4–8-hourly).
- *Hiccough* (due to diaphragmatic spasm). Where this is intractable and exhausting, chlorpromazine (or other phenothiazine) or metoclopramide may help. Alternatively, baclofen, nifedipine or sodium valproate may be used.

Mental disorders include:

- *Delirium (acute confusional state)*. Drugs are used only if symptoms are marked or accompanied by restlessness. Haloperidol (1.5–5 mg) p.o. or s.c. is useful when delirium is accompanied by restlessness or when psychotic symptoms such as hallucinations or paranoia are prominent. Severe agitation that is accompanied by delirium in patients who are imminently dying may be treated with levomepromazine (a phenothiazine tranquilliser with analgesic and antiemetic effect) and midazolam.
- *Insomnia*. Benzodiazepines and other hypnotics are generally recommended for short-term use owing to concerns regarding tolerance, dependence and addiction. These concerns may be less relevant in the palliative care population for whom life expectancy is limited. In the elderly, the use of hypnotics is associated with falls, fractures and cognitive impairment. If the occasional use of hypnotics is necessary, a short-acting hypnotic without active metabolites (e.g. zolpidem) should be chosen.

Other symptoms that are commonly encountered in palliative care include:

- *Urinary frequency, urgency and incontinence*. Flavoxate, tolterodine, oxybutynin (antimuscarinics) may be useful in the treatment of urgency or bladder spasms. These drugs may cause retention of urine if there is anatomical obstruction.
- *Pruritus*. A plethora of systemic medications have been used in the treatment of pruritus. Opioid antagonists (naloxone, naltrexone) may relieve itch caused by spinal opioids, cholestasis and possibly uraemia. Other treatments for pruritus include thalidomide (in uraemia), rifampicin or colestyramine (cholestasis).
- *Fungating* tumours and ulcers may smell distressingly owing to anaerobic bacterial growth. Benefit may be gained by topical providone–iodine or metronidazole gel.

MIGRAINE HEADACHE

Classical migraine is a primary episodic headache disorder characterised by various combinations of neurological, gastrointestinal and autonomic changes. In Europe and the USA, about 18% of women and 6% of men suffered at least one migraine attack in the past year. Migraine has been ranked among the world's most disabling medical illnesses. Its socio-economic impact is substantial; an estimated annual cost of US$17 billion for treatment costs alone.

The pathophysiology of migraine is complex and may involve abnormal cortical activity, in which sensory input from dural and cerebrovascular sensory fibres is amplified and perceived as pain. Migraine possesses features of inflammatory and functional pain, as well as objective neurological dysfunction. The migraine aura of visual or sensory disturbance probably originates in the occipital or sensory cortex; the throbbing headache is due to dilatation of pain-sensitive arteries outside the brain, including scalp arteries. Diagnosis is based on the headache's characteristics and associated symptoms.[8]

[8]Iovino M et al 2004 International Headache Society: international classification of headache disorders. Cephalalgia 24(Suppl 1):1–160.

MANAGEMENT OF MIGRAINE

Migraine is best thought of, and managed, as a chronic pain syndrome. Non-pharmacological management of migraine involves helping patients to identify and avoid triggering factors such as stress, foods containing vasoactive amines (e.g. chocolate, cheese), bright lights, loud noises, hormonal changes and hypoglycaemia. Various behavioural and psychological preventive interventions include relaxation training, thermal biofeedback combined with relaxation training, electromyography biofeedback and cognitive behavioural therapy.

Pharmacotherapy of migraine is either abortive or preventive. Drugs used to *abort* an acute attack of migraine are either non-specific (analgesics) or specific (triptans and ergots). With frequent use, most of these medications tend to increase headache frequency and may cause a state of refractory daily or near-daily headache, called 'analgesic-associated chronic daily headache' (CDH). Codeine-containing compound analgesics are notorious and their use requires careful monitoring for worsening symptoms. Patients who require regular analgesics may be treated more easily with some of the standard preventive medications described below.

Treatment may start with simple analgesics with an antiemetic (below). Alternatively, choice of treatment can be guided by the likelihood of response. For example, patients with greater disability may benefit from having early access to triptans.

Aspirin (900 mg) and paracetamol (1000 mg) by mouth can provide effective analgesia, and oral domperidone (10 mg) or metoclopramide (10 mg) reduce nausea. NSAIDs, such as naproxen (500–1000 mg p.o. or p.r. with an antiemetic), ibuprofen (400–800 mg p.o.) or tolfenamic acid (200 mg p.o.) can be effective, when tolerated.

When simple measures fail, or more aggressive and specific drug treatment is required.

SELECTIVE 5-HT$_1$ AGONISTS (TRIPTANS)

In patients without cardiovascular contraindications, triptans are safe, effective and appropriate first-line treatments for patients who have a moderate to severe headache, or for whom analgesics have failed to provide adequate relief. The severity of headache and its rapidity of onset and duration are important factors when deciding the triptan or route of administration to be used. Headache that intensifies rapidly, or severe nausea and emesis, are features that call for early parenteral therapy.

Sumatriptan

Sumatriptan (Imigran) selectively stimulates a subtype of 5-HT$_1$ receptor (called 5-HT$_{1B/1D}$) that exists in cranial blood vessels, causing them to constrict. It is rapidly absorbed after oral administration and undergoes extensive presystemic metabolism such that systemic availability is only 16%. The $t_{1/2}$ is 2 h.

The oral dose is 50–100 mg, and should not exceed 300 mg in a 24-h period. This route can be avoided (because of disagreeable taste) by sumatriptan 20 mg given intranasally and repeated once after 2 h, but no more than 40 mg should be given in 24 h. When a rapid response is required, sumatriptan 6 mg is given s.c. (systemic availability by this route is 96%) and, again, can be repeated once in 24 h.

Sumatriptan is generally well tolerated. Malaise, fatigue, dizziness, vertigo and sedation are associated with oral use. Nausea and vomiting may follow oral or subcutaneous administration. The most important adverse effects are feelings of chest pressure, tightness and pain, which are probably due to coronary artery spasm and occur in about 5% of cases, and have been known to be accompanied by cardiac arrhythmia and myocardial infarction. Patients with ischaemic heart disease, unstable angina or previous myocardial infarction should not receive sumatriptan.

Other triptans include *zolmitriptan, naratriptan, rizatriptan, almotriptan, frovatriptan* and *eletriptan*. They have similar safety profiles but the therapeutic response to, and adverse effects of, different triptans are often idiosyncratic, and trial of different drugs may be necessary to find one that offers relief with minimal unwanted events.

Ergotamine

Although ergotamine is a useful antimigraine compound, it is no longer considered a first-line drug for migraine because of its adverse effects. Ergots have much greater receptor affinity at serotonergic (5-HT$_{1A}$, 5-HT$_2$), adrenergic and dopaminergic receptors compared with triptans. Peripheral vasoconstriction from ergotamine administration can persist for as long as 24 h, and repeated doses lead to cumulative effects long outlasting the migraine attack. Ergotamine may precipitate angina pectoris, probably by increasing cardiac pre- and after-load. Ergotamine should never be used for prophylaxis of migraine.

Ergotamine is incompletely absorbed from the gastrointestinal tract and rectal administration may be preferred in an acute migraine attack. It is extensively metabolised in the liver and, therefore, contraindicated when liver function is significantly impaired.

PREVENTIVE TREATMENT FOR MIGRAINE

Criteria for preventive treatment include:

- Migraine that substantially interferes with the patient's daily routine despite acute treatment.
- Failure of, contraindication to, or troublesome adverse events from acute drugs.
- Acute drug overuse.
- Very frequent headaches (more than two per week) (risk of drug overuse).
- Patient preference.
- Special circumstances, such as hemiplegic migraine or attacks with a risk of permanent neurological injury.

Drugs used include β-adrenergic blockers, antidepressants, calcium-channel antagonists, serotonin antagonists, anticonvulsants and NSAIDs. Those with the best documented effectiveness are β-adrenergic blockers, pizotifen (below) and the anticonvulsant drugs, sodium valproate and topiramate. The choice is based on effectiveness, experience of adverse events, and coexistent and co-morbid conditions.

Women of child-bearing potential should be made aware of the risk of drugs in pregnancy. All drugs for migraine prophylaxis, especially those that cause drowsiness, should be started at a low dose and increased slowly until the intended outcome results or the maximum dose is reached; a full therapeutic trial may take 2–6 months. Patients should try to avoid overusing drugs for acute attacks during the trial period. If headaches are well controlled, treatment can be tapered down and may be discontinued if the patient remains symptom free.

Pizotifen

Pizotifen is an antihistamine drug with serotonin antagonist activity. It is structurally related to the tricyclic antidepressant drugs and shares their potential for antimuscarinic adverse effects such as dry mouth, urinary retention and constipation. The antihistamine action produces drowsiness, and the drug also causes weight gain. Treatment is usually started with 500 micrograms at night and increased to the desired effect. It is rare to exceed 1 mg t.i.d. (or as a single 3-mg dose at night).

GUIDE TO FURTHER READING

Carroll I, Angst M S, Clark J D R 2004 Management of perioperative pain in patients chronically consuming opioids. Regional Anesthesia and Pain Medicine 29(6):576–591

Colvin L, Forbes K, Fallon M 2006 Difficult pain. British Medical Journal 332:1081–1083

Fallon M (ed.) 2006 Palliative care. Clinical Medicine 6:133–150 (a series of articles on this subject)

Fallon M, Hanks G, Cherny N 2006 Principles of control of cancer pain. British Medical Journal 332:1022–1024

Kehlet H, Jensen T S, Woolf C J 2006 Persistent postsurgical pain: risk factors and prevention. Lancet 367:1618–1625

Nestler E J 2004 Historical review: molecular and cellular mechanisms of opiate and cocaine addiction. Trends in Pharmacological Sciences 25(4):210–218

Silberstein S D 2004 Migraine. Lancet 363:381–391

Woolf C J 2004 Pain: moving from symptom control toward mechanism-specific pharmacologic management. Annals of Internal Medicine 140(6):441–451

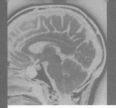

18

Anaesthesia and neuromuscular block

SYNOPSIS

The administration of general anaesthetics and neuromuscular blocking drugs is generally confined to trained specialists. Nevertheless, non-specialists are involved in perioperative care and will benefit from an understanding of how these drugs act. Doctors from a variety of specialties use local anaesthetics and the pharmacology of these drugs is discussed in detail.

- General anaesthesia
- Pharmacology of anaesthetics
- Inhalation anaesthetics
- Intravenous anaesthetics
- Muscle relaxants: neuromuscular blocking drugs
- Local anaesthetics
- Obstetric analgesia and anaesthesia
- Anaesthesia in patients already taking drugs
- Anaesthesia in the diseased, the elderly and children; sedation in intensive therapy units

GENERAL ANAESTHESIA

Until the mid-19th century such surgery as was possible had to be undertaken at tremendous speed. Surgeons did their best for terrified patients by using alcohol, opium, cannabis, hemlock or hyoscine.[1] With the introduction of general anaesthesia, surgeons could operate for the first time with careful deliberation. The problem of inducing quick, safe and easily reversible unconsciousness for any desired length of time in humans began to be solved only in the 1840s when the long-known substances nitrous oxide, ether and chloroform were introduced in rapid succession.

The details surrounding the first use of surgical anaesthesia were submerged in bitter disputes on priority following an attempt to take out a patent for ether. The key events around this time were:

- 1842 – W E Clarke of Rochester, New York, administered ether for a dental extraction; however, the event was not made widely known at the time.
- 1844 – Horace Wells, a dentist in Hartford, Connecticut, introduced nitrous oxide to produce anaesthesia during dental extraction.
- 1846 – On October 16 William Morton, a Boston dentist, successfully demonstrated the anaesthetic properties of ether.
- 1846 – On December 21 Robert Liston performed the first surgical operation in England under ether anaesthesia.[2]
- 1847 – James Y Simpson, professor of midwifery at the University of Edinburgh, introduced chloroform for the relief of labour pain.

The next important developments in anaesthesia were in the 20th century when the appearance of new drugs, both as primary general anaesthetics and as adjuvants (muscle relaxants), new apparatus and clinical expertise in rendering prolonged anaesthesia safe enabled surgeons to increase their range. No longer was the duration and type of surgery determined by patients' capacity to endure pain.

---

[1] A Japanese pioneer in about 1800 wished to test the anaesthetic efficacy of a herbal mixture including solanaceous plants (hyoscine-type alkaloids). His elderly mother volunteered as subject as she was anyway expected to die soon. But the pioneer administered it to his wife for, 'as all three agreed, he could find another wife, but could never get another mother' (Journal of the American Medical Association 1966; 197:10).

[2] Frederick Churchill, a butler from Harley Street, had his leg amputated at University College Hospital, London. After removing the leg in 28 s, a skill necessary to compensate for the previous lack of anaesthetics, Robert Liston turned to the watching students, and said, 'This Yankee dodge, gentlemen, beats mesmerism hollow'. That night he anaesthetised his house surgeon in the presence of two women (Merrington W R 1976 University College Hospital and its Medical School: a history. Heinemann, London).

PHASES OF GENERAL ANAESTHESIA

Balanced surgical anaesthesia (*hypnosis, analgesia* and *muscle relaxation*) with a single drug would require high doses that would cause adverse effects such as slow and unpleasant recovery, and depression of cardiovascular and respiratory function. In modern practice, different drugs are used to attain each objective so that adverse effects are minimised.

The perioperative period may be divided into three phases, and several factors determine the choice of drugs given in each of these. In brief:

Before surgery, an assessment is made of:

- the patient's physical and psychological condition
- any concurrent illness
- the relevance of any existing drug therapy.

All of these may influence the choice of anaesthetic drugs.

During surgery, drugs will be required to provide:

- unconsciousness
- analgesia
- muscular relaxation when necessary
- control of blood pressure, heart rate and respiration.

After surgery, drugs will play a part in:

- reversal of neuromuscular block
- relief of pain, and nausea and vomiting
- other aspects of postoperative care, including intensive care.

Patients are often already taking drugs affecting the central nervous and cardiovascular systems, and there is considerable potential for interaction with anaesthetic drugs.

The techniques for giving anaesthetic drugs and the control of ventilation and oxygenation are of great importance, but are outside the scope of this book.

Before surgery (premedication)

The principal aims are to provide:

Anxiolysis and amnesia. A patient who is going to have a surgical operation is naturally apprehensive; this anxiety is reduced by reassurance and a clear explanation of what to expect. Very anxious patients will secrete a lot of adrenaline (epinephrine) from the suprarenal medulla and this may make them more liable to cardiac arrhythmias with some anaesthetics. In the past, sedative premedication was given to virtually all patients undergoing surgery. This practice has changed dramatically because of the increasing proportion of operations undertaken as 'day cases' (in the USA 75% of all surgical procedures and undertaken as day cases) and the recognition that sedative premedication prolongs recovery. Sedative premedication is now reserved for those who are particularly anxious or those undergoing major surgery.

Benzodiazepines, such as temazepam (10–30 mg for an adult), provide anxiolysis and amnesia for the immediate presurgical period.

Analgesia is indicated if the patient is in pain before surgery, or the analgesia can be given pre-emptively to prevent postoperative pain. Severe preoperative pain is treated with a parenteral opioid such as morphine. Non-steroidal anti-inflammatory drugs (NSAIDs) and paracetamol are commonly given orally before operation to prevent postoperative pain after minor surgery. For moderate or major surgery, these drugs are supplemented with an opioid towards the end of the procedure.

Drying of bronchial and salivary secretions using antimuscarinic drugs to inhibit the parasympathetic autonomic system is rarely undertaken these days. The exceptions include those patients who are expected to require an awake fibreoptic intubation or those undergoing bronchoscopy. Glycopyrronium is the antimuscarinic of choice for this purpose, and atropine and hyoscine are alternatives.

Timing. Premedication is given about an hour before surgery.

Gastric contents. Pulmonary aspiration of gastric contents can cause severe pneumonitis. Patients at risk of aspiration are those with full stomachs, in the third trimester of pregnancy or with an incompetent gastro-oesophageal sphincter. A single dose of an antacid, e.g. sodium citrate, may be given before a general anaesthetic to neutralise gastric acid in high-risk patients. Alternatively or additionally, a histamine H_2-receptor blocker, e.g. ranitidine, or proton pump inhibitor, e.g. omeprazole, will reduce gastric secretion volume as well as acidity. Metoclopramide usefully hastens gastric emptying, increases the tone of the lower oesophageal sphincter and is an antiemetic.

During surgery

The aim is to induce *unconsciousness, analgesia* and *muscle relaxation* – the anaesthetic triad. Total muscular relaxation (paralysis) is required for some surgical procedures, e.g. intra-abdominal surgery, but most surgery can be undertaken without neuromuscular blockade.

A typical general anaesthetic consists of:

Induction

1. Usually intravenous: pre-oxygenation followed by a small dose of an opioid, e.g. fentanyl or alfentanil to provide analgesia and sedation, followed by propofol or, less commonly, thiopental or etomidate to induce anaesthesia. Airway patency is maintained with an oral airway and face-mask, a laryngeal mask airway (LMA) or a tracheal tube. Insertion of a tracheal tube usually requires paralysis with a neuromuscular blocker and is undertaken if there is a risk of pulmonary aspiration from regurgitated gastric contents or from blood.
2. Inhalational induction, usually with sevoflurane, is undertaken less commonly. It is used in children, particularly if intravenous access is difficult, and in patients at risk from upper airway obstruction.

Maintenance

1. Most commonly with oxygen and air, or nitrous oxide and oxygen, plus a volatile agent, e.g. sevoflurane or isoflurane. Additional doses of a neuromuscular blocker or opioid are given as required.
2. A continuous intravenous infusion of propofol can be used to maintain anaesthesia. This technique of *total intravenous anaesthesia* is becoming more popular because the quality of recovery may be better than after inhalational anaesthesia. The propofol infusion is often combined with an infusion of remifentanil, an ultra-short-acting opioid.

When appropriate, peripheral nerve block with a local anaesthetic, or neural axis block, e.g. spinal or epidural, provides intraoperative analgesia and muscle relaxation. These local anaesthetic techniques provide excellent postoperative analgesia.

After surgery

The anaesthetist ensures that the effects of neuromuscular blocking drugs and opioid-induced respiratory depression have either worn off or have been adequately reversed by an antagonist; the patient is not left alone until conscious, with protective reflexes restored, and in a stable circulation.

Relief of pain after surgery can be achieved with several techniques. An *epidural infusion* of a mixture of local anaesthetic and opioid provides excellent pain relief after major surgery such as laparotomy. *Parenteral morphine*, given intermittently by a nurse or a patient-controlled system, will also relieve moderate or severe pain but has the attendant risk of nausea, vomiting, sedation and respiratory depression. The addition of regular paracetamol and a NSAID, given orally or rectally, will provide additional pain relief and reduce the requirement for morphine. Paracetamol can be also given intravenously.

Postoperative nausea and vomiting (PONV) is common after laparotomy and major gynaecological surgery, e.g. abdominal hysterectomy. The use of propofol, particularly when given to maintain anaesthesia, has dramatically reduced the incidence of PONV. Antiemetics, such as cyclizine, metoclopramide and ondansetron, may be helpful. Dexamethasone also reduces the incidence of PONV. Combinations of these drugs are particularly effective.

SOME SPECIAL TECHNIQUES

Dissociative anaesthesia is a state of profound analgesia and anterograde amnesia with minimal hypnosis during which the eyes may remain open; it can be produced by ketamine (see p. 319). It is particularly useful where modern equipment is lacking or where access to the patient is limited, e.g. at major accidents or on battlefields.

Sedation and amnesia without analgesia are provided by intravenous midazolam or, less commonly nowadays, by diazepam. These drugs can be used alone for procedures causing mild discomfort, e.g. endoscopy, and with a local anaesthetic where more pain is expected, e.g. removal of impacted wisdom teeth. Benzodiazepines produce anterograde, but not retrograde, amnesia. By definition, the sedated patient remains responsive and cooperative. (For a general account of benzodiazepines and the competitive antagonist flumazenil, see Chapter 19.)

Benzodiazepines can cause respiratory depression and apnoea, especially in the elderly and in patients with respiratory insufficiency. The combination of an opioid and a benzodiazepine is particularly dangerous. Benzodiazepines depress laryngeal reflexes and place the patient at risk of inhalation of oral secretions or dental debris.

Entonox, a 50:50 mixture of nitrous oxide and oxygen, is breathed by the patient using a demand valve. It is particularly useful in the prehospital environment and for brief procedures, such as splinting limbs.

PHARMACOLOGY OF ANAESTHETICS

All successful general anaesthetics are given intravenously or by inhalation because these routes enable closest control over blood concentrations and thus of effect on the brain.

MODE OF ACTION

General anaesthetics act on the brain, primarily on the midbrain reticular activating system, and the spinal cord. Many anaesthetics are lipid soluble and there is good correlation between this and anaesthetic effectiveness (the Overton–Meyer hypothesis); the more lipid soluble tend to be the more potent anaesthetics, but such a correlation is not invariable. Some anaesthetic agents are not lipid soluble and many lipid-soluble substances are not anaesthetics.

Until recently it was thought that the principal site of action of general anaesthetics was relatively non-specific action in the neuronal lipid bilayer membrane. The current view is that anaesthetic agents interact with proteins to alter the activity of specific neuronal ion channels, particularly the fast neurotransmitter receptors such as nicotinic acetylcholine, γ-aminobutyric acid (GABA) and glutamate receptors. The suppression of motor responses to painful stimuli by anaesthetics is mediated mainly by the spinal cord, whereas hypnosis and amnesia are mediated within the brain.

Comparison of the efficacy of inhalational anaesthetics is made by measuring the minimum alveolar concentration (MAC) in oxygen required to prevent movement in response to a standard surgical skin incision in 50% of subjects. The MAC of the volatile agent is reduced by the co-administration of nitrous oxide.

INHALATION ANAESTHETICS

The preferred inhalation anaesthetics are those that are minimally irritant and non-flammable, and comprise nitrous oxide and the fluorinated hydrocarbons, e.g. isoflurane.

PHARMACOKINETICS (VOLATILE LIQUIDS, GASES)

The level of anaesthesia is correlated with the tension (partial pressure) of anaesthetic drug in brain tissue. This is driven by the development of a series of tension gradients from the high partial pressure delivered to the alveoli and decreasing through the blood to the brain and other tissues. The gradients are dependent on the blood/gas and tissue/gas solubility coefficients, as well as on alveolar ventilation and organ blood flow.

An anaesthetic that has *high* solubility in blood, i.e. a high blood/gas partition coefficient, will provide a slow induction and adjustment of the depth of anaesthesia. Here, the blood acts as a reservoir (store) for the drug so that it does not enter the brain readily until the blood reservoir is filled. A rapid induction can be obtained by increasing the concentration of drug inhaled initially and by hyperventilating the patient.

Anaesthetics with *low* solubility in blood, i.e. a low blood/gas partition coefficient (nitrous oxide, desflurane, sevoflurane), provide rapid induction of anaesthesia because the blood reservoir is small and anaesthetic is available to pass into the brain sooner.

During induction of anaesthesia the blood is taking up anaesthetic selectively and rapidly, and the resulting loss of volume in the alveoli leads to a flow of anaesthetic into the lungs that is independent of respiratory activity. When the anaesthetic is discontinued the reverse occurs and it moves from the blood into the alveoli. In the case of nitrous oxide, this can account for as much as 10% of the expired volume and so can significantly lower the alveolar oxygen concentration. Mild hypoxia occurs and lasts for as long as 10 min. Oxygen is given to these patients during the last few minutes of anaesthesia and the early postanaesthetic period. This phenomenon, *diffusion hypoxia*, occurs with all gaseous anaesthetics, but is most prominent with gases that are relatively insoluble in blood, for they will diffuse out most rapidly when the drug is no longer inhaled, i.e.

just as induction is faster, so is elimination. Nitrous oxide is especially powerful in this respect because it is used at concentrations of up to 70%.

NITROUS OXIDE

Nitrous oxide (1844) is a gas with a slightly sweetish smell that is neither flammable nor explosive. It produces light anaesthesia without demonstrably depressing the respiratory or vasomotor centre provided that normal oxygen tension is maintained.

Advantages. Nitrous oxide reduces the requirement for other more potent and intrinsically more toxic anaesthetics. It has a strong analgesic action; inhalation of 50% nitrous oxide in oxygen (Entonox) may have similar effects to standard doses of morphine. Induction is rapid and not unpleasant, although transient excitement may occur, as with all anaesthetics. Recovery time rarely exceeds 4 min even after prolonged administration.

Disadvantages. Nitrous oxide is expensive to buy and to transport. It must be used in conjuction with more potent anaesthetics to produce full surgical anaesthesia.

Uses. Nitrous oxide is used to maintain surgical anaesthesia in combination with other anaesthetic agents, e.g. isoflurane or propofol, and, if required, muscle relaxants. Entonox provides analgesia for obstetric practice and for emergency treatment of injuries.

Dosage and administration. For the maintenance of anaesthesia, nitrous oxide must always be mixed with at least 30% oxygen. For analgesia, a concentration of 50% nitrous oxide with 50% oxygen usually suffices.

Contraindications. Any closed, distensible, air-filled space expands during administration of nitrous oxide, which moves into it from the blood. It is therefore contraindicated in patients with: demonstrable collections of air in the pleural, pericardial or peritoneal spaces; intestinal obstruction; arterial air embolism; decompression sickness; severe chronic obstructive airway disease; emphysema. Nitrous oxide will cause pressure changes in closed, non-compliant spaces such as the middle ear, nasal sinuses and the eye.

Precautions. Continued administration of oxygen may be necessary during recovery, especially in elderly patients (see diffusion hypoxia, above).

Adverse effects. The incidence of nausea and vomiting increases with the duration of anaesthesia. Exposure to nitrous oxide for more than 4 h can cause megaloblastic changes in the bone marrow. Because prolonged and repeated exposure of staff, as well as of patients, may be associated with bone marrow depression and teratogenic risk, scavenging systems are used to minimise ambient concentrations in operating theatres.

HALOGENATED ANAESTHETICS

Halothane was the first halogenated agent to be used widely, but in the developed world it has been largely superseded by isoflurane and sevoflurane. A description of isoflurane is provided, and of the others in so far as they differ. The MAC in oxygen of some volatile anaesthetics is:

Isoflurane   1.2%
Enflurane   1.7%
Sevoflurane   2.0%
Desflurane   6.0%
Halothane   0.74%.

Isoflurane

Isoflurane is a volatile colourless liquid that is not flammable at normal anaesthetic concentrations. It is relatively insoluble and has a lower blood/gas coefficient than halothane or enflurane, which enables rapid adjustment of the depth of anaesthesia. It has a pungent odour and can cause bronchial irritation, making inhalational induction unpleasant. Isoflurane is minimally metabolised (0.2%), and none of the breakdown products has been related to anaesthetic toxicity.

Respiratory effects. Isoflurane causes respiratory depression and diminishes the ventilatory response to carbon dioxide. Although it irritates the upper airway, it is a bronchodilator.

Cardiovascular effects. Anaesthetic concentrations of isoflurane, i.e. 1–1.5 MAC, cause only slight impairment of myocardial contractility. Isoflurane causes peripheral vasodilation and reduces blood pressure. It does not sensitise the heart to catecholamines. In low concentrations (<1 MAC), cerebral blood flow, intracranial pressure and cerebral auto-regulation are maintained. Isoflurane is a potent coronary vasodilator and in the presence of a coronary artery stenosis it may cause redistribution of blood away from an area of inadequate perfusion to one of normal perfusion. This phenomenon of 'coronary steal' may cause regional myocardial ischaemia.

Other effects. Isoflurane relaxes voluntary muscles and potentiates the effects of non-depolarising muscle relaxants. Isoflurane depresses cortical EEG activity and does not induce abnormal electrical activity or convulsions.

Sevoflurane

Sevoflurane is less chemically stable than the other volatile anaesthetics in current use. About 2.5% is metabolised in the body and it is degraded by contact with carbon dioxide absorbents, such as soda lime. The reaction with soda lime causes the formation of a vinyl ether (Compound A), which may be nephrotoxic. Sevoflurane is less soluble than isoflurane and is very pleasant to breathe, which makes it an excellent choice for inhalational induction of anaesthesia, particularly in children. The respiratory and cardiovascular effects of sevoflurane are very similar to isoflurane, but sevoflurane does not cause 'coronary steal'.

Enflurane

Enflurane is more soluble than isoflurane. It causes more respiratory depression than the other volatile anaesthetics and hypercapnia is almost inevitable in patients breathing spontaneously. More cardiovascular depression develops than with isoflurane and cardiac arrhythmias may occur. Some 2% of enflurane is metabolised, and prolonged administration or use in enzyme-induced patients may generate sufficient free inorganic fluoride from the drug molecule to cause polyuric renal failure. Jaundice and hepatatoxicity have been associated with enflurane but the incidence (about 1 in 1–2 million anaesthetics) is lower than with halothane.

Desflurane

Desflurane has the lowest blood/gas partition coefficient of any inhaled anaesthetic agent and thus gives particularly rapid onset and offset of effect. As it undergoes negligible metabolism (0.03%), any release of free inorganic fluoride is minimised; this characteristic favours its use for prolonged anaesthesia. Desflurane is extremely volatile and cannot be administered with conventional vaporisers. It has a very pungent odour and causes airway irritation to an extent that limits its rate of induction of anaesthesia.

Halothane

Halothane has the highest blood/gas partition coefficient of the volatile anaesthetic agents and recovery from halothane anaesthesia is comparatively slow. It is pleasant to breathe. Halothane reduces cardiac output more than any of the other volatile anaesthetics. It sensitises the heart to the arrhythmic effects of catecholamines and hypercapnia; arrhythmias are common, in particular atrioventricular dissociation, nodal rhythm and ventricular extrasystoles. Halothane can trigger malignant hyperthermia in those who are genetically predisposed (see p. 316).

About 20% of halothane is metabolised and it induces hepatic enzymes, including those of anaesthetists and operating theatre staff. Hepatic damage occurs in a small proportion of exposed patients. Typically fever develops 2–3 days after anaesthesia accompanied by anorexia, nausea and vomiting. In more severe cases this is followed by transient jaundice or, very rarely, fatal hepatic necrosis. Severe hepatitis is a complication of repeatedly administered halothane anaesthesia (incidence of 1 in 50 000) and follows immune sensitisation to an oxidative metabolite of halothane in susceptible individuals. This serious complication, along with the other disadvantages of halothane and the popularity of sevoflurane for inhalational induction, has almost eliminated its use in the developed world. It remains in common use in other parts of the world because it is comparatively inexpensive.

OXYGEN IN ANAESTHESIA

Supplemental oxygen is always used with inhalational anaesthetics to prevent hypoxia, even when air is used as the carrier gas. The concentration of oxygen in inspired anaesthetic gases is usually at least 30%, but oxygen should not be used for prolonged periods at a greater concentration than is necessary to prevent hypoxaemia. After prolonged administration, concentrations greater than 80% have a toxic effect on the lungs, which presents initially as a mild substernal irritation progressing to pulmonary exudation and atelectasis. Use of unnecessarily high concentrations of oxygen in incubators causes retrolental fibroplasia and permanent blindness in premature infants.

INTRAVENOUS ANAESTHETICS

Intravenous anaesthetics should be given only by those fully trained in their use and who are experienced with a full range of techniques of managing the airway, including tracheal intubation.

PHARMACOKINETICS

Intravenous anaesthetics enable an extremely rapid induction because the blood concentration can be raised quickly, establishing a steep concentration gradient and expediting diffusion into the brain. The rate of transfer depends on the lipid solubility and arterial concentration of the unbound, non-ionised fraction of the drug. After a single induction dose of an intravenous anaesthetic, recovery occurs quite rapidly as the drug is redistributed around the body and the plasma concentration reduces. Recovery from a single dose of intravenous anaesthetic is thus dependent on redistribution rather than rate of metabolic breakdown. With the exception of propofol, repeated doses or infusions of intravenous anaesthetics will cause considerable accumulation and prolong recovery. Attempts to use thiopental as the sole anaesthetic in war casualties led to it being described as an ideal form of euthanasia.[3]

It is common practice to induce anaesthesia intravenously and then to use a volatile anaesthetic for maintenance. When administration of a volatile anaesthetic is stopped, it is eliminated quickly through the lungs and the patient regains consciousness. The recovery from propofol is rapid, even after repeated doses or an infusion. This advantage, and others, has resulted in propofol displacing thiopental as the most popular intravenous anaesthetic.

Propofol

Induction of anaesthesia with 1.5–2.5 mg/kg occurs within 30 s and is smooth and pleasant with a low incidence of excitatory movements. Some preparations of propofol cause pain on injection, but adding lidocaine 20 mg to the induction dose eliminates

this. The recovery from propofol is rapid, and the incidence of nausea and vomiting is extremely low, particularly when propofol is used as the sole anaesthetic. Recovery from a continuous infusion of propofol is relatively rapid as the plasma concentration decreases by both redistribution and metabolic clearance (predominantly as the glucuronide). Special syringe pumps incorporating pharmacokinetic algorithms enable the anaesthetist to select a target plasma propofol concentration (e.g. 4 micrograms/mL for induction of anaesthesia) once details of the patient's age and weight have been entered. This technique of target-controlled infusion (TCI) provides a convenient method for giving a continuous infusion of propofol.

Central nervous system. Propofol causes dose-dependent cortical depression and is an anticonvulsant. It depresses laryngeal reflexes more than barbiturates, which is an advantage when inserting a laryngeal mask airway.

Cardiovascular system. Propofol reduces vascular tone, which lowers systemic vascular resistance and central venous pressure. The heart rate remains unchanged and the result is a fall in blood pressure to about 70–80% of the preinduction level and a small reduction in cardiac output.

Respiratory system. Unless it is undertaken very slowly, induction with propofol causes transient apnoea. On resumption of respiration there is a reduction in tidal volume and increase in rate.

Thiopental

Thiopental is a very short-acting barbiturate[4] that induces anaesthesia smoothly, within one arm-to-brain circulation time. The typical induction dose is 3–5 mg/kg. Rapid distribution (initial $t_{1/2}$ 4 min) allows swift recovery after a single dose. The terminal $t_{1/2}$ of thiopental is 11 h and repeated doses or continuous infusion lead to significant accumulation in fat and very prolonged recovery. Thiopental is metabolised in

---

[3]Halford J J 1943 A critique of intravenous anaesthesia in war surgery. Anesthesiology 4:67.

[4]Johan Adolf Bayer discovered malonylurea (the parent compound of barbiturates) on 4 December 1863. That same day he visited a tavern patronised by artillery officers and it transpired that 4 December was also the feast day of Saint Barbara, the patron saint of artillery officers, so he named the new compound 'barbituric acid' (Cozanitis D A 2004 One hundred years of barbiturates and their saint. Journal of the Royal Society of Medicine 97:594–598).

the liver. The incidence of nausea and vomiting after thiopental is slightly higher than that after propofol. The pH of thiopental is 11 and extravasation causes considerable local damage. Accidental intra-arterial injection will also cause serious injury distal to the injection site.

Central nervous system. Thiopental has no analgesic activity and may be antanalgesic. It is a potent anticonvulsant. Cerebral metabolic rate for oxygen consumption ($CMRO_2$) is reduced, causing cerebral vasoconstriction, reduction in cerebral blood flow and intracranial pressure.

Cardiovascular system. Thiopental reduces vascular tone, causing hypotension and a slight compensatory increase in heart rate. Antihypertensives or diuretics may augment the hypotensive effect.

Respiratory system. Thiopental reduces respiratory rate and tidal volume.

Methohexitone
Methohexitone is a barbiturate similar to thiopental but its terminal $t_{1/2}$ is considerably shorter. Since the introduction of propofol, its use is confined almost entirely to inducing anaesthesia for electroconvulsive therapy (ECT). Propofol shortens seizure duration and may reduce the efficacy of ECT.

Etomidate
Etomidate is a carboxylated imidazole. It causes pain on injection and excitatory muscle movements are common on induction of anaesthesia. There is a 20–50% incidence of nausea and vomiting associated with its use. Etomidate causes adrenocortical suppression by inhibiting 11β- and 17β-hydroxylase, and for this reason is not used for prolonged infusion. Despite all of these disadvantages it remains in common use, particularly for emergency anaesthesia, because it causes less cardiovascular depression and hypotension than thiopental or propofol.

Ketamine
Ketamine is a phencyclidine (hallucinogen) derivative and an antagonist of the NMDA receptor.[5] In anaesthetic doses it produces a trance-like state

known as *dissociative anaesthesia* (sedation, amnesia, dissociation, analgesia; see p. 314).

Advantages. Anaesthesia persists for up to 15 min after a single intravenous injection and is characterised by profound analgesia. Ketamine may be used as the sole analgesic for diagnostic and minor surgical interventions. In contrast to most other anaesthetic drugs, ketamine usually causes a tachycardia and increases blood pressure and cardiac output, making it a popular choice for inducing anaesthesia in shocked patients. Because pharyngeal and laryngeal reflexes are only slightly impaired, the airway may be less at risk than with other general anaesthetic techniques. It is a potent bronchodilator and is sometimes used to treat severe bronchospasm in asthmatics requiring mechanical ventilation.

Disadvantages. Ketamine produces no muscular relaxation. It increases intracranial and intraocular pressure. Hallucinations with delirium can occur during recovery (the emergence reaction), but are minimised if ketamine is used solely as an induction drug and followed by a conventional inhalational anaesthetic. Their incidence is reduced by giving a benzodiazepine both as a premedication and after the procedure. Ketamine causes salivary secretions, which are reduced by premedication with atropine.

Uses. Subanaesthetic doses of ketamine can be used to provide analgesia for painful procedures of short duration such as the dressing of burns, radiotherapeutic procedures, marrow sampling and minor orthopaedic procedures. Ketamine can be used for induction of anaesthesia before giving inhalational anaesthetics, or for both induction and maintenance of anaesthesia for short-lasting diagnostic and surgical interventions that do not require skeletal muscle relaxation. It is of particular value for children requiring frequent, repeated anaesthetics.

Dosage and administration
Induction. A dose of 2 mg/kg i.v. over a period of 60 s produces surgical anaesthesia within 1–2 min, lasting for 5–10 min; alternatively 5–10 mg/kg by deep intramuscular injection produces surgical anaesthesia within 3–5 min, lasting for up to 25 min.

Maintenance. Serial doses of 50% of the original intravenous dose or 25% of the intramuscular

---

[5]*N*-methyl-ᴅ-aspartate.

dose are given to prevent movement in response to surgical stimuli. Tonic and clonic movements resembling seizures occur in some patients but do not indicate a light plane of anaesthesia or a need for additional doses of the anaesthetic.

Recovery of consciousness is gradual. Emergence reactions (above) are lessened by benzodiazepine premedication and by avoiding unnecessary disturbance of the patient during recovery.

Contraindications include: moderate to severe hypertension, congestive cardiac failure or a history of stroke; acute or chronic alcohol intoxication, cerebral trauma, intracerebral mass or haemorrhage, or other causes of raised intracranial pressure; eye injury and increased intraocular pressure; psychiatric disorders such as a schizophrenia and acute psychoses.

Use in pregnancy. Ketamine is contraindicated in pregnancy before term, as it has oxytocic activity. It is also contraindicated in patients with eclampsia or pre-eclampsia. It may be used for assisted vaginal delivery by an experienced anaesthetist. Ketamine is better suited for use during caesarean section; it causes less fetal and neonatal depression than other anaesthetics.

MUSCLE RELAXANTS

NEUROMUSCULAR BLOCKING DRUGS

A lot of surgery, especially of the abdomen, requires that voluntary muscle tone and reflex contraction be inhibited. This could be attained by deep general anaesthesia (but with risk of cardiovascular depression, respiratory complications and slow recovery) or by regional nerve blockade (which may be difficult to do or contraindicated, e.g. if there is a haemostatic defect).

Selective relaxation of voluntary muscle with neuromuscular blocking drugs enables surgery under light general anaesthesia with analgesia; it also facilitates tracheal intubation, quick induction and quick recovery. However, mechanical ventilation and technical skill are required. Neuromuscular blocking drugs should be given only after induction of anaesthesia.

Neuromuscular blocking drugs first attracted scientific notice because of their use as arrow poisons by the natives of South America, who used the most

famous of all, curare, for killing food animals[6] as well as enemies. In 1811 Sir Benjamin Brodie smeared 'woorara paste' on wounds of guinea-pigs and noted that death could be delayed by inflating the lungs through a tube introduced into the trachea. Though he did not continue until complete recovery, he did suggest that the drug might be of use in tetanus.

Despite attempts to use curare for a variety of diseases including epilepsy, chorea and rabies, the lack of pure and accurately standardised preparations, as well as the absence of convenient techniques of mechanical ventilation if overdose occurred, prevented it from gaining any firm place in medical practice until 1942, when these difficulties were removed.

Drugs acting at the myoneural junction produce complete paralysis of all voluntary muscle so that movement is impossible and mechanical ventilation is needed. It is plainly important that a paralysed patient should be unconscious during surgery.[7]

---

[6]Curare was obtained from several sources but most commonly from the vine *Chondrodenron tomentosum*. The explorers Humboldt and Bonpland in South America (1799–1804) reported that an extract of its bark was concentrated as a tar-like mass and used to coat arrows. The potency was designated 'one tree' if a monkey, struck by a coated arrow, could make only one leap before dying. A more dilute ('three tree') form was used to paralyse animals so that they could be captured alive – an early example of a dose–response relationship.

[7]The introduction of tubocurarine into surgery made it desirable to decide once and for all whether the drug altered consciousness. Doubts were resolved in a single experiment: A normal subject was slowly paralysed (curarised) after arranging a detailed and complicated system of communication. Twelve minutes after beginning the slow infusion of curare, the subject, having artificial respiration, could move only his head. He indicated that the experience was not unpleasant, that he was mentally clear and did not want an endotracheal tube inserted. After 22 min, communication was possible only by slight movement of the left eyebrow, and after 35 min paralysis was complete and direct communication lost. An airway was inserted. The subject's eyelids were then lifted for him and the resulting inhibition of alpha rhythm of the electroencephalogram suggested that vision and consciousness were normal. After recovery, aided by neostigmine, the subject reported that he had been mentally 'clear as a bell' throughout, and confirmed this by recalling what he had heard and seen. The insertion of the endotracheal airway had caused only minor discomfort, perhaps because of the prevention of reflex muscle spasm. During artificial respiration he had 'felt that (he) would give anything to be able to take one deep breath' despite adequate oxygenation (Smith S M et al 1947 Anesthesiology 8:1). *Note*: a randomised controlled trial is not required for this kind of investigation.

Using modern anaesthetic techniques and monitoring, awareness while paralysed for a surgical procedure is extremely rare. In the UK, general anaesthesia using volatile agents should always be monitored with agent analysers, which measure and display the end-tidal concentration of volatile agent. In the past, misguided concerns about the effect of volatile anaesthetics on the newborn led many anaesthetists to use little, if any, volatile agent when giving general anaesthesia for caesarean section. Under these conditions some mothers were conscious and experienced pain while paralysed and therefore unable to move. Despite its extreme rarity nowadays[8], fear of awareness under anaesthesia is still a leading cause of anxiety in patients awaiting surgery.

Mechanisms

When an impulse passes down a motor nerve to voluntary muscle it causes release of acetylcholine from the nerve endings into the synaptic cleft. This activates receptors on the membrane of the motor endplate, a specialised area on the muscle fibre, opening ion channels for momentary passage of sodium, which depolarises the endplate and initiates muscle contraction.

Neuromuscular blocking drugs used in clinical practice interfere with this process. Natural substances that prevent the release of acetylcholine at nerve endings exist, e.g. *Clostridium botulinum* toxin (see p. 181) and some venoms.

There are two principal mechanisms by which drugs used clinically interfere with neuromuscular transmission:

1. *By competition* with acetylcholine (atracurium, cisatracurium, mivacurium, pancuronium, rocuronium, vecuronium). These drugs are competitive antagonists of acetylcholine. They do not cause depolarisation themselves but protect the endplate from depolarisation by acetylcholine. The result is a flaccid paralysis. Reversal of this type of neuromuscular block can be achieved with anticholinesterase drugs, such as neostigmine, which prevent the destruction by cholinesterase of acetylcholine released at nerve endings, enable the concentration to build

up and so reduce the competitive effect of a blocking agent.

2. *By depolarisation* of the motor endplate (suxamethonium). Such agonist drugs activate the acetylcholine receptor on the motor endplate; at their first application voluntary muscle contracts but, as they are not destroyed immediately, like acetylcholine, the depolarisation persists. It might be expected that this prolonged depolarisation would cause muscles to remain contracted, but this is not so (except in chickens). With prolonged administration, a depolarisation block changes to a competitive block (dual block). Because of the uncertainty of this situation, a competitive blocking drug is preferred for anything other than short procedures.

COMPETITIVE ANTAGONISTS

Atracurium is unique in that it is altered spontaneously in the body to an inactive form ($t_{\frac{1}{2}}$ 30 min) by a passive chemical process (Hofmann elimination). The duration of action (15–35 min) is thus uninfluenced by the state of the circulation, the liver or the kidneys, a significant advantage in patients with hepatic or renal disease and in the aged. It has very little direct effect on the cardiovascular system but at doses of greater than 0.5–0.6 mg/kg histamine release may cause hypotension and bronchospasm.

Cisatracurium is a stereoisomer of atracurium; it is less prone to cause histamine release.

Vecuronium is a synthetic steroid derivative that produces full neuromuscular blockade about 3 min after a dose of 0.1 mg/kg, lasting for 30 min. It has no cardiovascular side-effects and does not cause histamine release.

Rocuronium is another steroid derivative that has the advantage of a rapid onset of action, such that 0.6 mg/kg allows tracheal intubation to be achieved after 60 s. It has negligible cardiovascular effects and a similar duration of action to vecuronium.

Mivacurium belongs to the same chemical family as atracurium and is the only non-depolarising neuromuscular blocker that is metabolised by plasma cholinesterase. It is comparatively short acting (10–15 min), depending on the initial dose. Mivacurium can cause some hypotension because of histamine release.

---

[8]In a prospective series of 11 785 general anaesthetics, 18 patients recalled awareness during surgery (Sandin R H, Enlund G, Samuelsson P et al 2000 Awareness during anaesthesia: a prospective case study. Lancet 355:707–711).

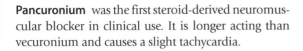
Pancuronium was the first steroid-derived neuromuscular blocker in clinical use. It is longer acting than vecuronium and causes a slight tachycardia.

Tubocurarine is now obsolete and no longer available in the UK. It is a potent antagonist at autonomic ganglia and causes significant hypotension.

Antagonism of competitive neuromuscular block: neostigmine

The action of competitive acetylcholine blockers is antagonised by anticholinesterase drugs, which enable accumulation of acetylcholine. Neostigmine (see p. 396) is given intravenously, mixed with glycopyrronium to prevent bradycardia caused by the parasympathetic autonomic effects of the neostigmine. It acts in 4 min and its effects last for about 30 min. Too much neostigmine can cause neuromuscular block by depolarisation, which will cause confusion unless there have been some signs of recovery before neostigmine is given. Progress can be monitored with a nerve stimulator.

DEPOLARISING NEUROMUSCULAR BLOCKER

Suxamethonium (succinylcholine)

Paralysis is preceded by muscle fasciculation, and this may be the cause of the muscle pain experienced commonly after its use. The pain may last for 1–3 days and can be minimised by preceding the suxamethonium with a small dose of a competitive blocking agent.

Suxamethonium is the neuromuscular blocker with the most rapid onset and the shortest duration of action. Tracheal intubation is possible in less than 60 s and total paralysis lasts for up to 4 min with 50% recovery in about 10 min ($t_{1/2}$ for effect). It is indicated particularly for rapid sequence induction of anaesthesia in patients who are at risk of aspiration – the ability to secure the airway rapidly with a tracheal tube is of the utmost importance. If intubation proves impossible, recovery from suxamethonium and resumption of spontaneous respiration is relatively rapid. Unfortunately, if it is impossible to ventilate the paralysed patient's lungs, recovery may not be rapid enough to prevent the onset of hypoxia.

Suxamethonium is destroyed by *plasma pseudocholinesterase* and so its persistence in the body is increased by neostigmine, which inactivates that enzyme, and in patients with hepatic disease or severe malnutrition whose plasma enzyme concentrations are lower than normal. Approximately 1 in 3000 of the European population have hereditary defects in amount or kind of enzyme, and cannot destroy the drug as rapidly as normal individuals.[9] Paralysis can then last for hours and the individual requires ventilatory support and sedation until recovery occurs spontaneously.

Repeated injections of suxamethonium can cause bradycardia, extrasystoles and even ventricular arrest. These are probably due to activation of cholinoceptors in the heart and are prevented by atropine. It can be used in caesarean section as it does not cross the placenta readily. Suxamethonium depolarisation causes a release of potassium from muscle, which in normal patients will increase the plasma potassium by 0.5 mmol/L. This is a problem only if the patient's plasma potassium concentration was already high, for example in acute renal failure. In patients with spinal cord injuries and those with major burns, suxamethonium may cause a grossly exaggerated release of potassium from muscle, sufficient to cause cardiac arrest.

USES OF NEUROMUSCULAR BLOCKING DRUGS

Only those who are competent at tracheal intubation and ventilation of the patient's lungs should use these drugs. The drugs are used:

■ to provide muscular relaxation during surgery, to enable intubation in the emergency department, and occasionally to assist mechanical ventilation in intensive therapy units; and
■ during electroconvulsive therapy to prevent injury to the patient from excessive muscular contraction.

OTHER MUSCLE RELAXANTS

Drugs that reduce spasm of the voluntary muscles without impairing voluntary movement can be useful in spastic states, low back syndrome and rheumatism with muscle spasm.

Baclofen is structurally related to γ-aminobutyric acid (GABA), an inhibitory central nervous system

---

[9]There are wide inter-ethnic differences. When cases are discovered the family should be investigated for low plasma cholinesterase activity and affected individuals warned.

(CNS) transmitter; it inhibits reflex activity resides mainly in the spinal cord. Baclofen reduces spasticity and flexor spasms, but, as it has no action on voluntary muscle power, function is commonly not improved. Ambulant patients may need their leg spasticity to provide support, and reduction of spasticity may expose the weakness of the limb. It benefits some cases of trigeminal neuralgia. Baclofen is given orally ($t_{1/2}$ 3 h).

Dantrolene acts directly on muscle and prevents the release of calcium from sarcoplasm stores (see malignant hyperthermia, p. 135).

ANAPHYLAXIS

Anaphylactic reactions are caused by the interaction of antigens with specific immunoglobulin (Ig) E antibodies, which have been formed by previous exposure to the antigen. *Anaphylactoid* reactions are clinically indistinguishable from anaphylaxis but are not caused by previous exposure to a triggering agent, do not involve IgE and may involve the sudden release of autacoids. Intravenous anaesthetics and muscle relaxants can cause anaphylactic or anaphylactoid reactions; rarely, they are fatal. Muscle relaxants are responsible for 70% of anaphylactic reactions during anaesthesia, and suxamethonium accounts for almost half of these.

LOCAL ANAESTHETICS

Cocaine had been suggested as a local anaesthetic for clinical use when Sigmund Freud investigated the alkaloid in Vienna in 1884 with Carl Koller. The latter had long been interested in the problem of local anaesthesia in the eye, for general anaesthesia has disadvantages in ophthalmology. Observing that numbness of the mouth occurred after taking cocaine orally, Koller realised that this was a local anaesthetic effect. He tried cocaine on animals' eyes and introduced it into clinical ophthalmological practice, whilst Freud was on holiday. Freud had already thought of this use and discussed it but, appreciating that sex was of greater importance than surgery, he had gone to see his fiancée. The use of cocaine spread rapidly and it was soon being used to block nerve trunks. Chemists then began to search for less toxic substitutes, with the result that procaine was introduced in 1905.

DESIRED PROPERTIES

Innumerable compounds have local anaesthetic properties, but few are suitable for clinical use. Useful substances must be water soluble, sterilisable by heat, have a rapid onset of effect, a duration of action appropriate to the operation to be performed, be non-toxic, both locally and when absorbed into the circulation, and leave no local after-effects.

MODE OF ACTION

Local anaesthetics prevent the initiation and propagation of the nerve impulse (action potential). By reducing the passage of sodium through voltage-gated sodium ion channels they raise the threshold of excitability; in consequence, conduction is blocked at afferent nerve endings, and by sensory and motor nerve fibres. The fibres in nerve trunks are affected in order of size, the smallest (autonomic, sensory) first, probably because they have a proportionately greater surface area, and then the larger (motor) fibres. Paradoxically the effect in the CNS is stimulation (see below).

PHARMACOKINETICS

The distribution rate of a single dose of a local anaesthetic is determined by diffusion into tissues with concentrations approximately in relation to blood flow (plasma $t_{1/2}$ of only a few minutes). By injection or infiltration, local anaesthetics are usually effective within 5 min and have a useful duration of effect of 1–1.5 h, which in some cases may be doubled by adding a vasoconstrictor (below).

Most local anaesthetics are used in the form of the acid salts, as these are both soluble and stable. The acid salt (usually the hydrochloride) dissociates in the tissues to liberate the free base, which is biologically active. This dissociation is delayed in abnormally acid, e.g. inflamed, tissues, but the risk of spreading infection makes local anaesthesia undesirable in infected areas.

Absorption from mucous membranes on topical application varies according to the compound. Those that are well absorbed are used as surface anaesthetics (cocaine, lidocaine, prilocaine). Absorption of topically applied local anaesthetic can be extremely rapid and give plasma concentrations comparable to those obtained by injection. This has led to deaths from overdosage, especially via the urethra.

For topical effect on intact skin for needling procedures, a eutectic[10] mixture of bases of prilocaine or lidocaine is used (EMLA – *eutectic mixture of local anaesthetics*). Absorption is very slow and a cream is applied under an occlusive dressing for at least 1 h. Tetracaine gel 4% (Ametop) is more effective than EMLA cream and enables pain-free venepuncture 30 min after application.

Ester compounds (cocaine, procaine, tetracaine, benzocaine) are hydrolysed by liver and plasma esterases, and their effects may be prolonged where there is a genetic enzyme deficiency.

Amide compounds (lidocaine, prilocaine, bupivacaine, levobupivacaine, ropivacaine) are dealkylated in the liver.

Impaired liver function, whether caused by primary cellular insufficiency or low liver blood flow as in cardiac failure, may both delay elimination and cause higher peak plasma concentrations of both types of local anaesthetic. This is likely to be important only with large or repeated doses or infusions.

PROLONGATION OF ACTION BY VASOCONSTRICTORS

The effect of a local anaesthetic is terminated by its removal from the site of application. Anything that delays its absorption into the circulation will prolong its local action and can reduce its systemic toxicity when large doses are used. Most local anaesthetics, with the exception of cocaine, cause vascular dilation. The addition of a vasoconstrictor such as adrenaline (epinephrine) reduces local blood flow, slows the rate of absorption of the local anaesthetic, and prolongs its effect; the duration of action of lidocaine is doubled from 1 h to 2 h. Normally, the final concentration of adrenaline should be 1 in 200 000, although dentists use up to 1 in 80 000.

Do not use a vasoconstrictor for nerve block of an extremity (finger, toe, nose, penis). For obvious anatomical reasons, the whole blood supply may be cut off by intense vasoconstriction so that the organ may be damaged or even lost. Enough adrenaline can be absorbed to affect the heart and circulation, and reduce the plasma potassium concentration.

This can be dangerous in cardiovascular disease, and with co-administered tricyclic antidepressants and potassium-losing diuretics. An alternative vasoconstrictor is *felypressin* (synthetic vasopressin), which, in the concentrations used, does not affect the heart rate or blood pressure and may be preferable in patients with cardiovascular disease.

OTHER EFFECTS

Local anaesthetics also have the following clinically important effects in varying degree:

- Excitation of parts of the CNS, which may manifest as anxiety, restlessness, tremors, euphoria, agitation and even convulsions, which are followed by depression.
- Quinidine-like actions on the heart.

USES

Local anaesthesia is generally used when loss of consciousness is neither necessary nor desirable, and also as an adjunct to major surgery to avoid high-dose general anaesthesia and to provide postoperative analgesia. It can be used for major surgery, with sedation, although many patients prefer to be unconscious. It is invaluable when the operator must also be the anaesthetist, which is often the case in some parts of the developing world.

Local anaesthetics may be used in several ways to provide:

- Surface anaesthesia, as solution, jelly, cream or lozenge.
- Infiltration anaesthesia, to block the sensory nerve endings and small cutaneous nerves.
- Regional anaesthesia.

Regional anaesthesia

Regional anaesthesia requires considerable knowledge of anatomy and attention to detail for both success and safety.

Nerve block means the anaesthetising of a region, small or large, by injecting the drug around, not into, the appropriate nerves, usually either a peripheral nerve or a plexus. Nerve block provides its own muscular relaxation as motor fibres are blocked as well as sensory fibres, although with care differential block, affecting sensory more than motor fibres, can be achieved. There are various specialised forms: brachial plexus, paravertebral, paracervical block.

---

[10]A mixture of two solids that becomes a liquid because the mixture has a lower melting point than either of its components.

Sympathetic nerve blocks may be used in vascular disease to induce vasodilation.

Intravenous. A double cuff is applied to the arm, inflated above arterial pressure after elevating the limb to drain the venous system, and the veins filled with local anaesthetic, e.g. 0.5–1% lidocaine without adrenaline (epinephrine). The arm is anaesthetised in 6–8 min, and the effect lasts for up to 40 min if the cuff remains inflated. The cuff must not be deflated for at least 20 min. The technique is useful in providing anaesthesia for the treatment of injuries speedily and conveniently, and many patients can leave hospital soon after the procedure. The technique must be meticulously conducted, for sudden release of the full dose of local anaesthetic accidentally into the general circulation may cause severe toxicity and even cardiac arrest. Bupivacaine is no longer used for intravenous regional anaesthesia as cardiac arrest caused by it is particularly resistant to treatment.

Extradural (epidural) anaesthesia is used in the thoracic, lumbar and sacral (caudal) regions. Lumbar epidurals are used widely in obstetrics and low thoracic epidurals provide excellent analgesia after laparotomy. The drug is injected into the *extradural space* where it acts on the nerve roots. This technique is less likely to cause hypotension than spinal anaesthesia. Continuous analgesia is achieved if a local anaesthetic, often mixed with an opioid, is infused through an epidural catheter.

Subarachnoid (intrathecal) block (spinal anaesthesia). The drug is injected *into the cerebrospinal fluid (CSF)* and, by using a solution of appropriate specific gravity and tilting the patient, it can be kept at an appropriate level. Sympathetic nerve blockade causes hypotension. Headache due to CSF leakage is virtually eliminated by using very narrow atraumatic 'pencil point' needles.

Serious local neurological complications, e.g. infection and nerve injury, are extremely rare.

Opioid analgesics are used intrathecally and extradurally. They diffuse into the spinal cord and act on its opioid receptors (see p. 298); they are highly effective in skilled hands for postsurgical and intractable pain. Respiratory depression may occur. The effect begins in 20 min and lasts for up to 12 h.

Diamorphine or other more lipid-soluble opioids, such as fentanyl, may be used.

ADVERSE REACTIONS

Excessive absorption causes paraesthesiae (face and tongue), anxiety, tremors and even convulsions. The latter are very dangerous, are followed by respiratory depression, and may require diazepam or thiopental for control. Cardiovascular collapse and respiratory failure occur with higher plasma concentrations of the local anaesthetic; the cause is direct myocardial depression compounded by hypoxia associated with convulsions. Cardiopulmonary resuscitation must be started immediately.

Anaphylactoid reactions are very rare with *amide* local anaesthetics and some of those reported have been due to preservatives. Most reported reactions to amide local anaesthetics are due to co-administration of adrenaline (epinephrine), intravascular injection or psychological effects (vasovagal episodes). Reactions with *ester* local anaesthetics are more common.

INDIVIDUAL LOCAL ANAESTHETICS

See Table 18.1.

Amides
Lidocaine is a first choice drug for surface use as well as for injection, combining efficacy with comparative lack of toxicity; the $t_{1/2}$ is 1.5 h. It is also useful in cardiac arrhythmias although it has been largely replaced by amiodarone for this purpose.

Prilocaine is used similarly to lidocaine ($t_{1/2}$ 1.5 h), but it is slightly less toxic. It used to be the preferred drug for intravenous regional anaesthesia but it is no longer available as a preservative-free solution and most clinicians now use lidocaine instead. Crystals of prilocaine and lidocaine base, when mixed, dissolve in one another to form a eutectic emulsion that penetrates skin and is used for dermal anaesthesia (EMLA; see p. 315), e.g. before venepuncture in children.

Bupivacaine is long acting ($t_{1/2}$ 3 h) (see Table 18.1) and is used for peripheral nerve blocks, and for epidural and spinal anaesthesia. Although onset of effect is comparable to that of lidocaine, peak effect occurs later (30 min).

Table 18.1 Licensed doses for three widely used amide local anaesthetics

	Solution	Dose by volume	Duration of effect (adult)
Lidocaine			1.5 h
Infiltration	0.25–0.5% + adrenaline (epinephrine)	up to 60 mL	
Nerve block	1% + adrenaline (epinephrine)	up to 50 mL	
(peripheral)	2% + adrenaline (epinephrine)	up to 25 mL	
Surface anaesthesia	2%	up to 20 mL	
	4%	up to 5 mL	
Bupivacaine			3–4 h
Infiltration	0.25%	up to 60 mL	
Nerve block	0.25%	up to 60 mL	
(peripheral)	0.5%	up to 30 mL	
Prilocaine			1.5–3 h
Infiltration	0.5%	up to 80 mL	
Nerve block	1%	up to 40 mL	
(peripheral)	2%	up to 20 mL	
	3% + felypressin (dental use)	up to 20 mL	

Notes:

1. Time to peak effect is about 5 min, except bupivacaine (see text).
2. Maximum doses of local anaesthetic plus vasoconstrictor are toxic in absence of the vasoconstrictor and so substantially less should be used. All doses are only approximate; larger amounts may be safe, but deaths have occurred with smaller amounts, so that the minimum dose that will suffice should be used.
3. Maximum dose of adrenaline (epinephrine) is 500 micrograms (see below).
4. Concentrations of solutions and dose of drug: errors of calculation occur with sometimes fatal results.
   1% means 1 g in 100 mL = 1000 mg in 100 mL = 10 mg/mL; 2% = 20 mg/mL; and so on.
   It is traditional to express adrenaline concentrations as 1 in 200 000, or 1 in 80 000, or 1 in 1000.
   1 in 1000 means 1000 mg (1.0 g) in 1000 mL = 1 mg/mL.
   1 in 200 000 means 1000 mg (1.0 g) in 200 000 mL = 5 micrograms/mL.
   Thus the maximum dose of adrenaline, 500 micrograms (see above), is contained in 100 mL of 1 in 200 000 solution.

Levobupivacaine is the *S*-enantiomer of racemic bupivacaine. The relative therapeutic ratio (levobupivacaine : racemic bupivacaine) for CNS toxicity is 1.03, indicating that levobupivacaine is marginally less toxic.

Ropivacaine may provide better separation of motor and sensory nerve blockade; effective sensory blockade can be achieved without causing motor weakness. The rate of onset of ropivacaine is similar to that of bupivacaine, but its absolute potency and duration of effect are slightly lower. The indications for ropivacaine are similar to those of bupivacaine.

Esters

Cocaine (alkaloid) is used medicinally solely as a surface anaesthetic (for abuse toxicity, see p. 167) usually as a 4% solution, because adverse effects are both common and dangerous when it is injected. Even as a surface anaesthetic, sufficient absorption may take place to cause serious adverse effects and cases continue to be reported; only specialists should use it and the dose must be checked and restricted.

Cocaine prevents the uptake of catecholamines (adrenaline, noradrenaline) into sympathetic nerve endings, thus increasing their concentration at receptor sites, so that cocaine has a built-in vasoconstrictor action, which is why it retains a (declining) place as a surface anaesthetic for surgery involving mucous membranes, e.g. nose. Other local anaesthetics do not have this action; indeed, most are vasodilators and added adrenaline (epinepehrine) is not so efficient.

OBSTETRIC ANALGESIA AND ANAESTHESIA

Although this soon ceased to be considered immoral on religious grounds, it has been a technically controversial topic since 1853 when it was announced that Queen Victoria had inhaled chloroform during the birth of her eighth child. *The Lancet* recorded 'intense astonishment … throughout the profession' at this use of chloroform, 'an agent which has unquestionably caused instantaneous death in a considerable number of cases'. But the Queen (perhaps ignorant of these risks) took a different view, writing in her private journal of 'that blessed chloroform' and adding that 'the effect was soothing, quieting and delightful beyond measure'.

The ideal drug must relieve labour pain without making the patient confused or uncooperative. It must not interfere with uterine activity nor must it influence the fetus, e.g. to cause respiratory depression by a direct action, by prolonging labour or by reducing uterine blood supply. It should also be suitable for use by a midwife without supervision.

Pethidine is used widely. There is little difference between the effects of equipotent doses of morphine and pethidine on analgesia, respiratory depression, and nausea and vomiting. All opioids have the potential to cause respiratory depression of the newborn but this can be reversed with naloxone if necessary. The popular choice of pethidine for analgesia during labour in the UK is not because of any clear pharmacological advantage, but because it remains the only opioid licensed for use by midwives.

Nitrous oxide and oxygen (50% of each: Entonox) may be administered for each contraction from a machine the patient works herself or supervised by a midwife (about 10 good breaths are needed for maximal analgesia).

Epidural local anaesthesia provides the most effective pain relief, but the technique should be undertaken only after adequate training. In the UK, only anaesthetists insert epidural anaesthetics.

Spinal anaesthesia is now used more commonly than epidural anaesthesia for caesarean section. The vast majority of caesarean sections are now undertaken with regional rather than general anaesthesia.

General anaesthesia during labour presents special problems. Gastric regurgitation and aspiration are a particular risk (see p. 658). The safety of the fetus must be considered; all anaesthetics and analgesics in general use cross the placenta in varying amounts and, apart from respiratory depression, produce no important effects except that high doses interfere with uterine contraction and may be followed by uterine haemorrhage. Neuromuscular blocking agents can be used safely.

ANAESTHESIA IN PATIENTS ALREADY TAKING MEDICATION

Anaesthetists are in an unenviable position. They are expected to provide safe service to patients in any condition, taking any drugs. Sometimes there is opportunity to modify drug therapy before surgery, but often there is not. Anaesthetists require a particularly detailed drug history from the patient.

DRUGS THAT AFFECT ANAESTHESIA

Adrenal steroids. Chronic corticosteroid therapy with the equivalent of prednisolone 10 mg daily within the previous 3 months suppresses the hypothalamic–pituitary–adrenal (HPA) system. Without corticosteroid supplementation perioperatively the patient may fail to respond appropriately to the stress of surgery and become hypotensive (see Chapter 34). A single dose of *etomidate* depresses the HPA axis for up to 24 h, but the clinical significance of this is unknown.

Antibiotics. Aminoglycosides, e.g. neomycin, gentamicin, potentiate neuromuscular blocking drugs.

Anticholinesterases can potentiate suxamethonium.

Antiepilepsy drugs. Continued medication is essential to avoid status epilepticus. Drugs must be given parenterally (e.g. phenytoin, sodium valproate) or rectally (e.g. carbamazepine) until the patient can absorb enterally.

Antihypertensives of all kinds; hypotension may complicate anaesthesia, but it is best to continue therapy. Hypertensive patients are particularly liable to excessive increase in blood pressure and heart rate during intubation, which can be dangerous if there is ischaemic heart disease. After surgery, parenteral therapy may be needed for a time.

β-Adrenoceptor blocking drugs can prevent the homeostatic sympathetic cardiac response to cardiac depressant anaesthetics and to blood loss.

Diuretics. Hypokalaemia, if present, will potentiate neuromuscular blocking agents and perhaps general anaesthetics.

Oral contraceptives containing oestrogen, and post-menopausal hormone replacement therapy, predispose to thromboembolism (see p. 521).

Psychotropic drugs. Neuroleptics potentiate or synergise with opioids, hypnotics and general anaesthetics.

Antidepressants. Monoamine oxidase inhibitors can cause hypertension when combined with certain amines, e.g. pethidine, or indirectly acting sympathomimetics, e.g. ephedrine. Tricyclics potentiate catecholamines and some other adrenergic drugs.

ANAESTHESIA IN THE DISEASED, AND IN PARTICULAR PATIENT GROUPS

The normal response to anaesthesia may be greatly modified by disease. Some of the more important aspects include:

Respiratory disease and smoking predispose the patient to postoperative pulmonary complications, principally infective. The site of operation, e.g. upper abdomen, chest, and the severity of pain influence the impairment to ventilation and coughing.

Cardiac disease. The aim is to avoid the circulatory stress (with increased cardiac work, which can compromise the myocardial oxygen supply) caused by hypertension and tachycardia. Intravenous drugs are normally given slowly to reduce the risk of overdosage and hypotension.

Patients with fixed cardiac output, e.g. with aortic stenosis or constrictive pericarditis, are at special risk from reduced cardiac output with drugs that depress the myocardium and vasomotor centre, for they cannot compensate. Induction with propofol or thiopental is particularly liable to cause hypotension in these patients. Hypoxia is obviously harmful. Skilled technique rather than choice of drugs on pharmacological grounds is the important factor.

Hepatic or renal disease is generally liable to increase drug effects and should be taken into account when selecting drugs and their doses.

Malignant hyperthermia (MH) is a rare pharmaco-genetic syndrome with an incidence of between 1 in 15 000 and 1 in 150 000 in North America, exhibiting autosomal dominant inheritance with variable penetrance. The condition occurs during or immediately after anaesthesia and may be precipitated by potent inhalation agents (halothane, isoflurane, sevoflurane) or suxamethonium. The patient may have experienced an uncomplicated general anaesthetic previously. The mechanism involves an abnormally increased release of calcium from the sarcoplasmic reticulum, often caused by an inherited mutation in the gene for the ryanodine receptor, which resides in the sarcoplasmic reticulum membrane. High calcium concentrations stimulate muscle contraction, rhabdomyolysis and a hypermetabolic state. Malignant hyperthermia is a life-threatening medical emergency. Oxygen consumption increases by up to three times the normal value, and body temperature may increase as fast as 1°C every 5 min, reaching as high as 43°C. Rigidity of voluntary muscles may not be evident at the outset or in mild cases.

Dantrolene 1 mg/kg i.v. is given immediately. Further doses are given at 10-min intervals until the patient responds, to a cumulative maximum dose of 10 mg/kg. Dantrolene ($t_\frac{1}{2}$ 9 h) probably acts by preventing the release of calcium from the sarcoplasm store that ordinarily follows depolarisation of the muscle membrane.

Non-specific treatment is needed for the hyperthermia (cooling, oxygen), and insulin and dextrose are given for hyperkalaemia caused by potassium release from contracted muscle. Hyperkalaemia and acidosis may trigger severe cardiac arrhythmias.

Once the immediate crisis has resolved, the patient and all immediate relatives should undergo investigation for MH. This involves a muscle biopsy, which is tested for sensitivity to triggering agents.

Anaesthesia in MH-susceptible patients is achieved safely with total intravenous anaesthesia using propofol and opioids. Dantrolene for intravenous use must be available immediately in every location where general anaesthesia is given. The relation of malignant hyperthermia syndrome with neuroleptic malignant syndrome (for which dantrolene may be used as adjunctive treatment, see p. 323) is uncertain.

Muscle diseases. Patients with myasthenia gravis are very sensitive to (intolerant of) competitive but not to depolarising neuromuscular blocking drugs.

Those with myotonic dystrophy may recover less rapidly than normal from central respiratory depression and neuromuscular block; they may fail to relax with suxamethonium.

Sickle cell disease. Hypoxia and dehydration can precipitate a crisis.

Atypical (deficient) pseudocholinesterase. There is delay in the metabolism of suxamethonium and mivacurium. The duration of neuromuscular block depends on the level of pseudocholinesterase activity.

Raised intracranial pressure will be made worse by high expired concentration inhalation agents, e.g. more than 1% isoflurane, by hypoxia or hypercapnia, and in response to intubation if anaesthesia is inadequate. Without support from a mechanical ventilator, excessive doses of opioids will cause hypercapnia and increase intracranial pressure.

The elderly (see p. 109) are liable to become confused by cerebral depressants, especially by hyoscine. Atropine also crosses the blood–brain barrier and can cause confusion in the elderly; glycopyrronium is preferable. In general, elderly patients require smaller doses of all drugs than the young. The elderly tolerate hypotension poorly; they are prone to cerebral and coronary ischaemia.

Children (see p. 108). The problems with children are more technical, physiological and psychological than pharmacological.

Sedation in critical care units is used to reduce patient anxiety and improve tolerance to tracheal tubes and mechanical ventilation. Whenever possible, patients are sedated only to a level that enables them to open their eyes to verbal command; oversedation is harmful. Commonly used drugs include propofol and midazolam, and opioids such as fentanyl, alfentanil, morphine or remifentanil.

Neuromuscular blockers are required only rarely to assist mechanical ventilation. If pain is treated properly and patient-triggered modes of ventilation are used, many patients in the critical care unit will not require sedation. Reassurance from sympathetic nursing staff is extremely important and far more effective than drugs.

Diabetes mellitus. See page 608.

Thyroid disease. See page 633.

Porphyria. See page 120.

GUIDE TO FURTHER READING

Campagna J A, Miller K W, Forman S A 2003 Mechanisms of actions of inhaled anesthetics. New England Journal of Medicine 348(21):2110–2124

Carter A J 1999 Dwale: an anaesthetic from old England. British Medical Journal 319:1623–1626 (concerns the use of medicinal herbs to render a patient unconscious for surgery before modern general anaesthesia)

Harper N 2001 Inhalational anaesthetics. Anaesthesia and Intensive Care Medicine 2:241–244

Hemmings H C, Akabas M A, Goldstein P A et al 2005 Emerging molecular mechanisms of general anaesthetic action. Trends in Pharmacological Sciences 26(10):503–510

Lagan G, McClure H A 2004 Review of local anaesthetic agents. Current Anaesthesia and Critical Care 15:247–254

Pollard B J 2001 Neuromuscular blocking agents. Anaesthesia and Intensive Care Medicine 2:281–284

Royston D, Cox F 2003 Anaesthesia: the patient's point of view. Lancet 362:1648–1658 (and the subsequent articles in this series published in later issues on pp. 1749–1757, 1838–1846, 1921–1928)

Sneyd J R 2004 Recent advances in intravenous anaesthesia. British Journal of Anaesthesia 93(5):725–736

Stern V 2000 Operations: spinal versus general anaesthetics – a patient's view. British Medical Journal 321:1606–1607

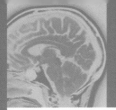

19

Psychotropic drugs

SYNOPSIS

Psychiatric disorders are some of the most common illnesses. Advances in drug treatment have revolutionised the practice of psychiatry over the past six decades. This chapter considers the following drug groups:

■ Antidepressants
■ Antipsychotics ('neuroleptics')
■ Mood stabilisers
■ Drugs for anxiety and sleep disorders
■ Drugs for dementia
■ Drugs for attention deficit/hyperactivity disorder

DIAGNOSTIC ISSUES

Older classifications of psychiatric disorder divided diseases into 'psychoses' and 'neuroses'. The term 'psychosis' is still widely used to describe a severe mental illness with hallucinations, delusions, extreme abnormalities of behaviour including marked overactivity, retardation and catatonia, usually with lack of insight. Psychotic disorders include schizophrenia, severe depression and mania. Psychosis may also be due to illicit substances or organic conditions. Clinical features of schizophrenia are subdivided into 'positive symptoms', which include hallucinations, delusions and thought disorder, and 'negative symptoms' such as apathy, flattening of affect and poverty of speech.

Disorders formerly grouped under 'neuroses' include anxiety disorders (e.g. panic disorder, generalised anxiety disorder, obsessive–compulsive disorder, phobias and post-traumatic stress disorder), eating disorders (e.g. anorexia nervosa and bulimia nervosa), depression (provided there are no 'psychotic' symptoms) and sleep disorders.

Also falling within the scope of modern psychiatric diagnostic systems are organic mental disorders (e.g. dementia in Alzheimer's disease), disorders due to substance misuse (e.g. alcohol and opiate dependence; see Chapter 10), personality disorders, disorders of childhood and adolescence (e.g. attention deficit/hyperactivity disorder, Tourette's syndrome), and mental retardation (learning disabilities).

DRUG THERAPY IN RELATION TO PSYCHOLOGICAL TREATMENT

No account of drug treatment strategies for psychiatric illness is complete without considering psychological therapies. Psychotherapies range widely, from simple counselling (supportive psychotherapy) through psychoanalysis to newer techniques such as cognitive behavioural therapy.

As a general rule, *psychotic illnesses* (e.g. schizophrenia, mania and depressive psychosis) require drugs as first-line treatment, with psychotherapy being adjunctive, for instance in promoting drug compliance, improving family relationships and helping individuals cope with distressing symptoms. By contrast, for *depression* and *anxiety disorders*, such as panic disorder and obsessive–compulsive disorder, forms of psychotherapy are available that provide alternative first-line treatment to medication. The choice between drugs and psychotherapy depends on treatment availability, previous history of response, patient preference and the ability of the patient to work appropriately with the chosen therapy. In many cases there is scope and sometimes advantage to the use of drugs and psychotherapy in combination.

Taking depression as an example, an extensive evidence base exists for the efficacy of several forms of *psychotherapy*. These include cognitive therapy (which normalises depressive thinking), interpersonal therapy (which focuses on relationships and roles), brief dynamic psychotherapy (a time-limited version of psychoanalysis) and cognitive analytical therapy (a structured time-limited therapy that combines the best points of cognitive therapy and traditional analysis).

All doctors who prescribe drugs engage in a 'therapeutic relationship' with their patients. A depressed person whose doctor is empathic, supportive and appears to believe in the efficacy of the drug prescribed is more likely to take the medication and to adopt a hopeful mindset than if the doctor seemed aloof and ambivalent about the value of psychotropic drugs. Remembering that placebo response rates of 30–40% are common in double-blind trials of antidepressants, we should never underestimate the importance of our relationship with the patient in enhancing the pharmacological efficacy of the drugs we use.

ANTIDEPRESSANT DRUGS

Antidepressants can be broadly divided into four main classes (Table 19.1), *tricyclics* (TCA, named after their three-ringed structure), *selective serotonin reuptake inhibitors* (SSRIs), *monoamine oxidase inhibitors* (MAOIs) and *novel compounds*, some of which are related to TCAs or SSRIs. Clinicians who wish to have a working knowledge of antidepressants would be advised to be familiar with the use of at least one drug from each of the four main categories tabulated. A more thorough knowledge base would demand awareness of differences between individual TCAs and of the distinct characteristics of the novel compounds. As antidepressants are largely similar in their therapeutic efficacy, awareness of profiles of unwanted effects is of particular importance.

An alternative categorisation of antidepressants is based solely on mechanism of action (Fig. 19.1). The majority of antidepressants, including TCAs, SSRIs and related compounds, are *reuptake inhibitors*. Certain novel agents including trazodone and mirtazapine are *receptor blockers*, whereas MAOIs are *enzyme inhibitors*.

The first TCAs (imipramine and amitriptyline) and MAOIs appeared between 1957 and 1961 (see Fig. 19.1). The MAOIs were developed from antituberculous agents that unexpectedly improved mood. Imipramine was a chlorpromazine derivative that showed antidepressant rather than antipsychotic properties. Over the next 25 years the TCA class enlarged to more than 10 agents with heterogeneous pharmacological profiles, and further modifications of the original three-ringed structure gave rise to the related (but pharmacologically distinct) antidepressant trazodone.

Table 19.1	Classification of antidepressants	
Tricyclics	**Selective serotonin reuptake inhibitors**	**Monoamine oxidase inhibitors**
dothiepin	fluoxetine	phenelzine
amitriptyline	paroxetine	isocarboxazid
lofepramine	sertraline	tranylcypromine
clomipramine	citalopram[a]	moclobemide (RIMA)
imipramine	escitalopram[a]	
trimipramine	fluvoxamine	
doxepin		
nortriptyline		
protriptyline		
desipramine		
Novel compounds		
Mainly noradrenergic	**Mainly serotonergic**	
reboxetine (NaRI)	trazodone[b]	
	nefazodone[b,c]	
Mixed		
venlafaxine (SNRI)		
mirtazapine (NaSSA)[b]		
duloxetine (SNRI)		
milnacipran (SNRI)[d]		

Within each class or subclass, drugs are listed in order of frequency of prescription in the UK (1997 data).
RIMA, reversible inhibitor of monoamine oxidase; NaRI, noradrenaline reuptake inhibitor; SNRI, serotonin and noradrenaline reuptake inhibitor; NaSSA, noradrenaline and specific serotonergic antidepressant.
[a]Escitalopram is the active *S*-enantiomer of citalopram.
[b]Trazodone, nefazodone and mirtazapine have been classed as 'receptor blocking' antidepressants based on their antagonism of postsynaptic serotonin receptors (trazodone, nefazodone, mirtazapine) and presynaptic α_2-receptors (trazodone, mirtazapine).
[c]Nefazodone has additional weak SSRI activity but has now been withdrawn due to risk of hepatitis.
[d]Not available in the UK.

In the 1980s an entirely new class of antidepressant arrived with the SSRIs: first, fluvoxamine, followed immediately by fluoxetine (Prozac®). Within 10 years, the SSRI class accounted for half of antidepressant prescriptions in the UK. Further developments in the evolution of antidepressants have been novel compounds such as venlafaxine, reboxetine and mirtazapine, and a reversible MAOI, moclobemide.

MECHANISM OF ACTION

The monoamine hypothesis proposes that, in depression, there is deficiency of the neurotransmitters *noradrenaline* and *serotonin* in the brain which can

331

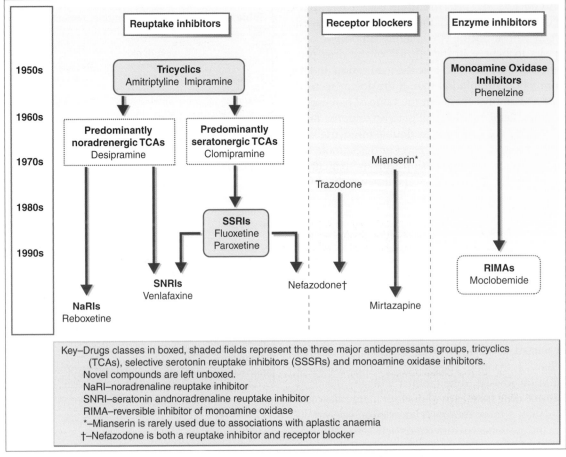

Fig. 19.1 Flow chart of the evolution of antidepressant drugs, and classification by mechanism of action.

be restored by antidepressants. Drugs that alleviate depression also enhance amine storage, release or uptake (Fig. 19.2), increasing activity at postsynaptic receptors. It is relevant that (older) antihypertensive agents, e.g. reserpine and clonidine which reduce the availability of noradrenaline, caused depression.

SSRIs act, as their name indicates, predominantly by preventing serotonin reuptake; they have little or no effect on noradrenaline reuptake.

Tricyclic antidepressants in general inhibit noradrenaline reuptake, but effects on serotonin reuptake vary widely; desipramine and protriptyline have no effect, whereas clomipramine is about five times more potent at blocking serotonin than noradrenaline reuptake. Venlafaxine is capable of inhibiting reuptake of both transmitters, although noradrenaline uptake blocking requires doses over 150 mg/day. Similarly duloxetine inhibits uptake of both neurotransmitters. Mirtazapine also achieves an increase in noradrenergic and serotonergic neuro-

transmission, but through antagonism of presynaptic α$_2$-autoreceptors (receptors that mediate negative feedback for transmitter release, i.e. an autoinhibitory feedback system).

MAOIs increase the availability of noradrenaline and serotonin by preventing their destruction by the monoamine oxidase type A enzyme in the presynaptic terminal (see Chapter 20, Table 20.3). The older MAOIs, phenelzine, tranylcypromine and isocarboxazid, bind irreversibly to monamine oxidase by forming strong (covalent) bonds. The enzyme is thus rendered permanently ineffective such that amine metabolising activity can be restored only by production of fresh enzyme, which takes weeks. These MAOIs are thus called 'hit and run' drugs as their effects greatly outlast their detectable presence in the body.

But how do changes in monoamine transmitter levels produce an eventual elevation of mood? Raised neurotransmitter concentrations produce immediate alterations in postsynaptic receptor activation, leading

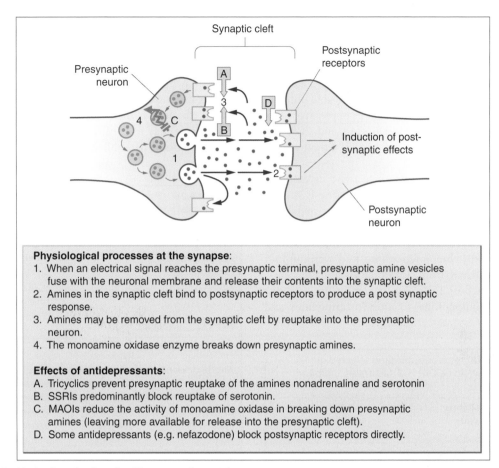

Fig. 19.2 Mechanism of action of antidepressant drugs at the synapse.

In the figure:

Synaptic cleft

Presynaptic neuron

Postsynaptic receptors

Induction of post-synaptic effects

Postsynaptic neuron

Physiological processes at the synapse:
1. When an electrical signal reaches the presynaptic terminal, presynaptic amine vesicles fuse with the neuronal membrane and release their contents into the synaptic cleft.
2. Amines in the synaptic cleft bind to postsynaptic receptors to produce a post synaptic response.
3. Amines may be removed from the synaptic cleft by reuptake into the presynaptic neuron.
4. The monoamine oxidase enzyme breaks down presynaptic amines.

Effects of antidepressants:
A. Tricyclics prevent presynaptic reuptake of the amines nonadrenaline and serotonin
B. SSRIs predominantly block reuptake of serotonin.
C. MAOIs reduce the activity of monoamine oxidase in breaking down presynaptic amines (leaving more available for release into the presynaptic cleft).
D. Some antidepressants (e.g. nefazodone) block postsynaptic receptors directly.

to changes in second-messenger (intracellular) systems and to gradual modifications in cellular protein expression. Antidepressants increase a cyclic AMP response element binding (CREB) protein, which in turn is involved in regulating the transcription of genes that influence survival of other proteins, including brain-derived neurotrophic factor (BDNF), which exerts effects on neuronal growth.

Although the monoamine hypothesis of depression is conceptually straightforward, it is in reality an oversimplification of a complicated picture. Other systems that are implicated in the aetiology of depression (and which provide potential targets for drug therapy) include the hypothalamic–pituitary–thyroid axis and the hypothalamic–pituitary–adrenal (HPA) axis. The finding that 50% of depressed patients have raised plasma cortisol concentrations constitutes evidence that depression may be associated with increased HPA drive.

Drugs with similar modes of action to antidepressants find other uses in medicine. Bupropion (amfeb-utamone) inhibits reuptake of both dopamine and noradrenaline, and was originally developed and used as an antidepressant; it is now used to assist smoking cessation (see p. 157). Sibutramine, licensed as an anorectic agent, is a serotonin and noradrenaline reuptake inhibitor (see Fig. 19.1).

PHARMACOKINETICS

The antidepressants listed in Table 19.1 are generally well absorbed after oral administration. Steady-state plasma concentrations of TCAs show great individual variation but correlate with therapeutic effect, and measurement of plasma concentration can be useful especially where there is apparent failure of response (though it is often not available). Antidepressants in general are metabolised principally by hepatic cytochrome P450 (CYP; see p. 343) enzymes. Of the many isoenzymes identified, the most important in antidepressant metabolism are CYP P450 2D6 (Table 19.2A) and CYP 3A4 (Table 19.2B). Other important P450 enzymes are

CYP 1A2 (inhibited by the SSRI fluvoxamine, induced by cigarette smoking, substrates include caffeine and the atypical antipsychotics clozapine and olanzapine) and the CYP 2C group (inhibition by fluvoxamine and fluoxetine, involved in breakdown of moclobemide). Sometimes several CYP enzymes are capable of mediating the same metabolic step. For example, at least six isoenzymes, including CYP 2D6, 3A4 and 2C9, can mediate the desmethylation of the SSRI sertraline to its major metabolite.

Several of these drugs produce active metabolites that prolong their action (e.g. fluoxetine is metabolised to norfluoxetine, $t_{1/2}$ 200 h). The metabolic products of certain TCAs are antidepressants in their own right, e.g. nortriptyline (from amitriptyline), desipramine (from lofepramine and imipramine) and imipramine (from clomipramine).

Half-lives of TCAs lie generally in a range from 15 h (imipramine) to 100 h (protriptyline), and those for SSRIs from 15 h (fluvoxamine) to 72 h (fluoxetine).

Around 7% of the Caucasian population have very limited CYP 2D6 enzyme activity. Such 'poor metabolisers' may find standard doses of TCAs intolerable, and it is often worth prescribing them at a very low dose. If the drug is then tolerated, plasma concentration assay may to confirm the suspicion that the patient is a poor metaboliser.

Table 19.2A Psychotropic (and selected other) drugs known to be CYP 2D6 substrates, inhibitors and inducers

CYP 2D6 inhibitors
Antidepressants
paroxetine
fluoxetine

CYP 2D6 substrates

Antidepressants	Antipsychotics	Miscellaneous
paroxetine	chlorpromazine	dexfenfluramine
fluoxetine	haloperidol	**Opioids**
citalopram	thioridazine	codeine
sertraline	zuclopenthixol	hydrocodone
venlafaxine[a]	perphenazine	dihydrocodeine
amitriptyline	risperidone	tramadol
clomipramine		ethyl morphine
desipramine		MDMA (ecstasy)
imipramine		bupropion
nortriptyline		**Beta-blockers**
		propranolol
		metoprolol
		timolol
		bufaralol

[a]CYP 2D6 is involved only in the breakdown of venlafaxine to its active metabolite and therefore implications of 2D6 interactions for efficacy are of limited significance.

A *substrate* is a substance that is acted upon and changed by an enzyme. Where two substrates of the same enzyme are prescribed together, they will compete and, if present in sufficient quantities, the metabolism of one or other, or both, drugs may also be inhibited, resulting in increased plasma concentration and possibly in enhanced therapeutic or adverse effects. An enzyme *inducer* accelerates the metabolism of co-prescribed drugs that are substrates of the same enzyme, reducing their effects. An enzyme *inhibitor* retards metabolism of co-prescribed drugs, increasing their effects.

Table 19.2B Psychotropic (and selected other) drugs known to be CYP 3A4 substrates, inhibitors and inducers

CYP 3A4 inhibitors

Antidepressants	Other drugs
fluoxetine	cimetidine
nefazodone	erythromycin
	ketoconazole
	(grapefruit juice)

CYP 3A4 substrates

Antidepressants	Anxiolytics, hypnotics and antipsychotics	Miscellaneous
fluoxetine	alpraxolam	buprenorphine
sertraline	aripiprazole	carbamazepine
amitriptyline	buspirone	cortisol
imipramine	diazepam	dexamethasone
nortriptyline	midazolam	methadone
trazodone[a]	triazolam	testosterone
	zopiclone	**Calcium channel blockers**
	haloperidol	diltiazem
	quetiapine	nifedipine
	sertindole	amlodipine
		Other drugs
		amiodarone
		omeprazole
		oral contraceptives
		simvastatin

CYP 3A4 inducers

Antidepressants	Miscellaneous
St John's wort	carbamazepine
	phenobarbital
	phenytoin

[a] mCPP (meta-chlorophenylpiperazine), the active metabolite of trazodone, is a CYP 2D6 substrate; observe for unwanted effects when trazodone is co-administered with the 2D6 inhibitors fluoxetine or paroxetine.

A *substrate* is a substance that is acted upon and changed by an enzyme. Where two substrates of the same enzyme are prescribed together, they will compete and, if present in sufficient quantities, the metabolism of one or other, or both, drugs may also be inhibited, resulting in increased plasma concentration and possibly in enhanced therapeutic or adverse effects. An enzyme *inducer* accelerates the metabolism of co-prescribed drugs that are substrates of the same enzyme, reducing their effects. An enzyme *inhibitor* retards metabolism of co-prescribed drugs, increasing their effects.

THERAPEUTIC EFFICACY

Provided antidepressant drugs are prescribed at an adequate dose and taken regularly, 60–70% of patients with depression should respond within 3–4 weeks. Meta-analyses have shown little evidence that any particular drug or class of antidepressant is more efficacious than others, but there are four possible exceptions to this general statement:

- *Venlafaxine*, in high dose (>150 mg/day) may have greater efficacy than other antidepressants.
- *Amitriptyline* appears to be slightly more effective than other TCAs and also SSRIs, but this advantage is compromised by its poor tolerability relative to more modern agents.
- The older MAOIs (e.g. *phenelzine*) may be more effective than other classes in 'atypical' depression, a form of depressive illness where mood reactivity is preserved, lack of energy may be extreme and biological features are the opposite of the normal syndrome, i.e. excess sleep and appetite with weight gain.
- Evidence suggests that in patients hospitalised with *severe* depression, TCAs as a class (also venlafaxine) may be slightly more effective than either SSRIs or MAOIs.

SELECTION

An antidepressant should be selected to match individual patients' requirements, such as the need or otherwise for a sedative effect, or the avoidance of antimuscarinic effects (especially in the elderly). In the absence of special factors, the choice rests on tolerability, safety in overdose and the likelihood of an effective dose being reached. *SSRIs, lofepramine, mirtazapine, reboxetine* and *venlafaxine* are highlighted as best fulfilling these needs.

MODE OF USE

Antidepressants usually require 3–4 weeks for effect. When a minimal response is seen, an antidepressant can usefully be extended to 6 weeks to see whether further benefit is achieved. By contrast, patients may experience unwanted drug effects immediately on starting treatment (they should be warned), but such symptoms often diminish with time. Titrating from a generally tolerable starting dose, e.g. amitriptyline 30–75 mg/day (25–50 mg/day for imipramine), with weekly increments to a recognised 'minimum therapeutic' dose, usually around 125 mg/day

(140 mg/day for lofepramine), lessens the impact of adverse symptoms before a degree of tolerance (and therapeutic benefit) develops. Low starting doses are particularly important for elderly patients. Only when the drug has reached the minimum therapeutic dose and been taken for at least 4 weeks can response or non-response be considered adequate.

Some patients do achieve response or remission at subtherapeutic doses, for reasons of drug kinetics and limited capacity to metabolise, the self-limiting nature of depression, or by a placebo effect (reinforced by the experience of side-effects suggesting that the drug must be having some action). TCAs are given either in divided doses or, for the more sedative compounds, as a single evening dose.

SSRIs have advantages over tricyclics in simplicity of introduction and use. Dose titration is often unnecessary as the minimum therapeutic dose can usually be tolerated as a starting dose. Divided doses are not required, and administration is by a single morning or evening dose. Evidence suggests that patients commencing treatment on SSRIs are more likely to reach an effective dose than those starting on TCAs.

Of the novel compounds, trazodone usually requires titration to a minimum therapeutic dose of at least 200 mg/day. Response to reboxetine, venlafaxine and mirtazapine may occur at the starting dose, but some dose titration is commonly required. Venlafaxine is licensed for treatment-resistant depression by gradual titration from 75 to 375 mg/day. There is some need for dose titration when using MAOIs. Unlike other drug classes, reduction to a lower maintenance dose is recommended after a response is achieved if unwanted effects are problematical.

CHANGING AND STOPPING ANTIDEPRESSANTS

When an antidepressant fails through lack of efficacy despite an adequate trial or due to unacceptable adverse effects, a change to a drug of a different class is generally advisable. For a patient who has not responded to an SSRI it is logical to try a TCA or a novel compound such as venlafaxine, reboxetine or mirtazapine. Any of these options may offer a greater increase in synaptic noradrenaline than the ineffective SSRI.

Evidence also suggests that patients failing on one SSRI may respond to a different drug within the class, an approach that is particularly useful where other antidepressant classes have been unsuccessful previously, are contraindicated, or have characteristics that the patient or doctor feels are undesirable. For example, a patient who is keen to avoid putting on weight may prefer to try a second SSRI after an initial failure than to switch to a TCA or MAOI, as both of these classes commonly cause weight gain. Awareness of differences between drugs within a class may also be helpful, e.g. the greater serotonergic enhancing effects of clomipramine compared with other tricyclics may be advantageous in a patient who cannot tolerate any other drug class.

When changing between SSRIs and/or TCAs, doses should be reduced progressively over 2–4 weeks, and where a new drug is to be introduced it should be 'cross-tapered', i.e. the dose increased gradually as that of the substituted drug is reduced. Changes to or from MAOIs must be handled with great caution due to the dangers of interactions between antidepressants (see below). Therefore MAOIs cannot safely be introduced within 2 weeks of stopping SSRIs and TCAs (3 weeks for imipramine and clomipramine; combination of the latter with tranylcypramine is particularly dangerous), and not until 5 weeks after stopping fluoxetine due to the long $t_{1/2}$ of the active metabolite (6 days). Similarly, TCAs and SSRIs should not be introduced until 2–3 weeks have elapsed from discontinuation of MAOI (as these are irreversible inhibitors; see p. 332). No washout period is required when using the reversible MAOI, moclobemide.

When a patient achieves remission, the antidepressant should be continued for at least 9 months at the dose that returned mood to normal. Premature dose reduction or withdrawal is associated with increased risk of relapse. In cases where three or more depressive episodes have occurred, evidence suggests that long-term continuation of an antidepressant offers protection, as further relapse is almost inevitable in the next 3 years.

When ceasing use of an antidepressant, the dose should be reduced gradually to avoid a discontinuation syndrome (symptoms include anxiety, agitation, nausea and mood swings). Discontinuation of SSRIs and venlafaxine are associated additionally with dizziness, electric shock-like sensations and paraesthesia. Short $t_{1/2}$ drugs that do not produce active metabolites (e.g. paroxetine, venlafaxine) and TCAs are most likely to cause such problems.

AUGMENTATION

Augmentation, i.e. the addition of another drug, is used to enhance the effects of standard antidepressants when two or more have successively failed to alleviate depressive symptoms despite treatment at an adequate dose for an adequate time. The therapeutic efficacy of new agents, e.g. venlafaxine, has provided clinicians with further options, which now tend to be employed before augmentation, but the following may be used.

The most common augmentation is with the mood stabiliser, *lithium carbonate*. Controlled trials suggest that up to 50% of patients who have not responded to standard antidepressants can respond after lithium augmentation. Addition of lithium requires careful titration of the plasma concentration up to the therapeutic range, with periodic checks thereafter and monitoring for toxicity (see p. 350).

Tri-iodothyronine (T3) also aids antidepressant action, and most evidence points to added benefit with TCAs. When co-prescribing TCAs with thyroid hormone derivatives, be aware that the combination of lofepramine with the *levo*-isomer of thyroxine is contraindicated. The amino acid L-*tryptophan* and the β-adrenoceptor blocker *pindolol* may also be used to augment. Tryptophan increases 5-hydroxytryptamine (5HT) production, and pindolol may act by blocking negative feedback of 5HT on to $5HT_{1A}$-autoreceptors. More recently augmentation with atypical antipsychotics was effective in clinical trials of olanzapine, quetiapine and risperidone.

OTHER INDICATIONS FOR ANTIDEPRESSANTS

Antidepressants may benefit most forms of *anxiety disorder*, including panic disorder, generalised anxiety disorder, post-traumatic stress disorder, obsessive–compulsive disorder and social phobia (see p. 354).

Fluoxetine is effective in milder cases of the eating disorder *bulimia nervosa*, in higher doses (60 mg/day) than are required for depression. This effect is independent of that on depression (which may coexist), and may therefore involve a different mode of action. Antidepressants appear to be ineffective in anorexia nervosa.

ADVERSE EFFECTS

As most antidepressants have similar therapeutic efficacy, the decision regarding which drug to select often rests on adverse effect profiles and potential to cause toxicity.

Tricyclic antidepressants

The commonest unwanted effects are those of antimuscarinic action, i.e. dry mouth (predisposing to tooth decay), blurred vision and difficulty with accommodation, raised intraocular pressure (glaucoma may be precipitated) and bladder neck obstruction (may lead to urinary retention in older males).

Patients may also experience: postural hypotension (through inhibition of α-adrenoceptors), which is often a limiting factor in the elderly; interference with sexual function; weight gain (through blockade of histamine H_1 receptors); prolongation of the QTc interval of the ECG, which predisposes to cardiac arrhythmias especially in overdose (use after myocardial infarction is contraindicated).

Some TCAs (especially trimipramine and amitriptyline) are heavily sedating through a combination of antihistaminergic and α_1-adrenergic blocking actions, and this presents special problems to those whose lives involve driving vehicles or performing skilled tasks. In selected patients, sedation may be beneficial, e.g. a severely depressed person who has a disrupted sleep pattern or marked agitation.

There is great heterogeneity in adverse-effect profiles between TCAs. Imipramine and lofepramine cause relatively little sedation, and lofepramine is associated with milder antimuscarinic effects (but is contraindicated in patients with severe liver disease).

Overdose. Depression is a risk factor for both parasuicide and completed suicide, and TCAs are commonly taken by those who deliberately self-harm. *Dothiepin* and *amitriptyline* are particularly toxic in overdose, being responsible for up to 300 deaths per year in the UK despite the availability of many alternative antidepressants. Lofepramine is at least 15 times less likely to cause death from overdose; clomipramine and imipramine occupy intermediate positions.

Clinical features of overdose reflect the pharmacology of TCAs. Antimuscarinic effects result in warm, dry skin from vasodilatation and inhibition of sweating, blurred vision from paralysis of accommodation, papillary dilatation, and urinary retention.

Consciousness is commonly dulled, and respiration depression and hypothermia may develop. Neurological signs including hyperreflexia, myoclonus,

divergent strabismus and extensor plantar responses may accompany lesser degrees of impaired consciousness and provide scope for diagnostic confusion, e.g. with structural brain damage. Convulsions occur in a proportion of patients. Hallucinations and delirium occur during recovery of consciousness, often accompanied by a characteristic plucking at bedclothes.

Sinus tachycardia (due to vagal blockade) is a common feature but abnormalities of cardiac conduction accompany moderate to severe intoxication and may proceed to dangerous tachyarrhythmias or bradyarrhythmias. Hypotension may result from a combination of cardiac arrhythmia, reduced myocardial contractility and dilatation of venous capacitance vessels.

Supportive treatment suffices for the majority of cases. Activated charcoal by mouth is indicated to prevent further absorption from the alimentary tract and may be given to the conscious patient in the home prior to transfer to hospital. Convulsions are less likely if unnecessary stimuli are avoided, but severe or frequent seizures often precede cardiac arrhythmias and arrest, and their suppression with diazepam is important. Cardiac arrhythmias do not need intervention if cardiac output and tissue perfusion are adequate. Correction of hypoxia with oxygen, and acidosis by intravenous infusion of sodium bicarbonate are reasonable first measures and usually suffice.

Reboxetine is not structurally related to tricyclic agents and acts predominantly by noradrenergic reuptake inhibition. Pseudo-antimuscarinic effects trouble only a minority of patients, postural hypotension may occur, and impotence in males. It is relatively safe in overdose.

Selective serotonin reuptake inhibitors

SSRIs have a range of unwanted effects including nausea, anorexia, dizziness, gastrointestinal disturbance, agitation, akathisia (motor restlessness) and anorgasmia (failure to experience an orgasm). They lack direct sedative effect, an advantage in patients who need to drive motor vehicles. SSRIs can disrupt the pattern of sleep with increased awakenings, transient reduction in the amount of rapid eye movement (REM) and increased REM latency, but eventually sleep improves due to improved mood. This class of antidepressant does not cause the problems of postural hypotension, antimuscarinic or antihistaminergic effects seen with TCAs. Their use is not associated with weight gain, although conversely they may induce weight loss through their anorectic effects. SSRIs are relatively safe in overdose.

The serotonin syndrome is a rare but dangerous complication of SSRI use and features restlessness, tremor, shivering and myoclonus, possibly leading on to hyperpyrexia, convulsions and delirium.

The risk is increased by co-administration with drugs that enhance serotonin transmission, especially MAOIs, the antimigraine triptan drugs and St John's wort.

When comparing SSRIs and TCAs for dropouts (a surrogate endpoint for tolerability), most meta-analyses show a slight benefit in favour of SSRIs. Lofepramine, the second most prescribed TCA in the UK and the one TCA that causes little sedation, has few antimuscarinic effects and is as safe as SSRIs in overdose, is rarely used as a comparator in trials and patients deriving benefit from this drug are therefore under-represented in meta-analyses.

Novel compounds

Venlafaxine produces unwanted effects that resemble those of SSRIs with a higher incidence of nausea. Sustained hypertension (due to blockade of noradrenaline reuptake) is a problem in a small proportion of patients at high dose, and blood pressure should be monitored when more than 200 mg/day is taken. Venlafaxine appears to have some association with cardiac arrhythmias but whether this is to a degree that is clinically significant is unclear.

Duloxetine may cause early nausea, which tends to subside quickly. Other unwanted effects are somnolence, dizziness and constipation.

Mirtazapine has benefits in rarely being associated with sexual dysfunction and in improving sleep independent of mood but, like TCAs, it may cause unwanted sedation and weight gain.

Trazodone is an option for depressed patients where heavy sedation is required. It also has the advantages of lacking antimuscarinic effects and of being relatively safe in overdose. Males should be warned of the possibility of priapism (painful penile erections), attributable to the drug's blockade of α_1-adrenoceptors.

Monoamine oxidase inhibitors

Adverse effects include postural hypotension (especially in the elderly) and dizziness. Less common are headache, irritability, apathy, insomnia, fatigue, ataxia, gastrointestinal disturbances including dry mouth and constipation, sexual dysfunction (especially anorgasmia), blurred vision, difficult micturition, sweating, peripheral oedema, tremulousness, restlessness and hyperthermia. Appetite may increase inappropriately causing weight gain.

INTERACTIONS

Antidepressants use offers considerable scope for adverse interaction with other drugs and it is prudent always to check specific sources for unwanted outcomes whenever a new drug is added or removed to a prescription list that includes an antidepressant.

Pharmacodynamic interactions

- Many tricyclics cause sedation and therefore co-prescription with other sedative agents such as opioid analgesics, H_1-receptor antihistamines, anxiolytics, hypnotics and alcohol may lead to excessive drowsiness and daytime somnolence.
- The majority of tricyclics have undesirable cardiovascular effects, in particular prolongation of the QTc interval. Numerous other drugs also prolong the QTc interval, e.g. amiodarone, disopyramide, procainamide, propafenone, quinidine, terfenadine, and psychotropic agents such as pimozide, sertindole and thioridazine. Their use in combination with TCAs that prolonged QTc enhances the risk of ventricular arrhythmias. Giving thioridazine with any such tricyclic is particularly dangerous and is formally contraindicated.
- Tricylics potentiate the effects of catecholamines and other sympathomimetics, but not those of β_2-receptor agonists used in asthma. Even the small amounts of adrenaline (epinephrine) or noradrenaline (norepinephrine) in dental local anaesthetics may produce a serious rise in blood pressure.
- Both TCAs and SSRIs may cause central nervous system (CNS) toxicity if co-prescribed with the dopaminergic drugs entacapone and selegiline (for Parkinson's disease). SSRIs increase the risk of the serotonin syndrome when combined with drugs that enhance serotonin transmission, e.g. the antimigraine triptan drugs which are $5HT_1$-receptor antagonists, and the antiobesity drug sibutramine.

■ TCAs and SSRIs lower the convulsion threshold, complicate the drug control of epilepsy and lengthen seizure time in electroconvulsive therapy (ECT). The situation is made more complex by the capacity of carbamazepine to induce the metabolism of antidepressants and of certain antidepressants to inhibit carbamazepine metabolism (see below).

Pharmacokinetic interactions

Metabolism by cytochrome P450 enzymes provides ample opportunity for interaction of antidepressants with other drugs by inhibition of, competition for, or induction of enzymes. Tables 19.2A and 19.2B indicate examples of mechanisms by which interaction that may occur when relevant drugs are added to, altered in dose or discontinued from regimens that include antidepressants.

Enzyme inhibition. In depressive psychosis, antidepressants are commonly prescribed with antipsychotics and there is potential for enhanced drug effects with paroxetine + thioridazine (CYP 2D6), fluoxetine + sertindole (3A4) and fluvoxamine + olanzapine (1A2). Rapid tranquillisation with zuclopenthixol acetate (see p. 345) of an agitated patient who is also taking fluoxetine or paroxetine can result in toxic plasma concentrations with excessive sedation and respiratory depression due to inhibition of zuclopenthixol metabolism by CYP 2D6. P450 enzyme inhibition by SSRIs may also augment effects of alcohol, tramadol, methadone, terfenadine (danger of cardiac arrhythmia), -caine anaesthetics and theophylline.

Enzyme-inducing drugs, e.g. carbamazepine and several other antiepilepsy drugs, accelerate the metabolism of antidepressants, reducing their therapeutic efficacy and requiring adjustment of dose. Epilepsy is a particularly common co-morbid illness in patients who have both psychiatric illness and learning disabilities, and the combination of an anticonvulsant and an antidepressant or major psychotropic drug is to be anticipated. Depression and hypertension are both common conditions such that some co-morbidity is inevitable. Panic disorder (an indication for an antidepressant drug) is associated epidemiologically with hypertension.[1]

[1]Davies S J C, Ghahramani P, Jackson P R et al 1999 Association of panic disorder and panic attacks with hypertension. American Journal of Medicine 107:310–316.

An antidepressant that is an enzyme inhibitor may exaggerate antihypertensive effects of metoprolol (metabolised by CYP 2D6), or diltiazem or amlodipine (3A4).

Monoamine oxidase inhibitors

Hypertensive reactions. Patients taking MAOIs are vulnerable to highly dangerous hypertensive reactions. Firstly, as MAOIs increase catecholamine stores in adrenergic and dopaminergic nerve endings, the action of sympathomimetics that act indirectly by releasing stored noradrenaline is augmented. Secondly, patients taking a MAOI are deprived of the protection of the MAO enzyme present in large quantities in the gut wall and liver. Thus orally administered sympathomimetics that would normally be inactivated by MAO are absorbed intact. (Note that enhanced effects are not to be expected from adrenaline, noradrenaline and isoprenaline, which are chiefly destroyed by another enzyme, catechol-*O*-methyltransferase, in the blood and liver.)

Symptoms include severe, sudden throbbing headache with slow palpitation, flushing, visual disturbance, nausea, vomiting and severe hypertension. If headache occurs without hypertension it may be due to histamine release. The hypertension is due both to vasoconstriction from activation of α-adrenoceptors and to increased cardiac output consequent on activation of cardiac β-adrenoceptors. The mechanism is thus similar to that of the episodic hypertension in a patient with phaeochromocytoma.

The rational and effective treatment is an α-adrenoceptor blocker (phentolamine 5 mg i.v.), with a β-blocker later added in case of excessive tachycardia.

Patient education. It is essential to warn patients taking MAOIs of possible sources of the hypertensive reaction.

Many simple remedies sold direct to the public, e.g. for nasal congestion, coughs and colds, contain sympathomimetics (ephedrine, phenylpropanolamine).

Foods to avoid are those that contain sympathomimetics, most commonly *tyramine*, which acts by releasing tissue-stored noradrenaline. Degradation of the protein, casein, by resident bacteria in well matured cheese can produce tyramine from the amino acid tyrosine (hence the general term 'cheese reaction' to describe provocation of a hypertensive crisis).

Stale foods present a particular danger, as any food subjected to autolysis or microbial decomposition during preparation or storage may contain pressor amines resulting from decarboxylation of amino acids.

Foods likely to produce hypertensive effects in patients taking MAOIs include:

- cheese, especially if well matured
- red wines (especially Chianti) and some white wines; some beers (non- or low-alcohol varieties contain variable but generally low amounts of tyramine)
- yeast extracts (Marmite, Oxo, Bovril)
- some pickled herrings
- broad bean pods (contain dopa, a precursor of adrenaline)
- over-ripe bananas, avocados, figs
- game
- stale foods
- fermented bean curds including soy sauce
- fermented sausage, e.g. salami, shrimp paste
- flavoured textured vegetable protein (Vegemite).

This list may be incomplete and any partially decomposed food may cause a reaction. Milk and yoghurt appear safe.

The newer drug moclobemide offers the dual advantages of selective MAO-A inhibition; in theory, this should avoid the 'cheese' reaction by sparing the intestinal MAO, which is mainly MAO-B, and of being a competitive, reversible inhibitor. Whereas the irreversible inhibitors inactivate the MAO enzyme and can therefore continue to cause dangerous interactions in the 2–3 weeks after withdrawal, until more enzyme can be synthesised, the reversible nature of MAO inhibition means it is incomplete except during peak plasma concentrations. As the inhibition is competitive, tyramine can then displace the inhibitor from the active site of the MAO enzyme. Consequently there are fewer dietary restrictions for patients using moclobemide, although hypertensive reactions have been reported.

MAOI interactions with other drugs. The mechanisms of many of the following interactions are obscure, and some are probably due to inhibition of drug-metabolising enzymes other than MAO

enzyme, as MAOIs are not entirely selective in their action. Effects last for up to 2–3 weeks after discontinuing a MAOI.

Antidepressants. Combination with tricyclic antidepressants has the potential to precipitate a hypertensive crisis complicated by CNS excitation with hyperreflexia, rigidity and hyperpyrexia.

MAOI–SSRI combinations may provoke the life-threatening 'serotonin syndrome' (see above). Strict rules apply regarding washout periods when switching between MAOIs and other drugs (see above, Changing antidepressants, p. 335). Very occasionally, MAOIs are co-prescribed with other antidepressants, but as many combinations are highly dangerous such practice should be reserved for specialists only and then as a last resort.

Narcotic analgesics. With co-prescribed pethidine, respiratory depression, restlessness, even coma, and hypotension or hypertension may result (probably due to inhibition of its hepatic demethylation). Interaction with other opioids occurs but is milder.

Other drugs that cause minor interactions with MAOIs include antiepileptics (convulsion threshold lowered), dopaminergic drugs, e.g. selegeline (MAO-B inhibitor) may cause dyskinesias, antihypertensives and antidiabetes drugs (metformin and sulphonylureas potentiated). Concomitant use with bupropion/amfebutanone (smoking cessation), sibutramine (weight reduction) and $5HT_1$-agonists (migraine) should be avoided. Because of the use of numerous drugs during and around surgery, an MAOI is best withdrawn 2 weeks before, if practicable.

Overdose with MAOIs can cause hypomania, coma and hypotension or hypertension. General measures are used as appropriate with minimal administration of drugs: chlorpromazine for restlessness and excitement; phentolamine for hypertension; no vasopressor drugs for hypotension, because of risk of hypertension (use posture and plasma volume expansion).

ST JOHN'S WORT

The herbal remedy St John's wort (*Hypericum perforatum*) has found favour in some patients with mild to moderate depression. The active ingredients in the hypericum extract have yet to be identified, and their mode of action is unclear. Several of the known mechanisms of action of existing antidepressants are postulated including inhibition of monoamine reuptake and the MAO enzyme, as well as a stimulation of GABA receptors. Much of the original research into the efficacy of St John's wort was performed in Germany, where its use is well established. Several direct comparisons with tricyclic antidepressants have shown equivalent rates of response, but the interpretation of these studies is complicated by the fact that many failed to use standardised ratings for depressive symptoms, patients tended to receive TCAs below the minimum therapeutic dose, and sometimes received St John's wort in doses above the maximum recommended in commercially available preparations. Use of St John's wort is further complicated by the lack of standardisation of the ingredients. A large multicentre trial found only limited evidence of benefit for St John's wort over placebo in significant major depression.[2]

Despite these reservations, there is certainly a small proportion of patients who, when presented with all the available facts, express a strong desire to take only St John's wort, perhaps from a preference for herbally derived compounds over conventional medicine. For patients with mild depression, it seems reasonable on existing evidence to accede to this preference rather than impair the therapeutic alliance and risk prescribing a conventional antidepressant that will not be taken.

Adverse effects. Those who wish to take St John's wort should be made aware that it may cause dry mouth, dizziness, sedation, gastrointestinal disturbance and confusion. Importantly also, it induces hepatic P450 enzymes (CYP1A2 and CYP3A4) with the result that the plasma concentration and therapeutic efficacy of warfarin, oral contraceptives, some anticonvulsants, antipsychotics and HIV protease/reverse transcriptase inhibitors are reduced. Concomitant use of tryptophan and St John's wort may cause serotonergic effects including nausea and agitation.

[2]Shelton R C, Keller M B, Gelenberg A et al 2001 Effectiveness of St John's wort in major depression. A randomised control trial. Journal of the American Medical Association 285:1978–1986.

ELECTROCONVULSIVE THERAPY

ECT involves the passage of a small electrical charge across the brain by electrodes applied to the frontotemporal aspects of the scalp with the aim of inducing a tonic–clonic seizure. Reference to it is made here principally to indicate its place in therapy.

ECT requires the patient to be under a general anaesthetic, carrying the small risks equivalent to those associated with general anaesthesia in minor surgical operations. It may cause memory defect, although this is generally transient. For these reasons, as well as the relative ease of use of antidepressant drugs, ECT is usually reserved for psychiatric illness where pharmacological treatments have been unsuccessful or where the potential for rapid improvement characteristic of ECT treatment is important. This may arise where patients are in acute danger from their mental state, for instance the severely depressed patient who has stopped eating or drinking, or those with florid psychotic symptoms. Modern-day ECT is a safe and effective alternative to antidepressant treatment and remains a first-line option in clinical circumstances where a rapid response is desired, when it can be life saving.

ANTIPSYCHOTICS

CLASSIFICATION

Originally tested as an antihistamine, *chlorpromazine* serendipitously emerged as an effective treatment for psychotic illness in the 1950s. Chlorpromazine-like drugs were originally termed 'neuroleptics' or 'major tranquillisers', but the preferred usage now is 'antipsychotics'. Classification is by chemical structure, e.g. phenothiazines, butyrophenones. Within the large phenothiazine group, compounds are divided into three types on the basis of the side-chain, as this tends to predict adverse effect profiles (Table 19.3).

The continuing search for greater efficacy and better tolerability led researchers and clinicians to reinvestigate *clozapine*, a drug that was originally licensed in the 1960s but subsequently withdrawn because of toxic haematological effects. Clozapine appeared to offer greater effectiveness in treatment-resistant schizophrenia, to have efficacy against 'negative' in addition to 'positive' psychiatric symptoms (see Table 19.4), and to be less likely to cause extrapyramidal motor symptoms. It regained its licence in the early 1990s with strict requirements

Table 19.3	Antipsychotic drugs	
Atypical antipsychotics[a]	**Classical antipsychotics**	
clozapine	*Phenothiazines*	
olanzapine	Type 1	chlorpromazine
quetiapine		promazine
risperidone	Type 2	thioridazine[d,e]
ziprasidone		pericyazine
amisulpride[b]	Type 3	trifluoperazine
zotepine		prochlorperazine
sertindole[c]		fluphenazine
aripiprazole	*Butyrophenones*	haloperidol
		benperidol
	Substituted benzamide	sulpiride[b,e]
	Thioxanthines	flupentixol
		zuclopenthixol
	Other	pimozide
		loxapine

[a] No recognised classification system exists for atypical antipsychotics. Tentative terms based on receptor binding profiles have been applied to certain drug groupings, e.g. 'broad-spectrum atypicals' for clozapine, olanzapine and quetiapine, whereas risperidone and ziprasidone have been described as 'high-affinity serotonin–dopamine antagonists'.

[b] Amisulpride and sulpiride are structurally related.

[c] Sertindole is available only on a named-patient basis when at least one previous antipsychotic has failed owing to lack of efficacy or adverse effects.

[d] Licensed indications for thioridazine were severely restricted in 2000 after evidence emerged of cardiovascular toxicity.

[e] In some classifications thioridazine and sulpiride are considered to be 'atypical' due to their low propensity to cause extrapyramidal side-effects.

on dose titration and haematological monitoring. The renewed interest in clozapine and its unusual efficacy and tolerability stimulated researchers to examine similar 'atypical' antipsychotic drugs.

Thus the most important distinction in modern-day classification of antipsychotic drugs is between the *classical* (typical) agents, such as chlorpromazine, haloperidol and zuclopenthixol, and the *atypical* antipsychotics, which include clozapine and now risperidone, olanzapine, quetiapine and aripiprazole. These latter are 'atypical' in their mode of action, lack of extrapyramidal motor symptoms and adverse effect profiles. Categorisation of atypical agents by their chemical structure is of limited value clinically as they are very heterogeneous. A classification by receptor binding profiles is likely to emerge with growing evidence of the clinical importance of their actions on interrelated transmitter systems.

INDICATIONS

Antipsychotic drugs are used for the prophylaxis and acute treatment of psychotic illnesses including *schizophrenia* and *psychoses associated with depression and mania*. They also have an important role as an alternative or adjunct to benzodiazepines in the management of the *acutely disturbed patient*, for both tranquillisation and sedation. Antipsychotics have been given *short term in severe anxiety*, but this use is now only as a last resort. Certain antipsychotics have an antidepressant effect that is distinct from their ability to alleviate the psychosis associated with depression, but such use is difficult to justify given the many pharmacological options now available for treating depression. Antipsychotics have also proved useful in the tic disorder Tourette's syndrome, and for recurrent self-harming behaviour.

The threshold for seeking specialist involvement in starting antipsychotics is much lower than that when initiating antidepressant drugs. This reflects the complexity of diagnosis of psychotic illness, its chronicity, the increased likelihood of poor compliance without appropriate support and the potential toxicity of antipsychotic agents.

MECHANISM OF ACTION

The common action of all antipsychotics (except oxypertine and aripiprazo) is to decrease brain dopamine function by blocking the *dopamine D_2 receptors* (Fig. 19.3). The atypical drugs act on numerous receptors and modulate several interacting transmitter systems. All atypicals (except amisulpride) exhibit greater antagonism of *$5HT_2$ receptors* than of D_2 receptors, compared with the classical agents. Atypical drugs that do antagonise dopamine D_2 receptors appear to have affinity for those in the *mesolimbic system* (producing antipsychotic effect) rather than the *nigrostriatal system* (associated with unwanted motor effects). Clozapine and risperidone exert substantial antagonism of *α_2-adrenoceptors*, a property that may explain their benefits against negative symptoms. Blockade of *muscarinic* acetylcholine receptors as with chlorpromazine and clozapine reduces the occurrence of extrapyramidal effects. Aripiprazole is a unique drug because it is a partial dopamine D_2-receptor agonist that acts conversely as an antagonist in regions where dopamine is overactive, such as the limbic system. It increases dopamine function where it is low (such as in the frontal cortex) and has little motor effect.

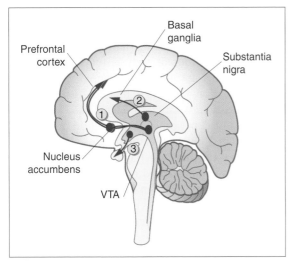

Fig. 19.3 Sagittal brain section illustrating dopaminergic pathways. (1) *Mesolimbic pathway* (thought to be overactive in psychotic illness according to the dopamine hypothesis of schizophrenia). (2) *Nigrostriatal pathway* (involved in motor control, underactive in Parkinson's disease and associated with extrapyramidal motor symptoms). (3) *Tuberoinfundibular pathway* (moderates prolactin release from the hypothalamus). VTA, ventrotegmental area.

PHARMACOKINETICS

Antipsychotics are well absorbed after oral administration and distribute widely. They are metabolised mainly by hepatic cytochrome P450 isoenzymes, e.g. CYP 2D6 (zuclopenthixol, risperidone; see Table 19.2A), CYP 3A4 (sertindole; see Table 19.2B), CYP 1A2 (olanzapine, clozapine). Metabolism of some compounds is complex, e.g. chlorpromazine, haloperidol, utilising several P450 enzymes and resulting in the production of many inactive metabolites. Amisulpride is an exception to the general rule as it is eliminated unchanged by the kidneys. Elimination $t_{1/2}$ values range from quetiapine 7h, clozapine 12h, haloperidol 18h to olazapine 33h. Depot preparations usefully release drug over 2–4weeks after intramuscular injection (see below).

EFFICACY

Symptoms in schizophrenia are defined as *positive* and *negative* (Table 19.4). Although a classical antipsychotic drug should provide adequate treatment of positive symptoms including hallucinations and delusions, at least 60% of patients may have unresolved negative symptoms such as apathy, flattening of affect and alogia. Evidence suggests that *clozapine*

Table 19.4 Symptoms of schizophrenia

Positive symptoms	Negative symptoms
Hallucinations: most commonly auditory (i.e. voices) in the third person, which patients may find threatening. The voices may also give commands. Visual hallucinations are rare	*Affective flattening* manifest by unchanging facial expression with lack of communication through expression, poor eye contact, lack of responsiveness, psychomotor slowing
Delusions: most commonly persecutory. 'Passivity phenomena' include delusions of thought broadcasting, thought insertion or thought withdrawal, made actions, impulses or feelings	*Alogia* (literally 'absence of words', manifesting clinically as a lack of spontaneous speech (poverty of speech)
Bizarre behaviours including agitation, sexual disinhibition, repetitive behaviour, wearing of striking but inappropriate clothing	*Anhedonia* (inability to derive pleasure from any activity) and *associality* (narrowing of repertoire of interests and impaired relationships)
Thought disorder manifest by failure in the organisation of speech such that it drifts away from the point (tangentiality), never reaches the point (circumstantiality), moves from one topic to the next illogically (loosened associations, knight's move thinking), breaks off abruptly only to continue on an unrelated topic (derailment) or moves from one topic to the next on the basis of a pun or words that sound similar (clang association)	*Apathy/avolution* involving lack of energy, lack of motivation to work, participate in activities or initiate any goal-directed behaviour, and poor personal hygiene
	Attention problems involving an inability to focus on any one issue or engage fully with communication

may have a significant advantage against negative symptoms. This drug has a further advantage over all other antipsychotics, whether classical or atypical, in that it is the most effective agent for 'resistant' schizophrenia, i.e. where other antipsychotics prescribed at adequate doses fail to produce improvement or are not tolerated.

Schizophrenia often runs a chronic relapsing and remitting course. Less than a quarter of patients avoid further episodes, with the most common reason for relapse being the stopping of medication against medical advice.

MODE OF USE

As the potency (therapeutic efficacy in relation to dose) of antipsychotic agents varies markedly between compounds, it is useful to think of the effective antipsychotic dose of classical agents in terms of *'chlorpromazine equivalents'* (see Table 19.5). For example, *haloperidol* has a relatively high antipsychotic potency, such that 2–3 mg is equivalent to chlorpromazine 100 mg, whereas 200 mg *sulpiride* (low potency) is required for equivalent antipsychotic effect.

Patients who are 'neuroleptic naive', i.e. have never previously taken any antipsychotic agent, should start at the lowest available dose, e.g. haloperidol 0.5 mg/day or chlorpromazine 25 mg/day, in case the patient is particularly susceptible to adverse, especially extrapyramidal motor, effects. Conservative starting doses are advisable for the elderly and patients with learning disabilities (who may require antipsychotics for psychosis or severe behavioural disturbance). The longer a psychosis is left untreated, the less favourable is the outcome and drug treatment should be instigated as soon as an adequate period of assessment has allowed a provisional diagnosis to be established. The dose is increased at intervals, until the desired effect on psychotic symptoms, calming disturbed behaviour or effecting sedation, is achieved, the urgency of the situation determining the interval between increments.

A licensed maximum dose is defined for each antipsychotic agent, e.g. chlorpromazine 1000 mg/day. Prescribing in excess of this requires specialist involvement. With co-prescribed antipsychotics, their total maximum antipsychotic dose should not exceed 1000 mg chlorpromazine equivalents per day, except under specialist supervision. The licensed maximum dose of some antipsychotics is considerably below 1000 mg chlorpromazine equivalents per day: that of *thioridazine* was reduced to 600 mg/day following concerns about its cardiovascular toxicity. Plasma electrolytes and electrocardiograms (ECGs) should be checked on introducing or increasing the dose of thioridazine, and ECGs should be seen before prescribing pimozide or sertindole.

Prescription of atypical antipsychotics follows similar rules to those for classical drugs, starting at low doses in neuroleptic-naive patients. Whereas there is a wide range of effective doses for many classical agents (e.g. chlorpromazine 25–1000 mg/day),

much narrower ranges have been defined for atypical agents (see Table 19.5). Although classical antipsychotics are licensed for the management of acutely disturbed behaviour as well as for schizophrenia, atypical agents are generally licensed only for the latter indication (although that for risperidone is broader). For most atypical agents used in schizophrenia, a brief period of dose titration by protocol up to a stated lowest therapeutic dose is usual, e.g. risperidone 4 mg/day, quetiapine 300 mg/day. Dose increases are indicated when there is no response after 2 weeks, and these may be repeated until the maximum licensed dose is achieved.

Clozapine may be initiated only under specialist supervision and usually after at least one other antipsychotic has failed through lack of efficacy or unacceptable adverse effects. Additionally, monitoring of leucocyte count is mandatory (danger of agranulocytosis) and blood pressure checking is required (for hypotensive effect). Patients are most vulnerable to agranulocytosis on initiation of therapy, with 75% of cases occurring in the first 18 weeks. The dose titration schedule must be followed strictly, starting with clozapine 12.5 mg nocte and working up over a period of 4 weeks to a target therapeutic dose of 450 mg/day.

Alternative administration strategies in acute antipsychotic use

Preparations of antipsychotics for intramuscular injection are advantageous in patients who are unable or unwilling to swallow tablets, a common situation in psychosis or severe behavioural disturbance; haloperidol is used most commonly. An intramuscular preparation of olanzapine is suitable for acute behavioural disturbance in schizophrenia, as is a formulation that dissolves rapidly on contact with the tongue and is rapidly absorbed in a disturbed and uncooperative patient.

Long-acting depot injections

Haloperidol, zuclopenthixol, fluphenazine, flupentixol, risperidone and *pipothiazine* are available as long-acting (2–4 weeks) depot intramuscular injections for maintenance treatment of patients with schizophrenia and other chronic psychotic disorders. Compliance is improved and there is less risk of relapse from ceasing to take medication. In view of the prolonged effect, it is prudent to administer a small initial test dose and review 5–10 days later for unwanted effects.

Rapid tranquillisation

Rapid tranquillisation protocols address the problem of severely disturbed and violent patients who have not responded to non-pharmacological approaches. The risks of administering psychotropic drugs (notably cardiac arrhythmia with high-dose antipsychotics) then greatly outweigh those of non-treatment.

A first step is to offer oral medication, usually haloperidol, olanzapine or respiridone with or without the benzodiazepine, lorazepam. If this is not accepted or fails to achieve control despite repeated doses, the intramuscular route is used to administer a benzodiazepine (e.g. lorazepam or midazolam) or an antipsychotic (e.g. haloperidol or olanzapine), or both (but intramuscular olanzapine should not be given with a benzodiazepeine). After emergency use of an intramuscular antipsychotic or benzodiazepine, pulse, blood pressure, temperature and respiration are monitored, and pulse oximetry (for oxygen saturation) if consciousness is lost.

Zuclopenthixol acetate i.m. has been favoured for patients who do not respond to two doses of haloperidol i.m. This usually induces a calming effect within 2 h, persisting for 2–3 days. Clinicians are now becoming reluctant to use this heavily sedating preparation other than for patients who have previously responded well to it, and never use it for neuroleptic-naive patients. Patients must be observed with care following administration. Some will require a second dose within 1–2 days.

Amylobarbitone and paraldehyde still have a role in emergencies when antipsychotic and benzodiazepine options have been exhausted.

ADVERSE EFFECTS (TABLE 19.5)

Active psychotic illnesses often cause patients to have poor insight into their condition, and adverse drug effects can compromise an already fragile compliance, leading to avoidable relapse.

Classical antipsychotics

It is rare for any patient taking classical antipsychotic agents completely to escape their adverse effects. Thus it is essential to discuss with patients the possibility of unwanted effects and regularly to review this aspect of their care.

Extrapyramidal symptoms. All classical antipsychotics produce these effects because they act by blocking dopamine receptors in the nigrostriatal pathway. Consequently some 75% of patients experience extrapyramidal symptoms shortly after starting the drug or increasing its dose (acute effects), or some time after a particular dose level has been established (tardive effects).

Acute extrapyramidal symptoms. Dystonias are manifest as abnormal movements of the tongue and facial muscles with fixed postures and spasm, including torticollis and bizarre eye movements ('oculogyric crisis'). *Parkinsonian symptoms* result in the classical triad of bradykinesia, rigidity and tremor. Both dystonias and parkinsonian symptoms are believed to result from a shift in favour cholinergic rather than dopaminergic neurotransmission in the nigrostriatal pathway (see p. 343). Anticholinergic (antimuscarinic) agents, e.g. procyclidine, orphenadrine or benzatropine, act to restore the balance in favour of dopaminergic transmission but are liable to provoke antimuscarinic effects (dry mouth, urinary retention, constipation, exacerbation of glaucoma and confusion) and they offer no relief for tardive dyskinesia, which may even worsen. They should be used only to treat established symptoms and not for prophylaxis. Benzodiazepines are an alternative.

Akathisia is a state of motor and psychological restlessness, in which patients exhibit persistent foot tapping, moving of legs repetitively and being unable to settle or relax. A strong association has been noted between its presence in treated schizophrenics and subsequent suicide. A β-adrenoceptor blocker, e.g. nadolol, is the best treatment, although anticholinergic agents may be effective where akathisia coexists with dystonias and parkinsonian symptoms. Differentiating symptoms of psychotic illness from adverse drug effects is often difficult: drug-induced akathisia may be mistaken for agitation induced by psychosis.

Tardive dyskinesia affects about 25% of patients taking classical antipsychotic drugs, the risk increasing with length of exposure. It was originally thought to be a consequence of up-regulation or supersensitivity of dopamine receptors, but a more recent view is that oxidative damage leads to increases in glutamate transmission.

Patients display a spectrum of abnormal movements from minor tongue protrusion, lip-smacking, rotational tongue movements and facial grimacing, choreoathetoid movements of the head and neck,

Table 19.5 Relative frequency of selected adverse effects of antipsychotic drugs

Drug	CPZ equiv. dose (mg)	Max. dose (mg/day)	Structure	Extrapyramidal effects	Anticholinergic effects	Hyperprolactinaemia	Weight gain	Cardiotoxicity	Blood dyscrasias	Sedation
Classical										
chlorpromazine	100	1000	Type 1: phenothiazine	++	++	+++	++	+	+	+++
thioridazine	50	300[a]	Type 2: phenothiazine	+	+++	+++	+++	++	+	+++
trifluoperazine	5	50	Type 3: phenothiazine	+++	+	+++	++	+	+	+
haloperidol	3	30	Butyrophenone	+++	+	+++	++	+	+	+
sulpiride	200	2400	Substituted benzamide	+	+	+++	+	–	+	–
zuclopenthixol	25	150	Thioxanthene	++	++	+++	++	+	+	++
	Min. eff. dose (mg/day)	Max. dose (mg/day)								
Atypical										
clozapine[b]	300	900	Dibenzodiazepine	–	+++	–	++	+	+++	+++
olanzapine	5–10	20	Theinobenzodiazepine	–	++	+	+++	+	+	++
quetiapine	300	750	Dibenzothiazepine	–	+	–	+	–	+	+++
risperidone	4	16	Benzisoxazole	+	+	++	+	+	+	+
amisulpride	800[c]	1200	Substituted benzamide	+	–	++	+	–	+	–
aripiprazole[d]	10–15	30		–	–	–	–	–	–	+

CPZ equiv. dose, Chlorpromazine equivalent dose. This concept is of value in comparing the potency of classical antipsychotics. Dose ranges are not specified as they are extremely wide and drugs are normally increased from low starting doses, e.g. chlorpromazine 25 mg or equivalent, until an adequate antipsychotic effect is achieved or the maximum dose reached. The chlorpromazine equivalent dose concept is of less value for atypical antipsychotics because minimum effective doses (Min. eff. dose) and narrower therapeutic ranges have been defined. Maximum dose (Max. dose) should be exceeded only under specialist supervision.

[a] The maximum dose of thioradazine has been reduced to 300 mg/day (or 600 mg/day in hospitalised patients) following concerns relating to QTc prolongation and risk of fatal cardiac arrhythmias at higher doses.

[b] A dose of clozapine 50 mg is considered equivalent to chlorpromazine 100 mg.

[c] Lower doses of amisulpride, e.g. 100 mg/day, are indicated only for patients with negative symptoms of schizophrenia.

[d] Aripiprazole appears to be free of most unwanted effects characteristically associated with antipsychotics, but may cause nausea, light-headedness, somnolence and akathisia.

and even to twisting and gyrating of the whole body. Remission on discontinuing the causative agent is less likely than are simple dystonias and parkinsonian symptoms. Any anticholinergic agent should be withdrawn immediately. Reduction of the dose of classical antipsychotic is an option, but psychotic symptoms may then worsen or be 'unmasked'. Alternatively, an atypical antipsychotic can provide rapid improvement whilst retaining control of psychotic symptoms. Atypicals, particularly at high doses, can cause extrapyramidal effects, so this strategy is not always helpful. Clozapine, which does not appear to cause tardive dyskinesia, may be used in severe cases where continuing antipsychotic treatment is required and symptoms have not responded to other medication strategies.

If the classical antipsychotic is continued, tardive dyskinesia remits spontaneously in around 30% of patients within 1 year, but the condition is difficult to tolerate and patients may be keen to try other medications even where evidence suggests that the success rates for remission are limited. These include vitamin E, benzodiazepines, β-blockers, bromocriptine and tetrabenazine.

Cardiovascular effects. Postural hypotension may result from blockade of α_1 adrenoceptors; it is dose related. Prolongation of the QTc interval in the cardiac cycle may rarely lead to ventricular arrhythmias and sudden death (particular warnings and constraints apply to the use of thioridazine and pimozide).

Prolactin increase. Classical antipsychotics raise plasma prolactin concentration by blocking dopamine receptors in the tuberoinfundibular pathway, causing gynaecomastia and galactorrhoea in both sexes, and menstrual disturbances in women. A change to an atypical agent such as quetiapine or olanzapine (but not risperidone or amisulpride) should minimise the effects. If continuation of the existing classical antipsychotic is obligatory, dopamine agonists such as bromocriptine and amantadine that reduce prolactin secretion may help.

Sedation. In the acute treatment of psychotic illness this may be a highly desirable property, but it may be undesirable as the patient seeks to resume work, study or relationships.

Classical antipsychotics may also be associated with:

- *weight gain* (a problem with almost all classical antipsychotics with the exception of loxapine, most pronounced with fluphenazine and flupentixol)
- *seizures* (chlorpromazine and thioridazine are especially likely to lower the convulsion threshold)
- *interference with temperature regulation* (hypothermia or hyperthermia, especially in the elderly)
- *skin problems* (phenothiazines, particularly chlorpromazine, may provoke photosensitivity necessitating advice about limiting exposure to sunlight); rashes and urticaria may also occur
- *sexual dysfunction* (ejaculatory problems through α-adrenoceptor blockade)
- *retinal pigmentation* (chlorpromazine, thioridazine, vision is affected if the dose is prolonged and high)
- *corneal and lens opacities* (especially thioridazine)
- *blood dyscrasias* (agranulocytosis and leucopenia)
- *osteoporosis* (associated with increased prolactin levels)
- *jaundice* (including cholestatic).

Atypical antipsychotics

Atypical drugs can provoke a range of adverse effects similar to those of the classical antipsychotics but generally of lesser degree. The following are the main differences.

Extrapyramidal effects are fewer (there is less blockade of dopamine D_2 receptors in the nigrostriatal pathway) but do occur with high doses of risperidone (8–12 mg/day) and olanzapine (>20 mg/day). Olanzapine and risperidone are also associated with a greater risk of stroke in elderly patients with dementia.

Anticholinergic (antimuscarinic) effects are most likely with clozapine and olanzapine, which are also more prone to cause *weight gain* and are second only to quetiapine in their *sedative effects*.

Galactorrhoea is as common with risperidone and amisulpride as with classical antipsychotics. Sexual dysfunction and skin problems are rare with atypical antipsychotics.

Clozapine warrants separate mention, given its value for patients with treatment-resistant schizophrenia or severe treatment-related extrapyramidal symptoms. Most important is the risk of *agranulocytosis* in up to 2% of patients (compared with 0.2% for classical antipsychotics). When clozapine was first licensed without requirement for regular blood counts, this problem caused appreciable mortality. With the introduction of strict monitoring, there have been no recorded deaths in the UK from agranulocytosis since clozapine was reintroduced, and internationally the death rate from agranulocytosis is now less than 1 in 1000.

Clozapine may cause postural hypotension and tachycardia, and provoke seizures in 3–5% of patients at doses above 600 mg/day.

Neuroleptic malignant syndrome

The syndrome may develop in up to 1% of patients using antipsychotics, both classical and atypical (although rarely with the latter); it is more prevalent with high doses. The elderly and those with organic brain disease, hyperthyroidism or dehydration are thought to be most susceptible. Clinical features include fever, confusion or fluctuating consciousness, rigidity of muscles which may become severe, autonomic instability manifest by labile blood pressure, tachycardia and urinary incontinence or retention.

Raised plasma creatine kinase concentration and white cell count are suggestive (but not conclusive) of neuroleptic malignant syndrome. There is some clinical overlap with the 'serotonin syndrome' (see p. 338) and concomitant use of SSRI antidepressants (or possibly TCAs) with antipsychotics may increase the risk.

When the syndrome is suspected, it is essential to discontinue the antipsychotic, and to be ready to undertake rehydration and body cooling. A benzodiazepine is indicated for sedation, tranquillising effect and may be beneficial where active psychosis remains untreated. Dopamine agonists (bromocriptine, dantrolene) are helpful in some cases. Even when recognised and treated, the condition carries a mortality rate of 12–15%, through cardiac arrhythmia, rhabdomyolysis or respiratory failure. The condition usually lasts for 5–7 days after the antipsychotic is stopped but may continue longer when a depot preparation has been used. Fortunately those who survive tend to have no long-lasting physical effects from their ordeal.

CLASSICAL VERSUS ATYPICAL ANTIPSYCHOTICS

Atypical antipsychotics may have advantages in three areas:

1. Tolerability and thus compliance appears to be better,[3] in particular with less likelihood of inducing extrapyramidal effects and hyperprolactinaemia (although the latter remains common with risperidone and amisulpride).
2. Greater efficacy against the negative symptoms of schizophrenia, which are particularly debilitating in chronic illness.
3. Clozapine (but not the newer atypicals) is more effective than classical agents in treatment-resistant schizophrenia.

In some countries finance may be the overriding factor in favour of retaining classical agents rather than atypicals as first choice in schizophrenia. However, the basis for any such decision must extend beyond crude drug costs and take account of the capacity of atypicals to lessen extrapyramidal symptoms, improve compliance, and thus prevent relapse of psychotic illness and protect patients from the lasting damage of periods of untreated psychosis. Additionally, greater efficacy in alleviating negative symptoms affords schizophrenic patients the opportunity to re-integrate into the community and make positive contributions to society, when the alternative is long-term residence in hospital. Recognising drugs as therapeutic entities as well as units of cost is an important element in deciding between classical and atypical drugs, and indeed about decision-making in the purchase of all drugs by institutions or countries.

MOOD STABILISERS

In bipolar affective disorder patients suffer episodes of mania, hypomania and depression, classically with periods of normal mood in between. *Manic episodes* involve greatly elevated mood, often associated with

---

[3]Whilst the advantages of atypicals over classical antipsychotics may seem clearcut, one analysis using only trials in which doses of classical antipsychotics were at or below a dose of haloperidol 12 mg/day or equivalent (now regarded as the upper limit for optimised use of these agents) produced rather different results. Although the atypicals retained their advantage in causing extrapyramidal effects less frequently, overall tolerability and efficacy appeared to be similar. Geddes J, Freemantle N, Harrison P, Bebbington P 2000 Atypical antipsychotics in the treatment of schizophrenia: systematic overview and meta-regression analysis. British Medical Journal 321:1371–1376.

irritability, loss of social inhibitions, irresponsible behaviour and grandiosity accompanied by biological symptoms (increased energy, restlessness, decreased need for sleep, and increased sex drive). Psychotic features may be present, particularly disordered thinking manifested by grandiose delusions and 'flight of ideas' (acceleration of the pattern of thought with rapid speech). *Hypomania* is a less dramatic and less dangerous presentation, but retains the features of elation or irritability and the biological symptoms, abnormalities in speech being limited to increased talkativeness and in social conduct to over-familiarity and mild recklessness. *Depressive episodes* may include any of the depressive symptoms described above, and may include psychotic features.

LITHIUM

Lithium salts were known anecdotally to have beneficial psychotropic effects as long ago as the middle of the 19th century, but scientific evidence of their efficacy was not obtained until 1949, when lithium carbonate was tried in manic patients; it was found to be effective in the acute state and, later, to prevent recurrent attacks.[4]

The mode of action is not fully understood. Its main effect is probably to inhibit hydrolysis of inositol phosphate, so reducing the recycling of free inositol for synthesis of phosphatidylinositides, which if present in excess may interfere with cell homeostasis by promoting uncontrolled cell signalling. Other putative mechanisms involve the cyclic AMP 'second messenger' system, and monoaminergic and cholinergic neurotransmitters.

Pharmacokinetics. The therapeutic and toxic plasma concentrations are close (low therapeutic index). Lithium is a small cation and, given orally, is rapidly absorbed throughout the gut. High peak plasma concentrations are avoided by using sustained-release formulations which deliver the peak plasma lithium concentrations in about 5 h. At first lithium is distributed throughout the extracellular water, but with continued administration it enters the cells and is eventually distributed throughout the total body water with a somewhat higher concentration in brain, bones and thyroid gland. Lithium is easily dialysable from the blood but the concentration gradient from cell to blood is relatively small and the intracellular concentration (which determines toxicity) falls slowly. Being a metallic ion it is not metabolised, nor is it bound to plasma proteins.

The kidneys eliminate lithium. Like sodium, it is filtered by the glomerulus and 80% is reabsorbed by the proximal tubule, but it is not reabsorbed by the distal tubule. Intake of sodium and water are the principal determinants of its elimination. In sodium deficiency lithium is retained in the body, and thus concomitant use of a diuretic can reduce lithium clearance by as much as 50%, and precipitate toxicity. Sodium chloride and water are used to treat lithium toxicity.

With chronic use the plasma $t_{1/2}$ of lithium is 15–30 h. It is usually given 12–24-hourly to avoid unnecessary fluctuation (peak and trough) and maintain plasma concentrations just below the toxic level. A steady-state plasma concentration will be attained after about 5–6 days (i.e. $5 \times t_{1/2}$) in patients with normal renal function. Old people and patients with impaired renal function will have a longer $t_{1/2}$ so that steady state will be reached later and dose increments must be adjusted accordingly.

Indications and use. Lithium carbonate is effective *treatment* in more than 75% of episodes of acute mania or hypomania. Because its therapeutic action takes 2–3 weeks to develop, lithium is generally used in combination with a benzodiazepine such as lorazepam or diazepam (or with an antipsychotic agent where there are also psychotic features).

For *prophylaxis*, lithium is indicated when there have been two episodes of mood disturbance in 2 years, although in severe cases prophylactic use is indicated after one episode. When an adequate dose of lithium is taken consistently, around 65% of patients achieve improved mood control.

Patients who start lithium only to discontinue it within 2 years have a significantly poorer outcome than matched patients who are not given any pharmacological prophylaxis. The existence of a 'rebound effect' (recurrence of manic symptoms) during withdrawal dictates that long-term treatment with the drug is of great importance.

Lithium salts are ineffective for prophylaxis of bipolar affective disorder in around 35% of patients. The search for alternatives has centred on anticonvulsants, notably carbamazepine and sodium valproate and lamotrigine.

---

[4]Cade J F 1970 The story of lithium. In: Ayd F J, Blackwell B (eds) Biological psychiatry. Lippincott, Philadelphia.

Lithium is also used to augment the action of antidepressants in treatment-resistant depression (see p. 336).

Pharmaceutics. The dose of lithium ions (Li⁺) delivered varies with the pharmaceutical preparation; thus it is vital for patients to adhere to the same pharmaceutical brand. For example, *Camcolit* 250-mg tablets each contain 6.8 mmol Li⁺, *Liskonium* 450-mg tablets contain 12.2 mmol Li⁺ and *Priadel* 200-mg tablets contain 5.4 mmol Li⁺. The proprietary name must be stated on the prescription.

Some patients cannot tolerate slow-release preparations because release of lithium distally in the intestine causes diarrhoea; they may be better served by the liquid preparation, lithium citrate, which is absorbed proximally. Patients who are naive to lithium should be started at the lowest dose of the preparation selected. Any change in preparation demands the same precautions as does initiation of therapy.

Monitoring. Dose is guided by monitoring of the plasma concentration once steady state has been reached. Increments are made at weekly intervals until the concentration lies within the range 0.4–1 mmol/L (maintenance at the lower level is preferred for elderly patients). The timing of blood sampling is important, and by convention a blood sample is taken prior to the morning dose, as close as possible to 12 h after the evening dose. Once the plasma concentration is at steady state and in the therapeutic range, it should be measured/assayed every 3 months. For toxicity monitoring, thyroid function (especially in women) and renal function (plasma creatinine and electrolytes) should be measured before initiation and every 3–6 months during therapy.

Patient education about the role of lithium in the prophylaxis of bipolar affective disorder is particularly important to achieve compliance with therapy; treatment cards, information leaflets and, where appropriate, video material are used.

Adverse effects are encountered in three general categories:

- Those occurring at plasma concentrations within the therapeutic range (0.4–1 mmol/L), which include fine tremor (especially involving the fingers; a β-blocker may benefit), constipation, polyuria, polydipsia, metallic taste in the mouth, weight gain, oedema, goitre, hypothyroidism, acne, rash, diabetes insipidus and cardiac arrhythmias. Mild cognitive and memory impairment also occur.
- Signs of intoxication, associated with plasma concentrations greater than 1.5 mmol/L, are mainly gastrointestinal (diarrhoea, anorexia, vomiting) and neurological (blurred vision, muscle weakness, drowsiness, sluggishness and coarse tremor, leading on to giddiness, ataxia and dysarthria).
- Frank toxicity, due to severe overdosage or rapid reduction in renal clearance, usually associated with plasma concentrations above 2 mmol/L, constitutes a medical emergency. Hyperreflexia, hyperextension of limbs, convulsions, hyperthermia, toxic psychoses, syncope, oliguria, coma and even death may result if treatment is not instigated urgently.

Overdose. Acute overdose may present without signs of toxicity but with plasma concentrations well exceeding 2 mmol/L. This requires only measures to increase urine production, e.g. by ensuring adequate intravenous and oral fluid intake whilst avoiding sodium depletion (and a diuretic is contraindicated; see above). Treatment is otherwise supportive with special attention to electrolyte balance, renal function and control of convulsions. Where toxicity is chronic, haemodialysis may be needed, especially if renal function is impaired. Plasma concentration may rise again after acute reduction, because lithium leaves cells slowly, and also due to continued absorption from sustained-release formulations. Whole bowel irrigation may be an option for significant ingestion (see p. 131), but specialist advice should be sought.

Interactions. Drugs that interfere with lithium excretion by the renal tubules cause the plasma concentration to rise. They include diuretics (thiazides more than loop type), angiotensin-converting enzyme (ACE) inhibitors and angiotensin-II antagonists, and non-steroidal anti-inflammatory analgesics. Theophylline and sodium-containing antacids reduce plasma lithium concentration. These effects can be important because lithium has a low therapeutic ratio. Diltiazem, verapamil, carbamazepine and phenytoin may cause neurotoxicity without affecting the plasma lithium level. Concomitant use of thioridazine should be avoided as ventricular arrhythmias may result.

CARBAMAZEPINE

Carbamazepine is licensed as an alternative to lithium for prophylaxis of bipolar affective disorder, although clinical trial evidence is actually stronger to support its use in the treatment of acute mania. Carbamazepine appears to be more effective than lithium for rapidly cycling bipolar disorders, i.e. with recurrent swift transitions from mania to depression. It is also effective in combination with lithium. (See also Epilepsy, p. 372.)

VALPROIC ACID

Valproic acid has become the drug of first choice for prophylaxis of bipolar affective disorder in the USA, despite the lack of robust supporting clinical trial evidence. Treatment with valproic acid is easy to initiate (especially compared to lithium), it is well tolerated and its use appears likely to extend if the evidence base expands. The semi-sodium salt of valproic acid (Depakote) is licensed for the treatment of acute mania unresponsive to lithium.

Treatment with carbamazepine or valproic acid appears not to be associated with the 'rebound effect' of relapse into manic symptoms that may accompany early withdrawal of lithium therapy.

OTHER DRUGS

Evidence is emerging for the efficacy of lamotrigine in prophylaxis of bipolar affective disorder and treatment of bipolar depression. Other drugs that have been used in augmentation of existing agents include the anticonvulsant gabapentin, the benzodiazepine clonazepam, and the calcium channel blocking agents verapamil and nimodipine.

DRUGS USED IN ANXIETY AND SLEEP DISORDERS

The disability and health costs caused by anxiety are high and comparable with those of other common medical conditions such as diabetes, arthritis or hypertension. People with anxiety disorders experience impaired physical and role functioning, more work-days lost due to illness, increased impairment at work and high use of health services. Our understanding of the nature of anxiety has increased greatly from advances in research in psychology and neuroscience. It is now possible to distinguish different types of anxiety with distinct biological and cognitive symptoms, and clear criteria have been accepted for the diagnosis of various anxiety disorders. The last decade has seen developments in both drug and psychological therapies such that a range of treatment options can be tailored to individual patients and their condition.

Anxiety does not manifest itself only as a psychic or mental state, there are also somatic or physical concomitants, e.g. consciousness of the action of the heart (palpitations), tremor, diarrhoea, which are associated with increased activity of the sympathetic autonomic system. These symptoms are not only caused by anxiety, they also add to the feeling of anxiety (positive feedback loop). Anxiety symptoms exist on a continuum and many people with a mild anxiety, perhaps of recent onset and associated with stressful life events but without much disability, tend to improve without specific intervention. The chronic nature and associated disability of many anxiety disorders means that most patients who fulfill diagnostic criteria for a disorder are likely to benefit from some form of treatment.

CLASSIFICATION OF ANXIETY DISORDERS

The diagnostic criteria of DSM-IV (Diagnostic and Statistical Manual) or ICD-10 (International Classification of Diseases) are generally used. Both divide anxiety into a series of sub-syndromes with clear operational criteria to assist in distinguishing them. At any one time many patients may have symptoms of more than one syndrome, but making the primary diagnosis is important as this can markedly influence the choice of treatment (Table 19.6).

The key features of each anxiety disorder follow, with a practical description of the preferred choice of medication, its dose and duration.

PANIC DISORDER (PD)

The main feature is recurrent, unexpected panic attacks. These are discrete periods of intense fear accompanied by characteristic physical symptoms such as skipping or pounding heart, sweating, hot flushes or chills, trembling/shaking, breathing difficulties, chest pain, nausea, diarrhoea and other gastrointestinal symptoms, dizziness or light-headedness. The first panic attack often occurs without warning but may subsequently become associated with specific situations, e.g. in a crowded

Table 19.6 Evidence-based treatments for anxiety disorders

	GAD	Panic	Social phobia	PTSD	OCD	Simple phobia
First-line treatment	SSRI	SSRI	SSRI	(Acute prevention – if feasible consider propanolol after major trauma. Routine debriefing not indicated). SSRI	SSRI	Psychological – exposure therapy
Psychotherapy treatments	CBT	CBT	CBT	Prevention – trauma-focused CBT. Trauma-focused CBT also prevents chronic PTSD in patients with symptoms at 1 month. Eye movement desensitisation and reprocessing (EMDR)	Exposure therapy, CBT (lower relapse rate after psychological than pharmacological therapy)	Exposure therapy
Pharmacological treatments	Most SSRIs, venlafaxine, alprazolam, imipramine, buspirone, hydroxyzine	All SSRIs, clomipramine, imipramine, some benzodiazepines (alprazolam, clonazepam, diazepam, lorazepam), venlafaxine, reboxetine	Most SSRIs, venlafaxine, phenelzine, moclobemide, some benzodiazepines (bromazepam, clonazepam) and anticonvulsants (gabapentin, pregabalin), olanzepine	Some SSRIs (fluoxetine, paroxetine, sertraline), some TCAs (amitriptyline, imipramine), phenelzine, mirtazapine, venlafaxine, lamotrigine	Clomipramine, SSRIs	
Duration of drug treatment	Further 6 months if response at 12 weeks	Further 6 months if response at 12 weeks	Further 6 months if response at 12 weeks	Further 12 months if response at 12 weeks	Further 12 months if response at 12 weeks	
Higher doses associated with better response	SSRIs, venlafaxine	SSRIs (limited evidence)	Individual patients may benefit	Individual patients may benefit	SSRIs	
Relapse prevention	SSRI	CBT with exposure; SSRI; imipramine	CBT with exposure; SSRI; clonazepam	SSRIs	SSRIs	

Strategies if resistant	If no response to SSRI, switch to venlafaxine or imipramine. Try BDZ after non-reponse to SSRI and SNRI. Combine drugs and CBT	If no response to SSRI, switch to another evidence-based treatment. If partial response to SSRI, add buspirone or paroxetine. Combine drugs and CBT	If no response to SSRI, switch to venlafaxine. If partial response to SSRI, add buspirone. Consider BDZs in patients who do not respond to other approaches. Add CBT to drug treatment	Switch to another evidence-based treatment; combine treatments; augment antidepressants with atypical antipsychotic	Increase dose of SSRI/clomipramine. Combine drug therapy with exposure therapy or CBT. Augment with antipsychotics or pindolol

General considerations for treatment of anxiety disorders include the need to discuss the benefits and risks of specific treatments with patients before treatment and take account of clinical features, patient needs and preference, and local service availability when choosing treatments. SSRIs are usually effective in anxiety disorders and are generally suitable for first-line treatment.

Benzodiazepines are effective in many anxiety disorders but their use should be short term except in treatment-resistant cases. TCAs, MAOIs, antipsychotics and anticonvulsants need to be considered in relation to their evidence base for specific conditions and their individual risks and benefits.

With all antidepressants, especially SSRIs and venlafaxine, there should be specific discussion and monitoring of possible adverse effects early in treatment, and also on stopping the drugs after a week of treatment – the latter also applies to benzodiazepines.

Specific psychological treatments are as good in acute treatment as pharmacological approaches in GAD, PD, SAD and OCD. Treatment effect is often slow, and it is advisable to wait 12 weeks to assess efficacy.

When initial treatments fail, one should consider switching to another evidence-based treatment, combining evidence-based treatments (only when there are no contraindications), and referring to regional or national specialist services in refractory patients.

BDZ, benzodiazepine; CBT, cognitive behavioural therapy.

shop, while driving. Anticipatory anxiety and avoidance behaviour develop in response to this chain of events. The condition must be distinguished from alcohol withdrawal, caffeinism, hyperthyroidism and (rarely) phaeochromocytoma.

Patients experiencing panic attacks often do not know what is happening to them and, because the symptoms are similar to those of cardiovascular, respiratory or neurological conditions, often present to non-psychiatric services, e.g. casualty departments, family doctors, medical specialists, where they may either be extensively investigated or given reassurance that there is nothing wrong. A carefully taken history reduces the likelihood of this occurrence.

Treatment. The choice lies between a fast-acting benzodiazepine such as lorazepam or alprazolam and one with delayed efficacy but fewer problems of withdrawal such as a tricyclic antidepressant (TCA), e.g. clomipramine or a serotonin selective reuptake inhibitor (SSRI), e.g. paroxetine. The different time-course of these two classes of agent in panic disorder is depicted in Figure 19.4 (see also Table 19.6).

Benzodiazepines rapidly reduce panic frequency and severity, and continue to be effective for months; significant tolerance to the therapeutic action is uncommon. On withdrawal of the benzodiazepine, even when it is gradual, increased symptoms of anxiety and panic attacks may occur, reaching a maximum when the final dose is stopped. Indeed, some patients find they are unable to withdraw and remain long term on a benzodiazepine.

Antidepressants (both SSRIs and TCAs) have a slower onset of action and may cause an initial increase in both anxiety and panic frequency, such that a patient may discontinue medication, even

after a single dose. This provoking reaction usually lasts for only 2–3 weeks, after which panic frequency and severity improve quickly, but patients need help to stay on treatment in the first weeks. The doctor needs to give a clear explanation of the likely course of events and the antidepressant should be started at half the usual initial dose to reduce the likelihood of exacerbation. A short course of a long-acting benzodiazepine (e.g. diazepam 5 mg up to t.i.d.) can provide benefit. The dose of antidepressant required to treat panic disorder is generally as high as or higher than that for depression, and maximal benefit may not emerge for 8–12 weeks. Patients should therefore receive as large a dose as can be tolerated for this length of time.

SOCIAL ANXIETY DISORDER (SAD)

The essential feature of social phobia is a marked and persistent fear of performance situations when patients feel they will be the centre of attention and will do something humiliating or embarrassing. The situations that provoke this fear can be quite specific, e.g. public speaking, or of a much more generalised nature involving fear of most social interactions, e.g. initiating or maintaining conversations, participating in small groups, dating, speaking to anyone in authority. Exposure to the feared situation almost invariably provokes anxiety with symptoms similar to those experienced by patients with panic attacks, but some seem to be particularly prominent and difficult, i.e. blushing, tremor, sweating and a feeling of 'drying up' when speaking.

Treatment. The drugs with established efficacy are the SSRIs (*paroxetine, escitalopram*), the MAOI *phenelzine* and the reversible inhibitor of MAO-A (RIMA) *moclobemide* in the same doses as for depression. These achieve equivalent degrees of improvement; *phenelzine* has a slightly faster onset of action but produces more adverse effects. Some benzodiazepines and other SSRIs are reported to provide benefit, but evidence for their therapeutic efficacy is less conclusive. β-Adrenoceptor blockers continue to be widely used despite their having no proven efficacy in social phobia. However, they have a place in the treatment of specific performance anxiety, e.g. in musicians, when management of the tremor is crucial.

The duration of treatment is as for depression or longer, for this can be a lifelong condition.

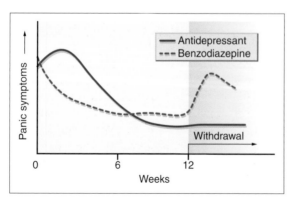

Fig. 19.4 Schematic representation of the time course of panic treatments.

POST-TRAUMATIC STRESS DISORDER (PTSD)

Symptoms characteristically follow exposure to an extremely traumatic stressor event. These include persistent re-experiencing of the traumatic event, persistent avoidance of stimuli associated with the trauma and numbing of general responsiveness, and persistent symptoms of increased arousal. In taking a history the association with the event is usually obvious. PTSD is differentiated from acute stress disorder (below) by its persistence – the symptoms of the latter resolve within about 4 weeks. Depression quite commonly coexists with PTSD and should be enquired for in the history.

Treatment is poorly researched; there have been no properly controlled trials and almost all open trials have been conducted on small numbers of patients long after the causative incident. The wide range of drugs that has been reported to provide benefit includes benzodiazepines, TCAs and MAOIs; *paroxetine* (SSRI) is now licensed for this indication in the UK. The preferred treatment immediately after the incident should probably be a short course of a hypnotic (or sedating antidepressant, e.g. *mirtazapine*) to promote sleep and help minimise mental rehearsal of the trauma that may lead to its perpetuation. Long-term therapy with antidepressants appears to be indicated at doses in the same range as for other anxiety disorders.

ACUTE STRESS DISORDER/ADJUSTMENT DISORDER

Acute stress disorder is anxiety in response to a recent extreme stress. Although in some respects it is a normal and understandable reaction to an event, the problems associated with it are not only the severe distress the anxiety causes but also the risk that it may evolve into a more persistent state.

Treatment. A benzodiazepine used for a short time is the preferred approach for treating overwhelming anxiety that needs to be brought rapidly under control. It particularly relieves the accompanying anxiety and sleep disturbance. A drug with a slow onset of action such as *oxazepam* (60–120 mg/day) causes less dependence and withdrawal, and is preferred to those that enter the brain rapidly, e.g. diazepam, lorazepam. Some patients find it hard to discontinue the benzodiazepine, so its use should be reserved for those in whom extreme distress disrupts normal coping strategies.

GENERALISED ANXIETY DISORDER (GAD)

The essential feature of this condition is chronic anxiety and worry. To the non-sufferer the focus of the worry often seems to be trivial, e.g. getting the housework done or being late for appointments, but to the patient it is insurmountable. The anxiety is often associated with other symptoms, which include restlessness, difficulty in concentrating, irritability, muscle tension and sleep disturbance. The course of the disorder is typically chronic with exacerbations at times of stress and is often associated with depression. Its chronic nature with worsening at times of stress helps to distinguish GAD from anxiety in the form of episodic panic attacks with associated anticipatory anxiety (panic disorder). Hyperthyroidism and caffeinism should also be excluded.

Treatment. Historically *benzodiazepines* have been seen as the most effective treatment for GAD for they rapidly reduce anxiety and improve sleep and somatic symptoms. Consequently patients like taking them, but the chronic nature of GAD raises issues of duration of treatment, tolerance, dependence and withdrawal reactions.

Buspirone is structurally unrelated to other anxiolytics and was the first non-benzodiazepine to demonstrate efficacy in GAD. Although its mode of action is not well understood, it is a $5HT_{1A}$-receptor partial agonist, and over time produces anxiolysis without undue sedation. Buspirone has a $t_{1/2}$ of 7 h and is metabolised in the liver; it has an active metabolite that may accumulate over weeks.

Buspirone is generally less effective and slower in action than benzodiazepines and does not improve sleep; it does not benefit benzodiazepine withdrawal symptoms. The advantages are that it does not seem to cause dependence or withdrawal reactions and does not interact with alcohol. It appears to be less effective in patients who have previously received benzodiazepines and is therefore probably best reserved for benzodiazepine-naive patients. A disadvantage is that useful anxiolytic effect is delayed for 2 weeks or more.

Adverse effects can include dizziness, headache, nervousness, excitement, nausea, tachycardia and drowsiness.

Paroxetine, escitalopram (SSRI) and *venlafaxine* (SNRI) are effective (and are licensed for GAD in the UK), and TCAs have also been shown to give benefit, and are probably more efficacious than buspirone or benzodiazepines. These drugs have a slower onset of action than benzodiazepines and are less well tolerated, but cause fewer problems of dependence and on withdrawal.

A delayed response in GAD is not as problematic as with acute situational anxiety. A sensible approach is to start with an antidepressant (SSRI or venlafaxine) for 6–8 weeks at least, increasing over 2–3 weeks to minimise unwanted actions; patients should be warned not to expect an immediate benefit. Those who do not respond should receive either buspirone for 6–8 weeks at full therapeutic dose (possibly as an add-on). There remain some patients, including those with a long history of benzodiazepine use, who fail to respond. A benzodiazepine may be the only medication that provides relief for such resistant cases, and can be used as the sole treatment.

The *duration of therapy* depends on the nature of the underlying illness. If symptoms are intermittent, i.e. triggered by anxiety-provoking situations, then intermittent use of a benzodiazepine (for a few weeks) may be sufficient. More typically GAD requires treatment over 6–8 months with gradual withdrawal of medication thereafter. This may suffice but some patients experience severe, unremitting anxiety and the best resort is to chronic maintenance treatment with a benzodiazepine (analogous to long-term drug use in epilepsy). Such clinically supervised benzodiazepine use is justified because, without treatment, patients often derive comfort from the most widely accessible, easily available anxiolytic – alcohol.

SIMPLE PHOBIA

A specific phobia is a fear of a circumscribed object or situation, for instance fear of spiders, of flying, of heights. The diagnosis is not usually in doubt. A course of treatment by a trained therapist, involving graded exposure to the feared stimulus is the treatment of choice and can be very effective. By its nature such therapy generates severe anxiety, and a *benzodiazepine* (or prior treatment with a SSRI, e.g. paroxetine) may be necessary to allow patients to engage in therapy.

OBSESSIVE–COMPULSIVE DISORDER (OCD)

Obsessive compulsive disorder has two main components:

1. The repetition of acts or thoughts that are involuntary, recognised by the sufferer to be generated by their own brain but are not in keeping with their usual thought processes, morals or values, and are therefore very distressing.
2. Anxiety provoked by the occurrence of such thoughts, or by prevention of the compulsive acts.

OCD on its own often starts in adolescence and has a chronic and pervasive course unless treated. OCD starting later on in life is often associated with affective or anxiety disorders. Symptoms often abate briefly if the individual is taken to a new environment.

Treatments are cognitive behavioural therapy and a *SSRI* or *clomipramine* (i.e. antidepressants that enhance serotonergic function), used at higher doses and for much longer periods than for depressive disorders. Neuroleptics, atypical antipsychotics in low dose and benzodiazepines can be used successfully to augment the SSRIs if they are not wholly effective, especially in patients with tics. Psychosurgery is still occasionally used for severe and treatment-resistant cases. Interestingly the brain pathways targeted by the surgeon are those that show abnormalities in neuroimaging (positron emission tomography; PET) studies of OCD, i.e. the basal ganglia/orbitofrontal pathways.

GENERAL COMMENTS ABOUT TREATING ANXIETY DISORDERS (TABLE 19.7)

- There is need to discuss the benefits and risks of specific treatments with patients before treatment and take account of their clinical features, needs, preferences and availability of local service when choosing treatments.
- SSRIs are usually effective in anxiety disorders and are generally suitable for first-line treatment.
- Benzodiazepines are effective in many anxiety disorders but their use should be short term except in treatment-resistant cases.
- TCAs, MAOIs, antipsychotics and anticonvulsants need to be considered in

Table 19.7 Properties of antianxiety drugs

	Benzodiazepines	Buspirone	Antidepressants	
			SSRIs	*TCAs*
Onset	Fast	Slow	Slow	Slow
Initial worsening of symptoms	No	Rarely	Sometimes (especially panic)	
Withdrawal symptoms				
Acute	Yes (~30%)	No	Sometimes	Sometimes
Chronic	?Yes (~10%)	No	No	No
Abuse potential	Low	Zero	Zero	Zero
Interactions with alcohol	Marked	Slight	Slight	Moderate
Adverse effects				
Sedation	Yes	No	No	Some TCAs
Amnesia	Yes	No	No	Some TCAs
Cardiovascular	No	No	No	Yes
Gastrointestinal	No	Slight	Yes, diarrhoea	Yes, constipa-tion
Sexual	No	No	Delay orgasm	Delay orgasm
Depression	Sometimes	No	No	No
Safety in overdose	Yes	Yes	Yes	No

relation to their evidence base for specific conditions and their individual risks and benefits.

- With all antidepressants, especially SSRIs and venlafaxine, there should be specific discussion and monitoring of possible adverse effects early in treatment, and also on stopping the drugs after a week of treatment; this latter also applies to benzodiazepines.
- Treatment effect is often slow, and it is advisable to wait 12 weeks to assess efficacy.
- In a first episode, patients may need medication for at least 6 months, withdrawing over a further 4–8 weeks if they are well. Those with recurrent illness may need treatment for 1–2 years to enable them to learn to put into place psychological approaches to their problems. In many cases the illnesses are lifelong and chronic maintenance treatment is justified if it has significantly improved their well-being and function.
- Specific psychological treatments are as good in acute treatment as pharmacological approaches in GAD, PD, SAD and OCD.
- When initial treatments fail, consider switching to another evidence-based treatment, combining evidence-based treatments (only when there are no contraindications) and referring to regional or national specialist services in refractory patients.

SLEEP DISORDERS

NORMAL SLEEP

Humans spend about a third of their lives asleep, but why we sleep is not yet fully understood. Sleep is a state of inactivity accompanied by loss of awareness and a markedly reduced responsiveness to environmental stimuli. When a recording is made of the electroencephalogram (EEG) and other physiological variables such as muscle activity and eye movements during sleep (a technique called polysomnography), a pattern of sleep emerges, consisting of five different stages. This varies from person to person, but usually consists of four or five cycles of *quiet* sleep alternating with *paradoxical*, or active, sleep, with longer periods of paradoxical sleep in the latter half of the night. A representation of these various stages and cycles over time is known as a *hypnogram*, and one of these derived from a normal subject is shown in Figure 19.5, with paradoxical sleep depicted as the shaded areas.

Quiet sleep is divided further into four stages, each with a characteristic EEG appearance, with progressive relaxation of the muscles and slower, more regular breathing as the deeper stages are reached. Most sleep in these deeper stages occurs in the first half of the night.

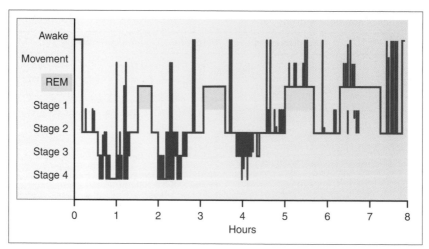

Fig. 19.5 Normal hypnogram.

During paradoxical sleep, the EEG appearance is similar to that of waking or drowsiness. There is irregular breathing, complete loss of tone of the skeletal muscles, and frequent phasic movements, particularly of the eyes, consisting of conjugate movements which are mostly lateral but can also be vertical. This stage of sleep is called *rapid eye movement* (REM) sleep; most dreaming takes place in this stage.

The length of total sleep in a day varies between 3 and 10 h in normal subjects, with an average of 7–8 h in those aged 20–45 years. Sleep time is decreased in older subjects, to about 6 h in people aged more than 70 years, with increased daytime napping reducing the actual night-time sleep even more. The amount of time spent in each of the five stages varies between subjects and particularly with age, with much less slow-wave sleep in older people. The number of awakenings after the onset of sleep also increases with advancing age. A normal subject has several short awakenings during the night, most of which are not perceived as awakenings unless they last for more than about 2 min. Probably there will not be clear consciousness, but subjects may have occasional brief thoughts of how comfortable they feel or how pleased that it's not yet time to get up, with an immediate return to sleep. If during the short period of waking some factor causes anxiety or anger, e.g. aircraft noise, partner's snores or dread of being awake, progress to full awakening and being remembered is much more likely. The more times this happens, the more subjects complain of an unrefreshing sleep. The time spent in sleep as a percentage of the time in bed is used as a measure of sleep efficiency (96% in the case shown in Figure 19.5).

One of the most common ways in which insomnia develops is by 'clock watching': subjects check the time on awakening, remember it and repeat this cycle many times during the night. Remembering the time of a transient awakening reinforces the subject's belief that they do sleep poorly (periods of sleep in between are neglected) and also produces anger and frustration, which in turn delay their return to sleep and may promote subsequent awakenings.

TYPES OF SLEEP DISORDER

Several types of sleep disorder are recognised, and their differentiation is important; a simplified summary is given below but reference to DSM, ICSD and ICD-10[5] will clarify the exact diagnostic criteria.

- *Insomnia*: not enough sleep or sleep of poor quality; problems of falling asleep (initial insomnia) or staying asleep (maintenance insomnia), or waking too early.
- *Hypersomnia*: excessive daytime sleepiness.

---

[5]DSM-IV: American Psychiatric Association 1994 Diagnostic and statistical manual of mental disorders (DSM IV), 1st edn. American Psychiatric Association, Washington, DC.
ICSD: American Sleep Disorders Association 1992 International Classification of Sleep Disorders: Diagnostic and Coding Manual.
ICD-10: World Health Organization 1994 Classification of Mental and Behavioural Disorders. WHO, Geneva.

- *Parasomnia*: unusual happenings in the night
  - nightmares
  - night terrors
  - sleepwalking
  - REM behaviour disorder.
- Other
  - sleep scheduling disorders (circadian rhythm disorder)
  - restless legs syndrome
  - periodic leg movements of sleep.

INSOMNIA

Insomnia characterised by the complaint of poor sleep, with difficulty either in initiating sleep or in maintaining sleep throughout the night. It can occur exclusively in the course of another physical disorder such as pain, mental disorder, e.g. depression, or sleep disorder, e.g. sleep apnoea. In a large proportion of patients it is a primary sleep disorder, and causes significant impairment in social, occupational or other important areas of functioning. One survey showed similar deficits in quality of life in insomniacs as in patients with long-term disorders such as diabetes.

About 60% of patients with insomnia have abnormal sleep when measured objectively, but the rest have no sleep abnormality that can be measured at present, yet are subjectively as disabled by their perceived symptoms as those with measurable sleep.

Insomnia may or may not be accompanied by daytime fatigue, but is not usually accompanied by subjective sleepiness during the day. Moreover, when sleep propensity in the daytime is measured by objective means (time to EEG sleep), these patients are in fact less sleepy (take longer to fall asleep) than normal subjects.

The time of falling asleep is determined by three factors, which in normal sleepers occur at bedtime. These are: (a) circadian rhythm, i.e. the body's natural clock in the hypothalamus triggers the rest/sleep part of the sleep–wake cycle; (b) 'tiredness', i.e. time since last sleep, usually about 16 h, which is in part mediated by the build-up of sleep-promoting chemicals in the brain; and (c) lowered mental and physical arousal. If one of these processes is disrupted then sleep initiation is difficult, and it is these three factors that are addressed by a standard *sleep hygiene programme* (see below). Early in the course of insomnia, rigorous adherence to sleep hygiene principles alone may restore the pre-morbid sleep pattern, but in some patients the circadian process is less stable and they are less responsive to these measures.

A summary of precipitating factors for insomnia is shown in Box 19.1.

Disruption of circadian rhythm

Shift work, jet lag and *irregular routine* can cause insomnia, in that patients cannot sleep when they wish to.

Timely treatment of short-term insomnia is valuable, as it may prevent progression to a chronic condition, which is much harder to alleviate. Psychological treatments are effective and pharmacotherapy may be either unnecessary, or used as a short-term adjunct. The approaches to sleep hygiene are:

- Treat any precipitating cause (see above).
- Educate and reassure.
- Establish good sleep habits
  - keep regular bedtimes and rising times
  - avoid daytime napping
  - daytime (but not evening) exercise and exposure to daylight
  - avoid stimulants alcohol and cigarettes in the evening
  - establish bedtime routine: 'wind-down' – a milk drink may be helpful
  - avoid dwelling on problems in bed – set aside a time early in the evening for planning
  - bed should be comfortable.
- Consider hypnotic medication.

In the treatment of long-term insomnia the most important factor is *anxiety about sleep*, arising from conditioning behaviours that predispose to heightened arousal and tension at bedtime. Thus the bedroom is associated with not sleeping, and automatic negative thoughts about the sleeping process occur in the evening. *Cognitive behavioural therapy*, if available, is helpful in dealing with 'psychophysiological' insomnia and, together with education and sleep hygiene measures, is the treatment of choice for long-term primary insomnia. Cognitive behavioural therapists help people to change their behaviour and thoughts about sleep, particularly concentrating on learned, sleep-incompatible behaviours and automatic negative thoughts at bedtime.

Drug therapy may:

- relieve short-term insomnia when precipitating causes cannot be improved
- prevent progression to a long-term problem by establishing a sleep habit
- interrupt the vicious cycle of anxiety about sleep itself.

Box 19.1   Precipitating factors for insomnia

Psychological

Hyperarousal due to:

- *stress*
- the need to be *vigilant* at night because of sick relatives or young children
- being '*on call*'.

Psychiatric

- Patients with *depressive illnesses* often have difficulty falling asleep at night and complain of restless, disturbed and unrefreshing sleep, and early morning waking. When their sleep is analysed by polysomnography, time to sleep onset is indeed prolonged, and there is a tendency for more REM sleep to occur in the first part of the night, with reduced deep quiet sleep in the first hour or so after sleep onset, and increased awakenings during the night. They may wake early in the morning and fail to get back to sleep again.
- *Anxiety* disorders may cause patients to complain about their sleep, either because there is a reduction in sleep continuity or because normal periods of nocturnal waking are somehow less well tolerated. Nocturnal panic attacks can make patients fearful of going off to sleep.
- *Bipolar* patients in the hypomanic or manic phase will sleep less than usual, and often changes in sleep pattern give early warning that an episode is imminent.

Pharmacological

- Non-prescription drugs such as *caffeine* or *alcohol*. Alcohol reduces the time to onset of sleep, but disrupts sleep later in the night. Regular and excessive consumption disrupts sleep continuity; insomnia is a key feature of alcohol withdrawal. Excessive intake of caffeine and theophylline, in tea, coffee or cola drinks, also contributes to sleeplessness, probably because caffeine acts as an antagonist to adenosine, the endogenous sleep-promoting neurotransmitter.
- Starting treatment with certain *antidepressants*, especially serotonin reuptake inhibitors (e.g. fluoxetine, fluvoxamine), or monoamine uptake inhibitors; sleep disruption is likely to resolve after 3–4 weeks.
- Other drugs that increase central noradrenergic and serotonergic activity include *stimulants*, such as amfetamine, cocaine and methylphenidate, and *sympathomimetics*, such as the β-adrenergic agonist salbutamol and associated substances.
- *Withdrawal* from hypnotic drugs; this is usually short lived.
- Treatment with *β-adrenoceptor blockers* may disrupt sleep, perhaps because of their serotonergic action; a β-blocking drug that crosses blood–brain barrier less readily is preferred, e.g. atenolol.

Physical

- *Pain,* in which case adequate analgesia will improve sleep.
- *Pregnancy.*
- *Coughing* or wheezing: adequate control of asthma with stimulating drugs as above, may paradoxically improve sleep by reducing waking due to breathlessness.
- *Respiratory and cardiovascular disorders.*
- *Need to urinate*; this may be affected by timing of diuretic medication.
- *Neurological disorders,* e.g. stroke, movement disorders.
- *Periodic leg movements of sleep* (frequent jerks or twitches during the descent into deeper sleep); rarely reduce subjective sleep quality but are more likely to cause them in the subject's sleeping partner.
- *Restless legs syndrome* (irresistible desire to move the legs), which is usually worse in the evening and early night, and can prevent sleep.

DRUGS FOR INSOMNIA

Most drugs used in insomnia act at the *GABA$_A$– benzodiazepine receptor,* and have effects other than their directly sedating action, including muscle relaxation, memory impairment and ataxia, which can impair performance of skills such as driving. Clearly those drugs with onset and duration of action confined to the night period will be most effective in insomnia and less prone to unwanted effects during the day. Those with longer duration of action are likely to affect psychomotor performance, memory and concentration; they will also have enduring anxiolytic and muscle-relaxing effects.

The GABA$_A$–benzodiazepine receptor complex

γ-Aminobutyric acid (GABA) is the most important inhibitory transmitter in the CNS, comprising up to 40% of all synapses. GABAergic neurones are distributed widely in the CNS, and GABA controls the state of neuronal excitability in all brain areas. The balance between *excitatory* inputs (mostly glutamatergic) and *inhibitory* GABAergic activity determines neuronal activity. If the balance swings in favour of GABA, then sedation, amnesia, muscle relaxation and ataxia appear, and nervousness and anxiety are reduced. The mildest reduction of GABAergic activity (or increase in glutamate) elicits arousal, anxiety, restlessness, insomnia and exaggerated reactivity.

When GABA binds with the GABA$_A$ receptor, the permeability of the central pore of the receptor complex opens, so allowing more chloride ions into the neurone and decreasing excitability. Classical benzodiazepines in clinical use bind to another receptor on the complex (the benzodiazepine receptor) and enhance the effectiveness of GABA, producing a larger inhibitory effect (Fig. 19.6). These drugs are agonists at the receptor and an antagonist,

flumazenil, prevents agonists from binding at the receptor site; it is used clinically to reverse benzodiazepine actions.

Benzodiazepines

A general account of the benzodiazepines is appropriate here, although their indications extend beyond use as hypnotics.

All *benzodiazepines* and newer *benzodiazepine-like* drugs are safe and effective for insomnia if the substance with the right timing of onset of action and elimination is chosen. They should not be used for patients with sleep-related breathing disorders such as obstructive sleep apnoea (see below), which is exacerbated by benzodiazepines. Objective measures of sleep show that benzodiazpines decrease time to sleep onset and waking during the night. They also improve subjective sleep, usually to a greater extent than the objective changes, probably by their anxiolytic actions (selectivity between anxiolytic and sedative effect is low). Other changes in sleep architecture are to some extent dependent on duration of action, with the very short-acting compounds having the least effect. Most commonly very light (stage 1) sleep is decreased, and stage 2 sleep is increased. Higher doses of longer-acting drugs partially suppress slow-wave sleep.

Occasionally the agonist (sedative) compounds in current use cause paradoxical effects, e.g. excitement, aggression and antisocial acts. Alteration of dose, up or down, may eliminate these, as may chlorpromazine in an acute situation.

Pharmacokinetics. Benzodiazepines are effective after administration by mouth but enter the circulation at very different rates as reflected in the speed of onset of action, e.g. alprazolam is rapid, oxazepam is slow (Table 19.8). The liver metabolises them, usually to inactive metabolises, some with a long $t_{1/2}$, which greatly extends drug action, e.g. chlordiazepoxide, clorazepate and diazepam all form desmethyldiazepam ($t_{1/2}$ 80 h).

Uses. Oral benzodiazepines are used for insomnia, anxiety, alcohol withdrawal states, muscle spasm due to a variety of causes, including tetanus and cerebral spasticity. Injectable preparations are used for rapid tranquillisation in psychosis (see previous section), anaesthesia and sedation for minor surgery and invasive investigations (see index).

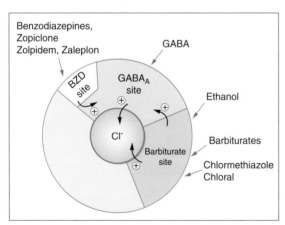

Fig. 19.6 Schematic representation of the binding sites on the GABA$_A$–benzodiazepine receptor complex. Note that drugs binding to the benzodiazepine (BZD) receptor site do not open the chloride channel directly, but rather augment the capacity of GABA to do so. Conversely agents such as the barbiturates both potentiate GABA and at higher concentrations have a direct effect on the chloride channel. This explains why barbiturates and alcohols are more toxic in overdose than the benzodiazepines.

Table 19.8 Properties of drugs used for insomnia

	Works selectively to enhance GABA	Rapid onset	$t_{1/2}$ (h)	Usual oral dose	Daytime (hangover) effects	Safety
zopiclone	√	+	3.5–6	7.5 mg	?Yes	√
zolpidem	√	++	1.5–3	10 mg	No	√
zaleplon[a]	√	++	1–2	10 mg	No	√
temazepam	√		5–12	20 mg	?Yes	√
loprazolam	√		5–13	1 mg	?Yes	√
lormetazepam	√	+	8–10	1 mg	?Yes	√
nitrazepam	√	+	20–48	5–10 mg	Yes	√
lorazepam	√	+	10–20	0.5–1 mg	Yes	√
diazepam	√	+	20–60	5–10 mg	Yes	√
oxazepam	√		5–20	15–30 mg	Yes	√
alprazolam	√	+	9–20	0.5 mg	Yes	√
clonazepam	√	+	18–50	0.5–1 mg	Yes	√
cloral hydrate/cloral betaine	X	+	8–12	0.7–1 g	?Yes	X
clomethiazole	X	+	4–8	192 mg	?Yes	X
Barbiturates	X	+			Yes	X
promethazine	X		7–14	25 mg	?Yes	X/√

[a] Can be taken during the night, until 5 h before needing to drive, etc.

The choice of drug as hypnotic and anxiolytic is determined by pharmacokinetic properties (see above and Table 19.8).

Doses. Oral doses can be seen in Table 19.8.

Tolerance to the *anxiolytic* effects does not seem to be a problem. In *sleep disorders* the situation is not so clear; studies of subjective sleep quality show enduring efficacy, but about half of the objective (EEG) studies indicate decreased effects after 4–8 weeks, implying that some tolerance develops. That said, the necessity for dose escalation in sleep disorders is rare.

Dependence. Both animal and human research has shown that brain $GABA_A$ receptors do change in function during chronic treatment with benzodiazepines, and therefore take time to return to premedication status after cessation. Features of withdrawal and dependence vary. Commonly there is a kind of psychological dependence based on the fact that the treatment works to reduce patients' anxiety or sleep disturbance, and therefore they are unwilling to stop. If they do stop, there can be *relapse*, where the original symptoms return. There can also be a *rebound of symptoms*, particularly after stopping hypnotics,

with a worsening of sleep disturbance for one or two nights, longer sleep-onset latency and increased waking during sleep – this is common. In anxiety disorders there may be a few days of increased anxiety and edginess, which then resolves, probably in 10–20% of patients.

More rarely, there is a *longer withdrawal syndrome* characterised by the emergence of symptoms not previously experienced, e.g. agitation, headache, dizziness, dysphoria, irritability, fatigue, depersonalisation, hypersensitivity to noise and visual stimuli. Physical symptoms include nausea, vomiting, muscle cramps, sweating, weakness, muscle pain or twitching, and ataxia. After prolonged high doses, abrupt withdrawal may cause confusion, delirium, psychosis and convulsions. The syndrome is ameliorated by resuming medication but resolves in weeks; in a very few patients it persists, and these people have been the subject of much research, mainly focusing on their personality and cognitive factors.

Withdrawal of benzodiazepines should be gradual after as little as 3 weeks' use, but for long-term users it should be very slow, e.g. about one-eighth of the dose every 2 weeks, aiming to complete it in 6–12 weeks. Withdrawal should be slowed if marked symptoms occur and it may be useful to substitute a drug with a long $t_{1/2}$ (diazepam) to minimise rapid fluctuations in plasma concentrations. Abandonment of the final dose may be particularly distressing. In difficult cases withdrawal may be assisted by concomitant use of an antidepressant.

Adverse effects. In addition to the above, benzodiazepines can affect memory and balance. Hazards with car driving or operating machinery can arise from amnesia and impaired psychomotor function. Amnesia for events subsequent to administration occurs with high doses given intravenously, e.g. for endoscopy, dental surgery (with local anaesthetic), cardioversion, and in these situations it can be regarded as a blessing.

Paradoxical behaviour effects (see above) and perceptual disorders, e.g. hallucinations, occur occasionally. Headache, giddiness alimentary tract upsets, skin rashes and reduced libido can occur. Extrapyramidal reactions, reversible by flumazenil, are rare.

Benzodiazepines in pregnancy. Benzodiazepines should be avoided in early pregnancy as far as possible, because their safety is not established with certainty. Safety in pregnancy is not only a matter of avoiding prescription during an established pregnancy, for individuals may become pregnant on long-term therapy. Benzodiazepines cross the placenta and can cause fetal cardiac arrhythmia, muscular hypotonia, poor suckling, hypothermia and respiratory depression in the newborn.

Interactions. The benzodiazepines offer scope for adverse interaction with numerous agents, but the underlying mechanisms can be summarised. The principal *pharmacodynamic* interaction of concern is exacerbation of *sedation* with other centrally depressant drugs, including antidepressants, H_1-receptor antihistamines, antipsychotics, alcohol and general anaesthetics. All are likely to exacerbate breathing difficulties where this is already compromised, e.g. in obstructive sleep apnoea. Unexpected *hypotension* may occur with any co-prescribed antihypertensive drug and with vasodilators, e.g. nitrates.

Pharmacokinetic interactions occur with drugs that slow metabolism by *enzyme inhibition*, e.g. ritonavir, indinavir, itraconazole, olanzapine, cimetidine, fluvoxamine, erythromycin, increasing benzodiazepine effect. By contrast, acceleration of metabolism, lowering of plasma concentration and reduced effect occur with *enzyme inducers*, e.g. rifampicin.

Overdose. Benzodiazepines are remarkably safe in acute overdose and even 10 times the therapeutic dose produces only deep sleep from which the subject is easily aroused. It is said that there is no reliably recorded case of death from a benzodiazepine taken alone by a person in good physical (particularly respiratory) health, which is a remarkable tribute to their safety (high therapeutic index); even if the statement is not absolutely true, death must be extremely rare. But deaths have occurred in combination with alcohol (which combination is quite usual in those seeking to end their own lives) and opiates, e.g. buprenorphine and methadone. Flumazenil selectively reverses benzodiazepine effects and is useful in diagnosis, and in treatment (see below).

Benzodiazepine antagonist. *Flumazenil* is a highly selective competitive antagonist at benzodiazepine receptors so does not oppose sedation due to non-benzodiazepines, e.g. barbiturates, alcohol.

Clinical uses include reversal of benzodiazepine sedation after endoscopy, dentistry and in intensive care. Heavily sedated patients become alert within 5 min. The $t_{1/2}$ of 1 h is much shorter than that of most benzodiazepines (see Table 19.8), so that repeated intravenous administration may be needed. Thus the recovery period needs supervision lest sedation should recur; if used in day surgery it is important to tell patients that they may not drive a car home. The dose is 200 micrograms by intravenous injection given over 15 s, followed by 100 micrograms over 60 s if necessary, to a maximum of 300–600 micrograms. Flumazenil is useful for diagnosis of self-poisoning, and also for treatment, when 100–400 micrograms are given by continuous intravenous infusion and adjusted to the degree of wakefulness.

Adverse effects can include brief anxiety, seizures in epileptics treated with a benzodiazepine and precipitation of withdrawal syndrome in dependent subjects.

Non-benzodiazepine hypnotics that act at the GABA$_A$–benzodiazepine receptor

Although structurally unrelated to the benzodiazepines, these drugs act on the same receptor; their effects can be blocked by flumazenil, the receptor antagonist. Those described below are all effective in insomnia and have a low propensity for tolerance, rebound insomnia, withdrawal symptoms and abuse potential. Data from long-term studies suggest that these agents are safe and effective over at least 12 months. Withdrawal effects similar to those of the benzodiazepines hypnotics occur, but to a lesser extent.

Zopiclone, a cyclopyrrolone, has an onset of action that is relatively rapid (about 1 h) and lasts for 6–8 h, making it suitable for both initial insomnia and maintenance insomnia. It may cause fewer problems on withdrawal than benzodiazepines. The duration of action is prolonged in the elderly and in hepatic insufficiency. About 40% of patients experience a metallic aftertaste (genetically determined). Care should be taken with concomitant medication that affects its metabolic pathway (see Table19.2A).

Zolpidem is an imidazopyridine that has a faster onset (30–60 min) and shorter duration of action. In patients aged over 80 years clearance is slower and action longer lasting.

Zaleplon, a pyrazolopyrimidine, has a fast onset and short duration of action. In volunteers, it appeared to have no effect on psychomotor (including driving) skills when taken at least 5 h before testing. When patients have tried unsuccessfully to fall asleep, this property would allow zaleplon to be taken during at least the early part of the night, without hangover effect.

Other drugs that act on the GABA$_A$–benzodiazepine receptor

Chloral hydrate, clomethiazole and barbiturates also enhance GABA function, but at high doses have the additional capacity directly to open the membrane chloride channel (see Fig. 19.6); this may lead to potentially fatal respiratory depression and explains their low therapeutic ratio. These drugs also have a propensity for abuse/misuse, and are thus very much second-line treatments.

Chloral hydrate has a fast (30–60 min) onset of action and 6–8 h duration of action. Chloral hydrate,

a pro-drug, is rapidly metabolised by alcohol dehydrogenase into the active hypnotic *trichloroethanol* ($t_{1/2}$ 8 h). Chloral hydrate is dangerous in serious hepatic or renal impairment, and aggravates peptic ulcer. Interaction with ethanol is to be expected as both are metabolised by alcohol dehydrogenase. Alcohol (ethanol) also appears to induce the formation of trichloroethanol, which attains higher concentrations if alcohol is co-administered, increasing sedation. Triclofos and cloral betaine are related compounds.

Clomethiazole is structurally related to vitamin B1 (thiamine) and is a hypnotic, sedative and anticonvulsant. When taken orally, it is subject to extensive hepatic first-pass metabolism (which is defective in the old and in liver-damaged alcoholics who exhibit higher peak plasma concentrations); the $t_{1/2}$ is 4 h. It may also be given intravenously. It is comparatively free from hangover but can cause nasal irritation and sneezing. Dependence occurs and use should always be brief.

Barbiturates are hardly ever used as they have a low therapeutic index, i.e. relatively small overdose may endanger life; they also cause dependence and have been popular drugs of abuse.

Other drugs used in insomnia

Antihistamines. Most proprietary (over the counter) sleep remedies contain H$_1$-receptor antihistamines with sedative action. Promethazine (Phenergan) has a slow (1–2 h) onset and long duration of action ($t_{1/2}$ 12 h). Sleep-onset latency and awakenings during the night are reduced after a single dose, but there have been no studies showing enduring action. It is sometimes used as a hypnotic in children. There are no controlled studies showing improvements in sleep after other antihistamines. *Alimemazine* (trimeprazine) is used for short-term sedation in children. Most antihistamine sedatives have a relatively long action and may cause daytime sedation.

Antidepressants. In the depressed patient, improvement in mood is almost always accompanied by improvement in subjective sleep, and therefore choice of antidepressant should usually not involve additional consideration of sleep effects.

Nevertheless, some patients are more likely to continue with medication if there is a short-term improvement, in which case *mirtazapine* or *trazodone* may provide effective antidepressant together with sleep-promoting effects.

Antidepressant drugs, particularly those with $5HT_2$-blocking effects, may occasionally be effective in long-term insomnia (but see Table 19.7).

Antipsychotics have been used to promote sleep in resistant insomnia occurring as part of another psychiatric disorder, probably because of the combination of $5HT_2$-antagonism, α_1-adrenoceptor antagonism and histamine H_1-receptor antihistamine effects in addition to their primary dopamine antagonist effects. Their long action leads to daytime sedation, and extrapyramidal movement disorders may result from their blockade of dopamine receptors (see above, Antipsychotics, p. 345). Nevertheless, modern antipsychotics, e.g. *quetiapine*, are being used for intractable insomnia, usually at a dose well below that required to treat psychosis, e.g. 25–50 mg/day.

Melatonin, the hormone produced by the pineal gland during darkness, has been investigated for insomnia, but is at best only weakly effective. Lack of light causes adrenergic stimulation of the pineal β receptors to cause melatonin production (an effect abolished by beta-blockers). The impressive nature of the diurnal rhythm in melatonin secretion (maximum at night) has resulted in its use therapeutically to reset circadian rhythm to prevent jet lag on long-haul flights, and for blind or partially sighted people who cannot use daylight to synchronise their natural rhythm.

Herbal preparations. Randomised trials have shown some effect of valerian in mild to moderate insomnia.

Summary of pharmacotherapy for insomnia

- Drug treatment is usually effective for a short period (2–4 weeks).
- Some patients may need long-term medication.
- Intermittent medication that is taken only on nights that symptoms occur is desirable and may often be possible with modern, short-acting compounds.

- Discontinuing hypnotic drugs is usually not a problem if the patient knows what to expect. There will be a short period (usually one or two nights) of rebound insomnia on stopping hypnotic drugs, which can be ameliorated by phased withdrawal.

HYPERSOMNIA

Sleep-related breathing disorders causing excessive daytime sleepiness are rarely treated with drugs. Sleepiness caused by the night-time disruption of sleep apnoea syndrome is sometimes not abolished completely by the standard treatment of continuous positive airway pressure overnight, and wake-promoting drugs, e.g. modafinil, may have a role in these patients.

Narcolepsy is a chronic neurological disorder, characterised by excessive daytime sleepiness (EDS) and sleep attacks, usually accompanied by *cataplexy* (attacks of muscle weakness on emotional arousal). These symptoms are often associated with the intrusion into wakefulness of other elements of rapid eye movement (REM) sleep, such as sleep paralysis and hypnagogic hallucinations, i.e. in a transient state preceding sleep.

Stimulants are effective in the treatment of EDS due to narcolepsy. *Modafinil* is usually preferred as it is not a controlled drug, failing which methylphenidate or dexamfetamine is added or substituted.

In *narcolepsy*, patients usually need a stimulant for their hypersomnia and an antidepressant for their cataplexy. Combining a SSRI antidepressant with modafinil has been shown to be safe, but dexamfetamine and methylphenidate must not be given with MAOIs.

Cataplexy is most effectively treated with 5HT uptake-blocking drugs such as clomipramine or fluoxetine, or other antidepressant drugs, e.g. reboxetine, selegiline.

Modafinil is a wake-promoting agent whose specific mechanism of action is not properly known; it does not appear to be overtly stimulant like the amfetamines. Its onset of action is slow and lasts 8–12 h. Potential for abuse is low. Modafinil is used in narcolepsy and other hypersomnias (e.g. that with sleep apnoea), and also promotes wakefulness in normal people who need to stay awake for long periods, e.g. military personnel. Its use is associated with a wide variety of gastrointestinal, CNS and other unwanted effects; contraindications to its use include moderate to severe hypertension, a history of left ventricular hypertrophy or cor pulmonale. Modafinil accelerates the metabolism of oral contraceptives, reducing their efficacy.

Amfetamines release dopamine and noradrenaline in the brain. This causes a behavioural excitation, with increased alertness, elevation of mood, increase in physical activity and suppression of appetite. *Dexamfetamine*, the dextrorotatory isomer of amfetamine, is about twice as active in humans as the laevo-isomer and is the main prescribed amfetamine. It is rapidly absorbed orally and acts for 3–24 h; most people with narcolepsy find twice-daily dosing optimal to maintain alertness during the day. About 40% of narcoleptic patients find it necessary to increase the dose, suggesting some tolerance. Although physical dependence does not occur, mental and physical depression may develop following withdrawal.

Unwanted effects include edginess, restlessness, insomnia and appetite suppression, weight loss, and increase in blood pressure and heart rate. Amfetamines are commonly abused because of their stimulant effect, but this is rare in narcolepsy. Contraindications to its use include moderate to severe hypertension, hyperthyroidism, and a history of drug or alcohol abuse.

Methylphenidate also promotes dopamine release but its principal action is to inhibit uptake of central neurotransmitters. Its effects and adverse effects resemble those of the amfetamines. Methylphenidate has a low systemic availability and slow onset of action, making it less liable to abuse. Its short duration of effect (3–4 h) requires that patients with narcolepsy need to plan the timing of tablets taking to fit with daily activities. Methylphenidate is also used in attention deficit/hyperactivity disorder (see below).

Unwanted effects include anxiety, anorexia and difficulty sleeping, which usually subside. Methylphenidate reduces expected weight gain and has been associated with slight growth retarda-

tion. Monitoring of therapy should include height and weight, also blood pressure and blood counts (thrombocytopenia and leucopenia occur). It should not be used in patients with hyperthyroidism, severe angina or cardiac arrhythmias.

PARASOMNIAS

Nightmares arise out of REM sleep and are reported by the patient as structured, often stereotyped, dreams that are very distressing. Usually the patient wakes up fully and remembers the dream. Psychological methods of treatment may be appropriate, e.g. a programme of rehearsing the dream and inventing a different pleasant ending. In a small number of cases where adverse events such as angina have been provoked by recurrent nightmares it may be appropriate to consider drug treatment with an antidepressant that markedly suppresses REM sleep, e.g. the MAOI phenelzine. Nightmares of a particularly distressing kind are a feature of post-traumatic stress disorder. Case reports indicate benefit from various pharmacological agents, but no particular drug emerges as superior. Many psychiatrists prefer to use a 5HT blocker such as trazodone or mirtazapine.

Night terrors and sleep-walking arise from slow-wave sleep, and they are often coexistent. There is usually a history dating from childhood, and often a family history. Exacerbations commonly coincide with periods of stress, and alcohol increases their likelihood. In a night terror patients usually sit or jump up from deep sleep (mostly in the first few hours of sleep) with a loud cry, look terrified and move violently, sometimes injuring themselves or others. They appear asleep and uncommunicative, often returning to sleep without being aware of the event. These terrors are thought to be a welling up of anxiety from deep centres in the brain that is normally inhibited by cortical mechanisms. If the disorder is sufficiently frequent or disabling, night terrors respond to the SSRI paroxetine (also effective in sleep-walkers) or the benzodiazepine, clonazepam.

REM behaviour disorder first described in 1986, consists of lack of paralysis during REM sleep which results in brief acting-out of dreams, often vigorously with injury to self or others. It can occur acutely as a result of drug or alcohol withdrawal, or in patients taking high doses of antidepressants such as clomipramine, venlafaxine or mirtazapine. Its chronic manifestation can be idiopathic or associated with neurological disorder. It is much commoner among older patients, with approximately 90% of patients being male. It is becoming increasingly clear that it may be a very early prodrome to the onset of Parkinson's disease or certain dementias many years after its onset. Successful symptomatic relief has been described with clonazepam or clonidine.

OTHER SLEEP DISORDERS

Restless legs syndrome (RLS) is a disorder characterised by disagreeable leg sensations usually prior to sleep onset, and an almost irresistible urge to move the legs. The sensation is described as 'crawling', 'aching' or 'tingling', and is partially or completely relieved with leg motion, returning after movement ceases. Most if not all patients with this complaint also have *periodic limb movements of sleep* (PLMS), which may occur independently of RLS. These periodic limb movements consist of highly stereotyped movements, usually of the legs, that occur repeatedly (typically every 20–40 s) during the night. They may wake the patient, in which case there may be a complaint of daytime sleepiness or occasionally insomnia, but often awaken only the sleeping partner, who is usually kicked. RLS and PLMS are considered to be movement disorders and may respond to formulations of levodopa.

Sleep scheduling disorders. Circadian rhythm disorders are often confused with insomnia and both can be present in the same patient. With such sleep scheduling disorders, sleep occurs at the 'wrong' time, i.e. at a time that does not fit with work, social or family commitments. A typical pattern may be a difficulty in initiating sleep for a few nights due to stress, whereupon, once asleep, the subject continues sleeping well into the morning to 'catch up' the lost sleep. Thereafter the 'time since last sleep' cue for sleep initiation is delayed, and the sleep period gradually becomes more delayed until the subject is sleeping in the day instead of at night. A behavioural programme with strategic light exposure is appropriate, with pharmacological treatment as an adjunct, e.g. melatonin, to help reset the sleep–wake schedule.

DRUGS FOR ALZHEIMER'S[6] DISEASE (DEMENTIA)

Dementia is described as a syndrome 'due to disease of the brain, usually of chronic or progressive nature in which there is disturbance of multiple higher cortical functions, including memory, thinking, orientation, comprehension, calculation, learning capacity, language and judgement, without clouding of consciousness.'[7] Deterioration in emotional control, social behaviour or motivation may accompany or precede cognitive impairment. Alzheimer's and vascular (multi-infarct) disease are the two most common forms of dementia, accounting for about 80% of presentations. Alzheimer's disease is associated with deposition of β-amyloid in brain tissue and abnormal phosphorylation of the intracellular tau (τ) proteins causing abnormalities of microtubule assembly and collapse of the cytoskeleton. Pyramidal cells of the cortex and subcortex are particularly affected.

In Western countries, the prevalence of dementia is less than 1% in those aged 60–64 years, but doubles with each 5-year cohort to a figure of around 16% in those aged 80–84 years. The emotional impact of dementia on relatives and carers, and the cost to society in social support and care facilities, are great. Hence the impetus for an effective form of treatment is compelling.

Evidence indicates that *cholinergic transmission* is diminished in Alzheimer's disease. All agents that benefit the condition act to enhance *acetylcholine* activity by inhibiting the *acetylcholinesterase* which metabolises and inactivates synaptically released acetylcholine. Consequently acetylcholine remains usable for longer. Individual drugs are categorised by the type of enzyme inhibition they cause. *Donepezil* is classed as a 'reversible' agent as binding to the acetylcholinesterase enzymes lasts only minutes, whereas *rivastigmine* is considered 'pseudoirreversible' as inhibition lasts for several hours. *Galantamine* is associated both with reversible inhibition and with enhanced acetylcholine action on

---

[6]Alois Alzheimer (1864–1915) German psychiatrist who studied the brains of demented and senile patients and correlated histological findings with clinical features.
[7]International Classification of Diseases, 10th edition, diagnostic system.

nicotinic receptors.[8] Clinical trials show that these agents produce an initial increase in patients' cognitive ability. There also may be associated global benefits, including improvements in non-cognitive aspects such as depressive symptoms. But the drugs do not alter the underlying process, and the relentless progress of the disease is paralleled by a reduction in acetylcholine production with a decline in cognition.

The beneficial effects of drugs are therefore to:

- *stabilise* the condition initially and sometimes improve cognitive function
- *delay* the overall pace of decline (and therefore the escalating levels of support required)
- *postpone* the onset of severe dementia.

The severity of cognitive deficits in patients suffering from, or suspected of having, dementia can be quantified by a simple 30-point schedule, the mini mental state examination (MMSE) of Folstein. A score of 21–26 denotes mild, 10–20 moderate and less than 10 severe Alzheimer's disease. The MMSE can also be used to monitor progress.

Given the limited evidence of overall benefit in relation to cost, the use of these drugs is the subject of continuing debate. The position adopted by the UK National Institute for Health and Clinical Excellence (NICE) in 2001–2005 was that donepezil, galantamine and rivastigmine should be available as adjuvant therapy for those with a MMSE score above 12 points, subject to the following conditions:

- Alzheimer's disease must be diagnosed and assessed in a specialist clinic; the clinic should also assess cognitive, global and behavioural functioning, activities of daily living, and the likelihood of compliance with treatment.
- Treatment should be initiated by specialists but may be continued by family practitioners under a shared-care protocol.
- The carers' views of the condition should be sought before and during drug treatment.
- The patient should be assessed 2–4 months after a maintenance dose is established; drug treatment should continue only if the MMSE score has improved or has not deteriorated *and* behavioural and functional assessment shows improvement.

- The patient should be assessed every 6 months and drug treatment should normally continue only if the MMSE score remains above 12 points and if treatment is considered to have a worthwhile effect on the global functional and behavioural condition.

Subsequent amendments to these guidelines suggest that the cost : benefit ratio is favourable only in those with moderate dementia (MMSE score between 10 and 20 points).

Doses are:

- donepezil 5–10 mg nocte increasing to 10 mg nocte after 1 month
- galantamine 4 mg b.d. increasing to 8–12 mg b.d. at 4-week intervals
- rivastigmine 1.5 mg b.d. increasing to 3–6 mg b.d. at 2-week intervals.

Adverse effects inevitably include cholinergic symptoms, with nausea, diarrhoea and abdominal cramps appearing commonly. There may also be bradycardia, sinoatrial or atrioventricular block. Additionally, urinary incontinence, syncope, convulsions and psychiatric disturbances occur. Rapid dose increase appears to make symptoms more pronounced. Hepatotoxicity is a rare association with donepezil.

The deterioration of function in dementia of Alzheimer's disease is often accompanied by acute behavioural disturbance and the development of psychotic symptoms, which may require therapy with antipsychotics.

Other substances. *Memantine*, a glutamate modulator, is now licensed in the UK for moderate to severe dementia in Alzheimer's disease. Other approaches include the antioxidant vitamin E, the monoamine oxidase type B inhibitor, selegeline and the plant extract *gingko biloba*, which is thought to have antioxidant and cholinergic activity. Oestrogens and non-steroidal anti-inflammatory agents may also have protective effects.

DRUGS IN ATTENTION DEFICIT/ HYPERACTIVITY DISORDER

Attention deficit hyperactivity disorder (ADHD) affects 5% of children in the UK and is characterised by inattention, impulsivity and motor overactivity. For

---

[8]Irreversible antagonists exist but, not surprisingly, are not used in therapeutics (sarin nerve gas is an example).

diagnostic purposes, these should be present before the age of 7 years and cause pervasive impairment across situations, especially school and home.

Methylphenidate (see above) is effective in children with ADHD, reducing each of the three principal symptoms. It should be initiated only by a specialist in these conditions and form part of a comprehensive treatment programme of psychological, educational and social measures. Periodic breaks in treatment once symptoms have been stabilised

('drug holidays') are recommended to determine continued efficacy.

Dexamfetamine (see above) is an alternative that has similar efficacy in ADHD and is the preferred drug in children with epilepsy. It has a greater potential for abuse.

Both methylphenidate and dexamfetamine are controlled drugs in the UK (class B schedule 2 of the Misuse of Drugs Act), so prescribing restrictions apply.

Table 19.9 Summary of indications for psychotropic drugs

	Antidepressants	Lithium and mood stabilisers	Antipsy-chotics	Benzodia-zepines	Other hypnotic and anxiolytic drugs	Other drug groups
Depressive disorders	*	*(1)				
Depressive disorders with psychotic symptoms	*	*(1)	*			
Bipolar affective disorder (prophylaxis)		*				
Bipolar affective disorder (acute manic episode)		*	*	*		
Anxiety disorders	*		*(2)	*	*(3)	
Schizophrenia			*			
Acute behavioural disturbance			*	*		
Alcohol withdrawal				*	*(4)	*(5)
Insomnia	*(6)			*	*	
Eating disorders	*(7)					
Dementia of Alzheimer's disease						*(8)
Attention deficit/ hyperactivity disorder			*(9)			*(9)

*Recognised indication; where numbers appear in the table, see notes below:
(1) Lithium augmentation may be used in depression. Lithium is given in combination with tricyclic, SSRI or novel antidepressants, usually when the symptoms have proved resistant to adequate trials of two or more antidepressants.
(2) Antipsychotics may be used short-term for management of severe anxiety, but only where other drug options have failed (due to adverse effects). Olanzapine may be useful as an adjunct to SSRIs in obsessive–compulsive disorder.
(3) Buspirone may be used in generalised anxiety disorder as an alternative to a benzodiazepine. It also has a role in treatment resistant social anxiety disorder. β-Adrenoceptor blockers may be helpful for performance anxiety, combating tremor and other symptoms of autonomic overactivity.
(4) Chlomethiazole was an alternative to a benzodiazepine for alcohol withdrawal, but is now rarely used due to concerns over respiratory suppression and abuse potential.
(5) Drugs for alcohol dependence and withdrawal are discussed in Chapter 10.
(6) When a patient complaining of insomnia also has depression, a sedative antidepressant such as trazodone, mirtazapine or trimpramine should be considered. SSRIs do not provide direct sedation in such patients but may improve the quality of sleep over a longer period as mood improves.
(7) Fluoxetine is licensed for the treatment of bulimia nervosa.
(8) Acetylcholinesterase inhibitors provide transient improvement in cognitive and global functioning in mild to moderate dementia of Alzheimer's disease. They delay the onset of severe illness but cannot ultimately halt or change the course of the disease.
(9) The CNS stimulants methylphenidate and dexamfetamine are drugs of choice for attention deficit/hyperactivity disorder. Atomoxetine is an alternative. Second-line treatment options include clonidine and the antipsychotic agents, risperidone, haloperidol and sulpiride.

Atomoxetine, a noradrenaline reuptake inhibitor (like reboxetine), is now licensed for ADHD. It is thought to act by increasing noradrenaline and dopamine availability in the frontal cortex (where dopamine is taken up into noradrenergic nerve terminals). It has no known abuse liability and is not a controlled drug.

Clonidine, tricyclic antidepressants (TCAs) and certain antipsychotic agents, e.g. risperidone, sulpiride, may have a role in ADHD where methylphenidate and dexamfetamine are contraindicated or have failed to produce benefit.

DRUGS FOR PSYCHIATRIC ILLNESS IN CHILDHOOD

Children do suffer psychiatric illnesses. Many drugs used in childhood psychiatric illness are not properly tested in young people. Now there are regulatory pressures for drugs (in general) to have safety tests in children subsequent to their licensing in adults. Some drugs are deemed not to have adequate risk:benefit ratios in children, e.g. in depression most SSRI drugs are not recommended (an exception is fluoxetine for which evidence of efficacy and safety in children does exist). Similar caveats apply to the use of TCAs in childhood. By contrast, there are good efficacy data for several SSRIs in obsessive–compulsive disorder, and for benefit of risperidone for aggression in children with autism.

SUMMARY

Table 19.9 summarises indications of the major groups of psychotropic drugs. Remember that psychiatric illnesses are often associated with co-morbid conditions, which may themselves require treatment; for example, schizophrenia may be associated with depression, so both antipsychotics and antidepressants may be required.

GUIDE TO FURTHER READING

Anderson I M, Nutt D J, Deakin J F W 2000 Evidence-based guidelines for treating depressive disorders with antidepressants: a revision of the 1993 British Association for Psychopharmacology guidelines. Journal of Psychopharmacology 14(1):3–20

Baldwin D S, Anderson I M, Nutt D J, Bandelow B, Bond A 2005 Evidence-based guidelines for the pharmacological treatment of anxiety disorders: recommendations from the British Association for Psychopharmacology. Journal of Psychopharmacology 19(6):567–596

Ballenger J C, Davidson J R T, Lecrubier Y et al 1998 Consensus statement on panic disorder from the International Consensus Group on Depression and Anxiety. Journal of Clinical Psychiatry 59:47–54

Ballenger J C, Davidson J R T, Lecrubier Y et al 1998 Consensus statement on social anxiety disorder from the International Consensus Group on Depression and Anxiety. Journal of Clinical Psychiatry 59:54–60

Ballenger J C, Davidson J R T, Lecrubier Y et al 2000 Consensus statement on posttraumatic stress disorder from the International Consensus Group on Depression and Anxiety. Journal of Clinical Psychiatry 61:60–66

Ballenger J C, Davidson J R T, Lecrubier Y et al 2001 Consensus statement on generalized anxiety disorder from the International Consensus Group on Depression and Anxiety. Journal of Clinical Psychiatry 62:53–58

Belmaker R H 2004 Bipolar disorder. New England Journal of Medicine 351(5):476–486

Biederman J, Faraone S V 2005 Attention-deficit hyperactivity disorder. Lancet 366:237–248

Blennow K, de Leon M J, Zetterberg H 2006 Alzheimer's disease. Lancet 368:387–403

Ebmeier K P, Donaghey C, Steele J 2006 Recent developments and current controversies in depression. Lancet 367:153–167

Fink M 2001 Convulsive therapy: a review of the first 55 years. Journal of Affective Disorders 63:1–15

Heyman I, Mataix-Cols D, Fineberg N A 2006 Obsessive–compulsive disorder. British Medical Journal 333:424–429

Lieberman J A, Mataix-Cols D, Fineberg N A for the Clinical Antipsychotic Trials of Intervention Effectiveness (CATIE) Investigators 2005 Effectiveness of antipsychotic drugs in patients with chronic schizophrenia. New England Journal of Medicine 353(12):1209–1223

Mann J J 2005 The medical management of depression. New England Journal of Medicine 353(17):1819–1834

Mueser K T, McGurk S R 2004 Schizophrenia. Lancet 363:2063–2072

Nutt D J, Malizia A L 2001 New insights into the role of the GABA-A–benzodiazepine receptor. British Journal of Psychiatry 179:390–396

Paykel E S 2001 Continuation and maintenance therapy in depression. British Medical Bulletin 57:145–160

Roth T, Hajak G, Ustün T B 2001 Consensus for the pharmacological management of insomnia in the new millennium. International Journal of Clinical Practice 55:42–52

Rush A J, Trivedi M, Fava M 2003 Depression, IV: STAR*D treatment trial for depression. American Journal of Psychiatry 160:237

Ryan N D 2005 Treatment of depression in children and adolescents. Lancet 366:933–940

Taylor C B 2006 Panic disorder. British Medical Journal 332:951–955

Wilson S J, Lillywhite A R, Potokar J P, Bell C J, Nutt D J 1997 Adult night terrors and paroxetine. Lancet 350:185

Wong I C K, Besag F M C, Santosh P J, Murray M L 2004 Use of selective serotonin reuptake inhibitors in children and adolescents. Drug Safety 27(13):991–1000

Yehuda R 2002 Post-traumatic stress disorder. New England Journal of Medicine 346:108–114

Zeman A (ed.) 2005 Clinical Medicine 5(2):97–101

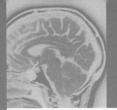

20

Epilepsy, parkinsonism and allied conditions

SYNOPSIS

- Antiepilepsy drugs: principles of management; withdrawal of therapy; pregnancy; teratogenic effects; epilepsy in children; status epilepticus
- Individual drugs: carbamazepine, phenytoin, sodium valproate, lamotrigine, vigabatrin, gabapentin, clonazepam, topiramate, levetiracetam
- Parkinsonism
- Objectives of therapy
- Drug therapy; problems of long-term treatment
- Other disorders of movement
- Tetanus

ANTIEPILEPSY DRUGS

Epilepsy affects 5–10 per 1000 of the general population.[1] It is due to sudden, excessive depolarisation of some or all cerebral neurones. This may remain localised (focal seizure) or may spread to cause a secondary generalised seizure, or affect all cortical neurones simultaneously (primary generalised seizure).[2]

Epilepsy was treated with bromide in 1857 and phenobarbital was introduced in 1912 to control patients resistant to bromides. The next significant advance came in 1938 with phenytoin (a hydantoin), which structurally resembles the barbiturates. Subsequent discoveries produced many other anticonvulsants, but phenytoin remains a drug of choice, particularly in the intensive care setting. Over the past 10 years there has been a dramatic increase in the number of new anticonvulsant drugs (vigabatrin, gabapentin, lamotrigine, topiramate, oxcarbazepine, levetiracetam), but none has been shown to be superior to the major standard anticonvulsants (phenytoin, carbamazepine and sodium valproate), although the newer agents are better tolerated.

MODE OF ACTION

Antiepilepsy (anticonvulsant) drugs inhibit the neuronal discharge or its spread, and do so in one or more of three ways to:

- reduce cell membrane permeability to ions, particularly the voltage-dependent sodium channels which are responsible for the inward current that generates an action potential. Cells that are firing repetitively at high frequency are blocked preferentially, which permits discrimination between epileptic and physiological activity.
- enhance the activity of γ-aminobutyric acid (GABA), the principal inhibitory transmitter of the brain; the result is increased membrane permeability to chloride ion, which reduces cell excitability.
- inhibit excitatory neurotransmitters, e.g. glutamate.

CLASSIFICATION OF EPILEPSIES

A generally accepted classification is given in Table 20.2 (see p. 377), together with drugs of choice for the various seizure disorders.

PRINCIPLES OF MANAGEMENT

These call for attention to conservative as well as drug measures:

---

[1] Some people with epilepsy make pilgrimages to Terni (Italy) to seek intercession from Saint Valentine to relieve their condition. There was more than one Saint Valentine and it is unclear whether he was also the patron saint of lovers.

[2] Epilepsy has been recognised since early times. A Babylonian medical text dated about 650 BC gives the following description: '…while he is sitting down, his left eye moves to the right, a lip puckers, saliva flows from his mouth, and his hand, leg and trunk on the left side jerk like a slaughtered sheep …' Because of its unusual manifestations epilepsy was known as the 'sacred disease'. Wilson J V K, Reynolds E H 1990 Medical History 34:192.

- Any causative factor must, of course, be treated, e.g. cerebral neoplasm.
- Educate the patient about the disease, duration of treatment and need for compliance.
- Avoid precipitating factors, e.g. alcohol, sleep deprivation, emotional stress.
- Anticipate natural variation, e.g. fits may occur particularly or exclusively around periods in women (catamenial[3] epilepsy).
- Give antiepilepsy drugs only if seizure type and frequency require it.

GENERAL GUIDE TO ANTIEPILEPSY DRUG THERAPY

The decision whether or not to initiate drug therapy after a single seizure must take into account the fact that approximately 25% of patients may not have another seizure. Evidence suggests that immediate treatment of single or infrequent seizures does not affect long-term remission but introduces the potential for adverse effects.[4]

1. Therapy should start with a single, well tried and safe drug. The majority of patients (70%) can be controlled on one drug (*monotherapy*).
2. Anticonvulsant drug treatment should be appropriate to the type of seizure disorder. Although some drugs have a wide spectrum of action against different seizure types, some are more specific and may even aggravate certain seizure types. Carbamazepine is a drug of first choice for focal and secondary generalised epilepsy but aggravates myoclonic and absence seizures. Sodium valproate and lamotrigine have a wide spectrum of action and are active against both primary and secondary generalised epilepsy.
3. *Age and sex* also determine the choice of drug. This is particularly true of women, who avoid drugs associated with teratogenesis, e.g. valproate, or that have adverse effects on their appearance, e.g. hirsutism from phenytoin.
4. If control of a patient's epilepsy with a single drug is unsuccessful, it should be replaced by a *second-line* drug, although these are effective in only about 10% of cases. There is little evidence

that three drugs are better than two, and not much that two are better than one. More drugs give scope for more adverse effects.
5. *Abrupt withdrawal.* Effective therapy must never be stopped suddenly either by the doctor (carelessness) or by the patient (carelessness, intercurrent illness or ignorance), for status epilepticus may occur. But if rapid withdrawal is required by the occurrence of toxicity, a substantial dose of another antiepilepsy drug should be given at once.
6. In cases where fits are liable to occur at a particular *time*, e.g. the menstrual period, adjust the dose to achieve maximal drug effect at this time or confine drug treatment to this time. For example, in catamenial epilepsy, clobazam can be useful given only at period time.
7. Once treatment is stable, patients should keep to a particular proprietary brand as different brands of the same generic agent may exhibit varying pharmacokinetics.

Dosage and administration

Generally, give drugs as a single or twice daily dose to facilitate compliance. Many patients dislike taking medication to the workplace or school and being seen to take it but, necessarily, drugs with short duration of action may require to be taken three or even four times a day.

Regimens for *initial dosing* tend to vary with different drugs. In general, commence drugs in a small dose and increase at 2-week intervals to the minimum effective dose. Monitor the patient's seizures and increase the dose only if seizures continue. The time interval for dosage increases should therefore be sufficiently wide apart, to relate changes in the seizure frequency accurately to changes in drug therapy; dose alterations are best avoided by doctors who are unfamiliar with the individual patient, e.g. in emergency departments.

It is important to consider the cause of fitting, whether it is non-compliance (which can be due to intercurrent disease), an inadequate drug regimen or an increase in the severity of the disease.

MONITORING BLOOD CONCENTRATIONS OF ANTICONVULSANTS

Many biochemistry laboratories no longer undertake routine measurement of the plasma concentration

---

[3]Greek *katamenios*, monthly.
[4]Marson A, Jacoby A, Johnson A, Kim L, Gamble C 2005 Lancet 365:2007–2013.

for most anticonvulsant drugs because plasma concentrations are insufficiently stable to serve as a useful guide to change of dose. The exception is phenytoin, for which a small increase in dose may lead to a disproportionate rise in the plasma drug concentration (see zero-order pharmacokinetics, p. 259).

DRUG WITHDRAWAL

After a period of several years free from seizures, it is reasonable to consider withdrawal of antiepilepsy drug therapy.[5,6] The prognosis of a seizure disorder is determined by a number of factors. Some remit spontaneously, e.g. benign rolandic epilepsy and petit mal, whereas others never remit, e.g. juvenile myoclonic epilepsy. In many types of epilepsy the outlook is less certain and only general indicators are available. The following can be important:

- The *type* of seizure disorder – major seizures are more easily controlled.
- The *time* to remission – early remission carries a better outlook.
- The *number* of drugs required to induce remission – rapid remission on a single drug is a favourable indicator for successful withdrawal.
- The presence of an *underlying lesion* – control is often difficult.
- The presence of an associated *neurological deficit* or learning difficulty – control is often difficult.
- The *length of time of seizure freedom* on treatment – the longer the period the better is the outlook for successful withdrawal.
- The desire to withdraw treatment – many patients prefer to continue on medication for social reasons (see Driving Regulations, below).
- The EEG findings – abnormal EEG disturbance is a predictor of poor outcome for drug withdrawal in idiopathic generalised epilepsy.

In general, if a patient with epilepsy has no neurological deficit or structural lesion and is of normal intelligence, there is a reasonable chance of continued remission, particularly if a single drug achieves this rapidly. For adult epilepsy, discontinuing the antiepilepsy drug is associated with about 20% relapse during withdrawal and a further 20% relapse over the following 5 years; after this period relapse is unusual. A general recommendation is to withdraw the antiepilepsy drug over a period of 6 months. If a fit occurs during this time, full therapy must recommence until the patient has been free from seizures for several years.

DRIVING REGULATIONS AND EPILEPSY

The UK allows patients to drive a car (but not a truck or bus) if they have not had a daytime fit for 1 year (or after 3 years if they continue to be subject to fits only whilst asleep). Any fit that occurs during or after drug withdrawal incurs loss of the driving licence for a year. Many patients prefer to remain on medication despite being seizure free because they perceive losing the right to drive to be a significant social disability.

PREGNANCY AND EPILEPSY

Pregnancy can affect seizure disorder, which worsens in about a third, improves in a third, and is unchanged in the remainder. Ideally, patients should have their seizure disorder properly investigated and treated before pregnancy, with the best control achieved on the lowest dose of the least teratogenic drug.

Major seizures are harmful to the developing fetus because of the possibility of anoxia and metabolic disorder. *Minor* seizures are probably harmless and therefore need not be eradicated. Advise patients of the necessity of taking folic acid supplements, as some antiepilepsy drugs affect folic acid metabolism and folic acid deficiency is a risk factor for neural tube defects. Hepatic enzyme inducing antiepilepsy drugs lower the mother's concentration of vitamin K, which can aggravate any postpartum haemorrhage. Give an oral vitamin K for the last 2 weeks of pregnancy.

Breast-feeding

Antiepilepsy drugs pass into breast milk (see p. 100): phenobarbital, primidone and ethosuximide in significant quantities, phenytoin and sodium valproate less so. There is a risk that the baby will become sedated or suckle poorly but, provided a watch is maintained for these effects, the balance of advantage favours breast-feeding whilst taking antiepilepsy drugs.

[5]Medical Research Council 1991 Antiepileptic Drug Withdrawal Study Group. Lancet 337:1175–1180.
[6]Medical Research Council 1993 Antiepileptic Drug Withdrawal Study Group. British Medical Journal 306:1374–1378.

Teratogenic effects

The features of what has collectively become known as *anticonvulsant embryopathy* comprise: major malformations (often cardiac), microcephaly, growth retardation, and hypoplasia of the midface and fingers (this definition excludes a number of malformations not considered to be major). Children of mothers taking antiepilepsy drugs have an approximately 2–3-fold increased chance of features of anticonvulsant embryopathy at birth. In a case–control study of pregnant women, the frequency of malformations was 20.6% in infants whose mothers took one anticonvulsant drug and 28.0% in those taking two or more such drugs, compared with 8.5% in matched controls.[7] The frequency of most malformations increased in infants exposed to phenytoin alone or phenobarbital alone. With current information, carbamazepine seems to be the safest drug for use during pregnancy. Other drugs (including lamotrigine) do not differ greatly amongst themselves in respect of teratogenicity, but sodium valproate has the worst profile.

When counselling whether or not to treat, and with which drug, factors such as the severity and type of seizure disorder also need to be taken into account, as control of major seizures is of fundamental importance.

Folic acid taken daily prior to conception and through the first trimester reduces teratogenic risk.

EPILEPSY AND ORAL CONTRACEPTIVES

Some antiepilepsy drugs (carbamazepine, phenytoin, barbituates, topiramate, oxcarbazepine) induce steroid-metabolising enzymes and can cause hormonal contraception to fail. Patients who are taking these drugs need a higher dose of oestrogen (at least 50 micrograms/day) if they wish to continue on the pill, although this does not guarantee complete protection from pregnancy with the associated risks to the fetus. Lamotrigine and sodium valproate are not enzyme inducers and their use is not reason to alter the dose of oral contraceptive, but, because valproate has a greater teratogenic risk, it may be wise to consider alternative medication, preferably prior to conception.

EPILEPSY IN CHILDREN

Fits in children are treated as in adults, but children may respond differently and become irritable, e.g. with sodium valproate or phenobarbital. Whether antiepilepsy drugs interfere with later mental and physical development remains uncertain, and it is unwise to assume they do not. The sensible course is to control the epilepsy with monotherapy in minimal doses and with special attention to precipitating factors, and to attempt drug withdrawal when it is deemed safe (see above).

When a child has *febrile convulsions,* the decision to embark on continuous prophylaxis has serious implications, and incorporates on an assessment of risk factors, e.g. age, nature and duration of the fits. Most children who have febrile convulsions do not develop epilepsy. Prolonged drug therapy, e.g. with phenytoin or phenobarbital, has been shown to interfere with cognitive[8] development, the effect persisting for months after the drug is withdrawn. Parents may be supplied with a specially formulated solution of diazepam for rectal administration (absorption from a suppository is too slow) for easy and early administration, and advised on managing fever, e.g. use paracetamol at the first hint of fever, and tepid sponging.

STATUS EPILEPTICUS

Generalised convulsive status epilepticus (GCSE) is a medical emergency. It comprises generalised epileptic convulsions continuing for 30 min or more, or repeated generalised seizures without recovery of consciousness. Initial treatment is with intravenous *lorazepam* or *diazepam.* Lorazepam has the advantage of longer duration of action, with less risk of seizure recurrence, but has slower brain penetration and may take longer to work. Both may cause hypotension and respiratory depression. Give *phenytoin* intravenously at the same time to suppress further seizures (with ECG and blood pressure monitoring, as cardiac arrhythmias and hypotension may result). Intravenous phenobarbital is an alternative, but carries a possibly higher risk of cardiorespiratory suppression than phenytoin if benzodiazepines are also given.

If resuscitation facilities are not immediately available, diazepam by rectal solution is a useful option.

[7]Holmes L B, Harvey E A, Coull B A et al 2001 The teratogenicity of anticonvulsant drugs. New England Journal of Medicine 344:1132–1138.

[8]Activities associated with thinking, learning and memory.

In some cases, midazolam (nasally) may be preferred, e.g. in children or those with severe learning disability. *There is no place for ward-based benzodiazepine infusions.* If GCSE continues for more than 30 min, the patient should be transferred to intensive care.

Always remember to investigate the cause of the GCSE, and ensure that maintenance anticonvulsive therapy is instituted/re-instituted. Details of further management appear in Table 20.1.

Magnesium sulfate is the treatment of choice for seizures related to eclampsia (see also p. 131).[9]

PHARMACOLOGY OF INDIVIDUAL DRUGS

The drugs used in the treatment of various forms of epilepsy are shown in Table 20.2.

Carbamazepine

Carbamazepine (Tegretol) has a range of actions, of which probably the most important is blockade of voltage-dependent sodium ion channels, reducing membrane excitability.

Pharmacokinetics. Carbamazepine is metabolised extensively; one of the main products, an epoxide (a chemically reactive form), has anticonvulsant activity similar to that of the parent drug but may also cause some of its adverse effects. The $t_{1/2}$ of carbamazepine falls from 35 h to 20 h over the first few weeks of therapy due to induction of hepatic enzymes that metabolise it as well as other drugs, including corticosteroids (adrenal and contraceptive), theophylline and warfarin. Cimetidine and valproate inhibit its metabolism. There are complex interactions with other antiepilepsy drugs, constituting a reason for monodrug therapy.

Uses. Carbamazepine finds use for secondary generalised and partial seizures, and primary generalised seizures. Because another antiepilepsy drug (phenytoin) was sometimes beneficial in trigeminal neuralgia, carbamazepine was tested in this condition, for which it is now the drug of choice.

Adverse effects include central nervous system (CNS) symptoms (reversible blurring of vision, diplopia, dizziness and ataxia) and depression of cardiac AV conduction. Alimentary symptoms, skin rashes, blood disorders, and liver and kidney dysfunction also occur. Osteomalacia by enhanced metabolism of vitamin D (enzyme induction) occurs over years; so also does folate deficiency. Enzyme induction reduces the efficacy of combined and progestogen-only contraceptives. Carbamazepine impairs cognitive function less than phenytoin.

OXYCARBAZEPINE

Oxcarbazepine, like its analogue carbamazepine, acts by blocking voltage-sensitive sodium channels. It is rapidly and extensively metabolised in the liver; the $t_{1/2}$ of the parent drug is 2 h, but that of its principal metabolite (which also has therapeutic activity) is 11 h. Unlike carbamazepine, it does not form an epoxide, which may explain its fewer unwanted effects. Oxcarbazepine is a selective inducer of a cytochrome isoenzyme that metabolises oral contraceptives and a 50-microgram oestrogen preparation is necessary for protection. It does not induce hepatic enzymes in general.

Oxcarbazepine is as effective as carbamazepine, sodium valproate and phenytoin in the treatment of partial and secondary generalised seizures; it is used either as monotherapy or add-on therapy.

The most common chronic adverse effect is hyponatraemia, but this is usually mild, asymptomatic and of no clinical significance. Routine monitoring of the plasma sodium is indicated only where there is special risk, e.g. patients taking diuretics, or the elderly.

Table 20.1	Treatment of status epilepticus in adults
Status	**Treatment**
Early	lorazepam 4 mg i.v., repeat once after 10 min if necessary, or clonazepam 1 mg i.v. over 30 s, repeat if necessary, or diazepam 10–20 mg over 2–4 min, repeat once after 30 min if necessary
Established	phenytoin 15–18 mg/kg i.v. at a rate of 50 mg/min, and/or phenobarbital 10–20 mg/kg i.v. at a rate of 100 mg/min
Refractory	thiopental or propofol or midazolam with full intensive care support

[9]Eclampsia Trial Collaborative Group 1995 Which anticonvulsant for women with eclampsia? Evidence from the Collaborative Eclampsia Trial. Lancet 345:1455–1463.

Table 20.2 Drugs of choice for the treatment of epilepsy

Seizure disorder	Drug	Usual daily oral dose	
		Adult	Child
Generalised seizures			
Primary generalised tonic–clonic (grand mal)	*Drugs of choice:*		
	sodium valproate	1–2 g	15–40 mg/kg
	lamotrigine	a	a
	Alternatives:		
	clonazepam	2–6 mg	<1 year: 0.5–1 mg
			1–5 years: 1–3 mg
			5–12 years: 3–6 mg
	topiramate	200–400 mg	5–9 mg/kg (2–16 years)
	carbamazepine[b]	0.8–1.2 g	<1 year: 100–200 mg
			1–5 years: 200–400 mg
			5–10 years: 400–600 mg
			10–15 years: 0.6–1 g
	phenytoin	200–400 mg	4–8 mg/kg
Absence (petit mal)	*Drugs of choice:*		
	ethosuximide	1–1.5 g	>6 years: 1–1.5 g
	sodium valproate	As above	As above
	Alternatives:		
	clonazepam	As above	As above
	lamotrigine	a	a
Atypical absence, myotonic, atonic	*Drugs of choice:*		
	sodium valproate	As above	As above
	clonazepam	As above	As above
	lamotrigine[c]	a	a
	phenytoin	As above	As above
	ethosuximide	As above	As above
	phenobarbital	60–90 mg	5–8 mg/kg
Myoclonic	*Drugs of choice:*		
	sodium valproate[d]	As above	As above
	clonazepam	As above	As above
	Alternatives:		
	lamotrigine	a	a
Partial and/or secondary generalised seizures	*Drugs of choice:*		
	carbamazepine	As above	As above
	sodium valproate	As above	As above
	Alternatives:		
	phenytoin	As above	As above
	lamotrigine	a	a
	gabapentin	0.9–1.2 g	0.9 g (26–36-kg body-wt.)
			1.2 g (37–50-kg body-wt.)
	vigabatrin[e]	2–3 g	0.5–1 g (10–15-kg body-wt.)
			1–1.5 g (15–30-kg body-wt.)
			1.5–3 g (30–50-kg body-wt.)
			2–3 g (>50-kg body-wt.)
	topiramate	As above	As above
	oxcarbazepine	0.6–2.4 g	
	levetiracetam	1–3 g	

[a]Varies with mono or adjunctive therapy; see manufacturer's recommendations.
[b]Avoid if major seizures are accompanied by absence seizures or myoclonic jerks.
[c]Lamotrigine may be effective, particularly if used with sodium valproate.
[d]Alone or in combination with clonazepam, which may be synergistic.
[e]In adults, used as a last resort; in children, used for infantile spasms (West's syndrome). Regular visual field monitoring is mandatory.

Phenytoin

Phenytoin (diphenylhydantoin, Epanutin, Dilantin) alters ionic fluxes but principally the voltage-dependent sodium ion channels in the neuronal membrane; this action is described as membrane stabilising, and discourages the spread (rather than the initiation) of seizure discharges.

Pharmacokinetics. Phenytoin provides a good example of the application of pharmacokinetics for successful prescribing.

Saturation kinetics. Phenytoin is hydroxylated extensively in the liver and this process becomes saturated at about the doses needed for therapeutic effect. Thus phenytoin at low doses exhibits first-order kinetics but saturation or zero-order kinetics develop as the therapeutic plasma concentration range (10–20 mg/L) is approached, i.e. the dose increments of equal size produce a *disproportional rise in steady-state plasma concentration*. Thus dose increments should become smaller as the dose increases (which is why there is a 25-mg capsule). Plainly, monitoring serial plasma concentration measurement will help.

Enzyme induction and inhibition. Phenytoin is a potent inducer of hepatic enzymes that metabolise other drugs (carbamazepine, warfarin), dietary and endogenous substances (including vitamin D and folate), and phenytoin itself. This latter causes a slight fall in steady-state phenytoin concentration over the first few weeks of therapy, though this may not be noticeable with progressive dose increments. Drugs that inhibit phenytoin metabolism (causing its plasma concentration to rise) include sodium valproate, cimetidine, co-trimoxazole, isoniazid, chloramphenicol, some non-steroidal anti-inflammatory drugs and disulfiram.

Phenytoin given orally is well absorbed but there have been pharmaceutical bioavailability problems in relation to the nature of the diluent in the capsule; patients should always use the same formulation.

Uses. Phenytoin is used to prevent all types of partial epilepsy, whether or not the seizures thereafter become generalised, and to treat generalised seizures and status epilepticus. It is not used for absence attacks.

Other uses. The membrane-stabilising effect of phenytoin has been used in cardiac arrhythmias and, rarely, in cases of resistant pain, e.g. trigeminal neuralgia.

Adverse effects of phenytoin, many of which can be very slow to develop, include impairment of cognitive function, which has led many physicians to prefer carbamazepine and valproate. Other nervous system effects range from sedation to delirium to acute cerebellar disorder to convulsions. Peripheral neuropathy also occurs. Cutaneous reactions include rashes (dose related), coarsening of facial features and hirsutism. Gum hyperplasia (due to inhibition of collagen catabolism) may develop and is more marked when gum hygiene is poor and in children.

Other effects include Dupuytren's contracture and pseudolymphoma. Some degree of macrocytosis is common but anaemia probably occurs only when dietary folate intake is inadequate. This responds to folate supplement (there is increased requirement for folate, which is a co-factor for some hydroxylation reactions that accelerate with enzyme induction by phenytoin). Osteomalacia due to increased metabolism of vitamin D occurs after years of therapy.

Overdose causes cerebellar symptoms and signs, coma and apnoea; treatment is according to general principles. The patient may remain unconscious for a long time because of saturation kinetics, but will recover with standard care (see p. 129).

Fosphenytoin, a pro-drug of phenytoin, is soluble in water, and easier and safer to administer; its conversion in the blood to phenytoin is rapid and it may be used as an alternative to phenytoin for status epilepticus (see Table 20.1).

Sodium valproate

Sodium valproate (valproic acid, Epilim) acts by inhibiting GABA transaminase, the enzyme responsible for the breakdown of the inhibitory neurotransmitter, GABA, so increasing its concentration at GABA receptors.

Sodium valproate is metabolised extensively in the liver ($t_{1/2}$ 13 h). It is a non-specific metabolic inhibitor, and indeed inhibits its own metabolism, and that of lamotrigine, phenobarbital, phenytoin and carbamazepine. Sodium valproate does not induce drug-metabolising enzymes but its metabolism is accelerated by enzyme-inducing drugs, including antiepileptics.

Sodium valproate is effective for a wide range of seizure disorders, including generalised and partial epilepsy, and for the prophylaxis of febrile convulsions and post-traumatic epilepsy.

Adverse effects can be troublesome. The main concerns, particularly to women, are weight gain, teratogenicity (see p. 126), polycystic ovary syndrome and loss of hair, which grows back curly.[10] Nausea may be a problem. Some patients exhibit a rise in liver enzymes, which is usually transient and without sinister import, but patients should be closely monitored until the biochemical tests return to normal as, rarely, liver failure occurs (risk maximal at 2–12 weeks); this is often indicated by anorexia, malaise and a recurrence of seizures. Other reactions include pancreatitis, and coagulation disorder due to inhibition of platelet aggregation (coagulation should be assessed before surgery).

Ketone metabolites may cause confusion in urine testing in diabetes.

Metabolic inhibition by valproate prolongs the action of co-administered antiepilepsy drugs (see above). The effect is significant and the dose of lamotrigine, for example, should be halved in patients who are also taking sodium valproate.

Barbiturates

Antiepilepsy members include *phenobarbital* ($t_{1/2}$ 100 h), *methylphenobarbital* and *primidone* (Mysoline), which latter is metabolised largely to phenobarbital, i.e. it is a pro-drug. These drugs still find use for generalised seizures; sedation is usual.

Clonazepam

Clonazepam (Rivotril) ($t_{1/2}$ 25 h) is a benzodiazepine used as a second-line drug for treatment of primary generalised epilepsy and for status epilepticus (see Table 20.1).

Vigabatrin

Vigabatrin (Sabril) ($t_{1/2}$ 6 h) is structurally related to the inhibitory CNS neurotransmitter GABA, and acts by irreversibly inhibiting GABA-transaminase so that GABA accumulates. GABA-transaminase is resynthesised over 6 days. The drug is not metabolised and does not induce hepatic drug-metabolising enzymes.

Vigabatrin is effective in partial, secondary generalised seizures that are not satisfactorily controlled by other anticonvulsants, and in infantile spasms, as monotherapy. It worsens absence and myoclonic seizures.

Unwanted effects from drugs sometimes become apparent only following prolonged use, and this is a case in point. Vigabatrin had been licensed for a number of years before there were reports of visual field constriction (up to 40% of patients), an effect that is insidious and leads to irreversible tunnel vision.[11] Its discovery emphasises the value of post-marketing drug surveillance programmes.[12] Vigabatrin is now indicated only for patients with the specific seizure disorders responsive to the drug (above), and no other. Patients should undergo visual field monitoring at 6-month intervals whilst taking the drug.

Other adverse effects on the CNS are similar to those of antiepilepsy drugs in general but include confusion and psychosis. Increase in weight also occurs in up to 40% of patients during the first 6 months of treatment.

Lamotrigine

Lamotrigine acts to stabilise presynaptic neuronal membranes by blocking voltage-dependent sodium channels (a property it shares with carbamazepine and phenytoin), and it reduces the release of excitatory amino acids, such as glutamate and aspartate. The $t_{1/2}$ of 24 h allows for a single daily dose.

Lamotrigine is effective as monotherapy and adjunctive therapy for partial and primary and secondarily generalised tonic–clonic seizures. It is generally well tolerated but may cause serious adverse effects on the skin, including Stevens–Johnson syndrome and toxic epidermal necrolysis (fatally, on rare occasions). The risk of cutaneous effects lessens if treatment begins with a low dose and escalates slowly. Concomitant use of valproate, which inhibits the metabolism and thus the inactivation

---

[10] 'We thought the change might be welcomed by the patients, but one girl preferred her hair to be long and straight, and one boy was mortified by his curls and insisted on a short hair cut.' (Jeavons P M, Clark J E, Harding G F 1977 Valproate and curly hair. Lancet i:359).

[11] Eke T, Talbot J F, Lawden M C 1997 Severe persistent visual field constriction associated with vigabatrin. British Medical Journal 314:180–181.

[12] Wilton L V, Stephens M D B, Mann R D 1999 Visual field defect associated with vigabatrin: observational cohort study. British Medical Journal 319:1165–1166.

of lamotrigine, adds to the hazard. Carbamazepine, phenytoin and primidone accelerate the metabolic breakdown of lamotrigine, which must be given in higher dose when combined.

Gabapentin

Gabapentin is an analogue of GABA that is sufficiently lipid soluble to cross the blood–brain barrier, but its mode of action is uncertain. It is excreted unchanged and, unlike many other antiepilepsy agents, does not induce or inhibit hepatic metabolism of other drugs.

Gabapentin is effective only for partial seizures and secondary generalised epilepsy (not absence or myoclonic epilepsy), in combination with established agents. It also finds use for neuropathic pain.

Gabapentin may cause somnolence, unsteadiness, dizziness and fatigue.

Topiramate

Topiramate possesses a range of actions that include blockade of voltage-sensitive sodium channels, enhancement of GABA activity and possibly weak blockade of glutamate receptors. The $t_{1/2}$ of 21 h allows once-daily dosing; it is excreted in the urine, mainly as unchanged drug.

Topiramate is used as adjunctive treatment for partial seizures, with or without secondary generalisation. Unwanted effects limit its use, particularly sedation, naming difficulty and weight loss. Acute myopia and raised intraocular pressure may occur.

Levetiracetam

Levetiracetam acts in a manner different to other antiepilepsy drugs. It has a potentially broad spectrum of use but is currently indicated for adjunctive treatment in partial seizures with or without secondary generalisation. It is rapidly and completely absorbed after oral administration, and is effective with twice-daily dosing. Its therapeutic index appears to be high and the commonest of the adverse effects are asthenia, dizziness and drowsiness.

Succinimides

Ethosuximide (Zarontin) ($t_{1/2}$ 55 h) differs from other antiepilepsy drugs in that it blocks a particular type of calcium channel that is active in absence seizures (petit mal), and it is used specifically for this condition. Adverse effects include gastric upset, CNS effects, and allergic reactions including eosinophilia and other blood disorders, and lupus erythematosus.

PARKINSONISM

A NOTE ON PATHOPHYSIOLOGY

Parkinson's disease[13] affects about 1 in 200 of the elderly population. In broad terms, it is caused by degeneration of the substantia nigra[14] in the midbrain, and consequent loss of dopamine-containing neurones in the nigrostriatal pathway (see Fig. 19.3, p. 343). There is no known cure but drug treatment can, if properly managed, dramatically improve quality of life in this progressive disease.

Two balanced systems are important in the extrapyramidal control of motor activity at the level of the corpus striatum and substantia nigra: in one the neurotransmitter is *acetylcholine*; in the other it is a *dopamine*. In Parkinson's disease, there is degenerative loss of nigrostriatal dopaminergic neurones and the symptoms and signs of the disease are due to *dopamine depletion*. Certain drugs also produce the features of Parkinson's disease (see below).

The symptom triad of the disease is *bradykinesia*, *rigidity* and *tremor*. Patients who have received levodopa for a long time may exhibit the 'on–off' phenomenon in which, abruptly and distressingly, dyskinesia (the 'on' phase) alternates with hypokinesia (the 'off 'phase). One sufferer, a physician, wrote about his condition:

> One of its most trying aspects is the extent to which it interferes with the trivial events in daily life. Nothing is easy in Parkinson's disease. There is no feature of any task that is not potentially out of control. A cuff-link refuses to find its way into a tuxedo shirt, my wife is out of town, and I miss the annual dinner. I am unable to stuff change from a $5 bill into my wallet, and the patrons in line behind the cash register fume. Bow ties won't tie and shoelaces won't lace. A cube of beef obstructs the glottis. In Parkinson's disease one must expect the unexpected … About five years ago, my disease began to close in on me, becoming more aggressive and difficult to handle. I had increasing discomfort from hyperkinesias. My voice was almost inaudible, and periods when my feet felt frozen to the floor became commonplace. I lost the advantage I

---

[13]James Parkinson (1755–1824), physician; he described paralysis agitans in 1817.
[14]*Substantia nigra* is (Latin) black substance. A coronal section at this point in the brain shows the distinctive black areas, visible with the naked eye in the normal brain, but absent from the brains of patients with Parkinson's disease.

had previously enjoyed of a comfortable margin between the effective dose and the dose with intolerable side effects. I had an 'off' spell … in a telephone booth…[15]

OBJECTIVES OF THERAPY

The following mechanisms act to restore the dopaminergic/cholinergic balance.

1. Enhancement of dopaminergic activity by drugs which may:
   - *replenish* neuronal dopamine by supplying levodopa, which is its natural precursor; administration of dopamine itself is ineffective as it does not cross the blood–brain barrier
   - act as *dopamine agonists* (bromocriptine, pergolide, cabergoline, apomorphine)
   - *prolong* the action of dopamine through selective inhibition of its metabolism (selegiline)
   - *release* dopamine from stores and inhibit reuptake (amantadine); or
2. Reduction of cholinergic activity by antimuscarinic (anticholinergic[16]) drugs; this approach is most effective against tremor and rigidity, and less effective in the treatment of bradykinesia (including iatrogenic, caused by dopamine receptor antagonists).

Both approaches are effective in therapy and are usefully combined. It therefore comes as no surprise that drugs that prolong the action of acetylcholine (anticholinesterases) or drugs that deplete dopamine stores (reserpine) or block dopamine receptors (antipsychotics, e.g. chlorpromazine) will exacerbate the symptoms of parkinsonism or induce a parkinson-like state.

Other parts of the brain in which dopaminergic systems are involved include the medulla (induction of vomiting), the hypothalamus (suppression of prolactin secretion) and certain paths to the cerebral cortex. Different effects of dopaminergic drugs can be explained by activation of these systems, namely emesis, suppression of lactation (mainly direct dopamine agonists) and occasionally psychotic illness.

Classical antipsychotics (see p. 348) used to manage psychotic behaviour act by blockade of dopamine D_2 receptors and, as is to be expected, they are also antinauseant, may sometimes cause galactorrhoea, and can induce parkinsonism. Drug-induced parkinsonism is alleviated by antimuscarinics, but not by levodopa or dopamine agonists, because the antipsychotics block dopamine receptors by which these drugs act. As many antipsychotics also have some antimuscarinic activity, those with greatest efficacy in this respect, e.g. thioridazine, are the least likely to cause parkinsonism.

DRUGS FOR PARKINSON'S DISEASE

DOPAMINERGIC DRUGS

Levodopa and dopa-decarboxylase inhibitors

Levodopa ('dopa' stands for dihydroxyphenylalanine) is a natural amino acid precursor of dopamine. The latter is unsuitable for treatment as it is rapidly metabolised in the gut, blood and liver by monoamine oxidase and catechol-*O*-methyltransferase; intravenously administered dopamine, or dopamine formed in peripheral tissues, is insufficiently lipid soluble to penetrate the CNS. But levodopa is readily absorbed from the upper small intestine by active amino acid transport and has a $t_{1/2}$ of 1.5 h. It can traverse the blood–brain barrier by a similar active transport, and within the brain it is decarboxylated (by dopa decarboxylase) to the neurotransmitter *dopamine*.

A major disadvantage is that levodopa is also extensively decarboxylated to dopamine in peripheral tissues so that only 1–5% of an oral dose of levodopa reaches the brain. Thus large quantities of levodopa would have to be given. These inhibit gastric emptying, delivery to the absorption site is erratic, and fluctuations in plasma concentration occur. The drug and its metabolites cause significant adverse effects by peripheral actions, notably nausea, but also cardiac arrhythmia and postural hypotension. This problem has been largely circumvented by the development of *decarboxylase inhibitors*, which do not enter the CNS, so that they prevent only the *extracerebral* metabolism of levodopa. The inhibitors are given in combination with levodopa and there is a range of formulations comprising a decarboxylase inhibitor with levodopa:

---

[15]Saltzman E W 1996 Living with Parkinson's disease. New England Journal of Medicine 334:114–116.

[16]The term *antimuscarinic* is now preferred (see p. 399).

- *co-careldopa* (carbidopa + levodopa in proportions 12.5/50, 10/100, 25/100 and 25 mg/250 mg) (Sinemet)
- *co-beneldopa* (benserazide + levodopa in proportions 12.5/50, 25/100, 50 mg/200 mg) (Madopar).

The combinations produce the same brain concentrations as with levodopa alone, but only 25% of the dose of levodopa is required, which smoothes the action of levodopa and reduces the incidence of adverse effects, especially nausea, from about 80% to less than 15%.

Dose management. Levodopa, alone and in combination (see above), is introduced gradually and titrated according to individual response.

Compliance is important. Abrupt discontinuation of therapy leads to dramatic relapse.

Adverse effects. *Postural hypotension* occurs. *Nausea* may be a limiting factor if the dose is increased too rapidly; it may be helped by cyclizine 50 mg taken 30 min before food or by domperidone (little of which enters the brain). Levodopa-induced *dyskinesias* take the form of involuntary limb jerking or head, lip or tongue movements and constitute a major constraint on how the drug is used (see below). *Mental changes* may be seen; these include depression, which is common (best controlled with a tricyclic antidepressant), dreams, and hallucinations and delusions (clozapine may help). *Agitation and confusion* occur but it may be difficult to decide whether these are due to drug or to disease. In these circumstances, the drugs most likely to be the cause of a toxic confusional state (antimuscarinics and direct dopamine agonists) are withdrawn.

Interactions. With non-selective monoamine oxidase inhibitors (MAOIs), the monoamine dopamine formed from levodopa is protected from destruction; it accumulates and also follows the normal path of conversion to noradrenaline (norepinephrine), by dopamine β-hydroxylase; *severe hypertension results*. The interaction with the selective MAO-B inhibitor, selegiline, is possibly therapeutic (see below).

Levodopa antagonises the effects of antipsychotics (dopamine receptor blockers). Tricyclic antidepressants are safe.

Dopamine agonists

These mimic the effects of dopamine, the endogenous agonist, which stimulates both of the main types of dopamine receptor, D_1 and D_2 (coupled respectively to adenylyl cyclase stimulation and inhibition). The D_2 receptor is the principal target in Parkinson's disease; chronic D_1-receptor stimulation appears to potentiate the response to the D_2 receptor. The main problems with dopamine (i.e. the pro-drug, levodopa) are its short $t_{1/2}$ and, possibly, the consequences of delivering large amounts of substrate to an oxidative pathway, MAO (see below). On the other hand, the problems of developing synthetic alternatives are:

- reproducing the right balance of D_1 and D_2 stimulation (dopamine itself is slightly D_1 selective, in test systems, but its net effect in vivo is determined also by the relative amounts and locations of receptors – which differ in parkinsonian patients from normal)
- avoiding the undesired effects of peripheral, mainly gastric, D_2 receptors
- synthesising a full, not partial, agonist.

Bromocriptine (a derivative of ergot) is a D_2-receptor agonist, but also a weak α-adrenoreceptor antagonist. It is commonly used with levodopa. The drug is rapidly absorbed after administration by mouth; the $t_{1/2}$ is 5 h, so that its action is smoother than that of levodopa, which can be an advantage in patients who develop end-of-dose deterioration with levodopa. Dosing should start very low (1–1.25 mg p.o. at night), increasing at approximately weekly intervals and according to clinical response.

Nausea and vomiting are the commonest adverse effects; these may respond to domperidone, but tend to become less marked as treatment continues. Postural hypotension may cause dizziness or syncope. In high dose, confusion, delusions or hallucinations may occur and, after prolonged use, pleural effusion and retroperitoneal fibrosis.

Lisuride ($t_{1/2}$ 2 h) and *pergolide* ($t_{1/2}$ 6 h) are similar to bromocriptine, though the latter also stimulates D_1 receptors. *Cabergoline*, also an ergot derivative, has a $t_{1/2}$ of more than 80 h. This long duration of action allows it to be used in a single daily (or even twice weekly) dose, which is appreciated by patients who are often taking other drugs every 2–3 h; it is also valuable for night-time problems due to lack of levodopa. *Pramipexole* is a non-ergot dopamine D_2-receptor agonist that is more effective against tremor than the others. *Ropinirole* is a direct D_2-receptor agonist, which is also a non-ergot derivative.

Apomorphine is a derivative of morphine having structural similarities to dopamine; it is a full agonist at D_1 and D_2 receptors. Its main use is in young patients with severe motor fluctuations and dyskinesias (the 'on–off' phenomenon, see above) when it is given by subcutaneous injection or infusion for patients with levodopa-resistant 'off'. The rapid onset of action by the subcutaneous route (self-administration can be taught) enables the 'off' component to be aborted without the patient waiting for 45–60 min to absorb another oral dose of levodopa.

Apomorphine may need to be accompanied by an antiemetic, e.g. domperidone (which does not cross the blood–brain barrier as does metoclopramide), to prevent its characteristic emetic action. Overdose causes respiratory depression; naloxone antagonises its action. Apomorphine can induce penile erection (without causing sexual excitement) and it enhances the penile response to visual erotic stimulation.

Inhibition of dopamine metabolism

Monoamine oxidase (MAO) enzymes have an important function in modulating the intraneuronal content of neurotransmitter. The enzymes exist in two principal forms, A and B, defined by specific substrates, some of which cannot be metabolised by the other form (Table 20.3). The therapeutic importance of recognising these two forms arises because they are to some extent present in different tissues, and the enzyme at these different locations can be selectively inhibited by the individual inhibitors: *moclobemide* for MAO-A (used for depression, see p. 330) and *selegiline* for MAO-B (Table 20.3).

Selegiline is a selective, irreversible inhibitor of MAO type B. The problem with non-selective MAO inhibitors is that they prevent degradation of dietary amines, especially tyramine, which is then able to act systemically as a sympathomimetic: the hypertensive 'cheese reaction' (see p. 340). As will be apparent from Table 20.3, selegiline does not cause the cheese reaction, because MAO-A is still present in the liver to metabolise tyramine. MAO-A also metabolises tyramine in the sympathetic nerve endings, so providing a further line of protection (tyramine is an indirectly acting amine which displaces noradrenaline from the nerve endings). In the CNS selegiline protects dopamine from intraneuronal degradation. It has no effect on synaptic cleft concentrations of those amines, such as serotonin and noradrenaline, which are normally potentiated by the MAOI used in depression; therefore selegiline has no antidepressant action.

Table 20.3 Isoforms of monoamine oxidase: MAO-A and MAO-B, an explanation
The table shows the definition of the isoforms by their specific substrates, and then their selectivity (or non-selectivity) towards a number of other substrates and inhibitors. Determination of therapeutic and adverse effects is a function of selectivity of the inhibitor and the tissue location of the enzyme.

Enzyme	MAO-A	MAO-A and B	MAO-B
Substrate	Serotonin (see footnote)	Noradrenaline (norepinephrine) (see footnote) Adrenaline (epinephrine) Dopamine Tyramine	Phenylethylamine
Inhibitors	moclobemide	tranylcypromine phenelzine iproniazid	selegiline
Tissues	Liver CNS (neurones) Sympathetic neurones	See MAO-A and MAO-B	Gut CNS (glial cells)

Explanation: The specific substrate for MAO-A is serotonin, whereas that for MAO-B is the non-endogenous amine, phenylethylamine (present in many brands of chocolate). Noradrenaline, tyramine and dopamine can be metabolised by both isoforms of MAO. MAO-A is the major form in liver and in neurones (both CNS and peripheral sympathetic); MAO-B is the major form in the gut, but is also present in the liver, lungs and glial cells of the CNS.

Combination of levodopa with selegiline is associated with excess mortality[17] and is not recommended.

Entacapone inhibits catechol-*O*-methyltransferase (COMT), one of the principal enzymes responsible for the metabolism of dopamine; the action of levodopa is thus prolonged. It is most effective for patients with early end-of-dose deterioration, and allows them to take levodopa at 3–4-hourly intervals, giving a more predictable and useful response. Entacapone is preferred to long-acting preparations of levodopa whose main disadvantage is their slow onset of action. It can increase the dyskinesias seen in the late stages of Parkinson's disease.

DOPAMINE RELEASE

Amantadine antedates the discovery of dopamine receptor subtypes, and its discovery as an antiparkinsonian drug was an example of serendipity. It is an antiviral drug which, given for influenza to a parkinsonian patient, was noticed to be beneficial. The two effects are probably unrelated. It appears to act by increasing synthesis and release of dopamine, and by diminishing neuronal reuptake. It also has slight antimuscarinic effect. The drug is much less effective than levodopa, whose action it enhances slightly. It is more effective than the standard antimuscarinic drugs, with which it has an additive effect. Amantadine is relatively free from adverse effects, which, however, include ankle oedema (probably a local effect on blood vessels), postural hypotension, livedo reticularis and CNS disturbances: insomnia, hallucinations and, rarely, fits.

ANTIMUSCARINIC (ANTICHOLINERGIC) DRUGS (SEE ALSO P. 399)

Antimuscarinic drugs benefit parkinsonism by blocking acetylcholine receptors in the CNS, thereby partially redressing the imbalance created by decreased dopaminergic activity. Their use originated when hyoscine was given to parkinsonian patients in an attempt to reduce sialorrhoea by peripheral effect, and it then became apparent that they had other beneficial effects in this disease. Synthetic derivatives are now used orally. These include benzhexol (trihexyphenidyl), orphenadrine, benzatropine, procyclidine, biperiden. There is little to choose between these. Antimuscarinics produce modest improvements in tremor, rigidity, sialorrhoea, muscular stiffness and leg cramps, but little in bradykinesia, the most disabling symptom of Parkinson's disease. They are also effective intramuscularly or intravenously in acute drug-induced dystonias.

Unwanted effects include dry mouth, blurred vision, constipation, urine retention, glaucoma, hallucinations, memory defects, toxic confusional states and psychoses (which should be distinguished from presenile dementia).

TREATMENT OF PARKINSON'S DISEASE

The main features that require alleviation are *tremor*, *rigidity* and *bradykinesia*.

General measures Are important and include the encouragement of regular physical activity and specific help such as physiotherapy, speech therapy and occupational therapy.

DRUG THERAPY

Drugs play the most important role in symptom relief. No agent yet found alters the progressive course of the disease.

Treatment should begin only when it is judged necessary in each individual case. For example, a young man with a physically demanding job will require treatment before an older retired person. Two conflicting objectives have to be balanced: the desire for satisfactory relief of current symptoms and the avoidance of adverse effects as a result of longcontinued treatment.

There is debate as to whether the treatment should commence with levodopa or a synthetic dopamine agonist. Levodopa provides the biggest improvement in motor symptoms but its use is associated with the development of dyskinesias, which are inevitable after some 5–10 years, although often dose related. Dopamine agonists have a much less powerful motor effect but are less likely to produce dyskinesias. Most neurologists therefore prefer a dopamine

---

[17]Ben-Sholomo Y, Churchyeard A, Head J et al 1998 Investigation by Parkinson's Disease Research Group of United Kingdom into excess mortality seen with combined levodopa and selegiline treatment in patients with early, mild Parkinson's disease: further results of randomised trial and confidential inquiry. British Medical Journal 316:1191–1196.

agonist alone as the initial choice. Unfortunately, only about 30% of patients obtain a satisfactory motor response. An alternative could be to begin treatment with levodopa in low dose to get a good motor response, and to add a dopamine agonist when the initial benefit begins to wane or to add the dopamine agonist simultaneously to the levodopa enabling the total dose of the latter to be reduced. With either approach, it seems likely that the position after 5 years of treatment may well be the same, but that by starting with levodopa the patient will have had the benefit of an earlier motor response. It does appear that the development of dyskinesia is related to the total levodopa dose, hence the desire to prescribe the lowest dose practical.

Antimuscarinic drugs are suitable only for younger patients predominantly troubled with tremor and rigidity. They do not benefit bradykinesia, the main disabling symptom. The unwanted effects of acute-angle glaucoma, retention of urine, constipation and psychiatric disturbance are general contraindications to the use of antimuscarinics in the elderly.

Amantadine can delay the use of either levodopa or a synthetic dopamine agonist in the early stages of the disease if mild symptomatic benefit is required, but this approach is seldom necessary.

A typical course is that for about 2–4 years on treatment with levodopa or a dopamine agonist the patient's disability and motor performance remain near normal despite progression of the underlying disease. After some 5 years, about 50% of patients exhibit the problems of long-term treatment (dose-related to exposure to levodopa), i.e. dyskinesia and end-of-dose deterioration with the 'on–off' phenomenon. After 10 years, virtually 100% of patients may be affected.

Dyskinesia comprises involuntary writhing movement of the face and limbs that may be biphasic (occurring at the start and end of motor response) or develop at the time of the maximum plasma levodopa concentration. It responds initially to reducing the dose of levodopa but at the cost of bradykinesia, and as time passes there is progressively less scope to obtain benefit without unwanted effects. Amantadine may be useful here.

End-of-dose deterioration is managed by increasing the frequency of dosing with levodopa (e.g. to 2–3-hourly), but this tends to result in the appearance, or worsening of the dyskinesia. The motor response then becomes more brittle with abrupt swings between hypermobility and hypomobility (the on–off phenomenon). Despite their unpredictable nature over the course of a single day, these changes are in fact dose related, an effect that becomes apparent only when the response is related to total medication taken over a week.

Various strategies exist to overcome these problems. Controlled-release preparations of levodopa tend to be associated with an inadequate initial response and disabling dyskinesia at the end of the dose. A more effective approach appears to be the use of a *COMT inhibitor*, e.g. entacapone, which can sometimes allay early end-of-dose deterioration without causing dyskinesia. This is now the main indication for its use.

Continuous subcutaneous infusion of *apomorphine* can transform the quality of life of younger patients with severe motor fluctuations and dyskinesia, but this may lead to neuropsychiatric effects. If drug treatment fails in young non-demented patients, stereotactic subthalamotomy or bilateral stereotactic subthalamic stimulation can be very successful, with only a small risk of surgical complications in experienced hands.

Some 20% of patients with Parkinson's disease, notably the older ones, develop impairment of memory and speech with a fluctuating confusional state and hallucinations. As these symptoms are often aggravated by medication, it is preferable gradually to reduce the antiparkinsonian treatment, even at the expense of lessened mobility.

DRUG-INDUCED PARKINSONISM

The classical antipsychotic drugs (see p. 348) block dopamine receptors and their antipsychotic activity relates closely to this action, which notably involves the D_2 receptor, the principal target in Parkinson's disease. It comes as no surprise, therefore, that these drugs can induce a state with clinical features very similar to those of idiopathic Parkinson's disease. The piperazine phenothiazines, e.g. trifluoperazine, and the butyrophenones, e.g. haloperidol, are most commonly involved. In one series[18] of 95 new cases of parkinsonism referred to a department of geriatric medicine, 51% were associated with prescribed drugs and half of these required hospital admission. After withdrawal of the offending drug, most cases resolved completely within 7 weeks.

[18]Stephen P J, Williamson J 1984 Drug-induced parkinsonism in elderly. Lancet ii:1082–1083.

When drug-induced parkinsonism is troublesome, an antimuscarinic drug, e.g. benzhexol, is beneficial. Atypical antipsychotics provoke fewer extrapyrimidal effects (see p. 345).

OTHER MOVEMENT DISORDERS

Essential tremor Is often, and with justice, called benign, but a few individuals may be incapacitated by it. Alcohol, through a central action, helps about 50% of patients but is plainly unsuitable for long-term use and a non-selective β-adrenoceptor blocker, e.g. propranolol 120 mg/day, will benefit about 50%; clonazepam or primidone is sometimes beneficial.

Drug-induced dystonic reactions are seen:

- as an acute reaction, often of the torsion type, and occur following administration of dopamine receptor-blocking antipsychotics, e.g. haloperidol, and antiemetics, e.g. metoclopramide. An antimuscarinic drug, e.g. biperiden or benzatropine, given intramuscularly or intravenously and repeated as necessary, provides relief
- in some patients who are receiving levodopa for Parkinson's disease
- in younger patients on long-term antipsychotic treatment, who develop tardive dyskinesia (see p. 345).

Hepatolenticular degeneration (Wilson's disease) is caused by a genetic failure to eliminate copper absorbed from food so that it accumulates in the liver, brain, cornea and kidneys. Chelating copper in the gut with penicillamine (see p. 132) or trientine can establish a negative copper balance (with some clinical improvement if treatment is started early). The patients may also develop cirrhosis, and the best treatment for both may be liver transplantation.

Chorea of any cause may be alleviated by dopamine receptor-blocking antipsychotics, and also by tetrabenazine, which inhibits neuronal storage of dopamine and serotonin.

Involuntary muscle spasm. Blepharospasm, hemifacial spasm, spasmodic torticollis and, indeed, the spasm of chronic anal fissure are treated with *botulinum toxin*. This irreversibly blocks release of acetylcholine from cholinergic nerve endings and is injected locally. Its effect lasts for about 3 months. Botulinum toxin is at least partially effective in up to 90% of patients with these conditions. Dysphagia may occasionally occur as a complication.

Spasticity results from lesions at various sites within the CNS and spinal cord. Drugs used include the GABA agonist baclofen, diazepam and tizanidine (an α_2-adrenoceptor agonist).

Myotonia, in which voluntary muscle fails to relax after contraction, may be symptomatically benefited by drugs that increase muscle refractory period, e.g. procainamide, phenytoin, quinidine.

Restless legs syndrome (RLS) is a condition in which the patient has an urge to move their legs because of an unpleasant sensation. Movement can provide temporary relief. The disorder occurs as a result of dopaminergic and opioidergic neurotransmitter system modulated by the metabolism of iron. A variety of medications have been tried including levodopa, bromocriptine and recently ropinorole has been licensed for its use.

MULTIPLE SCLEROSIS

Multiple sclerosis (MS) or disseminated sclerosis ('sclerose en plaques') affects the white matter of the CNS. Drugs are given to alleviate chronic muscle spasm or spasticity (see above) but, until recently, there has been no disease-modifying treatment in this relapsing and remitting condition, in which the placebo effect of most drugs can appear quite powerful. Although its cause remains unknown, the pathophysiology of MS is likely to include autoimmune and/or genetic factors. Drugs that might modify the immune response and release of cytokines have been therefore tested.

Corticosteroid therapy is the mainstay of pharmacological intervention for acute attacks in MS. Corticosteroid has been shown to reduce the length of time an attack lasts but has no effect on reducing recurrent attacks or the final disability. *Methylprednisolone* (0.5–1 g) is given intravenously over a 3–5-day period. Even though each daily dose is delivered in about 1 h, patients are usually hospitalised to allow multidisciplinary management, e.g. with physiotherapy. The use of corticosteroid for treating optic neuritis remains disputed.[19]

Interferon (IFN) β is the first treatment to show, in placebo-controlled trials, a reduction in the number of relapses (and cerebral 'lesion load' determined by magnetic resonance brain imaging). IFNβ may also have a modest effect in delaying disability by 12–18 months in relapsing/remitting disease. In a clinical trial 372 patients with relapsing/remitting disease, able to walk 100 metres without aid or rest, were randomised to receive 8 million IU or 1.6 million IU of IFNβ or placebo by subcutaneous injection on alternate days. After 2 years there was a reduction in the relapse rate from 1.27 per year in the placebo group to 0.84 per year in the patients receiving the higher dose.[20]

IFNβ is not indicated in patients with progressive forms of disease, or in severely disabled patients. The high cost per patient treated in relation to the benefit gained has prevented widespread access to this drug. In the UK, only designated neurologists can prescribe IFNβ.

Other proven treatments for acute relapse based on controlled clinical trials include adrenocorticotrophic hormone (ACTH), oral prednisolone, cyclophosphamide and mitoxantrone.

Urinary frequency and urgency (spastic bladder) is common and propantheline or oxybutynin can relax the detrusor muscle. Constipation should be treated as is appropriate. Muscle spasticity can be severe and disabling. Oral baclofen can reduce such spasticity but over-treatment may lead to flaccidity with its own rehabilitation problems. Very occasionally in severe spasticity intrathecal baclofen can be administered using an implanted pump. Fatigue is common in MS and may respond to amantadine (100 mg b.d.). The role of general supportive measures, such as ramps, wheelchairs, stairlifts, prevention of bedsores, cannot be overstated.

MOTOR NEURONE DISEASE

The cause of the progressive destruction of upper and lower motor neurones is unknown. The only drug available, riluzole, acts by inhibiting accumulation of the neurotransmitter, glutamate. In 959 patients, *riluzole* prolonged median survival time from 13 to 16 months, with no effect on motor function.[21] It may cause neutropenia. Its use in the UK is limited to neurologists

TETANUS

Tetanus remains a potentially fatal disease among underprivileged people in parts of the world where immunisation programmes are inadequate. Management involves:

- Immediate neutralisation of any toxin that has not yet become attached irreversibly to the CNS. Human tetanus immunoglobulin 150 units/kg should be given intramuscularly at multiple sites to neutralise unbound toxin.
- Wound debridement and destruction of *Clostridium tetani* with metronidazole (for alternatives, see p. 205).
- Control of convulsions whilst maintaining respiratory function. Midazolam or diazepam is given for spasms and rigidity, and tracheal intubation and mechanical ventilation for prolonged spasms with respiratory dysfunction (in severe cases, a neuromuscular blocking drug, e.g. intermittent doses of pancuronium, may be required).
- Control of cardiovascular function (tetanus toxin often causes disturbances in autonomic control, with sympathetic overactivity). First-line treatment is by sedation with a benzodiazepine and opioid; infusion of the short-acting β-blocker esmolol, or the $α_2$-adrenergic agonist clonidine, helps to control episodes of hypertension.
- Maintenance of fluid, electrolyte and nutritional status. Severe cases generally require admission to an intensive care unit for 3–5 weeks; weight loss is universal in tetanus and patients require enteral nutrition.
- Prevention of intercurrent infection (usually pulmonary), thromboembolism, pressure sores.

[19]Beck R W, Cleary P A, Anderson M M, Keltner J L, Shults W 1992 A randomized, controlled trial of corticosteroids in the treatment of acute optic neuritis. New England Journal of Medicine 326:581–588.

[20]The Interferon Beta Multiple Sclerosis Study Group and the University of British Columbia MS/MRI Analysis Group 1995 Neurology 45:1277–1285.

[21]Lacomblez L, Bensimon G, Leigh P N et al 1996 A controlled trial of Riluzole in ALS. Lancet 347: 1425–1431.

GUIDE TO FURTHER READING

Baker M G, Graham L 2004 The journey: Parkinson's disease. British Medical Journal 329:611–614

Chang B S, Lowenstein D H 2003 Epilepsy. New England Journal of Medicine 349(13):1257–1266

Compston A, Coles A 2002 Multiple sclerosis. Lancet 359:1221–1231

Cook T M, Protheroe R T, Handel J M et al 2001 Tetanus: a review of the literature. British Journal of Anaesthesia 87(3):477–487

Duncan J S, Sander J W, Sisodiya S M, Walker M C 2006 Adult epilepsy. Lancet 367:1087–1100

Kwan P, Brodie M J 2001 Neuropsychological effects of epilepsy and antiepileptic drugs. Lancet 357:216–222

Langgartner M, Langgartner I, Drlicek M 2005 The patient's journey: multiple sclerosis. British Medical Journal 330:885–888

Nutt J G, Wooten G F 2005 Diagnosis and initial management of Parkinson's disease. New England Journal of Medicine 353:1021–1027

Pirie A M 2005 Epilepsy in pregnancy. Journal of the Royal College of Physicians of Edinburgh 35:236–238

Samii A, Nutt J G, Ransom B R 2004 Parkinson's disease. Lancet 363:1783–1793

Shaw P J 1999 Motor neurone disease. British Medical Journal 318:1118–1121

Swift A 2003 The current uses of botulinum toxin. Symposium on botulinum toxin. British Journal of Hospital Medicine 64:450–451

Walker M 2005 Status epilepticus: an evidence based guide. British Medical Journal 331:673–677

Section 5

CARDIORESPIRATORY AND RENAL SYSTEMS

21

Cholinergic and antimuscarinic (anticholinergic) mechanisms and drugs

SYNOPSIS

Acetylcholine is a widespread chemotransmitter in the body, mediating a broad range of physiological effects. The two classes of receptor for acetylcholine are defined on the basis of their preferential activation by the alkaloids *nicotine* and *muscarine*.

Cholinergic drugs (acetylcholine receptor agonists) mimic acetylcholine at all sites, although the balance of nicotinic and muscarinic effects is variable.

Acetylcholine antagonists that block the nicotine-like effects (neuromuscular blockers and autonomic ganglion blockers) are described elsewhere (Chapter 18).

Acetylcholine antagonists that block the muscarine-like effects, e.g. atropine, are often imprecisely called anticholinergics. The more specific term 'antimuscarinic' is preferred here.

- Cholinergic drugs:
  – classification
  – sites of action
  – pharmacology
  – choline esters
  – alkaloids with cholinergic effects
  – anticholinesterases; organophosphate poisoning
  – disorders of neuromuscular transmission: myasthenia gravis
- Drugs that oppose acetylcholine action: –antimuscarinic drugs

CHOLINERGIC DRUGS (CHOLINOMIMETICS)

These drugs act on postsynaptic acetylcholine receptors (cholinoceptors) at all sites in the body where acetylcholine is the effective neurotransmitter. They initially stimulate and usually later block transmission. In addition, like acetylcholine, they act on the non-innervated receptors that relax peripheral blood vessels.

Uses of cholinergic drugs
- For myasthenia gravis, both to diagnose (edrophonium) and to treat symptoms (neostigmine, pyridostigmine, distigmine).
- To lower intraocular pressure in chronic simple glaucoma (pilocarpine).
- To bronchodilate patients with airflow obstruction (ipratropium, oxitropium).
- To improve cognitive function in Alzheimer's disease (rivastigmine, donepezil).

CLASSIFICATION

Direct-acting (receptor agonists)

- Choline esters (bethanechol, carbachol), which act at all sites, like acetylcholine, but are resistant to degradation by acetylcholinesterases (AChE; see Fig. 21.1). Muscarinic effects much more prominent than nicotinic (see p. 139).
- Alkaloids (pilocarpine, muscarine) act selectively on end-organs of postganglionic, cholinergic neurones. Effects are exclusively muscarinic.

Indirect-acting

Cholinesterase inhibitors, or anticholinesterases (physostigmine, neostigmine, pyridostigmine, distigmine, galantamine, rivastigmine, donepezil), block *acetylcholinesterase* (AChE), the enzyme that destroys acetylcholine, allowing endogenous acetylcholine to persist and produce intensified effects.

SITES OF ACTION

- Autonomic nervous system (Fig. 21.1, sites 1 and 2).
- Neuromuscular junction (Fig. 21.1, site 1).
- Central nervous system (CNS).
- Non-innervated sites: blood vessels, chiefly arterioles (Fig. 21.1, site 3).

Acetylcholine is released from nerve terminals to activate a postsynaptic receptor, except on blood

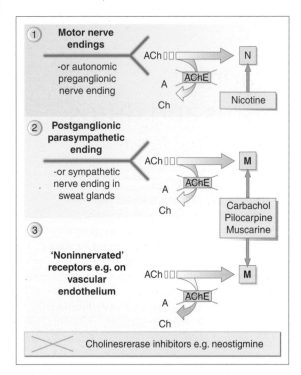

Fig. 21.1 Cartoon showing the different origins for acetylcholine (ACh) activating nicotinic (N) versus muscarinic (M) cholinergic receptors. The three sites (numbered 1–3) are referred to in the text.

vessels where the action of cholinergic drugs is unrelated to cholinergic 'vasodilator' nerves. It is also produced in tissues unrelated to nerve endings, e.g. placenta and ciliated epithelial cells, where it acts as a local hormone (autacoid) on local receptors.

A list of principal effects is given below. Not all occur with every drug and not all are noticeable at therapeutic doses. For example, CNS effects of cholinergic drugs are best seen in cases of anticholinesterase poisoning. Atropine antagonises all the effects of cholinergic drugs except nicotinic actions on autonomic ganglia and the neuromuscular junction, i.e. it has antimuscarinic but not antinicotinic effects (see below).

PHARMACOLOGY

Autonomic nervous system

There are two distinct classes of receptor for acetylcholine, defined on the basis of their preferential activation by the alkaloids *nicotine* (from tobacco) and *muscarine* (from a toxic mushroom, *Amanita muscaria*).

It was Henry Dale who, in 1914, first made this functional division, which remains a robust and useful way of classifying cholinergic drug effects. He noted that the actions of acetylcholine and substances acting like it at autonomic ganglia and the neuromuscular junction mimic the stimulant effects of nicotine (hence nicotinic). In contrast, the actions at postganglionic cholinergic endings (parasympathetic endings plus the cholinergic sympathetic nerves to the sweat glands) and non-innervated receptors on blood vessels resembled the alkaloid, muscarine (hence muscarinic).

Parasympathetic division. Stimulation of cholinoceptors in autonomic ganglia and at postganglionic endings affects chiefly the following organs:

- *Eye*: miosis and spasm of the ciliary muscle occur so that the eye is accommodated for near vision. Intraocular pressure falls.
- *Exocrine glands*: there is increased secretion most noticeably from salivary, lachrymal, bronchial and sweat glands. The last are cholinergic, but anatomically part of the sympathetic system; some sweat glands, e.g. axillary, may be adrenergic.
- *Heart*: bradycardia occurs with atrioventricular block, and eventually cardiac arrest.
- *Bronchi*: there is bronchoconstriction and mucosal hypersecretion that may be clinically serious in asthmatic subjects, in whom cholinergic drugs should be avoided if possible.
- *Gut*: motor activity is increased and may cause colicky pain. Exocrine secretion is also increased. Tone in sphincters falls which may cause defaecation (anal sphincter) or acid reflux/regurgitation (oesophageal sphincter).
- *Urinary bladder and ureters* contract and the drugs promote micturition.

Sympathetic division. Only the ganglia are stimulated and cholinergic nerves to the adrenal medulla. These effects are overshadowed by effects on the parasympathetic system and are usually seen only if atropine has been given to block the latter, when tachycardia, vasoconstriction and hypertension occur.

Neuromuscular (voluntary) junction

The neuromuscular junction has cholinergic nerve endings and so is activated when anticholinesterases allow acetylcholine to persist, causing muscle fasciculation. Prolonged activation leads to a secondary depolarising neuromuscular block.

Central nervous system

There is usually stimulation followed by depression but considerable variation between drugs is observed, possibly due to differences in CNS penetration. In overdose, mental excitement occurs, with confusion and restlessness, insomnia (with nightmares during sleep), tremors and dysarthria, and sometimes even convulsions and coma. Nicotinic receptor activation in the CNS is also thought to be important for cognitive processing, which appears to be impaired in schizophrenic subjects.

Blood vessels

There is stimulation of cholinergic vasodilator nerve endings in addition to the more important dilating action on arterioles and capillaries mediated through non-innervated muscarinic receptors. Activation of these receptors stimulates nitric oxide production from the vascular endothelium that relaxes the underlying smooth muscle.

CHOLINE ESTERS

Acetylcholine

As acetylcholine has such importance in the body it is not surprising that attempts have been made to use it therapeutically. But a substance with such a huge variety of effects and rapid destruction in the body is unlikely to be useful when given systemically, as its use in psychiatry illustrates.

Acetylcholine was first injected intravenously as a therapeutic convulsant in 1939, in the reasonable expectation that the fits would be less liable to cause fractures than those following therapeutic leptazol convulsions. Recovery rates of up to 80% were claimed in various psychotic conditions. Enthusiasm began to wane, however, when it was shown that the fits were due to anoxia resulting from cardiac arrest and not to pharmacological effects on the brain.[1]

The following description is typical:

A few seconds after the injection (which was given as rapidly as possible, to avoid total destruction in the blood) the patient sat up 'with knees drawn up to the chest, the arms flexed and the head bent forward. There were repeated violent coughs, sometimes with flushing. Forced swallowing and loud peristaltic rumblings could be heard'. Respiration was laboured and irregular. 'The coughing abated as the patient sank back in the bed. Forty seconds after the injection the radial and apical pulse were zero and the patient became comatose.' The pupils dilated, and deep reflexes were hyperactive. In 45 seconds the patient went into opisthotonos with brief apnoea.

Lachrymation, sweating and borborygmi were prominent. The deep reflexes became diminished. The patient then relaxed and 'lay quietly in bed – cold moist and gray. In about 90 seconds, flushing of the face marked the return of the pulse'. The respiratory rate rose and consciousness returned in about 125 seconds. The patients sometimes micturated but did not defaecate. They 'tended to lie quietly in bed after the treatment'. 'Most of the patients were reluctant to be retreated.'[2]

Other choline esters

Carbachol is not destroyed by cholinesterase; its actions are most pronounced on the bladder and gastrointestinal tract, so that the drug was used to stimulate these organs, e.g. after surgery. These uses are now virtually obsolete, e.g. catheterisation is preferred for bladder atony. It is occasionally applied topically (3% solution) to the eye as a miotic.

Bethanechol resembles carbachol in its actions but is some 10-fold less potent (it differs by a single β-methyl group) and has no significant nicotinic effects at clinical doses.

ALKALOIDS WITH CHOLINERGIC EFFECTS

Nicotine (see also p. 159) is a social drug that lends its medicinal use as an adjunct to stopping its own abuse as tobacco. It is available as either gum to chew, as dermal patches, a nasal spray or inhalator. These deliver a lower dose of nicotine than cigarettes and appear to be safe in patients with ischaemic heart disease. The patches are slightly better tolerated than the gum, which releases nicotine in a more variable fashion depending on the rate at which it is chewed and the salivary pH, which is influenced by drinking coffee and carbonated drinks. Nicotine treatment is reported to be nearly twice as effective as placebo in achieving sustained withdrawal from smoking (18% versus 11%

[1]Harris M et al 1943 Archives of Neurology and Psychiatry 50:304.

[2]Cohen L H et al 1944 Archives of Neurology and Psychiatry 51:171.

in one review).[3] Treatment is much more likely to be successful if it is used as an aid to, not a substitute for, continued counselling. *Bupropion* is possibly more effective than the nicotine patch[4] (see also p. 162).

Pilocarpine, from a South American plant (*Pilocarpus* spp.), acts directly on muscarinic receptors (see Fig. 21.1); it also stimulates and then depresses the CNS. The chief clinical use of pilocarpine is to lower intraocular pressure in primary open-angle glaucoma (also called chronic simple or wide-angle glaucoma), as an adjunct to a topical β-blocker; it produces miosis, opens drainage channels in the trabecular network and improves the outflow of aqueous humour. Oral pilocarpine is available for the treatment of xerostomia (dry mouth) in Sjögren's syndrome, or following irradiation of head and neck tumours. The commonest adverse effect is sweating, an effect actually exploited in a diagnostic test for cystic fibrosis.

Arecoline is an alkaloid in the betel nut, which is chewed extensively throughout India and South-East Asia. Presumably the lime mix in the 'chews' provides the necessary alkaline pH to maximise its buccal absorption. It produces a mild euphoric effect, like many cholinomimetic alkaloids.

Muscarine is of no therapeutic use but it has pharmacological interest. It is present in small amounts in the fungus *Amanita muscaria* (Fly agaric), named after its capacity to kill the domestic fly (*Musca domestica*); muscarine was so named because it was thought to be the insecticidal principle, but it is relatively non-toxic to flies (orally administered). The fungus may contain other antimuscarinic substances and γ-aminobutyric acid (GABA) receptor agonists (such as muscimol) in amounts sufficient to be psychoactive in humans. The antimuscarinic components may explain why the dried fungus was used previously to treat excessive sweating, especially in patients with tuberculosis.

Poisoning with these fungi may present with antimuscarinic, cholinergic or GABAergic effects. All have CNS actions. Happily, poisoning by *Amanita muscaria* is seldom serious, but species of *Inocybe* contain substantially larger amounts of muscarine

(see Chapter 9). The lengths to which humans are prepared to go in taking 'chemical vacations' when life is hard are shown by the inhabitants of eastern Siberia, who used *Amanita muscaria* recreationally for its cerebral stimulant effects. They were apparently prepared to put up with the autonomic actions to escape briefly from reality – so much so that when the fungus was scarce in winter they were even prepared to drink their own urine to prolong the experience. Sometimes, in generous mood, they would even offer their urine to others as a treat.

ANTICHOLINESTERASES

At cholinergic nerve endings and in erythrocytes there is a specific enzyme that destroys acetylcholine, true cholinesterase or *acetylcholinesterase*. In various tissues, especially plasma, there are other esterases that are not specific for acetylcholine but that also destroy other esters, e.g. suxamethonium, procaine (and cocaine) and bambuterol (a pro-drug that is hydrolysed to terbutaline). Hence, they are called *pseudocholinesterases*.

Chemicals that inactivate these esterases (anticholinesterases) are used in medicine and in agriculture as pesticides. They act by allowing naturally synthesised acetylcholine to accumulate instead of being destroyed. Their effects are explained by this accumulation in the CNS, neuromuscular junction, autonomic ganglia, postganglionic cholinergic nerve endings (which are principally in the parasympathetic nervous system) and in the walls of blood vessels, where acetylcholine has a paracrine[5] role not necessarily associated with nerve endings. Some of these effects oppose one another, e.g. the effect of anticholinesterase on the heart will be the resultant of stimulation at sympathetic ganglia and the opposing effect of stimulation at parasympathetic (vagal) ganglia and at postganglionic nerve endings.

Physostigmine is an alkaloid, obtained from the seeds of the West African Calabar bean (spp. *Physostigma*), which has had long use both as a weapon and as an ordeal poison.[6] It acts for a few hours. It has been shown to have some efficacy in improving cognitive function in Alzheimer-type dementia.

---

[3]Drug and Therapeutics Bulletin 1999; 37 (July issue).
[4]Jorenby D E , Leischow S J, Nides M A et al 1999
A controlled trial of sustained-release bupropion, a nicotine patch, or both for smoking cessation New England Journal of Medicine 340:685–692.

[5]A hormone function that is restricted to the local environment.
[6]To demonstrate guilt or innocence according to whether the accused died or lived after the judicial dose. The practice had the advantage that the demonstration of guilt provided simultaneous punishment.

Neostigmine ($t_{1/2}$ 2 h) is a synthetic reversible anti-cholinesterase whose actions are more prominent on the neuromuscular junction and the alimentary tract than on the cardiovascular system and eye. It is therefore used principally in myasthenia gravis and as an antidote to competitive neuromuscular blocking agents; its use to stimulate the bowels or bladder after surgery is now obsolete. Neostigmine is effective orally, and by injection (usually subcutaneous). But higher doses may be used in myasthenia gravis, often combined with atropine to reduce the unwanted muscarinic effects.

Pyridostigmine is similar to neostigmine but has a less powerful action that is slower in onset and slightly longer in duration, and perhaps with fewer visceral effects. It is used in myasthenia gravis.

Distigmine is a variant of pyridostigmine (two linked molecules as the name implies).

Edrophonium is structurally related to neostigmine but its action is brief and autonomic effects are minimal except at high doses. The drug is used to diagnose myasthenia gravis and to differentiate a myasthenic crisis (weakness due to inadequate anticholinesterase treatment or severe disease) from a cholinergic crisis (weakness caused by overtreatment with an anticholinesterase). Myasthenic weakness is substantially improved by edrophonium whereas cholinergic weakness is aggravated but the effect is transient; the action of 3 mg i.v. is lost in 5 min.

Carbaryl (carbaril) is another reversible carbamoylating anticholinesterase that closely resembles physostigmine in its actions. It is used widely as a garden insecticide and, clinically, to kill head and body lice. Sensitive insects lack cholinesterase-rich erythrocytes and succumb to the accumulation of acetylcholine in the synaptic junctions of their nervous system. Effective and safe use in humans is also probably due to the very limited absorption of carbaryl after topical application. The anticholinesterase *malathion* is effective against scabies, head and crab lice.

A more recent use of anticholinesterase drugs has been to improve cognitive function in patients with Alzheimer's disease, where both the degree of dementia and amyloid plaque density correlate with the impairment of brain cholinergic function. *Donepezil, galantamine* (which has additional nicotinic agonist properties) and *rivastigmine* are licensed

in the UK for this indication. They are all reversible inhibitors that are orally active and cross the blood–brain barrier readily (see p. 368).

Anticholinesterase poisoning

The anticholinesterases used in therapeutics are generally of the carbamate type that reversibly inactivates cholinesterase only for a few hours. This contrasts markedly with the very long-lived inhibition caused by inhibitors of the organophosphate (OP) type. In practice, the inhibition is so long that clinical recovery from organophosphate exposure is usually dependent on synthesis of new enzyme. This process may take weeks to complete, although clinical recovery is usually evident in days. Cases of acute poisoning are usually met outside therapeutic practice, e.g. after agricultural, industrial or transport accidents.

Substances of this type have also been developed and used in war, especially the three G agents: GA (tabun), GB (sarin) and GD (soman). Although called nerve 'gas', they are actually volatile liquids, which facilitates their use.[7] Where there is known risk of exposure, prior use of *pyridostigmine*, which occupies cholinesterases reversibly for a few hours (the lesser evil), competitively protects them from access by the irreversible warfare agent (the greater evil); soldiers during the Gulf Wars expecting attack were provided with preloaded syringes (of the same design as the Epipen for delivering adrenaline [epinephrine]) as antidote therapy (see below). Organophosphate agents are absorbed through the skin, the gastrointestinal tract and by inhalation. Diagnosis depends on observing a substantial part of the list of actions below.

Typical features of acute poisoning involve the gastrointestinal tract (salivation, vomiting, abdominal cramps, diarrhoea, involuntary defaecation), the respiratory system (bronchorrhoea, bronchoconstriction, cough, wheezing, dyspnoea), the cardiovascular system (bradycardia), the genitourinary system (involuntary micturition), the skin (sweating), the skeletal system (muscle weakness, twitching) and the nervous system (miosis, anxiety, headache, convulsions, respiratory failure). Death is due to a combination of

---

[7]In recent times, there have been major instances of use against populations by both military and terrorist bodies (in the field and in an underground transport system).

the actions in the CNS, to paralysis of the respiratory muscles by peripheral depolarising neuromuscular block, and to excessive bronchial secretions and constriction causing respiratory failure. At autopsy, ileal intussusceptions are commonly found.

Quite frequently and typically 1–4 days after resolution of symptoms of acute exposure, the *intermediate syndrome* may develop, characterised by a proximal flaccid limb paralysis that may reflect muscle necrosis. Even later, after a gap of 2–4 weeks, some exposed persons exhibit *delayed polyneuropathy*, with sensory and motor impairment usually of the lower limbs. Claims of chronic effects (subtle cognitive defects, peripheral neuropathy) following recurrent, low-dose exposure, as with organophosphate used as sheep dip, continues to be the subject of investigation but, as yet, there is no conclusive proof.

Treatment. As the most common circumstance of accidental poisoning is exposure to pesticide spray or spillage, contaminated clothing should be removed and the skin washed. Attendants should take care to ensure that they themselves do not become contaminated.

- *Atropine* is the mainstay of treatment; 2 mg is given i.m. or i.v. as soon as possible and repeated every 15–60 min until dryness of the mouth and a heart rate exceeding 70 beats per minute indicate that its effect is adequate. A poisoned patient may require 100 mg or more for a single episode. Atropine antagonises the muscarinic parasympathomimetic effects of the poison, i.e. due to the accumulated acetylcholine stimulating postganglionic nerve endings (excessive secretion and vasodilatation), but has no effect on the neuromuscular block, which is nicotinic.
- *Mechanical ventilation* may therefore be needed to assist the respiratory muscles; special attention to the airway is vital because of bronchial constriction and excessive secretion.
- *Diazepam* may be needed for convulsions.
- *Atropine eyedrops* may relieve the headache caused by miosis.
- *Enzyme reactivation.* The organophosphate (OP) pesticides inactivate cholinesterase by irreversibly phosphorylating the active centre of the enzyme. Substances that reactivate the enzyme hasten the destruction of the accumulated acetylcholine and, unlike atropine, they have both antinicotinic and antimuscarinic effects. The principal agent is *pralidoxime*, which should be given by slow intravenous injection (diluted) over 5–10 min, initially 30 mg/kg repeated every 4–6 h or by intravenous infusion, 8 mg/kg/h; usual maximum 12 g in 24 h. Its efficacy is greatest if administered within 12 h of poisoning, then falls off steadily as the phosphorylated enzyme is further stabilised by 'aging'. If significant reactivation occurs, muscle power improves within 30 min.

Poisoning with *reversible* anticholinesterases is appropriately treated by atropine and the necessary general support; it lasts only hours.

In poisoning with *irreversible* agents, erythrocyte or plasma cholinesterase content should be measured if possible, both for diagnosis and to determine when a poisoned worker may return to the task (should he or she be willing to do so). Return should not be allowed until the cholinesterase exceeds 70% of normal, which may take several weeks. Recovery from the intermediate syndrome and delayed polyneuropathy is slow and is dependent on muscle and nerve regeneration.

DISORDERS OF NEUROMUSCULAR TRANSMISSION

MYASTHENIA GRAVIS

In myasthenia gravis synaptic transmission at the neuromuscular junction is impaired; most cases have an autoimmune basis and some 85% of patients have a raised titre of autoantibodies to the muscle acetylcholine receptor. The condition is probably heterogeneous, as about 15% do not have receptor antibodies, or have antibodies to another neuromuscular junction protein (muscle specific kinase) and, rarely, it occurs with penicillamine used for rheumatoid arthritis.

Neostigmine was introduced in 1931 for its stimulant effects on intestinal activity. In 1934 it occurred to Dr Mary Walker that, as the paralysis of myasthenia had been (erroneously) attributed to a curare-like substance in the blood, physostigmine (eserine), an anticholinesterase drug known to antagonise curare, might be beneficial. It was, and she reported this important observation in a short letter.[8] Soon after this she used neostigmine by mouth, with greater benefit. The sudden appearance of an effective treatment for a hitherto untreatable chronic disease must always be a dramatic event for its victims. One patient described the impact of the discovery of the action of neostigmine, as follows:

> My myasthenia started in 1925, when I was 18. For several months it consisted of double vision and fatigue … An ophthalmic surgeon … prescribed glasses with a prism. However, soon more alarming symptoms began. [Her limbs became weak and she] 'was sent to an eminent neurologist. This was a horrible experience. He … could find no physical signs … declared me to be suffering from hysteria and asked me what was on my mind. When I answered truthfully, that nothing except anxiety over my symptoms, he replied 'my dear child, I am not a perfect fool…', and showed me out. [She became worse and at times she was unable to turn over in bed. Eating and even speaking were difficult. Eventually, her fiancé, a medical student, read about myasthenia gravis and she was correctly diagnosed in 1927.] There was at that time no known treatment and therefore many things to try. [She had gold injections, thyroid, suprarenal extract, lecithin, glycine and ephedrine. The last had a slight effect.] Then in February 1935, came the day that I shall always remember. I was living alone with a nurse … It was one of my better days, and I was lying on the sofa after tea … My fiancé came in rather late saying that he had something new for me to try. My first thought was 'Oh bother! Another injection, and another false hope'. I submitted to the injection with complete indifference and within a few minutes began to feel very strange … when I lifted my arms, exerting the effort to which I had become accustomed, they shot into the air, every movement I attempted was grotesquely magnified until I learnt to make less effort … it was strange, wonderful and at first, very frightening … we danced twice round the carpet. That was my first meeting with neostigmine, and we have never since been separated.[9]

Pathogenesis. The clinical features of myasthenia gravis are caused by specific autoantibodies to the nicotinic acetylcholine receptor. These antibodies accelerate receptor turnover, shortening their typical lifetime in the skeletal muscle membrane from around 7 days, to 1 day in a myasthenic. This process results in marked depletion of receptors from myasthenic skeletal muscle (about 90%), explaining its fatigability. The frequent finding of a specific human leucocyte antigen (HLA) haplotype (A1-B8-Dw3) in myasthenics and concurrent hyperplasia or tumours of the thymus support the autoimmune basis for the disease.

Diagnosis. Edrophonium dramatically and transiently (5 min) relieves myasthenic muscular weakness. A syringe is loaded with edrophonium 10 mg; 2 mg is given i.v. and if there is no improvement in weakness in 30 s the remaining 8 mg is injected. Adults without suitable veins may receive 10 mg by i.m. injection. Atropine should be at hand to block severe cholinergic autonomic (muscarinic) effects, e.g. bradycardia, should they occur.

Titres of acetylcholine receptor antibodies should also be measured to confirm the diagnosis.

Treatment involves immunosuppression, thymectomy (unless contraindicated) and symptom relief with drugs:

- *Immunosuppressive treatment* is directed at eliminating the acetylcholine receptor autoantibody. *Prednisolone* induces improvement or remission in 80% of cases. The dose should be increased slowly using an alternate-day regimen until the minimum effective amount is attained; an immunosuppressive improvement may take several weeks. *Azathioprine* may be used as a steroid-sparing agent. Prednisolone is effective for ocular myasthenia, which is fortunate, for this variant of the disease responds poorly to thymectomy or anticholinesterase drugs. Some acute and severe cases respond poorly to prednisolone with azathioprine and, for these, intermittent plasmapheresis or immunoglobulin i.v. (to remove circulating anti-receptor antibody) can provide dramatic short-term relief.
- *Thymectomy* should be offered to those with generalised myasthenia gravis under 40 years of age, once the clinical state allows and unless there are powerful contraindications to surgery. Most cases benefit and about 25% can discontinue drug treatment. Thymectomy should also be undertaken in all myasthenic patients who have a thymoma, but the main reason is to prevent local infiltration, as the procedure is less likely to relieve the myasthenia.
- *Symptomatic* drug treatment is decreasingly used. Its aim is to increase the concentration

---

[8]Walker M B 1934 Lancet i:1200.
[9]*Disabilities and How to Live with Them.* (1952) Lancet Publications, London.

of acetylcholine at the neuromuscular junction with anticholinesterase drugs. The mainstay is usually *pyridostigmine*, starting with 60 mg by mouth 4-hourly. It is preferred because its action is smoother than that of neostigmine, but the latter is more rapid in onset and can with advantage be given in the mornings to get the patient mobile. Either drug can be given parenterally if bulbar paralysis makes swallowing difficult. An antimuscarinic drug, e.g. propantheline (15–30 mg t.i.d.), should be added if muscarinic effects are troublesome.

Excessive dosing with an anticholinesterase can actually worsen the muscle weakness in myasthenics if the accumulation of acetylcholine at the neuromuscular junction is sufficient to cause depolarising blockade (*cholinergic crisis*). It is important to distinguish this type of muscle weakness from an exacerbation of the disease itself (*myasthenic crisis*). The dilemma can be resolved with a test dose of edrophonium 2 mg i.v. (best before next dose of anticholinesterase), which relieves a myasthenic crisis but worsens a cholinergic one. The latter may be severe enough to precipitate respiratory failure and should be attempted only with full resuscitation facilities, including mechanical ventilation, at hand.

A cholinergic crisis should be treated by withdrawing all anticholinesterase medication, mechanical ventilation if required, and atropine i.v. for muscarinic effects of the overdose. The neuromuscular block is a nicotinic effect and will be unchanged by atropine. A resistant myasthenic crisis may be treated by withdrawal of drugs and mechanical ventilation for a few days. Plasmapheresis or immunoglobulin i.v. may be beneficial by removing anti-receptor antibodies (see above).

LAMBERT–EATON SYNDROME

Separate from myasthenia gravis is the Lambert–Eaton syndrome, in which symptoms similar to those of myasthenia gravis occur in association with a carcinoma; in 60% of patients this is a small-cell lung cancer. The defect here is presynaptic with a deficiency of acetylcholine release due to an autoantibody directed against L-type voltage-gated calcium channels.

Patients with the Lambert–Eaton syndrome do not usually respond well to anticholinesterases. The drug 3,4-diaminopyridine (3,4-DAP) increases neurotransmitter release and also the action potential (by blocking potassium conductance), producing a non-specific enhancement of cholinergic neurotransmission. It should be taken orally, four or five times a day. Adverse effects due to CNS excitation (insomnia, seizures) can occur. An example of an orphan drug without a product licence, 3,4-DAP is available in the UK on a 'named patient' basis.

DRUG-INDUCED DISORDERS OF NEUROMUSCULAR TRANSMISSION

Quite apart from the neuromuscular blocking agents used in anaesthesia, a number of drugs possess actions that impair neuromuscular transmission and, in appropriate circumstances, give rise to:

- Postoperative respiratory depression in people with otherwise normal neuromuscular transmission.
- Aggravation or unmasking of myasthenia gravis.
- A drug-induced myasthenic syndrome.

These drugs include:

Antimicrobials. Aminoglycosides (neomycin, streptomycin, gentamicin), polypeptides (colistimethate sodium, polymyxin B) and perhaps the quinolones (e.g. ciprofloxacin) may cause postoperative breathing difficulty if they are instilled into the peritoneal or pleural cavity. It appears that the antibiotics both interfere with the release of acetylcholine and also have a competitive curare-like effect on the acetylcholine receptor.

Cardiovascular drugs. Those that possess local anaesthetic properties (quinidine, procainamide, lidocaine) and certain β-blockers (propranolol, oxprenolol) interfere with acetylcholine release and may aggravate or reveal myasthenia gravis.

Other drugs. *Penicillamine* causes some patients, especially those with rheumatoid arthritis, to form antibodies to the acetylcholine receptor and a syndrome indistinguishable from myasthenia gravis results. Spontaneous recovery occurs in about two-thirds of cases when penicillamine is withdrawn. Phenytoin may rarely induce or aggravate myasthenia gravis, or induce a myasthenic syndrome, possibly by depressing release of acetylcholine. Lithium may impair presynaptic neurotransmission by substituting for sodium ions in the nerve terminal.

DRUGS THAT OPPOSE ACETYLCHOLINE

These may be divided into:

- *Antimuscarinic drugs*, which act principally at postganglionic cholinergic (parasympathetic) nerve endings, i.e. atropine-related drugs (see Fig. 21.1). Muscarinic receptors can be subdivided according to their principal sites, namely in the brain (M_1), heart (M_2) and glandular, gastric parietal cells and smooth muscle cells (M_3). As with many receptors, the molecular basis of the subtypes has been defined together with two further cloned subtypes M_4 and M_5, the precise functional roles of which remain to be clarified.
- *Antinicotinic drugs:*
  - ganglion-blocking drugs (see Chapter 24)
  - neuromuscular blocking drugs (see Fig. 21.1 and Chapter 18).

ANTIMUSCARINIC DRUGS

Atropine is the prototype drug of this group and will be described first. Other named agents will be mentioned only in so far as they differ from atropine. All act as non-selective and competitive antagonists of the various muscarinic receptor subtypes (above). Atropine is a simple tertiary amine; certain others (see Summary) are quaternary nitrogen compounds, a modification that increases antimuscarinic potency in the gut, imparts ganglion-blocking effects and reduces CNS penetration.

Atropine

Atropine is an alkaloid from the deadly nightshade, *Atropa belladonna*.[10] It is a racemate (DL-hyoscyamine), and almost all of its antimuscarinic effects are attributable to the L-isomer alone. Atropine is more stable chemically as the racemate, which is the preferred formulation. In general, the effects of atropine are inhibitory but in large doses it stimulates the CNS

(see poisoning, below). Atropine also blocks the muscarinic effects of injected cholinergic drugs, both peripherally and on the CNS. The clinically important actions of atropine at parasympathetic postganglionic nerve endings are listed below; they are mostly the opposite of the activating effects on the parasympathetic system produced by cholinergic drugs.

Exocrine glands. All secretions except milk are diminished. Dry mouth and dry eye are common. Gastric acid secretion is reduced but so also is the total volume of gastric secretion, so that pH may be little altered. Sweating is inhibited (sympathetic innervation but releasing acetylcholine). Bronchial secretions are reduced and may become viscid, which can be a disadvantage, as removal of secretion by cough and ciliary action is rendered less effective.

Smooth muscle is relaxed. In the gastrointestinal tract there is reduction of tone and peristalsis. Muscle spasm of the intestinal tract induced by morphine is reduced, but such spasm in the biliary tract is not significantly affected. Atropine relaxes bronchial muscle, an effect that is useful in some asthmatics. Micturition is slowed and urinary retention may be induced, especially when there is pre-existing prostatic enlargement.

Ocular effects. Mydriasis occurs with a rise in intraocular pressure due to the dilated iris blocking drainage of the intraocular fluid from the angle of the anterior chamber. An attack of glaucoma may be induced in eyes predisposed to primary angle (also called acute closed-angle or narrow-angle) closure and is a medical emergency. There is no significant effect on pressure in normal eyes. The ciliary muscle is paralysed and so the eye is accommodated for distant vision. After atropinisation, normal pupillary reflexes may not be regained for 2 weeks. Atropine use is a cause of unequally sized and unresponsive pupils.[11]

---

[10]The first name commemorates its success as a homicidal poison, for it is derived from the senior of three legendary Fates, Atropos, who cuts with shears the thread of life spun out by her sister Clothos, of a length determined by her other sister Lachesis (there is a minor synthetic atropine-like drug called lachesine). The term belladonna (Italian: beautiful woman) refers to the once fashionable female practice of using an extract of the plant to dilate the pupils (incidentally blocking ocular accommodation) as part of the process of improving attractiveness.

[11]A doctor, after working in his garden greenhouse, was alarmed to find that the vision in his left eye was blurred and the pupil was grossly dilated. Physical examination failed to reveal a cause and the pupil gradually and spontaneously returned to normal, suggesting that the explanation was exposure to some exogenous agent. The doctor then recalled that his greenhouse contained flowering plants called 'angels' trumpet' (sp. *Brugmansia*, syn. *Datura*, of the nightshade family), and he may have brushed against them. Angels' trumpet is noted for its content of scopolamine (hyoscine), and is very toxic if ingested. The plant is evidently less angelic than the name suggests (Merrick J, Barnett S 2000 British Medical Journal 321:219).

Cardiovascular system. Atropine reduces vagal tone, thus increasing the heart rate and enhancing conduction in the bundle of His. As efficacy depends on the level of vagal tone, full atropinisation may increase heart rate by 30 beats/min in a young subject, but has little effect in the elderly.

Atropine has no significant effect on peripheral blood vessels in therapeutic doses but in overdose there is marked vasodilatation.

Central nervous system. Atropine is effective against both the tremor and rigidity of parkinsonism. It prevents or abates motion sickness.

Antagonism to cholinergic drugs. Atropine opposes the effects of muscarinic agonists on the CNS, at postganglionic cholinergic nerve endings and on peripheral blood vessels. It does not block cholinergic effects at the neuromuscular junction or significantly at the autonomic ganglia, i.e. atropine opposes the muscarine-like but not the nicotine-like effects of acetylcholine.

Pharmacokinetics. Atropine is readily absorbed from the gastrointestinal tract and may also be injected by the usual routes, including intratracheal instillation in an emergency setting. The occasional cases of atropine poisoning following use of eyedrops are due to the solution running down the lachrymal ducts into the nose and being swallowed. Atropine is in part destroyed in the liver and in part excreted unchanged by the kidney ($t_{1/2}$ 2 h).

Dose. 0.6–1.2 mg by mouth at night or 0.6 mg i.v., repeated as necessary to a maximum of 3 mg per day; for chronic use atropine has largely been replaced by other antimuscarinic drugs.

Poisoning with atropine (and other antimuscarinic drugs) presents with the more obvious peripheral effects: dry mouth (with dysphagia), mydriasis, blurred vision, hot, flushed, dry skin, and, in addition, hyperthermia (CNS action plus absence of sweating), restlessness, anxiety, excitement, hallucinations, delirium, mania. The cerebral excitation is followed by depression and coma or, as it has been described with characteristic American verbal felicity, 'hot as a hare, blind as a bat, dry as a bone, red as a beet and mad as a hen'.[12] Poisoning typically seen (especially in

children) following ingestion of the rather attractive berries of solanaceous plants, e.g. deadly nightshade and henbane. Treatment involves activated charcoal to adsorb the drug, sponging to cool the patient and diazepam for the central excitement.

Uses of antimuscarinic drugs

- **For their central actions** – some (benzhexol [trihexyphenidyl] and orphenadrine) are used against the rigidity and tremor of *parkinsonism*, especially drug-induced parkinsonism, where doses higher than the usual therapeutic amounts are often needed and tolerated. They are used as *antiemetics* (principally hyoscine, promethazine). Their sedative action is used in anaesthetic premedication (hyoscine).
- **For their peripheral actions** – atropine, homatropine and cyclopentolate are used in *ophthalmology* to dilate the pupil and to paralyse ocular accommodation. Patients should be warned of a transient, but unpleasant, stinging sensation, and that they cannot read or drive (at least without dark glasses) for at least 3–4 h. Tropicamide is the shortest acting of the mydriatics. If it is desired to dilate the pupil and to spare accommodation, a sympathomimetic, e.g. phenylephrine, is useful.

In anaesthesic premedication, atropine, and hyoscine* block the vagus and reduce mucosal secretions; hyoscine also has useful sedative effects. Glycopyrronium* is frequently used during anaesthetic recovery to block the muscarinic effects of neostigmine given to reverse a non-depolarising neuromuscular blockade.

In the respiratory tract, ipratropium* is a useful bronchodilator in chronic obstructive pulmonary disease and acute asthma.

- **For their actions on the gut,** against muscle spasm and hypermotility, e.g. against colic (pain due to spasm of smooth muscle) and to reduce morphine-induced smooth muscle spasm when the analgesic is used against acute colic.
- **In the urinary tract,** flavoxate, oxybutynin, propiverine, tolterodine, trospium and propantheline* are used to relieve muscle spasm accompanying infection in cystitis, and for detrusor instability.

---

[12]Cohen H L et al 1944 Archives of Neurology and Psychiatry 51:171.

- **In disorders of the cardiovascular system,** atropine is useful in bradycardia following myocardial infarction.
- **In cholinergic poisoning,** atropine is an important antagonist of both central nervous, parasympathomimetic and vasodilator effects, though it has no effect at the neuromuscular junction and will not prevent voluntary muscle paralysis. It is also used to block muscarinic effects when cholinergic drugs, such as neostigmine, are used for their effect on the neuromuscular junction in myasthenia gravis.

Disadvantages of the antimuscarinics include glaucoma and urinary retention, where there is prostatic hypertrophy.

*Quaternary ammonium compounds (see text).

Other antimuscarinic drugs

In the following accounts, the peripheral atropine-like effects of the drugs may be assumed; only differences from atropine are described.

Hyoscine (scopolamine) is structurally a close relative of atropine. It differs chiefly in being a CNS depressant, although it may sometimes cause excitement. Elderly patients are often confused by hyoscine and so it is avoided in their anaesthetic premedication. Mydriasis is also briefer than with atropine.

Hyoscine butylbromide (strictly *N*-butylhyoscine bromide, Buscopan) also blocks autonomic ganglia. If injected, it is an effective relaxant of smooth muscle, including the cardia in achalasia, the pyloric antral region and the colon, properties utilised by radiologists and endoscopists. It may sometimes be useful for colic.

Homatropine is used for its ocular effects (1% and 2% solutions as eye-drops). Its action is shorter than that of atropine, and it is therefore less likely to cause serious increases in intraocular pressure; the effect wears off in a day or two. Complete cycloplegia cannot always be obtained unless repeated instillations are made every 15 min for 1–2 h. Its effects are especially unreliable in children, in whom cyclopentolate or atropine is preferred. The

pupillary dilatation may be reversed by physostigmine eye-drops.

Tropicamide (Mydriacyl) and *cyclopentolate* (Mydrilate) are useful (as 0.5% or 1% solutions) for mydriasis and cycloplegia. They are quicker and shorter acting than homatropine. Both cause mydriasis in 10–20 min and cycloplegia shortly thereafter. The duration of action is 4–12 h.

Ipratropium (Atrovent) is used as an inhaled bronchodilator for both acute asthma and chronic obstructive pulmonary disease (COPD), and in chronic COPD. It has very limited efficacy in most chronic asthmatics.

Tiotropium (Spiriva) is a long-acting (>24 h) alternative to ipratropium, but only for patients with chronic COPD. It is not licensed for acute bronchoconstriction because of its slow onset of action.

Flavoxate (Urispas) is used for urinary frequency, tenesmus and urgency incontinence because it increases bladder capacity and reduces unstable detrusor contractions (see p. 491).

Oxybutynin is also used for detrusor instability, but antimuscarinic adverse effects may limit its value.

Glycopyrronium is used in anaesthetic premedication to reduce salivary secretion; given intravenously it causes less tachycardia than atropine.

Propantheline (Pro-Banthine) also has ganglion-blocking properties. It may be used as a smooth muscle relaxant, e.g. for irritable bowel syndrome and diagnostic procedures.

Dicyclomine (Merbentyl) is an alternative.

Benzhexol (*trihexyphenidyl*) and *orphenadrine*: see parkinsonism (p. 380).

Promethazine. See p. 50.

Propiverine, *tolterodine* and *trospium* diminish unstable detrusor contractions and are used to reduce urinary frequency, urgency and incontinence.

Oral antimuscarinics have occasional use in the treatment of hyperhidrosis.

Summary

- Acetylcholine is the most important receptor agonist neurotransmitter in both the brain and the peripheral nervous system.
- It acts on neurones in the CNS and at autonomic ganglia, on skeletal muscle at the neuromuscular junction, and at a variety of other effector cell types, mainly glandular or smooth muscle.
- The effector response is terminated rapidly through enzymatic destruction by acetylcholinesterase.
- Outside the CNS, acetylcholine has two main classes of receptor: those on autonomic ganglia and skeletal muscle responding to stimulation by nicotine, and the rest which respond to stimulation by muscarine.
- Drugs that mimic or oppose acetylcholine have a wide variety of uses. For instance, the muscarinic agonist pilocarpine lowers intraocular pressure and antagonist atropine reverses vagal slowing of the heart.
- The main use of drugs at the neuromuscular junction is to relax muscle in anaesthesia, or to inhibit acetylcholinesterase in diseases where nicotinic receptor activation is reduced, e.g. myasthenia gravis.

GUIDE TO FURTHER READING

1987 Medical manual of defence against chemical agents (no. 0117725692) (JSP 312) HMSO, London

Cohen L H et al 1944 Acetylcholine treatment of schizophrenia. Archives of Neurology and Psychiatry 51:171–175

Hawkins J R et al 1956 Intravenous acetylcholine therapy in neurosis. A controlled clinical trial. Journal of Mental Science 102:43 (in the same issue see also: Carbon dioxide inhalation therapy in neurosis. A controlled clinical trial (p. 52); The placebo response (p. 60).

Morita H, Yanigasawa T, Shimizu M et al 1995 Sarin poisoning in Matsumoto, Japan. Lancet 346:290–293

Morton H G et al 1939 Atropine intoxication: its manifestation in infants and children. Journal of Pediatrics 14(6):755–760

Report 1998 Organophosphate sheep dip: clinical aspects of long-term low-dose exposure. Royal College of Physicians and Royal College of Psychiatrists, London

Steenland K 1996 Chronic neurological effects of organophosphate pesticides. British Medical Journal 312:1312–1313

Vincent A, Palace J, Hilton-Jones D 2001 Myasthenia gravis. Lancet 357:2122–2128

Weitz G 2003 Love and death in Wagner's *Tristan und Isolde* – an epic anticholinergic crisis. British Medical Journal 327:1469–1471

22

Adrenergic mechanisms and drugs

SYNOPSIS

Anyone who administers drugs acting on cardiovascular adrenergic mechanisms requires an understanding of how they act in order to use them to the best advantage and with safety.

- Adrenergic mechanisms
- Classification of sympathomimetics: by mode of action and selectivity for adrenoceptors
- Individual sympathomimetics
- Mucosal decongestants
- Shock
- Chronic orthostatic hypotension

ADRENERGIC MECHANISMS

The discovery in 1895 of the hypertensive effect of adrenaline (epinephrine) was initiated by Dr Oliver, a physician in practice, who conducted a series of experiments on his young son into whom he injected an extract of bovine suprarenal and detected a 'definite narrowing of the radial artery'.[1] The effect was confirmed in animals and led eventually to the isolation and synthesis of adrenaline in the early 1900s. Many related compounds were examined and, in 1910, Barger and Dale invented the word sympathomimetic[2] and also pointed out that noradrenaline (norepinephrine) mimicked the action of the sympathetic nervous system more closely than did adrenaline.

Adrenaline, noradrenaline and dopamine are formed in the body and are used in therapeutics. The natural synthetic path is: tyrosine → dopa → dopamine → noradrenaline → adrenaline.

CLASSIFICATION OF SYMPATHOMIMETICS

BY MODE OF ACTION

Noradrenaline is synthesised and stored in vesicles within adrenergic nerve terminals (Fig. 22.1). The vesicles can be released from these stores by stimulating the nerve or by drugs (ephedrine, amfetamine). The noradrenaline stores can also be replenished by intravenous infusion of noradrenaline, and abolished by reserpine or by cutting the sympathetic nerve. Sympathomimetics may be classified on the basis of their sites of action (see Fig. 22.1) as acting:

1. **directly**: *adrenoceptor agonists*, e.g. adrenaline, noradrenaline, isoprenaline (isoproterenol), methoxamine, xylometazoline, metaraminol (entirely); and dopamine and phenylephrine (mainly)
2. **indirectly**: by causing a release of *noradrenaline* from stores at nerve endings[3], e.g. amfetamines, tyramine; and ephedrine (largely)
3. **by both mechanisms** (1 and 2, though often with a preponderance of one or other): *other synthetic agents*.

All of the above mechanisms operate in both the central and peripheral nervous systems, but discussion below will focus on agents that influence peripheral adrenergic mechanisms.

---

[1]Dale H 1938 Edinburgh Medical Journal 45:461.
[2]'Compounds which … simulate the effects of sympathetic nerves not only with varying intensity but with varying precision … a term … seems needed to indicate the types of action common to these bases. We propose to call it "sympathomimetic". A term which indicates the relation of the action to innervation by the sympathetic system, without involving any theoretical preconception as to the meaning of that relation or the precise mechanism of the action' (Barger G, Dale H H 1910 Journal of Physiology XLI:19–50).

[3]Fatal hypertension can occur when this class of agent is taken by a patient treated with monoamine oxidase inhibitor. In addition, remember that large amounts of tyramine are contained in certain food substances (cheese, red wine and marmite), forming the basis of the pressor 'cheese reaction' in these patients (see p. 339).

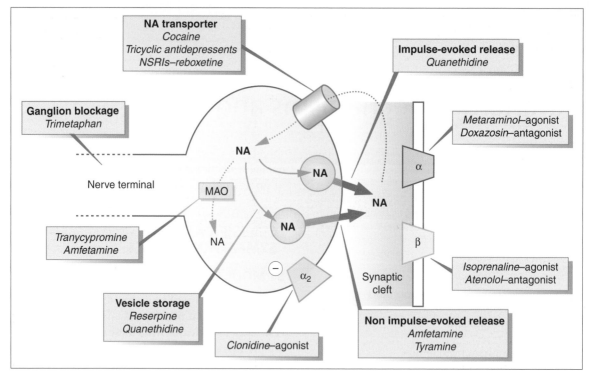

Fig. 22.1 Cartoon of a noradrenergic nerve terminal releasing noradrenaline (NA) to show the sites of action of drugs that impair or mimic adrenergic function. α and β refer to adrenergic receptor subtypes; MAO, monoamine oxidase.

Tachyphylaxis (rapidly diminishing response to repeated administration) is a particular feature of group 2 drugs. It reflects depletion of the 'releasable' pool of noradrenaline from adrenergic nerve terminals that makes these agents less suitable as, for example, pressor agents than drugs in group 1. Longer-term tolerance (see p. 80) to the effects of direct sympathomimetics is much less of a clinical problem and reflects an alteration in adrenergic receptor density or coupling to second messenger systems.

Interactions of sympathomimetics with other vasoactive drugs are complex. Some drugs block the reuptake mechanism for noradrenaline in adrenergic nerve terminals and potentiate the pressor effects of noradrenaline e.g. cocaine, tricyclic antidepressants or highly noradrenaline-selective reuptake inhibitors (NSRIs) such as reboxetine (see Fig. 22.1). Others deplete or destroy the intracellular stores within adrenergic nerve terminals (e.g. reserpine and guanethidine) and thus block the action of indirect sympathomimetics.

Sympathomimetics are also generally optically active drugs, with only one stereoisomer conferring most of the clinical efficacy of the racemate (a 50:50 mixture of stereoisomers); for instance, L-noradrenaline is at least 50 times as active as the D-form. Noradrenaline, adrenaline and phenylephrine are all used clinically as their L-isomers.

History. Up to 1948 it was known that the peripheral motor (vasoconstriction) effects of adrenaline were preventable and that the peripheral inhibitory (vasodilatation) and cardiac stimulant actions were not preventable by the then available antagonists (ergot alkaloids, phenoxybenzamine). That same year, Ahlquist hypothesised that this was due to two different sorts of adrenoceptors (α and β). For a further 10 years, only antagonists of α-receptor effects (α-adrenoceptor block) were known, but in 1958 the first substance selectively and competitively to prevent β-receptor effects (β-adrenoceptor block), dichloroisoprenaline, was synthesised. It was unsuitable for clinical use because it behaved as a partial agonist, and it was not until 1962 that pronethalol (an isoprenaline analogue) became the first β-adrenoceptor blocker to be used clinically. Unfortunately it had a low therapeutic index and was carcinogenic in mice; it was soon replaced by propranolol.

Table 22.1 Clinically relevant aspects of adrenoceptor functions and actions of agonists

α_1-adrenoceptor effects[a]	β-adrenoceptor effects
Eye:[b] mydriasis	
	Heart (β_1, β_2):[c]
	increased rate (SA node)
	increased automaticity (AV node and muscle)
	increased velocity in conducting tissue
	increased contractility of myocardium
	increased oxygen consumption decreased refractory period of all tissues
Arterioles:	**Arterioles:**
constriction (only slight in coronary and cerebral)	dilatation (β_2)
	Bronchi (β_2): relaxation
	Anti-inflammatory effect:
	inhibition of release of autacoids (histamine, leukotrienes) from mast cells, e.g. asthma in type I allergy
Uterus: contraction (pregnant)	**Uterus** (β_2): relaxation (pregnant)
	Skeletal muscle: tremor (β_2)
Skin: sweat, pilomotor	
Male ejaculation	
Blood platelet: aggregation	
Metabolic effect:	**Metabolic effects:**
hyperkalaemia	hypokalaemia (β_2)
	hepatic glycogenolysis (β_2)
	lipolysis (β_1, β_2)
Bladder sphincter: contraction	**Bladder detrusor:** relaxation
Intestinal smooth muscle relaxation is mediated by α and β adrenoceptors.	
α_2-adrenoceptor effects:[a] α_2 receptors on the nerve ending, i.e. presynaptic autoreceptors, mediate negative feedback which inhibits noradrenaline release	

[a]For the role of subtypes (α_1 and α_2), see prazosin.
[b]Effects on intraocular pressure involve both α and β adrenoceptors as well as cholinoceptors.
[c]Cardiac β_1 receptors mediate effects of sympathetic nerve stimulation. Cardiac β_2 receptors mediate effects of circulating adrenaline, when this is secreted at a sufficient rate, e.g. following myocardial infarction or in heart failure. Both receptors are coupled to the same intracellular signalling pathway (cyclic AMP production) and mediate the same biological effects.
Use of the term cardioselective to mean β_1-receptor selective only, especially in the case of β-receptor blocking drugs, is no longer appropriate. Although in most species the β_1 receptor is the only cardiac β receptor, this is not the case in humans. What is not generally appreciated is that the endogenous sympathetic neurotransmitter noradrenaline has about a 20-fold selectivity for the β_1 receptor – similar to that of the antagonist atenolol – with the consequence that under most circumstances, in most tissues, there is little or no β_2-receptor stimulation to be affected by a non-selective β-blocker. Why asthmatics should be so sensitive to β-blockade is paradoxical: all the bronchial β receptors are β_2, and the bronchi themselves are not innervated by adrenergic fibres; the circulating adrenaline levels are, if anything, low in asthma.

It is evident that the site of action has an important role in selectivity, e.g. drugs that act on end-organ receptors directly and stereospecifically may be highly selective, whereas drugs that act indirectly by discharging noradrenaline indiscriminately from nerve endings, e.g. amfetamine, will have a wider range of effects.

Subclassification of adrenoceptors is shown in Table 22.1.

Consequences of adrenoceptor activation

All adrenoceptors are members of the G-coupled family of receptor proteins, i.e. the receptor is coupled to its effector protein through special transduction proteins called G-proteins (themselves a large protein family). The effector protein differs amongst adrenoceptor subtypes. In the case of β-adrenoceptors, the effector is adenylyl cyclase and hence cyclic AMP is the second messenger molecule. For α-adrenoceptors, phospholipase C is the commonest effector protein and the second messenger here is inositol trisphosphate (IP_3). It is the cascade of events initiated by the second messenger molecules that produces the variety of tissue effects shown in Table 22.1. Hence, specificity is provided by the receptor subtype, not the messengers.

SELECTIVITY FOR ADRENOCEPTORS

The following classification of sympathomimetics and antagonists is based on selectivity for receptors and on use. But selectivity is relative, not absolute; some agonists act on both α and β receptors, some are partial agonists and, if sufficient drug is administered, many will extend their range. The same applies to selective antagonists (receptor blockers), e.g. a β_1-selective adrenoceptor blocker can cause severe exacerbation of asthma (a β_2 effect), even at low dose. It is important to remember this because patients have died in the hands of doctors who have forgotten or been ignorant of it.[4]

Adrenoceptor agonists (see Table 22.1)

α + β effects, non-selective: *adrenaline* is used as a vasoconstrictor (α) with local anaesthetics, as a mydriatic (α), and in the emergency treatment of anaphylactic shock (see p. 122).

α_1 effects: *noradrenaline* (with slight β effect on the heart) is selectively released physiologically, but as a therapeutic agent it is used for hypotensive states, excepting septic shock where dopamine and dobutamine are preferred (for their cardiac inotropic effect). Other agents with predominantly α_1 effects are imidazolines (xylometazoline, oxymetazoline), metaramitnol, phenylephrine, phenylpropanolamine, ephedrine and pseudoephedrine; some are used solely for topical vasoconstriction (nasal decongestants).

α_2 effects in the central nervous system: *clonidine*.

β Effects, non-selective (i.e. β_1 + β_2): *isoprenaline* (isoproterenol). Its uses as a bronchodilator (β_2), positive cardiac inotrope and to enhance conduction in heart block (β_1, β_2) have largely been superseded by more selective agents. Other non-selective β agonists (ephedrine and orciprenaline) are also obsolete.

β_1 effects, with some α effects: *dopamine*, used in cardiogenic shock.

β_1 effects: *dobutamine*, used for cardiac inotropic effect.

β_2 effects, used in *asthma*, or to relax the uterus, include: salbutamol, terbutaline, fenoterol, pirbuterol, reproterol, rimiterol, isoxsuprine, orciprenaline, ritodrine.

Adrenoceptor antagonists (blockers)

See page 76.

Effects of a sympathomimetic

The overall effect of a sympathomimetic depends on the site of action (receptor agonist or indirect action), on receptor specificity and on dose; for instance adrenaline ordinarily dilates muscle blood vessels (β_2; mainly arterioles, but veins also) but in very large doses constricts them (α). The end-results are often complex and unpredictable, partly because of the variability of homeostatic reflex responses and partly because what is observed, e.g. a change in blood pressure, is the result of many factors, e.g. vasodilatation (β) in some areas, vasoconstriction (α) in others, and cardiac stimulation (β).

To block all the effects of adrenaline and noradrenaline, antagonists for both α and β receptors must be used. This can be a matter of practical importance, e.g. in phaeochromocytoma (see p. 76).

Physiological note. The termination of action of noradrenaline released at nerve endings is by:

- reuptake into nerve endings where it is stored or subject to monoamine oxidase (MAO) degradation (see Fig. 22.1)
- diffusion away from the area of the nerve ending and the receptor (junctional cleft)
- metabolism (by extraneuronal MAO and catechol-*O*-methyltransferase, COMT).

These processes are slower than the rapid destruction of acetylcholine at the neuromuscular junction by extracellular acetylcholinesterase seated alongside the receptors. This reflects the differing signalling requirements: almost instantaneous (millisecond) responses for voluntary muscle movement versus the much more leisurely contraction of arteriolar muscle to control vascular resistance.

---

[4]Although it is simplest to regard the selectivity of a drug as relative, being lost at higher doses, strictly speaking it is the benefits of the receptor selectivity of an agonist or antagonist that are dose dependent. A 10-fold selectivity of an agonist at the β_1 receptor, for instance, is a property of the agonist that is independent of dose, and means simply that 10 times less of the agonist is required to activate this receptor compared with the β_2 subtype.

Synthetic non-catecholamines in clinical use have a $t_{1/2}$ of hours, e.g. salbutamol 4 h, because they are more resistant to enzymatic degradation and conjugation. They may be given orally, although much higher doses are then required. They penetrate the central nervous system (CNS) and may have prominent effects, e.g. amfetamine. Substantial amounts appear in the urine.

Pharmacokinetics

Catecholamines (adrenaline [epinephrine], noradrenaline [norepinephrine], dopamine, dobutamine, isoprenaline) (plasma $t_{1/2}$ approx. 2 min) are metabolised by MAO and COMT. These enzymes are present in large amounts in the liver and kidney, and account for most of the metabolism of injected catecholamines. MAO is also present in the intestinal mucosa (and in peripheral and central nerve endings). Because of these enzymes catecholamines are ineffective when swallowed, but non-catecholamines, e.g. salbutamol and amfetamine, are effective orally.

Adverse effects

These may be deduced from their actions (Table 22.1, Fig. 22.2). Tissue necrosis due to intense vasoconstriction (α) around injection sites occurs as a result of leakage from intravenous infusions. The effects on the heart (β_1) include tachycardia, palpitations, cardiac arrhythmias including ventricular tachycardia and fibrillation, and muscle tremor (β_2). Sympathomimetic drugs should be used with great caution in patients with heart disease.

The effect of the sympathomimetic drugs on the pregnant uterus is variable and difficult to predict, but serious fetal distress can occur, due to reduced placental blood flow as a result both of contraction of the uterine muscle (α) and arterial constriction (α). β_2-Agonists are used to relax the uterus in premature labour, but unwanted cardiovascular actions can be troublesome. Sympathomimetics were particularly likely to cause cardiac arrhythmias (β_1 effect) in patients who received halothane anaesthesia (now rarely used). The oxytocin antagonist, atosiban, does not have these unwanted effects.

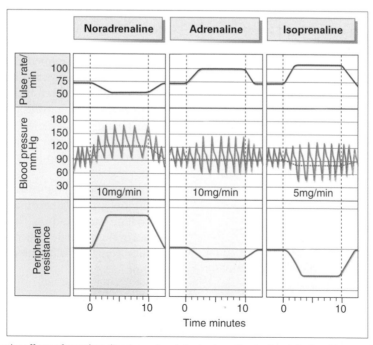

Fig. 22.2 Cardiovascular effects of noradrenaline (norepinephrine), adrenaline (epinephrine) and isoprenaline (isoproterenol): pulse rate (beats/min), blood pressure in mmHg (dotted line is mean pressure), peripheral resistance in arbitrary units. The differences are due to the differential α- and β-agonist selectivities of these agents (see text). (By permission, after Ginsburg J, Cobbold A F 1960 In: Vane J R, Wolstenholme G E W, O'Connor M O (eds) Adrenergic mechanisms. Churchill, London, p. 173–179.)

Sympathomimetics and plasma potassium. Adrenergic mechanisms have a role in the physiological control of plasma potassium concentration. The Na/K pump that shifts potassium into cells is activated by β_2-adrenoceptor agonists (adrenaline [epinephrine], salbutamol, isoprenaline) and can cause hypokalaemia. β_2-Adrenoceptor antagonists block the effect.

The hypokalaemic effect of administered (β_2) sympathomimetics may be clinically important, particularly in patients with pre-existing hypokalaemia, e.g. due to intense adrenergic activity such as occurs in myocardial infarction,[5] in fright (admission to hospital is accompanied by transient hypokalaemia), or with previous diuretic therapy, and patients taking digoxin. In such subjects the use of a sympathomimetic infusion or of an adrenaline-containing local anaesthetic may precipitate cardiac arrhythmia. Hypokalaemia may occur during treatment of severe asthma, particularly where the β_2-receptor agonist is combined with theophylline.

β-Adrenoceptor blockers, as expected, enhance the hyperkalaemia of muscular exercise, and one of their benefits in preventing cardiac arrhythmias after myocardial infarction may be due to block of β_2 receptor-induced hypokalaemia.

Overdose of sympathomimetics is treated according to rational consideration of mode and site of action (see Adrenaline, below).

INDIVIDUAL SYMPATHOMIMETICS

The actions are summarised in Table 22.1. The classic, mainly endogenous, substances will be described first despite their limited role in therapeutics, and then the more selective analogues that have largely replaced them.

CATECHOLAMINES

Traditionally catecholamines have had a dual nomenclature (as a consequence of a company

patenting the name Adrenalin), broadly European and North American. The latter has been chosen by the World Health Organization as recommended international non-proprietary names (rINNs) (see Chapter 6), and the European Union has directed member states to use rINNs. By exception, adrenaline and noradrenaline are the terms used in the titles of monographs in the *European Pharmacopoeia* and are thus the official names in the member states. Because uniformity has not yet been achieved, and because of the scientific literature, we use both names.

For pharmacokinetics, see above.

Adrenaline (epinephrine)

Adrenaline (α- and β-adrenoceptor effects) is used:

- as a vasoconstrictor with local anaesthetics (1 in 80 000 or weaker) to prolong their effects (about two-fold)
- as a topical mydriatic (sparing accommodation; it also lowers intraocular pressure)
- for severe allergic reactions, i.e. anaphylactic shock, intramuscularly or intravenously. The route must be chosen with care (for details, see p. 412). The subcutaneous route is not recommended as the intense vasoconstriction slows absorption.

Adrenaline is used in anaphylactic shock because of its mix of actions, cardiovascular and bronchial; it may also stabilise mast cell membranes and reduce release of vasoactive autacoids (see p. 408). Patients who are taking non-selective β-blockers may not respond to adrenaline (use intravenous salbutamol) and indeed may develop severe hypertension (see below).

Adrenaline (topical) decreases intraocular pressure in chronic open-angle glaucoma, as does dipivefrine, an adrenaline ester pro-drug. These drugs are contraindicated in closed-angle glaucoma because they are mydriatics. Hyperthyroid patients are intolerant of adrenaline.

Accidental overdose with adrenaline occurs occasionally. It is rationally treated with propranolol to block the cardiac β effects (cardiac arrhythmia) and phentolamine or chlorpromazine to control the α effects on the peripheral circulation that will be prominent when the β effects are abolished. Labetalol (α + β blockade) is a good alternative.

---

[5]Normal subjects, infused with intravenous adrenaline in amounts that approximate to those found in the plasma after severe myocardial infarction, show a fall in plasma potassium concentration of about 0.8 mmol/L (Brown M J, Brown D C, Murphy M B 1983 Hypokalemia from beta2-receptor stimulation by circulating epinephrine. New England Journal of Medicine 309:1414–1419).

β-Adrenoceptor block alone is hazardous as the then unopposed α-receptor vasoconstriction causes (severe) hypertension (see Phaeochromocytoma, p. 445). Use of other classes of antihypertensives is irrational and may even cause adrenaline release.

Noradrenaline (norepinephrine) (chiefly α and β₁ effects)

Noradrenaline (norepinephrine) (chiefly a and β, effects)

The main effect of administered noradrenaline is to raise the blood pressure by constricting the arterioles and so increasing the total peripheral resistance, with reduced blood flow (except in coronary arteries which have few α_1 receptors). Though it does have some cardiac stimulant (β_1) effect, the tachycardia of this is masked by the profound reflex bradycardia caused by the hypertension. Noradrenaline is given by intravenous infusion to obtain a gradual sustained response; the effect of a single intravenous injection would last only a minute or so. It is used where peripheral vasoconstriction is specifically desired, e.g. vasodilatation of septic shock. Adverse effects include peripheral gangrene and local necrosis; tachyphylaxis occurs and withdrawal must be gradual.

Isoprenaline (isoproterenol)

Isoprenaline (isopropylnoradrenaline) is a nonselective β-receptor agonist, i.e. it activates both β_1 and β_2 receptors. It relaxes smooth muscle, including that of the blood vessels, and has negligible metabolic or vasoconstrictor effects, but a vigorous stimulant effect on the heart. This latter is its main disadvantage in the treatment of bronchial asthma. It may still find use in complete heart block, massive overdose of β-blocker, and occasionally in cardiogenic shock (hypotension).

Dopamine

Dopamine activates different receptors depending on the dose used. At the lowest effective dose it stimulates specific dopamine (D_1) receptors in the CNS and the renal and other vascular beds (dilator); it also activates presynaptic autoreceptors (D_2) which suppress release of noradrenaline. As dose is increased, dopamine acts as an agonist on β_1 adrenoceptors in the heart (increasing contractility and rate); at high doses it activates α adrenoceptors (vasoconstrictor). It is given by continuous intravenous infusion because, like all catecholamines, its $t_{1/2}$ is short (2 min). An intravenous infusion (2–5 micrograms/kg/min) increases renal blood flow (partly through an effect on cardiac output). As the dose rises the heart is stimulated, resulting in tachycardia and increased cardiac output. At these higher doses, dopamine is referred to as an 'inoconstrictor'.

Dopamine is stable for about 24 h in sodium chloride or dextrose. Subcutaneous leakage causes vasoconstriction and necrosis, and should be treated by local injection of an α-adrenoceptor blocking agent (phentolamine 5 mg, diluted).

It may be mixed with dobutamine.

For CNS aspects of dopamine, agonists and antagonists, see Neuroleptics (p. 306) and Parkinsonism (p. 345).

Dobutamine

Dobutamine is a racemic mixture of D- and L-dobutamine. The racemate behaves primarily as a β_1-adrenoceptor agonist with greater inotropic than chronotropic effects on the heart; it has some α-agonist effect, but less than dopamine. It is useful in shock (with dopamine) and in low-output heart failure (in the absence of severe hypertension).

Dopexamine

Dopexamine is a synthetic catecholamine whose principal action is as an agonist for the cardiac β_2 adrenoceptors (positive inotropic effect). It is also a weak dopamine agonist (thus causing renal vasodilatation) and inhibitor of noradrenaline uptake, thereby enhancing stimulation of cardiac β_1 receptors by noradrenaline. It is used occasionally to optimise the cardiac output, particularly perioperatively.

NON-CATECHOLAMINES

Salbutamol, fenoterol, rimiterol, reproterol, pirbuterol, salmeterol, ritodrine and terbutaline are β-adrenoceptor agonists that are relatively selective for β_2 receptors, so that cardiac (chiefly β_1-receptor) effects are less prominent. Tachycardia still occurs because of atrial (sinus node) β_2-receptor stimulation; the β_2 adrenoceptors are less numerous in the ventricle and there is probably less risk of serious ventricular arrhythmias than with the use of non-selective catecholamines. The synthetic agonists are also longer acting than isoprenaline because they are not substrates for catechol-*O*-methyltransferase, which methylates catecholamines in the liver. They are used principally in asthma, and to reduce uterine contractions in premature labour.

Salbutamol (see also Asthma)

Salbutamol (Ventolin) ($t_{1/2}$ 4 h) is taken orally, 2–4 mg up to four times per day; it also acts quickly by inhalation and the effect can last for 4–6 h, which makes it suitable for both prevention and treatment of asthma. Of an inhaled dose less than 20% is absorbed and can cause cardiovascular effects. It can also be given by injection, e.g. in asthma, premature labour (β_2 receptor) and for cardiac inotropic (β_1) effect in heart failure (where the β_2-vasodilator action is also useful). Clinically important hypokalaemia can also occur (the shift of potassium into cells). The other drugs above are similar.

Salmeterol (Serevent) is a variant of salbutamol that has an additional binding site adjacent to the β_2 adrenoceptor; this results in slow onset and long duration of action (12–18 h) (see p. 432).

Ephedrine

Ephedrine ($t_{1/2}$ approx. 6 h) is a plant alkaloid[6] with indirect sympathomimetic actions that resemble those of adrenaline peripherally. Centrally (in adults) it produces increased alertness, anxiety, insomnia, tremor and nausea; children may be sleepy when taking it. In practice central effects limit its use as a sympathomimetic in asthma.

Ephedrine is well absorbed when given orally and, unlike most other sympathomimetics, undergoes relatively little first-pass metabolism in the liver; it is excreted largely unchanged by the kidney. It differs from adrenaline principally in that its effects come on more slowly and last longer. Tachyphylaxis occurs on repeated dosing. It can be given by mouth for reversible airways obstruction, topically as a mydriatic and mucosal vasoconstrictor or by slow intravenous injection to reverse hypotension from spinal or epidural anaesthesia. Newer drugs that are better suited for these purposes have largely replaced it. It is sometimes useful in myasthenia gravis (adrenergic

---

[6]Ephedra alkaloids are found in Chinese herbal remedies (ma hunag) and in guarana-derived caffeine products which are widely consumed as appetite suppressants or for energy enhancement. These have been associated with stroke and seizures only rarely. The relationship of phenylpropanolamine consumption and haemorrhagic stroke seems clearer and has led to the suspension of its sale in the USA (Fleming G A 2000 The FDA, regulation, and the risk of stroke. New England Journal of Medicine 243:1886–1887).

agents enhance cholinergic neuromuscular transmission). *Pseudoephedrine* is similar.

Phenylpropanolamine (norephedrine) is similar but with fewer CNS effects. Prolonged administration of phenylpropanolamine to women as an anorectic has been associated with pulmonary valve abnormalities and stroke, leading to its withdrawal in some countries.[6]

Amfetamine (Benzedrine) and *dexamfetamine* (Dexedrine) act indirectly. They are seldom used for their peripheral effects, which are similar to those of ephedrine, but usually for their effects on the CNS (narcolepsy, attention deficit in children). (For a general account of amfetamine, see p. 168).

Phenylephrine has actions qualitatively similar to those of noradrenaline but of longer duration, up to several hours. It can be used as a nasal decongestant (0.25–0.5% solution), but sometimes irritates. In the doses usually given, the CNS effects are minimal, as are the direct effects on the heart. It is also used as a mydriatic and briefly lowers intraocular pressure.

MUCOSAL DECONGESTANTS

Nasal and bronchial decongestants (vasoconstrictors) are widely used in allergic rhinitis, colds, coughs and sinusitis, and to prevent otic barotrauma, as nasal sprays or taken orally. All of the sympathomimetic vasoconstrictors, i.e. with α effects, have been used for the purpose, with or without an antihistamine (H_1 receptor), and there is little to choose between them. Ischaemic damage to the mucosa is possible if they are used excessively (more often than 3-hourly) or for prolonged periods (more than 3 weeks), and is a common problem for regular users of cocaine. The occurrence of rebound congestion is also liable to lead to overuse.

The least objectionable drugs are ephedrine 0.5% and phenylephrine 0.5%. Xylometazoline 0.1% (Otrivine) should be used, if at all, for only a few days because longer application reduces the ciliary activity and leads to rebound congestion. Oily drops and sprays, used frequently and long term, may also enter the lungs and eventually cause lipoid pneumonia. They interact with antihypertensives and can be a cause of unexplained failure of therapy unless enquiry into patient self-medication is made. Fatal hypertensive crises have occurred when patients treated for depression with a monoamine oxidase inhibitor have taken these preparations.

SHOCK

Definition. Shock is a state of inadequate organ perfusion (oxygen deficiency) to an extent that adversely affects cellular metabolism causing malfunction, including release of enzymes and vasoactive substances,[7] i.e. it is a *low flow* or *hypoperfusion* state.

The blood pressure is low in fully developed cases. With the exception of septic shock, the cardiac output is usually low. In septic shock the cardiac output is typically high, but a maldistribution of blood (due to constriction, dilatation, shunting) and poor oxygen utilization causes tissue injury (warm shock).

The essential element, hypoperfusion of vital organs, is present whatever the cause, whether pump failure (myocardial infarction), maldistribution of blood (septic shock) or loss of intravascular volume (bleeding or increased permeability of vessels damaged by bacterial cell products, burns or anoxia). Function of vital organs, such as the brain (consciousness, respiration) and kidney (urine formation) are clinical indicators of adequacy of perfusion of these organs.

Treatment may be summarised:

- *Treatment of the cause*: bleeding, infection, adrenocortical deficiency.
- *Replacement of any fluid lost* from the circulation.
- *Perfusion of vital organs* (brain, heart, kidneys) and maintenance of the mean blood pressure.

Blood flow (oxygen delivery) rather than blood pressure is of the greatest immediate importance for the function of vital organs. A reasonable blood pressure is needed to ensure organ perfusion, but peripheral vasoconstriction may maintain a normal mean arterial pressure despite a very low cardiac output. Under these circumstances, blood flow to vital organs will be inadequate and multiple organ failure will ensue unless the patient is resuscitated adequately.

The decision on how to treat shock depends on assessment of the pathophysiology:

- whether cardiac output, and thus peripheral blood flow, is inadequate (low pulse volume, cold-constricted periphery)
- whether cardiac output is normal or high and peripheral blood flow is adequate (good pulse volume and warm dilated periphery), but there is maldistribution of blood
- whether the patient is hypovolaemic or not, or needs a cardiac inotropic agent, a vasoconstrictor or a vasodilator.

Types of shock

In poisoning by a cerebral depressant or after spinal cord trauma, the principal cause of hypotension is low peripheral resistance due to reduced vascular tone. The cardiac output can be restored by infusing fluid and/or giving vasoactive drugs (e.g. noradrenaline, metaraminol).

In central circulatory failure (cardiogenic shock, e.g. after myocardial infarction) the cardiac output and blood pressure are low because of pump failure; myocardial perfusion is dependent on aortic pressure. Venous return (central venous pressure) is normal or high. The low blood pressure may trigger the sympathoadrenal mechanisms of peripheral circulatory failure summarised below.

Not surprisingly, the use of drugs in low-output failure caused by acute myocardial damage is disappointing. Vasoconstriction (by an α-adrenoceptor agonist) may raise the blood pressure by increasing peripheral resistance, but the additional burden on the damaged heart can further reduce the cardiac output. Cardiac stimulation with a β_1-adrenoceptor agonist may fail; it increases myocardial oxygen consumption and may cause an arrhythmia. Dobutamine or dopamine offers a reasonable choice if a drug is judged necessary; dobutamine is preferred as it tends to vasodilate, i.e. it is an 'inodilator'. A selective phosphodiesterase inhibitor such as enoximone may also be effective, unless its use is limited by hypotension.

If there is bradycardia (as sometimes complicates myocardial infarction), cardiac output can be increased by accelerating the heart rate by vagal block with atropine.

---

[7] In fact, a medley of substances (autacoids) – kinins, prostaglandins, leukotrienes, histamine, endorphins, serotonin, vasopressin – has been implicated. In endotoxic shock, the toxin also induces synthesis of nitric oxide, the endogenous vasodilator, in several types of cell other than the endothelial cells that are normally its main source.

Septic shock is severe sepsis with hypotension that is not corrected by adequate intravascular volume replacement. It is caused by lipopolysaccharide (LPS) endotoxins from Gram-negative organisms and other cell products from Gram-positive organisms; these initiate host inflammatory and procoagulant responses through the release of cytokines, e.g. interleukins, and the resulting diffuse endothelial damage is responsible for many of the adverse manifestations of shock. The procoagulant state, in particular, predisposes to the development of microvascular thrombosis that leads to tissue ischaemia and organ hypoperfusion. Activation of nitric oxide production by LPS and cytokines worsens the hypoperfusion by decreasing arterial pressure. This initiates a vigorous sympathetic discharge that causes constriction of arterioles and venules; the cardiac output may be high or low according to the balance of these influences.

There is a progressive peripheral anoxia of vital organs and acidosis. The veins (venules) dilate and venous pooling occurs so that blood is sequestered in the periphery; effective circulatory volume decreases because of this and fluid loss into the extravascular space from endothelial damage caused by bacterial products.

When septic shock is recognised, appropriate antimicrobials should be given in high dose immediately after taking blood for culture (see p. 178). Beyond that, the prime aim of treatment is to restore cardiac output and vital organ perfusion by increasing venous return to the heart, and to reverse the maldistribution of blood. Increasing intravascular volume will achieve this, guided by the central venous pressure to avoid overloading the heart. Oxygen is essential as there is often uneven pulmonary perfusion.

After adequate fluid resuscitation has been established, inotropic support is usually required. *Noradrenaline* is the vasoactive drug of choice for septic shock: its potent α-adrenergic effect increases the mean arterial pressure and its modest β_1 effect may raise cardiac output, or at least maintain it as the peripheral vascular resistance increases. *Dobutamine* may be added to augment cardiac output further. Some clinicians use adrenaline, in preference to noradrenaline plus dobutamine, on the basis that its powerful α and β effects are appropriate in the setting of septic shock; it may exacerbate splanchnic ischaemia and lactic acidosis.

Hypotension in (atherosclerotic) occlusive vascular disease is particularly serious, for these patients are dependent on pressure to provide the necessary blood flow in vital organs whose supplying vessels are less able to dilate. It is important to maintain an adequate mean arterial pressure, whichever inotrope is selected.

Choice of drug in shock

On present knowledge the best drug would be one that both stimulates the myocardium and selectively modifies peripheral resistance to increase flow to vital organs.

- *Dobutamine* is used when cardiac inotropic effect is the primary requirement.
- *Adrenaline* is used when a more potent inotrope than dobutamine is required, e.g. when the vasodilating action of dobutamine compromises mean arterial pressure.
- *Noradrenaline* is used when vasoconstriction is the first priority, plus some cardiac inotropic effect, e.g. septic shock.

Additionally, *recombinant activated protein C (APC) drotrecogin α* can be given to reverse the procoagulant state of septic shock. Inflammatory conditions such as septic shock inhibit the generation of endogenous APC, which normally inactivates factors Va and VIIIa, with the result that production of these procoagulant factors is unchecked. Recombinant human APC improved survival of patients with septic shock and multi-organ failure in a large randomised controlled trial.[8]

Monitoring drug use

Modern monitoring by both invasive and noninvasive techniques is complex and is undertaken in units dedicated to, and equipped for, this activity. The present comment is an overview. Monitoring normally requires close attention to heart rate and rhythm, blood pressure, fluid balance and urine flow, pulmonary gas exchange and central venous pressure. The use of drugs in shock is secondary to accurate assessment of cardiovascular state (especially of peripheral flow) and to other essential management, treatment of infection and maintenance of intravascular volume.

[8]Bernard G D, Vincent J L, Laterre P F et al 2001 Efficacy and safety of recombinant human activated protein C for severe sepsis. New England Journal of Medicine 344:699–709.

Restoration of Intravascular volume[9]

In an emergency, speed of replacement is more important than its nature. *Crystalloid* solutions, e.g. isotonic saline, Hartmann's, Plasma-Lyte, are immediately effective, but they leave the circulation quickly. (Note that dextrose solutions are completely ineffective because they distribute across both the extracellular and intracellular compartments.) Macromolecules (*colloids*) remain in the circulation longer. The two classes (crystalloids and colloids) may be used together.

The choice of crystalloid or colloid for fluid resuscitation remains controversial. However, a recent large prospective randomised controlled trial of albumin versus saline in critically ill patients showed no difference in survival or in the number of organ failures in the two groups.[10]

Artificial colloidal solutions include dextrans (glucose polymer), gelatin (hydrolysed collagen) and hydroxyethyl starch.

Dextran 70 (mol. wt. 70 000) has a plasma restoring effect lasting for 5–6 h. Dextran 40 is used to decrease blood sludging and so to improve peripheral blood flow.

Gelatin products (e.g. Haemaccel, Gelofusine) have a plasma restoring effect of 2–3 h (at best).

Etherified starch. Several hydroxyethyl starch solutions are available, with widely differing effects on plasma volume. The high molecular weight (450 000) solutions have a volume restoring effect for 6–12 h, whereas the effect of medium molecular weight (200 000) starches lasts for 4–6 h.

Adverse effects include anaphylactoid reactions; dextran and hydroxyethyl starch can impair haemostatic mechanisms.

CHRONIC ORTHOSTATIC HYPOTENSION

Chronic orthostatic hypotension occurs most commonly with increasing age, in primary progressive autonomic failure, and secondary to parkinsonism and diabetes. The clinical features can be mimicked by saline depletion. The two conditions are clearly separated by measurement of plasma concentrations of noradrenaline (supine and erect) and rennin, which are raised in saline depletion, but depressed in most causes of hypotension due to autonomic failure.

As blood pressure can be considered a product of 'volume' and 'vasoconstriction', the logical initial treatment of orthostatic hypotension is to expand blood volume using a sodium-retaining adrenocortical steroid (fludrocortisone[11]) or desmopressin (see p. 640), plus elastic support stockings to reduce venous pooling of blood when erect.

It is more difficult to reproduce the actions of the endogenous vasoconstrictors, and especially their selective release on standing, in order to achieve erect normotension without supine hypertension. Because of the risk of hypertension when the patient is supine, only a modest increase in erect blood pressure should be sought; fortunately a systolic blood pressure of 85–90 mmHg is usually adequate to maintain cerebral perfusion in these patients. Few drugs have been formally tested or can be recommended with confidence.

Clonidine and pindolol are partial agonists at, respectively, α and β receptors, and may therefore be more effective agonists in the absence of the endogenous agonist, noradrenaline, than in normal subjects. Midodrine, an α-adrenoceptor agonist, is the only vasoconstrictor drug to receive UK regulatory approval for the treatment of postural hypotension. It is given at doses of 5–15 mg t.i.d.

Postprandial fall in blood pressure (probably due to redistribution of blood to the splanchnic area) is characteristic of this condition; it occurs especially after breakfast (blood volume is lower in the morning). Substantial doses of caffeine (two large cups of coffee) can mitigate this, but they need to be taken before or early in the meal. The action may be due to block of splanchnic vasodilator adenosine receptors. Administration of the somatostatin analogue, octreotide, also prevents postprandial hypotension, but twice-daily subcutaneous injections are often not attractive; long-acting formulations of somatostatin (and its relative lanreotide) are available which can be given as subcutaneous or intramuscular depots monthly – this may be more tolerable.

Some of the variation reported in drug therapy may be due to differences in adrenergic function

[9]Nolan J 2001 Fluid resuscitation for the trauma patient. Resuscitation 48:57–69.

[10]Finfer S, Bellomo R, Boyce N et al 2004 A comparison of albumin and saline for fluid resuscitation in the intensive care unit. New England Journal of Medicine 350:2247–2256.

[11]Effective doses may not restore blood volume and may work by sensitising vascular adrenocept ors.

dependent on whether the degeneration is central, peripheral, preganglionic, postganglionic or due to age-related changes in the adrenoceptors on end-organs. In central autonomic degeneration – 'multi-system atrophy' – noradrenaline is still present in peripheral sympathetic nerve endings. In these patients, an indirect-acting amine may be successful, and one patient titrated the amount of Bovril (a tyramine-rich meat extract drink) she required in order to stand up.[12]

Erythropoietin has also been used with success (it increases haematocrit and blood viscosity).

Summary

- The adrenergic arm of the autonomic system uses noradrenaline (norepinephrine) as its neurotransmitter.
- Adrenaline (epinephrine), unlike noradrenaline, is a circulating hormone.
- These two catecholamines act on the same adrenoceptors: α_1 and α_2, which are blocked by phenoxybenzamine but not by propranolol, and β_1 and β_2, which are blocked by propranolol but not phenoxybenzamine. Noradrenaline is a 20-fold weaker agonist at β_2 receptors than is adrenaline.
- Distinction between receptor classes is made initially by defining the differing ability of two agonists (or antagonists) to mimic (or block) the effects of catecholamines.
- Often these differences correlate with a difference in receptor type on two different tissues: e.g. stimulation of cardiac contractility by β_1 receptors, and bronchodilatation by β_2 receptors.
- The distinction between α_1 and α_2 receptors corresponds to their principal location on blood vessels (causing vasoconstriction) and neurones respectively.
- Catecholamines themselves can be used in therapy when rapid onset and offset are desired. Selective mimetics at each of the four main receptor subtypes are used for individual locations, e.g. α_1 for nasal decongestion, α_2 for systemic hypotension, α_1 for septic shock, β_2 for bronchoconstriction.
- Both α- and β-blockade are used in hypertension; selective β-blockade is used in angina and heart failure.

GUIDE TO FURTHER READING

Ahlquist R P 1948 A study of adrenotropic receptors. American Journal of Physiology 153:586–600

Brown M J 1995 To β-block or better block? British Medical Journal 311:701–702

Brown S G 2005 Cardiovascular aspects of anaphylaxis: implications for treatment and diagnosis. Current Opinion Allergy Clinical Immunology 5(4):359–364

Bunn F, Alderson P, Hawkins V 2003 Colloid solutions for fluid resuscitation. Cochrane Library of Systematic Reviews (1) CD001319

Evans T W, Smithies M 1999 ABC of intensive care. Organ dysfunction. British Medical Journal 318:1606–1609

Hotchkiss R S, Karl I E 2003 The pathophysiology and treatment of sepsis. New England Journal of Medicine 348:138–150

Insel P A 1996 Adrenergic receptors – evolving concepts and clinical implications. New England Journal of Medicine 334:580–585

Moore F A, McKinley B A, Moore E E et al 2004 The next generation in shock resuscitation. Lancet 363:1988–1996

Polderman K H, Girbes A R J 2004 Drug intervention trials in sepsis. Lancet 363:1721–1723

Rice T W, Bernard G R 2005 Therapeutic intervention and targets for sepsis. Annual Review of Medicine 56:225–248

---

[12]Karet F E, Dickerson J E C, Brown J et al 1994 Bovril and moclobemide: a novel therapeutic strategy for central autonomic failure. Lancet 344:1263–1265.

23

Arterial hypertension, angina pectoris, myocardial Infarction

SYNOPSIS

Hypertension and coronary heart disease (CHD) are of great importance. Hypertension affects more than 20% of the total population of the USA, with its major impact on those aged over 50 years. CHD is the cause of death in 30% of males and 22% of females in England and Wales. Management requires attention to detail, both clinical and pharmacological.

The way in which drugs act in these diseases is outlined and the drugs are described according to class.

- Hypertension and angina pectoris: how drugs act
- Drugs used in both hypertension and angina
  - diuretics
  - vasodilators: organic nitrates, calcium channel blockers, ACE inhibitors, angiotensin II receptor antagonists
  - adrenoceptor-blocking drugs, α and β
  - peripheral sympathetic nerve terminal
  - autonomic ganglion-blocking drugs
  - central nervous system
  - treatment of angina pectoris
- Acute coronary syndromes and myocardial infarction
- Arterial hypertension
- Sexual function and cardiovascular drugs
- Phaeochromocytoma

HYPERTENSION: HOW DRUGS ACT

Consider the following relationship:

Blood pressure = cardiac output × peripheral resistance

This being true, drugs can lower blood pressure by:

- Dilatation of arteriolar *resistance vessels*. Dilatation can be achieved through direct relaxation of vascular smooth muscle cells, by stimulation of nitric oxide (NO) production, or by blocking (suppressing) endogenous vasoconstrictors, noradrenaline (norepinephrine) and angiotensin.
- Dilatation of venous *capacitance vessels*; reduced venous return to the heart (preload) leads to reduced cardiac output, especially in the upright position.
- Reduction of cardiac *contractility* and *heart rate*.
- Depletion of *body sodium*. This reduces plasma volume (transiently), and reduces arteriolar response to noradrenaline (norepinephrine).
- Modern antihypertensive drugs lower blood pressure with minimal interference with homeostatic control, i.e. change in posture, exercise.

ANGINA PECTORIS: HOW DRUGS ACT

Angina can be viewed as a problem of supply and demand. Drugs used in angina pectoris are those that either increase supply of oxygen and nutrients, or reduce the demand for these, or both.

The supply of myocardial oxygen can be increased by:

- dilating coronary arteries
- slowing the heart (coronary flow, uniquely, occurs in diastole, which lengthens as heart rate falls).

Demand can be decreased by:

- reducing afterload, (i.e. peripheral resistance), so reducing the work of the heart in perfusing the tissues
- reducing preload (i.e. venous filling pressure); according to Starling's law of the heart, workload and therefore oxygen demand varies with stretch of cardiac muscle fibres
- slowing the heart rate.

DRUGS USED IN HYPERTENSION AND ANGINA

Two groups of drugs, β-adrenergic blockers and calcium channel blockers, are used in both hypertension and angina. Several drugs for hypertension are also used in the treatment of heart failure.

DIURETICS (see also Chapter 26)

Diuretics, particularly the thiazides, are useful antihypertensives. They cause an initial loss of sodium with a parallel contraction of the blood and extracellular fluid volume. The effect may reach 10% of total body sodium, but it is not maintained. After several months of treatment, the main blood pressure-lowering effect appears to reflect a reduced responsiveness of resistance vessels to endogenous vasoconstrictors, principally noradrenaline. Although this hyposensitivity may be a consequence of the sodium depletion, thiazides are generally more effective antihypertensive agents than loop diuretics, despite causing less salt loss, and evidence suggests an independent action of thiazides on an unidentified ion channel on vascular smooth muscle cell membranes. Maximal effect on blood pressure is delayed for several weeks and other drugs are best added after this time.

Adverse metabolic effects of thiazides on serum potassium, blood lipids, glucose tolerance and uric acid metabolism led to suggestions that they should be replaced by newer agents without these effects. It is now recognised that unnecessarily high doses of thiazides were used in the past and that with low doses, e.g. bendrofluazide (bendroflumethiazide) 1.25–2.5 mg/day or less (or hydrochlorothiazide 12.5–25 mg), thiazides are both effective and well tolerated. Moreover, they are by far the least costly antihypertensive agents available worldwide and have proved to be the most effective in several outcome trials in preventing the major complications of hypertension, myocardial infarction and stroke. The characteristic reduction in renal calcium excretion induced by thiazides may, in long-term therapy, also reduce the occurrence of hip fractures in older patients and benefit women with postmenopausal osteoporosis.

VASODILATORS

ORGANIC NITRATES

Organic nitrates (and nitrite) were introduced into medicine in the 19th century.[1] De-nitration in the smooth muscle cell releases nitric oxide (NO), which is the main physiological vasodilator, normally produced by endothelial cells. *Nitrodilators* (a generic term for drugs that release or mimic the action of NO) activate the soluble guanylate cyclase in vascular smooth muscle cells and cause an increase in intracellular cyclic guanosine monophosphate (GMP) concentrations. This is the second messenger which alters calcium fluxes in the cell, decreases stored calcium and induces relaxation. The result is a generalised dilatation of venules (capacitance vessels) and to a lesser extent of arterioles (resistance vessels), causing a fall of blood pressure that is postural at first; the larger coronary arteries especially dilate. Whereas some vasodilators can 'steal' blood away from atheromatous arteries, with their fixed stenoses, to other, healthier arteries, nitrates probably have the reverse effect as a result of their supplementing the endogenous NO. Atheroma is associated with impaired endothelial function, resulting in reduced release of NO and, possibly, its accelerated destruction by the oxidised low-density lipoprotein (LDL) in atheroma (see Chapter 25).

The venous dilatation causes a reduction in venous return and a fall in left ventricular filling pressure with reduced stroke volume, but cardiac output is sustained by the reflex tachycardia induced by the fall in blood pressure.

Pharmacokinetics. The nitrates are generally well absorbed across skin and the mucosal surface of the mouth or gut wall. Nitrates absorbed from the gut are subject to extensive first-pass metabolism in the liver, as shown by the substantially higher doses required by that route compared with sublingual application (and explains why swallowing a sublingual tablet of glyceryl trinitrate terminates its effect). They are first de-nitrated and then conjugated with glucuronic acid. The $t_{1/2}$ periods vary (see below), but for glyceryl trinitrate (GTN) it is 1–4 min.

---

[1]Murrell W 1879 Nitroglycerin as a remedy for angina pectoris. Lancet i:80–81. Nitroglycerin was actually first synthesised by Sobrero in 1847 who noted that, when he applied it to his tongue, it caused a severe headache.

Tolerance to the characteristic vasodilator headache comes and goes quickly (hours).[2] Ensuring that a continuous steady-state plasma concentration is avoided prevents tolerance. This is easy with occasional use of GTN, but with nitrates having longer $t_{1/2}$ (see below) and sustained-release formulations it is necessary to plan the dosing to allow a low plasma concentration for 4–8 h, e.g. overnight; alternatively transdermal patches may be removed for a few hours if tolerance is suspected.

Uses. Nitrates are chiefly used to relieve angina pectoris and sometimes left ventricular failure. An excessive fall in blood pressure will reduce coronary flow as well as cause fainting due to reduced cerebral blood flow, so it is important to avoid accidental overdosing. Patients with angina should be instructed on the signs of overdose – palpitations, dizziness, blurred vision, headache and flushing following by pallor – and what to do about it (see below).

The discovery that coronary artery occlusion by thrombosis is itself 'stuttering' – developing gradually over hours – and associated with vasospasm in other parts of the coronary tree has made the use of isosorbide dinitrate (Isoket) by continuous intravenous infusion adjusted to the degree of pain, a logical, and effective, form of analgesia for unstable angina.

Transient relief of pain due to spasm of other smooth muscle (colic) can sometimes be obtained, so that relief of chest pain by nitrates does not prove the diagnosis of angina pectoris.

Nitrates are contraindicated in angina due to anaemia.

Adverse effects. Collapse due to fall in blood pressure resulting from overdose is the commonest side-effect. The patient should remain supine with the legs raised above the head to restore venous return to the heart. The patient should also spit out or swallow the remainder of the tablet.

Nitrate headache, which may be severe, is probably due to the stretching of pain-sensitive tissues around the meningeal arteries resulting from the increased pulsation that accompanies the local vasodilatation. If headache is severe the dose should be halved. Methaemoglobinaemia can occur with heavy dosage.

Interactions. An important footnote to the use of nitrates (and NO dilators generally) has been the marked potentiation of their vasodilator effects observed in patients taking phosphodiesterase (PDE) inhibitors, such as sildenafil (Viagra) and tadalafil (Cialis). These agents target an isoform of PDE (PDE-5) expressed in the blood vessel wall. Other methylaxanthine PDE inhibitors, such as theophylline, do not cause a similar interaction because they are rather weak inhibitors of PDE-5, even at the doses effective in asthma. A number of pericoital deaths reported in patients taking sildenafil have been attributed to the substantial fall in blood pressure that occurs when used with a nitrate. This is an ironic twist for an agent in first-line use in erectile dysfunction that was originally developed as a drug to treat angina.[3]

GLYCERYL TRINITRATE (see also above)

Glyceryl trinitrate (1879) (trinitrin, nitroglycerin, GTN) ($t_{1/2}$ 3 min) is an oily, non-flammable liquid that explodes on concussion with a force greater than that of gunpowder. Physicians meet it mixed with inert substances and made into a tablet, in which form it is both innocuous and fairly stable. But tablets more than 8 weeks old or exposed to heat or air will have lost potency by evaporation and should be discarded. Patients should also be warned to expect the tablet to cause a burning sensation under the tongue if it still contains active GTN. An alternative is to use a nitroglycerin spray (see below), which,

---

[2]Explosives factory workers exposed to a nitrate-contaminated environment lost it over a weekend and some chose to maintain their intake by using nitrate-impregnated headbands (transdermal absorption) rather than have to accept the headaches and re-acquire tolerance so frequently. A recent study has also reported that patients with angina who develop a headache with GTN are less likely to have obstructive coronary artery disease (His D H, Roshandel A, Singh N, Szombathy T, Meszaros Z S 2005 Headache response to glyceryl trinitrate in patients with and without obstructive coronary artery disease. Heart 91:1164–1166).

[3]It has been argued that deaths on sildenafil largely reflect the fact that it is used by patients at high cardiovascular risk. But postmarketing data shows that death is 50 times more likely after sildenafil taken for erectile failure than alprostadil, the previous first-line agent (Mitka M 2000 Some men who take Viagra die – why? Journal of the American Medical Association 283:590–593).

formulated as a pressurised liquid GTN, has a shelf-life of at least 3 years.

GTN is the drug of choice in the treatment of an attack of angina pectoris. The tablets should be chewed and dissolved under the tongue, or placed in the buccal sulcus, where absorption is rapid and reliable. Time spent ensuring that patients understand the way to take the tablets, and that the feeling of fullness in the head is harmless, is time well spent. The action begins in 2 min and lasts for up to 30 min. The dose in the standard tablet is 300 micrograms, and 500- or 600-microgram strengths are also available; patients may use up to 6 mg daily in total, but those who require more than two or three tablets per week should take a long-acting nitrate preparation. GTN is taken at the onset of pain and as a prophylactic immediately before any exertion likely to precipitate the pain. Sustained-release buccal tablets are available (Suscard), 1–5 mg. Absorption from the gastrointestinal tract is good, but extensive hepatic first-pass metabolism renders the sublingual or buccal route preferable; an oral metered aerosol that is sprayed under the tongue (nitrolingual spray) is an alternative.

For prophylaxis, GTN can be given as an oral (buccal, or to swallow, Sustac) sustained-release formulation or via the skin as a patch (or ointment); these formulations can be useful for sufferers from nocturnal angina.[4]

Venepuncture. The ointment can assist difficult venepuncture and a transdermal patch adjacent to an intravenous infusion site can prevent extravasation and phlebitis, and prolong infusion survival.

Isosorbide dinitrate (Cedocard) ($t_{1/2}$ 20 min) is used for prophylaxis of angina pectoris and for congestive heart failure (tablets sublingual, and to swallow). An intravenous formulation, 500 micrograms/mL (Isoket), is available for use in left ventricular failure and unstable angina.

Isosorbide mononitrate (Elantan) ($t_{1/2}$ 4 h) is used for prophylaxis of angina (tablets to swallow). Hepatic first-pass metabolism is much less than for the dinitrate so that systemic bio-availability is more reliable.

Pentaerithrityl tetranitrate (Peritrate) ($t_{1/2}$ 8 h) is less efficacious than its metabolite pentaerithrityl trinitrate ($t_{1/2}$ 11 h).

CALCIUM CHANNEL BLOCKERS

Calcium is involved in the initiation of smooth muscle and cardiac cell contraction, and in the propagation of the cardiac impulse. Actions on cardiac pacemaker cells and conducting tissue are described in Chapter 24.

Vascular smooth muscle cells. Contraction of these cells requires an influx of calcium across the cell membrane. This occurs through voltage-operated ion channels (VOCs) and this influx is able to trigger further release of calcium from intracellular stores in the sarcoplasmic reticulum. The VOCs have relatively long opening times and carry large fluxes; hence they are usually referred to as L-type channels.[5] The rise in intracellular free calcium results in activation of the contractile proteins, myosin and actin, with shortening of the myofibril and contraction of smooth muscle. During relaxation calcium is released from the myofibril and either pumped back into the sarcoplasm or lost through Na/Ca exchange at the cell surface.

There are three structurally distinct classes of calcium channel blocker:

- Dihydropyridines (the most numerous).
- Phenylalkylamines (principally verapamil).
- Benzothiazepine (diltiazem).

The differences between their clinical effects can be explained in part by their binding to different parts of the L-type calcium channel. All members of the group are vasodilators, and some have negative inotropic and negative chronotropic effects on the heart via effects on pacemaker cells in the conducting tissue. The attributes of individual drugs are described below.

---

[4]Useful, but not always safe. Defibrillator paddles and nitrate patches make an explosive combination, and it is not always in the patient's interest to have the patch as unobtrusive as possible (see Canadian Medical Association Journal 1993; 148:790).

[5]Several calcium-selective channels have been described in different tissues, e.g. the N (present in neuronal tissue) and T (transient, found in brain, neuronal and cardiovascular pacemaker tissue); the drugs discussed here selectively target the L-channel for its cardiovascular importance.

The therapeutic benefit of the calcium blockers in hypertension and angina is due mainly to their action as vasodilators. Their action on the heart gives non-dihydropyridines an additional role as class 4 antiarrhythmics.

Pharmacokinetics. Calcium channel blockers in general are well absorbed from the gastrointestinal tract and their systemic bio-availability depends on the extent of first-pass metabolism in the gut wall and liver, which varies between the drugs. All undergo metabolism to less active products, predominantly by cytochrome P450 CYP3A, which is the source of interactions with other drugs by enzyme induction and inhibition. As their action is terminated by metabolism, dose adjustments for patients with impaired renal function are therefore either minor or unnecessary.

Indications for use

- *Hypertension*: amlodipine, isradipine, nicardipine, nifedipine, verapamil.
- *Angina*: amlodipine, diltiazem, nicardipine, nifedipine, verapamil.
- *Cardiac arrhythmia*: verapamil.
- *Raynaud's disease*: nifedipine.
- *Prevention* of ischaemic neurological damage following subarachnoid haemorrhage: nimodipine.

Adverse effects. Headache, flushing, dizziness, palpitations and hypotension may occur during the first few hours after dosing, as the plasma concentration is increasing, particularly if the initial dose is too high or increased too rapidly. Ankle oedema may also develop. This is probably due to a rise in intracapillary pressure as a result of the selective dilatation by calcium blockers of the precapillary arterioles. Thus the oedema is not a sign of sodium retention. It is not relieved by a diuretic but disappears after lying flat, e.g. overnight. Bradycardia and arrhythmia may occur, especially with the non-dihydropyridines. Gastrointestinal effects include constipation, nausea and vomiting; palpitation and lethargy may be experienced.

There has been some concern that the shorter-acting calcium channel blockers may adversely affect the risk of myocardial infarction and cardiac death. The evidence is based on case–control studies which cannot escape the possibility that sicker patients, i.e. with worse hypertension or angina, received

calcium channel blockade. The safety and efficacy of the class has been strengthened by the recent findings of two prospective comparisons with other antihypertensives.[6]

Interactions are numerous. Generally, the drugs in this group are extensively metabolised, and there is risk of decreased effect with enzyme inducers, e.g. rifampicin, and increased effect with enzyme inhibitors, e.g. ketoconazole or cimetidine. Conversely, calcium channel blockers decrease the plasma clearance of several other drugs by mechanisms that include delaying their metabolic breakdown. The consequence, for example, is that diltiazem and verapamil cause increased exposure to carbamazepine, quinidine, statins, ciclosporin, metoprolol, theophylline and (HIV) protease inhibitors. Verapamil increases plasma concentration of digoxin, possibly by interfering with its biliary excretion. β-Adrenoceptor blockers may exacerbate atrioventricular block and cardiac failure. Grapefruit juice raises the plasma concentration of dihydropyridines (except amlodipine) and verapamil, while St John's wort as an inducer of CYP3A can reduce bio-availability of verapamil and dihydropyridines.

Individual calcium blockers

Nifedipine ($t_{1/2}$ 2 h) is the prototype dihydropyridine. It selectively dilates arteries with little effect on veins; its negative myocardial inotropic and chronotropic effects are much less than those of verapamil. There are sustained-release formulations of nifedipine that permit once-daily dosing, minimising peaks and troughs in plasma concentration so that adverse effects due to rapid fluctuation of

---

[6]Both the NORDIL and INSIGHT trials confirmed that a calcium channel blocker (diltiazem and nifedipine respectively) had the same efficacy as older therapies (diuretics and/or β-blockers) in hypertension, with no evidence of increased sudden death (Hansson L, Hedner T, Lund-Johansen P et al 2000 Randomised trial of effects of calcium antagonists compared with diuretics and beta-blockers on cardiovascular morbidity and mortality in hypertension: the Nordic Diltiazem [NORDIL] study. 356:359–365; Brown M J, Palmer C R. Castaigne A et al 2000 Morbidity and mortality in patients randomised to double-blind treatment with a long-acting calcium-channel blocker or diuretic in the International Nifedipine GITS study: Intervention as a Goal in Hypertension Treatment [INSIGHT]. Lancet 356:355–372).

concentrations are lessened. Various methods have been used to prolong, and smooth, drug delivery, and bio-equivalence between these formulations cannot be assumed; prescribers should specify the brand to be dispensed. The adverse effects of calcium blockers with a short duration of action may include the hazards of activating the sympathetic system each time a dose is taken. The dose range for nifedipine is 30–90 mg daily. In addition to the adverse effects listed above, gum hypertrophy may occur. Nifedipine can be taken 'sublingually', by biting a capsule and squeezing the contents under the tongue. In point of fact, absorption is still largely from the stomach after this manoeuvre, and it should not be used in a hypertensive emergency because the blood pressure reduction is unpredictable and sometimes large enough to cause cerebral ischaemia (see p. 444).

Amlodipine has a $t_{1/2}$ (40 h) sufficient to permit the same benefits as the longest-acting formulations of nifedipine without requiring a special formulation. Its slow association with L-channels and long duration of action render it unsuitable for emergency reduction of blood pressure where frequent dose adjustment is needed. On the other hand an occasional missed dose is of little consequence. Amlodipine differs from all other dihydropyridines listed in this chapter in being safe to use in patients with cardiac failure (the PRAISE study).[7]

Verapamil ($t_{1/2}$ 4 h) is an arterial vasodilator with some venodilator effect; it also has marked negative myocardial inotropic and chronotropic actions. It is given thrice daily as a conventional tablet or daily as a sustained-release formulation. Because of its negative effects on myocardial conducting and contracting cells it should not be given to patients with bradycardia, second- or third-degree heart block, or patients with Wolff–Parkinson–White syndrome to relieve atrial flutter or fibrillation. Amiodarone and digoxin increase the AV block. Verapamil increases plasma quinidine concentration and this interaction may cause dangerous hypotension.

Diltiazem ($t_{1/2}$ 5 h) is given thrice daily, or once or twice daily if a slow-release formulation is prescribed. It causes less myocardial depression and prolongation of AV conduction than does verapamil but should not be used where there is bradycardia, second- or third-degree heart block or sick sinus syndrome.

Nimodipine has a moderate cerebral vasodilating action. Cerebral ischaemia after subarachnoid haemorrhage may be partly due to vasospasm; clinical trial evidence indicates that nimodipine given after subarachnoid haemorrhage reduces cerebral infarction (incidence and extent). Although the benefit is small, the absence of any more effective options has led to the routine administration of nimodipine (60 mg every 4 h) to all patients for the first few days after subarachnoid haemorrhage. No benefit has been found in similar trials following other forms of stroke.

Other members include felodipine, isradipine, lacidipine, lercanidipine, nisoldipine.

ANGIOTENSIN CONVERTING ENZYME (ACE) INHIBITORS AND ANGIOTENSIN (AT) II RECEPTOR BLOCKERS (ARBS)

Renin is an enzyme produced by the kidney in response to a number of factors, but principally adrenergic (β_1 receptor) activity and sodium depletion. Renin converts a circulating glycoprotein (angiotensinogen) into the biologically inert angiotensin I, which is then changed by *angiotensin-converting enzyme* (ACE or kininase II) into the highly potent vasoconstrictor *angiotensin II*. ACE is located on the luminal surface of capillary endothelial cells, particularly in the lungs; and there are also renin–angiotensin systems in many organs, e.g. brain, heart, the relevance of which is uncertain.

Angiotensin II acts on two G-protein-coupled receptors, of which the angiotensin 'AT$_1$' subtype accounts for all the classic actions of angiotensin. As well as vasoconstriction these include stimulation of aldosterone (the sodium-retaining hormone) production by the adrenal cortex. It is evident that angiotensin II can have an important effect on blood pressure. In addition, it stimulates cardiac and vascular smooth muscle cell growth, probably contributing to the progressive amplification in hypertension once the process is initiated. The AT$_2$-receptor subtype is coupled to inhibition of muscle growth or proliferation, but appears of minor importance in

---

[7]PRAISE = Prospective Randomised Amlodipine Survival Evaluation (see Packer M, O'Connor C M, Ghali J K et al 1996 The effect of amlodipine on morbidity and mortality in severe chronic heart failure. New England Journal of Medicine 335:1107–1114).

the adult cardiovascular system. The recognition that the AT_1-receptor subtype is the important target for drugs that antagonise angiotensin II has led, a little confusingly, to alternative nomenclatures for these drugs: either angiotensin II blockers or AT_1-receptor blockers (ARBs), which latter abbreviation is used here for consistency.

Bradykinin (an endogenous vasodilator found in blood vessel walls) is also a substrate for ACE. Potentiation of bradykinin contributes to the blood pressure-lowering action of ACE inhibitors in patients with low-renin causes of hypertension. Either bradykinin or one of the neurokinin substrates of ACE (such as substance P) may stimulate cough (below). The ARBs differ from the ACE inhibitors in having no effect on bradykinin and they do not cause cough. Those that achieve complete blockade of the receptor are slightly more effective than ACE inhibitors at preventing angiotensin II vasoconstriction. ACE inhibitors are more effective at suppressing aldosterone production in patients with normal or low plasma renin levels.

Uses

Hypertension. The antihypertensive effect of ACE inhibitors and ARBs results primarily from vasodilatation (reduction of peripheral resistance) with little change in cardiac output or rate; renal blood flow may increase (desirable). A fall in aldosterone production may also contribute to the blood pressure-lowering action of ACE inhibitors. Both classes slow progression of glomerulopathy. Whether the long-term benefit of these drugs in hypertension exceeds that to be expected from blood pressure reduction alone remains controversial.

ACE inhibitors and ARBs are most useful in hypertension when the raised blood pressure results from excess renin production, e.g. renovascular hypertension, or where concurrent use of another drug (diuretic or calcium blocker) renders the blood pressure renin dependent. The fall in blood pressure can be rapid, especially with short-acting ACE inhibitors, and low initial doses of these should be used in patients at risk: those with impaired renal function or suspected cerebrovascular disease. These patients may be advised to omit any concurrent diuretic treatment for a few days before the first dose. The antihypertensive effect increases progressively over weeks with continued administration (as with other antihypertensives) and the dose may be increased at intervals of 2 weeks.

Cardiac failure (see p. 483). ACE inhibitors have a useful vasodilator and diuretic-sparing (but not diuretic-substitute) action that is critical to the treatment of all grades of heart failure. Mortality reduction here may result from their being the only vasodilator that does not reflexly activate the sympathetic system.

The ARBs are at least as effective as ACE inhibitors in patients with heart failure and they can be substituted if patients are intolerant of an ACE inhibitor. Based on the Candesartan in Heart Failure Assessment of Reduction in Mortality and Morbidity (CHARM) trial, they may also benefit patients with heart failure and a low ejection fraction when added to treatment with a β-blocker and ACE inhibitor.[8]

Diabetic nephropathy. In patients with type I (insulin dependent) diabetes, hypertension often accompanies the diagnosis of frank nephropathy, and aggressive blood pressure control is essential to slow the otherwise inexorable decline in renal function that follows. ACE inhibitors appear to have a specific renoprotective effect, probably because of the role of angiotensin II in driving the underlying glomerular hyperfiltration.[9] These drugs are now first-line treatment for hypertensive type I diabetics, although most patients will need a second or third agent to reach the rigorous blood pressure (BP) targets for this condition (see below). There is evidence that ACE inhibitors have a proteinuria-sparing effect in type I diabetics with 'normal' BP, but whether this extends beyond a simple BP-lowering effect is less clear.[10] For hypertensive type 2 diabetics with early nephropathy, ARBs clearly provide better renoprotection than antihypertensive regimes lacking either an AT_1-receptor blocker or ACE inhibitor.[11] The Diabetics

[8]Demers C, McMurray J J V, Swedberg K et al for the CHARM investigators 2005 Impact of candesartan on nonfatal myocardial infarction and cardiovascular death in patients with heart failure. Journal of the American Medical Association 294:1794–1798.

[9]For a review see: Cooper M E 1998 Pathogenesis, prevention and treatment of diabetic nephropathy. Lancet 352:213–219.

[10]The EUCLID study group 1997 The EUCLID study. Randomised, placebo-controlled trial of lisinopril in normotensive patients with insulin-dependent diabetes and normoalbuminuria or microalbuminuria. Lancet 349:1787–1792.

[11]This is based on three trials: RENAAL (Reduction in ENdpoints with the Angiotensin Antagonist Losartan), IRMA (IRbesartan MicroAlbuminuric type 2 diabetes in hypertensive patients) II and IDNT (Irbesartan in Diabetic Nephropathy Trial). A useful review on PowerPoint slides of these trials is available: http://www.hypertensiononline.org/slides2

Exposed to Telmisartan And enaprIL (DETAIL) trial comparing an ARB against an ACE inhibitor showed equal renoprotective effect.[12] Whether combining the two classes of drugs ('dual block') confers additional benefit is not yet known.

Myocardial infarction (MI). Following a myocardial infarction, the left ventricle may fail acutely from the loss of functional tissue or in the long-term from a process of 'remodelling' due to thinning and enlargement of the scarred ventricular wall (see p. 467). Angiotensin II plays a key role in both of these processes and an ACE inhibitor given after MI markedly reduces the incidence of heart failure. The effect is seen even in patients without overt signs of cardiac failure, but who have low left ventricular ejection fractions (<40%) during the convalescent phase (3–10 days) following the MI. Such patients receiving captopril in the SAVE trial,[13] had a 37% reduction in progressive heart failure over the 60-month follow-up period compared with placebo. The benefits of ACE inhibition after MI are additional to those conferred by thrombolysis, aspirin and β-blockers. ARBs also prevent remodelling and heart failure in post-MI patients, but there is no additional benefit from 'dual blockade'.[14]

Cautions

Certain constraints apply to the use of ACE inhibitors:

- *Heart failure*: severe hypotension may result in patients taking diuretics, or who are hypovolaemic, hyponatraemic, elderly, have renal impairment or with systolic blood pressure of less than 100 mmHg. A test dose of captopril

6.25 mg by mouth may be given because its effect lasts for only 4–6 h. If tolerated, the preferred long-acting ACE inhibitor may then be initiated in low dose.

- *Renal artery stenosis* (RAS, whether unilateral, bilateral renal or suspected from the presence of generalised atherosclerosis): an ACE inhibitor may cause renal failure and is contraindicated. ARBs are not necessarily any safer in this situation, because angiotensin II-mediated constriction of the efferent arteriole is thought to be crucial to the maintenance of glomerular perfusion in RAS.
- *Aortic stenosis/left ventricular outflow tract obstruction*: an ACE inhibitor may cause severe, sudden hypotension and, depending on severity, is relatively or absolutely contraindicated.
- *Pregnancy* represents an absolute contraindication (see below).
- *Angio-oedema* may result (see below).

Adverse effects

ACE Inhibitors:

- *Persistent dry cough* occurs in 10–15% of patients.
- *Urticaria and angio-oedema* (less than 1 in 100 patients) are much rarer, occurring usually in the first weeks of treatment. The angio-oedema varies from mild swelling of the tongue to life-threatening tracheal obstruction, when subcutaaneous adrenaline (epinephrine) should be given. The basis of the reaction is probably pharmacological rather than allergic, due to reduced breakdown of bradykinin.
- *Impaired renal function* may result from reduced glomerular filling pressure, systemic hypotension or glomerulonephritis, and plasma creatinine levels should be checked before and during treatment.
- *Hyponatraemia* may develop, especially where a diuretic is also given; clinically significant hyperkalaemia (see effect on aldosterone above) is confined to patients with impaired renal function.
- ACE inhibitors cause major malformations in the first trimester and are *fetotoxic* in the second trimester, causing reduced renal perfusion, hypotension, oligohydramnios and fetal death (see Pregnancy hypertension, p. 443).
- *Neutropenia* and other blood dyscrasias occur. Other reported reactions include rashes, taste disturbance (dysguesia), musculoskeletal pain, proteinuria, liver injury and pancreatitis.

---

[12]The DETAIL study randomised type 2 diabetics to telmisartan or enalapril and followed their renal function over 5 years. The loss of GFR was the same in both groups (Barnett A H, Bain S C, Bouter P et al 2004 Angiotensin-receptor blockade versus converting-enzyme inhibition in type 2 diabetes and nephropathy. New England Journal of Medicine 351:1952–1961).

[13]Pfeffer M A, Braunwald E, Moye L A et al 1992 Effect of captopril on mortality and morbidity in patients with left ventricular dysfunction after myocardial infarction. Results of the survival and ventricular enlargement trial. The SAVE Investigators. New England Journal of Medicine 327:669–677.

[14]Pfeffer M A, McMurray J V C, Velaquez E J et al for the Valsartan in Acute Myocardial Infarction Trial Investigators 2004 Valsartan, captopril, or both in myocardial infarction complicated by heart failure, left ventricular dysfunction, or both. New England Journal of Medicine 349:1893–1906.

ARBs are contraindicated in pregnancy by implication with ACE inhibitors, but avoid the other complications of these drugs – especially the cough and angio-oedema. They are, in fact, the only antihypertensive drugs for which there is no 'typical' side-effect.

Interactions. Hyperkalaemia can result from use with potassium-sparing diuretics. Renal clearance of lithium is reduced and toxic concentrations of plasma lithium may follow. Severe hypotension can occur with diuretics (above), and with chlorproma-zine, and possibly other phenothiazines.

Individual drugs

Captopril (Capoten) has a $t_{1/2}$ of 2 h and is partly metabolised and partly excreted unchanged; adverse effects are more common when renal function is impaired; it is given twice or thrice daily. Captopril is the shortest acting of the ACE inhibitors, one of the few that is itself active by mouth, not requiring de-esterification after absorption.

Enalapril (Innovace) is a pro-drug ($t_{1/2}$ 35 h) that is converted to the active enalaprilat ($t_{1/2}$ 10 h). Effective 24-h control of blood pressure probably requires twice-daily administration.

Other members include *cilazapril, fosinopril, imi-dapril, lisinopril, moexipril, perindopril, quinapril, ramipril* and *trandolapril*. Of these, lisinopril has a marginally longer $t_{1/2}$ than enalapril (it is the lysine analogue of enalaprilat), probably justifying its pop-ularity as a once-daily ACE inhibitor. Some of the others are longer acting, with quinapril and ramipril also having a higher degree of binding to ACE in vas-cular tissue. The clinical significance of these differ-ences is disputed. In the Heart Outcomes Prevention Evaluation (HOPE) Study of 9297 patients, ramipril reduced, by 20–30%, the rates of death, myocardial infarction and stroke in a broad range of high-risk patients who were not known to have a low ejection fraction or heart failure.[15] The authors considered (probably erroneously) that the results could not be explained entirely by blood pressure reduction.

Losartan was the first ARB to be licensed in the UK. It is a competitive blocker with a non-competitive active metabolite. The drug has a short $t_{1/2}$ (2 h) but the metabolite is much longer lived ($t_{1/2}$ 10 h), per-mitting once-daily dosing.

Other ARBs in clinical use include *candesartan, eprosartan, irbesartan, telmisartan* and *valsartan*. Some of these appear to be more effective than losartan, which is generally used in combination with hydro-chlorothiazide. In a landmark study this combi-nation was 25% more effective than atenolol plus hydrochlorothiazide in preventing stroke.[16]

This class of drug is very well tolerated; in clini-cal trials the side-effect profiles are indistinguish-able or even better than those of placebo. Unlike the ACE inhibitors they do not produce cough, and are a valuable alternative for the 10–15% of patients who thereby discontinue their ACE inhib-itor. ARBs are used to treat hypertension, left ven-tricular (LV) failure after MI and established heart failure. With the possible exception of chronic heart failure, they do not appear to be superior to ACE inhibitors.

The cautions listed for the use of ACE inhibitors (above) apply also to AT_1-receptor blockers.

OTHER VASODILATORS

Several older drugs are powerfully vasodilating, but precluded from routine use in hypertension by their adverse effects. Minoxidil and nitroprusside still have special indications.

Minoxidil is a vasodilator selective for arterioles rather than for veins, similar to diazoxide and hydralazine. Like the former, it acts through its sul-phate metabolite as an ATP-dependent potassium channel opener. It is highly effective in severe hyper-tension, but in common with all potent arterial vasodilators its hypotensive action is accompanied by a compensatory baroreceptor-mediated sympa-thetic discharge, causing tachycardia and increased cardiac output. There is also renin release with sec-ondary salt and water retention, which antago-nises the hypotensive effect (so-called 'tolerance' on

[15]Yusuf S, Sleight P, Pogue J, Bosch J, Davies R, Dagenais G 2000 Effects of an angiotensin-converting-enzyme inhibitor, ramipril, on cardiovascular events in high-risk patients. The Heart Outcomes Prevention Evaluation Study Investigators. New England Journal of Medicine 342:145–153.

[16]Dahlof B et al 2002 Cardiovascular morbidity and mortality in the Losartan Intervention For Endpoint reduction in hypertension study (LIFE): a randomised trial against atenolol. Lancet 359:995–1010.

long-term use). Therefore, it is used in combination with a β-blocker and loop diuretic (as is hydralazine; see below). *Hypertrichosis* is perhaps the most notorious side-effect of minoxidil. The hair growth is generalised when taken orally and, although a cosmetic problem in women, it has been exploited as a 2–5% topical solution for the treatment of male-pattern baldness (Regaine).

Sodium nitroprusside is a highly effective antihypertensive agent when given intravenously. Its effect is almost immediate and lasts for 1–5 min. Therefore it must be given by a precisely controllable infusion. It dilates both arterioles and veins, which would cause collapse were the patient to stand up, e.g. for toilet purposes. There is a compensatory sympathetic discharge with tachycardia and tachyphylaxis to the drug.

The action of nitroprusside is terminated by metabolism within erythrocytes. Specifically, electron transfer from haemoglobin iron to nitroprusside yields methaemoglobin and an unstable nitroprusside radical. This breaks down, liberating cyanide radicals capable of inhibiting cytochrome oxidase (and thus cellular respiration). Fortunately most of the cyanide remains bound within erythrocytes but a small fraction does diffuse out into the plasma and is converted to thiocyanate. Hence, monitoring plasma thiocyanate concentrations during prolonged (days) nitroprusside infusion is a useful marker of impending systemic cyanide toxicity. Poisoning may be obvious as a progressive metabolic acidosis, or may manifest as delirium or psychotic symptoms. Intoxicated subjects are also reputed to have the characteristic bitter almond smell of hydrogen cyanide. Clearly nitroprusside infusion must be used with caution, and outside specialist units it may be safer overall to choose another more familiar drug.

Sodium nitroprusside is used in hypertensive emergencies, refractory heart failure and for controlled hypotension in surgery. An infusion[17] may begin at 0.3–1.0 micrograms/kg/min, and control of blood pressure is likely to be established at 0.5–6.0 micrograms/kg/min; close monitoring of blood pressure is mandatory, usually by direct arterial monitoring; rate changes of infusion may be made every 5–10 min.

Diazoxide reduces peripheral arteriolar resistance through activation of the ATP-dependent potassium channel (cf. nicorandil and minoxidil), with little effect on veins. The $t_{1/2}$ is 36 h. Diazoxide was used formerly as an intravenous bolus for the emergency treatment of severe hypertension, but the dangers of excessive hypotension are now recognised to outweigh the benefit, and its emergency use is obsolete.

As diazoxide activates the same potassium channel in the pancreatic islet cells that is blocked by sulphonylureas, it causes hyperglycaemia and is a useful drug for patients with chronic hypoglycaemia from excess endogenous insulin secretion, either from an islet cell tumour or islet cell hyperplasia. Long-term use causes the same problems of hair growth seen with minoxidil.

Hydralazine is now little used for hypertension except for that related to pregnancy (owing to its established lack of teratogenicity), but it may have a role as a vasodilator (plus nitrates) in heart failure. It reduces peripheral resistance by directly relaxing arterioles, with negligible effect on veins; the mechanism of vasorelaxation is unclear. The $t_{1/2}$ is 1 h.

In most hypertensive emergencies (except for dissecting aneurysm) hydralazine 5–20 mg i.v. may be given over 20 min, when the maximum effect will be seen in 10–80 min; it can be repeated according to need and the patient transferred to oral therapy within 1–2 days.

Prolonged use of hydralazine at doses above 50 mg/day may cause a systemic lupus-like syndrome, more commonly in white than in black races, and in those with the slow acetylator phenotype.

Three other vasodilators find a role outside hypertension:

Nicorandil is effective through two actions: it acts as a nitrate by activating cyclic GMP (see above) but also opens the ATP-dependent potassium channel to allow potassium efflux and hyperpolarisation of the membrane, which reduces calcium ion entry and induces muscular relaxation. It is indicated for use in angina, where it has similar efficacy to β-blockade, nitrates or calcium channel blockade. It is administered orally and is an alternative to nitrates when tolerance is a problem, or to the other classes

---

[17]Light causes sodium nitroprusside in solution to decompose; hence solutions should be made fresh and immediately protected by an opaque cover, e.g. metal foil. The fresh solution has a faint brown colour; if the colour is strong it should be discarded.

when these are contraindicated by asthma or cardiac failure. Adverse effects to nicorandil are similar to those of nitrates, with headache reported in 35% of patients. It is the only antianginal drug for which at least one trial has demonstrated a beneficial influence on outcome.[18]

Papaverine is an alkaloid present in opium, but is structurally unrelated to morphine. It inhibits phosphodiesterase and its principal action is to relax smooth muscle throughout the body, especially in the vascular system. It is occasionally injected into an area where local vasodilatation is desired, especially into and around arteries and veins to relieve spasm during vascular surgery and when setting up intravenous infusions. It is also used to treat male erectile dysfunction (see p. 492).

Alprostadil is a stable form of prostaglandin E_1. It is effective in psychogenic and neuropathic penile erectile dysfunction by direct intracorporeal injection (see p. 493) and is used intravenously to maintain patency of the ductus arteriosus in the newborn with congenital heart disease.

VASODILATORS IN HEART FAILURE

See page 416.

VASODILATORS IN PERIPHERAL VASCULAR DISEASE

The aim has been to produce peripheral arteriolar vasodilatation without a concurrent significant drop in blood pressure, so that an increased blood flow in the limbs will result. Drugs are naturally more useful in patients in whom the decreased flow of blood is due to spasm of the vessels (Raynaud's phenomenon) than where it is due to organic obstructive changes that may make dilatation in response to drugs impossible (arteriosclerosis, intermittent claudication, Buerger's disease).

Intermittent claudication. Patients should 'stop smoking and keep walking', i.e. take frequent exercise within their capacity. Other risk factors should be treated vigorously, especially hypertension and hyperlipidaemia. Patients should also receive low-dose aspirin (75 mg daily) as an antiplatelet agent. Most patients with intermittent claudication succumb to ischaemic or cerebrovascular disease, and therefore a major objective of treatment should be prevention of such outcomes. Vasodilators such as naftidrofuryl (Praxilene) and oxpentifylline (pentoxifylline) (Trental) increase blood flow to skin rather than muscle; they have been used successfully in the treatment of venous leg ulcers (varicose and traumatic). A trial of these drugs for intermittent claudication is worthwhile but they should be withdrawn if there is no benefit within a few weeks.

Naftidrofuryl has several actions. It is classed as a metabolic enhancer because it activates the enzyme succinate dehydrogenase, increasing the supply of ATP and reducing lactate concentrations in muscle. It also blocks $5HT_2$ receptors and inhibits serotonin-induced vasoconstriction and platelet aggregation.

Oxpentifylline is thought to improve oxygen supply to ischaemic tissue by improving erythrocyte deformability and reducing blood viscosity, in part by reducing plasma fibrinogen. Neither of these drugs is a direct vasodilator, as is the third drug used for intermittent claudication, *inositol nicotinate*. The evidence in favour of any benefit is stronger for the first two, for which meta-analyses provide some evidence of efficacy (increase in walking distance). Most vasodilators act selectively on healthy blood vessels, causing a diversion ('steal') of blood from atheromatous vessels.

Night cramps occur in the disease and quinine has a somewhat controversial reputation in their prevention. Nevertheless, meta-analysis of six double-blind trials of nocturnal cramps (not necessarily associated with peripheral vascular disease) shows that the number, but not severity or duration of episodes, is reduced by a night-time dose.[19] The benefit may not be seen for 4 weeks.

[18]The Impact Of Nicorandil in Angina (IONA) study was a double-blind, randomised, placebo-controlled trial conducted in the UK, in which high-risk patients with stable angina were assigned placebo or nicorandil 10–20 mg. Over a mean follow-up of 1.6 years significantly more placebo-treated patients suffered an acute coronary syndrome or coronary death (15.5% versus 13.1%, $P=0.01$) (The IONA Study Group 2002 Effect of nicorandil on coronary events in patients with stable angina: the Impact Of Nicorandil in Angina (IONA) randomised trial. Lancet 359:1269–1275).

[19]Man-Son-Hing M, Wells G 1995 Meta-analysis of efficacy of quinine for treatment of nocturnal cramps in elderly people. British Medical Journal 310:13–17.

Raynaud's phenomenon may be helped by nifedipine, reserpine (effectively an α-adrenoceptor blocker, in low doses) and also by topical glyceryl trinitrate; indeed any vasodilator is worth trying in resistant cases; enalapril (an ACE inhibitor) seems to lack efficacy. In severe cases, especially patients with ulceration, intermittent infusions over several hours of the endogenous vasodilator, prostacyclin (epoprostenol), achieves long-lasting improvements in symptoms.

β-Adrenoceptor blockers exacerbate peripheral vascular disease and Raynaud's phenomenon by reducing perfusion of a circulation that is already compromised. Switching to a β_1-selective blocker is unhelpful, because the adverse effect is due to reduced cardiac output rather than unopposed α receptor-induced vasoconstriction.

ADRENOCEPTOR BLOCKING DRUGS

Adrenoceptor blocking drugs occupy the adrenoceptor in competition with adrenaline (epinephrine) and noradrenaline (norepinephrine) (and other sympathomimetic amines) whether released from stores in nerve terminals or injected. There are two principal classes of adrenoceptor, α and β: for details of receptor effects see Table 22.1.

α-ADRENOCEPTOR BLOCKING DRUGS

There are two main subtypes of α adrenoceptor:

- 'Classic' α_1 adrenoceptors, on the effector organ (postsynaptic), mediate vasoconstriction.
- α_2 adrenoceptors are present both on some effector tissues (postsynaptic) and on the nerve ending (presynaptic). The presynaptic receptors (or autoreceptors) inhibit release of chemotransmitter (noradrenaline), i.e. they provide negative feedback control of transmitter release. They are also present in the CNS.

The first generation of α-adrenoceptor blockers were imidazolines (e.g. phentolamine), which blocked both α_1 and α_2 receptors. When subjects taking such a drug stand from the lying position or take exercise, the sympathetic system is physiologically activated (via baroreceptors). The normal vasoconstrictive (α_1) effect (to maintain blood pressure) is blocked by the drug and the failure of this response causes further sympathetic activation and the release

of additional transmitter. This would normally be restrained by negative feedback through α_2 autoreceptors, but these are blocked too.

The β adrenoceptors, however, are not blocked and the excess transmitter released at adrenergic endings is free to act on them, causing a tachycardia that may be unpleasant. Hence, non-selective α-adrenoceptor blockers are not used on their own in hypertension.

An α_1-adrenoceptor blocker that spares the α_2 receptor, so that negative feedback inhibition of noradrenaline release is maintained, is more useful in hypertension (less tachycardia and postural and exercise hypotension); prazosin is such a drug (see below).

For use in prostatic hypertrophy, see page 491.

Uses of α-adrenoceptor blocking drugs
- Hypertension
  - essential: doxazosin, labetalol
  - phaeochromocytoma: phenoxybenzamine; phentolamine (for crises)
- Peripheral vascular disease
- Benign prostatic hypertrophy (to relax capsular smooth muscle that may contribute to urinary obstruction)

Adverse effects. The converse of the benefit in the treatment of prostatism is the adverse effect of micturition incontinence in women. Other adverse effects of α-adrenoceptor blockade are postural hypotension, nasal stuffiness, red sclerae and, in the male, failure of ejaculation. They may also exacerbate symptoms of angina.[20] Effects peculiar to each drug are mentioned below.

Notes on individual drugs

Prazosin blocks postsynaptic α_1 receptors but not presynaptic α_2 autoreceptors. It has a curious adverse 'first-dose effect': within 2 h of the first dose (rarely after another) there may be a brisk fall in blood pressure sufficient to cause loss of consciousness. Hence the first dose should be small (0.5 mg) and given

---

[20]It can be the reflex sympathetic activation, as much as hypotension itself, that causes problems. Many cardiologists have had their efforts at controlling angina in elderly patients sabotaged when the patient visits a urologist for his prostatic symptoms, and is treated with a powerful α_1-blocker.

before going to bed. This unwanted effect, together with a rather short duration of action ($t_{1/2}$ 3 h) leads to longer-acting drugs being preferred.

Doxazosin ($t_{1/2}$ 8 h) was the first α-adrenoceptor blocker suitable for once-daily prescribing. The first-dose effect is also much less marked, although it is still advisable to start patients at a lower dose than is intended for maintenance. It is convenient, for instance, to prescribe 1 mg daily, increasing after 1 week to double this dose without repeating the blood pressure measurement at this stage. A slow-release formulation, Cardura XL, can be started at the maintenance dose of 4 mg daily.

Other α-adrenoceptor blockers used for prostatic symptoms are *alfuzosin* and *terazosin*.

Indoramin is an older $α_1$-blocker, which is a less useful antihypertensive but still used for prostatic symptoms. It is taken twice or thrice daily.

Phentolamine is a non-selective α-adrenoceptor blocker. It is given intravenously for brief effect in adrenergic hypertensive crises, e.g. phaeochromocytoma or the monoamine oxidase inhibitor–sympathomimetic interaction. In addition to α-receptor block it has direct vasodilator and cardiac inotropic actions. The dose for hypertensive crisis is 2–5 mg i.v. repeated as necessary (in minutes to hours). The use of phentolamine as a diagnostic test for phaeochromocytoma is appropriate only when biochemical measurements are impracticable, as it is less reliable.

Phenoxybenzamine is an irreversible non-selective α-adrenoceptor blocking drug whose effects may last for 2 days or longer. The daily dose must therefore be increased slowly. It is impossible to reverse the circulatory effects by secreting noradrenaline (norepinephrine) or other sympathomimetic drugs because its effects are insurmountable. This makes it the preferred α-blocker for treating phaeochromocytoma (see p. 445).

It is wise to observe the effects of a single test dose closely before starting regular administration.

Indigestion and nausea can occur with oral therapy, which is best given with food.

Thymoxamine (moxisylyte) is a non-selective α-blocker for which Raynaud's phenomenon is the only extant indication.

Labetalol has both α- and β-receptor blocking actions that are due to different isomers (see β-adrenoceptor block, below). Its parenteral preparation is valuable in the treatment of hypertension emergencies (see p. 442).

Chlorpromazine and amitriptyline, amongst their other actions, can both produce clinically significant α-blockade, which may be sufficient to cause postural hypotension and falls in the elderly.

β-ADRENOCEPTOR BLOCKING DRUGS

Actions

These drugs selectively block the β-adrenoceptor effects of noradrenaline (norepinephrine) and adrenaline (epinephrine). They may be pure antagonists or may have some agonist activity in addition (when they are described as partial agonists).

Intrinsic heart rate. Sympathetic activity (through $β_1$ adrenoceptors) accelerates, and parasympathetic activity (through muscarinic M_2 receptors) slows, the heart. If the sympathetic and the parasympathetic drives to the heart are simultaneously and adequately blocked by a β-adrenoceptor blocker plus atropine, the heart will beat at its 'intrinsic' rate. The intrinsic rate at rest is usually about 100 beats/min, as opposed to the usual rate of 80 beats/min, i.e. normally there is parasympathetic vagal 'tone', which decreases with age.

The *cardiovascular* effects of β-adrenoceptor block depend on the amount of sympathetic tone present. The chief effects result from reduction of sympathetic drive:

- Reduced automaticity (heart rate).
- Reduced myocardial contractility (rate of rise of pressure in the ventricle).
- Reduced renin secretion from the juxtaglomerular apparatus in the renal cortex.

With reduced rate the cardiac output per minute is reduced and the overall cardiac oxygen consumption falls. The results are more evident on the response to exercise than at rest. With acute administration of a pure β-adrenoceptor blocker, i.e. one with no intrinsic sympathomimetic activity (ISA), *peripheral vascular resistance* tends to rise. This is probably a reflex response to the reduced cardiac output, but also occurs because the β-adrenoceptor (vasoconstrictor) effects are no longer partially opposed by β_2-adrenoceptor (dilator) effects; peripheral flow is reduced. With chronic use peripheral resistance returns to about pre-treatment levels or a little below, varying according to presence or absence of ISA. But peripheral blood flow remains reduced. The cold extremities that accompany chronic therapy are probably due chiefly to reduced cardiac output with reduced peripheral blood flow, rather than to the blocking of peripheral (β_2) dilator receptors.

Hepatic blood flow may be reduced by as much as 30%, prolonging the $t_{1/2}$ of the lipid-soluble drugs whose metabolism is dependent on hepatic flow, i.e. whose first-pass metabolism is so extensive that it is actually limited by the rate of blood delivery to the liver; these include propranolol, verapamil and lidocaine, which may be used concomitantly for cardiac arrhythmias.

Effects

Within hours of starting treatment with a β-blocker, blood pressure starts to fall. The mechanism(s) remain uncertain, and the consistency of antihypertensive response in many different types of hypertension may reflect a contribution from a variety of mechanisms. β-Blockers are most effective in patients who respond also to ACE inhibitors; blockade of renin secretion is likely therefore to be the main cause of blood pressure reduction. An additional contributor may be the two- to three-fold increase in natriuretic peptide secretion caused by β-blockade.

Most of the blood pressure effect occurs quickly (hours, days) but there is often a modest further decrease over several weeks.

A substantial advantage of β-blockade in hypertension is that physiological stresses such as exercise, *upright posture* and *high environmental temperature* are not accompanied by hypotension, as they are with agents that interfere with α-adrenoceptor-mediated homeostatic mechanisms. With β-blockade these necessary adaptive α-receptor constrictor mechanisms remain intact.

At first sight the cardiac effects might seem likely to be disadvantageous rather than advantageous, and indeed maximum exercise capacity is reduced. But the heart has substantial functional reserves so that use may be made of the desired properties in the diseases listed below, e.g. angina, without inducing heart failure. Indeed, β-blockade is now routine practice in patients with established mild to moderate heart failure. But heart failure can occur in patients with seriously diminished cardiac reserve.

For the effect on plasma potassium concentration, see page 408.

β-Adrenoceptor selectivity

Some β-adrenoceptor blockers have higher affinity for cardiac β_1 receptors than for cardiac and peripheral β_2 receptors (Table 23.1). The ratio of the amount of drug required to block the two receptor subtypes is a measure of the *selectivity* of the drug. (See note to Table 22.1, p. 405, regarding the use of the terms 'β_1 selective' and '*cardioselective*'.) The question is whether the differences between selective and non-selective β-blockers confer clinical advantages. In theory β_1-blockers are less likely to cause bronchoconstriction, but in practice few available β_1-blockers are sufficiently selective to be safely recommended in asthma. Bisoprolol and nebivolol may be exceptions that can be tried at low doses in patients with mild asthma and a strong indication for β-blockade. There are unlikely ever to be satisfactory safety data to support such use. The main practical use of β_1-selective blockade is in diabetics, where β_2 receptors mediate both the symptoms of hypoglycaemia and the counter-regulatory metabolic responses that reverse the hypoglycaemia.

Some β-blockers (antagonists) also have agonist action or ISA, i.e. they are *partial agonists*. These agents cause less fall in resting heart rate than do the pure antagonists and may thus be less effective in severe angina pectoris where reduction of heart rate is particularly important. The fall in cardiac output may be less, and fewer patients may experience unpleasantly cold extremities. Intermittent claudication may be worsened by β-blockade whether or not there is partial agonist effect. Both classes of drug can *precipitate* heart failure, and indeed no important difference is to be expected because patients with heart failure already have high sympathetic drive (but note that β-blockade can be used to *treat* cardiac failure, pp. 483, 465).

Abrupt withdrawal may be less likely to lead to a rebound effect if there is some partial agonist action, as there may be less up-regulation of receptors, such as occurs with prolonged receptor block.

Some β-blockers have a membrane stabilising (quinidine-like or local anaesthetic) effect, a property that is unimportant at clinical doses but relevant in overdose (see below). Additionally, agents having this effect will anaesthetise the eye (undesirable) if applied topically for glaucoma (timolol is used in the eye and does not have this action).

Table 23.1 β-Adrenoceptor blocking drugs: properties at therapeutic doses

Drug		Partial agonist effect (intrinsic sympathomimetic effect)	Membrane stabilising effect (quinidine-like effect)
Division I: non-selective (β₁ + β₂) blockade			
Group I	oxprenolol	+	+
Group II	propranolol	−	+
Group III	pindolol	+	−
Group IV	sotalol	−	−
	timolol	−	−
	nadolol	−	−
Division II: β₁-('cardio')ᵃ-selective blockadeᵇ			
Group I	acebutolol	+	+
Group III	esmolol	+	+
Group IV	atenolol	−	−
	bisoprolol	−	−
	metoprolol	−	−
	nebivolol	−	−
	betaxolol	−	−
	celiprololᶜ	−	−
Division III: non-selective β-blockade + α₁-blockade			
Group II	carvedilol	−	+
Group IV	labetalolᶜ	−	−

ᵃSee Table 22.1, page 405 regarding use of the term 'cardioselective'. *Note*: hybrid agents having β-receptor block plus vasodilatation unrelated to adrenoceptor have been developed, e.g. nebivolol releases nitric oxide.

ᵇβ₁-selective drugs are considered to be up to 300 times (nebivolol) as effective against β₁-receptors compared with β₂-receptors. What selectivity really means is that 300 times more of the blocker is required to achieve the same blockade of the β₂-receptor as for the β₁-receptor. Therefore, as the dose (concentration at receptors) rises, the benefit of selectivity is gradually lost.

ᶜCeliprolol and labetalol both have partial β₂-selective agonist activity.

The ankle jerk relaxation time is prolonged by β₂-adrenoceptor block, which may be misleading if the reflex is being relied on in diagnosis and management of hypothyroidism.

Pharmacokinetics

The plasma concentration of a β-adrenoceptor blocker may have a complex relationship with its effect, for several reasons. First-order kinetics usually apply to elimination of drug from plasma, but the decline in receptor block is zero order. The practical application is important: within 4 h of giving propranolol 20 mg i.v. the plasma concentration falls by 50%, but the receptor block (as measured by exercise-induced tachycardia) falls by only 35%. The relationship between the concentration of the parent drug in plasma and its effect is further obscured if pharmacologically active metabolites are also present. Additionally, for some of the lipid-soluble β-blockers, especially timolol, plasma $t_{1/2}$ may not reflect the duration of β-blockade, because the drug remains bound to the tissues near the receptor when the plasma concentration is negligible.

Most β-adrenoceptor blockers can be given orally once daily in either ordinary or sustained-release formulations because the $t_{1/2}$ of the pharmacodynamic effect exceeds the elimination $t_{1/2}$ of the parent substance in the blood.

Lipid-soluble agents are extensively metabolised (hydroxylated, conjugated) to water-soluble substances that can be eliminated by the kidney. Plasma concentrations of drugs subject to extensive hepatic first-pass metabolism vary greatly between subjects (up to 20-fold) because the process itself is dependent on two highly variable factors: speed of absorption and hepatic blood flow, with latter being the rate-limiting factor.

Lipid-soluble agents readily cross cell membranes and so have a high apparent volume of distribution. They also readily enter the central nervous system (CNS), e.g. propranolol reaches concentrations in the brain 20 times those of the water-soluble atenolol.

Water-soluble agents show more predictable plasma concentrations because they are less subject to liver metabolism, being excreted unchanged by the kidney; thus their half-lives are greatly prolonged in renal failure, e.g. atenolol $t_{1/2}$ is increased from 7 to 24 h. Drugs (of any kind) having a long $t_{1/2}$ and an action terminated by renal elimination are best avoided in patients with renal disease. Water-soluble agents are less widely distributed and may have a lower incidence of effects attributed to penetration of the CNS, e.g. nightmares.

- The most lipid-soluble agents are propranolol, metoprolol, oxprenolol and labetalol.
- The least lipid-soluble (and most water-soluble) agents are atenolol, sotalol and nadolol.
- Others are intermediate.

Classification of β-adrenoceptor blocking drugs

- *Pharmacokinetic*: lipid soluble, water soluble, see above.
- *Pharmacodynamic* (see Table 23.1). The associated properties (partial agonist action and membrane stabilising action) have only minor clinical importance with current drugs at doses ordinarily used and may be insignificant in most cases. But it is desirable that they be known, for they can sometimes matter and they may foreshadow future developments.

β-Adrenoceptor blockers not listed in Table 23.1 include:

- *Non-selective*: carteolol, bufuralol.
- *$β_1$-receptor selective*: betaxolol, esmolol (ultra-short acting: minutes).
- *β- and α-receptor block*: bucindolol.

Uses of β-adrenoceptor blocking drugs

Cardiovascular uses:

Angina pectoris: β-blockade reduces cardiac work and oxygen consumption.

Hypertension: β-blockade reduces renin secretion and cardiac output; there is little interference with homeostatic reflexes.

Cardiac tachyarrhythmias: β-blockade reduces drive to cardiac pacemakers: subsidiary properties (see Table 24.1, p. 451) may also be relevant.

Myocardial infarction and β-adrenoceptor blockers: There are two modes of use that reduce acute mortality and prevent recurrence: the so-called 'cardioprotective' effect.

- *Early use* within 6 h (or at most 12 h) of onset (intravenously for 24 h then orally for 3–4 weeks). Benefit has been demonstrated only for atenolol. Cardiac work is reduced, resulting in a reduction in infarct size by up to 25% and protection against cardiac rupture. Surprisingly, tachyarrhythmias are not less frequent, perhaps because the cardiac $β_2$ receptor is not blocked by atenolol. Maximum benefit is in the first 24–36 h, but mortality remains lower for up to 1 year. Contraindications to early use include bradycardia (<55 beats/min), hypotension (systolic <90 mmHg) and left ventricular failure. A patient already taking a β-blocker may be given additional doses.
- *Late use* for secondary prevention of another myocardial infarction. The drug is started between 4 days and 4 weeks after the onset of the infarct and is continued for at least 2 years.[21]
- *Choice of drug.* The agent should be a pure antagonist, i.e. without ISA.

Aortic dissection and after subarachnoid haemorrhage: by reducing force and speed of systolic ejection (contractility) and blood pressure.

Obstruction of ventricular outflow where sympathetic activity occurs in the presence of anatomical abnormalities, e.g. Fallot's tetralogy (cyanotic attacks): hypertrophic subaortic stenosis (angina); some cases of mitral valve disease.

Hepatic portal hypertension and oesophageal variceal bleeding: reduction of portal pressure (see p. 585).

Cardiac failure (see also Chapter 24): there is now clear evidence from prospective trials that β-blockade is beneficial in terms of mortality for patients with all grades of moderate heart failure. Data support the use of both non-selective (carvedilol,

---

[21]In the first major study, sudden death occurred in 13.9% of placebo-treated and 7.7% of timolol-treated patients (The Norwegian Multicentre Study Group 1981 Timolol-induced reduction in mortality and reinfarction in patients surviving myocardial infarction. New England Journal of Medicine 304:801–807).

α-blocker as well) and β_1-selective (metoprolol and bisoprolol) agents. Survival benefit exceeds that provided by ACE inhibitors over placebo. The negative inotropic effects can still be significant, so the starting dose is low (e.g. bisoprolol 1.25 mg p.o. daily in the morning or carvedilol 3.125 mg twice daily, with food) and may be tolerated only with additional anti-failure therapy, e.g. diuretic.

Endocrine uses

Hyperthyroidism: β-blockade reduces unpleasant symptoms of sympathetic overactivity; there may also be an effect on metabolism of thyroxine (peripheral de-iodination from T4 to T3). A non-selective agent (propranolol) is preferred to counteract both the cardiac (β_1 and β_2) effects, and tremor (β_2).

Phaeochromocytoma: blockade of β-agonist effects of circulating catecholamines always in combination with adequate α-adrenoceptor block. Only small doses of a β-blocker are required.

Other uses

- Central nervous system
  - *anxiety* with somatic symptoms (non-selective β-blockade may be more effective than β_1-selective)
  - *migraine* prophylaxis (see p. 309)
  - essential tremor, some cases
  - *alcohol and opioid acute withdrawal* symptoms.
- Eyes
  - *glaucoma*: carveolol, betaxolol, levobunolol and timolol eye-drops act by altering production and outflow of aqueous humour.

Adverse reactions due to β-adrenoceptor blockade

Bronchoconstriction (β_2 receptor) occurs as expected, especially in patients with asthma[22] (in whom even eye-drops are dangerous[23]). In elderly chronic bronchitics there may be gradually increasing bronchoconstriction over weeks (even with eye-drops). Plainly, risk is greater with non-selective agents, but β_1 receptor-selective members can still have significant β_2-receptor occupancy and may precipitate asthma.

Cardiac failure may arise if cardiac output is dependent on high sympathetic drive (but β-blockade can be introduced at very low dose to treat cardiac failure; see above). The degree of heart block may be made dangerously worse.

Incapacity for vigorous exercise due to failure of the cardiovascular system to respond to sympathetic drive.

Hypotension when the drug is given after myocardial infarction.

Hypertension may occur whenever blockade of β receptors allows pre-existing α effects to be unopposed, e.g. phaeochromocytoma.

Reduced peripheral blood flow, especially with non-selective members, leading to cold extremities which, rarely, can be severe enough to cause necrosis; intermittent claudication may be worsened.

Reduced blood flow to liver and kidneys, reducing metabolism and biliary and renal elimination of drugs, is liable to be important if there is hepatic or renal disease.

Hypoglycaemia: β_2 receptors mediate both the symptoms of hypoglycaemia and the counter-regulatory metabolic responses that restore blood glucose. Non-selective β-blockers, by blocking β_2 receptors, impair the normal sympathetic-mediated homeostatic

---

[22]A 36-year-old patient with asthma collected, from a pharmacy, chlorphenamine for herself and oxprenolol for a friend. She took a tablet of oxprenolol by mistake. Wheezing began in 1 h and worsened rapidly; she experienced a convulsion, respiratory arrest and ventricular fibrillation. She was treated with positive-pressure ventilation (for 11 h) and intravenous salbutamol, aminophylline and hydrocortisone, and survived (Williams I P, Millard F J 1980 Severe asthma after inadvertent ingestion of oxprenolol. Thorax 35:160). There is a logical – or rather pharmacological – link between the use of timolol as eye-drops and the risk of asthma. For local

administration, a drug needs high potency, so that a high degree of receptor blockade is achieved using a physically small (and therefore locally administrable) dose of drug. Nevertheless, timolol is used topically as a 0.25–0.5% solution, which means the initial concentration of timolol in the tear film is up to 5 mg/mL (or >10 mmol/L). As the majority of this will be swallowed and a few milligrams orally will block systemic β_2 receptors, it is apparent why one drop of timolol down the lachrymal duct (of the wrong patient) is hazardous.

[23]Müller M E, van der Velde N, Krulder J W M, van der Cammen T J M 2006 Syncope and falls due to timolol eye drops. British Medical Journal 332:960–961.

mechanism for maintaining blood glucose levels, and recovery from hypoglycaemia is delayed; this is important in diabetes and after substantial exercise. Further, as α adrenoceptors are not blocked, hypertension (which may be severe) can occur as the sympathetic system discharges in an 'attempt' to reverse the hypoglycaemia. The symptoms of hypoglycaemia, in so far as they are mediated by the sympathetic nervous system (anxiety, palpitations), will not occur, except (cholinergic) sweating, and the patient may miss the warning symptoms of hypoglycaemia and slip into coma. β_1-selective drugs are preferred in diabetes.

Plasma lipoproteins: HIgh-density lipoprotein (HDL)-cholesterol falls and triglycerides rise during chronic β-blockade with non-selective agents. β_1-selective agents have much less impact overall. Patients with hyperlipidaemia needing a β-blocker should generally receive a β_1-selective one.

Sexual function: interference is unusual and generally not supported in placebo-controlled trials.

Abrupt withdrawal of therapy can be dangerous in angina pectoris and after myocardial infarction, and withdrawal should be gradual, e.g. reduce to a low dose and continue this for a few days. The existence and cause of a β-blocker withdrawal phenomenon is debated, but probably occurs due to up-regulation of β_2 receptors. It is particularly inadvisable to initiate an α-blocker at the same time as withdrawing a β-blocker in patients with ischaemic heart disease, because the β-blocker causes reflex activation of the sympathetic system. The β-blocker withdrawal phenomenon appears to be least common with partial agonists and most common with β_1-selective antagonists. Rebound hypertension is insignificant.

Adverse reactions not certainly due to β-adrenoceptor blockade

These include loss of general well-being, tired legs, fatigue, depression, sleep disturbances including insomnia, dreaming, feelings of weakness, gut upsets, rashes.

Oculomucocutaneous syndrome occurred with chronic use of practolol (now obsolete) and even occasionally after cessation of use.[24] Other members

either do not cause it, or so rarely do so that they are under suspicion only and, properly prescribed, the benefits of their use far outweigh such a very low risk. The mechanism of the syndrome is uncertain but appears immunological.

Overdose

Overdose, including self-poisoning, causes bradycardia, heart block, hypotension and low-output cardiac failure that can proceed to cardiogenic shock; death is more likely with agents that have a membrane stabilising action (see Table 23.1). Bronchoconstriction can be severe, even fatal, in patients subject to any bronchospastic disease; loss of consciousness may occur with lipid-soluble agents that penetrate the CNS. Receptor blockade will outlast the persistence of the drug in the plasma.

Rational treatment includes:

- *Atropine* (1–2 mg i.v. as one or two bolus doses) to eliminate the unopposed vagal activity that contributes to bradycardia. Most patients also require direct cardiac pacing.
- *Glucagon*, which has cardiac inotropic and chronotropic actions independent of the β-adrenoceptor (dose 50–150 micrograms/kg in glucose 5% i.v., repeated if necessary) to be used at the outset in severe cases (an unlicensed indication).
- If there is no response, intravenous injection or infusion of a β-adrenoceptor agonist is an alternative, e.g. isoprenaline (4 micrograms/min, increasing at 1–3-min intervals until the heart rate is 50–70 beats/min).
- Other sympathomimetics may be used as judgement counsels, according to the desired receptor agonist actions (β_1, β_2, α) required by the clinical condition, e.g. dobutamine, dopamine, dopexamine, noradrenaline, adrenaline.

which time there had accumulated about 200 000 patient-years of experience with the drug. It then became apparent that a small proportion of patients taking practolol could develop a bizarre syndrome that included conjunctival scarring, nasal and mucosal ulceration, fibrous peritonitis, pleurisy and cochlear damage (oculomucocutaneous syndrome). The condition was first recognised by an alert ophthalmologist who ran a special clinic for external eye diseases. (See Wright P 1975 Untoward effects associated with practolol administration: oculomucocutaneous syndrome. British Medical Journal i:595–589.)

[24]Practolol was developed to the highest current scientific standards; it was marketed in 1970 as the first cardioselective β-blocker, and only after independent review by the UK drug regulatory body. All seemed to go well for about 4 years, by

- For bronchoconstriction, salbutamol may be used; aminophylline has non-adrenergic cardiac inotropic and bronchodilator actions and should be given intravenously very slowly to avoid precipitating hypotension.
- A cardiac pacemaker may be used to increase the heart rate.

Treatment may be needed for days. With prompt treatment, death is unusual.

Interactions

Pharmacokinetic. β-blockers that are metabolised in the liver exhibit higher plasma concentrations when co-administered with drugs that inhibits hepatic metabolism, e.g. cimetidine. Enzyme inducers enhance the metabolism of this class of β-blockers. β-Adrenoceptor blockers themselves reduce hepatic blood flow (with fall in cardiac output) and reduce the metabolism of β-blockers and other drugs whose metabolic elimination is dependent on the rate of delivery to the liver, e.g. lidocaine, chlorpromazine.

Pharmacodynamic. The effect on the blood pressure of sympathomimetics having both α- and β-receptor agonist actions is increased by block of β receptors, leaving the α-receptor vasoconstriction unopposed (even adrenaline added to local anaesthetics may cause hypertension); the pressor effect of abrupt clonidine withdrawal is enhanced, probably by this action. Other cardiac antiarrhythmic drugs are potentiated, e.g. hypotension, bradycardia, heart block. Combination with verapamil (i.v.) is hazardous in the presence of atrioventricular nodal or left ventricular dysfunction because the latter has stronger negative inotropic and chronotropic effects than do other calcium channel blockers.

Most non-steroidal anti-inflammatory drugs (NSAIDs) attenuate the antihypertensive effect of β-blockers (but not perhaps of atenolol), presumably due to inhibition of formation of renal vasodilator prostaglandins, leading to sodium retention.

β-Adrenoceptor blockers potentiate the effect of other antihypertensives, particularly when an increase in heart rate is part of the homeostatic response (calcium channel blockers and α-adrenoceptor blockers).

Non-selective β-receptor blockers potentiate hypoglycaemia of insulin and sulphonylureas.

Pregnancy

β-Adrenoceptor blocking agents are used in pregnancy-related hypertension, including pre-eclampsia. Both lipid- and water-soluble members enter the fetus and may cause neonatal bradycardia and hypoglycaemia. They are not teratogenic in pregnancy, but some studies have suggested they cause intrauterine growth retardation.

Notes on some individual β-adrenoceptor blockers

(For general pharmacokinetics, see p. 80.)

Propranolol is available in standard (b.d. or t.i.d.) and sustained-release (once daily) formulations. When given i.v. (1 mg/min over 1 min, repeated every 2 min up to 10 mg) for cardiac arrhythmia or thyrotoxicosis it should be preceded by atropine (1–2 mg i.v.) to prevent excessive bradycardia; hypotension may occur.

Atenolol has a $\beta_1 : \beta_2$ selectivity of 1 : 15. It is widely used for angina pectoris and hypertension, in a dose of 25–100 mg orally once a day. The tendency in the past has been to use higher than necessary doses. When introduced, atenolol was considered not to need dose ranging, unlike propranolol, but this was in part because the initial dose was already at the top of the dose–response curve. Some 90% of absorbed drug is excreted by the kidney and the dose should be reduced when renal function is impaired, e.g. to 50 mg/day when the glomerular filtration rate (GFR) is 15–35 mL/min. It is best avoided in patients with GFR of less than 10 mL/min. The $t_{1/2}$ is 7 h.

Bisoprolol is more β_1 selective than atenolol (ratio 1 : 50). Although a relatively lipid-soluble agent, its $t_{1/2}$ (11 h) is one of the longest and there is not the wide range of dose requirement seen with propranolol. It is worth starting at a low dose (5 mg), to avoid causing unnecessary tiredness and obtain the maximum benefit of its selectivity. There is no need to alter doses when renal or hepatic function is reduced.

Nebivolol resembles bisoprolol in terms of lipophilicity and $t_{1/2}$ (10 h) but is more β_1 selective (ratio 1 : 300). Its unique feature is a direct vasodilator action (due to the D-isomer of the racemate, the L-isomer being the β_1 antagonist). The mechanism appears to be through direct activation of nitric oxide production by vascular endothelium.

COMBINED β_1- AND α-ADRENOCEPTOR BLOCKING DRUG

Labetalol is a racemic mixture: one isomer is a β-adrenoceptor blocker (non-selective), another blocks α adrenoceptors. Its dual effect on blood vessels minimises the vasoconstriction characteristic of non-selective β-blockade so that, for practical purposes, the outcome is similar to that of a β_1-selective β-blocker (see Table 23.1). It is less effective than drugs such as atenolol or bisoprolol for the routine treatment of hypertension, but is useful for some specific indications.

The β-blockade is 4 to 10 times greater than the α-blockade, varying with dose and route of administration. Labetalol is useful as a parenterally administered drug in the emergency reduction of blood pressure. Ordinary β-blockers may lower blood pressure too slowly, in part because reflex stimulation of unblocked α receptors opposes the fall in blood pressure. In most patients, even those with severe hypertension, a gradual reduction in blood pressure is desirable to avoid the risk of cerebral or renal hypoperfusion, but in the presence of a great vessel dissection or of fits, a more rapid effect is required (below).

Postural hypotension (characteristic of α-receptor blockade) is liable to occur at the outset of therapy and if the dose is increased too rapidly. But with chronic therapy when the β-receptor component is largely responsible for the antihypertensive effect, it is not a problem.

Labetalol reduces the hypertensive response to orgasm in women.

The $t_{1/2}$ is 4 h; it is extensively metabolised in the hepatic first-pass. The drug is given twice daily in a dose of 100–800 mg b.d.

For emergency control of severe hypertension (including pregnancy), the most convenient regimen is to initiate infusion at 1 mg/min, and titrate upwards at half-hourly intervals as required. If bradycardia is a problem, then intravenous atropine should be given (as 600-microgram boluses). The labetalol infusion is stopped as blood pressure control is achieved (up to 200 mg may be required), and re-initiated as frequently as required until regular oral therapy has been successfully introduced.

PERIPHERAL SYMPATHETIC NERVE TERMINAL

ADRENERGIC NEURONE BLOCKING DRUGS

Adrenergic neurone blocking drugs are taken up into adrenergic nerve endings by the active noradrenaline reuptake mechanism (uptake 1) (see Fig. 22.1). Their action within the nerve terminal is complex. They accumulate in the noradrenaline storage vesicles displacing noradrenaline, hence reducing the amount of noradrenaline released in response to nerve impulses (a 'false transmitter' effect); they also block the vesicle mechanism directly. The overall effect is to abolish presynaptic sympathetic function completely. This explains the severe postural hypotension in their (now obsolete) use to control hypertension (although guanethidine is still licensed in the UK for the rapid control of blood pressure). It is also used for regional intravenous sympathetic blockade in patients with intractable Raynaud's disease.

Meta-iodobenzylguanidine (MIBG) is used diagnostically as a radio-iodinated tracer, to locate chromaffin tumours (mainly phaeochromocytoma), which accumulate drugs in this class (see p. 445).

DEPLETION OF STORED TRANSMITTER (NORADRENALINE)

Reserpine is an alkaloid from plants of the genus *Rauwolfia*, used in medicine since ancient times for insanity; more recently, reserpine was extensively used in psychiatry but is now obsolete. Reserpine depletes adrenergic nerves of noradrenaline, primarily by blocking the transport of noradrenaline into storage vesicles (see Fig. 22.1). Its antihypertensive action is chiefly a peripheral action, but it enters the CNS and depletes central catecholamine stores; this explains the sedation, depression and parkinsonian side-effects that can accompany its use. These effects persist for days to weeks after it is withdrawn. Reserpine is rarely used in Europe but its low cost means it is still an attractive agent to treat hypertension in some parts of the world.

INHIBITION OF SYNTHESIS OF TRANSMITTER

Metirosine (α-methyl-*p*-tyrosine) is a competitive inhibitor of the enzyme *tyrosine hydroxylase*, which converts tyrosine to dopa; as dopa is converted to noradrenaline and adrenaline, both are depleted by metirosine. It is used as an adjuvant (with phenoxybenzamine) to treat phaeochromocytomas that cannot be removed surgically. Catecholamine synthesis is reduced by up to 80% over 3 days. It also enters the CNS and depletes brain noradrenaline and dopamine, causing reserpine-like adverse effects (see above). Hence, if life expectancy is threatened more by tumour invasion than hypertension, the need for the drug should be weighed carefully.

AUTONOMIC GANGLION BLOCKING DRUGS

Hexamethonium was the first orally active drug to treat hypertension, but the blockade of both sympathetic and parasympathetic systems caused severe side-effects. They are of historical interest only in hypertension therapy.

Trimetaphan, a short-acting agent, is given intravenously for the emergency control of hypertension; pressure may be adjusted by tilting the body to provide 'minute to minute' control, when the lack of selectivity is useful.

CENTRAL NERVOUS SYSTEM

α_2-ADRENOCEPTOR AGONISTS

Clonidine (Catapres) is an imidazoline that is an agonist to α_2 adrenoceptors (postsynaptic) in the brain, stimulation of which suppresses sympathetic outflow and reduces blood pressure. Drugs of this type are said to be selective for an imidazoline receptor (I_1), rather than the α_2 receptor. In fact, no such receptor has been identified at the molecular level, and genetic knockout experiments have shown that it is the α_2 receptor that is required for the blood pressure-lowering action of imidazoline drugs. At high doses clonidine activates peripheral α_2 adrenoceptors (presynaptic autoreceptors) on the adrenergic nerve ending; these mediate negative feedback suppression of noradrenaline release.

Clonidine was discovered to be hypotensive, not by the pharmacologists who tested it in the laboratory but by a physician who used it on himself as nose drops for a common cold. The $t_{1/2}$ is 6 h. Clonidine reduces blood pressure with little postural or exercise-related drop.

Its most serious handicap is that abrupt or even gradual withdrawal causes rebound hypertension. This is characterised by plasma catecholamine concentrations as high as those seen in hypertensive attacks of phaeochromocytoma. The onset may be rapid (a few hours) or delayed for as long as 2 days; it subsides over 2–3 days. The treatment is either to reinstitute clonidine, intramuscularly if necessary, or to treat as for a phaeochromocytoma (see below). Clonidine should never be used with a β-adrenoceptor blocker that exacerbates withdrawal hypertension (see phaeochromocytoma, p. 445). Other common adverse effects include sedation and dry mouth.

Tricyclic antidepressants antagonise the antihypertensive action and increase the rebound hypertension of abrupt withdrawal. Low-dose clonidine (Dixarit 50–75 mg b.d.) also has a minor role in migraine prophylaxis, menopausal flushing and choreas.

Rebound hypertension is a less important problem with longer-acting imidazolines, e.g. moxonidine, and a single dose can be omitted without rebound.

FALSE TRANSMITTER

Chemotransmitters and receptors in the CNS are similar to those in the periphery, and the drug in this section also has peripheral actions, as is to be expected.

Methyldopa (Aldomet) probably acts primarily in the brainstem vasomotor centres. It is a substrate (in the same manner as L-dopa) for the enzymes that synthesise noradrenaline. The synthesis of α-methylnoradrenaline results in tonic stimulation of CNS α_2 receptors because α-methylnoradrenaline cannot be metabolised by monoamine oxidase, and selectively stimulates the α_2 adrenoceptor. Stimulation of this receptor in the hindbrain nuclei concerned with blood pressure control results in a fall in blood pressure, i.e. methyldopa acts in the same way as clonidine. α-Methylnoradrenaline is also produced at peripheral adrenergic endings, but to a lesser extent and peripheral action is clinically insignificant. Methyldopa is reliably absorbed from the gastrointestinal tract and readily enters the CNS. The $t_{1/2}$ is 1.5 h.

Adverse effects, largely expected from its mode of action, include: sedation (frequent), nightmares, depression, involuntary movements, nausea, flatulence, constipation, score or black tongue, positive Coombs' test with occasionally haemolytic anaemia, leucopenia, thrombocytopenia, hepatitis.

Gynaecomastia and lactation occur due to interference with dopaminergic suppression of prolactin secretion. Any failure of male sexual function is probably secondary to sedation. Methyldopa is no longer a drug of first choice in routine long-term management of hypertension, but remains popular with obstetricians for the hypertension of pregnancy because of its safety profile.

DRUG TREATMENT OF ANGINA, MYOCARDIAL INFARCTION AND HYPERTENSION

ANGINA PECTORIS[25]

An attack of angina pectoris[26] occurs when myocardial demand for oxygen exceeds supply from the coronary circulation. The principal forms relevant to choice of drug therapy are angina of exercise (commonest) and its worsening form, unstable (preinfarction or crescendo) angina (see below), which occurs at rest. Variant (Prinzmetal) angina (very uncommon) results from spasm of a large coronary artery.

Antiangina drugs act as follows:

- *Organic nitrates* reduce preload and afterload and dilate the main coronary arteries (rather than the arterioles).
- β-*Adrenoceptor blocking drugs* reduce myocardial contractility and slow the heart rate. They may increase coronary artery spasm in variant angina.
- *Calcium channel blocking drugs* reduce cardiac contractility, dilate the coronary arteries (where there is evidence of spasm) and reduce afterload (dilate peripheral arterioles).

These classes of drug complement one another and can be used together. The combined nitrate and potassium channel activator, *nicorandil*, is an alternative when any of the other drugs is contraindicated.

---

[25]Angina pectoris: *angina*, a strangling; *pectoris*, of the chest.
[26]For a personal account by a physician of his experiences of angina pectoris, coronary bypass surgery, ventricular fibrillation and recovery, see Swyer G I M 1986 Personal view. British Medical Journal 292:337. Compelling and essential reading.

SUMMARY OF TREATMENT

- Any contributory cause is treated when possible, e.g. anaemia, arrhythmia.
- Lifestyle is changed so as to reduce the number of attacks. Weight reduction can be very helpful; stop smoking.
- For immediate pre-exertional prophylaxis: glyceryl trinitrate sublingually or nifedipine (bite the capsule and hold the liquid in the mouth or swallow it).
- For an acute attack: glyceryl trinitrate (sublingual) or nifedipine (bite capsule, as above).

For long-term prophylaxis:

- A *β_1-adrenoceptor blocking drug*, e.g. bisoprolol, is given regularly (not merely when an attack is expected). Dosage is adjusted by response. Some put an arbitrary upper limit to dose, but others recommend that, if complete relief is not obtained, the dose should be raised to the maximum tolerated, provided the resting heart rate is not reduced below 55 beats/min; or raise the dose to a level at which an increase causes no further inhibition of exercise tachycardia. In severe angina a pure antagonist, i.e. an agent lacking partial agonist activity, is preferred, as the latter may not slow the heart sufficiently. Warn the patient of the risk of abrupt withdrawal.
- A *calcium channel blocking drug*, e.g. nifedipine or diltiazem, is an alternative to a β-adrenoceptor blocker; use especially if coronary spasm is suspected or if the patient has myocardial insufficiency or any reversible airflow obstruction. It can also be used with a β-blocker, or
- A *long-acting nitrate*, isosorbide dinitrate or mononitrate: use so as to avoid tolerance (see p. 416).
- *Nicorandil*, a long-acting potassium channel activator, does not cause tolerance like the nitrates.
- Drug therapy may be adapted to the time of attacks, e.g. nocturnal (transdermal glyceryl trinitrate, or isosorbide mononitrate orally at night).
- Antiplatelet therapy (aspirin or clopidogrel) reduces the incidence of fatal and non-fatal myocardial infarction in patients with unstable angina, used alone or with low-dose heparin.
- Surgical revascularisation in selected cases.

In treating angina, it is important to remember not only the objective of reducing symptoms but also that of preventing complications, particularly myocardial infarction and sudden death. This requires vigorous treatment of all risk factors (hypertension, hyperlipidaemia, diabetes mellitus) and, of course, cessation of smoking. There is little evidence that the symptomatic treatments, medical or surgical, themselves affect outcome except in patients with stenosis of the main stem of the left coronary artery, who require surgical intervention. Although aspirin has not been studied specifically in patients with stable angina, it is now reasonable therapy, by extrapolation from the studies of aspirin in other patient groups.

MYOCARDIAL INFARCTION (MI)

(see also Chapter 28)

AN OVERVIEW

The *acute coronary syndromes* (ACSs) are now classified on the basis of the ECG and plasma troponin measurements into: (1) patients with ST elevation myocardial infarction (STEMI), (2) non-ST elevation myocardial infarction (non-STEMI, by ECG and a positive troponin test) and (3) unstable angina (by ECG and negative troponin test). The present account recognises that this is a rapidly evolving field, but therapeutic strategies are likely to evolve according to these forms of ACS.

A general practitioner or paramedic can administer the initial treatment appropriately before a definite diagnosis is established or the patient reaches hospital, namely:

- morphine or diamorphine (2.5 or 5 mg i.v. because of the certainty of haematoma formation when intramuscular injections are followed by thrombolytic therapy)
- aspirin 150–300 mg orally
- 60% oxygen.

The immediate objectives are relief of pain and initiation of treatment demonstrated to reduce mortality. Subsequent management of proven MI is concerned with treatment of complications, *arrhythmias*, *heart failure* and *thromboemboli*, and then *prevention* of further infarctions.

When STEMI is diagnosed, instituting myocardial reperfusion as early as possible provides the greatest benefit. Most commonly, the basis of this is *thrombolysis* (although its benefit will be increasingly compared with angioplasty, with or without stenting). This is initiated after arrival at hospital, preferably directly to the coronary care unit to avoid further delay, and provided there are no contraindications to thrombolysis (see below). Patients with non-STEMI may still benefit, especially those with left bundle branch block. Several trials have shown that patients without ECG changes (or with ST depression), and patients with unstable angina, benefit only slightly if at all from thrombolytic therapy.

The choice of thrombolytic is in most places dictated first by a wealth of comparative outcome data from well designed trials, and second by relative costs. For a first MI, patients should receive streptokinase 1 500 000 units infused over 1 h, unless they are in cardiogenic shock. For subsequent infarcts, the presence of antistreptokinase antibodies dictates the use of the recombinant tissue plasminogen activator (rtPA), *alteplase* (or *reteplase*). Both alteplase and streptokinase bind plasminogen and convert it to plasmin, which lyses fibrin. Alteplase has a much higher affinity for plasminogen bound to fibrin than in the circulation. This selectivity does not confer any therapeutic advantage as was originally anticipated, as severe haemorrhage following thrombolysis is almost always due to lysis of an appropriate clot at previous sites of bleeding or trauma. Indeed, the tendency for some lysis of circulating fibrinogen as well as fibrin gives streptokinase anticoagulant activity, which is lacking with alteplase, use of which needs to be accompanied and followed by heparin (for further details of thrombolytics, see p. 523).

For a discussion about the role of *aspirin*, see p. 260.

A third treatment reduces mortality in MI, namely β-blockade. In the ISIS-1 study,[27] atenolol 5 mg was given intravenously followed by 50 mg orally. The reduction in mortality is due mainly to prevention of cardiac rupture, which appears interestingly to remain the only complication of MI that is not reduced by thrombolysis. The usual contraindications to β-blockade apply, but most patients with a first MI should be able to receive this treatment.

Other antiplatelet agents. The final common pathway to platelet aggregation and thrombus

[27]First International Study of Infarct Survival Collaborative Group 1986 Randomised trial of intravenous atenolol among 16 027 cases of suspected acute myocardial infarction: ISIS-1. Lancet ii:57–66.

formation involves the expression of the glycoprotein IIb/IIIa receptor at the cell surface. This receptor binds fibrinogen with high affinity and can be blocked using either a specific monoclonal antibody (*abciximab*) or one of a rapidly expanding class of specific antagonists, e.g. *eptifibatide* and *tirofiban*. Another agent, *clopidogrel*, acts by inhibiting ADP-dependent platelet aggregation. It is more effective than aspirin for the prevention of ischaemic stroke or cardiovascular death in patients at high risk (see p. 524).

These drugs are useful adjuncts for the treatment of unstable angina, and in the prevention of thrombosis following percutaneous revascularisation procedures such as angioplasty and coronary artery stenting. Their role in preventing infarction in patients with acutely compromised myocardium is likely to expand rapidly.

Principal contraindications to thrombolysis

- Haemorrhagic diathesis
- Pregnancy
- Recent symptoms of peptic ulcer, or gastrointestinal bleeding
- Recent stroke (previous 3 months)
- Recent surgery (previous 10–14 days), especially neurosurgery
- Prolonged cardiopulmonary resuscitation (during current presentation)
- Proliferative diabetic retinopathy
- Severe, uncontrolled hypertension (diastolic BP >120 mmHg)

Unstable angina necessitates admission to hospital, the objectives of therapy being to relieve pain, and avert progression to MI and sudden death. Initial management is with aspirin 150–300 mg chewed or dispersed in water, followed by heparin or one of the low molecular weight preparations, e.g. dalteparin or enoxaparin. Nitrate is given preferably as isosorbide dinitrate by intravenous infusion until the patient has been pain free for 24 h. A β-adrenoceptor blocker, e.g. metoprolol, should be added orally or intravenously unless it is contraindicated, when a calcium channel blocker is substituted, e.g. diltiazem or verapamil. Patients perceived to be at high risk may also receive a glycoprotein IIb/IIIa inhibitor, e.g. eptifibatide or tirofiban.

SECONDARY PREVENTION

(See also Chapter 28.)

The best predictor of the risk of MI is to have had previous infarction. After the measures instituted in the first few hours, the principal objective of treatment therefore becomes prevention of future infarcts. Patients should receive advice about exercise and diet before discharge, and most enter a formal rehabilitation programme after leaving hospital. In particular, patients need to reduce saturated fat intake, and there is increasing evidence of the benefit of increased intake of fish and olive oil.

Drugs for secondary prevention

All patients should receive *aspirin* (see Chapter 4, Fig. 4.3) and a *β-blocker* for at least 2 years, unless contraindicated. The commonest contraindication to β-blockade after MI is *transient* heart failure, which should now be uncommon after a first MI. In such patients an *ACE inhibitor* should replace the β-blocker (but note that β-blockade may become necessary for the subsequent *long-term* management of *left ventricular failure*; see below).

Any of these agents, aspirin, a β-blocker or an ACE inhibitor[28], will reduce the incidence of reinfarction by 20–25%, although their benefit has not been shown to be additive.

In addition to these drugs, most patients should receive a statin, regardless of their plasma cholesterol concentration. Long-term benefit from LDL reduction after MI has been shown for simvastatin (20–40 mg/day) and pravastatin (40 mg/day).[29]

---

[28]In the SAVE (Survival and Ventricular Enlargement) study, captopril 50 mg t.i.d. or placebo was started 3–16 days after MI in 2231 patients without overt cardiac failure but with a left ventricular ejection fraction of less than 40%. The captopril group had a lower incidence of recurrent myocardial infarction (133) and death (228) than the placebo group (170 and 275 respectively) (Rutherford J D, Moye L A, Pfeffer M A et al for the SAVE investigators 1994 Effects of captopril on ischemic events after myocardial infarction. Results of the Survival and Ventricular Enlargement trial. SAVE Investigators. Circulation 90:1731–1738). Several other trials of ACE inhibitors have provided similar results.

[29]In the Heart Protection Study of 20 536 high-risk patients (one-third had previous MI), those randomly assigned to simvastatin 40 mg daily (compared with placebo) had a 12% reduction in all-cause mortality, and 24% reduction in strokes and coronary heart disease. The authors estimated that 5 years of statin treatment will prevent 100 major vascular events in every 1000 patients with previous MI, or 70 to 80 events in patients with other forms of coronary

There is no place for routine antiarrhythmic prophylaxis, and long-term anticoagulation is similarly out of place, except when indicated by arrhythmias or poor left ventricular function.

ARTERIAL HYPERTENSION

Clinical evaluation of antihypertensive drugs seeks to answer two types of question:

1. Whether long-term reduction of blood pressure benefits the patient by preventing complications and prolonging life; these studies take years, require enormous numbers of patients and are extremely costly.
2. Whether a drug is capable of effective, safe and comfortable control of blood pressure for about 1 year. There is now sufficient evidence of the benefit of reducing raised blood pressure that regulatory authorities do not demand trials of the first kind for all new drugs. Shorter studies are therefore deemed sufficient to allow the introduction of a new drug. Such trials may not reveal the long-term consequences of some metabolic effects, e.g. on blood glucose, which may adversely affect the risk of coronary heart disease. Placebo effects are prominent in these shorter trials and must be carefully controlled in trial design.

AIM OF TREATMENT

The principal long-term aim in most patients is the prevention of stroke and MI; reduction in the latter also requires attention to other risk factors such as smoking and plasma cholesterol. The more immediate aim of treatment is to reduce the blood pressure as near to normal as possible without causing symptomatic hypotension or otherwise impairing wellbeing (quality of life).

When this aim is achieved in severe cases there is great symptomatic improvement: retinopathy clears and vision improves; headaches are abolished. A variable amount of irreversible damage has often been done by the high blood pressure before treatment is started; so renal failure may progress despite treatment, left ventricular hypertrophy may not fully reverse, and arterial damage leads to ischaemic events (stroke and MI).

It is obviously desirable to start treatment before irreversible changes occur, and in mild and moderately severe cases this usually means advising treatment for symptom-free people whose hypertension was revealed by screening.

THRESHOLD AND TARGETS FOR TREATMENT

The British Hypertension Society guidelines[30] require that antihypertensive drug therapy be *initiated*:

- when sustained BP exceeds 160/100 mmHg, or
- when BP is in the range 140–159/90–99 mmHg and there is evidence of target organ damage, cardiovascular disease or a 10-year cardiovascular risk greater than 20%
- for diabetics when BP exceeds 140/90 mmHg.

The optimal *target* is to lower BP to 140/85 mmHg or less in all patients except those with renal impairment, diabetics or established cardiovascular disease where there is a lower target of less than 130/80 mmHg.

Effective treatment reduces the risk of all complications: strokes and MI, but also heart failure, renal failure and possibly dementia. It is easier in individual trials to demonstrate the benefits of treatment in preventing stroke, because the curve relating risk of stroke to blood pressure is almost twice as steep as that for MI. This raises issues of relative and absolute risk.

Relative risk refers to the increased likelihood of a patient having a complication, compared with a normotensive patient of the same age and sex. *Absolute* risk refers to the number of patients out of 100, with the same age, sex and blood pressure, predicted to have a complication over the next 10 years (see p. 56). So, the *relative* risk of MI due to hypertension is irreversible, but substantial reduction in the *absolute* risk of MI needs attention to hypercholesterolaemia as well as hypertension, i.e. both factors contribute independently to the risk of MI

heart disease or diabetes. There was no upper age limit to this benefit, and no lower limit to the level of LDL at which benefit was seen (Heart Protection Study Collaborative Group 2002 MRC/BHF Heart Protection Study of cholesterol lowering with simvastatin in 20 536 high-risk individuals. Lancet 360:7–22).

[30]The British Hypertension Society Guidelines (BHS-IV) are available in summary form in the British Medical Journal 2004; 328:634–640 or online at http://www.bhsoc.org

whereas hypertension is a more important risk factor for stroke than hypercholesterolaemia.

Treatment will almost always be lifelong for essential hypertension, because discontinuation of therapy leads to prompt restoration of pre-treatment blood pressures. If it does not, one should suspect the original diagnosis of hypertension, which should not be made unless blood pressure is increased on at least three occasions over 3 months.

The relative risks of hypertension and the benefits of treating the condition in the elderly are less than in those aged under 65 years, but the absolute risks and benefits are greater. Given the large choice of treatments available, doctors cannot cite improved quality of life as an excuse for not treating hypertension in the elderly. Starting doses should often be halved and, pending further evidence, less challenging targets for blood pressure reduction may be acceptable.

It is obvious that adverse effects of therapy are important in that very large numbers of patients must be treated so that a few may gain; this is a salient feature of the use of drugs to prevent disease.

PRINCIPLES OF ANTIHYPERTENSIVE THERAPY

General measures may be sufficient to control mild cases as follows:

- Obesity: reduce it.
- Alcohol: stay within recommended limits, e.g. 14 units/week for women, 21 units/week for men.
- Smoking: stop it.
- Diet: of proven value for the short-term reduction in blood pressure is reduction in fat content, and increase in fruit, vegetables and fibre. There is additional benefit from reducing intake of salt (<6 g/day): avoidance of highly salted foods, and omission of added salt from freshly prepared food.[31]
- Relaxation therapy: worth considering for highly motivated borderline patients.

DRUG THERAPY

Blood pressure may be reduced by any one or more of the actions listed at the beginning of this chapter

(see p. 415). (see p. 415). The large number of different drug classes for hypertension reduces, paradoxically, the likelihood of a randomly selected drug being the best for an individual patient. Patients and drugs can be divided broadly into two groups depending on their renin status and drug effect on this (Fig. 23.1).

- Type 1, or *high-renin* patients, are the younger caucasians (aged <55 years); they respond better to a β-blocker or ACE inhibitor.
- Type 2, or *low-renin* patients, in whom diuretics or calcium blockers are more likely to be effective as single agents.

As each drug acts on only one or two of the blood pressure control mechanisms, the factors that are uninfluenced by monotherapy are liable to adapt (homeostatic mechanism), to oppose the useful effect and to restore the previous state. There are two principal mechanisms of such adaptation or tolerance:

1. *Increase in blood volume*: this occurs with any drug that reduces peripheral resistance (increases intravascular volume) or cardiac output (reduces glomerular flow) due to activation of the renin–angiotensin system. The result is that cardiac output and blood pressure rise. Adding a diuretic in combination with the other drug can prevent this compensatory effect.

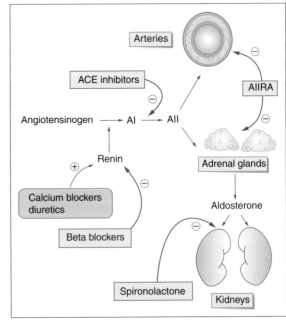

Fig. 23.1 Effects of drugs on the renin–angiotensin system. ARB, angiotensin II receptor blocker; ATI/II, angiotensin I/II.

---

[31]DASH-Sodium Collaborative Research Group 2001 Effects on blood pressure of reduced dietary sodium and the Dietary Approaches to Stop Hypertension (DASH) diet. New England Journal of Medicine 344:3–10.

2. *Baroreceptor reflexes*: A fall in blood pressure evokes reflex activity of the sympathetic system, causing increased peripheral resistance and cardiac activity (rate and contractility).

Therefore, whenever high blood pressure is proving difficult to control and whenever a number of anti-hypertensives are used in combination, the drugs chosen should between them act on all three main determinants of blood pressure, namely:

- *blood volume*
- *peripheral resistance*
- *cardiac output*.

Such combinations will:

- maximise antihypertensive efficacy by exerting actions at three different points in the cardiovascular system
- minimise the opposing homeostatic effects by blocking the compensatory changes in blood volume, vascular tone and cardiac function
- minimise adverse effects by permitting smaller doses of each drug each acting at a different site and having different unwanted effects.

First-dose hypotension is now uncommon and occurs mainly with drugs having an action on veins (α-adrenoceptor blockers, ACE inhibitors) when baroreflex activation is impaired, e.g. old age or with a contracted intravascular volume following diuretics.

TREATING HYPERTENSION

A simple stepped regimen in keeping with the 2006 revision of the National Institute for Health and Clinical Excellence (NICE)/British Hypertension Society guidelines[32] is the 'A/CD' schema illustrated in Figure 23.2.[33]

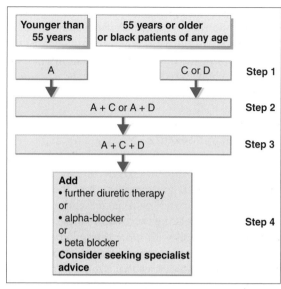

Fig. 23.2 ACD scheme for escalation of antihypertensive therapy. A, ACE inhibitor; C, calcium channel blocker; D, diuretic (see text). (From Williams B W, Poulter N R, Brown M J et al 2004 British Hypertension Society guidelines for hypertension management 2004 (BHS-1V): summary. British Medical Journal 328:634–640).

1. If the patient is young (age <55 years) or non-black, use either an ACE inhibitor (or ARB) (**A**). For older patients start with either a Calcium channel blocker or thiazide Diuretic as first-line therapy (**C** or **D**). If a drug is effective but not tolerated, switch to the other member of the pair.
2. If the blood pressure is not controlled at 4 weeks, a second agent should be added, using the opposite pair to the first drug, e.g. if the patient is on an ACE inhibitor add a Calcium channel blocker or thiazide Diuretic (**A+C** or **A+D**), as both vasodilatation or diuresis will stimulate the renin–angiotensin system and turn non-renin-dependent hypertension into renin-dependent hypertension.
3. If blood pressure control is still inadequate on dual therapy, **A+C+D** is the ideal triple regimen.
4. If additional therapy is required, α-blockade is effective at this stage by blocking the vasoconstrictor component of the baroreflex response to some of the other drugs. A very small number of patients may need reversion to an older class of drug such as minoxidil (provided that a loop diuretic and β-blocker can also be given to block the severe fluid retention and tachycardia) or methyldopa.

---

[32]Online. Available: http://www.nice.org.uk/CG034

[33]The original schema included β-blockers, i.e. four drug groups AB/CD (Dickerson J E C, Hingorani A D, Ashby M J, Palmer C R, Brown M J 1999 Optimisation of anti-hypertensive treatment by crossover rotation of four major classes. Lancet 353:2008–2013). This is revised in the light of clinical trial evidence that β-blockers are usually less effective than other antihypertensives at reducing major cardiovascular events, particularly stroke, and are associated with an unacceptably high risk of diabetes especially in combination with diuretics. Hence they are no longer recommended either as monotherapy (B in the original schema) or in combination with diuretics (B+D) unless there is a second indication for prescribing the β-blocker, e.g. angina.

5. Patients whose blood pressure remains substantially above target on triple therapy are likely to have aldosterone-sensitive hypertension that responds well to spironolactone. A particularly effective combination is spironolactone with a second-generation ARB, e.g. irbesartan or candesartan.

Treatment and severity

A single drug may adequately treat mild hypertension. The treatment target blood pressures of <140/<85 mmHg suggested by the British Hypertension Society[27] will increase the proportion of patients needing two or more drugs. The vast majority of patients with more severe hypertension can be treated by the stepped regimen (above); only rarely are there indications that a more rapid reduction in blood pressure is necessary. This is important so that the efficacy and tolerability of individual drugs can be assessed in each patient.

MONITORING

The blood pressure must be monitored by a doctor or specialist nurse (particularly important in the elderly) and also sometimes by the patient. A 24-h ambulatory blood pressure monitoring (ABPM) system is the 'gold standard', but the devices are too expensive to be recommended for most patients. Nevertheless, the 24-h blood pressure profile does predict outcome better than clinic blood pressure and can indicate whether a difficult or high-risk patient does need additional medication. Home monitoring is a cheaper alternative, provided the sphygmomanometer is validated. The easy-to-use wrist monitors are unfortunately unreliable in patients receiving drug treatment.

Diuretics and potassium. The potassium-losing (kaliuretic) diuretics used in hypertension deplete body potassium by 10–15%. Potassium chloride supplements are not required routinely, but hypokalaemia will occasionally occur (and should raise suspicion of Conn's syndrome). Uncomplicated patients may not need monitoring if the lowest possible doses are used, e.g. no more than bendroflumethiazide 2.5 mg/day. Vulnerable patients, e.g. the elderly, should be monitored for potassium loss at 3 months and thereafter every 6–12 months. In general a potassium-retaining diuretic (amiloride) in a fixed-dose combination with a thiazide (co-amilozide) is preferred over the use of fixed-dose diuretic/potassium chloride formulations (most supplements, typically 8 mmol KCl, are in any case inadequate).

Control of potassium balance is particularly important if the patient is also taking digoxin (hypokalemia potentiates its action). Because of the risk of hyperkalaemia, amiloride should usually be avoided in patients taking ACE inhibitors unless renal function is normal.

Compliance. Multi-drug therapy poses a substantial problem of compliance. As treatment will be lifelong, it is worthwhile taking the trouble to find the most convenient regimen for each individual and then to transfer to a fixed-dose combination that provides this. A single daily dose would be ideal, and to achieve this sustained-release formulations and fixed-dose combinations are useful. Examples include: Tenoretic (atenolol + chlortalidone), Tenif (atenolol + nifedipine), Zestoretic (lisinopril + hydrochlorothiazide), Co-Diovan (valsartan + hydrochlorothiazide).

TREATMENT OF HYPERTENSIVE EMERGENCIES

It is important to distinguish three circumstances that may exist separately or together; see the Venn diagram (Fig. 23.3)[34] which emphasises the following:

- *Severe hypertension* is not on its own an indication for urgent (or large) reductions in blood pressure.
- Blood pressure (BP) can occasionally require urgent (emergency) reduction even when the hypertension is not severe, especially where the BP has risen rapidly.
- *Accelerated phase* (malignant) *hypertension* rarely requires urgent reduction, and should instead be regarded as an indication for slow reduction in blood pressure during the first few days.

---

[34] J Venn (1834–1923), an English logician who 'adopted the diagrammatic method of illustrating propositions by inclusive and exclusive circles' (Dictionary of National Biography). A medical pilgrimage to Cambridge, where Venn worked, should take in Gonville and Caius College (named after its founder, Dr Caius, physician to the Tudor Court and early president of the London College of Physicians in the 16th century); as well as stained glass windows celebrating Venn's circles, the visitor can see a portrait of the most famous medical Caian, William Harvey. A picture is also available on the College website: http://www.cai.cam.ac.uk/rota.php?count=4.

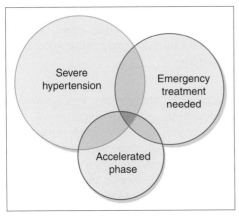

Fig. 23.3 Venn diagram illustrating intersections of three overlapping clinical states defined in the text.

The indications for *emergency reduction* of blood pressure are rare. They are:

- Hypertensive encephalopathy (including eclampsia).
- Acute left ventricular failure (due to hypertension).
- Dissecting aortic aneurysm.

In these conditions, BP should be reduced over the course of an hour. In patients with a dissecting aneurysm, where the BP may have been completely normal prior to dissection, the target is a BP of about 110/70 mmHg. Otherwise even small reductions will usually remove the emergency.

Accelerated phase hypertension was previously called 'malignant' hypertension because the lack of treatment heralded death within a year of diagnosis. It is characterised pathologically by fibrinoid necrosis of the small arteries. An important consequence is the loss of autoregulation of the cerebral and renal circulation, so that any reduction in BP causes a proportional fall in perfusion of these organs. It is therefore vital not to reduce diastolic BP by more than 20 mmHg on the first day of treatment. To ignore this is to risk cerebral infarction.

Treatment. Unless contraindicated, the best treatment for all circles in the Venn diagram is β-blockade, e.g. atenolol 25 or 50 mg orally. In emergencies, a vasodilator should be given intravenously, in addition.

A theoretically preferable, but often impractical, alternative is intravenous infusion of the vasodilator,

nitroprusside (see p. 446). In dissecting aneurysm, vasodilators should not be used unless patients are first β-blocked because any increase in the rate of rise of the pulse stroke is undesirable. *Labetalol* provides a convenient method of treating all patients within the three circles (except asthmatics), using either oral or parenteral therapy as appropriate. That said, it is not the most effective therapy and should be combined with a long-acting formulation of nifedipine, orally, where further blood pressure reduction is required.

Low doses of all drugs should be used if other antihypertensive drugs have recently been taken or renal function is impaired.

Oral maintenance treatment for severe hypertension should be started at once if possible; parenteral therapy is seldom necessary for more than 48 h.

PREGNANCY HYPERTENSION

Effective treatment of pregnancy-induced hypertension improves fetal and perinatal survival. There is a lack of good clinical trial evidence on which to base recommendations. Instead, drug selection reflects longevity of use without obvious harm to the fetus and methyldopa is still the drug of choice for many obstetricians. Calcium channel blockers (especially nifedipine) are common second-line drugs; parenteral hydralazine is reserved for emergency reduction of blood pressure in late pregnancy, preferably in combination with a β-blocker to avoid unpleasant tachycardia.

β-Blockers (labetalol and atenolol) are often effective and are probably the drugs of choice in the third trimester; there is anecdotal evidence to suggest growth retardation with β-blockade used in first and second trimester. Diuretics reduce the chance of developing pre-eclampsia, but are avoided in pre-eclampsia itself because these patients already have a contracted circulatory volume.

ACE inhibitors [and by implication angiotensin II receptor blockers (ARBs)] are absolutely contraindicated during pregnancy. They cause major malformations after first-trimester exposure[35] and fetal death, typically mid-trimester. There is no definite evidence that ACE inhibitors – or any of the

[35]Cooper W O, Hernandez-Diaz S, Arbogast P G et al 2006 Major congenital malformations after first-trimester exposure to ACE inhibitors. New England Journal of Medicine 354:2443–2451.

commonly used antihypertensive drugs – are tera-togenic, and women who become pregnant while receiving these should be reassured but should then discontinue the ACE inhibitor or ARB.

Raised blood pressure and proteinuria (pre-eclampsia) complicates 2–8% of pregnancies and may proceed to fitting (eclampsia), a major cause of mortality in mother and child. Magnesium sulphate halves the risk of progress to eclampsia (typically 4 g i.v. over 5–10 min followed by 1 g/h by i.v. infusion for 24 h after the last seizure).[36] Additionally, if a woman has one fit (treat with diazepam), then the magnesium regimen is superior to diazepam or phenytoin in preventing further fits.[37]

Aspirin, in low dose, was reported in early studies to reduce the incidence of pre-eclampsia in at-risk patients, but a more recent meta-analysis has not supported this. Consequently, it is not routinely recommended.

UNWANTED INTERACTIONS WITH ANTIHYPERTENSIVE DRUGS

Specific interactions are described in the accounts of individual drugs. The following are general examples for this diverse group of drugs.

Alcohol intake is the commonest contributing factor, or even cause, of hypertension, and should always be considered as a cause of erratic or failed responses to treatment (measurement of the γ-glutamyl trans-peptidase and red cell mean corpuscular volume may be useful).

Prostaglandin synthesis. NSAIDs, e.g. indometacin, attenuate the antihypertensive effect of β-adreno-ceptor blockers and of diuretics, perhaps by inhibiting the synthesis of vasodilator renal prostaglandins. This effect can also be important when a diuretic is used for severe left ventricular failure.

Enzyme inhibition. Ciprofloxacin and cimetidine inhibit hepatic metabolism of lipid-soluble

β-adrenoceptor blockers, e.g. metoprolol, labetalol, propranolol, increasing their effect. Methyldopa plus an MAO inhibitor may cause excitement and hallucinations.

Pharmacological antagonism. Sympathomimetics, e.g. amfetamine, phenylpropanolamine (present in anorectics and cold and cough remedies), may lead to loss of antihypertensive effect, and indeed to a *hypertensive reaction* when taken by a patient already on a β-adrenoceptor blocker, due to unopposed α-adrenergic stimulation.

Surgical anaesthesia may lead to a brisk fall in blood pressure in patients taking antihypertensives. Antihypertensive therapy should not be routinely altered before surgery, although it obviously can complicate care both during and after the operation. Anaesthetists must be informed.

SEXUAL FUNCTION AND CARDIOVASCULAR DRUGS

All drugs that interfere with sympathetic autonomic activity can potentially interfere with male sexual function, expressed as a failure of ejaculation or difficulty in sustaining an erection. Nevertheless, placebo-controlled trials have emphasised how common a symptom this is in the untreated male population (sometimes approaching 20–30%). It is also likely that hypertension itself is associated with an increased risk of sexual dysfunction since loss of nitric oxide production by the vascular endothelium is an early feature of the pathophysiology of this disease.

Laying the blame on antihypertensive medication is probably incorrect in most instances, especially with drugs from newer drug categories. Calcium channel blockers, ACE inhibitors and angiotensin II (AT_1) receptor blockers (ARBs) all have reported rates of sexual dysfunction that do not differ from placebo. If symptoms persist with these drugs other causes should be sought. It is important to listen to the patient but also to reassure them that the drug is not necessarily to blame; sexual dysfunction as a perceived adverse drug effect is a potent cause of compliance failure. Sildenafil (Viagra) can be used safely in patients receiving any of the commonly used antihypertensive drugs.

[36]The Magpie Trial Collaborative Group 2002 Do women with pre-eclampsia, and their babies, benefit from magnesium sulphate? The Magpie Trial: a randomised placebo-controlled trial. Lancet 359:1877–1890.

[37]The Eclampsia Trial Collaborative Group 1995 Which anticonvulsant for women with eclampsia? Evidence from the Collaborative Eclampsia Trial. Lancet 345:1455–1463.

As well as the concerns about sexual performance in treated hypertensives, there may be concerns about fitness per se to attempt intercourse. The real possibility that it is hazardous is compounded often by their age and concurrent coronary artery disease.

SEXUAL INTERCOURSE AND THE CARDIOVASCULAR SYSTEM

Normal sexual intercourse with orgasm is accompanied by transient but brisk physiological changes, e.g. tachycardia up to 180 beats/min, with increases of 100 beats/min over less than 1 min. Systolic blood pressure may rise by 120 mmHg and diastolic by 50 mmHg. Orgasm may be accompanied by transient pressure of 230/130 mmHg even in normotensive individuals. Electrocardiographic abnormalities may occur in healthy men and women. Respiratory rate may rise to 60 beats/min.

Such changes in the healthy might bode ill for the unhealthy (with hypertension, angina pectoris or after myocardial infarction). Sudden deaths do occur during or shortly after sexual intercourse (ventricular fibrillation or subarachnoid haemorrhage), usually in clandestine circumstances such as the bordello or the mistress's bed, especially when an older man and a younger woman are involved – although this may just reflect reporting bias in the press. In one series, 0.6% of all sudden deaths were (reportedly) attributable to sexual intercourse and in about half of these cardiac disease was present. Clearly, the older patient with coronary heart disease should aspire cautiously to the haemodynamic heights attainable in youth.

There are few, if any, records of sudden cardiovascular death amongst women under these circumstances.

If there is substantial concern about cardiovascular stress (hypertension or arrhythmia) during sexual intercourse in either sex, a dose of labetalol about 2 h before the event may well be justified (taking account of other therapy already in use). But patients taking a β-blocker long term for angina prophylaxis have shown reductions in peak heart rate during coitus from 122 to 82 beats/min.

Patients subject to angina pectoris should also use glyceryl trinitrate or isosorbide dinitrate as usual for pre-exertional prophylaxis 10 min before intercourse. *But they should be aware of the potentially fatal interaction of sildenafil (Viagra) with nitrates* (see p. 493).

Summary
- The treatment of both hypertension and angina requires drugs that reduce the work of the heart either directly or by lowering peripheral vascular resistance.
- β-Blockade, which acts mainly through reduced cardiac output, and calcium channel blockade, acting by selective arterial dilatation, may be used in either condition.
- Other vasodilators are suited preferentially to hypertension (ACE inhibitors, angiotensin [AT$_1$] receptor blockers [ARBs] and α-adrenoceptor blockers) or to angina (nitrates).
- The treatment of myocardial infarction requires thrombolysis, aspirin and β-adrenoceptor blockade acutely, with the latter two continued for at least 2 years as secondary prevention of a further infarction.
- Other important steps in secondary prevention include ACE inhibitors for cardiac failure and statins for hypercholesterolaemia in selected patients.

PULMONARY HYPERTENSION

Therapy is determined by the underlying cause. When the condition is secondary to hypoxia accompanying chronic obstructive pulmonary disease, *long-term oxygen therapy* improves symptoms and prognosis; anticoagulation is essential when the cause is multiple pulmonary emboli.

Primary pulmonary hypertension. Verapamil may give symptomatic benefit; also continuous intravenous infusion of prostaglandin. Evidence suggests that endothelin, a powerful endogenous vasoconstrictor, may play a pathogenic role, and *bosentan*, an endothelin receptor antagonist may improve exercise tolerance. Heart and lung transplantation is recommended for younger patients.

PHAEOCHROMOCYTOMA

This tumour of chromaffin tissue, usually arising in the adrenal medulla, secretes principally noradrenaline, but also variable amounts of adrenaline. Symptoms are related to this. Hypertension may be sustained or intermittent. If the tumour secretes only noradrenaline, which stimulates α and

445

β_1 adrenoceptors, rises in blood pressure are accompanied by reflex bradycardia due to vagal activation; this is sufficient to overcome the chronotropic effect of β_1-receptor stimulation. The recognition of *bradycardia* at the time of catecholamine-induced symptoms (e.g. anxiety, tremor or sweating) is useful in alerting the physician to the possibility of this rare syndrome, as physiological sympathetic nervous activation is coupled to vagal withdrawal and causes *tachycardia*. If the tumour also secretes adrenaline, which stimulates α, β_1 and β_2 adrenoceptors, blood pressure and heart rate change in parallel. This is because stimulation of the vasodilator β_2 receptor in resistance arteries attenuates the rise in diastolic pressure, and vagal activation is insufficient then to oppose the chronotropic effect of combined β_1- and β_2-receptor stimulation in the heart.

Diagnostic tests include measurement of catecholamines or their metabolites in urine followed by catecholamine concentrations in blood when the urine results are equivocal or high. With modern analytical techniques, interference by drugs and diet is less troublesome than formerly.

Antihypertensive drugs may alter catecholamine concentrations (particularly those that induce a reflex increase in sympathetic activity, e.g. vasodilators). False-positive tests can then occur and in the past patients have undergone unnecessary operations.[38]

A variety of pharmacological tests is now available, and these are best performed in specialist units to avoid erroneous results. Provocation tests are dangerous. A phaeochromocytoma may be stimulated to secrete and cause a hypertensive attack by metoclopramide and by any drug that releases histamine (opioids, curare, trimetaphan). The search for biochemical evidence for a phaeochromocytoma should always precede the imaging hunt for a tumour. Accurate measurement of adrenaline in plasma is invaluable in determining whether the tumour is likely to be adrenal or extra-adrenal. Only adrenal tumours can synthesise adrenaline because the enzyme that methylates noradrenaline to adrenaline needs to be induced by a concentration of cortisol higher than that which normally circulates; this is achieved within the normal adrenal gland by the portocapillary circulation from cortex to medulla. The circulation is progressively disrupted as the tumour grows, so that very large adrenal tumours may cease to secrete adrenaline.

Control of blood pressure before surgery or when the tumour cannot be removed is achieved by α-adrenoceptor blockade, which reverses peripheral vasoconstriction. β-Blockade may also be required to control tachycardia in patients with adrenaline-secreting tumours. As adrenaline secretion, as explained above, tends to fall as tumours enlarge, tachycardia is not usually a major problem. Initiation of α-blocker treatment can unmask tachycardia, because there is no longer baroreceptor-induced vagal activation to oppose β-receptor stimulation of the heart. A β-receptor blocker should never be given alone, because abolition of the peripheral vasodilator effects of adrenaline leaves the powerful α effects unopposed. A low dose of a β_1-selective agent (e.g. bisoprolol 5 mg) is safe in the presence of α-blockade.

For phaeochromocytoma the preferred α-blocker is not one of the selective α_1-blockers, as in essential hypertension, but the irreversible α-blocker, *phenoxybenzamine*, whose blockade cannot be overcome by a catecholamine surge. Treatment should be for several weeks, if possible, prior to surgery, to reverse intravascular volume depletion, which is always present in patients with phaeochromocytoma.

During surgical removal, *phentolamine* (or sodium nitroprusside) should be at hand to control rises in blood pressure when the tumour is handled. When the adrenal veins have been clamped, volume expansion is often required to maintain blood pressure even after adequate preoperative α-blockade. If a pressor infusion is still needed, isoprenaline is more use than the usual α agonists, to which the patient will be insensitive due to existing α-receptor blockade.

---

[38]On the other hand, a positive test must not be ignored. In 1954, a hospital clinical chemistry laboratory was asked to set up a biological assay for catecholamines in the urine. The head of the laboratory tested urine from the lab staff to obtain a reference range for the assay. All were negative except his own, which was strongly positive. He felt well and regarded the result as showing insufficient specificity of the test. Some 2 years later a fluorometric assay became available. The urines of the lab staff were tested again, with the same result. The head of the laboratory still felt well, but this time he decided to consult a physician colleague. A few days later, before the consultation, he was quietly reading a newspaper at home in the evening when he had a fatal cerebral infarction. Autopsy revealed a phaeochromocytoma (Robinson R 1980 Tumours that secrete catecholamines. Wiley, Chichester).

Metirosine (α-methyltyrosine) has been used with some success to block catecholamine synthesis in malignant phaeochromocytomas.

Meta-iodobenzylguanidine (MIBG, an analogue of guanethidine) is actively taken up by adrenergic tissue and is concentrated in phaeochromocytomas. Radio-iodinated MIBG ([^{123}I]MIBG) allows localisation of tumours and detection of metastases, and selective therapeutic irradiation of functioning metastases or other tumours of chromaffin tissue, e.g. carcinoid.

GUIDE TO FURTHER READING

Blood Pressure Lowering Treatment Trialists' Collaboration 2000 Effects of ACE inhibitors, calcium antagonists, and other blood-pressure-lowering drugs: results of prospectively designed overviews of randomised trials. Lancet 356:1955–1964

British Cardiac Society, British Hyperlipidaemia Association, British Hypertension Society, British Diabetic Association 2000 Joint British recommendations on prevention of coronary heart disease in clinical practice: summary. British Medical Journal 320:705–708

Brown M J 1995 Phaeochromocytoma. In: Weatherall D, Ledingham J, Warrell D (eds) Oxford textbook of medicine. Oxford University Press, Oxford, p. 2553–2557

Brown M J 2006 Hypertension and ethnic group. British Medical Journal 332:833–836

Gaziano T A, Opie L H, Weinstein M S et al 2006 Cardiovascular disease prevention with a multidrug regimen in the developing world: a cost–effectiveness analysis. Lancet 368:679–686

Guidelines Subcommittee, World Health Organization–International Society of Hypertension 1999 Guidelines for the management of hypertension. Journal of Hypertension 17:151–183

Hansson G K 2005 Inflammation, atherosclerosis, and coronary artery disease. New England Journal of Medicine 352:1685–1695

Kaplan N M, Opie L H 2006 Controversies in hypertension. Lancet 367:168–176

Lenders J W M, Eisenhofer G, Mannelli M, Pacak K 2005 Phaeochromocytoma. Lancet 366:665–675

Maynard S J, Scott G O, Riddell J W, Adgey A A J 2000 Management of acute coronary syndromes. British Medical Journal 321:220–223

Messerli F H 1995 This day 50 years ago. New England Journal of Medicine 332:(15):1038–1039 (an account of the hypertension and stroke suffered by US President F D Roosevelt)

O'Brien E, Coats A, Owens P et al 2000 Use and interpretation of ambulatory blood pressure monitoring: recommendations of the British Hypertension Society. British Medical Journal 320:1128–1134

Opie L H, Commerford P J, Gersh B J et al 2006 Controversies in stable coronary artery disease. Lancet 367:69–78

Pickering T G, Shimbo D, Haas D et al 2006 Ambulatory blood-pressure monitoring. New England Journal of Medicine 354:2368–2374

Redman C W G, Roberts J M 1993 Management of pre-eclampsia. Lancet 341:1451–1454

Safian R D, Textor S C 2001 Renal-artery stenosis. New England Journal of Medicine 344(6):431–442

Schmieder R E, Hilgers K F, Schlaich M P, Schmidt B M W 2007 Renin-angiotensin system and cardiovascular risk. Lancet 369:1208–1219

Staessen J A, Li Y, Richart T 2006 Oral renin inhibitors. Lancet 368:1449–1456

Vaughan C J, Delanty N 2000 Hypertensive emergencies. Lancet 356:411–417

Williams B, Poulter N R, Brown M J et al 2004 British Hypertension Society guidelines for hypertension management 2004 (BHS-IV): summary. British Medical Journal 328:634–640

24

Cardiac arrhythmia and heart failure

SYNOPSIS

The pathophysiology of cardiac arrhythmias is complex and the actions of drugs that are useful in stopping or controlling them may seem equally so. Nevertheless, many patients with arrhythmias respond well to therapy with drugs and a working knowledge of their effects and indications pays dividends, for irregularity of the heartbeat is at least inconvenient and at worst fatal. Drug therapy for arrhythmias has a place beside radiofrequency ablation or the use of implanted devices, e.g. pacemakers or implantable defibrillators (ICDs), which often provide the best treatment option.

There is now a better understanding of the mechanisms that sustain the failing heart. Carefully selected and monitored drugs can have a major impact on morbidity and mortality. Much of the risk that patients with heart failure encounter is due to ventricular arrhythmias, which are minimised with implantable devices (ICDs) and cardiac resynchronisation therapy (CRT)) rather than drugs.

- Drugs for cardiac arrhythmias
- Principal drugs by class
- Specific treatments, including those for cardiac arrest
- Drugs for cardiac failure

DRUGS FOR CARDIAC ARRHYTHMIAS

OBJECTIVES OF TREATMENT

In almost no other set of conditions is it so clearly obvious to remember the dual objectives, which are to reduce *morbidity* and *mortality*.

Arrhythmias are frequently a symptomatic but may be fatal. Indeed an estimated 70 000 deaths per year are ascribed to ventricular arrhythmias in the UK. In addition, all antiarrhythmics are also capable of generating arrhythmias and find use only in the presence of clear indications. In addition, antiarrhythmic agents are to a variable degree negatively inotropic (except for digoxin and amiodarone).

A second reason for a careful approach to antiarrhythmic treatment is the gulf between knowledge of their mechanism of action and their clinical uses. On the side of normal physiology, we can see the spontaneous generation and propagation of the cardiac impulse requiring a combination of specialised conducting tissue and inter-myocyte conduction. The heart also has backstops in case of problems with the variety of pacemakers. By contrast, the available drugs are at an early stage of evolution, and useful antiarrhythmic actions are yet discovered by chance, e.g. adenosine.

Doctors and drugs interfere with cardiac electrophysiology at their peril. In emergencies, the most junior doctor in the team often needs to take action, and some rote recommendations are then necessary. The diagnosis and elective treatment of chronic or episodic arrhythmias require greater skill to achieve the best balance between risk and benefit.

As will become clear, antiarrhythmic drugs have a hard time proving superior safety or efficacy over other therapeutic (non-drug) options.

SOME PHYSIOLOGY AND PATHOPHYSIOLOGY

There are broadly two types of cardiac tissue.

The *first type* is ordinary myocardial (atrial and ventricular) muscle, responsible for the pumping action of the heart.

The *second type* is specialised conducting tissue that initiates the cardiac electrical impulse and determines the order in which the muscle cells contract. The important property of being able to form impulses spontaneously (*automaticity*) is a feature of certain parts of the conducting tissue, e.g. the sinoatrial (SA) and atrioventricular (AV) nodes. The SA node has the highest frequency of spontaneous discharge, 70 times per minute, and thus controls the contraction rate of the heart, making the cells more distal in the system fire more rapidly than they would do spontaneously, i.e. it is the pacemaker. If the SA node fails to function, the next fastest part takes over. This is often the AV node (approx. 45 discharges per min) or a site in the His–Purkinje system (about 25 discharges per min).

Altered rate of automatic discharge or abnormality of the mechanism by which an impulse is generated from a centre in the nodes or conducting tissue, is one cause of cardiac arrhythmia, e.g. atrial fibrillation, flutter or tachycardia.

Ionic movements into and out of cardiac cells

Nearly all cells in the body exhibit a difference in electrical voltage between their interior and exterior, the membrane potential. Some cells, including the conducting and contracting cells of the heart, are excitable; an appropriate stimulus alters the properties of the cell membrane, ions flow across it and elicit an action potential. This spreads to adjacent cells, i.e. it is conducted as an electrical impulse and, when it reaches a muscle cell, causes it to contract; this is excitation–contraction coupling.

In the resting state the interior of the cell (conducting and contracting types) is electrically negative with respect to the exterior, owing to the disposition of ions (mainly sodium, potassium and calcium) across its membrane, i.e. it is *polarised*. The ionic changes of the action potential first result in a rapid redistribution of ions such that the potential alters to positive within the cell (*depolarisation*); subsequent and slower flows of ions then restore the resting potential (*repolarisation*). These ionic movements separate into phases, which are briefly described here and in Figure 24.1, for they help to explain the actions of antiarrhythmic drugs.[1]

CLASSIFICATION OF ANTIARRHYTHMIC DRUGS

This partially relates to the phases of the cardiac cycle depicted in Figure 24.1.

Phase 0 is the rapid depolarisation of the cell membrane that is associated with a fast inflow of sodium ions through channels that are selectively permeable to these ions.

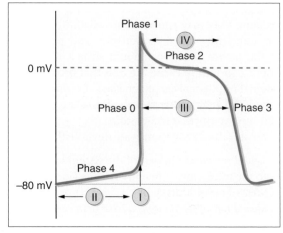

Fig. 24.1 The action potential of a cardiac cell that is capable of spontaneous depolarisation (SA or AV nodal, or His–Purkinje) indicating phases 0–4. The gradual increase in transmembrane potential (mV) during phase 4 is shown; cells that are not capable of spontaneous depolarisation do not exhibit increased voltage during this phase (see text). The modes of action of antiarrhythmic drugs of classes I, II, III and IV are indicated in relation to these phases.

Phase 1 is short initial period of rapid repolarisation brought about mainly by an outflow of potassium ions.

Phase 2 is a period when there is a delay in repolarisation caused mainly by a slow movement of calcium ions from the exterior into the cell through channels that are selectively permeable to these ions ('long-opening' or L-channels).

Phase 3 is a second period of rapid repolarisation during which potassium ions move out of the cell.

Phase 4 begins with the fully repolarised state. For cells that discharge *automatically*, potassium ions then progressively move back into, and sodium and calcium ions move out of, the cell. The result is that the interior becomes gradually less negative until a (threshold) potential is reached, which allows rapid depolarisation (phase 0) to occur, and the cycle is repeated; the prevailing sympathetic tone also influences automaticity. Cells that do not discharge spontaneously rely on the arrival of an action potential from another cell to initiate depolarisation.

In phases 1 and 2 the cell is in an *absolutely refractory* state and is incapable of responding further to any stimulus, but during phase 3, the *relative refractory period*, the cell will depolarise again if a stimulus is sufficiently strong. The orderly transmission of an electrical impulse (action potential) throughout the conducting system may be retarded in an area of disease, e.g. localised ischaemia or previous myocardial

[1]Grace A A, Camm A J 2000 Voltage-gated calcium channels and antiarrhythmic drug action. Cardiovascular Research 45:43–51.

infarction. An impulse travelling down a normal Purkinje fibre may spread to an adjacent fibre that has transiently failed to transmit, and pass up it in the *reverse* direction. Should such a retrograde impulse in turn re-excite the cells that provided the original impulse, *re-entrant excitation* becomes established and may cause an arrhythmia, e.g. paroxysmal supraventricular tachycardia.

Most cardiac arrhythmias are due to either:

- *slowed conduction* in part of the system leading to the formation of re-entry circuits (more than 90% of tachycardias), or
- *altered rate of spontaneous discharge* in conducting tissue. Some ectopic pacemakers appear to depend on adrenergic drive.

CLASSIFICATION OF DRUGS

The Vaughan–Williams[2] classification of antiarrhythmic drugs is the most commonly used and, despite its many peculiarities, it provides a sufficiently useful shorthand for referring to particular groups or actions of drugs.

Class I: sodium channel blockade. These drugs restrict the rapid inflow of sodium during phase 0 and thus slow the maximum rate of depolarisation. Another term for this property is *membrane stabilising activity*; it may contribute to stopping arrhythmias by limiting the responsiveness to excitation of cardiac cells. The class subdivides into drugs that:

- A. *lengthen* action potential duration and refractoriness (adjunctive class III action), e.g. quinidine, disopyramide, procainamide
- B. *shorten* action potential duration and refractoriness, e.g. lidocaine and mexiletine
- C. have *negligible effect* on action potential duration and refractoriness, e.g. flecainide, propafenone.

One value of the classification is that drugs in class 1B are ineffective for supraventricular arrhythmias, whereas they all have some action in ventricular arrhythmias. The classification is not useful in explaining why the classes differ anatomically in their efficacy.

Class II: catecholamine blockade. Propranolol and other β-adrenoceptor antagonists reduce background sympathetic tone in the heart, reduce automatic discharge (phase 4) and protect against adrenergically stimulated ectopic pacemakers.

Class III: lengthening of refractoriness (without effect on sodium inflow in phase 0). Prolongation of the cardiac action potential and increased cellular refractoriness beyond a critical point may stop a re-entrant circuit being completed and thereby prevent or halt a re-entrant arrhythmia (see above), e.g. amiodarone, sotalol. These drugs act by inhibiting I_{Kr}, the rapidly activating component of the delayed rectifier potassium current (phase 3). The gene *HERG* (the *human ether-à-go-go-related gene*) encodes a major subunit of the protein responsible for I_{Kr}. These are the most commonly used antiarrhythmic drugs at this time; newer agents in this class, e.g. dofetilide and azimilide, have not achieved wide use.

Class IV: calcium channel blockade. These drugs depress the slow inward calcium current (phase 2) and prolong conduction and refractoriness particularly in the SA and AV nodes, which helps to explain their effectiveness in terminating paroxysmal supraventricular tachycardia, e.g. verapamil.

Antiarrhythmic drugs are classified here according to a characteristic major action but most have other effects as well. For example, quinidine (class I) has major class III effects, propranolol (class II) has minor class I effects, and sotalol (class II) has major class III effects. Amiodarone has class I, II, III and IV effects but is usually classed under III.

PRINCIPAL DRUGS BY CLASS

For further data see Table 24.1.

CLASS 1A (SODIUM CHANNEL BLOCKADE WITH LENGTHENED REFRACTORINESS)

Quinidine

Quinidine is considered the prototype class I drug, although it is now used quite rarely.[3] In addition to its class IA activity, quinidine slightly enhances

---

[2]Roden D M 2003 Antiarrhythmic drugs: past, present and future. Journal of Cardiovascular Electrophysiology 14:1389–1396.

[3]In 1912 K F Wenckebach, a Dutch physician (who described 'Wenckebach block'), was visited by a merchant who wished to get rid of an attack of atrial fibrillation (he had recurrent attacks which, although they did not unduly inconvenience

Table 24.1 Drugs for cardiac arrhythmia

Class	Drug	Usual doses[a] and interval	Effect on ECG	Usually effective plasma concentration
1A	disopyramide	p.o.: 300–800 mg/day in divided doses i.v.: see specialist literature	Prolongs QRS, QTc and (±) PR	2–5 mg/L
IB	lidocaine	i.v. loading: 100 mg as a bolus over a few min i.v. maintenance: 1–4 mg/min	No significant change	1.5–6 mg/L
	mexiletine	p.o.: initial dose 400 mg, then after 2 h 200–250 mg × 6–8 h i.v.: see specialist literature	No significant change	0.5–2 mg/L
IC	flecainide	p.o.: 100–200 mg × 12 h i.v.: see specialist literature	Prolongs PR and QRS	0.2 mg/L
	propafenone	p.o.: see specialist literature	Prolongs PR and QRS	Active metabolite precludes establishment
II	propranolol	p.o.: 10–80 mg × 6 h i.v.: 1 mg over 1-min intervals to 10 mg max. (5 mg in anaesthesia)	Prolongs PR (±) No change in QRS Shortens QTc Bradycardia	Not established
	sotalol	80–160 mg × 2/day	Prolongs QTc and PR Sinus bradycardia	Not clinically useful
	esmolol	i.v.: infusion 50–200 micrograms/kg/min	As for propranolol	0.15–2 mg/L
III	amiodarone	p.o.: loading: 200 mg × 8 h for 1 week, then 200 mg × 12 h for 1 week; maintenance 200 mg/day	Prolongs PR, QRS and QTc Sinus bradycardia	Not established
IV	verapamil	p.o.: 40–120 mg × 8–12 h i.v.: see specialist literature	Prolongs PR	Not clinically useful
Other	digoxin	p.o.: initially 1–1.5 mg in divided doses over 24 h maintenance: 62.5–500 micrograms/day	Prolongs PR Depresses ST segment Flattens T wave	1–2 micrograms/L
	adenosine	i.v.: 6 mg initially; if no conversion after 1–2 min, give 12 mg and repeat once if necessary. Follow each bolus with saline flush	Prolongs PR Transient heart block	Not clinically useful

[a]Doses based on *British National Formulary* recommendations. Patients with decreased hepatic or renal function may require lower doses (see text). This table is adapted from that published in the *Medical Letter on Drugs and Therapeutics* (USA) 1996. We are grateful to the Chairman of the Editorial Board for allowing us to use this material.

him, offended his notions of good order in life's affairs). On receiving a guarded prognosis, the merchant inquired why there were heart specialists if they could not accomplish what he himself had already achieved. In the face of Wenckebach's incredulity he promised to return the next day with a regular pulse, which he did, at the same time revealing that he had done it with quinine (an optical isomer of quinidine). Examination of quinine derivatives led to the introduction of quinidine in 1918 (Wenckebach K F 1923 Journal of the American Medical Association 81:472).

contractility of the myocardium (positive inotropic effect) and reduces vagus nerve activity on the heart (antimuscarinic effect).

Pharmacokinetics. Absorption of quinidine from the gut is rapid; 75% of the drug is metabolised and the remainder is eliminated unchanged in the urine ($t_{1/2}$ 7 h). Active metabolites may accumulate when renal function is impaired.

Adverse reactions. Quinidine must not be used alone to treat atrial fibrillation or flutter as its antimuscarinic action enhances AV conduction and the heart rate may accelerate. Other cardiac effects include serious ventricular tachyarrhythmias associated with electrocardiographic QTc prolongation, i.e. torsades de pointes (Fig. 24.2), the cause of 'quinidine syncope'. Quinidine raises plasma digoxin concentration (by displacement from tissue binding and impairment of renal excretion); decrease the dose of digoxin when the drugs are used together. Noncardiac effects, called 'cinchonism', include diarrhoea and other gastrointestinal symptoms, rashes, thrombocytopenia and fever.

Disopyramide

Disopyramide was the most commonly used drug in this class but is much less so now. It has significant antimuscarinic activity.

Pharmacokinetics. Disopyramide is used orally (see Table 24.1) and is well absorbed. It is in part excreted unchanged and in part metabolised. The $t_{1/2}$ is 6 h.

Adverse reactions. The antimuscarinic activity is a significant problem causing dry mouth, blurred vision, glaucoma, and micturition hesitancy and retention. Gastrointestinal symptoms, rash and agranulocytosis can also occur. Effects on the cardiovascular system include hypotension and heart failure (negative inotropic effect).

CLASS IB (SODIUM CHANNEL BLOCKADE WITH SHORTENED REFRACTORINESS)

Lidocaine

Lidocaine finds use principally for ventricular arrhythmias, especially those complicating myocardial infarction. Its kinetics render it unsuitable for oral administration and its application is restricted to the treatment of acute arrhythmias.

Pharmacokinetics. Lidocaine is used intravenously, or occasionally intramuscularly; dosing by mouth is unsatisfactory because its $t_{1/2}$ is short (1.5 h) and the drug undergoes extensive pre-systemic (first-pass) elimination in the liver.

Adverse reactions are uncommon unless infusion is rapid or there is significant heart failure; they include hypotension, dizziness, blurred sight, sleepiness, slurred speech, numbness, sweating, confusion and convulsions.

Mexiletine is similar to lidocaine but is effective orally ($t_{1/2}$ 10 h). It has been used for ventricular arrhythmias, especially those complicating myocardial infarction, but is usually poorly tolerated.

Adverse reactions, almost universal and dose related, include nausea, vomiting, hiccough, tremor, drowsiness, confusion, dysarthria, diplopia, ataxia, cardiac arrhythmia and hypotension.

CLASS IC (SODIUM CHANNEL BLOCKADE WITH MINIMAL EFFECT ON REFRACTORINESS)

Flecainide

Flecainide slows conduction in all cardiac cells including the anomalous pathways responsible for the Wolff–Parkinson–White (WPW) syndrome.

The most common indication, indeed where it is the drug of choice, is atrioventricular (AV) re-entrant tachycardia, such as AV nodal tachycardia or in the tachycardias associated with the WPW syndrome or similar conditions with anomalous pathways. This should be as a prelude to definitive treatment with

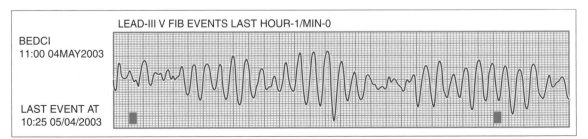

Fig. 24.2 Torsade de pointes ventricular arrhythmia. This patient had received the potassium channel blocking drug, amiodarone, which prolonged the QTc interval and produced this characteristic 'twisting about the points' pattern.

radiofrequency ablation, which is the treatment of choice. Flecainide may also be useful in patients with paroxysmal atrial fibrillation, used in conjunction with an agent that blocks the AV node to protect against rapid conduction to the ventricle. Following the salutary findings of the CAST study[4], flecainide is now restricted to patients without evidence of coronary or structural heart disease.

Pharmacokinetics. Metabolism in the liver and renal elimination of unchanged metabolites terminates its action. The $t_{1/2}$ is 14 h in healthy adults but may be over 20 h in patients with heart disease, in the elderly and in those with poor renal function.

Adverse reactions. Flecainide is contraindicated in patients with sick sinus syndrome, heart failure, and in those with a history of myocardial infarction who have ventricular arrhythmias. Minor adverse effects include blurred vision, abdominal discomfort, nausea, dizziness, tremor, abnormal taste sensations and paraesthesiae.

Propafenone

In addition to the defining properties of this class, propafenone has β-adrenoceptor blocking activity equivalent to a low dose of propranolol. It is occasionally used to suppress non-sustained ventricular arrhythmias in patients whose left ventricular function is normal.

Pharmacokinetics. Propafenone is metabolised by the liver and is a substrate for CYP 2D6 (see p. 107). Some 7% of caucasian patients are poor metabolisers who, for equivalent doses, thus have higher plasma concentrations than the remainder of the population.

---

[4]Flecainide, encainide and moricizine underwent clinical trial to establish whether suppression of asymptomatic premature beats with antiarrhythmic drugs would reduce the risk of death from arrhythmia after myocardial infarction. The study was terminated after preliminary analysis of 1727 patients revealed that the mortality rate in patients treated with flecainide or encainide was 7.7% compared with 3.0% in controls. The most likely explanation for the result was the induction of fatal ventricular arrhythmias, possibly due to ischaemia by flecainide and encainide, i.e. a proarrhythmic effect (Cardiac Arrhythmia Suppression Trial (CAST) Investigators 1989 Preliminary report: effect of encainide and flecainide on mortality in a randomized trial of arrhythmia suppression after myocardial infarction. New England Journal of Medicine 321:406–412).

Adverse reactions are similar to those of flecainide and are commoner in poor metabolisers. In addition, conduction block may occur, heart failure may worsen and ventricular arrhythmias may be exacerbated, and flecainide should not be used in patients with sustained ventricular tachycardia and poor left ventricular function.

CLASS II (CATECHOLAMINE BLOCKADE)

β-Adrenoceptor antagonists (see also Chapter 23)
β-Adrenoceptor blockers are effective probably because they counteract the arrhythmogenic effect of catecholamines. The following actions appear to be relevant:

- The rate of automatic firing of the SA node is accelerated by β-adrenoceptor activation and this effect is abolished by β-blockers. Some ectopic pacemakers appear to be dependent on adrenergic drive.
- β-Blockers prolong the refractoriness of the AV node, which may prevent re-entrant tachycardia at this site.
- Many β-blocking drugs (propranolol, oxprenolol, alprenolol, acebutolol, labetalol) also possess membrane stabilising (class I) properties. Sotalol prolongs cardiac refractoriness (class III effect) but has no class I effects; it is often preferred when a β-blocker is indicated for arrhythmias, but should be used with care. Esmolol (below) is a short-acting β_1-selective agent, whose sole use is in the treatment of arrhythmias. Its short duration and β_1 selectivity make it an option for some patients with contraindications to other β-blocking drugs.
- β-Adrenoceptor antagonists are effective for a range of supraventricular arrhythmias, in particular those associated with exercise, emotion or hyperthyroidism. Sotalol finds use to suppress ventricular ectopic beats and ventricular tachycardia, possibly in conjunction with amiodarone.

Pharmacokinetics. For long-term use, any of the oral preparations of β-blocker is suitable. In emergencies, esmolol is used (see Table 24.1), its short $t_{1/2}$ (9 min) rendering it suitable for administration by intravenous infusion with rapid alterations in dose, according to response.

Adverse reactions. Cardiac effects from overdosage include heart block or even cardiac arrest. Heart failure may be precipitated in a patient dependent on sympathetic drive to maintain cardiac output (see Chapter 23 for an account of other adverse effects).

Interactions. Concomitant intravenous administration of a calcium channel blocker that affects conduction (verapamil, diltiazem) increases the risk of bradycardia and AV block. In patients with depressed myocardial contractility, the combination of oral or intravenous β-blockade and calcium channel blockade (nifedipine, verapamil) may cause hypotension or heart failure.

CLASS III (LENGTHENING OF REFRACTORINESS DUE TO POTASSIUM CHANNEL BLOCKADE)

Amiodarone

Amiodarone is the most powerful antiarrhythmic drug available for the treatment and prevention of both atrial and ventricular arrhythmias. Even short-term use can cause serious toxicity, and its use should always follow a consideration or a trial of alternatives. Amiodarone prolongs the effective refractory period of myocardial cells, the AV node and of anomalous pathways. It also blocks β-adrenoceptors non-competitively.

Amiodarone is used in chronic ventricular arrhythmias; in atrial fibrillation it both slows the ventricular response and may restore sinus rhythm (chemical cardioversion). It may also be used to maintain sinus rhythm after cardioversion for atrial fibrillation or flutter. Amiodarone was used for the management of re-entrant supraventricular tachycardias associated with the Wolff–Parkinson–White syndrome, but radiofrequency ablation is now the treatment of choice.

Pharmacokinetics. Amiodarone is effective given orally; its enormous apparent distribution volume (70 L/kg) indicates that little remains in the blood. It is stored in fat and many other tissues and the $t_{1/2}$ of 54 days after multiple dosing signifies slow release from these sites (and slow accumulation to steady state means that a loading dose is necessary; see Table 24.1). The drug is metabolised in the liver and eliminated through the biliary and intestinal tracts.

Adverse reactions. Cardiovascular effects include bradycardia, heart block and induction of ventricular arrhythmia. Other effects include nausea, vomiting, taste disturbances and the development of corneal microdeposits, which may rarely cause visual haloes, night glare and photophobia; the latter are dose related, resolve on discontinuation and do not threaten vision. Plasma transaminase levels may rise (requiring dose reduction or withdrawal if accompanied by acute liver disorders). Amiodarone contains iodine, and both hyperthyroidism and hypothyroidism are quite common; monitoring thyroid function before and during therapy is essential.

Photosensitivity reactions are common, may be very severe and patients should be warned explicitly when starting the drug. Amiodarone may also cause a bluish discoloration on exposed areas of the skin (occasionally reversible on discontinuing the drug). Less commonly, pneumonitis and pulmonary fibrosis occur (X-ray chest before beginning treatment) and hepatitis, sometimes rapidly during short-term use of the drug; these may be fatal, so vigilance should be high. Cirrhosis is reported. Peripheral neuropathy and myopathy occur (usually reversible on withdrawal).

Interaction with digoxin (by displacement from tissue binding sites and interference with its elimination) and with warfarin (by inhibiting its metabolism) increases the effect of both these drugs. β-Blockers and calcium channel antagonists augment the depressant effect of amiodarone on SA and AV node function.

CLASS IV (CALCIUM CHANNEL BLOCKADE)

Calcium is involved in the contraction of cardiac and vascular smooth muscle cells, and in the automaticity of cardiac pacemaker cells. Actions of calcium channel blockers on vascular smooth muscle cells appear with the main account of these drugs in Chapter 23. Although the three classes of calcium channel blocker have similar effects on vascular smooth muscle in the arterial tree, their cardiac actions differ. The phenylalkylamine, verapamil, depresses myocardial contraction more than the others, and both verapamil and the benzothiazepine, diltiazem, slow conduction in the SA and AV nodes.

Calcium and cardiac cells

Cardiac muscle cells are normally depolarised by the fast inward flow of sodium ions, following which there is a slow inward flow of calcium ions through the L-type calcium channels (phase 2 in Fig. 24.1); the consequent rise in free intracellular calcium ions activates the contractile mechanism.

Pacemaker cells in the SA and AV nodes rely heavily on the slow inward flow of calcium ions (phase 4) for their capacity to discharge spontaneously, i.e. for their automaticity.

Calcium channel blockers inhibit the passage of calcium through the membrane channels; the result in myocardial cells is to depress contractility, and in pacemaker cells to suppress their automatic activity. Members of the group therefore may have negative cardiac inotropic and chronotropic actions, which can be separated: nifedipine, at therapeutic concentrations, acts almost exclusively on non-cardiac ion channels and has no clinically useful antiarrhythmic activity, whereas verapamil is an effective rate control agent.

Verapamil

Verapamil (see also p. 420) prolongs conduction and refractoriness in the AV node and depresses the rate of discharge of the SA node. If adenosine is not available, verapamil is a very attractive and, with due care, safe alternative for terminating narrow complex paroxysmal supraventricular tachycardia. Verapamil should not be given intravenously to patients with broad complex tachyarrhythmias, in whom it may be lethal.

Adverse effects include nausea, constipation, headache, fatigue, hypotension, bradycardia and heart block.

OTHER ANTIARRHYTHMICS

Digoxin and other cardiac glycosides[5]

Crude digitalis is a preparation of the dried leaf of the foxglove plant *Digitalis purpurea* or *lanata*. Digitalis contains a number of active glycosides (digoxin, lanatosides) whose actions are qualitatively similar, differing principally in rapidity of onset and duration; the pure individual glycosides are used. The following account refers to all the cardiac glycosides but digoxin is the principal one.

Mode of action. Cardiac glycosides affect the heart both directly and indirectly in a series of complex actions, some of which oppose one another. The *direct* effect is to inhibit the membrane-bound sodium–potassium adenosine triphosphatase (Na^+, K^+-ATPase) enzyme that supplies energy for the system that pumps sodium out of and transports potassium into contracting and conducting cells. By reducing the exchange of extracellular sodium with intracellular calcium, digoxin raises the store of intracellular calcium, which facilitates muscular contraction. The *indirect* effect is to enhance vagal activity by complex peripheral and central mechanisms.

The clinically important consequences are on:

- the contracting cells: increased contractility and excitability
- SA and AV nodes and conducting tissue: decreased generation and propagation.

Uses. Digoxin is not strictly an antiarrhythmic agent but rather it modulates the response to arrhythmias. Its most useful property, in this respect, is to slow conduction through the AV node. The main uses are in:

- *Atrial fibrillation*, benefiting chiefly by the vagal effect on the AV node, reducing conduction through it and thus slowing the ventricular rate.

---

[5]In 1775 Dr William Withering was making a routine journey from Birmingham (England), his home, to see patients at the Stafford Infirmary. Whilst the carriage horses were being changed half way, he was asked to see an old dropsical (oedematous) woman. He thought she would die and so some weeks later, when he heard of her recovery, was interested enough to enquire into the cause. Recovery was attributed to a herb tea containing some 20 ingredients, amongst which Withering, already the author of a botanical textbook, found it 'not very difficult … to perceive that the active herb could be no other than the foxglove'. He began to investigate its properties, trying it on the poor of Birmingham, whom he used to see without fee each day. The results were inconclusive and his interest flagged until one day he heard that the principal of an Oxford College had been cured by foxglove after 'some of the first physicians of the age had declared that they could do no more for him'. This put a new complexion on the matter and, pursuing his investigation, Withering found that foxglove extract caused diuresis in some oedematous patients. He defined the type of patient who might benefit from it and, equally importantly, he standardised his foxglove leaf preparations and was able to lay down accurate dosage schedules. His advice, with little amplification, served until relatively recently (Withering W 1785 An account of the foxglove. Robinson, London).

- *Atrial flutter*, benefiting by the vagus nerve action of shortening the refractory period of the atrial muscle so that flutter may occasionally be converted to fibrillation (in which state the ventricular rate is more readily controlled). Electrical cardioversion followed by radiofrequency ablation is preferred.
- *Heart failure*, benefiting chiefly by the direct action to increase myocardial contractility. Digoxin is still used occasionally in chronic heart failure due to ischaemic, hypertensive or valvular heart disease, especially in the short term. This is no longer a major indication following the introduction of other groups of drugs.

Pharmacokinetics. Digoxin is eliminated 85% unchanged by the kidney and the remainder is metabolised by the liver. The $t_{1/2}$ is 36 h. Digoxin is usually administered by mouth.

Dose and therapeutic plasma concentration. See Table 24.1. *Reduced* dose of digoxin is necessary in: renal impairment (see above); the elderly (probably from decline in renal clearance with age); electrolyte disturbances (hypokalaemia accentuates the potential for adverse effects of digoxin, as does hypomagnesaemia); hypothyroid patients (who are intolerant of digoxin).

Adverse effects. Abnormal cardiac rhythms usually take the form of ectopic arrhythmias (ventricular ectopic beats, ventricular tachyarrhythmias, paroxysmal supraventricular tachycardia) and heart block. Gastrointestinal effects include anorexia, which usually precedes vomiting and is a warning that dosage is excessive. Diarrhoea may also occur. Visual effects include disturbances of colour vision, e.g. yellow (xanthopsia) but also red or green vision, photophobia and blurring. Gynaecomastia may occur in men and breast enlargement in women with long-term use (cardiac glycosides have structural resemblance to oestrogen). Mental effects include confusion, restlessness, agitation, nightmares and acute psychoses.

Acute digoxin poisoning causes initial nausea and vomiting and hyperkalaemia because inhibition of the Na^+, K^+-ATPase pump prevents intracellular accumulation of potassium. The ECG changes (see Table 24.1) of prolonged use of digoxin may be absent. There may be exaggerated sinus arrhythmia, bradycardia and ectopic rhythms with or without heart block.

Treatment of overdose. For severe digoxin poisoning, infusion of the digoxin-specific binding (Fab) fragment (Digibind) of the antibody to digoxin neutralises digoxin in the plasma and is an effective treatment. Because it lacks the Fc segment, this fragment is non-immunogenic and it is sufficiently small to be eliminated as the digoxin–antibody complex in the urine. Intravenous phenytoin may be effective for ventricular arrhythmias, and atropine for bradycardia. Temporary electrical pacing may be needed, but direct current shock may cause ventricular fibrillation.

Interactions. Verapamil, nifedipine, quinidine and amiodarone raise steady-state plasma digoxin concentrations (see above) and the digoxin dose should be lowered when any of these is added. The likelihood of AV block due to digoxin is increased by verapamil and by β-adrenoceptor blockers.

Adenosine

Adenosine is an endogenous purine nucleotide that slows atrioventricular conduction and dilates coronary and peripheral arteries. It is rapidly metabolised by circulating adenosine deaminase and is also taken up by cells; hence its residence in plasma is brief ($t_{1/2}$ <2 s) and it must be given rapidly intravenously.

Administered as a bolus injection, adenosine is effective for terminating paroxysmal supraventricular (re-entrant) tachycardias, including episodes in patients with Wolff–Parkinson–White syndrome. The initial dose in adults is 6 mg over 2 s with continuous ECG monitoring, with doubling increments every 1–2 min. The average total dose is 125 micrograms/kg.

Adenosine is an alternative to verapamil for supraventricular tachycardia and possibly safer because adenosine is short acting and not negatively inotropic; verapamil is dangerous if used mistakenly in a ventricular tachycardia.

Adverse effects from adenosine are not serious because of the brevity of its action, but it may cause very distressing dyspnoea, facial flushing, chest pain and transient arrhythmias, e.g. bradycardia. Adenosine should not be given to asthmatics or to patients with second- or third-degree AV block or sick sinus syndrome (unless a pacemaker is in place).

Cardiac effects of the autonomic nervous system

Some drugs used for arrhythmias exert their actions through the autonomic nervous system by mimicking or antagonising the effects of the sympathetic or parasympathetic nerves that supply the heart. The neurotransmitters in these two branches of the autonomic system, noradrenaline and acetylcholine, are functionally antagonistic by having opposing actions on cyclic AMP production within the cardiomyocyte. Their receptors are coupled to the two trimeric GTP-binding proteins, Gs and Gi, which stimulate and inhibit adenylyl cyclase, respectively.

The sympathetic division (adrenergic component of the autonomic nervous system), when stimulated, has the following (receptor) effects on the heart:

- Tachycardia due to increased rate of discharge of the SA node.
- Increased automaticity in the AV node and His–Purkinje system.
- Increase in conductivity in the His–Purkinje system.
- Increased force of contraction.
- Shortening of the refractory period.

Isoprotenerol, a β-adrenoceptor agonist, finds use to accelerate the heart when there is extreme bradycardia due to heart block, prior to the insertion of an implanted pacemaker; this is now rarely needed. Adverse effects are those expected of β-adrenoceptor agonists and include tremor, flushing, sweating, palpitation, headache and diarrhoea.

The vagus nerve (*cholinergic, parasympathetic*), when stimulated, affects the heart in ways that are useful in the therapy of arrhythmias, by causing:

- bradycardia due to depression of the SA node
- slowing of conduction through and increased refractoriness of the AV node
- shortening of the refractory period of atrial muscle cells
- decreased myocardial excitability.

There is also reduced *force of contraction* of atrial and ventricular muscle cells.

Vagal stimulation can slow or terminate supraventricular arrhythmias, reflexly by physical manoeuvres (under ECG control, if possible).

Carotid sinus massage activates stretch receptors: external pressure is applied gently to one side at a time but never to both sides at once. Some individuals are very sensitive to the procedure and develop severe bradycardia and hypotension.

Other methods include the *Valsalva manoeuvre* (deep inspiration followed by expiration against a closed glottis, which both stimulates stretch receptors in the lung and reduces venous return to the heart); *the Müller procedure* (deep expiration followed by inspiration against a closed glottis); production of nausea and retching by inviting patients to put their own fingers down their throat.

The effects of vagus nerve activity are blocked by *atropine* (antimuscarinic action), an action that is used to accelerate the heart during episodes of sinus bradycardia as may occur after myocardial infarction. The dose is 600 micrograms i.v. and repeated as necessary to a maximum of 3 mg per day.

Adverse effects are those of muscarinic blockade, namely dry mouth, blurred vision, urinary retention, confusion and hallucination.

PROARRHYTHMIC DRUG EFFECTS

All antiarrhythmic drugs can also cause arrhythmia; they should be used with care and ideally only following advice from a specialist. Such proarrhythmic effects most commonly occur with drugs that prolong the QTc interval or QRS complex of the ECG; hypokalaemia aggravates the danger. Quinidine may cause tachyarrhythmias, torsade de pointes (see Fig. 24.2) in an estimated 4–6% of patients. The Cardiac Arrhythmia Suppression Trial (CAST) revealed a probable proarrhythmic effect of flecainide resulting in fatalities (see p. 453). Digoxin can induce a variety of bradyarrhythmias and tachyarrhythmias (see above).

CHOICE BETWEEN DRUGS AND ELECTROCONVERSION

Direct current (DC) electric shock applied externally is often the best way to convert cardiac arrhythmias to sinus rhythm. Many atrial or ventricular arrhythmias start from transiently operating factors but, once they have begun, the abnormal mechanisms are self-sustaining. With a successful electric shock, the heart is depolarised, the ectopic focus is extinguished and the SA node, the part of the heart with the highest automaticity, resumes as the dominant pacemaker.

Electrical conversion has the advantage that it is immediate, unlike drugs, which may take days or longer to act; also, the effective doses and adverse effects of drugs are largely unpredictable, and can be serious.[6]

Uses of electrical conversion: in supraventricular and ventricular tachycardia, ventricular fibrillation and atrial fibrillation and flutter. Drugs can be useful to prevent a relapse, e.g. sotalol, amiodarone.

See also UK Resuscitation Council guidelines (see Figs 24.3–24.5).

SPECIFIC TREATMENTS[7]

Sinus bradycardia

Acute sinus bradycardia requires treatment if it is symptomatic, e.g. where there is hypotension or escape rhythms; extreme bradycardia may allow a ventricular focus to take over and lead to ventricular tachycardia. The foot of the bed should be raised to assist venous return and atropine should be given intravenously. Chronic symptomatic bradycardia is an indication for the insertion of a permanent pacemaker.

Atrial ectopic beats

Reduction in the use of tea, coffee and other methylxanthine-containing drinks, and of tobacco, may suffice for ectopic beats not due to organic heart disease. For persistent symptoms, a small dose of a β-adrenoceptor blocker may be effective.

Paroxysmal supraventricular (AV re-entrant or atrial) tachycardia

For acute attacks, if vagal stimulation (by carotid massage, or swallowing ice) is unsuccessful, adenosine has the dual advantage of being effective in most such tachycardias, while having no effect on a ventricular tachycardia. The response to adenosine is therefore of diagnostic value. Intravenous verapamil is an alternative for the acute management of a narrow complex tachycardia. If the patient is in circulatory shock from the tachycardia, or drug treatment fails, DC conversion delivers immediate effect. Flecainide and sotalol are the drugs of choice for prophylaxis, but patients should be referred for radiofrequency ablation.

Atrial fibrillation (AF)

The therapeutic options are:

- Treatment or no treatment.
- Conversion or rate control.
- Immediate or delayed conversion.
- Drugs or DC conversion.

The information required is:

- Ventricular rate ('normal' or high).
- Haemodynamic state ('normal' or compromised).
- Atrial size ('normal' or enlarged).

In many patients, AF is an incidental finding on the background of some existing cardiovascular disease, and with a large atrium. With a very prolonged history of symptoms, *rate-controlling medication* such as a β-blocker, digoxin or calcium antagonist may suffice.

If the history appears shorter, and the atrium is of normal size, i.e. is unlikely to contain thrombus, or there has been recent onset of heart failure or shock, cardioversion should be attempted. Electrical (DC) conversion is favoured where treatment is either urgent or likely to be successful in holding the patient in sinus rhythm. Amiodarone can often provide pharmacological conversion over hours to days, and is also effective for patients who revert rapidly to AF after DC conversion. When conversion is not urgent, it should be delayed for a month to permit anticoagulation with warfarin, which should be continued for 4 weeks thereafter. If cardioversion is deemed urgent, then tranoesophageal echocardiography should be used to show there is no thrombus visible in the left atrium.

In patients who have reverted to AF after previous conversions, amiodarone is the drug of choice prior to further attempts at cardioversion. Amiodarone may also be used to suppress episodes of paroxysmal atrial fibrillation, but sotalol or flecainide are

---

[6]To the layperson, 'shock' treatment could be interpreted as frights (which stimulate the vagus, as described above), or as the electrical sort. Dr James Le Fanu quotes a Belfast doctor who reported a farmer with a solution that covered both possibilities. He had suffered from episodes of palpitations and dizziness for 30 years. When he first got them, he would jump from a barrel and thump his feet hard on the ground at landing. This became less effective with time. His next 'cure' was to remove his clothes, climb a ladder and jump from a considerable height into a cold water tank on the farm. Later, he discovered the best and simplest treatment was to grab hold of his high-voltage electrified cattle fence – although if he was wearing Wellington (rubber) boots he found he had to earth the shock, so besides grabbing the fence with one hand he simultaneously shoved a finger of the other hand into the ground.

[7]See also UK Resuscitation Council Guidelines (Figs 24.3-24.5).

preferred. Radiofrequency ablation is now emerging as the treatment of choice in many patients with both paroxysmal and persistent atrial fibrillation.

Additional treatments in chronic atrial fibrillation. Long-term treatment with warfarin is almost mandatory to reduce embolic complications. The efficacy of aspirin as an antiembolic agent is probably less in this group, but retains value in patients in whom warfarin is inappropriate.

Atrial flutter

It is doubtful whether this differs in any important way in its origins or sequelae from atrial fibrillation. The ventricular rate is usually faster (typically, half an atrial rate of 300 beats/min, where 2 : 1 block is present), which is too fast to leave without treatment. As, similarly, the patient is unlikely to have been in this rhythm for a prolonged period, there is less likelihood that atrial thrombus has accumulated. Previously, conversion without prior anticoagulation was undertaken occasionally, but transoesphageal echocardiography or anticoagulation is now mandatory. Patients should not remain in chronic atrial flutter, and DC conversion will usually either restore sinus rhythm or result in atrial fibrillation (treated as above). Patients who fail to convert, or who revert to atrial flutter, should be referred for radiofrequency ablation, which is highly effective and removes the cause of the atrial flutter in nearly all patients.

Atrial tachycardia with variable AV block

The atrial rate is 120–250 beats/min, and commonly there is AV block. Digoxin is a possible cause of the arrhythmia, and should be withdrawn. If the patient is not taking digoxin, it may be introduced to control the ventricular rate. These patients should be considered for radiofrequency ablation.

Heart block

In an emergency, antimuscarinic vagal block with atropine 600 micrograms i.v. or the β-adrenoceptor agonist, isoprenaline (0.5–10 micrograms/min i.v.) can improve AV conduction, but advanced heart block always requires implantation of a permanent pacemaker, possibly preceded by a temporary pacing wire.

Pre-excitation (Wolff–Parkinson–White) syndrome

This occurs in otherwise healthy individuals who possess an anomalous (accessory) atrioventricular (AV) pathway; they often experience attacks of paroxysmal AV re-entrant tachycardia or atrial fibrillation. Drugs that both suppress the initiating ectopic beats and delay conduction through the accessory pathway are used to prevent attacks, e.g. flecainide, sotalol or amiodarone. Do not use verapamil or digoxin, which may *increase* conduction through the anomalous pathway. Electrical conversion restores sinus rhythm when the ventricular rate is very rapid. Radiofrequency ablation of aberrant pathways provides a cure and is the treatment of choice.

Ventricular premature beats

These are common after myocardial infarction. Their particular significance is that the R-wave (ECG) of an ectopic beat, superimposed upon the early or peak phases of the T-wave of a normal beat, may precipitate ventricular tachycardia or fibrillation (the 'R-on-T' phenomenon). About 80% of patients with myocardial infarction who proceed to ventricular fibrillation have preceding ventricular premature beats. Lidocaine effectively suppresses ectopic ventricular beats but is not often used as its addition increases overall risk.

Ventricular tachycardia

Ventricular tachycardia demands urgent treatment because it frequently leads to ventricular fibrillation and circulatory arrest. A powerful thump of the fist on the mid-sternum or precordium may very occasionally stop a tachycardia. If there is rapid haemodynamic deterioration, electrical conversion is the treatment of choice. When the patient is in good cardiovascular condition, treatment may begin with intravenous lidocaine, failing which, intravenous amiodarone. For recurrent ventricular tachycardia, amiodarone or sotalol is preferred. Other Group 1A drugs (mexiletine, disopyramide, quinidine and propafenone) are not usually indicated. Patients should be considered for insertion of an implantable cardioverter defibrillator (ICD).

Ventricular fibrillation and cardiac arrest

Ventricular fibrillation is usually caused by myocardial infarction or ischaemia, or serious organic heart disease and is the main cause of *cardiac arrest*. Guidelines for the management of peri-arrest arrhythmias and cardiac arrest are issued by the UK Resuscitation Council and appear in Figures 24.3, 24.4 and 24.5. Patients suffering 'failed' sudden cardiac death (SCD) should be considered for the insertion of an ICD.

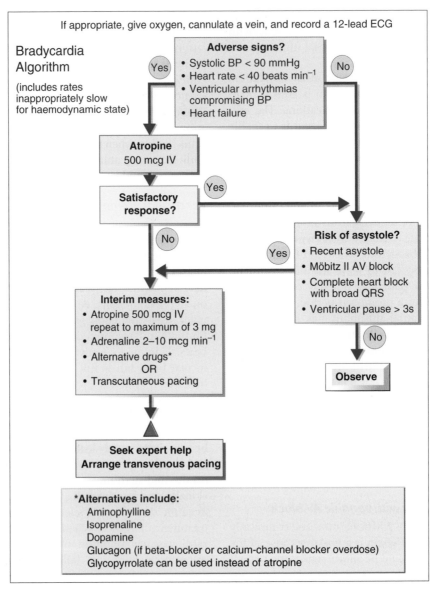

Fig. 24.3 Algorithm for the management of acute bradycardia. mcg, micrograms. With permission, UK Resuscitation Council. The latest version can be found at http://www.resus.org.uk

Long QTc syndromes

These are caused by malfunction of ion channels, leading to impaired ventricular repolarisation (expressed as prolongation of the QTc interval) and a characteristic ventricular tachycardia, torsade de pointes (see Fig. 24.2).[8] The symptoms range from episodes of syncope to cardiac arrest. Several drugs are responsible for the acquired form of the condition including antiarrhythmic drugs (see above), antimicrobials, histamine H_1-receptor antagonists and serotonin receptor antagonists; predisposing factors are female sex, recent heart rate slowing, and hypokalaemia.[9]

Congenital forms of the long QTc syndrome are due to mutations of the genes encoding ion channels, and exposure to drugs reveals some of these.

---

[8]French: *torsade*, twist; *pointe*, point. 'Twisting of the points', referring to the characteristic sequence of 'up' followed by 'down' QRS complexes. The appearance has been called a 'cardiac ballet'.

[9]Roden D M 2004 Drug-induced prolongation of the QT interval. New England Journal of Medicine 350:1013–1022.

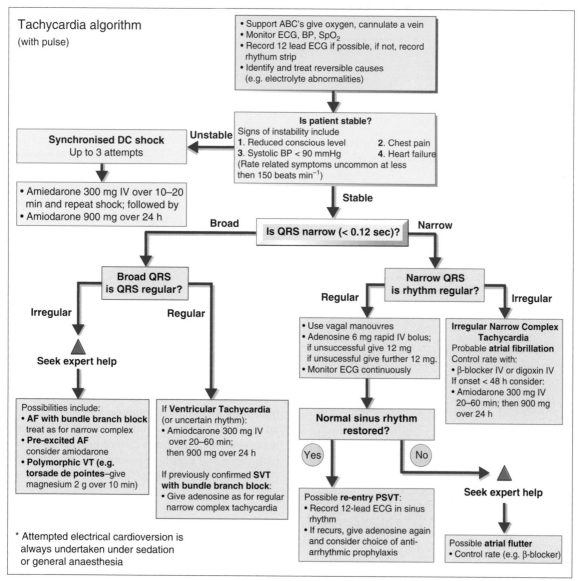

Tachycardia algorithm
(with pulse)

- Support ABC's give oxygen, cannulate a vein
- Monitor ECG, BP, SpO$_2$
- Record 12 lead ECG if possible, if not, record rhythum strip
- Identify and treat reversible causes (e.g. electrolyte abnormalities)

Is patient stable?
Signs of instability include
1. Reduced conscious level   **2.** Chest pain
3. Systolic BP < 90 mmHg   **4.** Heart failure
(Rate related symptoms uncommon at less then 150 beats min^{-1})

Unstable

Synchronised DC shock
Up to 3 attempts

- Amiedarone 300 mg IV over 10–20 min and repeat shock; followed by
- Amiodarone 900 mg over 24 h

Stable

Is QRS narrow (< 0.12 sec)?

Broad

Narrow

Broad QRS
is QRS regular?

Narrow QRS
is rhythm regular?

Irregular

Regular

Regular

Irregular

Seek expert help

- Use vagal manouvres
- Adenosine 6 mg rapid IV bolus; if unsuccessful give 12 mg if unsuccessful give further 12 mg.
- Monitor ECG continuously

Irregular Narrow Complex Tachycardia
Probable **atrial fibrillation**
Control rate with:
- β-blocker IV or digoxin IV
If onset < 48 h consider:
- Amiodarone 300 mg IV 20–60 min; then 900 mg over 24 h

Possibilities include:
- **AF with bundle branch block** treat as for narrow complex
- **Pre-excited AF** consider amiodarone
- **Polymorphic VT (e.g. torsade de pointes**–give magnesium 2 g over 10 min)

If **Ventricular Tachycardia** (or uncertain rhythm):
- Amiodcarone 300 mg IV over 20–60 min; then 900 mg over 24 h

If previously confirmed **SVT with bundle branch block**:
- Give adenosine as for regular narrow complex tachycardia

Normal sinus rhythm restored?

Yes

No

Seek expert help

* Attempted electrical cardioversion is always undertaken under sedation or general anaesthesia

Possible **re-entry PSVT**:
- Record 12-lead ECG in sinus rhythm
- If recurs, give adenosine again and consider choice of anti-arrhythmic prophylaxis

Possible **atrial flutter**
- Control rate (e.g. β-blocker)

Fig. 24.4 Algorithm for the management of acute tachycardia. With permission, UK Resuscitation Council. The latest version can be found at http://www.resus.org.uk

Summary

- The treatment of cardiac arrhythmias can be directly physical, electrical, pharmacological or surgical. Radiofrequency ablation and devices such as permanent pacemakers and ICDs are increasingly often the preferred procedures. The use of drugs alone is declining but they often constitute adjunctive treatments.
- The choice among drugs follows partly from theoretical predictions of their action on the cardiac cycle but substantially from short- and long-term observations of their efficacy and safety.
- All antiarrhythmics can be potentially dangerous, and should be used only in symptomatic or haemodynamically compromised patients.
- Adenosine is the treatment of choice for diagnosis and reversal of supraventricular arrhythmias. Verapamil is an alternative for the management of narrow complex tachycardias.
- Amiodarone is the most effective drug for reversing atrial fibrillation, and for preventing ventricular arrhythmias, but it has notable adverse effects.
- Digoxin retains a unique role as a positively inotropic antiarrhythmic, being most useful in slowing AV conduction in atrial fibrillation.

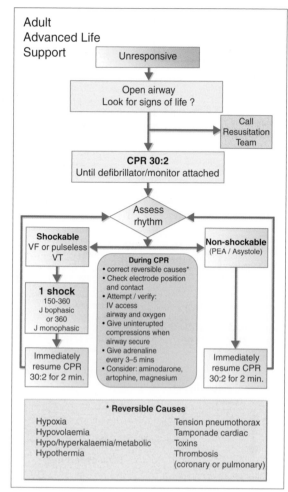

Fig. 24.5 Adult advanced life support. With permission, UK Resuscitation Council. The latest version can be found at http://www.resus.org.uk

HEART FAILURE AND ITS TREATMENT

SOME PHYSIOLOGY AND PATHOPHYSIOLOGY

Cardiac output (CO) depends on the rate of contraction of the heart (HR) and the volume of blood that is ejected with each beat, the stroke volume (SV); it is expressed by the relationship:

$$CO = HR \times SV$$

The three factors that regulate the stroke volume are preload, afterload and contractility:

- *Preload* is the load on the heart created by the volume of blood injected into the left ventricle by the left atrium (at the end of ventricular diastole) and that it must eject with each contraction. It can also be viewed as the amount of stretch to which the left ventricle is subject. As the preload rises so also do the degree of stretch and the length of cardiac muscle fibres. Preload is thus a *volume* load and can be excessive, e.g. when there is valvular incompetence.

- *Afterload* refers to the load on the contracting ventricle created by the resistance to the blood injected by the ventricle into the arterial system, i.e. the total peripheral resistance. Afterload is thus a *pressure* load and is excessive, e.g. in arterial hypertension.

- *Contractility* refers to the capacity of the myocardium to generate the force necessary to respond to preload and to overcome afterload.

DEFINITION OF CHRONIC HEART FAILURE

As the population ages and the treatment of acute myocardial infarction improves, this condition is becoming increasingly common and there is talk of an 'epidemic' of heart failure. Chronic heart failure is present when the heart cannot provide all organs with the blood supply appropriate to demand. This definition incorporates two elements: firstly, cardiac output may be normal at rest, but secondly, when demand is increased, perfusion of the vital organs (brain and kidneys) continues at the expense of other tissues, especially skeletal muscle. Overall, systemic arterial pressure is sustained until a late stage. These responses follow neuroendocrine activation when the heart begins to fail.

The therapeutic importance of recognising this pathophysiology is that many of the neuroendocrine abnormalities of heart failure – particularly the increased renin output and sympathetic activity – can be a consequence of drug treatment, as well as the disease. Renal perfusion is normal in early heart failure, whereas diuretics and vasodilators stimulate renin and noradrenaline production through actions at the juxtaglomerular apparatus in the kidney and on the arterial baroreflex, respectively. The earliest endocrine abnormality in almost all types of cardiac disease is increased release of the heart's own hormones, the natriuretic peptides ANP and BNP (A for atrial, B for brain, where it was first discovered). The concentration in plasma of BNP provides a strong prognostic indicator for patients with all stages of heart failure.[10] These peptides normally suppress renin and aldosterone production, but heart failure overrides this control, and measurement of BNP now aids the diagnosis of heart failure with a raised plasma concentration being a sensitive indicator of the disease.

THE STARLING CURVE AND HEART FAILURE

The Starling[11] curve originally described increased contractility of cardiac muscle fibres in response to increased stretch but, applied to the whole ventricle, it can explain the normal relationship between filling pressure and cardiac output (Fig. 24.6). Most patients with heart failure present in phase 'A' of the relationship, and before the 'decompensated' phase (B), in which there is gross dilatation of the ventricle. Diuretic therapy improves the congestive symptoms of heart failure, which are due to the increased filling pressure (preload), but actually *reduces* cardiac output in most patients. Depending on whether their predominant symptom is *dyspnoea* (due to pulmonary venous congestion) or *fatigue* (due to reduced cardiac output), patients feel better or worse. It is likely that a principal benefit of using angiotensin-converting enzyme (ACE) inhibitors in heart failure is their diuretic sparing effect.

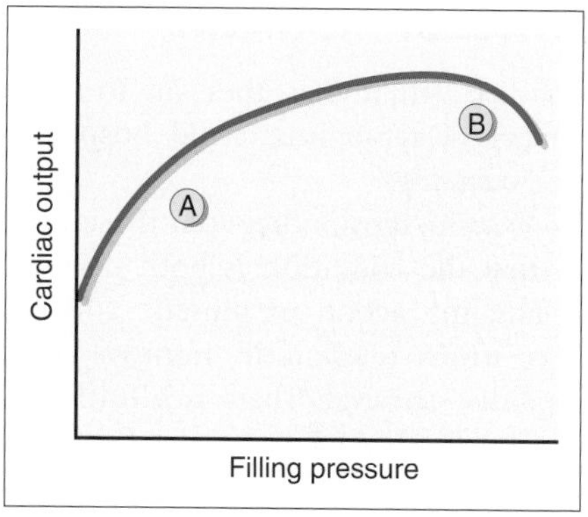

NATURAL HISTORY OF CHRONIC HEART FAILURE

Injury to the heart, e.g. myocardial infarction, hypertension, leads to adaptive ('compensatory') molecular, cellular and interstitial changes that alter its size, shape and function. Myocardial hypertophy and 'remodelling' takes place over weeks or months in response to haemodynamic load, neurohormonal activation and other factors, and the resulting pattern differs according to whether the stimulus is a pressure or volume overload. With passage of time, and with maladaption, the heart 'decompensates' and heart failure worsens. The process is outlined in Figure 24.7.

The degree of activity that the patient can undertake without becoming dyspnoeic offers a useful

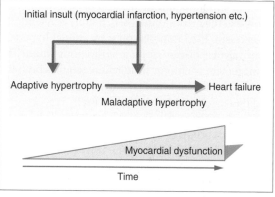

Fig. 24.6 The Starling curve of the relationship between cardiac filling pressure and cardiac output. In phase A, curve shows that lowering the blood volume (by diuretics) will reduce the filling pressure but the cardiac output will fall. In phase B, lowering the blood volume will reduce the filling pressure but the cardiac output will increase (see text).

Fig. 24.7 Progression of ventricular disease from hypertrophy through to failure following the initial insult. The process is generically referred to as 'cardiac remodelling' and the aim of much drug therapy in heart failure treatment is to try to place a brake on this process.

classification of the severity of heart failure. The New York Heart Association (NYHA)[12] classification offers also an approximate prognosis, with that of the worst grade (Class 4) being as bad as most cancers. Many patients with heart failure die from an arrhythmia, rather than from terminal decompensation, and drugs that avoid increasing the heart's exposure to increased catecholamine concentrations, as do some vasodilators (but see below), are best for improving prognosis.

---

[10]Doust J A, Pietrzak E, Dobson A, Glasziou P 2005 How well does B-type natriuretic peptide predict death and cardiac events in patients with heart failure: systematic review. British Medical Journal 330:625–627.

[11]Ernest Henry Starling 1866–1927, Professor of Physiology, University College, London. He also coined the word 'hormone'.

[12]NYHA Class 1, minimal dyspnoea (except after moderate exercise); Class 2, dyspnoea while walking on the flat; Class 3, dyspnoea on getting in/out of bed; Class 4, dyspnoea while lying in bed.

OBJECTIVES OF TREATMENT

As for cardiac arrhythmias, these are to reduce *morbidity* (relief of symptoms, avoid hospital admission) and *mortality*.

There is some tension between these two objectives in that the condition is both disabling and deadly, and the action of diuretic and vasodilator drugs, which temporarily improve symptoms, can jeopardise survival. There is a further tension between the needs of treating the features of *forwards* failure, or low output, and *backwards* failure, or the congestive features. The principal symptom of a low cardiac output, fatigue, is difficult to quantify, and patients have tended to have their treatment tailored more to the consequences of venous congestion.

Haemodynamic aims of drug therapy

Acute or chronic failure of the heart usually result from disease of the myocardium itself, mainly ischaemic, or an excessive load imposed on it by arterial hypertension, valvular disease or an arteriovenous shunt. The management of chronic heart failure requires both the relief of any treatable underlying or aggravating cause, and therapy directed at the failure itself.

The distinction between the capacity of the myocardium to pump blood and the load against which the heart must work is useful in therapy. The failing myocardium is so strongly stimulated to contract by increased sympathetic drive that therapeutic efforts to induce it to function yet more vigorously are in themselves alone unlikely to be of benefit. Despite numerous candidate drugs introduced over recent years, digoxin remains the only inotropic drug suitable for chronic oral use.

By contrast, agents that reduce preload or afterload are very effective, especially where the left ventricular volume is increased (less predictably so for failure of the right ventricle). The main hazard of their use is a drastic fall in cardiac output in those occasional patients whose output is dependent on a high left ventricular filling pressure, e.g. who are volume depleted by diuretic use or have severe mitral stenosis.

CLASSIFICATION OF DRUGS

Reduction of preload

Diuretics increase salt and water loss, reduce blood volume and lower excessive venous filling pressure (see Chapter 26). They are almost invariably required to relieve the congestive features of oedema, in the lungs and periphery; when the heart is grossly enlarged, cardiac output will also increase (see discussion of Starling curve, above). They are used flexibly, starting with a low dose; the usual sequence would be to begin with a thiazide, then move to furosemide, and in the most extreme cases then judiciously add metolazone.

Nitrates (see also Chapter 23) dilate the smooth muscle in venous capacitance vessels, increase the volume of the venous vascular bed (which normally may comprise 80% of the whole vascular system), reduce ventricular filling pressure, thus decreasing heart wall stretch, and reduce myocardial oxygen requirements. Their arteriolar dilating action is relatively slight. Glyceryl trinitrate provides benefit in acute left ventricular failure sublingually or by intravenous infusion. For chronic left ventricular failure nitrates have fallen out of favour, because the ACE inhibitors are more effective.

Reduction of afterload

Hydralazine (see also Chapter 23) relaxes arterial smooth muscle and reduces peripheral vascular resistance. Reflex tachycardia limits its usefulness and lupus erythematosus is a risk when the dose exceeds 100 mg per day.

Reduction of preload and afterload

ACE inhibitors and angiotensin receptor II blockers (ARBs) (see also Chapter 23) act by:

- reduction of afterload, by preventing the conversion of angiotensin I to the active form, angiotensin II, or blocking the effects of angiotensin II, which is a powerful arterioconstrictor and is present in the plasma in high concentration in heart failure
- reduction of preload, because the formation of aldosterone, and thus retention of salt and water (increased blood volume), is prevented by reducing the effects of angiotensin II.

ACE inhibitors are the only drugs that reduce peripheral resistance (afterload) without causing a reflex activation of the sympathetic system. The landmark CONSENSUS study compared enalapril with placebo in patients with NYHA class IV heart failure; after 6 months 26% of the enalapril group had died, compared with 44% in the control group. The reduction in mortality occurred among patients with progressive heart failure.[13] There is now strong evidence from long-term studies that ACE inhibitors[14] and ARBs[15] improve survival in and reduce hospital admissions for heart failure.

A common practice has been to give a test dose of a short-acting ACE inhibitor (e.g. captopril 6.25 mg by mouth) to patients who are in heart failure or on diuretic therapy for another reason, e.g. hypertension. Maintenance of blood pressure in such individuals may depend greatly on an activated renin–angiotensin–aldosterone system, and a standard dose of an ACE inhibitor or ARB can cause a catastrophic fall in blood pressure. That said, some of the many ACE inhibitors now available (see p. 420) have a sufficiently prolonged action that the initial doses have a cumulative effect on blood pressure over several days. Long-acting ACE inhibitors such as lisinopril ($t_{1/2}$ 12 h) and perindopril ($t_{1/2}$ 31 h) avoid the risk of sudden falls in blood pressure or renal function (glomerular filtration) after the first dose. Such drugs can be initiated outside hospital in patients who are unlikely to have a high plasma renin (absence of gross oedema or widespread atherosclerotic disease), although it is prudent to arrange for the first dose to be taken just before going to bed. Therapy begins with an ACE inhibitor, and an ARB is substituted if there is intolerance, or added if symptoms continue.

β-Adrenoceptor blockers. The realisation that activation of the renin–angiotensin–aldosterone and sympathetic nervous systems can adversely affect the course of chronic heart failure led to exploration of possible benefit from blockade of β adrenoceptors. Clinical trials have, indeed, shown that bisoprolol, carvedilol or metoprolol lower mortality and decrease hospitalisation when added to conventional treatment that is likely to include diuretics, digoxin and an ACE inhibitor (see below).

Spironolactone. Plasma aldosterone levels are raised in heart failure. Spironolactone acts as a diuretic by competitively blocking the aldosterone receptor, but in addition it has a powerful effect on outcome in heart failure (see below).

Stimulation of the myocardium

Digoxin improves myocardial contractility (*positive inotropic effect*) most effectively in the dilated, failing heart and, in the longer term, after an episode of heart failure has been brought under control. This effect occurs in patients in sinus rhythm and is distinct from its (*negative chronotropic*) action of reducing ventricular rate and thus improving ventricular filling in atrial fibrillation. Over 200 years after the first use of digitalis for dropsy, the DIG trial provided relief for doctors seeking evidence of long-term benefit.[16] Unlike all other positive inotropes, digoxin does not increase overall mortality or arrhythmias.

The phosphodiesterase inhibitors, *enoximone* and *milrinone*, have positive inotropic effects due to selective myocardial enzyme inhibition and may be used for short-term treatment of severe congestive heart failure. Evidence from longer-term use indicates that these drugs reduce survival.

Dopamine, dobutamine for shock: see page 409.

DRUG MANAGEMENT OF HEART FAILURE

CHRONIC HEART FAILURE

A scheme for the stepwise drug management of chronic heart failure appears in Figure 24.8. Points to emphasise in this scheme are that all patients, even those with mild heart failure, should receive an ACE inhibitor as first-line therapy. Several long-term

[13]Cooperative North Scandinavian Enalapril Survival Study (CONSENSUS) Trial Study Group 1987 Effects of enalapril on mortality in severe congestive heart failure. New England Journal of Medicine 316:1430–1435.

[14]Flather M D, Yusuf S, Kober L et al for the ACE-Inhibitor Myocardial Infarction Collaborative Group 2000 Long-term ACE-inhibitor therapy in patients with heart failure or left-ventricular dysfunction: a systematic overview of data from individual patients. Lancet 355:1575–1587.

[15]Demers C, McMurray J J V, Swedberg K et al for the CHARM investigators 2005 Impact of candesartan on nonfatal myocardial infarction and cardiovascular death in patients with heart failure. Journal of the American Medical Association 294:1794–1798.

[16]This prospective randomised trial compared digoxin with placebo in 7788 patients in NYHA Class II–III heart failure and sinus rhythm, most of whom also received an ACE inhibitor and a diuretic. Overall mortality did not differ between the groups but patients who took digoxin had fewer episodes of hospitalisation for worsening heart failure (Digitalis Investigation Group 1997 The effect of digoxin on mortality and morbidity in patients with heart failure. New England Journal of Medicine 336:525–532).

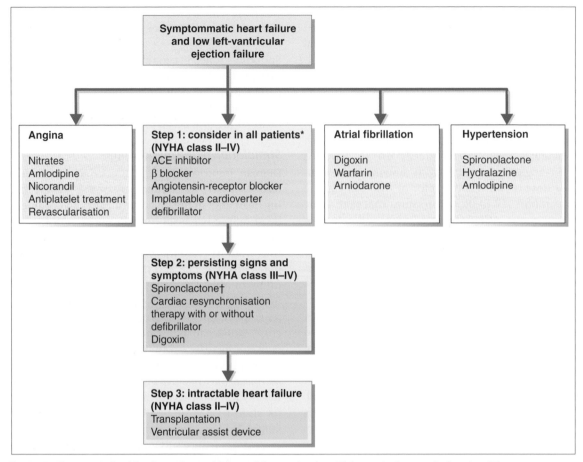

Fig. 24.8 Treatment algorithm for patients with heart failure and reduced left ventricular systolic function. *These treatments generally supplement existing diuretic drugs, with flexible dosing to maintain dry weight; consider hydralazine plus isosorbide dinitrate for black patients, as clinical trials indicate a favourable response in this subgroup. †The safety and efficacy of the combination of an ACE inhibitor, an ARB, and an aldosterone antagonist are unknown. NYHA, New York Heart Association. (Redrawn from McMurray J J, Pfeffer M A 2005 Heart failure. Lancet 365:1877–1889. Reproduced with permission from the Lancet.)

studies have demonstrated improved survival even when cardiac failure is mild.[17]

Diuretic therapy is very useful for symptom management but has no impact on survival. For most patients the choice will be a loop diuretic, e.g. furosemide starting at 20–40 mg/day. Because of the potassium-sparing effect of ACE inhibition, amiloride (also potassium sparing) is often not required, at least with low doses of a loop diuretic.

There is now overwhelming evidence for the benefit of β-blockers in chronic heart failure, despite the long-held belief that their negative intropic effect was a contraindication. Early trials were underpowered but a meta-analysis did suggest a 31% reduction in the mortality rate. Subsequently, the CIBIS-2 and MERIT-HF trials, have independently confirmed that chronic β-blockade has a survival effect of this size in moderate to severe (NHYA III/IV) heart failure.[18] Both studies confirmed the

[17]In the Studies of Left Ventricular Dysfunction (SOLVD, enalapril was compared with placebo in patients with either clinical features of heart failure or reduced left ventricular function in the absence of symptoms. Treatment reduced serious events (myocardial infarction and unstable angina) by approximately 20% and hospital admissions with progressive heart failure by up to 40%. (SOLVD Investigators 1991 Effect of enalapril on survival in patients with reduced left ventricular ejection fractions and congestive heart failure. New England Journal of Medicine 325:293–302).

one-third reduction in mortality. In MERIT-HF a life was saved for just 27 patient-years of treatment, i.e. it was unusually cost effective – more so than ACE inhibitor therapy. The action is probably a class effect of β-blockade, given the divergent pharmacology of the drugs used to date.

The reduction in mortality is additive to ACE inhibition and the survival benefit is largely through a decrease in sudden deaths as opposed to a reduction in progressive pump failure seen with ACE inhibitors. The only cautionary note is that patients must be β-blocked very gradually from low starting doses (e.g. bisoprolol 1.25 mg/day or carvedilol 3.125 mg b.d.) with regular optimisation of the dose of other drugs, especially the loop diuretic, to prevent decompensation of heart failure control.

The use of spironolactone has received considerable support from the RALES trial,[19] which implies that ACE inhibition even at high dose does not effectively suppress hyperaldosteronism in heart failure. The benefit occurs at a surprisingly low dose of spironolactone (25 mg/day); it probably reflects both improved potassium and magnesium conservation (both are antiarrhythmic) and reversal of fibrosis in the myocardium by aldosterone.

None of the available oral phosphodiesterase inhibitors is established in routine therapy, because

the short-term benefit of the increased contractility is offset by an increased mortality rate (presumably due to arrhythmias) on chronic dosing. Their use is restricted to short-term symptom control prior to, for example, transplantation.

ACUTE LEFT VENTRICULAR FAILURE

This is a common medical emergency, despite possible lessening in frequency with the advent of thrombolysis for myocardial infarction. The approach should be to reassure the anxious patient, who should sit upright with their legs dependent to reduce systemic venous return. A loop diuretic, e.g. furosemide 40–80 mg i.v., is the mainstay of therapy and provides benefit both by a rapid and powerful venodilator effect, reducing preload, and by the subsequent diuresis. Oxygen should be given, if the patient can tolerate a face mask, and diamorphine or morphine i.v. which, in addition to relieving anxiety and pain, have valuable venodilator effects.

Although there may be a case for short-term use of inotropic drugs (see Chapter 22) for heart failure where low output is a dominating feature, most such drugs substantially increase the risk of arrhythmias when the heart is hypoxic. The pharmacokinetics of digoxin does not favour emergency use. Aminophylline may be administered (5 mg/kg i.v. over 20 min), following with great care the precautions regarding dose and monitoring (see p. 507). By this stage, the possibility of assisted ventilation should be considered; where pulmonary oedema is the main problem, ventilation is likely to be both safer and more effective than inotropic drugs.

---

[18]Until 1997, 24 trials of β-blockade in heart failure provided just 3141 patients. MERIT-HF (1999 Effect of metoprolol CR/XL in chronic heart failure: Metoprolol CR/XL Randomised Intervention Trial in Congestive Heart Failure (MERIT-HF). Lancet 353:2001–2007) alone contained 3991 patients and CIBIS-2 (1999 The Cardiac Insufficiency Bisoprolol Study II (CIBIS-II): a randomised trial. Lancet 353:9–13) provided a further 2467.

[19]The RALES trial randomised 1663 patients with stable heart failure to either placebo or spironolactone. All patients maintained their 'optimised' therapy, which included ACE inhibitors. After 2 years of follow-up, the trial terminated prematurely following the demonstration of a 30% reduction in the mortality rate of spironolactone-treated patients, from sudden death as well as progressive pump failure. Gynaecomastia or breast discomfort occurred in 10% of patients receiving spironolactone (1% in controls), but significant hyperkalaemia occurred in surprisingly few patients. RALES was not adequately powered to decide whether the action of spironolactone was additive to that of a β-blocker (Pitt B, Zannad F, Remme W J et al 1999 The effect of spironolactone on morbidity and mortality in patients with severe heart failure. Randomized Aldactone Evaluation Study Investigators. New England Journal of Medicine 341(10):709–717).

SURGERY FOR HEART FAILURE

Although these options lie outside the scope of clinical pharmacology, an important element in meeting the objectives of treatment (see p. 464) is to recognise when further drug treatment is unlikely to improve symptoms or prognosis. Then, the physician must consider the possibility of a surgical intervention. Increasingly this may involve procedures short of transplantation itself, e.g. bypass grafting or stenting where stenosed vessels contribute to the heart failure or even a left ventricular assist device (LVAD). On occasion, it can help to make the patient aware that failure of both the heart and the drugs is not necessarily the end of the road.

Summary

- Heart failure is present when the heart cannot provide all organs with the blood supply appropriate to demand.
- Stroke volume is regulated by preload, afterload and contractility.
- In chronic heart failure, diuretics and nitrates reduce preload and provide symptomatic relief without affecting outcome.
- ACE inhibitors reduce both preload and afterload, and reduce morbidity and mortality by about one-third in all patients.
- β-Adrenoceptor blockers, gradually introduced, have an effect equivalent to that of ACE inhibitors in patients with moderate or severe heart failure (NYHA III or IV).
- Spironolactone, in low dose, adds further benefit.
- Digoxin improves myocardial contractility most effectively in the dilated, failing heart but also in the longer term, including in patients in sinus rhythm.
- The principal agents for treating acute left ventricular failure are furosemide, diamorphine and oxygen.

GUIDE TO FURTHER READING

Burnier M, Brunner H R 2000 Angiotensin II receptor antagonists. Lancet 355:637–645

Crystal E, Connolly S J 2004 Role of oral anticoagulation in management of atrial fibrillation. Heart 90:813–817

Delacretaz E 2006 Clinical practice. Supraventricular tachycardia. New England Journal of Medicine 354:1039–1051

Eisenberg M S, Mengery J 2001 Cardiac resuscitation. New England Journal of Medicine 344:1304–1313

Grace A A, Camm A J 1998 Quinidine. New England Journal of Medicine 338:35–45

Huikuri H V, Castellanos A, Myerburg R J et al 2001 Sudden death due to cardiac arrhythmias. New England Journal of Medicine 345(20):1473–1482

Jarcho J A 2005 Resynchronizing ventricular contraction in heart failure. New England Journal of Medicine 352:1594–1597

Jessup M, Brozena S 2003 Heart failure. New England Journal of Medicine 348(20):2007–2018

Mangrum J M, DiMarco J P 2000 The evaluation and management of bradycardia. New England Journal of Medicine 342(10):703–709

McMurray J J, Pfeffer M A 2005 Heart failure. Lancet 365:1877–1889

Morady F 2004 Catheter ablation of supraventricular arrhythmias: state of the art. Journal of Cardiovascular Electrophysiology 15(1):124–139

Neubauer S 2007 The failing heart – an engine out of fuel. New England Journal of Medicine 356:1140–1151

Page R L 2004 Newly diagnosed atrial fibrillation. New England Journal of Medicine 351(23):2408–2416

Page R L, Roden D M 2005 Drug therapy for atrial fibrillation: where do we go from here? Nature Reviews Drug Discovery 4(11):899–910

Peters N S, Schilling R J, Kanagaratnam P, Markides V 2002 Atrial fibrillation: strategies to control, combat and cure. Lancet 359:593–603

Schrier R W, Abraham W T 1999 Hormones and hemodynamics in heart failure. New England Journal of Medicine 341:577–585

25

Hyperlipidaemias

SYNOPSIS

Correction of blood lipid abnormalities offers scope for a major impact on cardiovascular disease. Drugs play a significant role and have a variety of modes of action. Dietary and lifestyle adjustment are components of overall risk prevention.

- Pathophysiology
- Primary (inherited) and secondary hyperlipidaemias
- Management: risk assessment, secondary and primary prevention, drugs, diet, lifestyle
- Drugs used in treatment: statins; ezetimibe, fibric acid derivatives, anion-exchange resins, nicotinic acid and derivatives

SOME PATHOPHYSIOLOGY

The normal function of lipoproteins is to distribute and recycle cholesterol. The pathways of lipid metabolism and transport and their *primary* (inherited) disorders are shown in Figure 25.1, and can be summarised thus:

- Cholesterol is absorbed from the *intestine* within chylomicrons. These are catabolised by lipoprotein lipase (LPL) to remnants, which are taken up by the hepatic low-density lipoprotein (LDL) receptor-related protein (LRP). A specific active transport mechanism also carries cholesterol across the gut mucosa (see below, ezetimibe).
- Cholesterol is synthesised de novo within the *liver* and *peripheral tissues* where, for example, it is converted to steroid hormones or used to form cell walls and membranes. Much of hepatic cholesterol enters the circulation as very-low-density lipoprotein (VLDL) and is metabolised to remnant lipoproteins after LPL removes triglyceride. The remnant lipoproteins are removed by the liver through apolipoprotein E receptors or LDL receptors (LDL-R), or further metabolised to LDL and then removed by peripheral tissues or the liver by LDL receptors.
- The quantity of cholesterol transported from the liver to peripheral tissues exceeds its catabolism there, and mechanisms exist to return about half of the cholesterol to the liver. Through this 'reverse transport', cholesterol is carried by high-density lipoprotein (HDL) from peripheral cells to the liver, where it is taken up by a process involving hepatic lipase. Cholesterol in the plasma is also recycled to LDL and VLDL by cholesterol-ester transport protein (CETP).
- Cholesterol in the liver is reassembled into lipoproteins, or secreted in bile and bile acids (essential for fat digestion and absorption), and then recycled by absorption or excreted in the faeces.

LIPID DISORDERS

Disorders of lipid metabolism are manifest by increased plasma concentrations of the various lipid and lipoprotein fractions (total and LDL cholesterol, VLDL, triglycerides, chylomicrons). They result, predominantly, in cardiovascular disease. This chapter addresses approaches (non-drug as well as drug) to correct abnormal lipid profiles and diminish vascular disease and its consequences.

Deposition of cholesterol in the arterial wall is central to the atherosclerotic process. Carriage of VLDL, remnant lipoprotein and LDL to arteries can thus be viewed as potentially *atherogenic*. In the reverse process, HDL carries cholesterol away from the arterial wall and can be regarded as *protective* against atherogenesis. Overproduction of VLDL in the liver raises plasma VLDL, remnant lipoprotein and LDL levels if the capacity to metabolise these lipoproteins is compromised by either a primary (inherited) and/or secondary (environmental) abnormality.

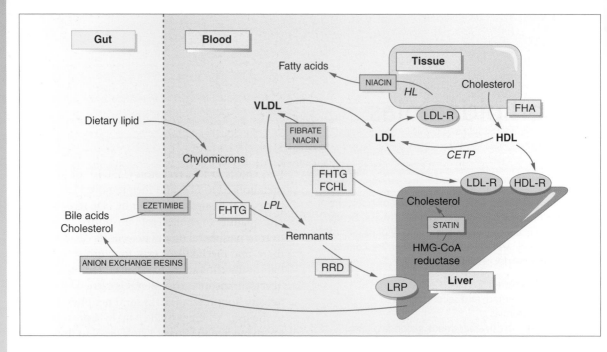

Fig. 25.1 Pathway of lipid transport and sites of drug action. CETP, cholesterol ester transfer protein; HL, hormone-sensitive lipase; LPL, lipoprotein lipase. See text for other abbreviations.

Raised levels of *LDL-cholesterol* are associated particularly with risk of coronary heart disease, but it is increasingly clear that moderately raised concentrations of *triglycerides*, *VLDL* or *remnants* in the presence of low HDL-cholesterol may also be atherogenic.

There are five *primary inherited lipoprotein disorders* that disturb lipid metabolism at the points indicated in Figure 25.1. These are:

- *Familial hypertriglyceridaemia* (FHTG) (rare), including lipoprotein lipase (LPL) deficiency, in which low LPL activity results in decreased removal, and thus increased levels of plasma *triglyceride*; there is increased hepatic secretion and thus a raised plasma concentration of *triglyceride-rich VLDL*. Patients are at risk of recurrent acute pancreatitis when plasma triglyceride exceeds 10 mmol/L, and especially when greater than 20 mmol/L.
- *Familial combined hyperlipidaemia* (FCHL) (common and most important) in which there is increased hepatic secretion of apolipoprotein B containing VLDL, and conversion to LDL; in consequence plasma *LDL* and *VLDL* levels are raised. Patients exhibit macrovascular disease (coronary heart, peripheral and cerebral).

- *Remnant removal disease* (RRD, also called remnant lipaemia, familial dysbetalipoproteinaemia) (uncommon) in which there is a defect of apolipoprotein E. This is the major ligand that allows internalisation and subsequent metabolism of remnant particles derived from VLDL and chylomicrons. The consequence is accumulation of VLDL remnants called intermediate-density lipoprotein (IDL), with cholesterol and triglycerides usually in the range 6–9 mmol/L. Patients experience severe macrovascular disease (as above).
- *Familial hypoalphalipoproteinaemia* (FHA, Tangier disease) (rare) in which the serum concentration of (protective) HDL is very low. Coronary heart and peripheral vascular disease result.
- *Familial hypercholesterolaemia* (FH) (common) is characterised by raised plasma levels of *total* and *LDL-cholesterol*. In the less severe heterozygous form, it affects about 1 in 500 of the population (one copy of the LDL-receptor protein is absent or defective). LDL-cholesterol levels are increased from childhood. Untreated, half the males will be dead by age 60 years, females 10 years later. The principal consequence is coronary heart, but occasionally also peripheral and cerebrovascular disease.

Secondary hyperlipidaemias results from liver and biliary disease, obesity, untreated hypothyroidism, diabetes, diet, alcohol excess, renal disease (nephrotic syndrome) and drugs (including etretinate, HIV protease inhibitors, thiazide diuretics, oral contraceptive steroids, glucocorticoids, β-adrenoceptor antagonists, ciclosporin).

Most commonly, patients present with more modestly increased levels of total and LDL-cholesterol which result from overproduction of VLDL in the liver due to a combination of high dietary saturated fat, obesity and individual (genetic) susceptibility; the secondary lipaemias thus aggravate underlying dislipaemic tendencies. The resulting picture is called *polygenic*, manifesting in adult life, with atherosclerosis occurring early but not as early as in FH.

The most severe hyperlipidaemias usually occur in patients with concurrent conditions, e.g. diabetes mellitus with one of the primary hyperlipidaemias, in this polygenic background.

SITES OF DRUG ACTION

In general, drugs act to reduce the concentration of cholesterol within hepatocytes, producing a compensatory increase in LDL receptors on their surface, and increased uptake of cholesterol-rich LDL particles from the bloodstream (see Fig. 25.1). *Statins* decrease the synthesis of cholesterol and hence secretion of VLDL, and increase the surface expression of hepatic LDL receptors. *Bile acid-binding (anion exchange) resins* deplete the bile acid and thus the cholesterol pool. *Fibrates* decrease the secretion of VLDL and increase the activity of LPL, thereby increasing the removal of triglycerides. *Nicotinic acid* decreases fatty acid production in the tissues and the secretion of VLDL and clearance of HDL. It also enhances LPL. *Ezetimibe* blocks the uptake of cholesterol from the gut by targeting a specific cholesterol transporter.

MANAGEMENT

The management of hyperlipidaemias should be viewed against the background of the following observations:

- Hyperlipidaemias are common; 66% of the adult UK population have a plasma cholesterol concentration in excess of 5.0 mmol/L, the lowest concentration generally associated with initiating drug treatment (in fact, statistical correlation with cardiovascular risk can be shown for cholesterol concentrations well below this value). The decision to treat an individual is made not just on the value for plasma lipids, but also on the absolute cardiovascular risk.

- Investigation of hyperlipidaemia must be directed initially at excluding contributory causes, i.e. secondary hyperlipidaemias (see above). None of these should be assumed to be the sole cause, even if present. Long-term decisions on management should be initiated only on the basis of at least two fasting blood samples.

- All patients (and their spouses/partners, if appropriate) should receive advice on lifestyle, diet and weight control, which are important components of overall macrovascular risk prevention. Dietary treatment of hypercholesterolaemia has a modest effect in the individual (at best an 8% reduction in LDL-cholesterol is possible), but diet and weight reduction are more effective for hypertriglyceridaemia. Intake of total fat, especially *saturated* fat, should be reduced (and partially replaced with monounsaturated and polyunsaturated fats); spreads containing plant sterols and stanols, e.g. Benecol and Flora Proactiv, taken as part of a *mixed meal* are useful as they can reduce plasma cholesterol by up to 10%. Increasing attention is now paid the *hydrogenated* fat content of food (hydrogen bubbled through liquid oils improves texture, flavour and shelf-life). In some individuals, especially those with *mixed hyperlipidaemia* (raised cholesterol and triglyceride levels, often due to secondary factors on a polygenic background), successful adherence to dietary advice and weight loss produce very significant improvements. Patients with remnant lipaemia (RRD hyperlipidaemia) may respond excellently to diet and weight loss (and, possibly, the addition of a fibrate).

- Much of the work of lipid clinics is taken up with attending to multiple interacting risk factors such as hypertension, diabetes, thyroid disease and smoking, as well as to the lipid abnormality. The Joint British Societies Guidelines[1] stress the importance of identifying

---

[1]JBS 2: Joint British Societies Guidelines on Prevention of Cardiovascular Disease in Clinical Practice. 2005 Heart 91(Suppl V).

the high-risk individuals who need intervention with diet and lifestyle changes and, if necessary, pharmacotherapy. *Equal* priority is given to: (1) patients with clinical atherosclerotic disease in any territory, (2) those with diabetes mellitus Types 1 and 2 (the most numerous), and (3) those without symptomatic vascular disease but whose 10-year risk of developing it is greater than 20%.

■ The decision to use lipid-lowering drugs is made on the basis of the overall absolute cardiovascular disease risk (CVD; see below and footnote 3), e.g. evidence of existing CVD, hypertension, diabetes mellitus and a positive family history. The justification is easiest in two cases. Firstly, for *primary prevention* in the relatively small number of patients who are asymptomatic but have significant abnormalities of their lipid profiles; patients with FH and remnant lipaemia are at high risk: the decision to treat is made on the patient's absolute risk as well as the degree of lipid abnormality. Secondly, for *secondary prevention* in patients who have evidence of CVD (previous myocardial infarction [MI], angina pectoris, stroke or transient ischaemic attack [TIA]), peripheral vascular disease or diabetes mellitus: in the landmark Scandinavian '4S' Study[2], 4444 patients with a total cholesterol concentration of 5.8–8.0 mmol/L after a MI were randomised to receive simvastatin (median dose 27 mg) or placebo. Those on active treatment showed a 30% reduction in the overall mortality rate, a 42% fall in deaths from coronary heart disease and a 34% fall in risk of recurrent MI. In terms of absolute risk, the authors estimated that addition of simvastatin to the treatment regimens of 100 patients with coronary heart disease would, over 6 years, preserve the lives of 4 of 9 patients who would otherwise die, and would prevent a non-fatal MI in 7 of an expected 21 cases.

■ *Consensus minimum targets* for primary and secondary prevention of CVD with statins are: a total plasma cholesterol of less than 5 mmol/L (or a reduction of 20–25% if the result is lower) or a LDL-cholesterol of less than 3 mmol/L (or a reduction of 30% if that is lower).[3] Recent guidelines from the UK and USA recommend more stringent levels: LDL-cholesterol of less than 2 mmol/L for the highest risk patients.[4]

■ There is evidence that statins protect against stroke. The benefit is seen in patients with plasma cholesterol levels greater than 5.0 mmol/L (or LDL-cholesterol above 3.0 mmol/L) who have a history of ischaemic stroke or TIA, or CVD or diabetes mellitus.

The issue about *primary prevention* (treatment of clinically unaffected patients with moderately raised cholesterol levels) is neither its effectiveness, nor its cost-effectiveness, both of which are proven, but the total proportion of the population to whom the effectiveness applies and the aggregate potential cost; these matters are for government.

Secondary prevention should start with diet and drugs when they are indicated. Dietary treatment can lower cholesterol levels in committed subjects, and is obviously less costly than drug treatment. Unfortunately numerous studies have shown that over any substantial period of time (e.g. 1 year) diet has no clinically significant influence on plasma cholesterol, and the wait for diet to have an effect often results in patients being lost from hospital follow-up after their initial MI.

Evidence comes from the WOSCOPS study[5] in which pravastatin 40 mg/day and placebo were compared in 6590 men aged 50–70 years with LDL-cholesterol levels of 4–6 mmol/L. Pravastatin reduced coronary heart disease (fatal and non-fatal events) by 31%. The authors estimated that treatment of 1000 such subjects each year would prevent 20 MIs. Meta-

[3]Wood D, Durrington P, Poulter N et al 1998 Joint British recommendations on prevention of coronary heart disease in clinical practice. Heart 80(Suppl):S1–29. (British Cardiac Society, British Hyperlipidaemia Association, British Hypertension Society [BHS], British Diabetic Association).
[4]BHS-IV guidelines: Williams B, Poulter N R, Brown M J 2004 Journal of Human Hypertension 18:139–185. NCEP III, revised: Grundy S M, Cleeman J I, Merz C N et al 2004 Circulation 110:227–239.
[5]West of Scotland Coronary Prevention Study: Shepherd J, Cobbe S M, Ford I et al 1995 Prevention of coronary heart disease with pravastatin in men with hypercholesterolemia. New England Journal of

[2]Scandinavian Simvastatin Survival Study Group 1994 Randomised trial of cholesterol lowering in 4444 patients with coronary heart disease: the Scandinavian Simvastatin Survival Study (4S). Lancet 344:1383–1389.

analysis of 14 randomised trials amply confirms the value of statin therapy.[6] Concerns that primary prevention could have a net adverse outcome (that cholesterol reduction increased the risk of cancer or violent deaths) have been laid to rest by a number of outcome trials.

The decision to offer a patient primary prophylaxis is influenced by the absolute risk for the individual, the potential risks from the statin therapy and costs to the health provider. As statins so far have an excellent safety record, costs will escalate with a decision to treat lower and lower levels of absolute risk. Current UK recommendations suggest treating all patients with a CVD risk of at least 30% over 10 years (this is the composite risk of non-fatal MI or stroke, fatal MI or stroke or new-onset angina); all diabetics should be assumed to be in this highest risk category. There is an aspiration to treat those with a 20–30% 10-year CVD risk if resources allow. The large number of additional patients involved by treating at the lower level raises issues of funding and resources (but not the cost-effectiveness of the treatment, which is clear). In the UK this has even prompted deregulation of simvastatin, so that it can be sold by pharmacists without a doctor's prescription but subject to certain restrictions.

The absolute CVD risk is computed using risk equations based on longitudinal cohorts such as those in the Framingham study; in reality this means consulting a simple colour-coded chart armed with data about the patient including age, sex, smoking status, pre-treatment blood pressure, and plasma levels of total and LDL-cholesterol.[7]

Management may proceed as follows:

1. *Any medical disorder* that may be causing hyperlipidaemia, e.g. diabetes, hypothyroidism, should be treated first.

---

[6]Keech A, Pollicino C, Kirby A, Sourjina T, Simes J on behalf of the Cholesterol Treatment Trialists' (CTT) Collaborators 2005 Efficacy and safety of cholesterol-lowering treatment: prospective meta-analysis of data from 90 056 participants in 14 randomised trials of statins. Lancet 366:1267–1278.
[7]The cardiac risk program (as an Excel spreadsheet) and risk assessment charts can be downloaded from the BHS website at http://www.bhsoc.org/. They may also be found in the *British National Formulary*. Note that they are not for use in patients with established CVD or renal failure, and an additional loading must be made for non-caucasians and those with a positive family history of premature CVD. The small print ought to be read with care. See also the footnote on the JBS 2 guidelines.

2. *Dietary adjustment.* The following applies to all patients:

- Those who are overweight should reduce their total calorie intake, ideally until they have returned to the weight that is appropriate for their height (i.e. body mass index, BMI), but realistically with an initial aim of reducing body-weight by 10% (see Appetite control, p. 624); this automatically assumes reduced intake of alcohol and total (especially animal) fat. Raised triglyceride concentrations may respond particularly well to alcohol withdrawal. Physical exercise assists weight reduction.
- Those who fail to achieve adequate weight reduction or who are already at their ideal weight should reduce their total fat intake; polyunsaturated and monounsaturated fats or oils may be taken partially to substitute for the reduction in animal fats. Reduction in dietary cholesterol is a much less important element of the diet. Benecol or Flora Proactiv should be added.

3. *Specific types of hyperlipidaemia* are treated thus:

- Familial hypertriglyceridaemia responds best to dietary modification and weight reduction (above) together with a fibrate; nicotinic acid may be added.
- Familial combined hyperlipidaemia should be treated with dietary modification and weight reduction (above) together with a statin; nicotinic acid and/or a fibrate may be added in resistant cases.
- Remnant removal disease (remnant lipaemia) responds to dietary modification and weight reduction (above) and a fibrate; a statin is an alternative and may be added where there is failure to respond.
- Familial or polygenic hypercholesterolaemia is treated by dietary modification and a statin, ezetimibe; an anion-exchange resin and/or a fibrate and/or nicotinic acid may be also be added.
- Familial hypoalphalipoproteinaemia may respond to exercise, weight loss and nicotinic acid; a fibrate and/or a statin may be added for a small HDL-raising effect, but primarily to lower LDL and triglycerides.

DRUGS USED IN TREATMENT

STATINS

These drugs block the rate-limiting enzyme for endogenous hepatic cholesterol synthesis, *hydroxymethylglutaryl coenzyme A* (HMG CoA) reductase. This results in increased synthesis of LDL receptors (up-regulation) in the liver and increased clearance of LDL from the circulation; plasma total cholesterol and LDL-cholesterol fall, with a maximum effect 1 month after commencing therapy. All statins cause a dose-dependent reduction in total and LDL-cholesterol, although there are differences in their therapeutic efficacy; for example, at their starting doses LDL-cholesterol falls after 1 month by an average of 17% with fluvastatin (20 mg/day), 28% with simvastatin (10 mg/day) and 38% with atorvastatin (10 mg/day). At higher doses, e.g. 80 mg/day atorvastatin or simvastatin, a 50% or greater reduction in LDL-cholesterol is possible. The effects of pravastatin are similar and so-called superstatins (e.g. rosuvastatin) may achieve this level of reduction at lower doses.[8]

There is no tolerance to continued administration of a statin, and because of a circadian rhythm to LDL-receptor synthesis, statins with short $t_{1/2}$ are slightly more effective if given in the evening rather than in the morning. Their efficacy in both primary and secondary prophylaxis of hypercholesterolaemia is probably a class effect, although long-term outcome studies may in time differentiate between the drugs. On current information, with no clear advantages or disadvantages between the different statins, the choice of agent to achieve the suggested total or LDL-cholesterol levels (see above) is heavily influenced by their relative cost, and the dose likely to achieve the target cholesterol concentration.

As a final caveat, there is growing interest in the possibility that some effects of statins may be 'lipid independent' and reflect actions on the inflammatory component of atheroma progression (so-called 'pleiotropic' effects).

Statins are well absorbed by mouth, and are metabolised in the liver. Except for rosuvastatin, they are metabolised through CYP pathways (usually 3A4), which is an important source of drug interactions particularly involving simvastatin and atorvastatin (some examples of drugs appear in Table 19.2B, p. 334). They are well tolerated, the commonest adverse effect being a transient, and usually minor, increase in serum transaminases in some 1% of patients. Asymptomatic increases in muscle enzymes (creatine phosphokinase, CPK) and myositis (with a generalised muscle discomfort) occur more rarely,[9] but are more frequent when statins are combined with other antihyperlidaemic drugs such as fibrates and nicotinic acid; patients should be counselled about myositis when these drugs are co-administered. Myositis is also more likely with co-administered anti-HIV protease inhibitors, e.g. ritonavir, and with drugs that interfere with metabolism of some statins, e.g. ciclosporin.

FIBRIC ACID DERIVATIVES (FIBRATES)

The class includes *bezafibrate, ciprofibrate, fenofibrate* and *gemfibrozil*; the original fibrate, clofibrate, is obsolete. The drugs partly resemble short-chain fatty acids and increase the oxidation of these acids in both liver and muscle. In the liver, secretion of triglyceride-rich lipoproteins falls, and in muscle the activity of lipoprotein lipase and fatty acid uptake from plasma are both increased. Fibrates act through a nuclear transcription factor (peroxisome proliferator-activated receptor (PPAR) α), which up-regulates expression of LPL and apolipoprotein A-1 genes, and down-regulates expression of the apolipoprotein C-11 gene. The result is that plasma levels of triglyceride decline by 20–30% and those of cholesterol by 10–15%; associated with this is a rise in the 'protective' HDL-cholesterol. The latter effect may have contributed

---

[8]The Heart Protection Study, which remains the largest statin intervention trial to date, randomised 20 536 patients to either placebo or simvastatin 40 mg for the secondary prophylactic effect on patients with coronary artery disease, occlusive arterial disease or diabetes. The simvastatin group had some 25% reduction in fatal/non-fatal MI, fatal/non-fatal stroke or revascularisation. This effect was seen across all groups and did not depend on cholesterol levels at entry or the reduction seen within the trial (averaging as a 1-mmol/L fall in LDL-cholesterol). The debate over cholesterol thresholds and targets lingers on. See: HPS Collaborative Group 2002 MRC/BHF Heart Protection Study of cholesterol lowering with simvastatin in 20 536 high-risk individuals: a randomised placebo-controlled trial. Lancet 360:7–22.

[9]In 30 641 patients in five major statin trials, myositis (serum creatinine kinase × 10 normal) occurred in 30 (control 29) and rhabdomyolysis in 2 (control 2) (Farmer J A 2001 Learning from the cerivastatin experience. Lancet 358: 1383–1385). There was also no significant excess of these events in the simvastatin arm of the Heart Protection Study.

to the reduction in non-fatal myocardial infarction with gemfibrozil in both the Helsinki Heart Study[10] and more recent Veterans Affairs HDL Intervention Trials (VA-HIT).[11]

Fibrates are the drugs of choice for *mixed hyperlipidaemia* (raised cholesterol plus triglycerides) but may be used in hypercholesterolaemia, alone or with anion exchange resins or (with care, see above) with statins. There is evidence of varying efficacy among the drugs both in cholesterol-lowering and in additional beneficial effects, such as reduction in blood fibrinogen and urate concentrations; the clinical significance of these differences is not yet known.

Fibric acid derivatives are well absorbed from the gastrointestinal tract, extensively bound to plasma proteins and excreted mainly by the kidney as unchanged drug or metabolites. They are contraindicated where hepatic or renal function is severely impaired (but gemfibrozil has been used in uraemic and nephrotic patients without aggravating deterioration in kidney function). Rarely, fibric acid derivatives may induce a myositis-like syndrome; the risk is greater in patients with poor renal function, and in those who are also receiving a statin; gemfibrizil in particular should *never* be used with a statin. Fibrates enhance the effect of co-administered oral anticoagulants.

ANION-EXCHANGE RESINS (BILE ACID SEQUESTRANTS)

Colestyramine is an oral anion-exchange resin;[12] it binds bile acids in the intestine and depletion of the bile acid pool stimulates conversion of cholesterol to bile acid. The result is a fall in intracellular cholesterol in hepatocytes, and an increase (upregulation) in both LDL receptors and cholesterol synthesis. Plasma LDL-cholesterol concentration falls by 20–25%. In many patients there is some compensatory increase in hepatic triglyceride output. Anion exchange resins may be used for *hypercholesterolaemia* but not when there is significant hypertriglyceridaemia.

Colestyramine is rather unpalatable and poorly tolerated, with up to 50% of patients experiencing constipation and some complain of anorexia, abdominal fullness and occasionally of diarrhoea – effects that may limit or prevent its use. Because the colestyramine binds anions, drugs such as warfarin, digoxin, thiazide diuretics, phenobarbital and thyroid hormones should be taken 1 h before or 4 h after colestyramine to avoid impairment of their absorption. Binding of fat-soluble vitamins in the gut may be sufficient to cause clinical deficiency, e.g. vitamin K-responsive prolongation of the prothrombin time.

Colestipol is similar to colestyramine but is available in capsule form to increase palatability.

Colesevalam is a bile acid sequestrant (not an anion-exchange resin) which binds bile acids and forms an insoluble complex that passes out in the faeces, taking with it bile acid-bound LDL-cholesterol.

EZETIMIBE

Some 30–70% of plasma cholesterol is attributable to cholesterol absorbed from the gut. Ezetimibe selectively blocks intestinal cholesterol absorption by inhibition of the Niemann–Pick C1-like 1 (NCPC1L1) transporter, which interrupts the enterohepatic cycling of cholesterol (see above). It is effective when used as monotherapy in a 10-mg dose, producing a 17% fall in LDL-cholesterol. Tolerability is similar to that with placebo. Ezetimibe is actually a pro-drug and metabolism in the liver produces the more effective blocker of cholesterol transport, ezetimibe glucuronide ($t_{1/2}$ 22 h).

The real promise of this drug is efficacy in combination with statins. Ezetimibe with a low dose of a statin, e.g. simvastatin 10 mg/day, produces a fall in plasma cholesterol similar to that with simvastatin 80 mg/day, providing a possible alternative treatment for patients unable to tolerate high-dose statin monotherapy. Ezetimibe may challenge resins as the agent of choice for patients with hypercholesterolaemia that is not controlled by a statin alone. There as yet are no long-term safety or outcome data.

[10]Frick M H, Elo O, Haapa K et al 1987 Helsinki Heart Study: primary-prevention trial with gemfibrozil in middle-aged men with dyslipidaemia. Safety of treatment, changes in risk factors, and incidence of coronary heart disease. New England Journal of Medicine 317:1237–1245.

[11]Rubins H B, Robins S J, Collins D et al for The Veterans Affairs High-Density Lipoprotein Cholesterol Intervention Trial Study Group 1999 Gemfibrozil for the secondary prevention of coronary heart disease in men with low levels of high-density lipoprotein cholesterol. New England Journal of Medicine 341:410–418.

[12]The resins consist of aggregations of large molecules carrying a fixed positive charge, which therefore bind negatively charged ions (anions).

NICOTINIC ACID AND DERIVATIVES

Nicotinic acid acts as an antilipolytic agent in adipose tissue, reducing the supply of free fatty acids and hence the availability of substrate for hepatic triglyceride synthesis and the secretion of VLDL. Nicotinic acid lowers plasma triglyceride and cholesterol concentrations, and raises HDL-cholesterol levels. It produces a modest reduction in plasma lipoprotein Lp(a), which may contribute to its overall protection against the complications of atheroma. The doses required to do this are well in excess of those required for its vitamin effect and are not shared by nicotinamide. Skin flushing (partially preventable by low-dose aspirin) and gastrointestinal upset are common side-effects of nicotinic acid; these are ameliorated by using a slow-release formulation and gradually building up the oral dose over 6 weeks, when tolerance emerges. Rarely there is major disturbance of liver function.

Acipimox is better tolerated than nicotinic acid and has a longer duration of action, but is less effective. Unlike nicotinic acid, it does not lower plasma Lp(a) levels.

OTHER DRUGS

Omega-3 marine triglycerides (Maxepa) contain the triglyceride precursors of two polyunsaturated fatty acids (eicosapentaenoic acid and docosahexaenoic acid) derived from oily fish. A related product, Omacor, contains omega 3-acid ethyl esters instead of triglycerides. They have no role in treating hypercholesterolaemia, but are taken for CHD prevention (when benefit may be due to an antithrombotic effect). Patients with moderate to severe hypertriglyceridaemia may respond to either agent, although LDL-cholesterol levels may rise.

Orlistat, a weight-reducing agent, lowers the glycaemia of diabetes mellitus to a degree that accords with the weight loss, and improves hyperlipidaemia to an extent greater than would be expected (see p. 469).

Rimonabant. See page 625.

α-Tocopherol acetate (vitamin E) has no effect on lipid concentrations but is a powerful antioxidant, and oxidation of LDL is an essential step in the development of atheroma. Interest thus focused on a possible role of both endogenous and therapeutic vitamin E in prevention of atheroma, but a recent overview of published outcome trials using vitamin E supplements found no compelling evidence for α-tocopherol in the treatment or prevention of atherosclerosis.

Summary

- The commonest and most important hyperlipidaemia is hypercholesterolaemia, which is one of the major risk factors for coronary heart disease.
- Most treatments work by reducing the intracellular concentration of cholesterol in hepatocytes, leading to a compensatory increase in low-density lipoprotein (LDL) receptors on their surface, and increased uptake of cholesterol-rich LDL particles from the bloodstream.
- The most effective cholesterol-reducing drugs are the statins, which inhibit the rate-limiting step in cholesterol synthesis.
- Additional agents may be required for mixed or severe hyperlipidaemia.
- In outcome trials with these drugs, reductions in blood cholesterol by 25–35% are associated with a 35–45% reduction in the risk of coronary heart disease.
- The main indications for their use are patients with even slightly increased levels of cholesterol (>5 mmol/L) after a myocardial infarction or any other macrovascular event, in patients with familial hypercholesterolaemia or diabetes, and in patients with a significant absolute CVD risk, especially where there is a family history of premature CVD.

GUIDE TO FURTHER READING

Amarenco P, Labreuche J, Lavallée P, Touboul P-J 2004 Statins in stroke prevention and carotid atherosclerosis: systematic review and up-to-date meta-analysis. Stroke 35(12):2902–2909

Ashen M D, Blumenthal R S 2005 Low HDL-cholesterol levels. New England Journal of Medicine 353:1252–1269

Davidson M H 2005 Clinical significance of statin pleiotropic effects: hypotheses versus evidence. Circulation 111:2280–2281

Hooper L, Summerbell C D, Higgins J P T et al 2001 Dietary fat intake and prevention of cardiovascular disease: systematic review. British Medical Journal 322:757–763

Keech A, Kirby A, Sourjina T et al on behalf of the Cholesterol Treatment Trialists' (CTT) Collaborators 2005 Efficacy and safety of cholesterol-lowering treatment: prospective meta-analysis of data from 90056 participants in 14 randomised trials of statins. Lancet 366:1267–1278

Knopp R H 1999 Drug treatment of lipid disorders. New England Journal of Medicine 341:498–511

Mozaffarian D, Katan M B, Ascherio A et al 2006 Trans fatty acids and cardiovascular disease. New England Journal of Medicine 354:1601–1613

Primatesta P, Poulter N 2000 Lipid concentrations and the use of lipid lowering drugs: evidence from a national cross sectional study. British Medical Journal 321:1322–1325

von Bergmann K, Sudhop T, Lutjohann D et al 2005 Cholesterol and plant sterol absorption: recent insights. American Journal of Cardiology 96:10–14

Kidney and genitourinary tract

The kidneys comprise only 0.5% of body-weight, yet they receive 25% of the cardiac output. Drugs that affect renal function have important roles in cardiac failure and hypertension. Disease of the kidney must be taken into account when prescribing drugs that are eliminated by it.

- Diuretic drugs: their sites and modes of action, classification, adverse effects and uses in cardiac, hepatic, renal and other conditions
- Carbonic anhydrase inhibitors
- Cation-exchange resins and their uses
- Alteration of urine pH
- Drugs and the kidney
- Adverse effects
- Drug-induced renal disease: by direct and indirect biochemical effects and by immunological effects
- Prescribing for renal disease: adjusting the dose according to the characteristics of the drug and to the degree of renal impairment
- Nephrolithiasis and its management
- Pharmacological aspects of micturition
- Benign prostatic hyperplasia
- Erectile dysfunction

DIURETIC DRUGS

(See also Chapter 23.)

Definition. A diuretic is any substance that increases urine and solute excretion. This wide definition includes substances not commonly thought of as diuretics, e.g. water. To be therapeutically useful a diuretic should increase the output of sodium as well as of water, because diuretics are normally required to remove oedema fluid, composed of water and solutes, of which sodium is the most important.

Diuretics are among the most commonly used drugs, perhaps because the evolutionary advantages of sodium retention have left an aging population without salt-losing mechanisms of matching efficiency.

Each day the body produces 180 L of glomerular filtrate which is modified in its passage down the renal tubules to appear as 1.5 L of urine. Thus, if reabsorption of tubular fluid falls by 1%, urine output doubles. Most clinically useful diuretics are organic anions, which are transported directly from the blood into tubular fluid. The following brief account of tubular function with particular reference to sodium transport will help to explain where and how diuretic drugs act; it should be read with reference to Figure 26.1.

SITES AND MODES OF ACTION

Proximal convoluted tubule

Some 65% of the filtered sodium is actively transported from the lumen of the proximal tubule by the sodium pump (Na^+, K^+-ATPase). Chloride is absorbed passively, accompanying the sodium; bicarbonate is also absorbed, through an action involving carbonic anhydrase. These solute shifts give rise to the iso-osmotic reabsorption of water, with the result that more than 70% of the glomerular filtrate is returned to the blood from this section of the nephron. The epithelium of the proximal tubule is described as 'leaky' because of its free permeability to water and a number of solutes.

Osmotic diuretics such as *mannitol* are non-resorbable solutes which retain water in the tubular fluid (**Site 1**, Fig. 26.1). Their effect is to increase water rather than sodium loss, and this is reflected in their special use acutely to reduce intracranial or intraocular pressure and not states associated with sodium overload.

Loop of Henle

The tubular fluid now passes into the loop of Henle where 25% of the filtered sodium is reabsorbed.

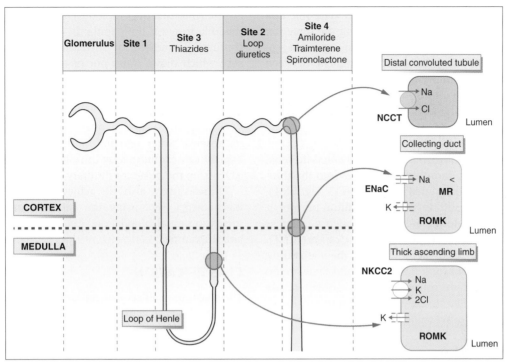

Fig. 26.1 Sites of action of diuretic drugs. Inset cartoons show the transporters and ion channels targeted in tubular cells at these sites. ENaC, epithelial sodium channel; NCCT, thiazide-sensitive Na–Cl co-transporter; NKCC2, Na–K–2Cl co-transporter; ROMK, rectifying outer medullary potassium channel.

There are two populations of nephron: those with short loops that are confined to the cortex, and the juxtamedullary nephrons whose long loops penetrate deep into the medulla and are concerned principally with *water* conservation;[1] the following discussion refers to the latter.

The physiological changes are best understood by considering first the *ascending* limb. In the thick segment (**Site 2**, Fig. 26.1), sodium and chloride ions are transported from the tubular fluid into the interstitial fluid by the three-ion co-transporter system (i.e. $Na^+/K^+/2Cl^-$ called NKCC2) driven by the sodium pump. The co-transport of these ions is dependent on potassium returning to the lumen through the rectifying outer medullary potassium (ROMK) channel; otherwise potassium would be rate limiting. As the tubule epithelium is 'tight' here, i.e. impermeable to water, the tubular fluid becomes dilute, the interstitium becomes hypertonic, and fluid in the adjacent *descending* limb, which is

permeable to water, becomes more concentrated as it approaches the tip of the loop, because the hypertonic interstitial fluid sucks water out of this limb of the tubule. The 'hairpin' structure of the loop thus confers on it the property of a *countercurrent multiplier*, i.e. by active transport of ions a small change in osmolality laterally across the tubular epithelium is converted into a steep vertical osmotic gradient.

The high osmotic pressure in the medullary interstitium is sustained by the descending and ascending vasa recta, long blood vessels of capillary thickness that lie close to the loops of Henle and act as *countercurrent exchangers*, for the incoming blood receives sodium from the outgoing blood.[2] *Furosemide,*

[1]Beavers and other freshwater mammals typically have nephrons with short loops, whereas desert-adapted mammals have long loops.

[2]The most easily comprehended counter-current exchange mechanism (in this case for heat) is that in wading birds in cold climates whereby the veins carrying cold blood from the feet pass closely alongside the arteries carrying warm blood from the body and heat exchange takes place. The result is that the feet receive blood below body temperature (which does not matter) and the blood from the feet, which is often very cold, is warmed before it enters the body so that the internal temperature is maintained more easily. The principle is the same for maintaining renal medullary hypertonicity.

bumetanide, piretanide, torasemide and *ethacrynic acid* act principally at Site 2 by inhibiting the three-ion transporter, thus preventing sodium ion reabsorption and lowering the osmotic gradient between cortex and medulla; this results in the formation of large volumes of dilute urine. Hence, these drugs are called 'loop' diuretics.

Distal convoluted tubule

The ascending limb of the loop then re-enters the renal cortex where its morphology changes into the thin-walled distal convoluted tubule (**Site 3**, Fig. 26.1). Here uptake is still driven by the sodium pump but sodium and chloride are taken through a different transporter, the Na–Cl co-transporter (called NCCT). Both ions are rapidly removed from the interstitium because cortical blood flow is high and there are no vasa recta present; consequently the urine becomes more dilute. *Thiazides* act principally at this region of the cortical diluting segment by blocking the NCCT.

Collecting duct

In the collecting duct (**Site 4**), sodium ions are exchanged for potassium and hydrogen ions. The sodium ions enter through the epithelial Na channel (called ENaC), which is stimulated by aldosterone. The aldosterone (mineralocorticoid) receptor is inhibited by the competitive receptor antagonist *spironolactone*, whereas the sodium channel is inhibited by *amiloride* and *triamterene*. All three of these diuretics are potassium sparing because potassium is normally secreted through the potassium channel, ROMK (see Fig. 26.1), down the potential gradient created by sodium reabsorption.

All other diuretics, acting proximal to Site 4, lose potassium, because they dump sodium into the collecting duct. Removal of this sodium through ENaC increases the potential gradient for potassium secretion through ROMK. The potassium-sparing diuretics are normally considered weak diuretics because Site 4 is normally responsible for 'only' 2–3% of sodium reabsorption, and they usually cause less sodium loss than thiazides or loop diuretics. Nevertheless, patients with genetic abnormalities of ENaC show salt wasting or retention to a degree that significantly affects their blood pressure, depending on whether the mutation causes respectively loss or gain of channel activity. Although ENaC clearly does not have the capacity to compensate for large sodium losses, e.g. during loop diuretic usage, it is the main site of physiological control (via aldosterone) over sodium loss.

The collecting duct then travels back through the medulla to reach the papilla; in doing so it passes through a gradient of increasing osmotic pressure which draws water out of tubular fluid. This final concentration of urine is under the influence of *antidiuretic hormone* (ADH) whose action is to increase water permeability by increasing the expression of specific water channels (or aquaporins); in its absence water remains in the collecting duct. *Ethanol* causes diuresis by inhibiting the release of ADH from the posterior pituitary gland.

Diuresis may also be achieved by extrarenal mechanisms, by raising the cardiac output and increasing renal blood flow, e.g. with dobutamine and dopamine.

CLASSIFICATION

The maximum efficacy in removing salt and water that any drug can achieve is dependent on its site of action, and it is appropriate to rank diuretics according to their natriuretic capacity, as set out below. The percentages refer to the highest fractional excretion of filtered sodium under carefully controlled conditions and should not be taken to represent the average fractional sodium loss during clinical use.

High efficacy

Furosemide and the other 'loop' diuretics can cause up to 25% of filtered sodium to be excreted. Their action impairs the powerful urine-concentrating mechanism of the loop of Henle and confers higher efficacy compared with drugs that act in the relatively hypotonic cortex (see below). Progressive increase in dose is matched by increasing diuresis, i.e. they have a high 'ceiling' of effect. In fact, they are so effective that over-treatment can readily dehydrate the patient. Loop diuretics remain effective at a glomerular filtration rate (GFR) below 10 mL/min (normal 120 mL/min).

Moderate efficacy

The thiazide family, including *bendrofluazide (bendroflumethiazide)* and the related *chlorthalidone, clopamide, indapamide, mefruside, metolazone* and *xipamide,* cause 5–10% of filtered sodium load to be excreted. Increasing the dose beyond a small range produces no added diuresis, i.e. they have a low 'ceiling' of effect. Such drugs cease to be effective once the GFR has fallen below 20 mL/min (except *metolazone*).

Low efficacy

Triamterene, amiloride and spironolactone cause 2–3% of the filtered sodium to be excreted. They are potassium sparing and combine usefully with more efficacious diuretics to prevent the potassium loss, which other diuretics cause.

Osmotic diuretics, e.g. *mannitol*, also fall into this category.

INDIVIDUAL DIURETICS

HIGH-EFFICACY (LOOP) DIURETICS

Furosemide

Furosemide (Lasix) acts on the thick portion of the ascending limb of the loop of Henle (Site 2) to produce the effects described above. Because more sodium is delivered to Site 4, exchange with potassium leads to urinary potassium loss and hypokalaemia. Magnesium and calcium loss are increased by furosemide to about the same extent as sodium; the effect on calcium is utilised in the emergency management of hypercalcaemia (see p. 665).

Pharmacokinetics. Furosemide is well absorbed from the gastrointestinal tract and is highly bound to plasma proteins. The $t_{1/2}$ is 2 h, but this rises to over 10 h in renal failure.

Uses. Furosemide is very successful for the relief of oedema. Urine production rises progressively with increasing dose. Taken orally it acts within an hour and diuresis lasts up to 6 h. Enormous urine volumes can result and over-treatment may lead to hypovolaemia and circulatory collapse. Given intravenously it acts within 30 min and can relieve acute pulmonary oedema, partly by a venodilator action which precedes the diuresis. An important feature of furosemide is that it retains efficacy even at a low GFR (10 mL/min or less). The dose is 20–120 mg by mouth per day; i.m. or i.v. 20–40 mg is given initially. For use in renal failure, special high-dose tablets (500 mg) are available, and a solution of 250 mg in 25 mL, which should be infused intravenously at a rate not greater than 4 mg/min.

Adverse effects are uncommon, apart from excess of therapeutic effect (electrolyte disturbance and hypotension due to low plasma volume) and those mentioned in the general account for diuretics (below). They include nausea, pancreatitis and, rarely, deafness, which is usually transient and associated with rapid intravenous injection in renal failure. Nonsteroidal anti-inflammatory drugs (NSAIDs), notably indometacin, reduce furosemide-induced diuresis, probably by inhibiting the formation of vasodilator prostaglandins in the kidney.

Bumetanide, piretanide and *ethacrynic acid* are similar to furosemide. Ethacrynic acid is less widely used as it is more prone to cause adverse effects, especially nausea and deafness. *Torasemide* is an effective antihypertensive agent at lower (non-natriuretic) doses (2.5–5 mg/day) than those used for oedema (5–40 mg/day).

MODERATE-EFFICACY DIURETICS

(See also Hypertension, Chapter 23.)

Thiazides

Thiazides depress salt reabsorption in the distal convoluted tubule (at Site 3) which is just proximal to the region of sodium-potassium exchange. These drugs thus raise potassium excretion to an important extent. Thiazides lower blood pressure, initially due to a reduction in intravascular volume but chronically by a reduction in peripheral vascular resistance. The latter is accompanied by diminished responsiveness of vascular smooth muscle to noradrenaline (norepinephrine); they may also have a direct action on vascular smooth muscle membranes, acting on an as yet unidentified ion channel.

Uses. Thiazides are given for mild cardiac failure and mild hypertension, or for more severe degrees of hypertension, in combination with other drugs.

Pharmacokinetics. Thiazides are generally well absorbed orally and most begin to act within an hour. Differences among the numerous derivatives lie principally in duration of action. The relatively water soluble, e.g. *cyclopenthiazide, chlorothiazide, hydrochlorothiazide*, are most rapidly eliminated, their peak effect occurring within 4–6 h and passing off by 10–12 h. They are excreted unchanged in the urine and active secretion by the proximal renal tubule contributes to their high renal clearance and $t_{1/2}$ of less than 4 h.

The relatively lipid-soluble members of the group, e.g. *polythiazide, hydroflumethiazide*, distribute more widely into body tissues and act for more than 24 h, which can be objectionable if the drug is used for diuresis, though useful for hypertension. With the exception of *metolazone*, thiazides are not effective when renal function is moderately impaired (GFR <20 mL/min), because they are not filtered in sufficient concentration to inhibit the NCCT.

Adverse effects in general are discussed below. Rashes (sometimes photosensitive), thrombocytopenia and agranulocytosis occur. Thiazide-type drugs increase total plasma cholesterol concentration, but in long-term use this is less than 5%, even at high doses. The questions about the appropriateness of thiazides for mild hypertension, of which ischaemic heart disease is a common complication, are laid to rest by their proven success in randomised outcome comparisons (see Chapter 23).

Bendroflumethiazide is a satisfactory member for routine use. For a diuretic effect the oral dose is 5–10 mg, which usually lasts less than 12 h, so that it should be given in the morning. It may be taken daily for the first few days then, say, 3 days a week. As an antihypertensive 1.25–2.5 mg is given daily; in the absence of a diuresis clinically important potassium depletion is uncommon, but plasma potassium concentration should be checked in potentially vulnerable groups such as the elderly (see Chapter 24).

Hydrochlorothiazide is a satisfactory alternative. Other members of the group include *benzthiazide, chlorothiazide, cyclopenthiazide, hydroflumethiazide* and *polythiazide*.

Diuretics related to the thiazides. Several compounds, although not strictly thiazides, share structural similarities with them and probably act at the same site on the nephron; they therefore exhibit moderate therapeutic efficacy. Overall, these substances have a longer duration of action, are used for oedema and hypertension, and their profile of adverse effects is similar to that of the thiazides. They are listed below.

Chlortalidone acts for 48–72 h after a single oral dose.

Indapamide is structurally related to chlortalidone but lowers blood pressure at subdiuretic doses, perhaps by altering calcium flux in vascular smooth muscle. It has less apparent effect on potassium, glucose or uric acid excretion (see below).

Metolazone is effective when renal function is impaired. It potentiates the diuresis produced by furosemide and the combination can be effective in resistant oedema, provided the patient's fluid and electrolyte loss are monitored carefully.

Xipamide is structurally related to chlortalidone and to furosemide. It induces a diuresis for about 12 h that is brisker than with thiazides; this may trouble the elderly.

LOW-EFFICACY DIURETICS

Spironolactone (Aldactone) is structurally similar to aldosterone and competitively inhibits its action in the distal tubule (Site 4; exchange of potassium for sodium); excessive secretion of aldosterone contributes to fluid retention in hepatic cirrhosis, nephrotic syndrome, congestive heart failure (see specific use in Chapter 24) and primary hypersecretion (Conn's syndrome). Spironolactone is also useful in the treatment of resistant hypertension, where increased aldosterone sensitivity is increasingly recognised as a contributory factor.

Spironolactone itself has a short $t_{1/2}$ (1.6 h), being extensively metabolised, and its prolonged diuretic effect is due to the most significant active product, canrenone ($t_{1/2}$ 17 h). Spironolactone is relatively ineffective when used alone but is more efficient when combined with a drug that reduces sodium reabsorption proximally in the tubule, i.e. a loop diuretic. Spironolactone (and amiloride and triamterene; see below) usefully reduces the potassium loss caused by loop diuretics, but its combination with another potassium-sparing diuretic must be avoided as hyperkalaemia will result. Dangerous potassium retention is particularly likely if spironolactone is given to patients with impaired renal function. It is given orally in one or more doses totalling 100–200 mg/day. Maximum diuresis may not occur for up to 4 days. If after 5 days the response is inadequate, the dose may be increased to 300–400 mg/day. Lower doses (0.5–1 mg/kg) are required to treat hypertension.

Adverse effects. Oestrogenic effects are the major limitation to its long-term use. They are dose dependent, but in the Randomized Aldactone Evaluation Study (RALES)[3] (see Chapter 24) even 25 mg/day caused breast tenderness or enlargement in 10%

---

[3]Pitt B, Zannad F, Remme W J et al 1999 The effect of spironolactone on morbidity and mortality in patients with severe heart failure. Randomized Aldactone Evaluation Study Investigators. New England Journal of Medicine 341:709–717.

of men. Women may also report breast discomfort or menstrual irregularities, including amenorrhoea. Minor gastrointestinal upset also occurs and there is increased risk of gastroduodenal ulcer and bleeding. These are reversible on stopping the drug. Spironolactone is reported to be carcinogenic in rodents, but many years of clinical experience suggest that it is safe in humans. Nevertheless, the UK licence for its use in essential hypertension was withdrawn (i.e. possible use long term in a patient group that includes the relatively young), but is retained for other indications.

Epleronone is a spironolactone analogue licensed for use in heart failure that appears to be free of the oestrogenic effects; probably because of its lower affinity for the oestrogen receptor. It is useful in patients who need an aldosterone-receptor blocking agent, but are intolerant of the endocrine effects of spironolactone.

Amiloride blocks the ENaC sodium channels in the distal tubule. This action complements that of the thiazides with which it is frequently combined to increase sodium loss and limit potassium loss. One such combination, co-amilozide (Moduretic; amiloride 2.5–5 mg plus hydrochlorothiazide 25–50 mg) is used for hypertension or oedema. The maximum effect of amiloride occurs about 6 h after an oral dose with a duration of action greater than 24 h ($t_{1/2}$ 21 h). The oral dose is 5–20 mg daily.

Triamterene (Dytac) is a potassium-sparing diuretic with an action and use similar to that of amiloride. The diuretic effect extends over 10 h. Gastrointestinal upsets occur. Reversible, non-oliguric renal failure may occur when triamterene is used with indometacin (and presumably other NSAIDs). It may also give the urine a blue coloration.

INDICATIONS FOR DIURETICS

- *Oedema states* associated with sodium overload, e.g. cardiac, renal or hepatic disease, and also without sodium overload, e.g. acute pulmonary oedema following myocardial infarction. Note that oedema may also be localised, e.g. angio-oedema over the face and neck or around the ankles with some calcium channel blockers, or due to low plasma albumin, or immobility in

the elderly; in none of these circumstances is a diuretic indicated.
- *Hypertension*, by reducing intravascular volume and probably by other mechanisms too, e.g. reduction of sensitivity to noradrenergic vasoconstriction.
- *Hypercalcaemia*. Furosemide reduces calcium reabsorption in the ascending limb of the loop of Henle, which action may be utilised in the emergency reduction of raised plasma calcium levels in addition to rehydration and other measures (see p. 665).
- *Idiopathic hypercalciuria*, a common cause of renal stone disease, may be reduced by thiazide diuretics.
- The *syndrome of inappropriate secretion of antidiuretic hormone secretion* (SIADH) may be treated with furosemide if there is a dangerous degree of volume overload (see also p. 641).
- *Nephrogenic diabetes insipidus*, paradoxically, may respond to diuretics which, by contracting vascular volume, increase salt and water reabsorption in the proximal tubule, and thus reduce urine volume.

THERAPY

Congestive Cardiac Failure

The main account appears in Chapter 24, where the emphasis is now on early use of angiotensin-converting enzyme (ACE) inhibitors and β-adrenoceptor antagonists that are specifically diuretic sparing. But oral diuretics are easily given repeatedly, and lack of supervision can result in insidious overtreatment. Relief at disappearance of the congestive features can mask exacerbation of the low-output symptoms of heart failure, such as tiredness and postural dizziness due to reduced blood volume. A rising blood urea level is usually evidence of reduced glomerular blood flow consequent on a fall in cardiac output, but does not distinguish whether the cause of the reduced output is over-diuresis or worsening of the heart failure itself. The simplest guide to the success or failure of diuretic regimens is to monitor *body-weight*, which the patient can do equipped with just bathroom scales. Fluid intake and output charts are more demanding of nursing time, and often less accurate.

Acute pulmonary oedema: left ventricular failure

(See page 467.)

Renal oedema

The chief therapeutic aims are to reduce dietary sodium intake and to prevent excessive sodium retention using diuretic drugs. Reduction of sodium reabsorption in the renal tubule by diuretics is most effective where glomerular filtration has not been seriously reduced by disease. Furosemide and bumetanide are effective even when the filtration rate is very low; furosemide may usefully be combined with metolazone but the resulting profound diuresis requires careful monitoring. Secondary hyperaldosteronism complicates the nephrotic syndrome because albumin loss causes plasma colloid pressure to fall, and the resulting diversion of intravascular volume to the interstitium activates the renin-angiotensin-aldosterone system; spironolactone may then be added usefully to potentiate a loop diuretic and to conserve potassium, loss of which can be severe.

HEPATIC ASCITES

(See also page 586.)

Ascites and oedema are due to portal venous hypertension together with decreased plasma colloid osmotic pressure causing hyperaldosteronism as with nephrotic oedema (above). Furthermore, diversion of renal blood flow from the cortex to the medulla favours sodium retention. In addition to dietary sodium restriction, spironolactone is the preferred diuretic to produce a gradual diuresis; too vigorous depletion of sodium with added potassium loss and hypochloraemic alkalosis may worsen hepatic encephalopathy. Abdominal paracentesis can be very effective if combined with human albumin infusion to prevent further aggravating hypoproteinaemia.

ADVERSE EFFECTS CHARACTERISTIC OF DIURETICS

Potassium depletion. Diuretics that act at Sites 1, 2 and 3 (see Fig. 26.1) cause more sodium to reach the sodium–potassium exchange site in the distal tubule (Site 4) and so increase potassium excretion. This subject warrants discussion because hypokalaemia may cause cardiac arrhythmia in patients at risk (e.g. receiving digoxin). The safe lower limit for plasma potassium concentration is normally quoted as 3.5 mmol/L. Whether or not diuretic therapy causes significant lowering of serum potassium

levels depends both on the drug and on the circumstances in which it is used.

- *The loop diuretics* produce a smaller fall in serum potassium concentration than do the thiazides, for equivalent diuretic effect, but have a greater capacity for diuresis, i.e. higher efficacy especially in large dose, and so are associated with greater decline in potassium levels. If diuresis is brisk and continuous, clinically important potassium depletion is likely to occur.
- *Low dietary intake* of potassium predisposes to hypokalaemia; the risk is particularly notable in the elderly, many of whom ingest less than 50 mmol per day (the dietary normal is 80 mmol).
- Hypokalaemia may be aggravated by other drugs, e.g. β_2-adrenoceptor agonists, theophylline, corticosteroids, amphotericin.
- Hypokalaemia during diuretic therapy is also more likely in *hyperaldosteronism*, whether primary or more commonly secondary to severe liver disease, congestive cardiac failure or nephrotic syndrome.
- Potassium loss occurs with diarrhoea, vomiting or small bowel fistula, and may be aggravated by diuretic therapy.
- When a thiazide diuretic is used for hypertension, there is probably no case for routine prescription of a potassium supplement if no predisposing factors are present (see Chapter 24).

Potassium depletion can be minimised or corrected by:

- Maintaining a good dietary potassium intake (fruits, fruit juices, vegetables).
- Combining a potassium-depleting with a potassium-sparing drug.
- Intermittent use of potassium-losing drugs, i.e. drug holidays.
- Potassium supplements: KCl is preferred because chloride is the principal anion excreted along with sodium when high-efficacy diuretics are used. Potassium-sparing diuretics generally defend plasma potassium more effectively than potassium supplements. All forms of potassium are irritant to the gastrointestinal tract, and in the oesophagus may even cause ulceration. The elderly, in particular, should be warned never to take such tablets dry but always with a large cupful of liquid and sitting upright or standing.

Hyperkalaemia may occur, especially if a potassium-sparing diuretic is given to a patient with impaired renal function. ACE inhibitors and angiotensin II receptor antagonists can also cause a modest increase in plasma potassium levels. They may cause dangerous hyperkalaemia if combined with KCl supplements or other potassium-sparing drugs, in the presence of impaired renal function. With suitable monitoring the combination can be used safely, as was well illustrated by the RALES trial.[4] Ciclosporin, tacrolimus, indometacin and possibly other NSAIDs may cause hyperkalaemia with the potassium-sparing diuretics.

Treatment of hyperkalaemia

Depends on the severity and the following measures are appropriate:

- Any potassium-sparing diuretic should be discontinued.
- A cation-exchange resin, e.g. polystyrene sulphonate resin (Resonium A, Calcium Resonium, see below) can be used orally (more effective than rectally), to remove body potassium by the gut.
- Potassium may be moved rapidly from plasma into cells by giving:
  - sodium bicarbonate, 50 mL 8.4% solution through a central line, and repeated in a few minutes if characteristic ECG changes persist
  - glucose, 50 mL 50% solution, plus 10 units soluble insulin by i.v. infusion
  - nebulised β_2-agonist, salbutamol 5–10 mg, is effective in stimulating the pumping of potassium into skeletal muscle.
- In the presence of ECG changes, calcium gluconate, 10 mL of 10% solution, should be given i.v. and repeated if necessary in a few minutes; it has no effect on the serum potassium but opposes the myocardial effect of a raised serum potassium level. Calcium may potentiate digoxin and should be used cautiously, if at all, in a patient taking this drug. Sodium bicarbonate and calcium salt must not be mixed in a syringe or reservoir because calcium precipitates.
- Dialysis may be needed in refractory cases and is highly effective.

---

[4]Pitt B, Zannad F, Remme W J et al 1999 The effect of spironolactone on morbidity and mortality in patients with severe heart failure. Randomized Aldactone Evaluation Study Investigators. New England Journal of Medicine 341:709–717.

Hypovolaemia can result from over-treatment. Acute loss of excessive fluid leads to postural hypotension and dizziness. A more insidious state of chronic hypovolaemia can develop, especially in the elderly. After initial benefit, the patient becomes sleepy and lethargic. Blood urea concentration rises and sodium concentration may be low. Renal failure may result.

Urinary retention. Sudden vigorous diuresis can cause acute retention of urine in the presence of bladder neck obstruction, e.g. due to prostatic enlargement.

Hyponatraemia may result if sodium loss occurs in patients who drink a large quantity of water when taking a diuretic. Other mechanisms are probably involved, including enhancement of antidiuretic hormone release. Such patients have reduced total body sodium and extracellular fluid and are oedema free. Discontinuing the diuretic and restricting water intake are effective. The condition should be distinguished from hyponatraemia with oedema, which develops in some patients with congestive cardiac failure, cirrhosis or nephrotic syndrome. Here salt and water intake should be restricted because extracellular fluid volume is expanded.

The combination of a potassium-sparing diuretic and ACE inhibitor can also cause severe hyponatraemia – more commonly than life-threatening hyperkalaemia.

Urate retention with hyperuricaemia and, sometimes, clinical gout occurs with thiazides and loop diuretics. The effect is unimportant or negligible with the low-efficacy diuretics, e.g. amiloride and spironolactone. Two mechanisms appear to be responsible. First, diuretics cause volume depletion, reduction in glomerular filtration and increased absorption of almost all solutes in the proximal tubule, including urate. Second, diuretics and uric acid are organic acids and compete for the transport mechanism that pumps such substances from the blood into the tubular fluid. Diuretic-induced hyperuricaemia can be prevented by allopurinol or probenecid (which also antagonises diuretic efficacy by reducing their transport into the urine).

Magnesium deficiency. Loop and thiazide diuretics cause significant urinary loss of magnesium; potassium-sparing diuretics probably also cause magnesium retention. Magnesium deficiency brought about by diuretics is rarely severe enough to induce the classic picture of neuromuscular irritability and tetany but cardiac arrhythmias, mainly of ventricular origin, do occur and respond to repletion of magnesium (8 mmol of Mg^{2+} is given as 4 mL 50% magnesium sulphate infused i.v. over 10–15 min followed by up to 72 mmol infused over the next 24 h).

Carbohydrate intolerance is caused by those diuretics that produce prolonged hypokalaemia, i.e. the loop and thiazide type. It appears that intracellular potassium is necessary for the formation of insulin, and glucose intolerance is probably due to insulin deficiency. Insulin requirements thus increase in established diabetics and the disease may become mainifest in latent diabetics. The effect is generally reversible over several months.

Calcium homeostasis. Renal calcium loss is increased by the loop diuretics; in the short term this is not a serious disadvantage and indeed *furosemide* may be used in the management of hypercalcaemia after rehydration has been achieved. In the long term, hypocalcaemia may be harmful especially in elderly patients, who tend in any case to be in negative calcium balance. *Thiazides*, by contrast, decrease renal excretion of calcium and this property may influence the choice of diuretic in a potentially calcium-deficient or osteoporotic individual, for thiazide use is associated with a reduced risk of hip fracture in the elderly. The hypocalciuric effect of the thiazides has also been used effectively in patients with idiopathic hypercalciuria, the commonest metabolic cause of renal stones.

INTERACTIONS

Loop diuretics (especially as intravenous boluses) potentiate ototoxicity of aminoglycosides and nephrotoxicity of some cephalosporins. NSAIDs tend to cause sodium retention, which counteracts the effect of diuretics; the mechanism may involve inhibition of renal prostaglandin formation. Diuretic treatment of a patient taking lithium can precipitate toxicity from this drug (the increased sodium loss is accompanied by reduced lithium excretion). Other drugs that may induce hyperkalaemia, hypokalaemia, hyponatraemia or glucose intolerance with diuretics are described above.

ABUSE OF DIURETICS

Psychological abnormality sometimes takes the form of abuse of diuretics and/or purgatives. The subject usually desires to slim to become more attractive, or may have anorexia nervosa. There can be severe depletion of sodium and potassium, with renal tubular damage due to chronic hypokalaemia.

OSMOTIC DIURETICS

Osmotic diuretics are small molecular weight substances that are filtered by the glomerulus but not reabsorbed by the renal tubule, and thus increase the osmolarity of the tubular fluid. Thus they prevent reabsorption of water (and also, by more complex mechanisms, of sodium) principally in the proximal convoluted tubule and probably also the loop of Henle. The result is that urine volume increases according to the load of osmotic diuretic.

Mannitol, a polyhydric alcohol (mol. wt. 452), is used most commonly; it is given intravenously. In addition to its effect on the kidney, mannitol encourages the movement of water from inside cells to the extracellular fluid, which is thus transiently expanded before diuresis occurs. These properties define its uses, which are for rapid reduction of intracranial or intraocular pressure, and to maintain urine flow to prevent renal tubular necrosis. Because it increases circulatory volume, mannitol is contraindicated in congestive cardiac failure and pulmonary oedema.

METHYLXANTHINES

The general properties of the methylxanthines (theophylline, caffeine) are discussed elsewhere (see p. 169). Their mild diuretic action probably depends in part on smooth muscle relaxation in the afferent arteriolar bed increasing renal blood flow, and in part on a direct inhibitory effect on salt reabsorption in the proximal tubule. Their uses in medicine depend on other properties.

CARBONIC ANHYDRASE INHIBITORS

The enzyme carbonic anhydrase facilitates the reaction between carbon dioxide and water to form carbonic acid (H_2CO_3), which then breaks down to hydrogen (H^+) and bicarbonate (HCO_3^-) ions. This process is fundamental to the production of either acid or alkaline secretions, and high concentrations of carbonic anhydrase are present in the gastric mucosa, pancreas, eye and kidney. Because the number of H^+ ions available to exchange with Na^+

in the proximal tubule is reduced, sodium loss and diuresis occur. But HCO_3^- reabsorption from the tubule is also reduced, and its loss in the urine leads within days to metabolic acidosis, which attenuates the diuretic response to carbonic anhydrase inhibition. Consequently, inhibitors of carbonic anhydrase are obsolete as diuretics, but still have specific uses. *Acetazolamide* is the most widely used carbonic anhydrase inhibitor.

Reduction of intraocular pressure.

This action is due not to diuresis (thiazides actually raise intraocular pressure slightly). The formation of aqueous humour is an active process requiring a supply of bicarbonate ions, which depends on carbonic anhydrase. Inhibition of carbonic anhydrase reduces the formation of aqueous humour and lowers intraocular pressure. This is a local action and is not affected by the development of acid–base changes elsewhere in the body, i.e. tolerance does not develop. In patients with acute glaucoma, acetazolamide can be taken either orally or intravenously. Acetazolamide is not recommended for long-term use because of the risk of hypokalaemia and acidosis, but *brinzolamide* or *dorzolamide* are effective as eye-drops, well tolerated, and thus suitable for chronic use in glaucoma.

High-altitude (mountain) sickness

may affect unacclimatised people at altitudes over 3000 metres, especially after rapid ascent; symptoms range from nausea, lassitude and headache to pulmonary and cerebral oedema. The initiating cause is hypoxia: at high altitude, the normal hyperventilatory response to falling oxygen tension is inhibited because alkalosis is also induced. Acetazolamide induces metabolic acidosis, increases respiratory drive, notably at night when apnoetic attacks may occur, and thus helps to maintain arterial oxygen tension. The usual dose is 125–250 mg b.d. given orally on the day before the ascent and continued for 2 days after reaching the intended altitude; 250 mg b.d. is used to treat established high-altitude sickness, combined with a return to a lower altitude. (Note that this is an unlicensed indication in the UK.) As an alternative or in addition to acetazolamide, dexamethasone may be used: 2 mg 6-hourly for prevention, and 4 mg 6-hourly for treatment.

The drug has two other uses. In *periodic paralysis*, where sudden falls in plasma K^+ concentration occur due to its exchange with Na^+ in cells, the rise in plasma H^+ caused by acetazolamide provides an alternative cation to K^+ for exchange with Na^+. Acetazolamide may be used occasionally as a second-line drug for *tonic–clonic* and *partial epileptic seizures*.

Adverse effects. High doses of acetazolamide may cause drowsiness and fever, rashes (it is a sulfonamido-type drug) and paraesthesiae may occur (from the acidosis). Blood disorders have been reported. Renal calculi may develop, because the urine calcium is in less soluble form owing to low citrate content of the urine, a consequence of metabolic acidosis.

Dichlorphenamide is similar, but a more potent, inhibitor of carbonic anhydrase.

CATION-EXCHANGE RESINS

Cation-exchange resins are used to treat hyperkalaemia by accelerating potassium loss through the gut, especially in the context of poor urine output or before dialysis (the most effective means of treating hyperkalaemia). The resins consist of aggregations of big insoluble molecules carrying fixed negative charges, which loosely bind positively charged ions (cations); these readily exchange with cations in the fluid environment to an extent that depends on their affinity for the resin and their concentration.

Resins loaded with sodium or calcium exchange these cations preferentially with potassium cations in the intestine (about 1 mmol potassium per g resin); the freed cations (calcium or sodium) are absorbed and the resin plus bound potassium is passed in the faeces. The resin does not merely prevent absorption of ingested potassium, but it also takes up the potassium normally secreted into the intestine and ordinarily reabsorbed.

In hyperkalaemia, oral administration or retention enemas of a polystyrene sulphonate resin may be used. A sodium-phase resin (Resonium A) should obviously not be used in patients with renal or cardiac failure as sodium overload may result. A calcium-phase resin (Calcium Resonium) may cause hypercalcaemia and should be avoided in predisposed patients, e.g. those with multiple myeloma, metastatic carcinoma, hyperparathyroidism and sarcoidosis. Orally they are very unpalatable, and as enemas patients rarely manage to retain them for as long as necessary (at least 9 h) to exchange potassium at all available sites on the resin.

ALTERATION OF URINE PH

Alteration of urine pH by drugs is sometimes desirable. The most common reason is in the treatment of poisoning (a fuller account is given on page 129). A summary of the main indications appears below.

Alkalinisation of urine:

■ increases the elimination of salicylate, phenobarbital and chlorophenoxy herbicides, e.g. 2,4-D, MCPA
■ reduces irritation of an inflamed urinary tract
■ discourages the growth of certain organisms, e.g. *Escherichia coli.*

The urine can be made alkaline by sodium bicarbonate i.v., or by potassium citrate by mouth. Sodium overload may exacerbate cardiac failure, and sodium or potassium excess are dangerous when renal function is impaired.

Acidification of urine:

■ is used as a test for renal tubular acidosis
■ increases elimination of amfetamine, methylene dioxymethafetamine (MDMA or 'Ecstasy'), dexfenfluramine, quinine and phencyclidine, although it is very rarely needed.
■ Oral NH_4Cl, taken with food to avoid vomiting, acidifies the urine. It should not be given to patients with impaired renal or hepatic function. Other means include arginine hydrochloride, ascorbic acid and calcium chloride by mouth.

DRUGS AND THE KIDNEY

ADVERSE EFFECTS

The kidneys comprise only 0.5% of body-weight, yet they receive 25% of the cardiac output. It is hardly surprising that drugs can damage the kidney and that disease of the kidney affects responses to drugs.

DRUG-INDUCED RENAL DISEASE

Drugs and other chemicals damage the kidney by:

1. *Direct biochemical effect.* Substances that cause such toxicity include:
   – heavy metals, e.g. mercury, gold, iron, lead
   – antimicrobials, e.g. aminoglycosides, amphotericin, cephalosporins
   – iodinated radiological contrast media, e.g. agents for visualising the biliary tract
   – analgesics, e.g. NSAID combinations and paracetamol (actually its metabolite, NABQI, in overdose, see p. 259)
   – solvents, e.g. carbon tetrachloride, ethylene glycol.
2. *Indirect biochemical effect*
   – cytotoxic drugs and uricosurics may cause urate to be precipitated in the tubule
   – calciferol may cause renal calcification by inducing hypercalcaemia
   – diuretic and laxative abuse can cause tubular damage secondary to potassium and sodium depletion
   – anticoagulants may cause haemorrhage into the kidney.
3. *Immunological effect.* A wide range of drugs produces a wide range of injuries:
   – drugs include phenytoin, gold, penicillins, hydralazine, isoniazid, rifampicin, penicillamine, probenecid, sulphonamides
   – injuries include arteritis, glomerulitis, interstitial nephritis, systemic lupus erythematosus.

A drug may cause damage by more than one of the above mechanisms, e.g. gold. The sites and pathological types of injury are as follows:

Glomerular damage. The large surface area of the glomerular capillaries renders them susceptible to damage from circulating immune complexes; glomerulonephritis, proteinuria and nephrotic syndrome may result, e.g. following treatment with penicillamine when the patient has made an immune response to the drug. The degree of renal impairment is best reflected in the creatinine clearance, which measures the GFR because creatinine is eliminated entirely by this process.

Tubule damage. By concentrating 180 L glomerular filtrate into 1.5 L urine each day, renal tubule cells are exposed to much greater amounts of solutes and environmental toxins than are other cells in the body. The proximal tubule, through which most water is reabsorbed, experiences the greatest concentration and so suffers most drug-induced injury. Specialised transport processes concentrate acids, e.g. salicylate (aspirin), cephalosporins and bases, e.g. aminoglycosides, in renal tubular cells. Heavy metals and radiographic contrast media also cause damage at this site. Proximal tubular toxicity is manifested by leakage of glucose, phosphate, bicarbonate and amino acids into the urine.

The counter-current multiplier and exchange systems of urine concentration (see p. 133) cause some drugs to accumulate in the renal medulla. Analgesic nephropathy is often first evident at this site, partly because of high tissue concentration and partly, it is believed, because of ischaemia through inhibition of locally produced vasodilator prostaglandins by NSAIDs. The distal tubule is the site of lithium-induced nephrotoxicity; damage to the medulla and distal nephron is manifested by failure to concentrate the urine after fluid deprivation and by failure to acidify urine after ingestion of ammonium chloride.

Tubule obstruction. Given certain physicochemical conditions, crystals can deposit within the tubular lumen. Methotrexate, for example, is relatively insoluble at low pH and can precipitate in the distal nephron when the urine is acid. Similarly the uric acid produced by the metabolism of nucleic acids released during rapid tumour cell lysis can cause a fatal urate nephropathy. This was a particular problem with the introduction of chemotherapy for leukaemias until the introduction of allopurinol, which is now routinely given before the start of chemotherapy to block xanthine oxidase so that the much more soluble uric acid precursor, hypoxanthine, is excreted instead. A recent and highly effective alternative to allopurinol for high-risk patients is recombinant uric acid oxidase (Rasburicase), which catalyses conversion of uric acid to the more soluble allantoin. Crystal nephropathy is also a problem with the widely used antiretroviral agent indinavir.

Other drug-induced lesions of the kidney include:

- Vasculitis, caused by allopurinol, isoniazid, sulphonamides.
- Allergic interstitial nephritis, caused by penicillins (especially), thiazides, allopurinol, phenytoin, sulphonamides.
- Drug-induced lupus erythematosus, caused by hydralazine, procainamide, sulfasalazine.

Drugs may thus induce any of the common clinical syndromes of renal injury, namely:

- *Acute renal failure*, e.g. aminoglycosides, cisplatin.
- *Nephrotic syndrome*, e.g. penicillamine, gold, captopril (only at higher doses than now recommended).

- *Chronic renal failure*, e.g. NSAIDs.
- *Functional impairment*, i.e. reduced ability to dilute and concentrate urine (lithium), potassium loss in urine (loop diuretics), acid–base imbalance (acetazolamide).

PRESCRIBING IN RENAL DISEASE

Drugs may:

- exacerbate renal disease (see above)
- be ineffective, e.g. thiazide diuretics in moderate or severe renal failure; uricosurics
- be potentiated by accumulation due to failure of renal excretion.

Clearly, the first option is to seek an alternative drug that does not depend on renal elimination. Problems of safety arise for patients with impaired renal function who must be treated with a drug that is potentially toxic and that is wholly or largely eliminated by the kidney.

A knowledge of, or at least access to, sources of pharmacokinetic data is essential for safe therapy for such patients, e.g. manufacturers' data, formularies and specialist journals.

The profound influence of impaired renal function on the elimination of some drugs is illustrated in Table 26.1.

The $t_{1/2}$ of other drugs, where activity is terminated by metabolism, is unaltered by renal impairment, but many such drugs produce *pharmacologically active metabolites* that are more water soluble than the parent drug, rely on the kidney for their elimination, and accumulate in renal failure, e.g. acebutolol, diazepam, warfarin, pethidine.

Table 26.1 Drug $t_{1/2}$ (h) in normal and severely impaired renal function

	Normal	Severe renal impairment[a]
captopril	2	25
amoxicillin	2	14
gentamicin	2.5	>50
atenolol	6	100
digoxin	36	90

[a]Glomerular filtration rate <5 mL/min (normal value is 120 mL/min). These values illustrate the major effect of impaired renal function on the elimination of certain drugs. Depending on the circumstances, alternative drugs must be found or special care exercised when prescribing drugs that depend significantly on the kidney for elimination.

The majority of drugs fall into an intermediate class and are partly metabolised and partly eliminated unchanged by the kidney.

Administering the correct dose to a patient with renal disease must therefore take into account both the extent to which the drug normally relies on renal elimination, and the degree of renal impairment; the best guide to the latter is the *creatinine clearance* and not the serum creatinine level itself[5], which can be notoriously misleading in the elderly and at extremes of body mass.

DOSE ADJUSTMENT FOR PATIENTS WITH RENAL IMPAIRMENT

- Adjustment of the *initial* dose (or where necessary the *priming* or *loading* dose, see p. 101) is generally unnecessary, as the volume into which the drug has to distribute should be the same in the uraemic as in the healthy subject. There are exceptions to this rule-of-thumb; for example, the volume of distribution of digoxin is contracted in uraemic patients due to altered tissue binding of the drug.
- Adjustment of the *maintenance* dose involves either reducing each dose given or lengthening the time between doses.
- Special caution is needed when the patient is *hypoproteinaemic* and the drug is usually extensively plasma protein bound, or in advanced renal disease when accumulated metabolic products may compete for protein binding sites. Careful observation is required in the early stages of dosing until response to the drug can be gauged.

General rules

1. Drugs that are *completely* or *largely* excreted by the kidney, or drugs that produce *active, renally eliminated metabolites*: give a normal or, if there is special cause for caution (see above), a slightly reduced initial dose, and lower the maintenance dose or lengthen the dose interval in proportion to the reduction in creatinine clearance.

2. Drugs that are *completely* or *largely metabolised* to inactive products: give normal doses. When the note of special caution (see above) applies, a modest reduction of initial dose and the maintenance dose rate are justified while drug effects are assessed.

3. Drugs that are *partly* eliminated by the kidney and partly metabolised: give a normal initial dose and modify the maintenance dose or dose interval in the light of what is known about the patient's renal function and the drug, its dependence on renal elimination and its inherent toxicity.

Recall that the time to reach steady-state blood concentration (see p. 373) is dependent only on drug $t_{1/2}$, and a drug reaches 97% of its ultimate steady-state concentration in $5 \times t_{1/2}$. Thus, if $t_{1/2}$ is prolonged by renal impairment, so also will be the time to reach steady state.

Schemes for modifying drug dosage for patients with renal disease diminish but do not remove their increased risk of adverse effects; such patients should be observed particularly carefully throughout a course of drug therapy. Where the service is available, dosing should be monitored by drug plasma concentration measurements.

NEPHROLITHIASIS

Calcareous stones result from hypercalciuria, hyperoxaluria and hypocitraturia. Hypercalciuria and hyperoxaluria render urine supersaturated in respect of calcium salts; citrate makes calcium oxalate more soluble and inhibits its precipitation from solution.

Non-calcareous stones occur most commonly in the presence of urea-splitting organisms, which create conditions in which magnesium ammonium phosphate (struvite) stones form. Urate stones form when urine is unusually acid (pH <5.5).

Management. Recurrent stone-formers should maintain a urine output exceeding 2.5 L/day. Some benefit from restricting dietary calcium or reducing the intake of oxalate-rich foods (rhubarb, spinach, tea, chocolate, peanuts).

- Thiazide diuretics reduce the excretion of calcium and oxalate in the urine, and reduce the rate of stone formation.

---

[5]The creatinine clearance can be predicted from the serum creatinine concentration, sex, age and weight using formulae such as the Cockcroft–Gault equation. Others are also used and a helpful conversion calculator to run on a PDA (personal digital assistant) can be downloaded from: http://www.ClinRx.com.

- Sodium cellulose phosphate (Calcisorb) binds calcium in the gut, reduces urinary calcium excretion and may benefit calcium stone-formers.
- Allopurinol is effective in those who have high excretion of uric acid in the urine.
- Potassium citrate, which alkalinises the urine, should be given to prevent formation of pure uric acid stones.

PHARMACOLOGICAL ASPECTS OF MICTURITION

SOME PHYSIOLOGY

The detrusor, whose smooth muscle fibres comprise the body of the bladder, is innervated mainly by parasympathetic nerves, which are excitatory and cause the muscle to contract. The internal sphincter, a concentration of smooth muscle at the bladder neck, is well developed only in the male and its principal function is to prevent retrograde flow of semen during ejaculation. It is rich in α_1 adrenoceptors, activation of which causes contraction. There is an abundant supply of oestrogen receptors in the distal two-thirds of the female urethral epithelium, which degenerates after the menopause causing loss of urinary control.

When the detrusor relaxes and the sphincters close, urine is stored; this is achieved by central inhibition of parasympathetic tone accompanied by a reflex increase in α-adrenergic activity. Voiding requires contraction of the detrusor, accompanied by relaxation of the sphincters. These acts are coordinated by a micturition centre, probably in the pons.

FUNCTIONAL ABNORMALITIES

The main abnormalities that require treatment are:

- *Unstable bladder* or detrusor instability, characterised by uninhibited, unstable contractions of the detrusor which may be of unknown aetiology or secondary to an upper motor neurone lesion or bladder neck obstruction.
- *Decreased bladder activity* or hypotonicity due to a lower motor neurone lesion or over-distension of the bladder, or both.
- Urethral sphincter dysfunction which is due to various causes including weakness of the muscles and ligaments around the bladder neck, descent of the urethrovesical junction and periurethral fibrosis; the result is stress incontinence.

- Atrophic change affects the distal urethra in females.

Drugs that may be used to alleviate abnormal micturition

Antimuscarinic drugs such as *oxybutynin* and *flavoxate* are used to treat urinary frequency; they increase bladder capacity by diminishing unstable detrusor contractions. Both drugs may cause dry mouth and blurred vision, and may precipitate glaucoma. Oxybutynin has a high level of unwanted effects; the dose needs to be carefully assessed, particularly in the elderly. Flavoxate has less marked side-effects but is also less effective. *Propiverine, tolterodine* and *trospium* are also antimuscarinic drugs used for urinary frequency, urgency and incontinence. Propantheline was formerly used widely in urinary incontinence but had a low response rate and a high incidence of adverse effects; it is now used mainly for adult enuresis. The need for continuing antimuscarinic drug therapy should be reviewed after 6 months.

Tricyclic antidepressants. Imipramine, amitriptyline and nortriptyline are effective, especially for nocturnal but also for daytime incontinence. Their parasympathetic blocking (antimuscarinic) action is probably in part responsible, but imipramine may also benefit by altering the patient's sleep profile.

Oestrogens either applied locally to the vagina or taken by mouth may benefit urinary incontinence due to atrophy of the urethral epithelium in post-menopausal women.

Parasympathomimetic drugs, e.g. bethanechol, carbachol and distigmine, may be used to stimulate the detrusor when the bladder is hypotonic, e.g. due to an upper motor neurone lesion. Distigmine, which is an anticholinesterase, is preferred but, as its effect is not sustained, intermittent catheterisation is also needed when the hypotonia is chronic.

BENIGN PROSTATIC HYPERPLASIA (BPH)

One of the commonest problems in men older than 50 years, BPH was for a long time helped only by surgical intervention. The prostate gland is a mixture of capsular and stromal tissue, rich in α_1 adrenoceptors, and glandular tissue under the influence of androgens. Both these, the α receptors and androgens, are targets for drug therapy. Because the bladder itself has few α receptors, it is possible to use selective α_1-blockade without affecting bladder contraction.

α-Adrenoceptor antagonists. Prazosin, alfuzosin, indoramin, terazosin and doxazosin are all α-adrenoceptor blockers with selectivity for the α_1 subtype. They cause significant increases (compared to placebo) in objective measures such as maximal urine flow rate, and drugs also improve semi-objective symptom scores. In normotensive men, falls in blood pressure are generally negligible; in hypertensive patients, the decline in pressure can be regarded as an added bonus (provided concurrent treatment is adjusted). These drugs can cause dizziness and asthenia, even in the absence of marked changes in blood pressure. Nasal stuffiness can be a problem – especially in patients who resort to α-agonists (e.g. pseudoephedrine) for rhinitis.

These adverse events are avoided by using *tamsulosin*, which selectively blocks the α_{1A} subclass[6] of adrenoceptors and is therefore less likely to affect blood pressure, provided the single 400-microgram daily dose of tamsulosin is not exceeded.

Finasteride. An alternative drug for such prostatic symptoms is the type II 5α-reductase inhibitor, finasteride, which inhibits conversion of testosterone to its more potent metabolite, dihydrotestosterone. Finasteride does not affect serum testosterone, or most non-prostatic responses to testosterone. It reduces prostatic volume by about 20% and increases urinary flow rates by a similar degree. These changes translate into modest clinical benefits, which are generally inferior to those of an α_1 antagonist.

Finasteride ($t_{1/2}$ 6 h) is taken as a single 5-mg tablet each day. The improvement in urine flow appears over 6 months (as the prostate shrinks in size), and in 5–10% of patients may be at the cost of some loss of libido. The serum concentration of prostate-specific antigen is approximately halved. Although this may reflect a real reduction in risk of prostatic cancer,

in patients receiving finasteride it is safer to regard values of the antigen in the upper half of the usual range as abnormal. Lower doses of finasteride have also been used successfully to halt the development of baldness.[7] Other antiandrogens, such as the gonadorelin agonists, are used in the treatment of prostatic cancer, but the need for parenteral administration makes them less suitable for BPH.

ERECTILE DYSFUNCTION

Erectile dysfunction (ED), the inability to achieve or maintain a penile erection sufficient to permit satisfactory sexual intercourse, is estimated to affect over 100 million men worldwide, with a prevalence of 39% in those aged 40 years.[8]

Its numerous causes include cardiovascular disease, diabetes mellitus and other endocrine disorders, alcohol and substance abuse, and psychological factors (14%). Although the evidence is not conclusive, drug therapy is thought to underlie 25% of cases, reputedly from antidepressants (selective serotonin-reuptake inhibitors [SSRIs] and tricyclics), phenothiazines, cyproterone acetate, fibrates, levodopa, histamine H_2-receptor blockers, phenytoin, carbamazepine, allopurinol, indometacin and, possibly, β-adrenoceptor blockers and thiazide diuretics.

Sexual arousal releases from the endothelial cells of penile blood vessels neurotransmitters that relax the smooth muscle of the arteries, arterioles and trabeculae of its erectile tissue, greatly increasing penile blood flow and facilitating rapid filling of the sinusoids and expansion of the corpora cavernosa. The venous plexus that drains the penis thus becomes compressed between the engorged sinusoids and the surrounding and firm tunica albuginea, causing the near-total cessation of venous outflow. The penis becomes erect, with an intracavernous pressure of 100 mmHg. The principal neurotransmitter is nitric oxide, which acts by raising intracellular concentrations of cyclic guanosine monophosphate (cGMP) to relax vascular smooth

---

[6]There are three cloned subtypes for the α_1-adrenoceptor: α_{1A}, α_{1B} and α_{1D}. The α_{1A} is the predominant subtype in the bladder base and prostatic urethra, whereas contraction of vascular smooth muscle is largely mediated by the α_{1B} subtype. Hence, α_{1A} selectivity would confer, at least in principle, 'prostatic' selectivity. But selectivity determined in vitro against cloned α_1 receptors only poorly predicts in vivo 'uroselectivity', which also diminishes as dose is increased (cf. the discussion of β-adrenoceptor selectivity with β-blocking drugs, Chapter 23, page 415).

[7]It has also been used as a treatment for hirsutism in women. Scalp follicles (of both sexes) contain type II 5α-reductase and the levels are increased in balding scalps (Tartagni M, Schonauer M, Cicinelli E et al 2004 Intermittent low-dose finasteride is as effective as daily administration for the treatment of hirsute women. Fertility and Sterility 82(3):752–755).

[8]Feldman H A, Goldstein I, Hatzichristou D G et al 1994 Impotence and its medical and psychological correlates: results of Massachusetts male aging study. Journal of Urology 151:54–61.

muscle. The isoenzyme phosphodiesterase type 5 (PDE5) is selectively active in penile smooth muscle and terminates the action of cGMP by converting it to the inactive non-cyclic GMP.

Sildenafil (Viagra) is a highly selective inhibitor of PDE5 (70-fold more so than isoenzymes 1, 2, 3 and 4 of PDE), prolonging the action of cGMP, and thus the vasodilator and erectile response to normal sexual stimulation. Its emergence as an agent for erectile dysfunction is an example of serendipity in drug development. Sildenafil was originally being developed for another indication but when the clinical trials ended the volunteers declined to return surplus tablets for they had discovered that the drug conferred unexpected benefits on their sexual lives. Its development for erectile dysfunction followed.

Sildenafil is well absorbed orally, reaches a peak in the blood after 30–120 min and has a $t_{1/2}$ of 4 h. The drug should be taken 1 h before intercourse in an initial dose of 50 mg (25 mg in the elderly); thereafter 25–100 mg may be taken according to response, with a maximum of one 100-mg dose per 24 h. Food may delay the onset and offset of effect. Sildenafil is effective in 80% of patients with erectile dysfunction.

Adverse effects are short lived, dose related, and comprise headache, flushing, nasal congestion and dyspepsia. High doses can inhibit PDE6, which is needed for phototransduction in the retina, and some patients report a transient blue coloration to their vision.[9] Some patients experience non-arteritic anterior ischaemic optic neuropathy (NAION), consisting of blurred vision and/or visual field loss generally within 24 h of taking sildenafil. Priapism[10] has been reported.

Interactions. Sildenafil is *contraindicated* in patients who are taking organic nitrates, for their metabolism is blocked and severe and acute hypotension result. Patients with recent stroke or myocardial infarction, or whose blood pressure is known to be less than 90/50 mmHg,

should not use it. Sildenafil is a substrate for the P450 isoenzyme CYP 3A4 (and to a lesser extent CYP 2C9), which gives scope for drug–drug interactions. The metabolic inhibitors erythromycin, saquinavir and ritonavir (protease inhibitors used for AIDS), and cimetidine produce substantial rises in the plasma level of sildenafil. More selective PDE5 inhibitors now available include vardenafil, which has a kinetic profile similar to that of sildenafil, and taladafil which has a very long $t_{1/2}$ (17h). This latter could be viewed as a mixed blessing in erectile dysfunction, but may be important if drugs of this class are developed for pulmonary hypertension.

Alprostadil is a stable form of prostaglandin E_1, a powerful vasodilator (see p. 416), and is effective for psychogenic and neuropathic erectile dysfunction. Alprostadil increases arterial inflow and reduces venous outflow by contracting the corporal smooth muscle that occludes draining venules. It is injected along the dorsolateral aspect of the proximal third of the penis, alternating sides and varying sites for each injection. The duration and grade of erection are dose related. The patient package insert from the manufacturer provides some helpful drawings. The dose is arrived at by titration (5–20 micrograms) initially in the doctor's surgery, aiming for an erection lasting for not more than 1 h. It may also be introduced through the urethra (0.125–1 mg). Painful erection is the commonest adverse effect.

Papaverine, an alkaloid (originally extracted from opium but devoid of narcotic properties[11]), is also a non-specific phosphodiesterase inhibitor. It is effective (up to 80%) for psychogenic and neurogenic erectile dysfunction by self-injection into the corpora cavernosa of the penis shortly before intercourse (efficacy may be increased by also administering the α-adrenoceptor blocker, phentolamine).[12] A physician who prescribes papaverine for this purpose must be ready to treat the occasional case of priapism by aspirating the corpora cavernosa and injecting an α-adrenoceptor agonist, e.g. metaraminol.

Apomorphine, a dopamine antagonist, is given by subcutaneous injection. Nausea can occur.

---

[9] The problem seems to be much less frequent with the newer and more PDE5-specific taladafil and vardenafil. This very unusual drug effect is reminiscent of the disturbed colour perception caused by digoxin (in overdose), except here patients report yellowed vision (xanthopsia). This may not be an adverse effect in all cases, as it has been suggested that xanthopsia is the explanation for the predominance of yellow in Van Gogh's art.

[10] Persistent erection (>4 h) of the penis, with pain and tenderness. In Greek mythology, Priapus was a god of fertility. He was also a patron of seafarers and shepherds.

[11] Papaveretum, whose actions are principally those of its morphine content, has occasionally been supplied in error, to the surprise, distress and hazard of the subject.

[12] Brindley G S 1986 Pilot experiments on the actions of drugs injected into the human corpus cavernosum penis. British Journal of Pharmacology 87:495 – an account of self-experimentation with 17 drugs.

Summary

- The actions of drugs on the kidney are of an importance disproportionate to the low prevalence of kidney disorders.
- The kidney is the main site of loss, or potential loss, of all body substances. It is among the functions of drugs to help reduce losses of desirable substances and increase losses of undesired substances.
- The kidney is also at increased risk of toxicity from foreign substances because of the high concentrations these can achieve in the renal medulla.
- Diuretics are among the most commonly used drugs, perhaps because the evolutionary advantages of sodium retention have left an aging population without salt-losing mechanisms of matching efficiency.
- Loop diuretics, acting on the ascending loop of Henle, are the most effective, and are used mainly to treat the oedema states. Potassium is lost as well as sodium.
- Thiazides, acting on the cortical diluting segment of the tubule, have lower natriuretic efficacy, but slightly greater antihypertensive efficacy than loop diuretics. Potassium loss is rarely a significant problem with thiazides, and thiazides reduce loss of calcium.
- Potassium retention with hyperkalaemia can occur with potassium-sparing diuretics, which block sodium transport in the last part of the distal tubule, either directly (e.g. amiloride) or by blocking aldosterone receptors (spironolactone).
- Drugs have little ability to alter the filtering function of the kidney when this is reduced by nephron loss.
- Prostatic enlargement is the main disease of the lower urinary tract; drugs can be used to postpone, or avoid, surgery. The symptoms of benign prostatic hyperplasia are partially relieved either by α_1-adrenoceptor blockade or by inhibiting synthesis of dihydrotestosterone in the prostate.
- Drugs are effective for the relief of erectile dysfunction, notably sildenafil, a highly specific phosphodiesterase inhibitor.

GUIDE TO FURTHER READING

Basnyat B, Murdoch D R 2003 High-altitude illness. Lancet 361:1967–1974

Brater D C 1998 Diuretic therapy. New England Journal of Medicine 339:387–395

Lameire N, Van Biesen W, Vanholder R et al 2005 Acute renal failure. Lancet 365:417–430

McMahon C N, Smith C J, Shabsigh R et al 2006 Treating erectile dysfunction when PDE5 inhibitors fail. British Medical Journal 332:589–592

Moe O W 2006 Kidney stones: pathophysiology and medical management. Lancet 367:333–344

Morgentaler A 1999 Male impotence. Lancet 354:1713–1718

Moynihan R 2005 The marketing of a disease: female sexual dysfunction. British Medical Journal 330:192–194

Ouslander J G 2004 Management of overactive bladder. New England Journal of Medicine 350(8):786–799

Thorpe A, Neal D 2003 Benign prostatic hyperplasia. Lancet 361:1359–1367

Vidal L, Shavit M, Fraser A, Paul M, Leibovici L 2005 Systematic comparison of four sources of drug information regarding adjustment of dose for renal function. British Medical Journal 331:263–266

27

Respiratory system

SYNOPSIS

- Cough: modes of action and uses of antitussives
- Respiratory stimulants: their place in therapy
- Pulmonary surfactant
- Oxygen therapy: its uses and dangers
- Histamine, antihistamines and allergies
- Bronchial asthma: types, modes of prevention, agents used for treatment and their use in asthma of varying degrees of severity
- Infections (see Chapter 13)

COUGH

There are two sorts of cough: the useful and the useless. Cough is useful when it effectively expels secretions or foreign objects from the respiratory tract, i.e. when it is *productive*; it is useless when it is unproductive and persistent. Useful cough should be allowed to serve its purpose and suppressed only when it is exhausting the patient or is dangerous, e.g. after eye surgery. Useless persistent cough should be stopped. Asthma, rhinosinusitis (causing postnasal drip) and oesophageal reflux are the commonest causes of persistent cough. Recently, *eosinophilic bronchitis* has been recognised as a possibly significant cause; it responds well to inhaled or oral corticosteroid. Clearly the overall approach to persistent cough must involve attention to underlying factors. The British Thoracic Society publishes guidelines on cough and its management.[1]

SITES OF ACTION FOR TREATMENT

Peripheral sites

On the *afferent* side of the cough reflex: by reducing input of stimuli from throat, larynx, trachea, a warm moist atmosphere has a demulcent effect on the pharynx.

On the *efferent* side of the cough reflex: measures to render secretions more easily removable (mucolytics, postural drainage) will reduce the amount of coughing needed, by increasing its efficiency.

The best antitussive of all is removal of the cause of the cough itself, i.e. treatment of underlying conditions (above). In patients with hypertension or cardiac failure, a common cause of a dry cough is treatment with an angiotensin-converting enzyme (ACE) inhibitor. This can be stopped by switching to an angiotensin II receptor blocker (ARB), e.g. losartan.

Central nervous system

Agents may act on the:

- medullary paths of the cough reflex (opioids)
- cerebral cortex
- subcortical paths (opioids and sedatives in general).

Cough is also under substantial voluntary control and can be inducible by psychogenic factors (e.g. the anxiety not to cough during the quiet parts of a musical concert) and reduced by a placebo. Considerations such as these are relevant to practical therapeutics.

COUGH SUPPRESSION

Antitussives that act peripherally

Smokers should stop smoking.

Cough originating above the larynx often benefits from syrups and lozenges that glutinously and soothingly coat the pharynx (demulcents[2]), e.g. simple linctus (mainly sugar-based syrup). Small children are prone to swallow lozenges, so a sweet on a stick may be preferred.

Linctuses are demulcent preparations that can be used alone and as vehicles of other specific antitussive agents. That their exact constitution is not critical was known and taught to medical students in 1896.

---

[1]http://www.brit-thoracic.org.uk.

[2]Latin: *demulcere*, to caress soothingly.

Many of you know that this (simple) linctus used to be very much thicker than it is now, and very likely the thicker linctus was more efficacious. The reason why it was made thinner was this. It was discovered that a large number of children came to the surgery complaining of cough, and they were given the linctus, but instead of their using it as a medicine, they took it to an old woman out in Smithfield, who gave them each a penny, took their linctus, and made jam tarts with it.[3]

Cough originating below the larynx is often relieved by water aerosol inhalations and a warm environment – the archetypal 'steam' inhalation. Compound benzoin tincture[4] may be used to give the inhalation a therapeutic smell (aromatic inhalation). This manoeuvre may have more than a placebo effect by promoting secretion of a dilute mucus that gives a protective coating to the inflamed mucous membrane. Menthol and eucalyptus are alternatives.

Local anaesthetics can also be used topically in the airways to block the mucosal cough receptors (modified stretch receptors and C-fibre endings) directly. Nebulised lidocaine, for example, reduces coughing during fibreoptic bronchoscopy and is also effective in the intractable cough that may accompany bronchial carcinoma.

Antitussives that act centrally

The most consistent means of suppressing cough irrespective of its cause is blockade of the *medullary cough centre* itself. *Opioids*, such as methadone and codeine, are very effective, although part of this antitussive effect could reflect their sedatory effect on higher nervous centres; nevertheless antitussive potency of an opiate is generally poorly correlated with its potency at causing respiratory depression.

As *dextromethorphan* (the D-isomer of the codeine analogue levorphanol) and *pholcodine* also have an antitussive effect that is not blocked by naloxone, non-μ-type opiate receptors are probably involved (and dubbed σ-type). It is not surprising, then, that these opiates also have no significant analgesic or respiratory-depressant effects at the doses required for their antitussive action.

Opioids are usually formulated as *linctuses* for antitussive use. Deciding on which agent to use depends largely on whether sedation and analgesia may be useful actions of the linctus. Hence methadone or diamorphine linctus may be preferred in patients with advanced bronchial carcinoma. In contrast, pholcodine, being non-sedating and non-addictive, is widely incorporated into over-the-counter linctuses.

Sedation generally reduces the sensitivity of the cough reflex. Hence older sedating antihistamines, e.g. diphenhydramine, can suppress cough by non-H_1-receptor actions; often the doses needed cause substantial drowsiness so that combination with other drugs, such as pholcodine and dextromethorphan, is common in over-the-counter cough remedies.

MUCOLYTICS AND EXPECTORANTS

Normally about 100 mL fluid is produced from the respiratory tract each day and most of it is swallowed. Respiratory mucus consists largely of water and its slimy character is due to glycoproteins cross-linked together by disulphide bonds. In pathological states much more mucus may be produced; an exudate of plasma proteins that bond with glycoproteins and form larger polymers results in the mucus becoming more viscous. Patients with chest diseases such as cystic fibrosis (CF) and bronchiectasis have difficulty in clearing their chest of viscous sputum by cough because the bronchial cilia are rendered ineffective. Drugs that liquefy mucus can provide benefit.

Mucolytics

Carbocisteine and *mecysteine* have free sulphydryl groups that open disulphide bonds in mucus and reduce its viscosity. They are given orally or by inhalation (or instillation) and may be useful chiefly where particularly viscous secretion is a problem (cystic fibrosis, care of tracheostomies). Mucolytics may cause gastrointestinal irritation and allergic reaction.

Water inhalation via an aerosol (breathing over a hot basin) is a cheap and effective expectorant therapy in bronchiectasis. Simply hydrating a dehydrated patient can also have a beneficial effect in lowering sputum viscosity.

Dornase α is phosphorylated glycosylated recombinant human deoxyribonuclease. It is given daily by inhalation of a nebulised solution containing 2500 units (2.5 mg). It is of modest value only in patients with cystic fibrosis, whose genetic defect

---

[3]Brunton L 1897 Lectures on the action of medicines. Macmillan, London.
[4]Friar's Balsam.

in chloride transport causes particularly viscous sputum. The blocked airways, as well as the sputum itself, are a trap for pathogens, and the lysis of invading neutrophils leads to substantial levels of free and very viscous DNA within the CF airways.

Expectorants

These are said to encourage productive cough by increasing the volume of bronchial secretion; there is little clinical evidence to support this, and they may be of no more value than placebo. The group includes squill, guaiphenesin, ipecacuanha, creosotes and volatile oils.

Cough mixtures

Every formulary is replete with combinations of antitussives, expectorants, mucolytics, bronchodilators and sedatives. Although choice is not critical, knowledge of the active ingredients is important, as some contain sedative antimuscarinic antihistamines or phenypropanolamines (which may antagonise antihypertensives). Use of glycerol or syrup as a demulcent cough preparation, or of simple linctus (citric acid), is probably defensible.

Choice of drug therapy for cough

As always, it is necessary to have a clear idea of the underlying problem before starting any therapy. For example, the approach to cough due to invasion of a bronchus by a neoplasm differs from that due to postnasal drip from chronic sinusitis or to that due to chronic bronchitis. The following are general recommendations.

Simple suppression of useless cough

Codeine, pholcodine, dextromethorphan and methadone linctuses can be used in large, infrequent doses. In children, cough is nearly always useful and sedation at night is more effective to give rest. A sedative antihistamine is convenient (e.g. promethazine), although sputum thickening may be a disadvantage. In pertussis infection (whooping cough), codeine and atropine methonitrate may be tried.

To increase bronchial secretion slightly and to liquefy what is there

Water aerosol with or without menthol and benzoin inhalation, or menthol and eucalyptus inhalation may provide comfort harmlessly.

Carbocysteine or another mucolytic orally may occasionally be useful.

Preparations containing any drug with antimuscarinic action are undesirable because this thickens bronchial secretion. Oxygen inhalation dries secretions, so rendering them even more viscous; oxygen must be bubbled through water, and patients having oxygen may need measures to liquefy sputum.

Cough originating in the pharyngeal region

Glutinous sweets or lozenges (demulcents), incorporating a cough suppressant or not, as appropriate, are used.

RESPIRATORY STIMULANTS

The drugs used (analeptics) are central nervous system (CNS) stimulants capable of causing convulsions in doses just above those used therapeutically. Hence, their use must be monitored carefully.

Doxapram increases the rate and depth of respiration by stimulating the medullary respiratory centres both directly and reflexly through the carotid body. A continuous i.v. infusion of 1.5–4.0 mg/min is given according to the patient's response. Coughing and laryngospasm that develop after its use may represent a return of normal protective responses.

Adverse effects include restlessness, twitching, itching, vomiting, flushing, bronchospasm and cardiac arrhythmias, and in addition doxapram causes patients to experience a feeling of perineal warmth; in high doses it raises blood pressure.

Aminophylline (a complex of theophylline and EDTA) in addition to its other actions (see also p. 170) is a respiratory stimulant and may be infused slowly i.v. (500 mg in 6 h).

USES

Respiratory stimulants have a much reduced role in the management of acute ventilatory failure, following the increased use of nasal positive-pressure ventilation for respiratory failure. Situations where they may still be encountered are:

■ Acute exacerbations of chronic lung disease with *hypercapnia*, drowsiness and inability to cough or to tolerate low (24%) concentrations of inspired oxygen (air is 21% oxygen). A respiratory stimulant can arouse the patient sufficiently to allow effective physiotherapy and, by stimulating respiration, can improve ventilation–perfusion matching. As a short-term measure, this may be used in conjunction with assisted ventilation without tracheal intubation (BIPAP[5]), and thereby 'buy time' for chemotherapy to control infection and avoid full tracheal intubation and mechanical ventilation.

■ *Apnoea* in premature infants; aminophylline and caffeine may benefit some cases.

Avoid respiratory stimulants in patients with epilepsy (risk of convulsions). Other relative contraindications include ischaemic heart disease, acute severe asthma ('status asthmaticus'), severe hypertension and thyrotoxicosis.

Irritant vapours, to be inhaled, have an analeptic effect in fainting, especially if it is psychogenic, e.g. aromatic solution of ammonia (Sal Volatile). No doubt they sometimes 'recall the exorbitant and deserting spirits to their proper stations'.[6]

PULMONARY SURFACTANT

The endogenous surfactant system produces stable low surface tension in the alveoli, preventing their collapse. Failure of production of natural surfactant occurs in respiratory distress syndrome (RDS), including that in the neonate. Synthetic phospholipids are now available for intratracheal instillation to act as surfactants: *colfosceril palmitate*, *poractant* α and *beractant*. These need to be stored chilled, and the manufacturers' instructions followed carefully because on reaching body temperature their physicochemical properties change rapidly. Their function is to coat the surface of the alveoli and maintain their patency, and their administration to premature neonates with RDS is a key part in reducing mortality and long-term complications in this condition.

OXYGEN THERAPY

Oxygen used in therapy should be prescribed with the same care as any drug; there should be a well defined purpose and its effects should be monitored objectively.

The absolute indication to supplement inspired air is *inadequate tissue oxygenation*. As clinical signs may be imprecise, arterial blood gases should be measured whenever suspicion arises. Tissue hypoxia can be assumed when the Pa_{O_2} falls below 6.7 kPa (50 mmHg) in a previously normal acutely ill patient, e.g. with myocardial infarction, acute pulmonary disorder, drug overdose, musculoskeletal or head trauma. Chronically hypoxic patients may maintain adequate tissue oxygenation with a Pa_{O_2} below 6.7 kPa by compensatory adaptations, including an increased red cell mass and altered haemoglobin–oxygen binding characteristics. Oxygen therapy is used as follows:

■ *High concentration* oxygen therapy is reserved for a state of low Pa_{O_2} in association with a *normal* or *low* Pa_{CO_2} (*type I respiratory failure*), as in: pulmonary embolism, pneumonia, pulmonary oedema, myocardial infarction and young patients with acute severe asthma. Concentrations of oxygen up to 100% may be used for short periods, as there is little risk of inducing hypoventilation and carbon dioxide retention.

■ *Low concentration* oxygen therapy is reserved for a state of low Pa_{O_2} in association with a *raised* Pa_{CO_2} (*type II failure*), typically seen during exacerbations of chronic obstructive pulmonary disease. The normal stimulus to respiration is an increase in Pa_{CO_2}, but this control is blunted in chronically hypercapnic patients whose respiratory drive comes from *hypoxia*. Increasing the Pa_{O_2} in such patients by giving them high concentrations of oxygen removes their stimulus to ventilate, exaggerates carbon dioxide retention and may cause fatal respiratory acidosis. The objective of therapy in such patients is to provide just enough oxygen to alleviate hypoxia without exaggerating the hypercapnia and respiratory acidosis; normally the inspired oxygen concentration should not exceed 28%, and in some 24% may be sufficient.

■ *Continuous long-term domiciliary oxygen therapy* (LTOT) is given to patients with severe persistent hypoxaemia and cor pulmonale due to chronic obstructive pulmonary disease (see below). Patients are provided with an oxygen concentrator. Clinical trial evidence indicates that taking oxygen for more than 15 h per day improves survival.

---

[5]Bi-level positive airways pressure. Air (if necessary enriched with oxygen 24% or 28%) is administered through a close-fitting facemask at a positive pressure of 14–18 cmH$_2$O to support inspiration, then at a pressure of 4 cmH$_2$O during expiration to help maintain patency of small airways and increase gas exchange in alveoli.

[6]Thomas Sydenham (1624–1689). He was referred to as the 'English Hippocrates' due to his classic description of diseases.

HISTAMINE, ANTIHISTAMINES AND ALLERGIES

Histamine is a naturally occurring amine that has long fascinated pharmacologists and physicians. It is found in most tissues in an inactive bound form, and pharmacologically active free histamine, released in response to stimuli such as physical trauma or immunoglobulin (Ig) E-mediated activation, is an important component of the acute inflammatory response.

The physiological functions of histamine are suggested by its *distribution in the body*, in:

- *body epithelia* (the gut, the respiratory tract and in the skin), where it is released in response to invasion by foreign substances
- *glands* (gastric, intestinal, lachrymal, salivary), where it mediates part of the normal secretory process
- *mast cells* near blood vessels, where it plays a role in regulating the microcirculation.

Actions. Histamine acts as a local hormone (autacoid) similarly to serotonin or prostaglandins, i.e. it functions within the immediate vicinity of its site of release. With gastric secretion, for example, stimulation of receptors on the histamine-containing cell causes release of histamine, which in turn acts on receptors on parietal cells which then secrete hydrogen ions (see Gastric secretion, Chapter 31). The actions of histamine that are clinically important are those on:

Smooth muscle. In general, histamine causes smooth muscle to contract (excepting arterioles, but including the larger arteries). Stimulation of the pregnant human uterus is insignificant. A brisk attack of bronchospasm may be induced in subjects who have any allergy, particularly asthma.

Blood vessels. Arterioles are dilated, with a consequent fall in blood pressure. This action is due partly to nitric oxide release from the vascular endothelium of the arterioles in response to histamine receptor activation. Capillary *permeability* also increases, especially at postcapillary venules, causing oedema. These effects on arterioles and capillaries represent the *flush* and the *wheal* components of the triple response described by Thomas Lewis.[7]

The third part, the *flare*, is arteriolar dilatation due to an axon reflex releasing neuropeptides from C-fibre endings.

Skin. Histamine release in the skin can cause itch.

Gastric secretion. Histamine increases the acid and pepsin content of gastric secretion.

As may be anticipated from the above actions, *anaphylactic shock*, which is due in large part to histamine release, is characterised by circulatory collapse and bronchoconstriction. The most rapidly effective antidote is adrenaline (epinephrine) (see below), and an antihistamine (H$_1$ receptor) may be given as well.

Various chemicals can cause release of histamine. The more powerful of these (proteolytic enzymes and snake venoms) have no place in therapeutics, but a number of useful drugs, such as D-tubocurarine and morphine, and even some antihistamines, cause histamine release. This *anaphylactoid* (i.e. IgE independent) effect is usually clinically mild with a transient reduction in blood pressure or a local skin reaction, but significant bronchospasm may occur in asthmatics.

Metabolism. Histamine is formed from the amino acid histidine and is inactivated largely by deamination and methylation. In common with other local hormones, this process is extremely rapid.

Histamine receptors. Histamine binds to H$_1$, H$_2$ and H$_3$ receptors, all of which are G-protein coupled. The H$_1$ receptor is largely responsible for mediating its pro-inflammatory effects, including the vasomotor changes, increased vascular permeability and up-regulation of adhesion molecules on vascular endothelium (see p. 425), i.e. it mediates the oedema and vascular effects of histamine. H$_2$ receptors mediate release of gastric acid (see p. 561). Blockade of histamine H$_1$ and H$_2$ receptors has substantial therapeutic utility.

H$_3$ receptors are expressed in a wide range of tissues including brain and nerve endings, and function as feedback inhibitors for histamine and other neurotransmitters. More recently identified is the H$_4$ receptor, which is involved in leucocyte chemotaxis.

HISTAMINE ANTAGONISM AND H$_1$- AND H$_2$-RECEPTOR ANTAGONISTS

The effects of histamine can be opposed in three ways:

---

[7]Lewis T et al 1924 Heart 11:209.

■ *By using a drug with opposing effects.* Histamine constricts bronchi, causes vasodilatation and increases capillary permeability; adrenaline (epinephrine), by activating α and β$_2$ adrenoceptors, produces opposite effects – referred to as *physiological antagonism.*

■ *By blocking histamine binding* to its site of action (receptors), i.e. using competitive H$_1$- and H$_2$-receptor antagonists.

■ *By preventing the release of histamine from storage cells.* Glucocorticoids and sodium cromoglicate can suppress IgE-induced release from mast cells; β$_2$ agonists have a similar effect.

Drugs that competitively block H$_1$-histamine receptors were the first to be introduced and are conventionally called the 'antihistamines'. They effectively inhibit the components of the triple response and partially prevent the hypotensive effect of histamine, but they have no effect on histamine-induced gastric secretion which is suppressed by blockade of histamine H$_2$ receptors. Thus, histamine antagonists are classified as:

■ histamine H$_1$-receptor antagonists (see below)
■ histamine H$_2$-receptor antagonists: cimetidine, famotidine, nizatidine, ranitidine (see Chapter 31)
■ histamine H$_1$-receptor antagonists.

The selectivity implied by the term 'antihistamine'is unsatisfactory because the older first-generation antagonists (see below) show considerable blocking activity against muscarinic receptors, and often serotonin and α-adrenergic receptors as well. These features are a disadvantage when H$_1$ antihistamines are used specifically to antagonise the effects of histamine, e.g. for allergies. Hence the appearance of second-generation H$_1$ antagonists that are more selective for H$_1$ receptors and largely free of antimuscarinic and sedative effects (see below) has been an important advance. They can be discussed together.

Actions. H$_1$-receptor antihistamines oppose, to varying degrees, the effects of liberated histamine. They are generally competitive, surmountable inhibitors and strongly block all components of the triple response (a pure H$_1$-receptor effect), but only partially counteract the hypotensive effect of high-dose histamine (a mixed H$_1$- and H$_2$-receptor effect). H$_1$ antihistamines are of negligible use in asthma, in which non-histamine mediators, such as the cysteinyl-leukotrienes, are the predominant constrictors.

They are more effective if used before histamine has been liberated, and reversal of effects of free histamine is more readily achieved by physiological antagonism with adrenaline (epinephrine), which is used first in life-threatening allergic reactions.

The older *first-generation* H$_1$ antihistamines cause drowsiness and patients should be warned of this, e.g. about driving or operating machinery, and about additive effects with alcohol. Paradoxically, they can increase seizure activity in epileptics, especially children, and can cause seizures in non-epileptic subjects if taken in overdose. The newer *second-generation* H$_1$ antihistamines penetrate the blood–brain barrier less readily and are largely devoid of such central effects. Antimuscarinic effects of first-generation H$_1$ antihistamines are sometimes put to therapeutic advantage in parkinsonism and motion sickness.

Pharmacokinetics. H$_1$ antihistamines taken orally are readily absorbed. They are metabolised mainly in the liver. Excretion in the breast milk may be sufficient to cause sedation in infants. They are generally administered orally and can also be given intramuscularly or intravenously.

Uses. The H$_1$ antihistamines are used for symptomatic relief of allergies such as hay fever and urticaria (see below). They are of broadly similar therapeutic efficacy.

INDIVIDUAL H$_1$-RECEPTOR ANTIHISTAMINES

Non-sedative second-generation drugs

These newer drugs are relatively selective for H$_1$ receptors, enter the brain less readily than do the earlier antihistamines, and lack the unwanted antimuscarinic effects. Differences lie principally in their duration of action.

Cetirizine ($t_{\frac{1}{2}}$ 7 h), *loratadine* ($t_{\frac{1}{2}}$ 15 h) and *terfenadine* ($t_{\frac{1}{2}}$ 20 h) are effective taken once daily and are suitable for general use. *Acrivastine* ($t_{\frac{1}{2}}$ 2 h) is so short acting that it is best reserved for intermittent therapy, e.g. when breakthrough symptoms occur in a patient using topical therapy for hay fever. Other non-sedating antihistamines are desloratadine, fexofenadine, levocetirizine and mizolastine.

Adverse effects. The second-generation antihistamines are well tolerated but a noteworthy effect occurs with terfenadine. This drug can prolong the

QTc interval on the surface ECG by blocking a potassium channel in the heart (the rapid component of delayed rectifier potassium current, I_{Kr}), which triggers a characteristic ventricular tachycardia (torsade de pointes, see p. 459) and probably explains the sudden deaths reported during early use of terfenadine. The event is prone to occur with high dose or when metabolism of terfenadine is inhibited. Terfenadine depends solely on the 3A4 isoform of cytochrome P450, and inhibiting drugs include erythromycin, ketoconazole and even grapefruit juice. Fexofenadine, the active metabolite of terfenadine, has a much lower affinity for the I_{Kr} channel and appears safe in this respect.

Sedative first-generation agents

Chlorphenamine ($t_{1/2}$ 20 h) is effective when urticaria is prominent, and its sedative effect is then useful.

Diphenhydramine ($t_{1/2}$ 32 h) is strongly sedative and has antimuscarinic effects; it is also used in parkinsonism and motion sickness.

Promethazine ($t_{1/2}$ 12 h) is so strongly sedative that it is used as an hypnotic in adults and children.

Alimemazine, azatadine, brompheniramine, clemastine, cyproheptadine, diphenylpyraline, doxylamine, hydroxyzine and *triprolidine* are similar.

Adverse effects. Apart from sedation, these include: dizziness, fatigue, insomnia, nervousness, tremors and antimuscarinic effects, e.g. dry mouth, blurred vision and gastrointestinal disturbance. Dermatitis and agranulocytosis can occur. Severe poisoning due to overdose results in coma and sometimes in convulsions.

DRUG MANAGEMENT OF SOME ALLERGIC STATES

Histamine is released in many allergic states, but it is not the sole cause of symptoms, other chemical mediators, e.g. leukotrienes and prostaglandins, also being involved. Hence the usefulness of H_1-receptor antihistamines in allergic states is variable, depending on the extent to which histamine, rather than other mediators, is the cause of the clinical manifestations.

Note also that H_2-receptor antagonists (separate from their role in reducing gastric acid secretion) can be used to reduce the effects of a type I hypersensitivity response, e.g. rhinitis, urticaria and conjunctivitis.

Hay fever. If symptoms are limited to rhinitis, a glucocorticoid (beclometasone, betamethasone, budesonide, flunisolide or triamcinolone), ipratropium or sodium cromoglicate applied topically as a spray or insufflation is often all that is required. Ocular symptoms alone respond well to sodium cromoglicate drops. When both nasal and ocular symptoms occur, or there is itching of the palate and ears as well, a systemic non-sedative H_1-receptor antihistamine is indicated. Sympathomimetic vasoconstrictors, e.g. ephedrine, are immediately effective when applied topically, but rebound swelling of the nasal mucous membrane occurs when medication is stopped. Rarely, a systemic glucocorticoid, e.g. prednisolone, is justified for a severely affected patient to provide relief for a short period, e.g. during academic examinations.[8]

Hyposensitisation, by subcutaneous injection of graded and increasing amounts of grass and tree pollen extracts, is an option for seasonal allergic hay fever due to pollens (which has not responded to antiallergy drugs), and of bee and wasp allergen extracts for people who exhibit allergy to these venoms (exposure to which can be life threatening). If hyposensitisation is undertaken, facilities for immediate cardiopulmonary resuscitation must be available because of the risk of anaphylaxis. An emerging strategy is to use a monoclonal antibody against IgE (omalizumab), which causes a rapid, dose-related and sustained fall in plasma IgE concentrations in patients with atopic and extrinsic asthma. The antibody is designed to bind to the part of the IgE molecule that interacts with the high-affinity IgE receptor (FcRI) on mast cells and basophils, thus preventing the activation of these cells by cross-linking of bound IgE.

Urticaria. See page 288.

Anaphylactic shock. See page 122.

BRONCHIAL ASTHMA

Asthma affects 10–15% of the UK population; this incidence is increasing.

---

[8] A man with severe hay fever who received at least one depot injection of corticosteroid each year for 11 years developed avascular necrosis of both femoral heads, an uncommon but serious complication of exposure to corticosteroid (Nasser S M S, Ewan P W 2001 Lesson of the week: depot corticosteroid treatment for hay fever causing avascular necrosis of both hips. British Medical Journal 322:1589–1591).

SOME PATHOPHYSIOLOGY

The bronchi become hyperreactive as a result of a persistent *inflammatory* process in response to a number of stimuli that include biological agents, e.g. allergens, viruses, and environmental chemicals such as ozone and glutaraldehyde. Inflammatory mediators are liberated from mast cells, eosinophils, neutrophils, monocytes and macrophages. Some mediators such as histamine are preformed and their release causes an immediate bronchial reaction. Others are formed after activation of cells and produce more sustained bronchoconstriction; these include metabolites of arachidonic acid from both the cyclo-oxygenase, e.g. prostaglandin D_2 and lipo-oxygenase, e.g. cysteinyl-leukotrienes C_4 and D_4, pathways. In addition platelet activating factor (PAF) is being recognised increasingly as an important mediator (see Chapter 15, p. 250).

The relative importance of many of the mediators is not defined precisely but they interact to produce mucosal oedema, mucus secretion and damage to the ciliated epithelium. Breaching of the protective epithelial barrier allows hyperreactivity to be maintained by bronchoconstrictor substances or by local axon reflexes through exposed nerve fibres. Wheezing and breathlessness result. The bronchial changes also obstruct access of inhaled drug to the periphery, which is why they can fail to give full relief.

Asthma, like many of the common chronic disorders (hypertension, diabetes mellitus), is a polygenic disorder, and already genetic loci linked to either increased production of IgE or bronchial hyperreactivity have been reported in some families with an increased incidence of asthma.

Early in an attack there is hyperventilation so that Pao_2 is maintained and $Paco_2$ is lowered, but with increasing airways obstruction the Pao_2 declines and $Paco_2$ rises, signifying a serious asthmatic episode.

TYPES OF ASTHMA

Asthma associated with specific allergic reactions

This *extrinsic* type is the commonest and occurs in patients who develop allergy to inhaled antigenic substances. They are also frequently atopic, showing positive responses to skin prick testing with the same antigens. The hypersensitivity reaction in the lung (and skin) is of the immediate type (Type 1) involving IgE-mediated mast cell activation. Allergen avoidance is particularly relevant to managing this type of asthma.

Asthma not associated with known allergy

Some patients exhibit wheeze and breathlessness in the absence of an obvious allergen or atopy. They are considered to have *intrinsic* asthma and, because of a lack of an identifiable allergen, allergen avoidance has no place in their management.

Exercise-induced asthma

Some patients develop wheeze that regularly follows within a few minutes of exercise. A similar response occurs following the inhalation of cold air, as the common mechanism appears to be airway drying. Inhalation of a β_2-adrenoceptor agonist, sodium cromoglicate (see below) or one of the newer leukotriene receptor antagonists (see below) prior to either challenge prevents bronchoconstriction.

Asthma associated with chronic obstructive pulmonary disease

A number of patients with persistent airflow obstruction exhibit substantial variation in airways resistance and in the extent to which they benefit from bronchodilator drugs. It is important to recognise that asthma may coexist with chronic obstructive pulmonary disease, and to assess their responses to bronchodilators or glucocorticoids over a period of time (as formal tests of respiratory function may not reliably predict clinical response in this setting).

APPROACHES TO TREATMENT

With the foregoing discussion in mind, the following approaches to treatment are logical:

- Prevention of exposure to allergen(s)
- Reduction of the bronchial inflammation and hyperreactivity
- Dilatation of narrowed bronchi.

These objectives may be achieved as follows:

Prevention of exposure to allergen(s)

This approach is appropriate for extrinsic asthmatics. Identification of an allergen may be aided by the patient's history (wheezing in response to contact with grasses, pollens, animals), by intradermal skin prick injection of selected allergen or by demonstrating specific IgE antibodies in the patient's serum, i.e. the RAST test (RadioAllergoSorbent Test). Avoiding an allergen may be feasible when it is related to some specific situation, e.g. occupation, but is less feasible if it is widespread, as with house-dust mite.

Reduction of the bronchial inflammation and hyperreactivity

As persistent inflammation is central to bronchial hyperreactivity, the use of anti-inflammatory drugs is logical.

Glucocorticoids (see p. 594) bring about a gradual reduction in bronchial hyperreactivity. They are the mainstay of asthma treatment. The exact mechanisms are still disputed but probably include: inhibition of the influx of inflammatory cells into the lung after allergen exposure; inhibition of the release of mediators from macrophages and eosinophils; and reduction of the microvascular leakage that these mediators cause. Glucocorticoids used in asthma include *prednisolone* (orally), and *beclometasone, fluticasone* and *budesonide* (by inhalation) (see Chapter 34).

Sodium cromoglicate (cromolyn, Intal) impairs the immediate response to allergen and was formerly thought to act by inhibiting the release of mediators from mast cells. Evidence now suggests that the late allergic response and bronchial hyperreactivity are also inhibited, and points to effects of cromoglicate on other inflammatory cells and also on local axon reflexes. Cromoglicate is poorly absorbed from the gastrointestinal tract but well absorbed from the lung, and it is given by inhalation (as powder, aerosol or nebuliser); it is eliminated unchanged in the urine and bile.

As it does not antagonise the bronchoconstrictor effect of the mediators after they have been released, cromoglicate is not effective at terminating an existing attack, i.e. it *prevents* bronchoconstriction rather than inducing bronchodilation. Special formulations are used for *allergic rhinitis* and *allergic conjunctivitis.*

Sodium cromoglicate is effective in extrinsic (allergic) asthma, including asthma in children and exercise-induced asthma, but its use has declined since the efficacy and safety of low-dose inhaled corticosteroid have become apparent.

It is remarkably non-toxic. Apart from cough and bronchospasm induced by the powder it may rarely cause allergic reactions. Application to the eye may produce a local stinging sensation and the oral form may cause nausea.

Nedocromil sodium (Tilade) is structurally unrelated to cromoglicate but has a similar profile of actions and can be used by metered aerosol in place of cromoglicate.

Other drugs. Ketotifen is a histamine H_1-receptor blocker that may also have some antiasthma effects but its benefit has not been demonstrated conclusively. In common with other antihistamines it causes drowsiness.

Dilatation of narrowed bronchi

This is achieved most effectively by *physiological antagonism* of bronchial muscle contraction, namely by stimulation of adrenergic bronchodilator mechanisms. Pharmacological antagonism of specific bronchoconstrictors is less effective, either because individual mediators are not on their own responsible for a large part of the bronchoconstriction (acetylcholine, adenosine, leukotrienes) or because the mediator is not even secreted during asthma attacks (histamine).

β_2-Adrenoceptor agonists. The predominant adrenoceptors in bronchi are of the β_2 type and their stimulation causes bronchial muscle to relax. β_2-Adrenoceptor activation also stabilises mast cells. Agonists in widespread use include *salbutamol, terbutaline, fenoterol, eformoterol* and *salmeterol,* and are discussed in Chapter 22. Salmeterol is longer acting because its lipophilic side-chain anchors the drug in the membrane adjacent to the receptor, slowing tissue washout.

Less selective adrenoceptor agonists such as adrenaline (epinephrine), ephedrine, isoetharine, isoprenaline and orciprenaline are less safe, being more likely to cause cardiac arrhythmias. α-Adrenoceptor activity contributes to bronchoconstriction, but α-adrenoceptor antagonists have not proved effective in practice.

Theophylline, a methylxanthine, relaxes bronchial muscle, although its precise mode of action is still debated. Inhibition of phosphodiesterase (PDE), especially its type 4 isoform, now seems the most likely explanation for its bronchodilating and more recently reported anti-inflammatory effects. Blockade of adenosine receptors is probably unimportant. Other actions of theophylline include chronotropic and inotropic effects on the heart and a direct effect on the rate of urine production (diuresis).

Absorption of theophylline from the gastrointestinal tract is usually rapid and complete. Some 90% is metabolised by the liver and there is evidence that the process is saturable at therapeutic doses. The $t_{1/2}$ is 8 h, with substantial variation. It is prolonged in patients with severe cardiopulmonary disease and cirrhosis; obesity and prematurity are associated with reduced rates of elimination; tobacco smoking enhances theophylline clearance by inducing hepatic P450 enzymes. These pharmacokinetic factors and the low therapeutic index render necessary the therapeutic monitoring of the plasma theophylline to achieve the best outcome; the desired concentration range is 10–20 mg/L (55–110 micromol/L).

Theophylline is relatively insoluble and is formulated either as a salt with choline (choline theophyllinate) or complexed with EDTA (aminophylline). *Aminophylline* is sufficiently soluble to permit intravenous use of theophylline in acute severe asthma (status asthmaticus). Rapid intravenous injection will induce unwanted effects (below) by exposing the heart and brain to high concentrations before distribution is complete. Intravenous injection must be slow (a loading dose of 5 mg/kg over 20 min followed by an infusion of 0.9 mg/kg/h, adjusted according to subsequent plasma theophylline concentrations). The loading dose should be avoided in any patient who is already taking a methylxanthine preparation (always enquire about this before injecting).

There are numerous sustained-release oral forms for use in chronic asthma, but because they are not bio-equivalent patients should not switch between them once they are stabilised on a particular preparation.

Adverse effects. At high therapeutic doses some patients experience nausea and diarrhoea, and plasma concentrations above the recommended range risk cardiac arrhythmia and seizures. Enzyme inhibition by erythromycin, ciprofloxacin, allopurinol or oral contraceptives increases the plasma concentration of theophylline; enzyme inducers such as carbamazepine, phenytoin and rifampicin reduce the concentration.

Overdose with theophylline has assumed greater importance with the advent of sustained-release preparations that prolong toxic effects, with peak plasma concentrations being reached 12–24 h after ingestion. Vomiting may be severe but the chief dangers are cardiac arrhythmia, hypotension, hypokalaemia and seizures. Activated charcoal should be given every 2–4 h until the plasma concentration is below 20 mg/L. Potassium replacement is important to prevent arrhythmias, and diazepam is used to control convulsions.

Antimuscarinic bronchodilators. Release of acetylcholine from vagal nerve endings in the airways activates muscarinic (M_3) receptors on bronchial smooth muscle causing bronchoconstriction. Blockade of these receptors with atropine causes bronchodilatation, although the preferred antimuscarinics in clinical practice are inhaled *ipratropium, oxitropium* or the recently introduced long-acting *tiotropium* (its effects last for up to 24 h). These synthetic compounds, unlike atropine, are permanently charged molecules that resist significant absorption after inhalation and thus minimise antimuscarinic effects outside of the lung. They are used mostly in older patients with chronic obstructive pulmonary disease, but are useful in acute severe asthma when combined with β_2-adrenoceptor agonists. Vagally mediated bronchoconstriction appears to be important in acute asthma, but relatively unimportant for most chronic stable asthmatics.

Leukotriene receptor antagonists, e.g. *montelukast* and *zafirlukast*, competitively prevent the bronchoconstrictor effects of cysteinyl-leukotrienes (C_4, D_4 and E_4) by blocking their common cysLT1 receptor. They have similar efficacy to low-dose inhaled glucocorticoid. The scarcity of comparisons with established medications consigns them to a second- or third-line role in treatment. They could be substituted at Step 2 or later stages of the current five-step regimen for asthma (see Fig. 27.1). There are no studies to justify their use as steroid-sparing (far less, replacement) therapy. When used occasionally in this way in patients unwilling or unable to use metered-dose inhalers, serial monitoring of spirometry is essential.

Montelukast is given once per day and zafirlukast twice daily. Leukotriene receptor antagonists are generally well tolerated, although Churg–Strauss syndrome has been reported rarely with their use. This probably represents unmasking of the disease as glucocorticoids are withdrawn following addition of the leukotriene receptor antagonist. Alerting features to this development are vasculitic rash, eosinophilia, worsening respiratory symptoms, cardiac complications and peripheral neuropathy.

DRUG THERAPY BY INHALATION

The inhaled route has been developed to advantage because the undesirable effects of systemic exposure to drugs, especially glucocorticoids, are substantially reduced. The pharmacokinetic advantages of using the inhaled versus the oral route are apparent from the substantially reduced dose requirement: salbutamol 100 micrograms from an aerosol inhaler will provide bronchodilatation similar to 2000 micrograms by mouth.

Before a drug can be inhaled, it must first be converted into particulate form; the optimum particle size to reach and be deposited in the small bronchi is around 2 μm. Such particles are delivered to the lung as an aerosol, i.e. dispersed in a gas, which can be produced in a number of different ways:

Pressurised aerosol. Drug is dissolved in a low boiling point liquid in a canister under pressure. Opening the valve releases a metered dose of liquid that is ejected into the atmosphere; the carrier liquid evaporates instantly leaving an aerosol of the drug that is inhaled. Until recently the vehicle has been a CFC (chlorofluorocarbon), but due to concerns over depletion of atmospheric ozone these are being replaced by hydrofluoroalkanes (HFAs), which are ozone friendly. This switch has introduced a noticeable change in the taste of some inhalers, but more importantly it has changed the bio-equivalence of inhaled glucocorticoids. HFA-based glucocorticoid inhalers are generally more potent than a CFC-based inhaler delivering the same dose at the lips (typically the efficacy is doubled).

To ensure optimal drug delivery, it is necessary to coordinate activation of the inhaler with inspiration and a final hold of breath. Many patients, especially the young and the elderly, find this very difficult and 'spacer' devices are often used between the inhaler and lips; these act as an aerosol reservoir and also reduce impaction of aerosol in the oropharynx. Topical deposition can cause local side-effects in the mouth, particularly candida with inhaled glucocorticoids; a spacer abolishes this problem.

Nebulisers convert a solution or suspension of drug into an aerosol. Jet nebulisers require a driving gas, usually air from a compressor unit for home use, or oxygen in hospital; the solution in the nebulising chamber is broken into droplets by the jet and the larger droplets are filtered off leaving the smaller ones to be inhaled. Ultrasonic nebulisers convert a solution into particles of uniform size by vibrations created by a piezo-electric crystal (which converts electricity into mechanical vibration). With either method the aerosol is delivered to the patient by a mouthpiece or facemask, so no coordination is called for, and the dose can be altered by changing the strength of the solution. Much larger doses can be administered by nebuliser than by pressurised aerosol.

Dry powder inhalers. The drug is formulated as a micronised powder and placed in a device, e.g. a spinhaler or diskhaler, from which it is inhaled. Patients can often use these when they fail with metered-dose aerosols. Inhalation of powder occasionally causes transient bronchoconstriction.

DRUG TREATMENT

This varies with the severity and type of asthma. It is a general rule that the effectiveness of changes in drug and dose should be monitored by serial measurements of the simple respiratory function tests such as peak expiratory flow rate (PEFR) or forced expiratory volume in 1 s (FEV_1). Neither the patient's feelings nor physical examination are alone sufficient to determine whether there is still room for improvement. When an asthmatic attack is severe, arterial blood gases must also be measured.

Constant and intermittent asthma

The 2003 British Thoracic Society guidelines recommend a five-step approach[9] (summarised in Fig. 27.1) to the drug management of chronic asthma. The scheme starts with a patient requiring occasional β_2-adrenoceptor agonist and follows an escalating plan of add-on anti-inflammatory treatment. Points to emphasise are:

1. Short-acting β_2-adrenoceptor agonists are used throughout as rescue therapy for acute symptoms.
2. Patients must be reviewed regularly as they can move up or down the scheme.

[9]British Thoracic Society 2003 Guidelines on the management of asthma. Thorax 58(Suppl 1). Online. Available: http://www.brit-thoracic.org.uk/Guidelinessince%201997_asthma_html.

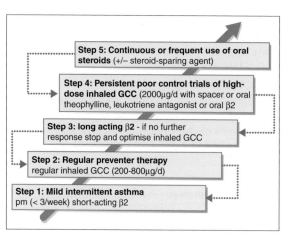

Fig. 27.1 A five-step management scheme for chronic asthma (British Thoracic Society 2003). β_2, β_2-Adrenoceptor agonist; GCC, glucocorticoid, e.g. beclometasone, budesonide or fluticasone.

3. Particular attention should be paid to inhaler technique, as this is an important cause of treatment failure. Patients who cannot manage inhaled therapy, even with the addition of a spacer device or use of a dry-powder device, can be given oral therapy, although this will be accompanied by more systemic side effects.

An inhaled β_2-adrenoceptor agonist should be used initially. *Salbutamol* or *terbutaline* (1–2 puffs up to four times daily) are typical short-acting β_2-adrenoceptor agonists whose bronchodilator effect is prompt in onset (within a few minutes) and lasts 4–6 h. *Salmeterol* and *eformoterol* have a much longer duration of effect (12–24 h), making them useful for nocturnal symptoms; they should not be used as 'rescue' bronchodilator (salmeterol in particular, because its bronchodilating action takes 15–30 min to emerge) nor as a replacement for inhaled glucocorticoid (see Step 3). β_2-Adrenoceptor agonists all cause dose-dependent tremor especially if given orally rather than inhaled.

Anti-inflammatory agents can commence either with *sodium cromoglicate* or low-dose inhaled glucocorticoid (Step 2). The inhaled glucocorticoids in current use (*beclometasone, budesonide* and *fluticasone*) are characterised by low oral bio-availability because of high first-pass metabolism in the liver (almost 100% for fluticasone). This property is important, as it minimises the systemic effects of inhaled glucocorticoid, 80–90% of which is actually

swallowed. Precisely for this reason, prednisolone or hydrocortisone would have less advantage (over oral administration) if inhaled, because they are absorbed from the gut and enter the circulation with relatively little pre-systemic metabolism. Low-dose inhaled glucocorticoids also exhibit higher lipid solubility and potency than those usually administered orally. Potency (the physical mass of drug in relation to its effect, see p. 79) is generally unimportant in comparisons of oral drugs, but is essential for locally administered drugs.

Inhaled glucocorticoids are generally safe at low doses. Topical effects (oral candida and hoarseness) are eliminated by using a spacer device and rinsing the mouth. High doses (>2000 micrograms/day) are reported to carry a slightly increased risk of cataract and glaucoma; this may reflect local aerosol deposition rather than a true systemic effect. Bone turnover is also increased in adults, suggesting a long-term risk of accelerated osteoporosis, and bone growth may be reduced in children (although evidence indicates that normal adult height can be attained[10]). Therefore, it is important that patients are maintained on the minimum dose of inhaled glucocorticoid necessary for symptom control.

Oral prednisolone is very effective for severe exacerbations and short courses (e.g. 30 mg daily for 5–7 days) are frequently given. Provided symptoms and peak flows respond promptly, more prolonged courses or prolonged reduction of dose is unnecessary. When oral glucocorticoids are used long term (Step 5), doses should be adjusted much more slowly. Adverse corticosteroid effects may also be minimised by administering a single morning dose to coincide with the normal peak cortisol concentration (and thus the least suppression of feedback to the hypothalamic–adrenal axis). This is possible because of the long duration of their biological effect (18–36 h) compared with plasma $t_{1/2}$ (3 h for prednisolone). Morning dosing with inhaled glucocorticoid may also have a prednisolone-sparing effect. Some patients may get further prednisolone-sparing by addition of nebulised high-dose budesonide, 1–2 mg b.d. or fluticasone 500 micrograms b.d.

---

[10]Agertoft L, Pedersen S 2000 Effect of long-term treatment with inhaled budesonide on adult height in children with asthma. New England Journal of Medicine 343:1064–1069.

Chest infections in asthma

Antimicrobials are over-prescribed for exacerbations of asthma. Respiratory tract infections do cause increased airflow obstruction and bronchial hyperresponsiveness, but viral not bacterial pathogens are the commonest culprits. Antimicrobials should be prescribed only if there is high suspicion of a bacterial respiratory tract infection, e.g. purulent sputum. Note that macrolide antibiotics, such as erythromycin and clarithromycin, interfere with theophylline metabolism.

Acute severe asthma ('status asthmaticus')

This is a life-threatening emergency requiring rapid aggressive treatment. The airways may become refractory to β_2-adrenoceptor agonists after 36–48 h, partly for pharmacological reasons (possibly receptor desensitisation) and partly due to the prolonged respiratory acidosis. The mucous plugs, which are the hallmark of the condition, may also prevent inhaled drugs from reaching the distal airways.

The following lists, with some explanation, the recommendations of the British Thoracic Society[9] for managing acute severe asthma:

Immediate treatment

- *Oxygen* by mask (humidified, to help liquefy mucus). Carbon dioxide narcosis is rare in asthma and 60% can be used if the diagnosis is not in doubt. In older patients, or when there is any concern about chronic carbon dioxide retention, start with 28% oxygen and to check that the Pa_{CO_2} has not risen before delivering 35% oxygen.
- *Salbutamol* by nebuliser in a dose of 2.5–5 mg over about 3 min, repeated in 15 min. Terbutaline 5–10 mg is an alternative.
- *Prednisolone* 30–60 mg p.o. or hydrocortisone 100 mg i.v.
- *Avoid sedation* of any kind.
- Chest radiography is required to exclude pneumothorax.

If life-threatening features are present (absent breath sounds, cyanosis, bradycardia, exhausted appearance, PEFR <33% predicted or best, arterial oxygen saturation of <92%):

- Ipratropium 0.5 mg should be added to the nebulised β_2 agonist.

- Consider i.v. magnesium sulphate (1.2–2 g over 20 min).[11]
- Alert the intensive care unit.

Subsequent management. If the patient is *improving*, continue:

- 40–60% oxygen.
- Prednisolone 30–60 mg daily or hydrocortisone 100–200 mg 6-hourly.
- Nebulised salbutamol or terbutaline 4-hourly.

If the patient is *not improving* after 15–30 min:

- Continue oxygen and glucocorticoid.
- Give *nebulised* β_2-adrenoceptor agonist more frequently, e.g. salbutamol up to 10 mg/h.
- Add ipratropium 0.5 mg to nebuliser and repeat 6-hourly until patient is improving.

If the patient is *still not improving*:

- Consider intravenous infusion of aminophylline (0.9 micrograms/kg/min)[11]; or
- Consider as an alternative *intravenous* β_2-adrenoceptor agonist (as above), e.g. salbutamol 250 micrograms over 10 min, then up to 20 micrograms/min as an infusion (as nebulised salbutamol may not be reaching the distal airways).
- Contact the intensive care unit to discuss intubation and mechanical ventilation.

Monitoring response to treatment

- By peak expiratory flow rate (PEFR) every 15–30 min.
- Oxygen saturation: maintain >92%.
- Repeat blood gas measurements if initial Pa_{O_2} <8 kPa (60 mmHg) and/or initial Pa_{CO_2} is normal or raised (the tachypnoea is expected to reduce Pa_{CO_2} in most patients).

Treatment in intensive care unit. Transfer (accompanied by doctor with facilities for intubation) is required if:

---

[11]This intervention is generally safe but not proven to affect outcome. The British Thoracic Society guideline no longer recommends intravenous aminophylline without consultation with a senior physician. Doubtless, this reflects an equal lack of evidence base for benefit and the very clear potential for harm if given to patients already taking oral theophyllines.

- any of the above deteriorates, despite maximal treatment
- the patient becomes exhausted, drowsy, or confused
- coma or respiratory arrest occurs.

Treatment at discharge from hospital. Patients should:

- continue high-dose inhaled glucocorticoid and complete course of oral prednisolone
- be instructed to monitor their own PEFR and not to reduce dose if the PEFR falls, or there is a recurrence of early morning dipping in the reading (patients should not generally be discharged until there is less than 25% diurnal variation in PEFR readings).

Warnings

Asthma may be precipitated by β-adrenoceptor blockade and the use of β-adrenoceptor antagonists is *contraindicated* in asthmatics; fatal asthma has been precipitated by β-blocker eye-drops, even allegedly β_1-selective agents.

Overuse of β_2-adrenergic agonists is dangerous. In the mid-1960s, there was an epidemic of sudden deaths in young asthmatics outside hospital. It was associated with the introduction of a high-dose, metered aerosol of isoprenaline (β_1 and β_2 agonist); it did not occur in countries where the high concentration was not marketed.[12] The epidemic declined in Britain when the profession was warned, and the aerosols were restricted to prescription only. Though the relationship between the use of β_2-receptor agonists and death is presumed to be causal, the actual mechanism of death is uncertain; overdose causing cardiac arrhythmia is not the sole factor. The subsequent development of selective β_2-receptor agonists was a contribution to safety, but a review in New Zealand during the 1980s found that the use of fenoterol (β_2 selective) by metered-dose inhalation was associated with increased risk of death in severe asthma,[13] and later analysis concluded that it was the most likely cause.[14] A further cause for

concern comes from a meta-analysis of 19 clinical trials which concluded that *long-acting* β agonists increased severe and life-threatening asthma exacerbations, as well as asthma-related deaths.[15]

CHRONIC OBSTRUCTIVE PULMONARY DISEASE (COPD)

Whereas asthma is characterised by *reversible* airways obstruction and bronchial hyperreactivity, COPD is characterised by *incompletely reversible* airways obstruction and *mucus hypersecretion*; it is predominantly a disease of the smaller airways. Nevertheless, distinguishing the two can be difficult in some patients,, and one view is that asthma predisposes smokers to COPD (the Dutch hypothesis). In practice, even though – indeed precisely because – most of the airway obstruction is fixed in COPD, it is important to maximise the reversible component. This can be assessed by measuring FEV_1 (forced expiratory volume in 1 s) before and after a course of oral prednisolone, e.g. at least 30 mg/day for 2 weeks; reversibility is arbitrarily defined as a rise in FEV_1 of more than 15% (and greater than 200 mL). An important caveat is that patients' symptoms sometimes improve despite little or no demonstrable reversibility, because FEV_1 measures large airways function, and in COPD mainly the small airways are affected.

Drugs used to treat COPD are exactly as for asthma, except that antimuscarinics, such as *ipratropium* or the longer-acting *tiotropium*, are often more effective bronchodilators than β_2 agonists. Patients with reversible airways obstruction should also receive an inhaled glucocorticoid and its combination with a long-acting β_2 agonist may improve control, especially in moderate or severe disease (FEV_1 <50% predicted), e.g. fluticasone + salmeterol (Seretide). This strategy is designed to reduce the frequency of disease exacerbations rather than affect the decline in lung function per se.[16]

[12]Stolley P D 1972 Why the United States was spared an epidemic of deaths due to asthma. American Review of Respiratory Diseases 105:833–890.

[13]Crane J, Pearce N, Flatt A, Burgess C, Jackson R 1989 Prescribed fenoterol and death from asthma in New Zealand: case control study. Lancet i:917–922.

[14]Pearce N, Beasley R, Crane J, Burgess C, Jackson R 1995 End of the New Zealand asthma mortality epidemic. Lancet 345:41–44.

[15]Salpeter S R, Buckley N S, Ormiston T M et al 2006 Meta-analysis: effect of long-acting β agonists on severe asthma exacerbations and asthma-related deaths. Annals of Internal Medicine 144:901–912.

[16]A trial in patients without reversibility found that inhaled glucocorticoid had no effect on the decline in their lung function (Pauwels R A, Lofdahl C G, Laitinen L A et al 1999 Long-term treatment with inhaled budesonide in persons with mild chronic obstructive pulmonary disease who continue smoking. New England Journal of Medicine 340:1948–1953).

A theophylline may also be effective in patients with severe disease, but requires special care in the elderly, including monitoring of plasma theophylline. Mucolytic drugs reduce acute episodes of COPD and days of illness; they are best reserved for patients with recurrent, prolonged or severe exacerbations of the disease. Quitting smoking remains the only action of proven benefit in preserving lung function in COPD.

Long-term oxygen therapy improves survival in hypoxic patients. It is indicated when:

- Pa_{O_2} is less than 7.3 kPa (56 mmHg) when stabilised on optimal medical treatment.
- Pa_{O_2} is 7.3–8.0 kPa and there is evidence of right-sided cardiac failure (cor pulmonale).

Summary

- Asthma is characterised by hypersensitivity to the endogenous bronchoconstrictors, acetylcholine and histamine, and by reversible obstruction of the airways.
- Drugs that block the actions of acetylcholine and histamine are weak or ineffective in the treatment of asthma.
- Most antiasthma treatment is therefore aimed either at reducing release of inflammatory cytokines (glucocorticoids and sodium cromoglicate) or at direct bronchodilatation by stimulation of the bronchial β_2 adrenoceptors.
- Aggressive use of glucocorticoids, especially by the inhaled route, is the keystone of the modern stepped approach to asthma management.
- Antihistamines conventionally refer to antagonists of the H_1 receptor, and have wide applications in the treatment of allergic disorders, and in anaphylaxis.
- The principal adverse effect of older first-generation antihistamines, sedation, is avoided by use of newer second-generation drugs which do not enter the CNS.
- Smoking cessation and long-term treatment with oxygen are the only interventions that are known to improve survival in chronic obstructive pulmonary disease.

GUIDE TO FURTHER READING

Devereux G 2006 ABC of chronic obstructive pulmonary disease. Definition, epidemiology, and risk factors. British Medical Journal 332:1142–1144 (the first in a series of 12 weekly articles on the subject)

Hendeles L, Colice G L, Meyer R J 2007 Withdrawal of albuterol inhalers containing chlorofluorocarbon propellants. New England Journal of Medicine 356:1344–1351

Holgate S T 2004 The epidemic of asthma and allergy. Journal of the Royal Society of Medicine 97:103–110

Holgate S T, Polosa R 2006 The mechanisms, diagnosis and management of severe asthma in adults. Lancet 368:780–793

Irwin R S, Madison J M 2000 The diagnosis and treatment of cough. New England Journal of Medicine 343(23):1715–1721

Kay A B 2001 Allergy and allergic diseases. New England Journal of Medicine 344:30–37 (part I); 109–113 (part 2)

National Institute for Clinical Excellence (NICE) 2004 Management of chronic obstructive pulmonary disease in adults in primary and secondary care. Clinical Guideline. Online. Available: http://www.nice.org.uk/pdf/CG012_niceguideline.pdf

O'Byrne P M, Parameswaran K 2006 Pharmacological management of mild or moderate persistent asthma. Lancet 368:794–803

Plaut M, Valentine M D 2005 Allergic rhinitis. New England Journal of Medicine 353:1934–1944

Poole P J, Black P N 2001 Oral mucolytic drugs for exacerbations of chronic obstructive pulmonary disease. British Medical Journal 322:1271–1273

Reynolds S M, Mackenzie A J, Spina D, Page C P 2004 The pharmacology of cough. Trends in Pharmacological Sciences 25:569–576

Simons F E R 2004 Advances in H_1-antihistamines. New England Journal of Medicine 351:2203–2217

Wedzicha J A, Muir J F 2002 Non-invasive ventilation in chronic obstructive pulmonary disease, bronchiectasis and cystic fibrosis. European Respiratory Journal 20(3):777–784

Weir E K, López-Barneo J, Buckler K J, Archer S L 2005 Acute oxygen-sensing mechanisms. New England Journal of Medicine 353(19):2042–2055

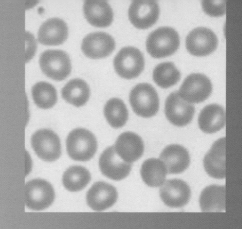

Section 6

BLOOD AND NEOPLASTIC DISEASE

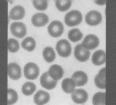

28

Drugs and haemostasis

SYNOPSIS

Occlusive vascular disease is a major cause of morbidity and mortality. There is now a better understanding of the mechanisms by which the haemostatic system maintains blood in a fluid state within vessels yet forms a solid plug when a vessel is breached, and of the ways in which haemostasis may be altered by drugs to prevent or reverse (lyse) pathological thrombosis.

- Coagulation system: the mode of action of drugs that promote coagulation and that prevent it (anticoagulants) and their uses
- Fibrinolytic system: the mode of action of drugs that promote fibrinolysis (fibrinolytics) and their uses to lyse arterial and venous thrombi (thrombolysis)
- Platelets: the ways that drugs that inhibit platelet activity benefit arterial disease

INTRODUCTION

It is essential that blood remains fluid within the circulation but clots at sites of vascular injury. The haemostatic system maintains the integrity of the vascular tree through a complex network of cellular, ligand–receptor and enzymatic interactions. In normal circumstances there is an equilibrium between the natural coagulant–anticoagulant and fibrinolytic–antifibrinolytic systems. In response to endothelial damage, there is rapid molecular switching to thrombin generation and antifibrinolysis at the site of injury, and enhanced natural anticoagulant activity and fibrinolytic activity at areas of adjacent healthy intact endothelium. Regulation of the haemostatic network in such a way results in localised thrombus formation with minimal loss of vascular patency.

Pathological disruption of the network results in thrombosis or bleeding, or both; the extreme example of haemostatic pathology is a complete breakdown as occurs in disseminated intravascular coagulation (DIC). Drugs that modulate the haemostatic system are valuable in the management of bleeding and thrombotic disorders. Drugs are classified according to the component of the system they affect and their perceived primary mode of action.

THE COAGULATION SYSTEM

Coagulation initiates with *tissue factor* (TF), a cell membrane protein that binds activated factor VII (indicated by adding the letter 'a', i.e. factor VIIa). Although there is a small fraction of circulating factor VII in the activated state, it has little or no enzymatic activity until it is bound to TF. Most non-vascular cells express TF in a constitutive[1] fashion, whereas de novo TF synthesis can be induced in monocytes and damaged endothelial cells. Injury to the arterial or venous wall exposes extravascular TF-expressing cells to blood. Lipid-laden macrophages in the core of atherosclerotic plaques are particularly rich in TF, thereby explaining the propensity for thrombus formation at sites of plaque disruption. Once bound to TF, factor VIIa activates factor IX and factor X (to IXa and Xa respectively) leading to thrombin generation and clot formation (Fig. 28.1).

The classical view of blood coagulation with separate 'extrinsic' and 'intrinsic' pathways initiated by either TF or contact with an anionic surface does not reflect physiological coagulation. It is now evident that coagulation does not occur as linear sequential enzyme activation pathways but rather by a network of simultaneous interactions, which undergo regulation and modulation during the thrombin generation process itself.

In the current model, blood coagulation starts with a transient release of *tissue factor* by damaged

---

[1]Genetically controlled by a constantly active promoter.

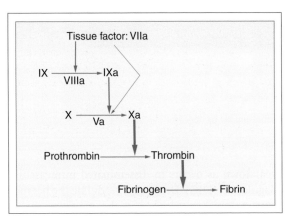

Fig. 28.1 The blood coagulation network (see text).

endothelium, resulting in the formation of sub-nanomolar amounts of *thrombin* via TF/VIIa-driven Xa formation (extrinsic-tenase). The initial thrombin activity is necessary to prime the system for a full thrombin explosion. Tissue factor pathway inhibitor (TFPI) rapidly shuts down this priming pathway and the full thrombin explosion is then dependent on Xa formation. Factor IXa-driven Xa formation (intrinsic-tenase) is amplified by the thrombin explosion itself, as thrombin forms a positive feedback loop by activating factor XIa (not shown in Fig. 28.1), which converts more IX to IXa.

Thrombin converts soluble fibrinogen into insoluble fibrin monomers, which spontaneously polymerise to form the fibrin mesh that is then stabilised and cross-linked by activated factor XIII (factor XIIIa), a thrombin-activated transglutaminase. Thrombin amplifies its own generation by:

- feedback activation of factor V and factor VIII
- activating platelet-bound factor XI, thereby leading to further factor Xa generation
- activating cells that provide the phospholipid surface required for assembly of the macromolecular enzymatic complexes.

PROCOAGULANT DRUGS

VITAMIN K

Vitamin K ('Koagulation' vitamin) is essential for normal coagulation. It occurs naturally in two forms. Vitamin K_1 (phylloquinone) is widely distributed in plants and K_2 includes vitamin synthesised in the alimentary tract by bacteria, e.g. *Escherichia coli* (menaquinones). Leafy green vegetables are a good

source of vitamin K_1. Bile is required for the absorption of the natural forms of vitamin K, which are fat soluble. The storage pool of vitamin K is modest and can be exhausted in 1 week, although gut flora will maintain suboptimal production of vitamin K dependent proteins. A synthetic analogue, *menadione* (K_3), is water soluble.

Vitamin K is necessary for the final stage in the synthesis of six coagulation-related proteins in the liver: the *coagulant* factors II (prothrombin), VII, IX and X, and *anticoagulant* regulatory proteins, proteins C and S. The vitamin allows γ-carboxylation of glutamic acid residues in their structure; this permits calcium to bind to the molecule, mediating the conformational change required for enzymatic activity, and binding to negatively charged phospholipid surfaces, e.g. platelets. Membrane binding is required for full enzymatic potential.

During γ-carboxylation of the proteins, the *reduced* and *active* form of vitamin KH_2, converts to an epoxide, an *oxidation* product. Subsequently vitamin K epoxide reductase and vitamin K reductase convert oxidised vitamin K back to the active vitamin K, i.e. there exists an interconversion cycle between vitamin K epoxide and reduced vitamin K (the vitamin K cycle; Fig. 28.2).

When the vitamin is deficient or where drugs inhibit its action, the coagulation proteins produced are unable to associate with calcium in order to form the necessary three-dimensional configuration and associated membrane-binding properties that are required for full enzymatic activity. Their physiologically critical binding to membrane surfaces

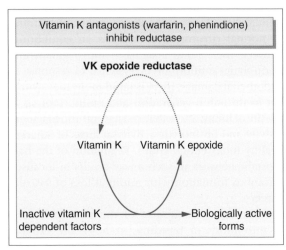

Fig. 28.2 The vitamin K cycle (see text)

fails to occur, and this impairs the coagulation mechanism. These proteins are called 'proteins induced in vitamin K absence' or PIVKAs.

Oral vitamin K antagonists exert an anticoagulant effect by interrupting the vitamin K cycle. There are two classes of drugs: the *coumarins*, including warfarin and acenocoumarol, and the *indanediones* such as phenindione. The anticoagulant effect of oral vitamin K antagonists is expressed as the International Normalised Ratio (INR).

Vitamin K deficiency may arise from:

- dietary deficiency
- bile failing to enter the intestine, e.g. obstructive jaundice or biliary fistula
- malabsorption syndromes, e.g. coeliac disease, or after extensive small intestinal resection
- reduced alimentary tract flora, e.g. in newborn infants and rarely after broad-spectrum antibiotics.

The following preparations of vitamin K are available:

Phytomenadione (Konakion), the naturally occurring fat-soluble vitamin K_1, acts within about 12 h and should reduce the anticoagulant effect of warfarin within 24–48 h when given orally in a dose of 5–10 mg. The intravenous formulation finds use in emergency and will begin to reverse a vitamin K-deficient coagulopathy by 6 h in a patient with normal liver function. Administer it slowly, lest an anaphylactoid reaction should occur: facial flushing, sweating, fever, chest tightness, cyanosis and peripheral vascular collapse. Otherwise phytomenadione may be given intramuscularly, subcutaneously or orally. The preferred route depends on the degree of coagulopathy and urgency of correcting the haemorrhagic tendency. The intramuscular route should not be used if the INR is increased, as local intramuscular haemorrhage may be induced; subcutaneous absorption is variable and, despite the risk of allergic reaction, the intravenous route ensures rapid delivery.

Menadiol sodium phosphate (vitamin K_3), the synthetic analogue of vitamin K, being water soluble, is preferred in intestinal malabsorption or in states in which bile flow is deficient. The main disadvantage is that it takes 24 h to act, but its effect lasts for several days. The dose is 5–40 mg daily, orally. Menadiol sodium phosphate in moderate doses causes haemolytic anaemia and, for this reason, neonates should not receive it, especially those that are deficient in glucose 6-phosphate dehydrogenase; their immature livers are unable to cope with the heavy bilirubin load and there is danger of kernicterus.

Fat-soluble analogues of vitamin K that are available in some countries include acetomenaphthone and menaphthone.

Vitamin K is used to treat:

- Haemorrhage or threatened bleeding due to the coumarin or indanedione anticoagulants. Phytomenadione is preferred for its more rapid action; dosage regimens vary according to the degree of urgency and the original indication for anticoagulation.
- Haemorrhagic disease of the newborn, which develops usually between 2 and 7 days, and late haemorrhagic disease that presents at 6–7 months. Prophylaxis is recommended during the period of vulnerability with vitamin K (phytomenadione, as Konakion) 1 mg by single i.m. injection at birth. Alternatively, give vitamin K by mouth as two doses of a colloidal (mixed micelle) preparation of phytomenadione in the first week. Breast-fed babies should receive a further 2 mg at 1 month of age. Formula-fed babies do not need this last supplement as the formula contains vitamin K. Fears that intramuscular vitamin K might cause childhood cancer have been dispelled.
- Hypoprothrombinaemia due to intestinal malabsorption syndromes; menadiol sodium phosphate should be used as it is water soluble.

COAGULATION FACTOR CONCENTRATES

Bleeding due to deficiency of specific coagulation factors is treated by either elevating the deficient factor, e.g. treatment of mild factor VIII deficiency with desmopressin (see below), or replacement of the missing factor. Recombinant factor VIII and IX are now available in some countries for patients with congenital deficiency of these factors. For patients with rare coagulation factor deficiencies or multiple acquired deficiencies (liver disease, massive blood loss with dilutional coagulopathy or DIC), replacement therapy still requires human-derived fresh frozen plasma (FFP).

Solvent–detergent virally inactivated FFP (Octaplas) is currently given to selected patients in the UK, for example those with rare bleeding disorders and patients with thrombotic thrombocytopenic purpura who require repeated exposure to FFP. Methylene blue-treated single donor unit FFP is also available as a virally inactivated product.

Use of coagulation factor concentrates

Management of haemophilia A and haemophilia B (deficiency of factor VIII and IX respectively) requires special expertise but the following points are notable:

- Superficial haemorrhage sometimes responds to local pressure.
- Minor bleeding can arrest with plasma factor concentrations of 25–30 units/dL, but severe bleeding requires at least 50 units/dL and surgical procedures or life-threatening haemorrhage require 75–100 units/dL by infusion of factor concentrate.
- In haemophilia A, *factor VIII concentrate* ($t_{1/2}$ 8–12 h) is used for bleeding that is more than minor. Repeat dosing is necessary to maintain haemostatic levels.
- *Factor IX* ($t_{1/2}$ 18–24 h) is used for bleeding that is more than minor in haemophilia B (Christmas disease).
- The speed of recovery of the affected joint or resolution of a haematoma determines the duration of therapy. After surgery, 7–14 days of replacement therapy is required to ensure adequate wound healing and to prevent secondary haemorrhage.
- Primary prophylaxis with factor concentrates two or three times weekly at doses sufficient to keep the factor above 1–2 units/dL reduces bleeding and hence chronic haemophilic arthropathy.

FEIBA is a human donor-derived factor concentrate for patients with inhibitory antibodies to factor VIII or IX. It contains a mixture of coagulation factors and produces thrombin generation even in the presence of inhibitors to factor VIII or IX.

Recombinant factor VIIa (NovoSeven) is effective for patients with inhibitory antibodies to factor VIII or IX or deficiency of factor VII. A pure synthetic activated coagulation factor, it generates thrombin even in the presence of inhibitors to factor VIII or IX. Owing to its short duration of action, three doses are usually necessary at 2-h intervals. It is used off licence for life-threatening haemorrhage that is not amenable to surgery.

DESMOPRESSIN (DDAVP)

Desmopressin is a vasopressin analogue that increases the plasma concentrations of factor VIII and von Willebrand factor, and directly activates platelets. DDAVP is usually given subcutaneously or intravenously, but unwanted effects (headache, flushing and tachycardia) are less severe after subcutaneous use. A concentrated form is available for intranasal use.

DDAVP is useful for treating patients with mild haemophilia A and von Willebrand's disease, especially for short-term therapy. For dental extraction, a single injection of 0.3 micrograms/kg 1–2 h before surgery, combined with the oral antifibrinolytic drug, tranexamic acid, for 5–7 days after the procedure (see Antifibrinolytic drugs, p. 524), will produce normal haemostasis and prevent secondary haemorrhage.

Patients with Type 3 (severe) or some forms of Type 2 von Willebrand's disease (VWD) and some with Type 1 with severe haemorrhage, or patients who require major surgery, need *replacement* therapy with human-derived intermediate-purity factor VIII concentrate known to contain high molecular weight von Willebrand factor (vWF) multimers. The larger multimers are required for normal haemostatic function. Cryoprecipitate that is rich in factor VIII and vWF is not virally inactivated and should no longer be used routinely for patients with VWD or mild to moderate factor VIII deficiency.

DDAVP shortens the bleeding time in patients with renal or liver failure.

Adverse effects. Water retention and hyponatraemia may complicate therapy and thus very young children must not receive DDAVP. Fluid intake should not exceed 1 L in the 24 h following treatment and with repeated doses the plasma sodium should be monitored. Tachyphylaxis (progressively diminishing response to the same dose) can occur.

OTHER AGENTS

Adrenaline (epinephrine) is effective as a topical agent for epistaxis, applied in ribbon gauze that is packed into the nostril; haemorrhage being arrested by local vasoconstriction.

Fibrin glue consists of fibrinogen and thrombin contained in two syringes, the tips of which form a common port that allows delivery of the two components to a bleeding point where fibrinogen converts to fibrin at a rate determined by the concentration of thrombin. Fibrin glue can be used to secure surgical haemostasis, e.g. on a large raw surface, and to prevent external oozing of blood in patients with haemophilia (see also above).

Sclerosing agents produce inflammation and thrombosis in veins to induce permanent obliteration, e.g. ethanolamine oleate injection, sodium tetradecyl sulphate (given intravenously for varicose veins) and oily phenol injection (given submucosaly for haemorrhoids). Local reactions and tissue necrosis may occur.

ANTICOAGULANT DRUGS

Anticoagulant drugs act principally to reduce the activity of *thrombin*, the enzyme that is mainly responsible for blood clotting. The following discussion will show that drugs do so by:

- *limiting thrombin generation*, either as a result of inhibiting other proteases (clotting factors) involved in its generation or by reducing the activity of zymogens (the precursor inactive forms of the enzymes); or
- *inhibiting (neutralising) thrombin activity*, either directly or indirectly, depending on whether or not they activate the natural serpin-dependent anticoagulant pathway.[2]

WARFARIN

Warfarin and other oral vitamin K antagonists (VKAs) reduce the activity of zymogens.

Mode of action. During the γ-carboxylation of factors II (prothrombin), VII, IX and X (and also the natural anticoagulant proteins C and S), active vitamin K (KH_2) is oxidised to an epoxide and must be reduced by the enzymes vitamin K epoxide reductase and vitamin K reductase to become active again (see the vitamin K cycle, p. 514).

Coumarins[3] are structurally similar to vitamin K and competitively inhibit vitamin K epoxide reductase and vitamin K reductase, so limiting availability of the active reduced form of the vitamin to form coagulant (and anticoagulant) proteins. The overall result is a shift in haemostatic balance in favour of anticoagulation because of the accumulation of clotting proteins with absent or decreased γ-carboxylation sites (PIVKAs).[4]

This shift does not take place until functioning vitamin K-dependent proteins, made before the drug was administered, have been cleared from the circulation. The process occurs at different rates for individual coagulation factors (VII $t_{1/2}$ 6 h, IX and X $t_{1/2}$ 18–24 h, prothrombin $t_{1/2}$ 72 h). The *anticoagulant* proteins C and S have a shorter $t_{1/2}$ than the *procoagulant* proteins and their more rapid decline in concentration may create a *transient hypercoagulable state*. This can be dangerous in individuals with inherited protein C or S deficiency who may develop thrombotic skin necrosis during initiation of oral anticoagulant therapy with vitamin K antagonists. Anticoagulation with heparin until the effect of warfarin is well established reduces the risk of skin necrosis when rapid induction of anticoagulation is required.

The therapeutic anticoagulant effect of warfarin develops only after 4–5 days. Furthermore, the INR does not reliably reflect anticoagulant protection during this initial phase, as the vitamin K-dependent factors diminish at different rates and the INR is particularly sensitive to the level of factor VII, which is not a principal determinant of thrombotic or bleeding risk.

Pharmacokinetics. Warfarin is readily absorbed from the gastrointestinal tract and, like all the current oral anticoagulants, is more than 90% bound to

---

[2]Serpin: serine protease inhibitors. Antithrombin is the principal serpin involved in regulating coagulation.

[3]Coumarins are present in many plants and are important in the perfume industry; the smell of new mown hay and grass is due to coumarins. Yellow Sweet Clover (King's Clover) is rich in coumarins and was used as a herbal medicine to reduce inflammation. It was a constituent of an ointment to 'cool and dry and comfort the Membre' of King Henry VIII of England, who enjoyed a particularly active sexual life (Cutler T 2003 College Commentary, May/June. Royal College of Physicians, London, p. 23). The discovery of coumarins as anticoagulants dates from investigation of an unexplained haemorrhagic disease of cattle that had eaten mouldy sweet clover. Subsequent research at the University of Wisconsin, USA, culminated in the isolation of the causative agent, dicoumarol (Stahmann M A, Huebner C F, Link K P 1941 Journal of Biological Chemistry 138:513–527).

[4]Warfarin is ten times more potent than dicoumarol and was originally used as a rodenticide. Its name is derived from the patent holder, Wisconsin Alumni Research Foundation, with the suffix from coumarin.

plasma proteins. Metabolism in the liver terminates its action. Warfarin ($t_{1/2}$ 36 h) is a racemic mixture of approximately equal amounts of two isomers, S ($t_{1/2}$ 27 h) and R ($t_{1/2}$ 40 h) warfarin, i.e. it is in effect two drugs. S warfarin is four times more potent than R warfarin. The isomers respond differently to drugs that interact with warfarin.

Uses. Warfarin is the oral anticoagulant of choice, for it is reliably effective and has the lowest incidence of adverse effects. Because of the delay in onset of anticoagulant effect with oral vitamin K antagonists (VKAs) there is a need for an immediate-acting anticoagulant, such as a heparin, in the first few days of therapy if rapid anticoagulation is required.

The response to warfarin, and other coumarins, varies within and between individuals and therefore regular monitoring of dose is essential. The pharmacokinetics (absorption and metabolism) and pharmacodynamics (haemostatic effect) are influenced by vitamin K intake and absorption, by heritable functional polymorphisms affecting metabolism such as P450 CYP2C9 polymorphisms, by rates of synthesis and clearance of coagulation proteins, and by drugs. The effectiveness of anticoagulant therapy with oral VKAs is determined by the INR (International Normalised Ratio), a standardised method derived from the prothrombin time that permits comparison between different laboratories.

Dose. There is much inter-individual variation in dose requirements. It is usual to initiate therapy with 10-mg doses, depending on the daily INR, with the maintenance dose then adjusted according to the INR using an established protocol.

The level of anticoagulation matches the perceived risk of thrombosis (see below). The target INR for deep vein thrombosis (DVT) is 2.5 (typical range 2.0–3.0).

Adverse effects. The major complication of treatment with warfarin is *bleeding*. As well as a risk of haemorrhage after trauma or surgery, spontaneous bleeding may occur. Each year a patient is on treatment there is a 1 in 20 (5%) risk of minor haemorrhage. The annual risk of major bleeding is 1 in 100, of which one-quarter are fatal. The risk of bleeding relates to the INR, not the dose of warfarin: the higher the INR, the greater the chance of bleeding. The risk of over-anticoagulation increases with intercurrent illness and interaction with other drugs,

and is more likely in patients whose anticoagulant control is unstable. Therefore, it is essential to:

- maintain as stable a level of anticoagulation as possible
- adopt the lowest effective target INR
- educate patients about risk, particularly that associated with additional drug use.

Warfarin is a small molecule that crosses the placenta and can produce harmful effects in the developing fetus.

Warfarin embryopathy develops only after exposure to oral anticoagulant during the first trimester of pregnancy. The most common feature is chondrodysplasia punctata, characterised by abnormal cartilage and bone formation (with stippling of epiphyses visible on radiography) in vertebrae and femur, and the bones of the hands and feet during infancy and early childhood; these disappear with age (warfarin is not the only cause of this abnormality). Other less common skeletal abnormalities include nasal hypoplasia and hypertelorism (wide-set eyes).

Bleeding into the central nervous system is a danger throughout pregnancy but particularly at the time of delivery.

As a consequence of the above, warfarin is contraindicated in the first 6–12 weeks of pregnancy and should be replaced by heparin before the anticipated date of delivery, as the action of the latter drug can be terminated rapidly prior to the birth.

Withdrawal of oral anticoagulant therapy. The balance of evidence is that abrupt, as opposed to gradual, withdrawal of oral anticoagulant therapy does not of itself add to the risk of thromboembolism, for renewed synthesis of functional vitamin K-dependent clotting factors takes several days.

Reversal of anticoagulation can be gradual or rapid depending on the circumstances, i.e. from undue prolongation of INR to frank bleeding. Vitamin K 5–10 mg is usually adequate for complete reversal, oral administration being less rapid than intravenous. Immediate reversal is more readily achieved with a factor concentrate than fresh frozen plasma. Detailed guidance on corrective therapy in relation to the degree of over-anticoagulation is available, e.g. from the *British National Formulary*.

Drug interactions. Oral anticoagulant control must be precise for safety and efficacy. If a drug that alters the action of warfarin is essential, monitor the INR frequently and adjust the dose of warfarin during the period of institution of the new drug until a new stable therapeutic dose of warfarin results; careful monitoring is also needed on withdrawal of the interacting drug.

Analgesics. Avoid, if possible, non-steroidal anti-inflammatory drugs (NSAIDs) including aspirin because of their irritant effect on gastric mucosa and action on platelets. Paracetamol is acceptable but doses above 1.5 g/day may raise the INR. Dextropropoxyphene inhibits warfarin metabolism, and compounds that contain it, e.g. co-proxamol, should be avoided. Codeine, dihydrocodeine and combinations with paracetamol, e.g. co-dydramol, are preferred. Concomitant use of misoprostol with a NSAID may reduce the risk of gastric bleeding and a selective cyclo-oxygenase (COX)-2 inhibitor may be associated with a lower bleeding risk in patients taking oral anticoagulants.

Antimicrobials. Aztreonam, cefamandole, chloramphenicol, ciprofloxacin, co-trimoxazole, erythromycin, fluconazole, itraconazole, ketoconazole, metronidazole, miconazole, ofloxacin and sulphonamides (including co-trimoxazole) increase anticoagulant effect by mechanisms that include interference with warfarin or vitamin K metabolism. Rifampicin and griseofulvin induce relevant hepatic enzymes and accelerate warfarin metabolism, reducing its effect. Intensive broad-spectrum antibiotics, e.g. eradication regimens for *Helicobacter pylori*, may increase sensitivity to warfarin by reducing the intestinal flora that provide vitamin K.

Anticonvulsants. Carbamazepine, phenobarbital and primidone accelerate warfarin metabolism (by enzyme induction); the effect of phenytoin is variable. Clonazepam and sodium valproate are safe.

Antiarrhythmics. Amiodarone, propafenone and possibly quinidine potentiate the effect of warfarin and dose adjustment is required, but atropine, disopyramide and lidocaine do not interfere.

Antidepressants. Serotonin-reuptake inhibitors may enhance the effect of warfarin, but tricyclics may be used.

Gastrointestinal drugs. Avoid cimetidine and omeprazole, which inhibit the clearance of R warfarin, and sucralfate, which may impair its absorption. Ranitidine may be used. Most antacids are safe.

Lipid-lowering drugs. Fibrates, and some statins, enhance anticoagulant effect. Avoid colestyramine as it may impair the absorption of both warfarin and vitamin K.

Sex hormones and hormone antagonists. The hormone antagonists danazol, flutamide and tamoxifen enhance the effect of warfarin.

Sedatives and anxiolytics. Benzodiazepines may be used.

USES OF ORAL ANTICOAGULANT DRUGS

Oral anticoagulant drugs are used to prevent and treat venous thrombosis and pulmonary embolus, and to prevent arterial thromboemboli in patients with atrial fibrillation or cardiac disease, including mechanical heart valves. The British Society for Haematology publishes recommended target INRs and duration of therapy for different thrombotic disorders, available at http://www.bcshguidelines.com. The following are general indications:

- *Target INR 2.5* is appropriate for treatment of DVT; pulmonary embolism (PE); systemic embolism; prevention of venous thromboembolism in myocardial infarction; mitral stenosis with embolism; transient ischaemic attacks; atrial fibrillation; mechanical prosthetic aortic valves.
- *Target INR 3.5* is preferred for recurrent DVT and PE when already on warfarin with target of 2.5, arterial disease and some mechanical prosthetic mitral valves.
- At least 6 weeks' anticoagulation is recommended after calf vein thrombosis and at least 3 months after proximal DVT or PE. For patients with temporary risk factors and a low risk of recurrence, 3 months of treatment may be sufficient. For patients with idiopathic venous thromboembolism or permanent risk factors, at least 6 months' anticoagulation is usual.

SURGERY IN PATIENTS RECEIVING ORAL ANTICOAGULANT

Elective surgery. Warfarin is withdrawn 3–5 days before the operation and recommenced when the patient resumes oral intake; heparin (low molecular weight heparin [LMWH] or unfractionated heparin [UFH]; see below) provides cover in the intervening period. In patients with mechanical mitral prosthetic valves, LMWH or UFH is added when the INR is subtherapeutic.

Emergency surgery. Proceed as for bleeding (above).

Dental extractions. Anticoagulation may continue for patients whose INR is less than 4.0. The INR is measured no more than 72 h before the procedure to ensure that the INR will be less than 4.0 on the day of the extraction.

OTHER VITAMIN K ANTAGONISTS

Acenocoumarol (nicoumalone) is similar to warfarin but seldom used; the kidney eliminates it mainly in unchanged form.

Indanedione anticoagulants are rarely used because of allergic reactions unrelated to coagulation; phenindione is still available.

HEPARIN

A medical student, J McLean, working at Johns Hopkins Medical School in 1916, discovered heparin. Seeking to devote 1 year to physiological research, he was set to study 'the thromboplastic (clotting) substance in the body'. He found that extracts of brain, heart and liver accelerated clotting but that activity deteriorated during storage. To his surprise, the extract of liver that he had kept longest not only failed to accelerate but actually retarded clotting. His personal account states:

> After more tests and the preparation of other batches of heparophosphatide, I went one morning to the door of Dr. Howell's office, and standing there (he was seated at his desk), I said 'Dr. Howell, I have discovered antithrombin'. He was most skeptical. So I had the Deiner, John Schweinhant, bleed a cat. Into a small beaker full of its blood, I stirred all of a proven batch of heparophosphatides, and I placed this on Dr. Howell's laboratory table and asked him to call me when it clotted. It never did clot. [*It was heparin*][5]

Heparin is a sulphated mucopolysaccharide that is found in the secretory granules of mast cells and

is prepared commercially from porcine intestinal mucosa to give preparations that vary in molecular weight from 3000 to 30 000 Da (average 15 000 Da). It is the strongest organic acid in the body and in solution carries an electronegative charge. The low molecular weight heparins (LMWH, mean mol. wt 4000–6500 Da) are prepared from standard unfractionated (UF) heparin by a variety of chemical techniques. Commercial preparations contain different fractions and display different pharmacokinetics. Some currently available in the UK include *bemiparin, dalteparin, enoxaparin, reviparin* and *tinzaparin.*

Mode of action. Heparin depends for its anticoagulant action on the presence in plasma of a single-chain glycoprotein called *antithrombin* (formerly antithrombin III), a naturally occurring inhibitor of activated coagulation proteases (factors) that include thrombin, factor Xa and factor IXa. Heparin binds to antithrombin, inducing a conformational change that leads to rapid inhibition of the proteases of the coagulation pathway. In the presence of heparin, antithrombin becomes approximately 1000-fold more active and inhibition is essentially instantaneous. Following destruction of the proteases, the affinity of antithrombin for heparin falls; heparin then dissociates from the antithrombin–protease complex and catalyses further antithrombin–protease interactions.

Factor Xa is critical to thrombin generation (see Fig. 28.1) and heparin has the capacity to inhibit factor Xa in small quantities by virtue of a specific pentasaccharide sequence. This provides the rationale for using low-dose subcutaneous heparin to *prevent* thrombus formation.

LMWHs inhibit factor Xa at a dose similar to that for UFH, but have much less antithrombin activity, the principal action of conventional heparin. Fibrin formed in the circulation binds to thrombin and protects it from inactivation by the heparin–antithrombin complex; this may provide a further explanation for the higher doses of heparin needed to stop *extension* of a thrombus than to *prevent* it.

Fondaparinux is a synthetic pentasaccharide that inhibits factor Xa by an antithrombin-dependent mechanism. It finds use for prevention and treatment of venous thromboembolism in the same way as traditional LMWHs. The risk of HIT(T) (see below) is probably lower, but the risk of bleeding may be greater than that associated with LMWHs.

---

[5]McLean gives a fascinating account of his struggles to pay his way through medical school, as well as his discovery of heparin in: McLean J 1959 Circulation XIX:75.

Pharmacokinetics. Heparin is poorly absorbed from the gastrointestinal tract and is given intravenously or subcutaneously; once in the blood its effect is immediate. Heparin binds to several plasma proteins, to endothelial cells, and is taken up by reticuloendothelial cells; the kidney excretes a proportion. Because of these different mechanisms, elimination of heparin from the plasma involves a combination of zero- and first-order processes. The result is that the plasma biological effect $t_{1/2}$ alters disproportionately with dose, being 60 min after 75 units/kg and increasing to 150 min after 400 units/kg.

LMW heparins are less protein bound and have a predictable dose–response profile when administered subcutaneously or intravenously. They also have a longer $t_{1/2}$ than standard heparin preparations.

Monitoring heparin therapy. Control of standard heparin therapy is by the activated partial thromboplastin time (APTT), the target therapeutic range being 1.5–2.5 times the control. An alternative method is to measure the plasma concentration of heparin by anti-Xa assay. Therapeutic amounts of LMWH do not prolong the APTT and, because the pharmacokinetics are predictable, a safe and effective dose can be calculated without laboratory monitoring, using an algorithm that is adjusted for body-weight.

Adverse effects. Bleeding is the main acute complication of heparin therapy. Patients with impaired hepatic or renal function, with carcinoma, and those aged over 60 years are most at risk. An APTT ratio greater than 3 is associated with an increased risk of bleeding.

Heparin-induced thrombocytopenia (HIT), sometimes accompanied by *thrombosis* (HIT/T), is due to an autoantibody against heparin in association with platelet factor 4, which activates platelets. It occurs most commonly with heparin derived from bovine lung and is more common with UFHs than with LMWHs. Suspect HIT in any patient in whom the platelet count falls by 50% or more after starting heparin. It usually occurs after 5 days or more of heparin exposure (or sooner if the patient has previously been exposed to heparin). Thrombosis occurs in less than 1% of patients treated with LMWHs but is associated with a mortality and limb amputation rate in excess of 30%. Patients with HIT/T should discontinue all heparin (UF and LMW) and receive an alternative thrombin inhibitor, such as danaparoid or lepirudin. Warfarin

should not be commenced until there is adequate anticoagulation with one of these agents and the platelet count has returned to normal.

Osteoporosis may complicate long-term heparin exposure. It is dose related and most frequently observed during pregnancy. The relative risk between LMWHs is not yet established but it appears to be less than with UFHs.

Hypersensitivity reactions and skin necrosis (similar to that seen with warfarin) occur but are rare. Transient alopecia may occur.

Heparin reversal. Protamine, a protein obtained from fish sperm, immediately reverses the anticoagulant action of heparin. It is as strongly basic as heparin is acidic, which explains its rapid action. The effect of UFH is short lived, and reversal with protamine sulphate is seldom required except after extracorporeal perfusion for heart surgery. Protamine sulphate, 1 mg by slow intravenous injection, neutralises 80–100 units UFH. The quantity of heparin given and its expected $t_{1/2}$ determine the amount required but the maximum must not exceed 50 mg. Protamine itself has some anticoagulant effect and overdosage is to be avoided. Its effectiveness in patients treated with LMWH is unknown.

Use of heparin

Treatment of established venous thromboembolism. Patients with acute venous thromboembolism are treated safely and effectively with LMWH as outpatients. Large-scale studies demonstrate that outpatient treatment of acute DVT with unmonitored, body-weight-adjusted LMWH is as safe and effective as inpatient treatment with adjusted-dose i.v. UFH. Further trials confirm the safety and efficacy of LMWH therapy in acute PE.

The traditional regimen for standard UFH is a bolus i.v. injection of 5000 units (or 10 000 units in major PE) followed by a constant-rate i.v. infusion of 1000–2000 units/h. The APTT should be measured 6 h after starting therapy and the administration rate adjusted to keep it in the optimal therapeutic range of 1.5–2.5; this usually requires daily measurement of APTT.

Coincident with commencing heparin, patients usually start taking an oral vitamin K antagonist, typically warfarin in the UK. The INR is monitored and loading doses of VKA are given according to a validated loading protocol in order to minimise the risk of over-anticoagulation and bleeding. Ideally the INR should be measured daily during the first 4 days of loading with a VKA; guidance is available at http://www.bcshguidelines.com.

Prevention of venous thromboembolism. LMWHs are preferred for perioperative prophylaxis because of their convenience. They are as effective and safe as UFH at preventing venous thrombosis. Once-daily subcutaneous administration suffices, as their duration of action is longer than that of UFH and no laboratory monitoring is required.

If UFH is used, 5000 units should be given s.c. every 8 or 12 h without monitoring (this dose does not prolong the APTT), or in pregnancy 5000–10 000 units s.c. every 12 h with monitoring (except for pregnant women with prosthetic heart valves, for whom specialist monitoring is needed).

Cardiac disease. LMWHs are at least as effective as standard heparin for unstable angina. Patients undergoing angioplasty may also receive LMWHs.

Heparin is used to reduce the risk of venous thromboembolism, and the size of emboli from mural thrombi following acute myocardial infarction.

Peripheral arterial occlusion. In the acute phase following thrombosis or arterial embolism, heparin may prevent extension of a thrombus and hasten its recanalisation. Long-term antithrombotic therapy for patients with ischaemic peripheral vascular disease generally requires specific antiplatelet therapy (see p. 527).

OTHER ANTICOAGULANT DRUGS

Heparinoids

Danaparinoid sodium is a mixture of several types of non-heparin glycosaminoglycans extracted from pig intestinal mucosa (84% heparan sulphate). It is an effective anticoagulant for the treatment of DVT, prophylaxis in high-risk patients and treatment of patients with heparin-associated thrombocytopenia (HIT/T).

Hirudin, a polypeptide originally isolated from the salivary glands of the medicinal leech *Hirudo medicalis*, is now produced by recombinant technology. It forms an almost irreversible complex with thrombin, causing a potent and specific inhibition of its action. The kidneys are principally responsible for clearing hirudin and the $t_{1/2}$ is 60 min after intravenous administration. No antidote is available for a bleeding patient. It has been used in patients with HIT, thromboprophylaxis in elective hip arthroplasty, unstable angina and myocardial infarction.

Bivalirudin is a bivalent direct thrombin inhibitor produced as a 20-amino-acid recombinant polypeptide. It is a relatively low-affinity inhibitor of thrombin and may thus present a lower bleeding risk, but clinical advantage remains to be shown.

Argatroban, a carboxylic acid derivative, binds non-covalently to the active site of thrombin and is an effective alternative to heparin in patients with HIT.

Anticoagulant drugs under development

Direct inhibitors of thrombin may prove effective as they inactivate fibrin-bound thrombin, which may promote thrombus extension. Heparin itself acts indirectly through antithrombin and may not inhibit clot-bound thrombin.

Other highly selective agents in clinical development include a variety of *blockers* of: (a) factor IXa (by active site-blocked factor IXa or monoclonal antibodies); (b) the factor VIIa/tissue factor pathway (with recombinant tissue factor pathway inhibitor, TFPI, the analogue of the natural inhibitor); and (c) factor Xa (by small peptidomimetics and NAPc2, a recombinant nematode anticoagulant peptide).

Novel delivery systems, using synthetic amino acids (e.g. SNAC) to facilitate absorption, allow the oral administration of unfractionated or LMW heparins.

FIBRINOLYTIC (THROMBOLYTIC) SYSTEM

The system acts to remove intravascular fibrin, thereby restoring blood flow.

Plasminogen activators that convert plasminogen to plasmin initiate the process. A trypsin-like protease, *plasmin*, then degrades fibrin into soluble *fibrin degradation products* (Fig. 28.3).

Two immunologically distinct plasminogen activators are found in blood, namely *tissue-type* (tPA) and *urokinase-type* (uPA), both of which are synthesised and released from endothelial cells. Intravascular plasminogen activation is initiated by tPA. In this process, plasminogen and tPA bind to fibrin and the enzymatic activity of tPA is enhanced by fibrin. The result is that plasmin formation takes

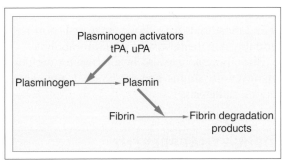

Fig. 28.3 The blood fibrinolytic system. tPA, tissue-type plasminogen activator; uPA, urokinase-type plasminogen activator.

place only on the *fibrin surface* and not generally in the circulation, where widespread defibrination would occur and compromise the whole coagulation mechanism. tPA is the plasminogen activator used for the treatment of coronary occlusion.

Plasminogen activator inhibitors. The most important is *endothelial cell-derived type 1 plasminogen activator inhibitor* (PAI-1), which blocks the action of tPA. Another inhibitor, α_2-*antiplasmin*, rapidly complexes with and inactivates *free* plasmin. Fibrin-bound plasmin is relatively protected from inactivation so that fibrinolysis can occur despite physiological plasma concentrations of this inhibitor.

An enzyme, known as *thrombin-activatable fibrinolysis inhibitor* (TAFI), attenuates fibrinolysis by cleaving carboxyl-terminal lysine residues from fibrin, the removal of which decreases plasminogen and plasmin binding to fibrin, retarding the lytic process. TAFI thus serves as a link between coagulation and fibrinolysis.

DRUGS THAT PROMOTE FIBRINOLYSIS

An important application of fibrinolytic drugs has been to dissolve thrombi in acutely occluded coronary arteries, thereby restoring blood flow to ischaemic myocardium and improving prognosis. The approach is to give a *plasminogen activator* by intravenous infusion or bolus injection in order to increase the formation of the fibrinolytic enzyme *plasmin*.

Recombinant thrombolytic proteins can be re-engineered to prolong $t_{1/2}$ and possibly reduce the induced systemic fibrinolytic state. Current drugs possess a broadly equivalent risk of inducing bleeding. Recombinant drugs of human origin are non-

antigenic, whereas those with a bacterial origin, whether purified from bacteria or produced by recombinant technology, can result in antibody formation and produce allergic reactions that preclude repeated treatment. The $t_{1/2}$ determines whether a drug is suitable for bolus i.v. injection or continuous i.v. infusion. Reteplase and tenecteplase are most appropriate for bolus injection.

Alteplase ($t_{1/2}$ 2–6 min) is a single-chain recombinant tissue-type plasminogen activator (rtPA) that is usually given by continuous i.v. infusion over 30–180 min, according to the indication, i.e. for acute myocardial infarction and acute ischaemic stroke. A bolus dose is recommended for pulmonary embolus.

Reteplase is a deletion mutant of tPA lacking a growth factor and the kringle-binding domain; it possesses a longer $t_{1/2}$ (1.6 h) than alteplase. This permits a double bolus regimen, with completion of treatment in 30 min, rather than the need for administration by infusion. It is licensed for acute myocardial infarction.

Tenecteplase is a tPA variant with amino acid substitutions that confer a longer $t_{1/2}$ (2 h), greater enzymatic efficiency and a more fibrin-specific profile. It is administered as a single i.v. injection over 5–10 s and is licensed for treatment of acute myocardial infarction.

Streptokinase, derived from culture filtrates of *Streptococcus haemolyticus*, is not an enzyme. It binds human plasminogen to produce a plasminogen activator that undergoes a time-dependent change of conformation to create an active site that autocatalytically converts plasminogen to plasmin. The plasmin-complexed streptokinase then decays by proteolytic degradation.

Streptokinase ($t_{1/2}$ 20 min) is given by i.v. infusion, e.g. for up to 72 h when treating patients with venous thromboembolism. It finds use for acute myocardial infarction, deep vein thrombosis and pulmonary embolism, acute arterial thromboembolism, and central retinal venous or arterial thrombosis. The rate of infusion may be limited by tachycardia, fever and muscle aches. Nausea and vomiting may also occur.

USES OF THROMBOLYTIC DRUGS

Coronary artery thrombolysis

The earlier thrombolysis starts, the better the outcome. Benefit is most striking in patients with anterior myocardial infarction treated within 4 h of onset. Contraindications to thrombolytic drug use are those that predispose to intracranial haemorrhage (haemorrhagic stroke, intracranial tumour, recent neurosurgery or brain trauma within the previous 10 days and uncontrolled hypertension) or massive haemorrhage (major surgery of thorax or abdomen within the previous 10 days, current major bleeding such as from the gastrointestinal tract or prolonged cardiopulmonary resuscitation).

Adverse effects. If bleeding occurs, thrombolytic therapy must cease. Depending on the timing of bleeding in relation to therapy, consider *antifibrinolytic* therapy with aprotonin (for longer-acting drugs) and raising the fibrinogen concentration with fresh frozen plasma or cryoprecipitate (more likely required after streptokinase therapy). Platelet transfusion may be given to correct the platelet function defect induced by plasmin proteolysis of platelet membrane receptors.

Following thrombolytic therapy intramuscular injections are contraindicated, any venepuncture requires at least 10 min of local compression, and arterial puncture must be avoided.

Hypotension can follow treatment with any thrombolytic drug but febrile allergic reactions are about six times more likely with use of a thrombolytic of bacterial origin. Some milder reactions can be managed with paracetamol, an H_1-receptor antihistamine and corticosteroid.

Non-coronary thrombolysis

Pulmonary embolism. Thrombolysis is used in patients with massive pulmonary emboli with cardiovascular compromise; its value in patients with submassive pulmonary embolus is uncertain.

Deep vein thrombosis. Thrombolysis is often not effective in patients with DVT but may be justified when the affected vessels are proximal and risk of pulmonary embolism is high.

Arterial occlusion. Systemic or local thrombolysis may be an option for arterial occlusions distal to the popliteal artery (thrombectomy is the usual therapeutic approach for occlusion of less than 24 h duration proximal to this site). Intravenous streptokinase will lyse 80% of occlusions if infusion begins within 12 h, and 60% if it is delayed for up to 3 days.

Ischaemic stroke. There is little evidence of benefit and most trials have shown increased short-term mortality in patients treated with thrombolysis.

Thrombolysis may also be effective for occluded arteriovenous shunts and for blocked, e.g. central venous, catheters.

DRUGS THAT PREVENT FIBRINOLYSIS

Antifibrinolytics are useful in a number of bleeding disorders.

Tranexamic acid competitively inhibits the binding of plasminogen and tPA to fibrin and effectively blocks conversion of plasminogen to plasmin; fibrinolysis is thus retarded. An intravenous bolus passes largely unchanged in the urine with a $t_{1/2}$ of 1.5 h. Oral and topical formulations are available.

Tranexamic acid is used principally to prevent the *hyperplasminaemic bleeding state* that results from damage to tissues rich in plasminogen activator, e.g. after prostatic surgery, tonsillectomy, uterine cervical cone biopsy and menorrhagia, whether primary or induced by an intrauterine contraceptive device. Tranexamic acid may also reduce bleeding after ocular trauma, and in von Willebrand's disease and haemophilia after dental extraction (normally combined with DDAVP or factor VIII respectively).

Some patients with *hereditary angio-oedema* may benefit, presumably by prevention of plasmin-induced activation of the complement system.

Tranexamic acid may be of value in *thrombocytopenia* (idiopathic or following cytotoxic chemotherapy). The natural fibrinolytic destabilisation of small platelet plugs is inhibited, reducing the risk of haemorrhage and requirement for platelet transfusion.

Adverse effects are rare but include nausea, diarrhoea and sometimes orthostatic hypotension. Tranexamic acid is contraindicated for patients with haematuria because clot lysis in the urinary tract is prevented and clot colic results.

Aprotinin is a naturally occurring inhibitor of plasmin and other proteolytic enzymes that has been used to limit bleeding following open heart surgery with extracorporeal circulation, and for the treatment of life-threatening haemorrhage due to hyperplasminaemia complicating liver transplantation surgery or thrombolytic therapy.

PLATELET FUNCTION

Platelets have a key role in maintaing vascular integrity. They aggregate at and adhere to exposed collagen to form a physical barrier at the site of vessel injury; they accelerate the activation of coagulation proteins; they release stored granules that promote vasoconstriction and wound healing.

Platelets have rightly been termed 'pharmacological packages'. To deliver the above functions, they must first undergo a process of *activation* that involves multiple agonists through numerous intracellular second-messenger pathways and complex networks (Fig. 28.4). These pathways converge on and activate the fibrinogen receptor, *glycoprotein IIbIIIa* (integrin αIIbβ3), inducing a conformational change that results in fibrinogen/fibrin binding. When fibrinogen occupies the receptor, outside-in signalling consolidates platelet activation by upregulating second-messenger pathways, so providing a positive feedback loop.

In the *coagulation process*, platelets provide an anionic phospholipid surface for assembly of the macromolecular enzymatic complexes required for thrombin generation. Phospholipids in the bilayer membrane of resting platelets are distributed asymmetrically, with anionic phospholipid held in the internal leaflet. Full platelet activation results in scrambling of the membrane with exposure of negatively charged phospholipid on the external leaflet. This lipid cooperates in the assembly of the thrombin-generating enzymatic complexes.

Receptors on the *platelet membrane* that are known to result in platelet activation through intracellular second messengers include those for thrombin, adenosine diphosphate (ADP), collagen, thromboxane and adrenaline (epinephrine).

Activation is enhanced by occupancy of glycoprotein IIbIIIa (the fibrinogen receptor) and glycoprotein Ib (a component of the Ib/IX/V receptor for von Willebrand protein). The process is mediated primarily through G-coupled second messengers in response to occupancy of the thrombin, ADP and collagen receptors (at high collagen concentration), and through phospholipases and consequent thromboxane generation in response to occupancy of the thromboxane, adrenaline and collagen receptors (at low collagen concentration).

Both thromboxane and ADP are produced in response to platelet activation, and recruit further platelets to activation sites, so providing a positive feedback loop to their respective receptors. There are several ADP receptors on the platelet membrane. Multiple second-messenger pathways are probably involved in their mechanism of activation, not just G-protein-coupled systems. Collagen-induced platelet activation involves at least three receptors with both thromboxane-dependent and thromboxane-independent second-messenger pathways.

High 'shear forces' also activate platelets but the mechanisms are unclear: fibrinogen and its receptor, GPIIbIIIa, are required at low shear rates, and von Willebrand factor and its receptor, GPIb, at high shear rates. ADP and adrenaline are synergistic at high shear and result in larger thrombi for a given rate of shear.

DRUGS THAT INHIBIT PLATELET ACTIVITY (ANTIPLATELET DRUGS)

(See also Myocardial infarction, p. 437.)

Aspirin (acetylsalicylic acid) acetylates and thus inactivates cyclo-oxygenase (COX), the enzyme responsible for the first step in the formation of prostaglandins, the conversion of arachidonic acid to prostaglandin H_2. As acetylation of COX is *irreversible* and the platelet is unable to synthesise new enzyme, COX activity is lost for the platelet lifetime (8–10 days).

Aspirin prevents formation of both thromboxane A_2 (TXA_2) and prostacyclin (PGI_2) (see Fig. 15.1,

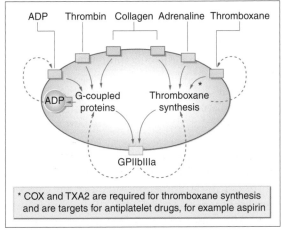

* COX and TXA2 are required for thromboxane synthesis and are targets for antiplatelet drugs, for example aspirin

Fig. 28.4 Mechanisms for the activation of platelets. ADP, adenosine diphosphate; GP, glycoprotein.

p. 251). Therapeutic interest in the antithrombotic effect of aspirin has centred on separating these actions by using a low dose. In general, 75–100 mg/day by mouth will abolish synthesis of TXA$_2$ without significant impairment of prostacyclin formation, i.e. amounts substantially below the 2.4 g/day used to control pain and inflammation. Laboratory testing of TXA$_2$ production or TXA$_2$-dependent platelet function can provide an assessment of the adequacy of aspirin dose. Amongst several causes of resistance to aspirin are genetic polymorphisms of COX-1 and other genes involved in thromboxane biosynthesis.[6]

Low-dose aspirin is not without risk: a proportion of peptic ulcer bleeds in people aged over 60 years occur from prophylactic low-dose aspirin.

Dipyridamole reversibly inhibits platelet phosphodiesterase, and consequently cyclic AMP concentration is increased and platelet activity reduced; evidence also suggests that its antithrombotic effect may derive from release of prostaglandin precursors by vascular endothelium. Dipyridamole is bound extensively to plasma proteins and has a $t_{1/2}$ of 12 h.

Clopidogrel is a thienopyridine derivative that inhibits ADP-dependent platelet aggregation. The $t_{1/2}$ of the parent drug is 40 h and metabolism by the liver converts it to its active form. Clopidogrel reduces the risk of the combined outcome of stroke, myocardial infarction (MI) or vascular death in patients with thromboembolic stroke. It decreases vascular death and MI in patients with unstable angina, reduces acute occlusion of coronary bypass grafts, and improves walking distance and decreases vascular complications in patients with peripheral vascular disease. Clopidogrel also finds use in the prevention of stroke in patients who are intolerant of aspirin.

Ticlopodine is also a thienopyridine derivative and is effective in preventing ischaemic stroke, MI or vascular death in patients at high risk. Neutropenia is the most serious adverse effect (risk 2.4%) and is greatest in the first 12 weeks of therapy; check the leucocyte counts every 2 weeks during this period. Diarrhoea and other gastrointestinal symptoms may occur in a third of patients.

Epoprostenol (prostacyclin) may be given as an anticoagulant during renal dialysis, with or without heparin; it is infused i.v. and s.c ($t_{1/2}$ 3 min). It is a potent vasodilator.

GLYCOPROTEIN (GP) IIB–IIIA ANTAGONISTS

The platelet glycoprotein IIb–IIIa complex is the predominant platelet integrin, a molecule restricted to megakaryocytes and platelets that mediates platelet aggregation by the binding of proteins such as fibrinogen and von Willebrand factor (vWF) (see Fig. 28.4). Hereditary absence of the GPIIb–IIIa complex (Glanzmann's thrombasthenia) results in platelets that are incapable of aggregation by physiological agonists.

GPIIb–IIIa antagonists have been developed as antiplatelet agents. As blockers of the *final common pathway* of platelet aggregation (the binding of fibrinogen or vWF to the GPIIb–IIIa complex) they are more complete inhibitors of platelets than either aspirin or clopidogrel which act only on the cyclooxygenase or ADP pathway respectively. GPIIb–IIIa antagonists also have an anticoagulant effect by reducing availability of platelet membrane anionic phospholipid. Inhibited of platelet aggregation is dose dependent.

Abciximab is a human–murine chimeric monoclonal antibody Fab fragment that binds to the GPIIb–IIIa complex with a high affinity and slow dissociation rate. Given intravenously, it is cleared rapidly from plasma ($t_{1/2}$ 20 min). Abciximab (0.25 mg/kg bolus then 0.125 micrograms/kg/min infusion for 12 h) produces immediate and profound inhibition of platelet activity that lasts for 12–36 h after termination of the infusion. The dose causes and maintains blockade of more than 80% of receptors, causing a greater than 80% reduction in aggregation. Patients may also receive heparin and an antiplatelet drug, e.g. aspirin. Abciximab is effective in acute coronary syndromes.

Eptifibatide is a cyclic heptapeptide based upon the Lys-Gly-Asp sequence. *Tirofiban* and *lamifiban* are non-peptide mimetics. All three are competitive inhibitors of the GPIIb–IIIa complex with lower affinities and higher dissociation rates than abciximab and relatively short plasma $t_{1/2}$ values (2–2.5 h). Platelet aggregation returns to normal from

[6]Hankey G J, Eikelboom J W 2006 Aspirin resistance. Lancet 367:606–617.

30 min to 4 h after discontinuation. Eptifibatide and tirofiban are effective in acute coronary syndromes.

Adverse effects. Platelet transfusion after cessation of abciximab is necessary for refractory or life-threatening bleeding. After transfusion, the antibody redistributes to the transfused platelets, reducing the mean level of receptor blockade and improving platelet function. Thrombocytopenia may occur from 1 h to days after commencing treatment in up to 1% of patients. This necessitates platelet counts 2–4 h after commencement and then daily; if severe, therapy must be stopped and, if necessary, platelets transfused. EDTA-induced pseudothrombocytopenia has been reported and a low platelet count should prompt examination of a blood film for agglutination before therapy is stopped.

OTHER DRUGS

Dextrans, particularly of mol. wt 70 000 Da (dextran 70), alter platelet function and prolong the bleeding time. Dextrans differ from the other antiplatelet drugs, which tend to be used for arterial thrombosis; dextran 70 reduces the incidence of postoperative venous thromboembolism if it is given during or just after surgery. The dose should not exceed 10% of the estimated blood volume. Dextrans are rarely used.

USES OF ANTIPLATELET DRUGS

Antiplatelet therapy protects at-risk patients against stroke, myocardial infarction or death. A meta-analysis of 145 clinical trials of prolonged (>1 month) antiplatelet therapy versus control, and trials between antiplatelet regimens, found that the chance of non-fatal myocardial infarction and non-fatal stroke fell by one-third, and that there was a one-sixth reduction in the risk of death from any vascular cause.[7] Expressed in another way, in the first month after an acute myocardial infarction (a vulnerable period) aspirin prevents death, stroke or a further heart attack in about 4 of every 100 patients treated. Continuing treatment from the end of year 1 to year 3 conferred further benefit.

Aspirin is by far the most commonly used antiplatelet agent. The optimal dose is not certain, but one not exceeding aspirin 325 mg/day is acceptable, and 75–100 mg/day may be as effective and preferred where there is gastric intolerance. Aspirin alone (mainly) or aspirin plus dipyridamole greatly reduced the risk of occlusion where vascular grafts or arterial patency were studied systematically.[8]

Many patients who take aspirin for vascular disease may also require a NSAID, e.g. for joint disease. Given their common mode of action by inhibiting prostaglandin synthesis, this raises the issue that NSAIDs may block access of aspirin to active sites on platelets, with loss of cardioprotection. Retrospective cohort[9] and case–control[10] studies suggest no adverse interaction with ibuprofen, but the issue remains unresolved and in the meantime it seems prudent to take aspirin 2 h before a NSAID, e.g. at bed-time.

Summary
- Coagulation does not occur as a consequence of linear sequential enzyme activation pathways but by a network of simultaneous interactions, with regulation and modulation of these interactions during the thrombin generation process itself.
- Vitamin K is necessary for the final stage in the synthesis of coagulant factors II (prothrombin), VII, IX and X, and anticoagulant regulatory proteins, proteins C and S.
- Vitamin K is used to treat haemorrhage or threatened bleeding due to the coumarin or indanedione anticoagulants, haemorrhagic disease of the newborn and hypoprothrombinaemia due to intestinal malabsorption syndromes.
- Desmopressin increases the plasma concentration of factor VIII and von Willebrand factor, directly activates platelets, and is useful in patients with mild haemophilia A and von Willebrand's disease.

(Continued)

[7]Antiplatelet Trialists' Collaboration 1994 Collaborative overview of randomised trials of antiplatelet therapy – I: Prevention of death, myocardial infarction and stroke by prolonged antiplatelet therapy and various categories of patients. British Medical Journal 308:81–106.

[8]Antiplatelet Trialists' Collaboration 1994 Collaborative overview of randomised trials of antiplatelet therapy – II: Maintenance of vascular grafts or arterial patency by antiplatelet therapy. British Medical Journal 308:159–168.

[9]García Rodríguez L A, Varas-Lorenzo C, Maguire A, González-Pérez A 2004 Nonsteroidal anti-inflammatory drugs and the risk of myocardial infarction in the general population. Circulation 109:3000–3006.

[10]Patel T N, Goldberg K C 2004 Use of aspirin and ibuprofen compared with aspirin alone and the risk of myocardial infarction. Archives of Internal Medicine 164:852–856.

Summary—Cont'd

- The predominant effect of anticoagulant drugs is to limit thrombin generation, or to neutralise thrombin.
- Warfarin and other oral vitamin K antagonists act by reducing the activity of vitamin K-dependent clotting factors (see above); they take 4–5 days to produce a therapeutic effect. Warfarin is the oral anticoagulant of choice, for it is reliably effective and has the lowest incidence of adverse effects.
- Oral anticoagulant drugs are used to prevent and treat venous thrombosis and pulmonary embolus, and to prevent arterial thromboemboli in patients with atrial fibrillation or cardiac disease, including mechanical heart valves.
- Heparin depends for its anticoagulant action on the presence in plasma of antithrombin, a naturally occurring inhibitor of activated coagulation proteases that include thrombin, factor Xa and factor IXa.
- Patients with acute venous thromboembolism can be treated safely and effectively with low molecular weight heparin as outpatients. LMWHs are the preferred drugs for perioperative prophylaxis and are at least as effective as standard heparin for unstable angina.
- Fibrinolytic drugs dissolve thrombi in acutely occluded coronary arteries, thereby restoring blood flow to ischaemic myocardium and improving prognosis. The earlier thrombolysis is given the better the outcome. Thrombolysis is also effective for massive pulmonary emboli with cardiovascular compromise.
- Aspirin acetylates and thus inactivates cyclo-oxygenase (COX), the enzyme responsible for the first step in the formation of prostaglandins, and in low dose reduces platelet activity by preventing the formation of thromboxane.
- Clopidogrel inhibits ADP-dependent platelet aggregation; it reduces the risk of stroke, myocardial infarction or vascular death.
- GPIIb–IIIa antagonists block the final common pathway of platelet aggregation (the binding of fibrinogen or vWF to the GPIIb–IIIa complex) and are more complete inhibitors of platelets than either aspirin or clopidogrel.
- Antiplatelet therapy protects at risk patients against stroke, myocardial infarction or death.

GUIDE TO FURTHER READING

Arepally G M, Ortel T L 2006 Heparin-induced thrombocytopenia. New England Journal of Medicine 355(8): 809–817

Blann A D, Lip G Y H 2006 Venous thromboembolism. British Medical Journal 332:215–219

Di Nisio M, Middeldorp S, Büller HR et al 2005 Direct thrombin inhibitors. New England Journal of Medicine 353:1028–1040

Ghorashian S, Hunt B J 2004 'Off-license' use of recombinant activated factor VII. Blood Reviews 18:245–259

Goldhaber S Z 2004 Pulmonary embolism. Lancet 363:1295–1305

Huntington J A, Baglin T P 2003 Targeting thrombin: rational drug design from natural mechanisms. Trends in Pharmacological Sciences 24:589–595

Kamali F, Pirmohamed M 2006 The future prospects of pharmacogenetics in oral anticoagulation therapy. British Journal of Clinical Pharmacology 61:746–751

Kelman C W, Kortt M A, Becker N G et al 2003 Deep vein thrombosis and air travel: record linkage study. British Medical Journal 327:1072–1075

Kyrle P A, Eichinger S 2005 Deep vein thrombosis. Lancet 365:1163–1174

Patrono C, Garcia Rodriguez L A, Landolfi R, Baigent C 2005 Low-dose aspirin for the prevention of atherothrombosis. New England Journal of Medicine 353(22):2373–2383

Toh C H, Dennis M 2003 Disseminated intravascular coagulation: old disease, new hope. British Medical Journal 327:974–977

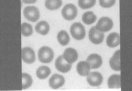

29

Cellular disorders and anaemias

SYNOPSIS

The rational use of haematinics is essential to the correction of anaemias. The emergence of haemopoietic growth factors opens the way to the successful management of many cellular, particularly erythrocyte, disorders.

- Iron deficiency, acute overdose and overload
- Vitamin B_{12} deficiency
- Folic acid deficiency
- Haemopoietic growth factors in haematological disease
- Sickle cell anaemia therapy
- Polycythaemia vera therapy
- Aplastic anaemia therapy

IRON

Iron is essential to erythrocyte oxygen transport and is a catalyst for oxidative metabolism in all cells. Iron symbolised strength in magical systems and, historically, was given for 'weakness'. Certainly, many benefited psychologically (placebo reactors) or because weakness was due to iron deficiency anaemia. The rational use of iron could not begin until both the presence of iron in blood's 'colouring matter' and iron deficiency anaemia had been recognised. Excess iron is toxic due to catalysis of free radical formation.

IRON KINETICS

Males have 40–50 mg iron/kg; females have less. Haemoglobin contains 30 mg/kg; muscle myoglobin and cellular enzymes comprise 6–7 mg/kg, and storage iron (ferritin and haemosiderin) in hepatocytes and macrophages is 5–6 mg/kg in females and 10–12 mg/kg in males. Transport iron (transferrin) is minute (<0.5%).

Iron balance reflects the difference between absorption and loss. Humans lack a mechanism to excrete excess iron, and physiological control is achieved by regulating absorption according to need: as stores decline, absorption increases and vice versa. Absorption can increase up to five-fold in iron deficiency, and also rises with increased erythropoiesis, anaemia and hypoxaemia; inflammation decreases absorption. Excess absorption relative to stores occurs in hereditary haemochromatosis.

Dietary iron is approximately 10–20 mg/day but only 5–10% is absorbed. At steady state, 1 mg/day of iron is required to compensate normal faecal loss. During the average menstrual cycle, women lose 10–15 mg iron.

Absorption occurs predominantly in the duodenum where an acid environment enhances solubility. Most iron in food is ferric (Fe^{3+}) hydroxide, ferric–protein complexes or haem–protein complexes. Iron is more readily absorbed in the ferrous (Fe^{2+}) state. Simultaneous ingestion of a reducing agent, e.g. ascorbic acid 50 mg, increases ferrous iron absorption 2–3-fold. Phytates, tannates and phosphates in food impair absorption.

Proximal small bowel mucosal cells have an important role in absorption. Many proteins are involved in iron absorption and the hormone *hepcidin* plays a regulatory role, as described in Fig. 29.1 *Ferroportin* facilitated by hephaestin transfers iron to plasma. Alternatively, iron may be stored intracellularly and excreted in faeces in shed mucosal cells.

Iron released into plasma binds to *transferrin*. Erythroid precursors express high levels of transferrin receptor 1, ensuring greatest uptake. Iron from senescent erythrocytes phagocytosed by macrophages is exported by ferroportin back to plasma transferrin. Hepatocytes store iron excess to requirements and, when demand increases, release it by ferroportin.

Hepcidin expression is regulated by iron stores, erythropoietic activity, haemoglobin, oxygen content and inflammation, and has an inverse relationship with iron absorption. Hepcidin binds to

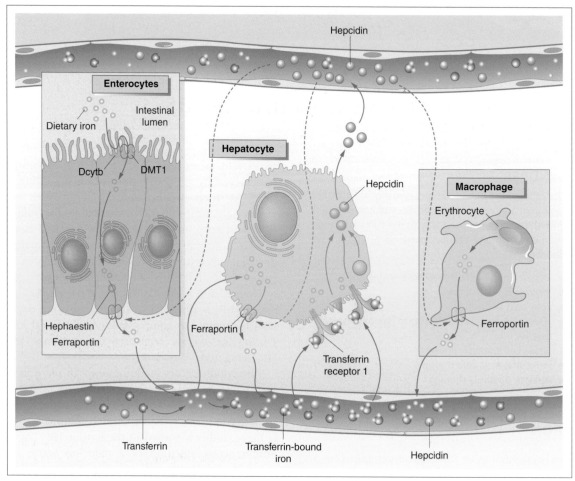

Fig. 29.1 Iron homeostasis. At the brush border, dietary iron is reduced to ferrous state by duodenal ferric reductase (Dcytb), transported into the mucosal cell by divalent metal transporter 1 (DMT1) and released via ferroportin into the circulation facilitated by hephaestin. Most absorbed iron is delivered to erythroid precursors. Hepatocytes take up iron from the circulation either as free iron or transferrin-bound iron via transferrin receptors 1 and 2. Hepcidin secretion by hepatocytes down-regulates ferroportin-mediated release of iron from enterocytes, macrophages and hepatocytes. (Reproduced with permission from Fleming R E, Bacon B R 2005 Orchestration of iron homeostasis. New England Journal of Medicine 352:1741–1744.)

ferroportin causing cellular internalisation and destruction. Increased hepcidin expression reduces intestinal iron absorption and increases iron stores in macrophages and hepatocytes. This occurs in the anaemia of chronic disease.

Iron is stored in hepatocytes and reticuloendothelial macrophages as *ferritin*, which is non-toxic and readily mobilised, and as its aggregate, *haemosiderin*. The serum ferritin (normally 20–300 mmol/L) provides a measure of iron stores. Ferritin is an acute-phase reactant and, in inflammatory states, serum ferritin is a misleading measure of stores. Measurement of serum soluble transferrin receptor (increased in iron deficiency but not

by inflammation) may differentiate iron deficiency from anaemia of chronic disease.

Small intestinal abnormalities may interfere with iron absorption, e.g. coeliac disease and other malabsorption syndromes, or with conversion of iron into the reduced form, e.g. from gastric hypoacidity.

Formation of insoluble iron salts (such as phosphate and phytate) in the alkaline environment of most of the small intestine explains why most ingested iron is not absorbed, even in severe iron deficiency. Prolonged excessive iron ingestion overwhelms regulatory mechanisms and results in haemosiderosis, as there is no physiological mechanism to increase excretion.

Interactions. Iron chelates in the gut with tetracyclines, penicillamine, methyldopa, levodopa, carbidopa, ciprofloxacin, norfloxacin and ofloxacin. Iron also forms stable complexes with thyroxine, captopril and biphosphonates. The resulting impairment of drug absorption can be clinically important and is largely avoided if ingestion is separated by 3 h.

Ascorbic acid increases absorption but its use is not clinically important in routine therapy; desferrioxamine binds iron and reduces absorption (see Poisoning, below); antacids, tea (tannins) and bran reduce absorption.

IRON THERAPY

Iron is indicated only for the treatment or prevention of iron deficiency. Making 25 mg iron/day available to iron-deficient bone marrow raises the haemoglobin concentration by 0.15 g/dL daily. A haemoglobin rise of 2 g/dL after 3 weeks' therapy is evidence of adequate response. Oral preparations are the treatment of choice due to effectiveness, safety and low cost. Parenteral preparations should be restricted to patients unable to absorb or tolerate oral preparations. Red cell transfusion is necessary only in patients with severe symptomatic anaemia or where chronic blood loss exceeds the capacity of oral or parenteral replacement.

Oral iron therapy

The goal of iron therapy is correction of anaemia and replenishment of stores. As about 30% of orally administered iron will be absorbed, 180 mg elemental iron daily for 1–3 months will correct anaemia, depending on severity. Oral therapy replenishes stores less easily and should be continued for 3–6 months (at lower dose) after correction of anaemia, until serum ferritin levels exceed 50 microgram/L or as long as blood loss continues.

Contraindications. It is illogical to give iron in the anaemia of chronic disease where iron utilisation is impaired. Such patients may also have iron deficiency, which is difficult to diagnose without visualisation of iron stores in bone marrow. Iron should not be given in haemolytic anaemias unless there is haemoglobinuria, for iron from lysed cells remains in the body. Moreover increased erythropoiesis associated with chronic haemolysis increases iron absorption and supplements may cause haemosiderosis.

Iron therapy is needed in

- Iron deficiency due to poor diet or chronic blood loss.
- Pregnancy. Extra iron required by mother and fetus totals 1000 mg, chiefly in the second half of pregnancy. The fetus takes iron even if the mother is deficient. Dietary iron is seldom adequate, and iron and folic acid (50–100 mg elemental iron plus folic acid 200–500 micrograms/day) should be given to pregnant women from second trimester. Opinions differ as to whether everyone should receive prophylaxis or only those identified as deficient. Warn parents not to allow children access to iron tablets.
- Abnormalities of the gastrointestinal tract that may reduce iron absorbtion, e.g. coeliac disease.
- Premature babies are born with low iron stores, and babies weaned late are at risk. There is very little iron in human milk and less in cow's milk.
- Patients on erythropoietin undergoing haemodialysis; haemoglobin rise requires iron reserves, which are depleted by dialysis.
- Early treatment of severe pernicious anaemia with hydroxocobalamin, as rapid erythropoiesis occasionally exhausts iron stores.

Oral iron preparations. There are many proprietary iron preparations (Table 29.1). Ferrous sulphate is as effective a source of elemental iron as more expensive preparations. It is important to avoid initial overdosage with iron as the resulting symptoms may cause the patient to abandon therapy. The objective is to give 100–200 mg elemental iron per day in an adult (3 mg/kg in a child). Iron given after food causes less gastrointestinal upset but less is absorbed than when given between meals. Nevertheless, administration with food is commonly preferred to improve compliance.

Table 29.1	Oral iron preparations		
	Tablet size (mg)	Daily dose (mg/day)	Elemental iron (mg/day)
Ferrous sulphate	200	200–600	65–195
Ferrous gluconate	300	300–1800	35–210
Ferrous fumarate	200	210–1260	68–408
Ferrous succinate	100	100–600	35–210

Choice of oral iron preparation. Oral iron is often used both for therapy and prophylaxis in people who feel little ill-health. Gastrointestinal upset is particularly important as it may cause the patient to discontinue treatment. No preparation clearly provides best iron absorption with fewest adverse effects. Gastrointestinal upset is minimal with a daily dose of less than 180 mg elemental iron, given with food.

A suggested strategy. Start a patient on ferrous sulphate taken after food once, then twice, then thrice daily. If gastrointestinal intolerance occurs, stop and reintroduce iron, increasing dosage weekly. If this causes gastrointestinal upset, try ferrous gluconate, succinate or fumarate. If simple preparations are unsuccessful, more expensive *sustained-release preparations* may be tried. These release iron slowly from resins, chelates (sodium feredetate) or plastic matrices only after passing the pylorus, e.g. Slow-Fe, Ferrograd, Feospan. Iron release occurs in the lower small intestine with less efficient absorption. The fewer unwanted effects reflect the small amount of iron available for absorption and these preparations have no therapeutic advantage.

Liquid formulations are available for adults and small children but they stain the teeth, e.g. Ferrous Sulphate Oral Solution, Paediatric: 5 mL contains 12 mg elemental iron. Polysaccharide–iron complex (Niferex): 5 mL contains 100 mg elemental iron.

Iron therapy blackens the faeces but does not generally interfere with modern tests for occult blood.

Failure of oral iron therapy is most commonly due to poor compliance, persistent bleeding or wrong diagnosis.

Adverse effects. Most patients tolerate oral iron therapy but 10–20% experience nausea, abdominal pain, and constipation or diarrhoea. Upper gastrointestinal effects appear to be dose related and are often improved by ingestion with or after food and/or reduction of dose (as above), prolonging the duration of treatment. Diarrhoea and constipation are treated symptomatically, usually without a change in regimen.

Parenteral iron therapy

This may be required if:

- Iron cannot be absorbed from the intestine.
- The patient experiences intolerable gut symptoms or cannot be relied on to take tablets.

Speed of haemopoietic response is no quicker than with full-dosage oral iron reliably taken and normally absorbed. Both provide as much iron as an active marrow can use. Parenterally administered iron is stored and utilised over months. Un-ionised iron complexes are used.

Iron dextran injection (ferric hydroxide complexed with dextrans, 50 mg/mL) is administered by deep intramuscular injection or by slow intravenous injection or infusion.

Iron sucrose injection (ferric hydroxide complexed with sucrose, 20 mg/mL) is delivered by slow intravenous injection or infusion (not recommended for children). The intravenous route is preferred as intramuscular iron has been associated with soft-tissue sarcomas. Iron sucrose appears to have a lower incidence of adverse reactions.

Cautions. Do not give oral iron preparations for 24 h before parenteral therapy or for 5 days after the last i.v. injection, as adverse reactions occur following saturation of transferrin binding capacity leading to a high, unbound plasma iron concentration. A history of allergic disorders including asthma, eczema and anaphylaxis is a contraindication to parenteral iron.

Dosage of parenteral preparations is determined from a formula using body-weight and haemoglobin deficit.

Adverse effects. Intramuscular iron can be painful and may stain the skin permanently.[1] Reactions include headache, dizziness, nausea, vomiting, disorientation, chest discomfort, myalgia, hypotension, metallic taste, urticaria and hypersensitivity. Intravenous iron may rarely cause anaphylactoid reactions, and facilities for cardiopulmonary resuscitation should be available.

Folate deficiency may be unmasked by effective iron therapy. Where there is a deficiency of both iron and folate, the latter may not be obvious until iron is administered. This is most likely in pregnancy due to

---

[1]Staining can be minimised by inserting the needle through the skin and then moving the subcutaneous tissue laterally before entering muscle, so that the needle track is disrupted when the needle is withdrawn (Z technique).

high fetal requirements for both haematinics, and folic acid is commonly given to anaemic pregnant women (see below). Combined deficiency may also occur in malabsorption syndromes.

Acute overdose: poisoning

Typically acute oral iron poisoning exhibits the phases listed in Box 29.1. Iron poisoning is commonest in children, usually accidental and particularly dangerous. Ferrous sulphate is most toxic. Sustained-release and chelated preparations cause less severe poisoning. Multivitamins with iron are commonly involved.

Poisoning is severe if the plasma iron concentration exceeds the total iron binding capacity (upper limit 75 mmol/L) or plasma becomes pink due to the formation of ferrioxamine.

Treatment is urgent and involves chelating iron in plasma. As an immediate measure, raw egg and milk help bind iron in the stomach. Chelation therapy consists of desferrioxamine by intravenous infusion not exceeding 15 mg/kg/h (maximum 80 mg/kg in 24 h).

Desferrioxamine (deferoxamine) (Desferal) ($t_{1/2}$ 6 h) is an iron-chelating agent (see Chelating agents, p. 131). An investigation of actinomycete metabolites revealed iron-containing substances (sideramines) including ferrioxamine. Removal of the iron produces desferrioxamine. When desferrioxamine is exposed to ferric iron, its straight-chain molecule twines around it and forms a non-toxic stable complex (ferrioxamine), which is excreted in urine (producing a red–orange colour) and in bile. It has a negligible affinity for other metals in the presence of iron excess.

Desferrioxamine is effective therapy in acute iron poisoning and in conditions associated with chronic iron accumulation. A topical formulation is available for ocular siderosis.

Serious adverse effects are uncommon but include rashes and anaphylactic reactions. With chronic use cataract, retinal damage and deafness can occur. Hypotension occurs with too rapid infusion. There is danger of potentially fatal adult respiratory distress syndrome if infusion proceeds beyond 24 h.[2]

Chronic iron overload

Humans are uniquely unable to excrete excess iron. Uncontrolled iron ingestion or excessive absorption (hereditary haemochromatosis) produces progressive accumulation. Grossly excessive parenteral iron therapy or many years of oral iron therapy or frequent transfusion (more than 100 as in thalassaemia[3]) can lead to *haemosiderosis*.

Treatment. The goals of therapy are the removal of excess iron and maintenance of normal stores to avoid tissue damage.

As there is no anaemia in *haemochromatosis* (cf. thalassaemia, below), iron is removed by venesection. A volume of 450 mL blood eliminates 200–250 mg iron and is repeated weekly until the plasma ferritin concentration is normal. Thereafter, occasional venesection keeps the plasma ferritin level at less than 50 micrograms/L. A small number of patients with cardiac failure may require chelator therapy.

Patients with *transfusion siderosis* require long-term chelation therapy. In patients who are transfusion dependent from infancy, e.g. thalassaemia major, chelation commences after 10 to 20 transfusions or about 3 years of age to avoid tissue damage. In older transfusion-dependent patients with anaemia, chelation is commenced after 20 transfusions or when the serum ferritin level is two to three times the normal value.

Box 29.1   Acute iron poisoning

Phase 1

0.5–1 h after ingestion there is abdominal pain, grey–black vomit, diarrhoea, leukocytosis and hyperglycaemia. Severe cases have acidosis and cardiovascular collapse which may proceed to coma and death.

Phase 2

Improvement occurs, lasting 6–12 h; may be sustained or may deteriorate to next phase.

Phase 3

Jaundice, hypoglycaemia, bleeding, encephalopathy, metabolic acidosis and convulsions are followed by cardiovascular collapse, coma and sometimes death 48–60 h after ingestion. Severe brain and liver damage is seen at autopsy.

Phase 4

1–2 months later: scarring and stricture may cause upper gastrointestinal obstruction.

---

[2]Tenenbein M, Kowalski S, Sienko A et al 1992 Lancet 339:699–701.
[3]A 26-year-old subject with β-thalassaemia major had been transfused with 404 units of blood over his lifetime. His iron stores were so high (estimated at above 100 g) that he triggered a metal detector at an airport security checkpoint (Jim R T S 1979 Lancet ii:1028 [letter]).

A negative iron balance is achieved by slow parenteral administration of desferrioxamine s.c. or i.v. (over 9–12 h 5 nights weekly). Compliance is a problem, typically during teenage years. Avoid simultaneous administration of ascorbic acid, which increases the availability of free iron for chelation but mobilises iron from relatively safe reticuloendothelial storage sites to a potentially toxic pool in parenchymal cells. Desferrioxamine therapy over a long period is costly and raises ethical problems in poor countries where thalassaemia is common.

A safe, effective, inexpensive, orally absorbed, iron chelating agent would improve compliance and quality of life. *Deferiprone* is the best of many agents tested. It is less effective than desferrioxamine and carries a risk of arthropathy and agranulocytosis but is an alternative in patients unwilling or unable to tolerate desferrioxamine.

VITAMIN B$_{12}$

A diagnosis of 'pernicious anaemia' was nearly equivalent to a death sentence in the early years of the 20th century, because it did not respond to iron salts, and hence its sinister name. Then in 1925 it was revealed that two factors were necessary for its cure: one in food (extrinsic factor) and one in gastric juice (intrinsic factor). Extrinsic factor (vitamin B$_{12}$) was isolated in 1948. Intrinsic factor (a glycoprotein secreted by gastric parietal cells) ensures cobalamin absorption by receptors in the terminal ileum.

COBALAMINS

Cobalamins are a family of compounds with a complex structure. When vitamin B$_{12}$ was originally isolated, an in vitro artefact placed a cyan group on the cobalt molecule, and it acquired the name *cyan*ocobalamin. Vitamin B$_{12}$ is an essential coenzyme for nucleic acid synthesis. Cobalamin is produced in nature only by microorganisms. Herbivores obtain it from plants contaminated with bacteria and faeces. Carnivores obtain it by ingesting animal tissue. Animal protein is the major dietary source in humans. Bacteria in the human colon synthesise cobalamin, but this is too distal for ileal absorption. Wild rabbits would suffer cobalamin deficiency if they did not eat their own faeces.

Deficiency of cobalamin leads to:
- Megaloblastic anaemia.
- Degeneration of the brain, spinal cord (subacute combined degeneration) and peripheral nerves, causing psychiatric or physical symptoms.
- Abnormalities of epithelial tissue, particularly the alimentary tract, e.g. sore tongue and malabsorption.

Absorption and transport

The daily requirement is about 3.0 micrograms. In the presence of intrinsic factor 70% of ingested cobalamin is absorbed, and without it less than 2%. At high dose, some absorption takes place by diffusion, independently of intrinsic factor.

The cobalamin–intrinsic factor complex binds to its receptor, cubulin, in the terminal ileum and undergoes endocytosis. In plasma, recently absorbed cobalamin binds to transcobalamin II, which is rapidly cleared from the circulation ($t_{1/2}$ 8 min). Hereditary deficiency of transcobalamin II causes severe cobalamin deficiency. Some 80% of circulating cobalamin is bound to transcobalamin I ($t_{1/2}$ 9–12 days), which may have a storage function (hereditary deficiency is of no consequence). Cobalamin in its reduced form, cob(I)alamin, is a coenzyme for methionine synthase, a reaction that generates tetrahydrofolate and is critical for DNA and RNA synthesis.

Cobalamin is not metabolised significantly, and passes into bile and urine. Intestinal disease interrupts this enterohepatic circulation and hastens the onset of deficiency. Body stores (about 5 mg, mainly in liver) are sufficient for 2–4 years after absorption ceases.

Indications

Indications for vitamin B$_{12}$ are the prevention and cure of deficiency. *Hydroxocobalamin* is preferred for clinical use (see below).

Dietary deficiency is virtually confined to vegans – particularly uncompromising vegetarians. Oral supplements are required.

Pernicious (Addisonian) anaemia. Autoimmune destruction of gastric parietal cells produces an atrophic gastric mucosa unable to produce intrinsic factor (or acid). Deficiency results from failure to absorb cobalamin in the terminal ileum. The prognosis of a patient treated with hydroxocobalamin is similar to that in the general population. The classical neurological complications, particularly spasticity, developing after prolonged severe deficiency, are rare today. Total gastrectomy or atrophy of the mucosa in a postgastrectomy remnant may lead, after several years, to a similar anaemia.

Malabsorption syndromes. In stagnant loop syndrome (bacterial overgrowth competes for available cobalamin and responds to broad-spectrum antimicrobials), ileal resection, Crohn's disease and chronic tropical sprue affecting the terminal ileum, cobalamin deficiency is common although megaloblastic anaemia occurs late. The fish tapeworm *Diphyllobothrum latum* may infest humans who eat raw or partially cooked freshwater fish roe, can grow to 10 m in length, and competes for ingested cobalamin.

Tobacco amblyopia has been attributed to cyanide intoxication from strong tobacco, which interferes with the coenzyme function of cobalamin; *hydroxocobalamin* (not cyanocobalamin) is given.

Diagnosis of cobalamin deficiency, in addition to assay of plasma vitamin B_{12} (normal level 170–925 nanograms/L) and characteristic peripheral blood and bone marrow signs, involves a test of vitamin B_{12} absorption, with and without intrinsic factor (Schilling test), to distinguish between gastric and intestinal causes.

Contraindications to cobalamin

Inconclusively diagnosed anaemia is an important contraindication. Therapy of pernicious anaemia is lifelong, and accurate diagnosis is essential. Even a single dose of vitamin B_{12} interferes with the haematological picture for weeks (megaloblastic haematopoiesis normalises within 12 h), although the Schilling test remains diagnostic.

Cobalamin therapy

Hydroxocobalamin is more tightly bound to transcobalamin II than is cyanocobalamin, less passes into the urine after injection, and longer dose intervals are therapeutic. Thus, hydroxocobalamin is preferred. As cyanocobalamin gives satisfactory results, it remains available.

The initial dose for pernicious anaemia is hydroxocobalamin 1 mg i.m. every 2–3 days for five doses. The maintenance dose is 1 mg every 3 months. Doses higher than this simply pass in to the urine but these are justified during renal or peritoneal dialysis (when hydroxocobalamin clearance is increased), and raised plasma methylmalonic acid and homocysteine levels signify an independent risk factor for vascular events.

Routine low-dose supplements of hydroxocobalamin, folate and pyridoxine fail to control hyperhomocysteinaemia in 75% of dialysis patients, but supraphysiological doses are effective: hydroxocobalamin 1 mg/day, folic acid 15 mg/day and pyridoxine 100 mg/day.

After starting therapy, patients feel better in 2 days, reticulocytes peak at 5–7 days, and the haemoglobin, red cell count and haematocrit rise after 1 week. These indices normalise within 2 months. Failure to respond implies a wrong or incomplete diagnosis (additional deficiency). Stimulation of haematopoiesis may deplete iron and folate stores, which may need supplementation. Hypokalaemia may occur at the height of the erythrocyte response in severe cases due to uptake of potassium by the rapidly increasing erythrocyte mass. Give oral potassium prior to initiating therapy in a patient with low or borderline plasma potassium levels.

Reversal of neurological damage is slow, rarely marked, and inversely related to the extent and duration of neuropathy.

If administration by injection is refused or impracticable (rare allergy, bleeding disorder), a snuff or aerosol may be effective, if less reliable. Large daily oral doses (1000 micrograms) are preferable but restoration of exhausted stores by parenteral cobalamin is necessary beforehand; patients must be compliant and frequent monitoring of response is advisable.

Adverse effects are virtually unknown. Use of vitamin B_{12} as a 'tonic' is an abuse of a powerful remedy, which may obscure the diagnosis of pernicious anaemia.

FOLIC ACID (PTEROYLGLUTAMIC ACID)

Folic acid[4] is one of the B vitamins and derives its name from being a bacterial growth factor present in spinach leaves.

---

[4]Latin: *folium*, a leaf.

OCCURRENCE AND REQUIREMENTS

Folate is widely distributed, notably in green vegetables, fruits, yeast and liver, and is found in nature conjugated with glutamate. Adult daily requirement is 50–100 micrograms and a diet containing 400 micrograms of polyglutamates provides this. In childhood the daily requirement is 50 micrograms, five times more on a weight basis. Body stores last for only 4 months.

FUNCTIONS

Folate is itself inactive. After absorption it is converted into the active coenzyme, tetrahydrofolic acid, essential for amino acid and DNA biosynthesis and cell division. The formyl derivative of tetrahydrofolic acid is folinic acid, which is used to bypass blockade of folic acid conversion (see folic acid antagonists, p. 537). Ascorbic acid protects active tetrahydrofolic acid from oxidation; the anaemia of scurvy, although usually normoblastic, may be megaloblastic due to deficiency of tetrahydrofolic acid.

Deficiency of folic acid causes megaloblastic anaemia because of impaired production of purines and pyrimidines, which are essential for DNA synthesis. The megaloblastic marrow of cobalamin deficiency is due to interference with folic acid metabolism, and the morphological changes of cobalamin deficiency are reversed by folic acid. It is vital to realise that folic acid does not provide adequate treatment for pernicious anaemia. When megaloblastic anaemia due to pernicious anaemia is incorrectly diagnosed as folate deficiency, folic acid supplements may accelerate progression of subacute combined degeneration of the spinal cord. Nor does vitamin B_{12} provide adequate treatment for the megaloblastic anaemia of folic acid deficiency, although a partial response may occur because vitamin B_{12} plays a role in folate metabolism.

INDICATIONS

Folic acid is used to prevent or cure deficiency of folate due either to decreased supply or to increased requirement.

Dietary deficiency. Folate deficiency is common in populations with malnutrition in developing countries and is a particular problem in childhood.

In Western countries, folate deficiency occurs in alcoholics, some slimming diets, the elderly, infirm and psychiatric patients.

Pregnancy. The increased daily requirement of 300–400 micrograms is not met by the normal diet in one-third of Western women. The problem is greater in developing countries where nutritional deficiency may be aggravated by increased requirements due to haemoglobinopathies and endemic malaria. Prophylaxis of anaemia in pregnancy therefore necessitates addition of folic acid to iron. The daily dose of 300 micrograms is insufficient to mask pernicious anaemia, which is very rare in women of reproductive age and probably incompatible with a successful pregnancy. Numerous preparations of iron plus folic acid are available but are suitable only for prophylaxis. Larger doses are used for therapy of anaemia during pregnancy (see below), which will remit spontaneously some weeks after delivery. Vigorous iron therapy in pregnancy may unmask folate deficiency. Increased requirements persist during lactation.

Prevention of fetal neural tube defect (spina bifida). Folic acid supplement taken before conception and during early pregnancy prevented the condition in pregnancies subsequent to an affected birth in an 8-year trial.[5] Women hoping to conceive, who have had an affected child, are advised to take folic acid 5 mg/day. To prevent a first occurrence, 400 micrograms/day should be taken before conception, or as soon as possible after diagnosis.[6] In both cases folate supplements should be taken for the first 12 weeks of pregnancy.

Premature infants need supplements because they miss the build-up of folate stores that normally occurs in the last few weeks of pregnancy.

Malabsorption syndromes. Poor absorption of folic acid from the duodenum and jejunum results in folate deficiency, particularly in gluten-sensitive enteropathy and tropical sprue.

[5]Hernández-Díaz S et al 1991 Lancet 338:131–137.
[6]A supplement of folic acid 5 mg/day is proposed for fuller risk reduction (Wald N J, Law M R, Morris J K, Walk D S 2001 Quantifying the effect of folic acid. Lancet 358:2069–2073).

Drugs. Antiepilepsy drugs, particularly phenytoin, primidone and phenobarbital, occasionally cause a macrocytic anaemia that responds to folic acid. This may be due to enzyme induction by the antiepileptics increasing the need for folic acid-mediated hydroxylation reactions (see Epilepsy, p. 372) but reduced absorption may be involved. Folate administration causes a recurrence of seizures in some patients. Some antimalarials, e.g. pyrimethamine, may interfere with conversion of folate to tetrahydrofolic acid, causing macrocytic anaemia. Methotrexate, another folate antagonist, may cause a megaloblastic anaemia especially when used long-term for leukaemia, rheumatoid arthritis or psoriasis.

Miscellaneous causes of excess utilisation or loss. Folate requirement increases in chronic haemolytic states, where erythropoiesis accelerates, and in myelofibrosis, where haematopoiesis is inefficient. Extensive shedding of skin cells in exfoliative dermatitis can lead to folate deficiency. Folate loss during chronic haemodialysis may be sufficient to require replacement.

CONTRAINDICATIONS

Imprecisely diagnosed megaloblastic anaemia is the principal contraindication (see vitamin B_{12}, above). Tumour cell proliferation in some cancers may be folate dependent and in malignant disease folic acid should be given only where there is confirmed folate deficiency anaemia.

PREPARATIONS AND DOSAGE

For therapy, give synthetic folic acid 5 mg/day by mouth for 4 months, or indefinitely if the cause of deficiency cannot be removed; 15 mg/day may be needed in malabsorption states, although 5 mg is usually adequate. There is no advantage in giving folinic acid instead of folic acid, except in the treatment of the toxic effects of folic acid antagonists such as methotrexate (folinic acid 'rescue', see p. 546).

- For prophylaxis, with iron, in pregnancy, see page 531.
- For prophylaxis in haemolytic diseases and in renal dialysis: 5 mg/day or per week depending on need.

Adverse reactions are rare: allergy occurs, and status epilepticus may be precipitated.

HAEMOPOIETIC GROWTH FACTORS

Recombinant DNA technology allows large-scale production of cytokines to stimulate erythroid and myeloid lineages. These agents are potentially useful for cytopenia due to disease or chemotherapy.[7]

ERYTHROPOIETIN

Erythropoietin is a glycoprotein encoded by a gene on chromosome 7 (7q), essential to red cell production. The kidneys produce 90% (the liver most of the remainder). Production increases with hypoxia and decreases with polycythaemia. The anaemia of chronic renal failure is largely due to failure of erythropoietin production.

Erythropoietin binds to receptors on erythrocyte progenitors and stimulates their survival, proliferation and differentiation.

Epoetin (recombinant human erythropoietin) must be given subcutaneously (which may be more effective) or intravenously; the $t_{1/2}$ is 4 h and is not affected by dialysis. The maximum reticulocyte response occurs in 4 days. Self-administration at home three times a week is practicable; dosage depends on response. Iron reserves must be adequate for optimal erythropoiesis, i.e. serum ferritin should exceed 100 micrograms/L. Epoetin is available as two preparations, *epoetin α* and *epoetin β*, which are interchangeable.

Epoetin is effective for the anaemia of chronic renal failure and significantly enhances quality of life of patients before dialysis and receiving dialysis. Patients become independent of blood transfusion. It has also been used successfully in anaemia due to cancer chemotherapy, notably in patients with a haemoglobin level lower than 10 g/dL and inadequate endogenous erythropoietin production.[8] Epoetin has also been effective for anaemia due to zidovudine treatment for HIV, prematurity, rheumatoid arthritis and myelodysplasia. In all of these settings

---

[7]Ozer H, Armitage J O, Bennett C L 2000 Update of recommendations for the use of haematopoietic colony-stimulating factors: evidence-based, clinical practice guidelines. Journal of Clinical Oncology 18:3558–3585.

[8]Rizzo J D, Lichtin A E, Woolf S H et al 2002 Use of epoietin in patients with cancer: evidence-based clinical practice guidelines of the American Society of Clinical Oncology and the American Society of Hematology. Blood 100:2303–2320.

higher doses of epoietin are required than are effective in renal patients. It may be used to reduce the need for blood transfusion in elective non-cardiac, non-vascular surgery, and can be considered before surgery in Jehovah's witnesses who decline blood transfusion.

Adverse effects. Transient influenza-like symptoms may accompany initial intravenous injections. In patients with renal failure, a dose-dependent increase in arterial blood pressure follows the rise in red cell mass, and encephalopathy may occur in some hypertensive patients. Arteriovenous shunts of dialysis patients, especially those that are compromised, may thrombose because of increased blood viscosity. Pure red cell aplasia due to development of antibodies may occur after epoietin α. As increased haematopoiesis outstrips iron stores, iron deficiency may develop, especially in dialysis patients, and provide an explanation for inadequate response, necessitating parenteral iron.

Darbepoietin is a hyperglycosylated erythropoietin derivative with a longer $t_{1/2}$ that allows administration once weekly or even less frequently for anaemia of renal failure and chemotherapy.

COLONY-STIMULATING FACTORS

Several cytokines stimulate the growth, differentiation and activity of myeloid cells. They have effects on multipotential stem cells, intermediate progenitors and mature cells.

Granulocyte colony-stimulating factors. G-CSF, an 18-kDa protein encoded by a gene on chromosome 17 (17q), stimulates proliferation of granulocyte progenitors and enhances neutrophil function.

A single dose of recombinant G-CSF increases the neutrophil count 4–5-fold within hours which persists for up to 72 h. The drug is rapidly cleared after intravenous injection ($t_{1/2}$ 2 h) and administration by intravenous infusion or subcutaneously is necessary to prolong plasma concentration. High concentrations of G-CSF are found in plasma, bone marrow and kidneys; it is degraded to amino acids and excreted in urine.

G-CSF is used to mobilise haematopoietic stem cells into peripheral blood for harvesting to support both autologous transplantation (from patients) and allogeneic transplantation (from donors). Mobilised progenitors from peripheral blood are associated with earlier neutrophil and platelet recovery, fewer transfusions and shorter hospitalisation than those from bone marrow.

G-CSF shortens the period of neutropenia and reduces infections in patients on cytotoxic chemotherapy but it does not improve survival despite allowing the oncologist to maintain intensity in chemotherapy dose. It improves neutrophil counts after autologous and allogeneic bone marrow transplantation, in aplastic anaemia and AIDS. G-CSF can improve the neutrophil count in myelodysplastic syndromes, and in some patients, in combination with epoetin, it improves the haemoglobin response, possibly by reduction of erythroid apoptosis.

G-CSF increases the neutrophil count substantially in congenital, cyclical and idiopathic neutropenia, reduces the risk of life-threatening infection and prolongs survival, but there is an increased risk of acute myeloid leukaemia in children with congenital neutropenia treated with G-CSF.

Adverse effect. Medullary bone pain occurs with high intravenous doses. Musculoskeletal pain, dysuria, splenomegaly, allergic reactions and raised liver enzymes also occur. Patients with sickle cell anaemia may develop painful crises.

Pegfilgrastim has polyethylene glycol covalently bound to G-CSF, which prolongs the $t_{1/2}$ to 40 h and allows less frequent dosing, e.g. once per chemotherapy cycle.

Thrombopoietin (TPO), a 36-kDa protein encoded by a gene on chromosome 3 (3q), regulates platelet production by stimulating growth and differentiation of megakaryocytes. It also primes platelets to respond to stimuli. TPO and similar small molecules with thrombopoietic activity are undergoing clinical evaluation.

SICKLE CELL ANAEMIA

In sickle cell disease, deoxygenated haemoglobin S (HbS) forms polymers that cause erythrocytes to become inflexible 'sickle-shaped' forms that obstruct blood flow and cause the clinical features, principally haemolysis, anaemia and painful bone crises. The observation that hereditary persistence of haemoglobin F (HbF) interferes with HbS polymerisation and inhibits erythrocyte sickling opened a therapeutic strategy.

Hydroxycarbamide (hydroxyurea), an antimetabolite, is the first widely available and affordable agent to provide real benefit. It promotes HbF production in maturating erythrocytes. The mode of action may be more complex: a fall in leucocyte counts may reduce vaso-occlusive events, and may lessen red cell and endothelial adhesiveness.[9]

Beneficial effects have been seen in adults, children and infants. Long-term daily administration of hydroxycarbamide at close to myelotoxic doses raises HbF to 15–20% (normally <1% in adults) and reduces the number of hospitalisations, pain, acute chest syndrome and need for blood transfusion. Neurological complications, e.g. stroke, may not be reduced. Long-term follow-up shows reduced mortality in patients taking hydroxycarbamide. Some 10–20% of patients fail to respond due to the condition of the bone marrow, or genetic effects (see also p. 667).

Adverse effects. The long-term risk of leukaemogenesis appears to be negligible. There appear to be no adverse effects on growth or development.

POLYCYTHAEMIA VERA

The clinical course of polycythaemia vera (PV) is marked by a risk of thrombotic complications and long-term transformation to myelofibrosis or acute myeloblastic leukaemia (AML). The object of treatment is to minimise the risk of thrombosis and to prevent transformation to AML. No treatment convincingly delays marrow fibrosis.

Venesection of 300–500 mL is performed weekly or twice weekly to attain a haematocrit of less than 0.45. Thereafter venesection is performed every 3–6 months to maintain a normal haematocrit. Iron deficiency may occur and requires cautious treatment. When a normal haematocrit can be maintained only by frequent venesection, or a raised platelet count indicates thrombotic risk, myelosuppressive

therapy is added. This reduces the risk of thrombosis during aggressive initial venesection, particularly in elderly patients. Low-dose aspirin (100 mg/day) reduces the rate of thrombosis and cardiac death in patients with PV.

Hydroxycarbamide (hydroxyurea) carries a lower risk of leukaemogenesis than busulfan or [32]P (see below) but concerns remain. Hydroxycarbamide 500–2000 mg/day inhibits myeloproliferation, normalises the platelet count and spleen size, reduces venesection requirements, reduces the incidence of thrombosis and ameliorates hypercatabolic symptoms. It is regarded as acceptable therapy for patients aged less than 60 years with PV or essential thrombocythaemia (ET).

Anagrelide, a prostaglandin synthetase inhibitor, lowers platelet counts by inhibiting megakaryocyte maturation. It is non-mutagenic and effectively controls thrombocytosis in polycythaemia and essential thrombocythaemia, but does not suppress other lineages or treat hypercatabolic symptoms. It is active orally.

Adverse effects are cardiovascular: headache, forceful heartbeats, fluid retention and cardiac arrhythmia.

Interferon α is a non-leukaemogenic alternative for younger patients. Doses of 3–5 megaunits s.c. three times weekly control blood counts, splenomegaly and constitutional symptoms; it may be used in pregnant women.

Busulfan is a radiomimetic cytotoxic agent that reduces vascular events and delays myelofibrosis in PV. Mutagenic potential restricts its use to older patients.

Radiophosphorus (^{32}P, sodium radiophosphate) is concentrated in bone and rapidly dividing cells. Erythroid precursors receive most of the β-irradiation. Accumulation in gonads always precluded use in younger patients with PV. Radiophosphorus is a palliative treatment option for elderly patients unable to tolerate other therapies, but otherwise is rarely used. Maximal therapeutic effect occurs 1–2 months after a single dose and usually provides control for 1–2 years. Excessive leukocytopenia and thrombocytopenia are the main adverse effects. Acute myeloid leukaemia occurs more frequently

[9]Steinberg M H, Barton F, Castro O et al 2003 Effect of hydroxyurea on mortality and morbidity in adult sickle cell anaemia: risks and benefits up to 9 years of treatment. Journal of the American Medical Association 289:1645–1651.

in patients treated with radiophosphorus especially when combined with hydroxycarbamide.

Other features. Pruritus is troublesome, unresponsive to venesection or antiplatelet therapy and difficult to relieve; it may be improved by H_1- and/or H_2-histamine receptor blockade, PUVA therapy, hydroxycarbamide or interferon-α. Hyperuricaemia, due to cell destruction, is corrected by allopurinol; iron and folate deficiency require replacement doses.

APLASTIC ANAEMIA

Aplastic anaemia may be idiopathic or secondary to chemicals, e.g. benzene, drugs or infection. Treatment is determined by the severity of the cytopenias, age, availability of a marrow donor and, less commonly, the cause. Good supportive treatment is important.

Therapeutic choice is between immunosuppression with antilymphocytic globulin and ciclosporin, and allogeneic bone marrow transplantation. The latter carries survival rates of 75–80% but chronic graft-versus-host disease causes continued morbidity.

Patients who are not candidates for bone marrow transplantation due to age or the lack of a donor (up to 70%) receive immunosuppression. Equine antithymocyte globulin (ATG) or rabbit antilymphocyte globulin (ALG) induce haematological responses, transfusion independence and freedom from infection in around 50%. Addition of ciclosporin to ATG or ALG improves response rates to 70–80%, and survival rates in responders to 90%. Treatment should be initiated within 14 days of diagnosis and responses generally occur within 4 months. Relapse occurs in 35% within 5 years but may respond to further immunosuppression (rabbit ALG after initial equine ATG).

Adverse effects of ATG and ALG include anaphylaxis, exacerbation of cytopenia and serum sickness. In refractory patients G-CSF and erythropoetin can improve blood counts.

GUIDE TO FURTHER READING

Abkowitz J L 2001 Aplastic anemia: which treatment? Annals of Internal Medicine 135(7):524–526

Botto L D, Moore C A, Khoury M J et al 1999 Neural tube defects. New England Journal of Medicine 341: 1509–1519

Carmel R 2000 Current concepts in cobalamin deficiency. Annual Reviews of Medicine 51:357–375

Castle W B 1966 Treatment of pernicious anemia: historical aspects. Clinical Pharmacology and Therapeutics 7(2): 147–161

Estey E, Döhner H 2006 Acute myeloid leukaemia. Lancet 368:1894–1907

Fleming R E, Bacon B R 2005 Orchestration of iron homeostasis. New England Journal of Medicine 352:1741–1744

Hehlmann R, Hochhaus A, Baccarani M On behalf of the European LeukemiaNet 2007 Chronic myeloid leukaemia. Lancet 370:342–350

Kaushansky K 2006 Lineage-specific hematopoietic growth factors. New England Journal of Medicine 354:2034–2045

Rund D, Rachmilewitz E 2005 β-thalassemia. New England Journal of Medicine 353:1135–1146

Spivak J L 2000 The blood in systemic disorders. Lancet 355:1707–1712

Tapiero H, Gate L, Tew K D et al 2001 Iron: deficiencies and requirements. Biomedicine and Pharmacotherapy 55:324–332

Tefferi A 2003 Polycythemia vera: a comprehensive review and clinical recommendations. Mayo Clinic Proceedings 78:174–194

Weatherall D J, Provan A B 2000 Red cells I: inherited anaemias. Lancet 355:1169–1175

Weatherall D J, Provan A B 2000 Red cells II: acquired anaemias and polycythaemia. Lancet 355:1260–1268

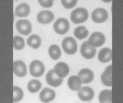

30

Neoplastic disease and immunosuppression

SYNOPSIS

In most cases, the cause of cancer is multifactorial. Most cancer incidences are sporadic, with fewer than 10% being familial. In about 75% of cases, environmental factors are recognised, some of which are within the control of the individual, e.g. tobacco smoking, diet, exposure to sunlight. The growing number and efficacy of systemic modalities available to treat patients with cancer are significantly improving disease outcomes. Immunosuppressive drugs are described here as they share many characteristics with anticancer drugs.

- Cancer treatments and outcomes
- Rationale for cytotoxic chemotherapy[1]
- Classes of cytotoxic chemotherapy drugs
- Chemotherapy in clinical practice
- Endocrine therapy
- Immunotherapy
- Targeted biological therapies
- Immunosuppression and immunosuppressive drugs

NEOPLASTIC DISEASE

CANCER TREATMENTS AND OUTCOMES

Cancers share some common characteristics:

- Growth that is not subject to normal restrictions for that tissue and fails to respond to apoptotic signals (see below) or in which a high proportion of cells are dividing, i.e. there is a high 'growth fraction'.

- Local invasiveness.
- Tendency to spread to other parts of the body (metastasise).
- Less differentiated cell morphology.
- Tendency to retain some characteristics of the tissue of origin.

Cancer treatment employs six established principal modalities:

1. surgery
2. radiotherapy
3. cytotoxic chemotherapy
4. endocrine therapy
5. immunotherapy
6. biological (or targeted) therapy.

This account describes the main groups of drugs (see p. 544) but it is important to understand the overall context in which systemic therapy is offered to patients.

SYSTEMIC CANCER THERAPY

Cancers originating from different organs of the body differ in their behaviour and in their response to treatments (Table 30.1). Primary surgery and/or radiotherapy to a *localised* cancer offer the best chance of *cure* for patients. Drug treatments offer cure only for certain types of cancer, often characterised by their high proliferative rate, e.g. lymphoma, testicular cancer, Wilms' tumour. More often, systemic therapy offers prolongation of life, although patients may ultimately die from their disease.

Use of drugs as *adjuvant therapy* attempts to eradicate residual microscopic cancer by treating patients usually after their primary surgery. This strategy has improved overall survival for patients after surgical resection of primary breast and colorectal cancer. In some situations, drugs are administered prior to surgery (*neoadjuvant therapy*), primarily to shrink large, locally advanced disease to enable surgical resection. Many patients with cancer are not cured

---

[1]Although not in strict accord with the definition of Chapter 11, the word 'chemotherapy' is in general use in this connection and it would be pedantic to avoid it. It arose because some malignant cells can be cultured and the disease transmitted by inoculation, as with bacteria. The more precise term 'cytotoxic chemotherapy' is adopted here.

Table 30.1 Degree of benefit achieved with systemic therapy for common cancers

Curable: chemosensitive cancers	Improved survival: some degree of chemosensitivity	Equivocal survival benefit: chemoresistant cancers
Teratoma	Colorectal cancer	Sarcoma
Seminoma	Small cell lung cancer	Bladder cancer
High-grade non-Hodgkin's lymphoma	Ovarian cancer	Melanoma
Hodgkin's lymphoma	Breast cancer	Renal cancer
Wilms' tumour	Cervical cancer	Primary brain cancers
Acute myeloblastic leukaemia	Endometrial cancer	Nasopharyngeal carcinoma
Acute lymphoblastic leukaemia in childhood	Gastro-oesophageal cancer	Cholangiocarcinoma
	Myeloma	Hepatoma
	Pancreatic cancer	
	Low-grade non-Hodgkin lymphoma	
	Non-small cell lung cancer	
	Adult acute lymphoblastic leukaemia	

by their primary treatment; the disease often returns months or years later even though at the time of completing their initial treatment there was no visible evidence of cancer. Clearly, this is a limitation of current standard (mainly radiological) techniques used to identify residual disease.

Palliative therapy, offered to patients with advanced, incurable cancer, aims both to increase survival and to improve quality of life by symptom control, at least in the short term. Despite significant improvements in cancer outcomes in the last 5–10 years, there remain a number of types of cancer that are poorly responsive to currently available drugs. Patients with *chemoresistant* cancers who are fit enough and willing may be offered experimental treatments within clinical trials.

Most treatments currently available are associated with unwanted effects of varying degrees of severity. The risk of causing harm must be weighed against the potential to do good in each individual case. *Systemic therapy* aims to kill malignant cells or modify their growth and leave those of the host unharmed or, and more usually, temporarily harmed but capable of recovery. When there is realistic expectation of cure or extensive life prolongation, then to risk more severe drug toxicity is justified. For example, the treatment of testicular cancer with potentially life-threatening platinum-based combination chemotherapy regimens offers a greater than 85% chance of cure, even for those with extensive, metastatic disease.

Where expectation is confined to palliation in terms of modest life prolongation of less certain quality, then the benefits and risks of treatment must be judged carefully. Palliative treatments should involve low risk of adverse effects, e.g. 5-fluorouracil-based chemotherapy for advanced colorectal cancer is well tolerated by most patients while improving survival by around 1–2 years.

Clearly, clinicians and nurses must explain the potential benefits and harm of treatment to patients and their families, who may themselves hold strong views about the quality and quantity of life.

RATIONALE FOR CYTOTOXIC CHEMOTHERAPY

The narrow therapeutic index of cytotoxic agents means that escalation of drug doses is constrained by damage to normal cells and the maximum doses that patients can tolerate are often suboptimal to achieve total cancer cell killing.

Even so, cytotoxic chemotherapy agents remain the mainstay of systemic anticancer treatment, as an understanding of their pharmacology has enabled clinicians to exploit the benefits of these drugs by various means (see below).

The very real limitations of cytotoxic chemotherapy have forced a concentration of much cancer research on trying to understand the carcinogenic process, the aim being to identify specific molecular targets that can be exploited to develop novel therapeutic approaches. So-called *targeted* therapies are now well established groups of anticancer drugs.

CLASSES OF CYTOTOXIC CHEMOTHERAPY DRUGS

Cytotoxic chemotherapy drugs exert their effect by inhibiting cell proliferation. All proliferating cells, whether normal and malignant, cycle through a series of phases of: *synthesis* of DNA (S phase), *mitosis* (M phase) and *rest* (G_1 phase). Non-cycling cells are quiescent in G_0 phase (Fig. 30.1).

Cytotoxic drugs interfere with cell division at various points of the cell cycle, in particular G1/S phase (e.g. synthesis of nucleotides from purines and pyrimidines), S phase (preventing DNA replication) and M phase (e.g. blocking the process of mitosis).

They are potentially mutagenic. Such drugs ultimately induce cell death by *apoptosis*[2], a process by which single cells are removed from the midst of living tissue by being fragmented into membrane-bound particles and phagocytosed by other cells. This occurs without disturbing the architecture or function of the tissue, or eliciting an inflammatory response. The instructions for the response are built into the cell's genetic material, i.e. 'programmed cell death'.[3]

In general, cytotoxics are most effective against actively cycling cells and least effective against resting or quiescent cells. The latter are particularly problematic in that, although inactive, they retain the capacity to proliferate and may start cycling again after a completed course of chemotherapy, often leading later to rapid regrowth of the cancer.

Cytotoxic drugs can be classified as either:

■ *Cell cycle non-specific*: these kill cells whether they are resting or actively cycling (as in a low growth fraction cancer such as solid tumours), e.g. alkylating agents, doxorubicin and allied anthracyclines.
■ *Cell cycle (phase) specific*: these kill only cells that are actively cycling, often because their site of action is confined to one phase of the cell cycle, e.g. antimetabolite drugs.

---

[2]Greek: *apo*, off; *ptosis*, a falling.
[3]Makin G, Dive C 2001 Apoptosis and cancer chemotherapy. Trends in Cell Biology 11:S22–26. (*Dysregulated* apoptosis is also involved in the pathogenesis of many forms of neoplastic disease, notably many lymphomas; understanding its mechanisms and the defective processes offers scope for novel approaches to the treatment of cancer.)

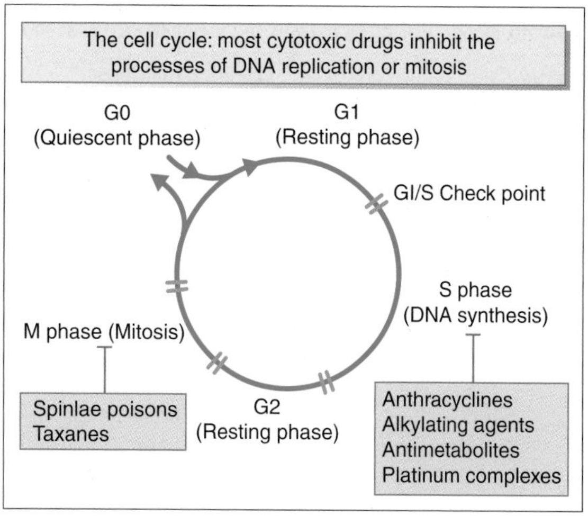

Fig. 30.1 The cell cycle. Most cytotoxic drugs inhibit the processes of DNA replication or mitosis.

Table 30.2 provides a summary of the key groups of anticancer drugs, their common toxicities and main treatment applications.

ADVERSE EFFECTS OF CYTOTOXIC CHEMOTHERAPY

Principal adverse effects are manifest as, or follow damage to, the following:

Nausea and vomiting may occur within hours of treatment or be delayed, and last for several days, depending on the agent. As emetogenicity is largely predictable, preventive action can be taken. The most effective drugs are competitive antagonists of serotonin (5-hydroxytryptamine type 3, $5HT_3$) receptors, e.g. ondansetron, and dexamethasone, which benefits by an unknown mechanism. Other effective antiemetics include cyclizine, prochlorperazine, domperidone and metoclopramide (see p. 568). Combinations of drugs may be used and routes of administration selected as commonsense counsels, e.g. prophylaxis may be oral, but when vomiting occurs the parenteral route and suppositories are available.

Suppression of bone marrow and the lymphoreticular system. Myelosuppression with depression of both antibody- and cell-mediated immunity is the single most important dose-limiting factor with cytotoxic agents, and carries life-threatening consequences.

Table 30.2 Principal classes of cytotoxic drug, their common toxicities and examples of clinical use

Drug class	Common toxicities	Examples of clinical use
Cytotoxic Drugs		
Alkylating agents	Nausea and vomiting, bone marrow depression (delayed with carmustine and lomustine), cystitis (cyclophosphamide, ifosfamide), pulmonary fibrosis (especially busulfan). Male infertility and premature menopause may occur. Myelodysplasia and secondary neoplasia	Widely used in the treatment of both haematological and non-haematological cancers, with varying degrees of success
Platinum drugs	Bone marrow depression, nausea and vomiting, allergy reaction (esp. carboplatin), nephrotoxicity, hypomagnesaemia; hypocalcaemia; hypokalaemia; hypophosphataemia; hyperuricaemia (all as a consequence of renal dysfunction, primarily associated with cisplatin); Raynaud's disease; sterility; teratogenesis; ototoxicity (cisplatin); peripheral neuropathy; cold dysaesthesia and pharyngolaryngeal dysaesthesia (oxaliplatin)	Testicular cancers, ovarian cancer; oxaliplatin acts synergistically with 5FU and is licensed in combination with 5FU to treat both advanced and early stages of colorectal cancer
Nucleoside analogues, e.g. cytarabine, gemcitabine, fludarabine	Bone marrow depression, mainly affecting platelets; mild nausea and vomiting; diarrhoea; anaphylaxis; sudden respiratory distress with high doses (cytarabine); rash, fluid retention and oedema; profound immunosuppression with fludarabine	Cytarabine is used in haematological regimens; gemcitabine is used for pancreatic cancer, bladder cancer and some other solid tumours; fludarabine is active in chronic lymphatic leukaemia and lymphoma
Taxanes	Nausea and vomiting, hypersensitivity reactions, bone marrow depression, fluid retention; peripheral neuropathy; alopecia; arthralgias; myalgias; cardiac toxicity; mild GI disturbances; mucositis	Breast and gynaecological cancers; recent evidence that docetaxel improves survival in advanced prostate cancer
Anthracyclines	Nausea and vomiting, bone marrow depression; cardiotoxicity (may be delayed for years); red-coloured urine; severe local tissue damage and necrosis on extravasation; alopecia; stomatitis; anorexia; conjunctivitis; acral (extremities) pigmentation; dermatitis in previously irradiated areas; hyperuricaemia	Common component of many chemotherapy regimens for both haematological and non-haematological malignancies
Antimetabolites, e.g. 5-fluorouracil, methotrexate	Nausea and vomiting; diarrhoea; mucositis, bone marrow depression, neurological defects, usually cerebellar; cardiac arrhythmias; angina pectoris, hyperpigmentation, hand–foot syndrome, conjunctivitis	Commonly used in haematological and non-haematological malignancies
Topoismerase I inhibitors	Nausea and vomiting; cholinergic syndrome; hypersensitivity reactions; bone marrow depression; diarrhoea; colitis; ileus; alopecia; renal impairment; teratogenic	Irinotecan is effective in advanced colorectal cancer; topotecan is used in gynaecological malignancies
Mitotic spindle inhibitors (vinca alkaloids)	Nausea and vomiting; local reaction and phlebitis with extravasation, neuropathy, bone marrow depression; alopecia; stomatitis; loss of deep tendon reflexes; jaw pain; muscle pain; paralytic ileus	Commonly used in haemato-oncology regimens
Hormones		
Tamoxifen	Hot flushes; transiently increased bone or tumour pain; vaginal bleeding and discharge; rash; thromboembolism; endometrial cancer	Oestrogen receptor positive, advanced and early stage breast cancer
Aromatase inhibitors	Nausea; dizziness; rash; bone marrow depression; fever; masculinisation	Equivalence with tamoxifen suggested

Drug class	Common toxicities	Examples of clinical use
Medroxyprogesterone acetate	Menstrual changes; gynaecomastia; hot flushes; oedema, weight gain; hirsutism; insomnia; fatigue; depression; thrombophlebitis and thromboembolism; nausea; urticaria; headache	Third-line therapy for slowly progressive breast cancer in postmenopausal women
Flutamide	Nausea; diarrhoea, gynaecomastia; hepatotoxicity	Prostate cancer
Goserelin	Transient increase in bone pain and urethral obstruction in patients with metastatic prostatic cancer; hot flushes; impotence; testicular atrophy; gynaecomastia	Prostate cancer
Leuprolelin (LHRH analogue)	Transient increase in bone pain and ureteral obstruction in patients with metastatic prostatic cancer; hot flushes, impotence; testicular atrophy; gynaecomastia; peripheral oedema	Prostate cancer
Immunotherapy		
BCG (bacille Calmette–Guérin)	Bladder irritation; nausea and vomiting; fever; sepsis, granulomatous pyelonephritis; hepatitis; urethral obstruction; epididymitis; renal abscess	Localised bladder cancer
Interferon-α	Fever; chills; myalgias; fatigue; headache; arthralgias, bone marrow depression; anorexia; confusion; depression; psychiatric disorders; renal toxicity; hepatic toxicity; rash	Renal cancer
Interleukin-2	Fever; fluid retention; hypotension; respiratory distress; rash; anaemia, thrombocytopenia; nausea and vomiting; diarrhoea, capillary leak syndrome, nephrotoxicity; myocardial toxicity; hepatotoxicity; erythema nodosum; neuropsychiatric disorders; hypothyroidism; nephrotic syndrome	Renal cancer
Trastuzumab (Herceptin)	Fever; chills; nausea and vomiting; pain; hypersensitivity and pulmonary reactions, bone marrow depression; cardiomyopathy; ventricular dysfunction; congestive cardiac failure; diarrhoea	Advanced and early stage breast cancer, combined with cytotoxic chemotherapy
Rituximab (MabThera)	Hypersensitivity reaction, bone marrow depression, angio-oedema, precipitation of angina or arrhythmia with pre-existing heart disease	Non-Hodgkin's lymphoma

Repeated blood monitoring is essential and transfusion of red cells and platelets may be necessary. Cell growth factors, e.g. the natural granulocyte colony-stimulating factor (filgrastim), are available to protect against or to resolve severe neutropenia.

Opportunistic infection by Gram-negative bacteria from the patient's own flora, e.g. from the gut that has been damaged by chemotherapy, may occur. Infections with virus (herpes zoster), fungus (candida) and protozoa (pneumocystis) are also increased. Fever in a patient receiving chemotherapy usually requires immediate hospitalisation, collection of samples for microbiological studies and urgent empirical initiation of antibiotic treatment. Where risk of neutropenia is high, antimicrobial prophylaxis may be used. High-dose chemoradiotherapy and allogeneic bone marrow transplant produce profound immunosuppression with significant risk of opportunistic infection and third-party graft-versus-host disease following unirradiated blood transfusion. Live vaccines are *contraindicated* in these patients.

Diarrhoea and mouth ulcers usually arise from drug damage to gut epithelium and other mucosal surfaces with a naturally rapid cell turnover.

Alopecia is due to an effect on the hair bulb; it recovers 2–6 months after ceasing treatment. Scalp cooling may prevent or limit this with certain drugs, e.g. vinca alkaloids.

Urate nephropathy is due to rapid destruction of malignant cells releasing purines and pyrimidines, which are metabolised to uric acid that may crystallise in and block the renal tubule (urate nephropathy). In practice this occurs only when there is a large cell mass or a tumour is very sensitive to drugs, e.g. acute leukaemias and high-grade lymphomas. High fluid intake, alkalinisation of the urine and use of allopurinol or rasburicase during the early stages of chemotherapy avert this outcome.

Local extravasation may damage surrounding tissues; it is a problem with certain vesicant cytotoxics, e.g. doxorubicin, dacarbazine. This is a medical emergency and policies for management (which may include debridement by a plastic surgeon) should be in place in every oncology centre.

Hypersensitivity reactions may occur with susceptible patients. These are more problematic with certain cytotoxic agents, e.g. paclitaxel, carboplatin, for which prophylactic corticosteroid and antihistamine are offered routinely.

Specific organ damage may result, e.g. lung toxicity with bleomycin, cardiotoxicity with anthracyclines, nephrotoxicity with platinum agents.

Delayed wound healing can be expected. Surgical wounds should be healed prior to commencing chemotherapy, wherever possible.

Germ cells and reproduction deserve special attention as chemotherapy may cause infertility. In addition, the mutagenic effects of cytotoxic drugs mean that reproduction is to be avoided during and for several months after therapy (although both men and women have reproduced normally whilst undergoing chemotherapy). When treatment may cause permanent sterility, men are offered the facility for prior storage of sperm. Cryopreservation of ovarian tissue is now also feasible. Prior contraceptive advice is necessary, as most cytotoxic drugs are teratogenic and are contraindicated during pregnancy.

Carcinogenicity may result in second malignancies and this becomes a more pressing issue where treatment improves life expectancy. Patients with Hodgkin's lymphoma are often young, and chemotherapy greatly prolongs survival but, by contrast, ovarian cancer does not. Many cytotoxic drugs are themselves carcinogenic, and a patient may be cured of the primary disease only to succumb to a second,

treatment-induced, cancer 5–20 years later. Whether this is due to a mutagenic effect, to immunosuppression, or to both, remains unclear. Alkylating agents are particularly incriminated, as are some antimetabolites (mercaptopurine) and anthracyclines (doxorubicin), and the risk can be as high as 10 to 20 times that for unexposed people. The cancers caused include leukaemia, lymphoma and squamous carcinoma.

CLASSES OF CYTOTOXIC AGENTS

ALKYLATING AGENTS

Alkylating agents (nitrogen mustards and ethylenimines) act by transferring alkyl groups to DNA in the N-7 position of guanine during cell division. Normal synthesis is prevented because of either DNA strand breakage or crosslinking of the two strands. Examples include: busulfan, carmustine, chlorambucil, cyclophosphamide, ifosfamide, lomustine, melphalan, mustine (mechlorethamine), thiotepa, treosulfan.

ANTIMETABOLITES

Antimetabolites are synthetic analogues of normal metabolites and act by competition to 'deceive' or 'defraud' bodily processes.

Methotrexate, a folic acid antagonist, competitively inhibits dihydrofolate reductase, preventing the synthesis of tetrahydrofolic acid (the co-enzyme that is important in synthesis of amino and nucleic acids). The drug also provides a cogent illustration of the need to exploit every possible means of enhancing selectivity. Where the desire is to maximise the effect of methotrexate, a potentially fatal dose is given, followed 24 h later by a dose of tetrahydrofolic (folinic) acid as calcium folinate (Ca Leucovorin) to bypass and terminate its action. This is called folinic acid 'rescue', because, if it is not given, the patient will die. The therapeutic justification for this manoeuvre is the cell kill obtained with very high plasma concentrations of methotrexate, allied to the fact that the bone marrow cells recover better than the tumour cells. The outcome is a useful degree of selectivity.

Pyrimidine antagonists: 5-fluorouracil (5FU) is metabolised intracellularly and its metabolite binds covalently with thymidilate synthase, thereby inhibiting DNA (and RNA) synthesis. 5FU has a short duration of action and addition of folinic acid in 5FU therapy improves its antitumour activity; protracted infusion can achieve the same outcome. Oral pro-drugs of 5FU include capecitabine and UFT (a mixture of ftorafur and uracil). These pro-drugs have a cytotoxic action equivalent to that of 5FU but cause less myelosuppression and stomatitis; the risk of hand–foot syndrome (damage to the palmar and plantar surfaces of the hands and feet causing reddening, soreness and blistering) is considerably higher.

Arabinosides (cytosine arabinoside, gemcitabine) and the *purine antagonists* (deoxycoformycin, fludarabine, 2-chloroadenisine) azathioprine, mercaptopurine and tioguanine are also converted intracellularly to active metabolites that inhibit DNA synthesis.

Antimetabolites find extensive use in anticancer therapy, either alone or in combination with other drugs. They remain the mainstay of treatment for haematological as well as common solid tumours such as breast and gastrointestinal tract cancers.

ANTHRACYCLINES AND RELATED COMPOUNDS

The original anthracyclines were antibiotics produced by microorganisms such as *Streptomycetes* spp. Daunorubicin and doxorubicin were the first compounds to be isolated and appear to interfere with both DNA and RNA synthesis. Other examples include bleomycin, dactinomycin, epirubicin, mitoxantrone, idarubicin, plicamycin (mithramycin), mitomycin and streptozotocin (most often used to treat the rare islet-cell pancreatic tumours).

TOPOISOMERASE INHIBITORS

Doxorubicin is a non-specific inhibitor of topoisomerase I and II. Topotecan and irinotecan selectively inhibit topoisomerase I, an enzyme required for DNA replication, and are effective in relapsed ovarian and colorectal cancer respectively. Bone marrow depression is dose limiting as, in the case of irinotecan, is delayed diarrhoea. Administration of irinotecan may be complicated by an acute cholinergic reaction, reversible by subcutaneous atropine. The epipodophyllotoxins (etoposide, teniposide) are the major inhibitors of topoisomerase II.

SPINDLE POISONS

The plant alkaloids (vincristine, vinblastine, vindesine and vinorelbine) and taxoids (paclitaxel, docetaxel) inhibit microtubule assembly and cause cell cycle arrest in mitosis. They particularly cause bone marrow depression and alopecia. Vincristine causes neuropathy.

PLATINUM DRUGS

This family of drugs (which include cisplatin, carboplatin and oxaliplatin) act by cross-linking DNA in a similar manner to alkylating agents. The parent drug, cisplatin, is associated with a variety of adverse effects, including severe emesis, nephrotoxicity and ototoxicity. Renal damage is ameliorated by carefully hydrating patients, and emetogenicity is effectively controlled with $5HT_3$ receptor (serotonin) antagonists. Second- (carboplatin) and third- (oxaliplatin) generation platinum agents have improved toxicity profiles, and offer effective treatment for germ cell, ovarian and colorectal cancers.

MISCELLANEOUS AGENTS

Asparaginase starves tumour cells dependent upon a supply of the amino acid, asparagine (except those able to synthesise it for themselves); its use is largely confined to acute lymphoblastic leukaemia.

CHEMOTHERAPY IN CLINICAL PRACTICE

DRUG USE AND TUMOUR CELL KINETICS

Evidence from leukaemia in laboratory animals shows that:

- Survival time is inversely related to the initial number of leukaemia cells, or to the number remaining after treatment.
- A single leukaemia cell is capable of multiplying and eventually killing the host.

Cytotoxic drugs act against all multiplying cells. Bone marrow, mucosal surfaces (gut), hair follicles, reticuloendothelial system and germ cells all divide more rapidly than many cancer cells and are damaged by cytotoxic drugs, leading to the particular adverse effects of chemotherapy. In contrast to haematological cancers, most solid tumours in humans divide slowly and recovery from cytotoxic agents is slow, whereas normal marrow and gut recover rapidly. This speed of recovery of normal tissues is exploited in devising intermittent courses of chemotherapy.

In cancer, the normal feedback mechanisms that mediate cell growth are defective and cell proliferation continues unchecked, cancer cells multiplying, at first, exponentially. Cancers with high growth fractions, e.g. acute leukaemias, high-grade lymphomas, may visibly enlarge at an alarming rate, but may also be highly sensitive to cytotoxic chemotherapy. In later stages, the growth rate of these cancers slows and the volume-doubling time lengthens due to several factors, most of which conspire to render the advanced cancer less susceptible to drugs, namely:

- increased cell cycle (division) time
- decrease in the number of cells actively dividing, with more in the resting state (decrease in growth fraction)
- increased cell death within the tumour as it ages
- overcrowding of cells leading to necrotic, avascular areas that cannot easily be penetrated by drugs.

Selectivity of drugs for cancer cells is generally low compared with the selectivity shown by antimicrobial agents but it can be substantial, e.g. in lymphoma, where tumour cell kill with some drugs is 10 000 times greater than that of marrow cells. Cell destruction by cytotoxic drugs follows first-order kinetics, i.e. a given dose of drug kills a constant *fraction* of cells (not a constant *number*) regardless of the number of cells present. Thus a treatment that reduces a cell population from 1 000 000 to 10 000 (a two-log cell kill) will reduce a cell population of 1000 to 10. Furthermore, cell chemosensitivity within a cancer is not homogeneous owing to random mutations as the tumour grows, the cells remaining after initial doses being more likely to resist further treatment. Therefore, combining several drugs may be more effective than a single agent given repeatedly to the limit of tolerance.

The selection of drugs in combination chemotherapy is influenced by:

- Choosing drugs that act at different biochemical sites in the cell.
- Using drugs that attack cells at different phases of the growth cycle (see Fig. 30.1). 'CHOP' is a standard combination chemotherapy regimen

for non-Hodgkin's lymphoma. The acronym stands for *c*yclophosphamide, doxorubicin (previously known as *h*ydroxydoxyrubicin), vincristine (previously called *o*ncovin) and *p*rednisolone. The first three cytotoxic drugs exert their antitumour effect on different aspects of cell proliferation. The antitumour effect of corticosteroid remains unclear.

- The desirability of attaining synchronisation of cell cycling to achieve maximum cell kill. Cells are killed or are arrested in mitosis by vincristine, which is then withdrawn. Cells then enter a new reproductive cycle more or less synchronously, and when most are judged to be in a phase sensitive to a particular phase-specific drug, e.g. methotrexate or cytarabine, it is given.
- Avoidance of cross-resistance (see below) between drugs. In some instances, use of one drug regimen *followed* by another rather than using them simultaneously in combination avoids drug resistance and improves therapeutic efficacy. For example, epirubicin given for four cycles followed by CMF (concomitant cyclophosphamide, methotrexate and 5-fluorouracil) for four cycles has largely replaced CMF alone as standard adjuvant chemotherapy for breast cancer, because the outcome is better.
- Non-overlapping toxicity profiles. Before establishing a combination regimen, trials are undertaken, frequently fixing the dose of one drug while escalating the dose of another, in small cohorts of carefully monitored patients, so that toxicity and patient safety can be monitored.
- Empirical evidence of efficacy against a particular tumour type. The antitumour activity of platinum complexes was a chance finding (see below).
- Enhanced cell killing in preclinical models when drugs are combined. Oxaliplatin on its own has limited cytotoxicity against colorectal cancer cell lines in vitro and in mouse xenograft models, but its combination with 5FU confers a more than additive, i.e. synergistic, killing effect on tumour cells.

Considerations of pharmacokinetics in relation to cell kinetics are of great importance, as drug treatment alters the behaviour of both malignant and normal cells.

DRUG RESISTANCE

Resistance to a cytotoxic chemotherapy agent may be present at the outset (primary resistance), or may develop with repeated drug exposure (acquired resistance). Increasing dosage is limited by toxicity, e.g. to bone marrow, which does not become tolerant. *Combination chemotherapy* is a strategy commonly used to address the problems of tumour resistance.

Multiple drug resistance (MDR) of a cancer is not uncommon. MDR is most frequently due to increased expression of an ATP-dependent membrane efflux pump called P-glycoprotein (Pgp), which is a member of a class of membrane proteins called the ATP-binding cassette superfamily. Pgp is an important protective mechanism possessed by many normal cells against environmental toxins and has broad specificity for hydrophobic compounds. Long-lived cells such as the haemopoietic stem cell, cells on excretory surfaces such as biliary hepatocytes, proximal renal tubule and intestinal cells, and the cells of the blood–brain barrier all have high expression of Pgp. A number of agents including immunosuppressants (ciclosporin) and calcium channel blockers (verapamil and nifedipine) block Pgp.

The MDR phenomenon illustrates how tumour cells adapt and enhance normal cell mechanisms to deal with the effects of chemotherapy, and how repeated cycles of chemotherapy select out a population of cells that have developed adaptive survival mechanisms, e.g. in myeloma where MDR proteins are rare at diagnosis but common at progression.

Cytotoxic drugs vary in their capacity to stimulate P-glycoprotein and some, e.g. cisplatin, do not induce this type of resistance.

In those tumours for which cures can be achieved by chemotherapy (acute lymphoblastic leukaemia in childhood, Hodgkin's lymphoma, choriocarcinoma) it is essential that optimal doses of chemotherapy be administered and dose intensity maintained in order to avoid the emergence of chemoresistance.

IMPROVING EFFICACY OF CHEMOTHERAPY

Methods that potentially widen the narrow therapeutic index of cytotoxic agents include:

- Regional (as opposed to systemic) administration of drugs: intrathecal, intra-arterial liver perfusion.

- Regional delivery of drug by altered formulation e.g. Caelyx is a formulation comprising high concentrations of doxorubicin encased in liposomes.
- High-dose (bone marrow ablative) chemotherapy is feasible by harvesting stem cells prior to drug exposure, and returning the cells to the patient on completion of treatment.
- Circadian rhythms exist in cell metabolism and proliferation, and those of leukaemic cells differ from normal leucocytes. The time of day at which therapy is administered can influence the outcome; for example, maintenance chemotherapy of some leukaemias is more effective if given in the evening (chronomodulation).
- In large solid tumours, the proportion of cells multiplying is often small. In ovarian cancer, for example, patients may undergo debulking surgery (cytoreduction) prior to cytotoxic drug therapy.

HAZARDS TO STAFF HANDLING CYTOTOXIC AGENTS

Urine from nurses and pharmacists who prepared infusions and injections of anticancer agents revealed drugs in concentrations that were mutagenic to bacteria. When they stopped handling the drugs, the contamination ceased. It can be assumed that absorption of even small amounts of these drugs is harmful (mutagenesis, carcinogenesis), especially when it occurs repeatedly over long periods. Pregnant staff should not handle these drugs.

A note of caution. Certain chemotherapy regimens require the simultaneous administration of *intrathecal* methotrexate and *intravenous* vincristine. In the UK until recently, each drug was presented in similar bolus volumes and the drug-filled syringes appeared very alike except that the syringe for intrathecal administration had a red stopper. Nevertheless, from 1985 in the UK inadvertent *intrathecal* administration of *vincristine* occurred on 14 occasions: 10 patients died and the remainder suffered paralysis.[4]

---

[4]As a consequence of the death of a patient following intrathecal administration of vincristine, two inexperienced doctors were charged with manslaughter (Dyer C 2001 Doctors suspended after injecting wrong drug into spine. British Medical Journal 322:257).

INTERACTIONS OF ANTICANCER AGENTS WITH OTHER DRUGS

The diverse modes of action of cytotoxic drugs offer ample scope for serious *unwanted drug–drug interactions,* and by different mechanisms. There is general cause for alertness. Drugs that inhibit enzymes and thus delay normal metabolic breakdown may cause harmful reactions to standard doses of cytotoxics, e.g. allopurinol (xanthine oxidase inhibitor) with mercaptopurine or cyclophosphamide. Enzyme-inducing drugs can reduce the therapeutic efficacy of anticancer drugs by accelerating metabolism. Competition with non-steroidal anti-inflammatory drugs (NSAIDs) reduces the renal tubular excretion of methotrexate, leading to methotrexate toxicity. A combination of cytotoxics causing a dangerous degree of immunosuppression represents an adverse pharmacodynamic reaction.

Therapeutic drug–drug interactions are an essential part of treatment, as witnessed by the many drug combinations used to treat cancer (see Drug use and tumour cell kinetics, p. 547).

ENDOCRINE THERAPY

HORMONAL INFLUENCE ON CANCER

The possibility of interfering with cancer other than by surgery, e.g. by endocrine manipulation, was first tested in 1895 when a Scottish surgeon, faced with a woman aged 33 years with advanced breast cancer:

> put it to her husband and herself as to whether she should have performed the operation of removal of the [fallopian] tubes and ovaries. Its nature was fully explained to them both, and also that it was a purely experimental one ... She readily consented ... as she knew and felt her case was hopeless. [*Eight months after operation*] all vestiges of her previous cancerous disease had disappeared. [*The surgeon concluded, after treating two further cases, that there may be ovarian influences in breast cancer and added that*] whether [*this is*] accepted or not, I am sure I shall be acquitted of having acted thoughtlessly or recklessly.[5]

The treatment had logic. The author, observing the weaning of lambs on a local farm, had noted a similarity between the proliferation of epithelial cells of the milk ducts in lactation and in cancer, and had conceived the idea that cancer of the breast might be due to an abnormal ovarian stimulus.

In 1941[6] it was shown that prostatic cancer with metastases was made worse by androgen and made better by oestrogen (diethylstilbestrol).

HORMONAL AGENTS

The growth of some cancers is hormone dependent and is inhibited by surgical removal of gonads, adrenals and/or pituitary. The same effect is achievable, at less cost to the patient, by administering hormones, or hormone antagonists, of oestrogens, androgens or progestogens and inhibitors of hormone synthesis.

Breast cancer cells may have receptors for oestrogen, progesterone and androgen, and hormonal manipulation benefits some 30% of patients with metastatic disease; when a patient's tumour is oestrogen-receptor positive the response is about 60%, and when negative it is only 10%. After treatment of the primary cancer, endocrine therapy with the *anti-oestrogen, tamoxifen,* is the adjuvant therapy of choice for postmenopausal women who have disease in the lymph nodes; both the interval before the development of metastases and overall survival are increased. Adjuvant therapy with cytotoxic drugs and/or tamoxifen is recommended for node-negative patients with large tumours or other adverse prognostic factors. Cytotoxic chemotherapy is more useful in younger women, with tamoxifen, increasingly, as adjuvant therapy. The optimal duration of dosing with tamoxifen is not yet established, but is likely to be 5 years or more.

Aromatase inhibitors cause 'medical adrenalectomy' in postmenopausal women by blocking conversion of adrenal androgens to oestrogens in peripheral fat by the enzyme aromatase. The first drug in this class, *aminoglutethimide,* causes significant adverse effects. More selective and less toxic aromatase inhibitors now include *anastrozole, letrozole* and *exemestane,* and find use after treatment with tamoxifen fails. Clinical trial data suggest that these drugs may rival tamoxifen in efficacy for both advanced and early breast cancer. *Progestogens,* e.g. *megestrol* or *medroxyprogesterone,* are third-line agents in postmenopausal women.

[5]Beatson G T 1896 Lancet ii:104, 162.

[6]Huggins C et al 1941 Cancer Research 1:293.

Prostatic cancer is androgen dependent and metastatic disease can be helped by *orchidectomy*, or by pituitary suppression of androgen secretion with a gonadorelin analogue, e.g. *buserelin, goserelin, leuprorelin* or *triptorelin* (see p. 639). These cause a transient stimulation of luteinising hormone and thus testosterone release, before inhibition occurs; some patients may experience exacerbation of tumour effects, e.g. bone pain, spinal cord compression. Where this can be anticipated, prior orchidectomy or *anti-androgen* treatment, e.g. with *cyproterone* or *flutamide*, is protective.

Benign prostatic hypertrophy is also androgen dependent, and drug therapy includes use of *finasteride*, an inhibitor of the enzyme (5α-reductase) that activates testosterone.

Adrenocortical steroids are used for their action on specific cancers and also to treat some of the complications of cancer, e.g. hypercalcaemia, raised intracranial pressure. In leukaemias, corticosteroid may reduce the incidence of complications, e.g. haemolytic anaemia and thrombocytopenia. A glucocorticoid is preferred, e.g. prednisolone, as doses are high, and the mineralocorticoid actions are not needed and cause fluid retention.

In general, endocrine therapy carries less serious consequences for normal tissues than do cytotoxic agents. In a sense, they represent the first generation of mechanism-driven targeted agents used to treat cancer.

IMMUNOTHERAPY

Immunotherapy (immunostimulation) derives from an observation in the 19th century that cancer sometimes regressed after acute bacterial infections, i.e. in response to non-specific immunostimulant effect. In general, it appears that the immune response is attenuated in cancer. Strategies to stimulate the host's own immune system to kill cancer cells more effectively are:

- *Non-specific stimulation* of active immunity with vaccines, e.g. BCG (bacille Calmette–Guérin[7]) instilled into the urinary bladder for bladder cancer. More modern approaches involve the injection of tumour cells or tumour cell extracts combined with an immune stimulant such as BCG.
- *Specific immunisation strategies*, where tumour-specific and tumour-associated antigens have been identified. Melanomas, for example, possess melanoma differentiation antigens (tyrosinase, gp100, MART1) as well as tumour-associated antigens (MAGE, BAGE, GAGE series of major histocompatibility complex (MHC)-associated peptides and a family of lipoproteins known as gangliosides). Both DNA and whole-protein vaccines derived from these antigens are being evaluated in melanoma.

Naturally occurring substances are increasingly used to treat cancer. Cytokines are produced in response to various stimuli, such as antigens, e.g. viruses. These peptides regulate cell growth, activation and differentiation, and immune responses (see p. 538) and can be synthesised by recombinant DNA technology. Examples include:

- *Interleukins* that stimulate proliferation of T lymphocytes and activate natural killer cells; interleukin-2 is used in metastatic renal cell carcinoma.
- *Interferons*. Interferon-α is used for chronic granulocytic leukaemia, hairy cell leukaemia, renal cell carcinoma and Kaposi's sarcoma.

Thalidomide was withdrawn in the 1960s following evidence of its teratogenic effects, including some on fetal limb development (see p. 62). These very effects prompted the notion that suppression of cell proliferation might actually provide benefit. Investigation revealed that thalidomide possessed immunomodulatory properties, anti-inflammatory actions, direct effects on tumour cells and their microenvironment, and actions on angiogenesis (see below). Thalidomide and analogues designed to reduce toxicity (immunomodulatory drugs: lenalidomide) have a therapeutic role in myeloma and are synergistic with dexamethasone and chemotherapeutic agents.

ATRA

All-*trans*-retinoic acid (ATRA) induces remission in newly diagnosed patients with promyelocytic leukaemia (APL), by leukaemic cell differentiation. APL is due to reciprocal translocation between chromosomes 15 and 17 producing a fusion gene

---

[7]An attenuated strain of *Mycobacterium bovis* used to prepare the BCG vaccine for immunisation against tuberculosis.

PML–RARa. The fusion protein blocks differentiation but is overcome by ATRA. Subsequent administration of anthracycline improves cure rates.

DEVELOPMENT OF ANTICANCER DRUG THERAPY

In general, anticancer drugs develop from:

- *Chance discovery: cisplatin*. In the 1960s, scientists studying the effect of an electric current on bacteria cultured in a Petri dish noted that the cells stopped dividing, instead forming long filamentous structures. Further investigation revealed that the inhibitor of cell division was in fact an ion formed in solution from the platinum electrodes used in the experiment. The platinum complex, *cis*-diammine-dichloroplatinum (II), later known as cisplatin, was isolated and subsequently developed for its potential to kill cancer cells. When given to patients with a variety of different types of cancer, germ cell tumours in particular were found to possess remarkable sensitivity to cisplatin treatment, and this drug remains in use for treating such patients today.[8]
- *Analogues*. Severe vomiting, renal and nerve damage, and deafness limit the therapeutic efficacy of cisplatin. Carboplatin and oxaliplatin, second- and third-generation compounds derived from cisplatin, combine enhanced toxicity towards cancer cells with improved tolerance.
- *Mass screening programmes*. See Chapter 3.
- *Rational drug design*. Academic institutions and commercial biotechnology companies involved in experimental therapeutics study the cancer process to identify key ('target') genes or gene products that regulate aspects of carcinogenesis and then try to find ways of blocking the function of these targets (see Table 30.3). Unlike conventional cytotoxic chemotherapy, many of these agents are cytostatic. In other words, a targeted biological agent may prevent tumour growth and enlargement, or delay recurrence, but may not induce tumour shrinkage, hitherto

the key conventional endpoint for evaluating cytotoxic drugs. Some examples follow to illustrate the opportunities created by this type of approach.

TARGETED BIOLOGICAL THERAPIES

PASSIVE IMMUNOTHERAPY USING MONOCLONAL ANTIBODIES RAISED AGAINST SPECIFIC TUMOUR-ASSOCIATED ANTIGENS ON THE CELL SURFACE

Targeted antibodies have the advantage of high cancer specificity and relatively low host toxicity.

- *Rituximab*, an anti-CD20 monoclonal antibody, is approved by the National Institute for Health and Clinical Excellence (NICE) in the UK for the treatment of low-grade follicular lymphomas and for use in combination with CHOP (see above) for high-grade lymphoma.
- Significant over-expression of the Her2/neu (erbB2) cell surface receptor occurs in approximately 20% of breast cancers and is associated with a far more aggressive form of breast cancer compared with non-Her2-expressing tumours. *Trastuzumab* (Herceptin), a humanised monocolonal antibody, binds specifically to the Her2/neu receptor, blocking its function in regulating intracellular processes, including cell proliferation. In combination with conventional cytotoxic chemotherapy, trastuzumab significantly improves the survival of patients with advanced or early breast cancer, compared with cytotoxic chemotherapy alone. A series of key adjuvant trials conducted across Europe and the USA showed that trastuzumab combined with chemotherapy provided the biggest survival gains ever recorded for this disease.[9–11]

[8]Rosenberg B, Van Camp L, Trosko J E et al 1969 Platinum compounds: a new class of potent antitumour agents. Nature 222:385–386.

[9]Bursetin H J 2005 The distinctive nature of HER2-positive breast cancers. New England Journal of Medicine 353:1652–1654.

[10]Piccard-Gebhart M J, Procter M, Leyland-Jones B et al for the Herceptin Adjuvant (HERA) Trial Study Team 2005 Trastuzumab after adjuvant chemotherapy in HER2-positive breast cancer. New England Journal of Medicine 353:1659–1672.

[11]Romond E H, Perez E A, Bryant J et al 2005 Trastuzumab plus adjuvant chemotherapy for operable HER2-positive breast cancer. New England Journal of Medicine 353:1673–1684.

Her2 is a member of the epidermal growth factor receptor (EGFR) family. EGFRs are highly expressed by about 85% of colorectal cancers and are important in regulating cell proliferation. Another monoclonal antibody, *cetuximab* (Erbitux), blocks EGFR function and is used for selected colorectal cancers.

■ *Vasculoendothelial growth factor* (VEGF) is a major angiogenic signal regulator for new blood vessel formation (angiogenesis). Angiogenesis, a process that is probably common to all cancers, is vital for the growth and establishment of secondary tumours, and blockade of VEGF and its receptor is proving a highly successful strategy for treating several types of neoplasm. The monoclonal antibody, *bevacizumab* (Avastin), improves survival when added to standard treatment for advanced colorectal, lung and breast cancers. This novel approach evokes a range of adverse drug reactions that differ from those of conventional cytotoxics: hypertension, proteinuria, bleeding, particularly from unhealed wounds, and increased risk of thromboembolic events.

Drugs that block effects of VEGF, e.g. pegatanib, ranibizumab, are being developed to treat neovascular age-related macular degeneration, a condition that causes loss of central vision on 2.3% of people >65 years.

Radioimmunotherapy

Monoclonal antibodies targeted against epitopes[12] on tumour cells, e.g. rituximab against CD20 in lymphoma, are conjugated to radionuclides such as yttrium-90 (ibritumomab) or iodine-131 (tositumomab) to deliver radiation directly to the cellular target; they produce durable responses in patients resistant to chemotherapy and unconjugated antibody.

Chemoimmunotherapy

Monoclonal antibodies conjugated to toxins deliver high concentrations of agents that are too toxic to give systemically, e.g. CD33 plus calcicheamycin (Gentuzumab ozogamicin) in AML.

Most therapeutic antibodies are monoclonal immunoglobulin (Ig) G antibodies produced in mammalian cell lines by recombinant DNA technology. Genetic engineering alters the molecular structure of key immunogenic portions of the antibody to generate 'humanised' chimeric[13] antibodies that avoid rejection by the human immune system (but hypersensitivity reactions may occur).

Signal transduction inhibitors

Tyrosine kinase activation of cell surface receptors and their downstream proteins is an important mechanism by which messages are translated to the nucleus to affect cell function. A family of small molecules called *tyrosine kinase inhibitors* (TKIs) is now showing significant promise as anticancer agents. These small molecules are active when taken orally. Multi-targeted kinase inhibitors are also attractive, as they may possess a wide spectrum of antitumour activity, but their potential for toxicity is a real concern.

■ Imatinib (Glivec) blocks the dysregulated tyrosine kinase hyperactivity produced by the Philadelphia chromosome (bcr-abl) that occurs in chronic myeloid leukaemia and some cases of acute lymphoblastic leukaemia; clinical trials support its therapeutic efficacy. This is an important example of a drug designed precisely to address the biological abnormality that causes a disease.

■ Tyrosine kinase inhibitors of VEGF receptor and its downstream effector pathways are also in clinical trial (see Fig. 30.2 & Table 30.3).

■ The EGFR tyrosine kinase inhibitors, gefitinib (Iressa) and erlotinib (Tarceva), now find use for variety of EGFR-expressing tumours.

Targeting the cell cycle

Recent advances in molecular biology have shown that the cell cycle is regulated by a series of proteins that include *cyclins, cyclin-dependent kinases* and *cyclin-dependent kinase inhibitors* (Fig. 30.3). Aberrations in these proteins are themselves implicated in uncontrolled progression through the cell cycle (and hence in carcinogenesis), but they also

---

[12]The simplest form of an antigenic determinant, on a complex antigenic molecule, that can combine with antibody or T-cell receptor (Steadman's Medical Dictionary).

[13]Composed of seemingly incompatible parts of different origin.

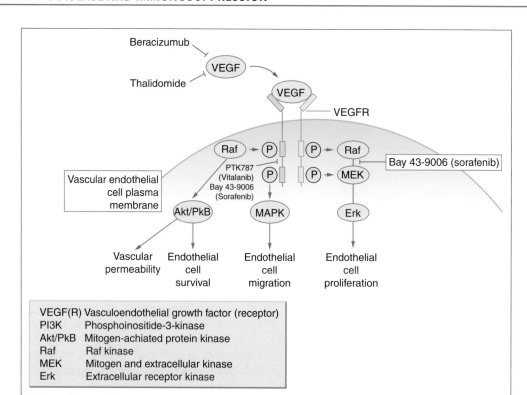

Fig. 30.2 Many new drugs target the vasculoendothelial growth factor (VEGF) pathway.

represent a new set of targets for anticancer therapy, e.g. flavopiridol, which has cyclin-dependent kinase inhibitor activity, and rapamycin, which inhibits mTor (mammalian target of rapamycin), another key regulator of cell cycle progression. Arsenic trioxide modulates cell growth and differentiation, and induces remission in relapsed refractory acute promyelocytic leukaemia in part through apoptosis induction and down-regulation of *Bcl-2*.

Protease inhibition

The ubiquitin–proteasome pathway is an intracellular proteolytic system that degrades cyclins and cyclin-dependent kinase inhibitors which regulate

Table 30.3 Some novel targets being exploited in anticancer drug development[a]

Target	Drug[b]	Examples of current clinical use
Her2/neu	trastuzumab (Herceptin)	Advanced and early stage breast cancer
CD20	rituximab (MabThera)	Non-Hodgkin's lymphoma
EGFR	cetuximab (Erbitux)	Improves survival in advanced colorectal cancer
EGFR	gefitinib (Iressa)	Advanced non-small cell lung cancer
EGFR	erlotinib (Tarceva)	Advanced non-small cell lung cancer, advanced pancreatic cancer
VEGF	bevacizumab (Avastin)	Advanced colorectal cancer; trials confirm efficacy in non-small cell lung cancer, renal cancer and probably many other tumours
Bcr-abl	imatinib (Glivec)	Chronic myeloid leukaemia
c-kit	imatinib (Glivec)	Gastrointestinal stromal tumours
Raf/MAPK	BAY 43–9006	Clinical trials ongoing in renal, breast cancer and melanoma
Cyclin-dependent kinase	flavopiridol	Undergoing clinical trial
mTor (a key regulator of cell cycle progression)	rapamycin	Undergoing clinical trial
Proteasome inhibitor	bortezomib	Active in myeloma; trials of combination therapy in progress

[a]Drugs at various stages in the process of obtaining a licence for use in the UK.
[b]The suffix 'mab' identifies a monoclonal antibody, whereas 'nib' identifies a tyrosine kinase inhibitor.

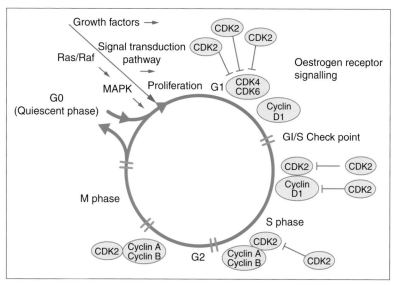

Fig. 30.3 The cell cycle is regulated by a series of proteins called cyclins, cyclin-dependent kinases (CDKs) and cyclin-dependent kinase inhibitors (CDKIs). Many CDKIs appear to be tumour-suppressing genes. These moieties are potential targets for anticancer therapy. MAPK, mitogen-activated protein kinase.

cell cycle progression. Bortezomib inhibits protea-some activity and, in myeloma, prevents degradation of nuclear factor κB inhibitor (IκB), resulting in a directly apoptotic effect, antiangiogenesis and inhibition of myeloma–stromal cell interaction. It has single-agent activity and restores chemosensitivity in resistant cells.

CHEMOPREVENTION OF CANCER

Because many cancers are currently incurable, cancer prevention is a logical objective. Individuals can change aspects of their lifestyle significantly to influence their risk of developing particular cancers, e.g. by ceasing to smoke tobacco.

Chemical interventions to reduce cancer risk are an option for the population as a whole, or for groups at high risk of a specific cancer. Vitamins and derivatives and dietary micronutrients that may inhibit the development of cancers are currently subject to large-scale trials, e.g. β-carotene, isotretinoin, folic acid, ascorbic acid, α-tocopherol. In a trial of antioxidant supplementation with ascorbic acid, vitamin E, β-carotene, selenium and zinc over 7.5 years, the

total cancer incidence was lower in men (who had a lower baseline antioxidant status) than in women.[14]

The anti-oestrogen, tamoxifen, used as an adjuvant therapy in women undergoing surgery for primary breast cancer, reduced the risk of cancer occurring in the contralateral breast. Tamoxifen and anastrozole (see above) are undergoing assessment for chemo-prevention in women at high risk of breast cancer.

See also aspirin (p. 260).

CANCER 'CURES': UNPROVEN REMEDIES

Conventional medicine cannot cure all cancers and inevitably some patients are prepared to try anything that seems to offer hope. This is perfectly understandable and many patients use unproven techniques, including medicines (see complementary and alternative medicine, p. 13).

Each decade seems to have had its own cancer 'cure' that achieved some prominence, only to fade away as new therapies emerged. Koch antitoxins (1940s), the Hoxie treatment (1950s), Krebiozen (1960s), laetrile (1970s), metabolic and immu-noaugmentative therapy (1980s) are prominent examples.[10]

Laetrile was a preparation of apricot seeds (pits, pips), which contained amygdalin (a β-glucoside) and incorporated cyanide. The claim was that it

[14]Hercberg S, Galan P, Preziosi P et al 2004 Randomized, placebo-controlled trial of the health effects of antioxidant vitamins and minerals. Archives of Internal Medicine 164:2335–2342.

relieved pain, prolonged survival and even induced complete remission of cancer. Benefit was reputed to result from release of cyanide in the body, killing cancer but not normal cells. Although it was said that laetrile had no toxic effects, an 11-month-old girl died after swallowing tablets (1–5) being used by her father. The toxicity arises from metabolic formation of hydrocyanic acid in the intestine. There is no serious evidence that laetrile is effective.

In the 1990s claims were made for 'Di Bella therapy' which

> ... consists of melatonin, bromocriptine, either somatostatin or octreotide, and retinoid solution (as well as cyclophosphamide and hydroxyurea in some cases) ... A retrospective matched pair comparison of 314 matched patients from Italian cancer registers showed a significantly shorter survival time for Di Bella's patients.[15]

As has so often been the case in the past, and no doubt will continue to be in the future, a mixture of emotionalism and exploitation obstructs the calm evaluation of claims.

Interestingly, despite criticism of over-permissive laxity of the drug regulatory authority (Food and Drug Administration, FDA) in the USA, the public is unwilling to accept the opinion of the FDA when it advises against the use of drugs such as laetrile. It is important to test these interventions for efficacy and toxicity in the same way as conventional drugs are subject to rigorous clinical trials.

There is a long and generally dishonourable history of the promotion of cancer 'cures'. As each new one appears the medical profession must yet again be willing to look dispassionately at the possibility that this time there really may be something in it, whilst avoiding the tragic raising of hopes that will not be realised – a sad and difficult task.

IMMUNOSUPPRESSION

Suppression of immune responses mediated via mononuclear cells (lymphocytes, plasma cells) is used in therapy of:

- Autoimmune, collagen, connective tissue and inflammatory disorders including systemic lupus erythematosus, rheumatoid arthritis, chronic

active hepatitis, inflammatory bowel disease, glomerulonephritis, nephrotic syndrome, some haemolytic anaemias and thrombocytopenias, uveitis, myasthenia gravis, polyarteritis, polymyositis, Behçet's syndrome.

- Organ or tissue transplantation: to prevent immune rejection.
- Cytotoxic cancer chemotherapeutic agents are immunosuppressive because they interfere with mononuclear cell multiplication and function. But they are generally too toxic for the above purposes and the following are principally used for intended immunosuppression:
  –adrenocortical steroids
  –azathioprine (see below)
  –ciclosporin, tacrolimus (see below)
  –some alkylating agents: cyclophosphamide and chlorambucil (see Table 30.2)
  –antilymphocyte immunoglobulin (see below).

With the exception of *ciclosporin* and *tacrolimus*, all of the above cause non-specific immunosuppression, so that the general defences of the body against infection are impaired.

Adrenal steroids destroy lymphocytes, reduce inflammation and impair phagocytosis (see Chapter 34).

Cytotoxic agents destroy immunologically competent cells. *Azathioprine*, a pro-drug for the purine antagonist mercaptopurine, is used in autoimmune disease because it provides enhanced immunosuppressive activity. Cyclophosphamide is a second choice; it depresses bone marrow, as is to be expected.

Ciclosporin

Ciclosporin is a polypeptide obtained from a soil fungus. It acts selectively and reversibly by preventing the transcription of interleukin-2 and other lymphokine genes, thus inhibiting the production of lymphokines by T lymphocytes (that mediate specific recognition of alien molecules). Ciclosporin spares non-specific function, e.g. of granulocytes, which are responsible for phagocytosis and metabolism of foreign substances. It does not depress haematopoiesis.

Pharmacokinetics. Ciclosporin is about 40% absorbed from the gastrointestinal tract and is metabolised extensively in the liver, mainly by the cytochrome P450 3A system ($t_{1/2}$ 27 h).

Uses. Ciclosporin is used to prevent and treat rejection of organ transplants (kidney, liver, heart–lung)

---

[15]Ernst E (ed.) 2001 The desktop guide to complementary and alternative medicine. Mosby, Edinburgh, pp. 229, 231.

and bone marrow transplants. For organ transplants, treatment continues indefinitely and requires careful monitoring of plasma concentration and renal function. In patients who have received a bone marrow transplant, ciclosporin is generally stopped after 6 months unless there is ongoing chronic graft-versus-host disease. It may be given orally or intravenously.

Ciclosporin also finds use for severe, resistant psoriasis in hospitalised patients.

Adverse reactions. Ciclosporin constricts the preglomerular afferent arteriole and reduces glomerular filtration; acute or chronic renal impairment may result if the trough plasma concentration consistently exceeds 250 mg/L. Generally, renal changes resolve when the drug is withdrawn. Hypertension develops in about 50% of patients, more commonly when a corticosteroid is co-administered but possibly due in part to mineralocorticoid action of ciclosporin. The blood pressure is controlled by standard antihypertensive therapy without the need to discontinue ciclosporin. Other adverse effects include gastrointestinal reactions, hepatotoxicity, hyperkalaemia, hypertrichosis, gingival hypertrophy, convulsions and, rarely, the clinical syndrome of thrombotic thrombocytopenic purpura.

Interactions. The plasma concentration of ciclosporin, and risk of toxicity, is increased by drugs including ketoconazole, erythromycin, chloroquine, cimetidine, oral contraceptives, anabolic steroids and calcium channel antagonists. Grapefruit juice also increases plasma ciclosporin concentrations (flavinoids in the juice inhibit the cytochrome that metabolises ciclosporin). Drugs that reduce the plasma concentration of ciclosporin, risking loss of effect, include enzyme-inducing antiepileptics, e.g. phenytoin, carbamazepine, phenobarbital, and rifampicin. Inherently nephrotoxic drugs add to the risk of renal damage with ciclosporin, e.g. aminoglycoside antibiotics, amphotericin, NSAIDs (diclofenac). Potassium-sparing diuretics add to the risk of hyperkalaemia.

Tacrolimus

Tacrolimus is a macrolide immunosuppressant agent that is isolated from a bacterium. It acts like ciclosporin, being used to protect and treat liver and kidney grafts when conventional immunosuppressants fail. Such rescue treatment may be graft or life saving. Tacrolimus may cause nephrotoxicity, neurotoxicity, disturbance of glucose metabolism, hyperkalaemia and hypertrophic cardiomyopathy.

Antilymphocyte immunoglobin

Antilymphocyte immunoglobin (ALG) is used in organ graft rejection, a process in which lymphocytes are involved. It is made by preparing antisera to human lymphocytes in animals (horses or rabbits), and allergic reactions are common. ALG largely spares the patient's response to infection. It is also used to treat severe aplastic anaemia, frequently producing a good partial response either as a single agent or in combination with ciclosporin. ALG is the treatment of choice for patients with severe aplastic anaemia for whom no bone marrow donor is available or who are too old or unfit for a bone marrow transplant.

Mycophenolate

Mycophenolate selectively blocks the proliferation of T and B lymphocytes and acts like azathioprine; it is being evaluated in combination immunosuppressive regimens for organ transplantation.

HAZARDS OF LIFE ON IMMUNOSUPPRESSIVE DRUGS

Impaired immune responses render the subject more liable to bacterial, viral and fungal infections. Treat all infection early and vigorously (using bactericidal drugs where practicable); use human γ-globulin to protect when there is exposure to virus infections, e.g. measles, varicella. Patients who have not had chickenpox and are receiving therapeutic (as opposed to replacement) doses of corticosteroid are at risk of severe chickenpox; they should receive varicella-zoster immunoglobulin if there has been contact with the disease within the previous 3 months.

Carcinogenicity is a hazard, generally after 4–7 years of therapy. The cancers most likely to occur are those thought to have viral origin (leukaemia, lymphoma, skin). Cytotoxic use creates the additional hazard of mutagenicity, which may induce cancer.

Hazards include those of long-term corticosteroid therapy, and of cytotoxics in general (bone marrow depression, infertility and teratogenesis).

Although such hazards may be justifiable to the patient who has life-endangering disease, there is more cause for concern when immunosuppressive regimens are an option in younger patients with a less serious disorder, e.g. rheumatoid arthritis, ulcerative colitis.

ACTIVE IMMUNISATION DURING IMMUNOSUPPRESSIVE THERAPY

Response to non-living antigens (tetanus, typhoid, poliomyelitis) is diminished, and giving one or two extra doses may be wise. *Living vaccines are contraindicated* in patients who are immunosuppressed by drug therapy or indeed by disease (AIDS, leukaemia, lymphoma) as there is a risk of serious generalised infection.

GUIDE TO FURTHER READING

A useful general account by several authors and covering all aspects of cancer therapy appears in Medicine 2004; 32:1–37

Arribas J 2005 Matrix metalloproteases and tumor invasion. New England Journal of Medicine 352:2020–2021

El-Shanawany T, Sewell W A C, Misbah S A, Jolles S 2006 Current uses of intravenous immunoglobulin. Clinical Medicine 6:356–359

Greenwald P 2002 Cancer chemoprevention. British Medical Journal 324:714–718

Kaur R 2005 Breast cancer: personal account. Lancet 365:1742

Key T J, Allen N E, Spencer E A, Travis R C 2002 The effect of diet on risk of cancer. Lancet 360:861–868

Khan S, Sewell W A C 2006 Oral immunosuppressive drugs. Clinical Medicine 6:252–355

Koon H, Atkins M 2006 Autoimmunity and immunotherapy for cancer. New England Journal of Medicine 354:758–760

Krause D S, Van Etten R A 2005 Tyrosine kinase as targets for cancer therapy. New England Journal of Medicine 353:172–187

Renehan A G, Booth C, Potten C S 2001 What is apoptosis, and why is it important? British Medical Journal 322:1536–1538

Roodman G D 2004 Mechanisms of bone metastasis. New England Journal of Medicine 350:1655–1664

Rosenberg S A, Yang J C, Restifo N P et al 2004 Cancer immunotherapy: moving beyond current vaccines. Nature Medicine 10:909–915

Turnbull C, Hodgson S 2005 Genetic predisposition to cancer. Clinical Medicine 5:491–498

Veronesi U, Boyle P, Goldhirsch A, Orecchia R, Vilae G 2005 Breast cancer. Lancet 365:1727–1741

Wooster R, Weber B 2003 Breast and ovarian cancer. New England Journal of Medicine 348:2339–2347

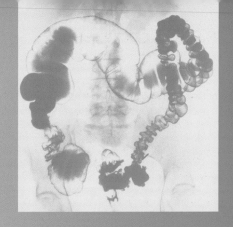

Section 7

GASTROINTESTINAL SYSTEM

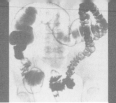

31

Oesophagus, stomach and duodenum

SYNOPSIS

Approximately one-third of the population in Western societies experience regular dyspepsia, although more than half self-medicate with over-the-counter antacid preparations and do not seek medical advice. Up to 50% of those who do will have demonstrable pathology, most commonly gastro-oesophageal reflux or peptic ulceration. The remainder, in whom no abnormality is found, are diagnosed as having non-ulcer dyspepsia. The pathophysiology and treatment differ for each of these three conditions.

- Drugs for peptic ulcer
  - neutralisation of secreted acid
  - reduction of acid secretion
  - enhancing mucosal resistance
  - eradication of *Helicobacter pylori*
  - NSAIDs and the stomach
- Gastro-oesophageal reflux and vomiting
  - antiemesis and pro-kinetic drugs
  - treatment of various forms of vomiting

PEPTIC ULCER

Peptic ulcer occurs when there is an imbalance between the damaging effects of gastric acid and pepsin, and the defence mechanisms that protect the gastric and duodenal mucosa from these substances (Fig. 31.1). The exact mechanisms are still poorly understood. A major cause of peptic ulcer is use of non-steroidal anti-inflammatory drugs (NSAIDs), particularly in the elderly.

For years, the treatment of peptic ulceration centred around measures to neutralise gastric acid, to inhibit its secretion or to enhance mucosal defences, but recognition of the central role of *Helicobacter pylori* revolutionised the approach. Additionally, smoking is a major environmental factor and patients who smoke should be advised to stop.

ACID SECRETION BY THE STOMACH

Gastric acid is secreted by the parietal cells in gastric mucosa (Fig. 31.2). The basolateral membranes of these cells contain receptors for the three main stimulants of acid secretion, namely *gastrin* (from antral G cells), *histamine* (from enterochromaffin-like cells) and *acetylcholine* (from vagal efferents). The action of all these is to stimulate the gastric acid (proton) pump, which is the *final common pathway* for acid secretion. The pump is a H^+/K^+-ATPase, and when stimulated it translocates from cytoplasmic vesicles to the secretory canaliculus of the parietal cell and uses energy, derived from hydrolysis of ATP, to transport H^+ out of parietal cells in exchange for K^+. Hydrogen ions combine with chloride ions to form hydrochloric acid (HCl), which is secreted into the gastric lumen.

INHIBITION AND NEUTRALISATION OF GASTRIC ACID

Healing of gastric and duodenal ulcers by antisecretory drugs and antacids is dependent upon:

- the degree of gastric acid suppression
- the duration of treatment.

Proton pump inhibitors, the most potent antisecretory drugs, heal the majority of peptic ulcers within

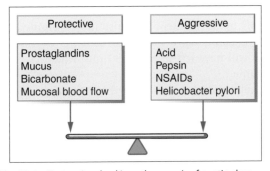

Fig. 31.1 Factors involved in pathogenesis of peptic ulcer.

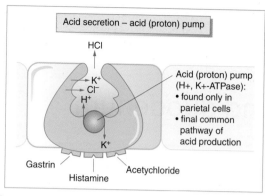

Fig 31.2   Secretion of acid by the parietal cell.

4 weeks, whereas the less powerful H_2-receptor antagonists require up to twice as long to achieve the same therapeutic effect. Antacids modify intragastric pH only transiently, yet relatively small daily doses (around 120 mmol) will heal ulcers if they are taken for long enough. Regardless of the treatment, 85% of peptic ulcers will have healed after 3 months but the stronger agents provide much more rapid symptom relief. In addition, numerous studies have shown a high rate of placebo response in ulcer healing.

ANTACIDS

Antacids are basic substances that reduce gastric acidity by neutralising hydrochloric acid. The hydroxide is the most common base, but trisilicate, carbonate and bicarbonate are also used. Therapeutic efficacy and adverse effects depend also on the metallic ion with which the base is combined, and this is usually aluminium, magnesium or sodium.

Antacids protect the gastric mucosa against acid (by neutralisation) and pepsin (which is inactive above pH 5, and which in addition is inactivated by aluminium and magnesium). Continuous increase of pH by intermittent administration is limited by gastric emptying. If the gastric contents are liquid, half will have left in about 30 min, whatever their volume.

Antacids are generally used to relieve dyspeptic symptoms and they are taken intermittently when symptoms occur. Side-effects and inconvenience limit their use as ulcer healing agents.

Individual antacids
Sodium bicarbonate reacts with acid and relieves pain within minutes. It is absorbed and causes

alkalosis, which in short-term use may not cause symptoms. Sodium bicarbonate can release sufficient carbon dioxide in the stomach to cause discomfort and belching, which may or may not have a psychotherapeutic effect, according to the circumstances.

Magnesium oxide and hydroxide react quickly, and magnesium trisilicate more slowly with gastric hydrochloric acid. All magnesium salts cause diarrhoea.

Aluminium hydroxide reacts with hydrochloric acid to form aluminium chloride; this in turn reacts with intestinal secretions to produce insoluble salts, especially phosphate. It tends to constipate.

Adverse effects of antacid mixtures
Those that apply to individual antacids are described above but the following general points are also relevant.

Some antacid mixtures contain *sodium*, which may not be readily apparent from the name of the preparation. Thus they may be dangerous for patients with cardiac or renal disease. For example, a 10-mL dose of magnesium carbonate mixture or of magnesium trisilicate mixture contains about 6 mmol sodium (normal daily dietary intake is approximately 120 mmol sodium).

Aluminium- and *magnesium*-containing antacids may interfere with the absorption of other drugs by binding with them or by altering gastrointestinal pH or transit time. It is probably advisable not to co-administer antacids with drugs that are intended for systemic effect by the oral route.

Choice and use of antacids
No single antacid is satisfactory for all circumstances and mixtures are often used. They may contain sodium bicarbonate for quickest effect, supplemented by magnesium hydroxide or carbonate. Sometimes magnesium trisilicate or aluminium hydroxide is added, but these are often used alone, although they are relatively slow acting.

Disturbed bowel habit can be corrected by altering the proportions of magnesium salts, which cause diarrhoea, and aluminium salts, which constipate.

Alginic acid may be combined with an antacid to encourage adherence of the mixture to the mucosa, e.g. for reflux oesophagitis.

Dimeticone is sometimes included in antacid mixtures as an antifoaming agent to reduce flatulence.

It is a silicone polymer that lowers surface tension and allows the small bubbles of froth to coalesce into large bubbles, which can more easily be passed up from the stomach or down from the colon. It helps distended mountaineers to belch usefully at high altitudes.

H$_2$-RECEPTOR ANTAGONISTS

These drugs bind selectively and competitively to the histamine H$_2$ receptor on the basolateral membrane of the parietal cell (see Fig. 31.2). As well as inhibiting gastric acid release by histamine, they inhibit acetylcholine- and gastrin-mediated acid secretion. The inhibitory effect can be overcome, particularly when gastrin levels are high, as occurs postprandially. In addition, tolerance may develop, probably as a result of down-regulation of receptors. Peptic ulcer healing with H$_2$-receptor antagonists correlates best with suppression of *nocturnal* acid secretion, and some prefer to give these drugs as a single evening dose. The usual ulcer-healing course is 8 weeks.

Cimetidine

Cimetidine was the first H$_2$-receptor antagonist to be used in clinical practice.

Adverse effects and interactions are few in short-term use. Cimetidine is a weak antiandrogen, and may cause gynaecomastia and sexual dysfunction in males. In the elderly, particularly, it may cause central nervous system (CNS) disturbances including lethargy, confusion and hallucinations. Cimetidine inhibits cytochromes P450, in particular CYP 1A2 and CYP 3A4, and there is potential for increased effect from any drug with a low therapeutic index that is inactivated by these isoenzymes, e.g. warfarin, phenytoin.

Ranitidine, famotidine, nizatidine

The modes of action, uses and therapeutic efficacy of these histamine H$_2$-receptor antagonists are essentially those of cimetidine. Ranitidine is 50%, famotidine is 25% and nizatidine is 10% metabolised, in each case the remainder being excreted unchanged by the kidney. The drugs do not inhibit hepatic microsomal enzymes and do not block androgen receptors.

H$_2$-receptor antagonists are available as over-the-counter preparations in the UK, albeit of lower strength than those available on prescription. The potential danger is that patients with serious pathology such as gastric carcinoma will self-medicate, allowing their disease to progress. Pharmacists are trained to advise patients to consult their doctor if they have recurrent symptoms or other worrying manifestations such as weight loss.

PROTON PUMP INHIBITORS (PPIS)

This class of drugs inactivates the H$^+$/K$^+$-ATPase (proton pump) in parietal cells, which is the final common pathway for acid production (see Fig. 31.2). *Omeprazole* was the first preparation to be used in clinical practice, and *esomeprazole, lansoprazole, pantoprazole* and *rabeprazole* were subsequently introduced. All are similar in efficacy and mode of action.

Omeprazole

Omeprazole is a pro-drug, in common with all PPIs. It enters the parietal cell from the blood by non-ionic diffusion but becomes ionised in the acid milieu around the secretory canaliculus, where it is trapped and concentrated. In this form it is a highly chemically reactive species which binds to sulphydryl groups on Na$^+$/K$^+$-ATPase. This irreversibly inactivates the enzyme causing profound inhibition of acid secretion: a single 20-mg dose reduces gastric acid output by 90% over 24 h. The Na$^+$/K$^+$-ATPase regenerates when the PPI is discontinued. Omeprazole is degraded at low pH and must be given in enteric-coated granules. Systemic availability increases with dose and also with time, owing to decreased inactivation of the pro-drug as gastric acidity is reduced.

Adverse effects include nausea, headache, diarrhoea, constipation and rash but are uncommon. Omeprazole inhibits the 2C family of the cytochrome P450 system, decreasing the metabolism of warfarin, diazepam, carbamazepine and phenytoin, and enhancing the effect of these drugs (but inhibition is less than with cimetidine).

Concern has arisen that long-term use of powerful antisecretory drugs may increase the risk of gastric neoplasia. Differing mechanisms have been proposed. When acid secretion is suppressed, gastrin is released as a normal homeostatic response. Gastrin stimulates growth of the gastric epithelium, including the enterochromaffin cells which could transform into carcinoid tumours; some rats developed these tumours after prolonged exposure to high doses of omeprazole. Furthermore, prolonged hypochlorhydria favours colonisation of the stomach by bacteria that have the potential to convert ingested nitrates into carcinogenic nitrosamines. Surveillance studies to date have not provided evidence that this is a real hazard in humans, and it is certainly unlikely with short-term use, e.g. up to 8 weeks.

Other theoretical concerns relate to reduced absorption of vitamin B_{12} and increased susceptibility to gastrointestinal infections as a result of prolonged hypochlorhydria. There is as yet no real evidence for these being a clinical problem.

PPIs are widely used and possible adverse effects from very long-term exposure, e.g. resistant symptoms from gastro-oesophageal reflux disease, are not yet known.

Antimuscarinic drugs

These agents (e.g. pirenzepine), formerly widely used to suppress acid secretion, are now obsolete.

ENHANCING MUCOSAL RESISTANCE

Drugs can increase mucosal resistance by:

- protecting the base of a peptic ulcer (bismuth chelate, sucralfate)
- 'cytoprotection' (misoprostol).

Bismuth chelate

Tripotassium dicitratobismuthate, bismuth subcitrate (De-Nol). This substance was originally thought to act mainly by chelating with protein in the ulcer base to form a coating that protects the ulcer from the adverse influences of acid, pepsin and bile. Subsequently, bismuth chelate was found to suppress growth of *Helicobacter pylori*, especially when combined with an antimicrobial (see below).

Bismuth chelate is used for benign gastric and duodenal ulcer, and has a therapeutic efficacy approximately equivalent to that of histamine H_2-receptor antagonists. Ulcers remain healed for longer after bismuth chelate than after H_2-receptor antagonists, and this may relate to the ability of the former but not the latter to eradicate *H. pylori*.

Adverse effects. Bismuth chelate, particularly as a liquid formulation, darkens the tongue, teeth and stool; the effect is less likely with the tablet, which is thus more acceptable. There is little systemic absorption of bismuth from the chelated preparation, but bismuth is excreted by the kidney and it is prudent to avoid giving the drug to patients with impaired renal function. Urinary elimination continues for months after bismuth is discontinued.

Sucralfate

This is a complex salt of sucrose sulphate and aluminium hydroxide. In the acid environment of the stomach, the aluminium moiety is released so that the compound develops a strong negative charge and binds to positively charged protein molecules that transude from damaged mucosa. The result is a viscous paste that adheres selectively and protectively to the ulcer base. It also binds to and inactivates pepsin and bile acids. Sucralfate has negligible acid-neutralising capacity, which explains why it is ineffective in gastro-oesophageal reflux disease (see below). Its therapeutic efficacy in healing gastric and duodenal ulcers is approximately equal to that of the histamine H_2-receptor antagonists.

Adverse effects. Sucralfate may cause constipation but is otherwise well tolerated. The concentration of aluminium in the plasma may be raised but this appears to be a problem only with long-term use by uraemic patients, especially those undergoing chronic intermittent haemodialysis. As the drug is effective only in acid conditions, an antacid should not be taken 30 min before or after a dose of sucralfate. Sucralfate interferes with absorption of co-administered ciprofloxacin, theophylline, digoxin, phenytoin and amitriptyline, possibly by binding due to its strong negative charge.

Misoprostol

Endogenous prostaglandins contribute importantly to the integrity of the gastrointestinal mucosa by a number of related mechanisms (see Chapter 15). Misoprostol is a synthetic analogue of prostaglandin E_1, which protects against the formation of gastric and duodenal ulcers in patients who are taking NSAIDs, presumably by these 'cytoprotective' mechanisms (see below). The drug also heals chronic gastric and duodenal ulcers unrelated to NSAID use, but here the mechanism appears related to its antisecretory properties rather than to a cytoprotective action.

Adverse effects. Diarrhoea and abdominal pain, transient and dose related, are the commonest. Women may experience gynaecological disturbances such as vaginal spotting and dysmenorrhoea; the drug is *contraindicated* in pregnancy or for women planning to become pregnant, as the products of conception may be aborted. Indeed, women have resorted to using misoprostol (illicitly) as an abortifacient in parts of the world where provision of contraceptive services is poor.[1]

Liquorice derivatives

Carbenoxolone and deglycyrrhizinised liquorice, formerly used for peptic ulcer, are now obsolete.

HELICOBACTER PYLORI ERADICATION

The association of *H. pylori* with peptic ulcer was first reported by Barry Marshall and Robin Warren.[2] The latter wrote: 'I was just doing my day-to-day pathology. I like looking for funny things and this day, I saw a funny thing and started wondering.' In a gastric biopsy he saw 'numerous bacteria in close contact with the surface epithelium … They appeared to be actively growing and not a contaminant'. The idea that this organism was causally related to peptic ulcer was initially greeted with a patronising response, disbelief, or sometimes hostility. 'Even the first major publication of their results[3] … was a difficult hurdle. The editors … [of the *Lancet*] … found it difficult to find reviewers who could agree the paper was important, general, and interesting enough to be published … The same year, in an act born to some extent of frustration, Marshall deliberately infected himself by drinking a solution swimming with the bacterium, as part of a successful and widely reported experiment to prove Koch's postulates.'[4] For their discovery that gastritis and peptic ulcer stem from an infection of the stomach caused by *H. pylori*, Warren and Marshall were jointly awarded the Nobel Prize in Physiology or Medicine in 2005.

Colonisation of the stomach with *H. pylori* is seen in virtually all patients with duodenal ulcer and in 70–80% of those with gastric ulcers. This close association is not seen in ulcers complicating NSAID therapy, in reflux oesophagitis or non-ulcer dyspepsia. In patients with duodenal ulcer there is an associated antral gastritis, whereas with gastric ulcer gastritis is more diffuse throughout the stomach. It is not known how *H. pylori* predisposes to peptic ulceration, but chronic infection with the organism, which establishes itself within and below the mucous layer, is associated with hypergastrinaemia and hyperacidity. With more extensive gastritis there is a reduction in parietal cell mass and decreased acid secretion. Although all patients colonised with *H. pylori* develop gastritis, only about 20% have ulcers or other lesions; host factors and differences in strain of the organism are likely to be important.

Other possible effects of long-term infection with *H. pylori* include gastric carcinoma and lymphoma, particularly of the MALT (mucosa-associated lymphoid tissue) type. Eradication of the organism may lead to resolution of the latter tumour.

H. pylori can be detected histologically from antral biopsies obtained at gastroscopy, or biochemically. In the CLO (campylobacter-like organism) test, an endoscopic biopsy specimen incubates in a medium containing urea and an indicator, which changes colour if ammonia is produced. Proton pump inhibitors and bismuth compounds suppress but do not eradicate *H. pylori*, and results may be falsely negative if any of these tests is carried out within 1 month of taking these drugs.

TREATMENT OF *HELICOBACTER PYLORI* INFECTION

Successful eradication of *H. pylori* infection usually results in long-term remission of the ulcer because reinfection rates are low, particularly in areas of low endemicity. The organism is sensitive to *metronidazole, amoxicillin, clarithromycin, tetracycline* and *bismuth salts*. The efficacy of antimicrobials can be increased considerably by co-administration of a proton pump inhibitor. The following regimens are recommended by NICE[5]:

[1]Gonzales C H, Marques-Dias M J, Kim C A et al 1998 Congenital abnormalities in Brazilian children associated with misoprostol misuse in first trimester of pregnancy. Lancet 351:1624–1627.

[2]Warren J R, Marshall B 1983 Unidentified curved bacilli on gastric epithelium in active chronic gastritis. Lancet i: 1273–1275 (letter).

[3]Marshall B J, Warren J R 1984 Unidentified curved bacillis in the stomach of patients with gastritis and peptic ulceration. Lancet i:1311–1315.

[4]Pincock S 2005 Nobel Prize winners Robin Warren and Barry Marshall. Lancet 366:1429.

[5]The UK National Institute for Health and Clinical Excellence.

- Proton pump inhibitor in full dose + clarithromycin 500 mg b.d. + amoxicillin 1 g b.d. for 7 days.
- Proton pump inhibitor in full dose+ clarithromycin 250 mg b.d. + metronidazole 400 mg b.d. for 7 days.

It is important that the full course of treatment is taken to avoid the emergence of antibiotic resistant strains of *H. pylori*.

Metronidazole resistance is a particular problem, with a prevalence of up to 80% in some countries, particularly sub-Saharan Africa. It is more common in women and probably reflects extensive use of this antimicrobial for pelvic and other infections. Resistance to clarithromycin is less common but may reach 20% of some communities.

It is not usually necessary to check for successful eradication unless the patient continues to have symptoms. Under these circumstances the urea breath test[6] is a useful non-invasive technique.

In summary, *Helicobacter pylori* eradication therapy is:

- *indicated* for gastric and duodenal ulcer not associated with NSAID use, and gastric lymphoma (especially MALT lymphoma)
- *not indicated* for reflux oesophagitis
- *equivocal* in value for nonulcer dyspepsia, after incidental detection, and for prophylaxis of gastric cancer.

NSAIDs AND THE STOMACH

Some 500 million prescriptions for NSAIDs are written each year in the UK, and 10–15% of patients develop dyspepsia while taking these drugs. Gastric erosions develop in up to 80%, but these are usually self-limiting. Gastric or duodenal ulcers occur in 1–5%. The incidence increases sharply with age in those over 60 years, and the risk of ulcers and their complications is doubled in patients aged more than 75 years and those with cardiac failure or a history of peptic ulceration or bleeding. Ibuprofen may be less prone to cause these problems than other NSAIDs.

---

[6]The urea breath test measures radiolabelled carbon dioxide in expired air after ingestion of labelled urea, exploiting the fact that the organism produces urease and can convert urea to ammonia.

MECHANISM OF GASTRIC MUCOSAL TOXICITY

Aspirin and the other NSAIDs exert their anti-inflammatory effect through inhibition of the enzyme cyclo-oxygenase (COX) (see Chapter 15). This enzyme is present in two isoforms. COX-1 is involved in the formation of prostaglandins, which *protect* the gastric mucosa, whereas COX-2 is induced in response to inflammatory stimuli and is involved in the formation of *cell-damaging cytokines*. Most NSAIDs inhibit both isoforms, so the beneficial anti-inflammatory effect is offset by the potential for gastric mucosal injury by depletion of prostaglandins. The harmful effects of the latter include reduction of mucosal blood flow and a diminished capacity to secrete protective mucus and bicarbonate ion. Aspirin is particularly potent in this respect, perhaps due to the fact that it inhibits COX irreversibly, unlike the other NSAIDs where inhibition is reversible and concentration dependent. Gastrointestinal bleeding can complicate use of low-dose aspirin.

NSAIDs are weak organic acids and the acid milieu of the stomach facilitates their non-ionic diffusion into gastric mucosal cells. Here the neutral intracellular pH causes the drugs to become ionised and they accumulate in the mucosa because they cannot diffuse out in this form. Nabumetone differs from other NSAIDs in that it is non-acidic and therefore not concentrated so avidly in gastric mucosa, which may partially explain why this drug is less likely to produce peptic ulceration.

TREATMENT OF NSAID-INDUCED PEPTIC ULCERS

Withdrawal of NSAIDs and acid suppression with standard doses of antisecretory drugs will allow prompt resolution of these ulcers, which should not recur unless the drugs are resumed. Many patients are prescribed NSAIDs inappropriately when their symptoms could be controlled by paracetamol or by local treatment. Topical NSAID creams applied over an affected joint may be helpful, but peptic ulcers can complicate therapy with NSAIDs administered as rectal suppositories. Prodrugs such as sulindac, which are metabolised to form anti-inflammatory derivatives, can also produce ulcers.

PREVENTION OF NSAID-INDUCED PEPTIC ULCERS

This is particularly relevant for the elderly and other high-risk patients (see above), but the optimal regimen remains to be established because data from current trials are conflicting. The synthetic prostaglandin misoprostol in a dose of 800 micrograms daily in two to four divided doses reduces the incidence of gastric and duodenal ulceration and their complications by about 40% when co-administered with NSAIDs. Abdominal pain and diarrhoea limit its use; halving the dose reduces the incidence of adverse effects, but at the expense of a reduced protective effect. The proton pump inhibitors, in healing doses, are similar in efficacy to the higher dose of misoprostol. H_2-receptor antagonists offer limited protection against duodenal ulcers but none against gastric ulcers.

There is no clear evidence that eradicating *Helicobacter pylori* is of benefit.

Selective inhibition of COX-2 has the objective of preserving anti-inflammatory activity whilst avoiding gastric mucosal toxicity. *Rofecoxib, celecoxib* and *meloxicam* vary in their selectivity for COX-2. The incidence of peptic ulcers and their complications with rofecoxib is similar to that seen when proton pump inhibitors are co-administered with non-selective NSAIDs. Unfortunately their use is limited by an increased incidence of cardiovascular side-effects (see Chapter 15).

GASTRO-OESOPHAGEAL REFLUX DISEASE (GORD)

Transient gastro-oesophageal reflux occurs in almost everybody and it is only when episodes become frequent, with prolonged exposure of the oesophageal mucosa to acid and pepsin, that problems develop. Factors contributing to pathological reflux include:

- Incompetence of the gastro-oesophageal sphincter.
- Delayed oesophageal clearance of acid.
- Delayed gastric emptying.

The commonest symptom is *heartburn*, and as many as 15% of people in Western populations experience this regularly. Approximately 50% will have oesophagitis, the severity of which does not correlate with symptoms. The other main complications are acute or chronic bleeding, oesophageal stricture and Barrett's metaplasia, which carries an increased risk of oesophageal carcinoma. There is no evidence that *Helicobacter pylori* is involved in the pathogenesis of GORD.

MANAGEMENT OF GORD

Patients should lose weight, if it is appropriate, and smokers should stop, because nicotine relaxes the gastro-oesophageal sphincter. Raising the head of the bed by 15–20 cm helps to diminish nocturnal reflux. Patients should avoid heavy meals and situations predisposing to reflux (such as lying down or prolonged bending within 3 h of a meal). Drugs that encourage reflux should be avoided if possible, e.g. those with antimuscarinic activity (tricyclic antidepressants), smooth muscle relaxants (nitrates and calcium channel blockers) or theophylline compounds.

Antacids are helpful in controlling mild reflux symptoms when taken regularly after meals with additional doses as needed. Preparations in which an antacid is combined with alginate are particularly useful: the alginate produces a viscous floating gel that blocks reflux and protectively coats the oesophagus.

Acid suppression. *H_2-receptor antagonists* in conventional peptic ulcer healing doses are useful in the short-term management of mild oesophagitis but are less effective in the longer term, and on maintenance treatment only one-third of patients will be in remission. *Proton pump inhibitors* are currently the most effective drugs. Conventional ulcer healing doses rapidly relieve reflux symptoms and heal oesophagitis in the majority of patients. Sometimes higher doses are needed, particularly for maintenance therapy. Over three-quarters of patients will still be in remission after 12 months' treatment with a proton pump inhibitor.

Pro-kinetic drugs. The antidopaminergic compounds *metoclopramide* and *domperidone* can alleviate GORD symptoms by increasing gastro-oesophageal sphincter tone and stimulating gastric emptying (actions that are additional to their central action as antiemetics, see below).

NON-ULCER DYSPEPSIA

Many patients with non-ulcer dyspepsia have abnormalities of gastric emptying and increased pain perception in the gastrointestinal tract, suggesting that the condition is part of the spectrum of irritable bowel syndrome (see Chapter 32). Patients with predominant *epigastric pain* or *reflux* symptoms may improve with simple antacids taken as needed. More severe symptoms may require antisecretory drugs, particularly a proton pump inhibitor, although the response rate is lower (40–50%) than in patients with documented pathology. Where the main symptom is *bloating*, a pro-kinetic agent (metoclopramide or domperidone, see below) is preferred.

Flatulent patients may benefit from *carminatives*, substances that are held to assist expulsion of gas from the stomach and intestines. Examples are dimethicone, peppermint, dill, anise and other herbs commonly included in liqueurs and (in non-alcoholic solutions) for babies. The problem is not new. The Roman Emperor Claudius (AD 10–54) planned an edict to legitimise the breaking of wind at table, either silently or noisily, after hearing about a man who was so modest that he endangered his health by an attempt to restrain himself (Suetonius [trans] R Graves).

The incidence of *Helicobacter pylori* colonisation in patients with non-ulcer dyspepsia is not significantly different from that in the general population, and eradication of the organism provides, at best, only one-quarter of patients with prolonged symptomatic improvement (a proportion that is similar to the placebo response for this condition).

VOMITING

SOME PHYSIOLOGY

Useful vomiting occurs as a protective mechanism for eliminating irritant or harmful substances from the upper gastrointestinal tract. The act of emesis is controlled by the *vomiting centre* in the medulla. Close to it lie other visceral centres, including those for respiration, salivation and vascular control, which give rise to the prodromal sensations of vomiting. These centres are not anatomically discrete but comprise interconnected networks within the nucleus of the tractus solitarius. The vomiting centre does not initiate, but rather coordinates, the act of emesis on receiving stimuli from various sources, namely:

- The chemoreceptor trigger zone (CTZ), a nearby area that is extremely sensitive to the action of drugs and other chemicals.
- The vestibular system.
- The periphery, e.g. distension or irritation of the gut, myocardial infarction, biliary or renal stone.
- Cortical centres.

The vomiting centre and the nucleus of the tractus solitarius contain many *muscarinic cholinergic* and *histamine H_1 receptors*, and the CTZ is rich in *dopamine D_2 receptors*; drugs that block these receptors are effective antiemetics. The precise role and location of $5HT_3$ receptors (see ondansetron, below) in relation to emesis remains to be defined but both central and peripheral mechanisms may be involved.

ANTIEMESIS DRUGS

These may be classified as shown in Table 31.1.

Metoclopramide

Metoclopramide acts *centrally* by blocking dopamine D_2 receptors in the CTZ, and *peripherally* by enhancing

Table 31.1 Classification of antiemesis drugs	
Drug	**Site of action/comment**
Dopalmine D_2 receptor antagonists	
domperidone	CTZ and gut
metoclopramide	CTZ and gut
haloperidol	CTZ
Phenothiazines, e.g. chlorpromazine, prochlorperazine, thiethylperazine	Vomiting centre and CTZ
$5HT_3$-receptor antagonists	
ondansetron	CTZ and gut
granisetron	
tropisetron	
Antimuscarinics	
hyoscine and some drugs also classed as histamine H_1-receptor antagonists, e.g. cyclizine, dimenhydrinate, promethazine	Vomiting centre and gut
Other agents	
Corticosteroids (dexamethasone, methylprednisolone)	Gut (vomiting due to cytotoxics)
Cannabinoids (nabilone)	
Benzodiazepines (lorazepam)	

the action of acetylcholine at muscarinic nerve endings in the gut. It raises the tone of the lower oesophageal sphincter, relaxes the pyloric antrum and duodenal cap, and increases peristalsis and emptying of the upper gut. The peripheral actions are utilised to empty the stomach before emergency anaesthesia and in labour. If an opioid has been given, metoclopramide may fail to overcome the opioid-induced inhibition of gastric emptying, and thus the risk of vomiting and inhaling gastric contents remains. The action of metoclopramide is terminated by metabolism in the liver ($t_{1/2}$ 4 h).

Uses. Metoclopramide is used for nausea and vomiting associated with gastrointestinal disorders, and with cytotoxic drugs and radiotherapy. It is also an effective antiemetic in migraine and is used as a pro-kinetic agent (see above).

Adverse reactions are characteristic of dopamine receptor antagonists and include extrapyramidal dystonia (torticollis, facial spasms, trismus, oculogyric crises), which occurs more commonly in children and young adults, and in those who are concurrently receiving other dopamine receptor antagonists, e.g. phenothiazine drugs. The antimuscarinic drug, benzatropine, given intravenously, rapidly abolishes the reaction. Long-term use of metoclopramide may cause tardive dyskinesia in the elderly. Metoclopramide stimulates prolactin release and may cause gynaecomastia and lactation. Restlessness and diarrhoea may also occur.

Domperidone

Domperidone is a selective dopamine D_2-receptor antagonist; unlike metoclopramide it does not possess an acetylcholine-like effect. Domperidone does not readily penetrate the blood–brain barrier; this does not limit its therapeutic efficacy, because the CTZ is functionally outside the barrier, but there is less risk of adverse effects in the CNS. Domperidone is used for nausea or vomiting associated with gastrointestinal disorders and with cytotoxic and other drug treatments. It can also be helpful in management of bloating in patients with non-ulcer dyspepsia (see above). It may cause gynaecomastia and galactorrhoea.

Ondansetron

Ondansetron is a selective $5HT_3$-receptor antagonist. Drugs with this activity appear to be highly effective against nausea and vomiting induced by cytotoxic agents and radiotherapy. Evidence suggests that such anticancer treatment releases serotonin (5HT) from enterochromaffin cells in the gut mucosa (where resides more than 80% of the serotonin in the body), thereby activating specific receptors in the gut and CNS to cause emesis.[7] The action of ondansetron is thus partly central and partly peripheral. Ondansetron may be given by intravenous injection or infusion immediately before cancer chemotherapy (notably with cisplatin), followed by oral administration for up to 5 days ($t_{1/2}$ 5 h). The drug appears to be well tolerated but constipation, headache and a feeling of flushing in the head and epigastrium may occur.

Granisetron and tropisetron are similar.

Nabilone

Nabilone is a synthetic cannabinoid and has properties similar to tetrahydrocannabinol (the active constituent of marijuana), which has an antiemetic action. It is used to relieve nausea or vomiting caused by cytotoxic drugs. Adverse effects include somnolence, dry mouth, decreased appetite, dizziness, euphoria, dysphoria, postural hypotension, confusion and psychosis. These may be reduced if prochlorperazine is given concomitantly.

TREATMENT OF VARIOUS FORMS OF VOMITING

MOTION SICKNESS

Motion sickness is more easily prevented than cured. It is due chiefly to over-stimulation of the vestibular apparatus (and does not occur if the labyrinth is destroyed). Other factors also contribute. Visually, a moving horizon can be most disturbing, as can the sensations induced by the gravitational inertia of a full stomach when the body is in vertical movement. It is a matter of common experience amongst all who have been on a rough sea that the environment, whether close and smelly or open and vivifying, is important. Psychological factors, including observation of the fate of one's companions, are also

---

[7]Cubeddu L X, Hoffmann I S, Fuenmayor N T, Finn A L 1990 Efficacy of ondansetron (GR 38032F) and the role of serotonin in cisplatin-induced nausea and vomiting. New England Journal of Medicine 322:810–816.

important. Tolerance to the motion occurs, generally over a period of days.

The pharmacology of vomiting was little studied until the world war of 1939–1945, when motion sickness attained military importance as a possible handicap for sea landings made in the face of resistance. The British military authorities and the Medical Research Council therefore organised an investigation. Whenever there was a prospect of sufficiently rough weather, about 70 soldiers were sent to sea in small ships, again and again, after being dosed with a drug or a dummy tablet and having had their mouths inspected to detect non-compliance. The ships returned to land when up to 40% of the soldiers vomited. 'On the whole the men enjoyed their trips'; some of them, however, being soldiers, thought the tablets were given in order to make them vomit and some 'believed firmly in the efficacy of the dummy tablets'. It was concluded that, of the remedies tested, hyoscine (0.6 or 1.2 mg) was the most effective.[8] This appears still to be the case.

Other drugs used for motion sickness include the antimuscarinic agents *cinnarizine, cyclizine, dimenhydrinate* and *promethazine*.

For prophylaxis an antiemetic is best taken 1 h before exposure to the motion. About 70% protection may be expected by the right dose given at the right time. Once motion sickness has started, oral administration of drugs may fail, and the intramuscular, subcutaneous or rectal route are required. Alternatively, hyoscine may be administered as a dermal patch, so avoiding the enteral route. Prevention of symptoms may therefore be possible only at the expense of troublesome unwanted effects: sleepiness, dry mouth, blurred vision.

DRUG-INDUCED VOMITING

If reducing the dose or withdrawing the offending drug is not an option then an attempt, often unsatisfactory, may be made to oppose it with another drug. In general, metoclopramide or a phenothiazine is best. Opioid-induced vomiting responds to one of the drugs used for motion sickness (see above); cyclizine and morphine are combined as Cyclimorph.

[8]Holling H E, McArdle B, Trotter W R 1944 Prevention of seasickness by drugs. Lancet i:127.

VOMITING DUE TO CYTOTOXIC DRUGS

Prevention and alleviation of this distressing and often very severe symptom of some forms of cancer treatment may allow an optimal chemotherapeutic regimen to be used, and avoid admitting the patient to hospital. Cisplatin is notably emetic. Ondansetron (see above) is highly effective as is dexamethasone, although its mode of action is unclear. Lorazepam, despite dose-limiting sedation and dysphoria, is a useful adjunct and provides amnesia, which may limit the development of anticipatory vomiting. For severe vomiting due to cytotoxics, ondansetron plus dexamethasone with or without lorazepam (all given intravenously) is an effective and well tolerated combination. Metoclopramide may be substituted for ondansetron where a less emetic regimen is used, especially in older patients who are less susceptible to its extrapyramidal reactions.

VOMITING AFTER GENERAL ANAESTHESIA

The condition affects some 30% of patients and routine prophylaxis seems warranted only where the risk is high, e.g. those with a history of postoperative vomiting or of motion sickness, or where vomiting carries special hazard, e.g. eye surgery. Metoclopramide or a $5HT_3$-receptor antagonist, e.g. ondansetron, or a butyrophenone, e.g. haloperidol, droperidol, may be used.

VOMITING IN PREGNANCY

This reaches a peak at 10–11 weeks and usually resolves by 13–14 weeks of gestation. Nausea alone does not require treatment. Much can be achieved by reassurance that the problem is transient and a discussion of diet, e.g. taking food before getting up in the morning. Rarely, a decision is taken to use a drug, and then a histamine H_1-receptor antagonist or a phenothiazine, e.g. promethazine (see above), is preferred. Although pyridoxine deficiency has not been shown to complicate simple pregnancy vomiting, it may occur in hyperemesis gravidarum, which requires intravenous fluids and multivitamin supplements.

VERTIGO

A great range of drugs has been recommended to treat vertigo and labyrinthine disorders but antimuscarinics and phenothiazines are generally preferred.

Cyclizine or prochlorperazine may be used to relieve an acute attack. Betahistine (a histamine analogue) is used in the hope of improving the blood circulation to the inner ear in Menière's syndrome; cinnarizine is also used.

GUIDE TO FURTHER READING

Chan F K L, Leung W K 2002 Peptic ulcer disease. Lancet 360:933–941

Costa S H, Vessey M P 1993 Misoprostol and illegal abortion in Rio de Janeiro, Brazil. Lancet 341:1258–1261

Fisher R S, Parkman H P 1998 Management of nonulcer dyspepsia. New England Journal of Medicine 339:1376–1381

Grunberg S M, Hesketh P J 1993 Control of chemotherapy-induced emesis. New England Journal of Medicine 329:1790–1796

Harvey R, Lane A J, Murray L J et al 2004 Randomised controlled trial of effects of Helicobacter pylori infection and its eradication on heartburn and gastro-oesophageal reflux. British Medical Journal 328:1417–1420

Hooper L, Brown T J, Elliott R A et al 2004 The effectiveness of five strategies for the prevention of gastrointestinal toxicity induced by nonsteroidal anti-inflammatory drugs; a systematic review. British Medical Journal 329:948–952

Huang J-Q, Sridhar S, Hunt R 2002 Role of Helicobacter pylori infection and non-steroidal anti-inflammatory drugs in peptic-ulcer disease: a meta-analysis. Lancet 359:14–22

Leontiadis G I, Sharma V K, Howden C W 2005 Systematic review and meta-analysis of proton pump inhibitor therapy in peptic ulcer bleeding. British Medical Journal 330:568–570

Megraud F 2004 Helicobacter pylori antibiotic resistance: prevalence, importance and advances in testing. Gut 53:1374–1384

Moayyedi P, Talley N 2006 Gastro-oesophageal reflux disease. Lancet 367:2086–2100

National Institute for Clinical Excellence 2004 Dyspepsia: management of dyspepsia in adults in primary care. Clinical Guideline 17. Online. Available: http://www.nice.org.uk/pdf/CG017NICEguideline.pdf

Richter J E 2001 Oesophageal motility disorders. Lancet 358:823–828

Suerbaum S, Michetti P 2002 Helicobacter pylori infection. New England Journal of Medicine 347:1175–1186

White P F 2004 Prevention of postoperative nausea and vomiting – a multimodal solution to a persistent problem. New England Journal of Medicine 350:2511–2515

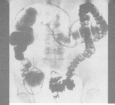

32

Intestines

SYNOPSIS

Problems of constipation, diarrhoea and irritable bowel syndrome are common. Infective diarrhoeal diseases are a significant cause of morbidity and mortality worldwide, especially in infants and children. The management of these conditions is reviewed.

- Constipation: mode of action and use of drugs
- Diarrhoea (drug treatment, importance of fluid and electrolyte replacement)
- Inflammatory bowel disease
- Irritable bowel syndrome

CONSTIPATION

The terms purgative, cathartic, laxative, aperient and evacuant are synonymous. They are medicines that promote defaecation largely by reducing the viscosity of the contents of the lower colon and are classified as follows:

- Stool bulking agents.
- Osmotic laxatives.
- Faecal softeners.
- Stimulant laxatives.

STOOL BULKING AGENTS

Dietary fibre comprises the cell walls and supporting structures of vegetables and fruits. Most of the fibre in our diet is in the form of non-starch polysaccharides (NSPs),[1] which are not digestible by human enzymes. Fibre may be soluble (pectins, guar, ispaghula) or insoluble (cellulose, hemicelluloses, lignin). Insoluble fibre has less effect than soluble fibre on the viscosity of gut contents but is a stronger laxative because it resists digestion in the small bowel and so enters the colon intact. In addition it has a vast capacity for retaining water; thus 1 g of carrot fibre can hold 23 g of water.[2] It has been proposed that as humans have refined the carbohydrates in their diet over the centuries, so they have deprived themselves of fibre, the ensuing under-filling of the colon being an important cause of constipation, haemorrhoids and diverticular disease. Stool bulking agents, which add fibre to the diet, are the treatment of choice for simple constipation. They act by increasing the volume and lowering the viscosity of intestinal contents to produce a soft bulky stool, which encourages normal reflex bowel activity. The mode of action of stool bulking agents is thus more physiological than other types of laxative. They should be taken with liberal quantities of fluid (at least 2 L daily).

Individual preparations

Bran is the residue left when flour is made from cereals; it contains between 25% and 50% of fibre. The fibre content of a normal diet can be increased by eating wholemeal bread and bran cereals but over-zealous supplementation may cause troublesome wind (from bacterial fermentation in the colon).

Viscous (soluble) fibres, e.g. ispaghula, are effective and more palatable than bran. Ispaghula husk contains mucilage and hemicelluloses, which swell rapidly in water. Methylcellulose takes up water to swell to a colloid about 25 times its original volume, and sterculia,[3] similarly, swells when mixed with water.

OSMOTIC LAXATIVES

These are but little absorbed and increase the bulk and reduce viscosity of intestinal contents to promote a fluid stool.

---

[1]The term 'unavailable complex carbohydrate' (UCC) is also used and refers to NSP plus undigested ('resistant') starch.

[2]McConnell A A, Eastwood M A, Mitchell W D 1974 Physical characteristics of vegetable foodstuffs that could influence bowel function. Journal of the Science of Food and Agriculture 25:1457–1464.

[3]Named after Sterculinus, a god of ancient Rome, who presided over manuring of agricultural land.

Some inorganic salts retain water in the intestinal lumen or, if given as hypertonic solution, withdraw it from the body. When constipation is mild, magnesium hydroxide will suffice but magnesium sulphate (Epsom[4] salts) is used when a more powerful effect is needed. Both magnesium salts act in 2–4 h.

Lactulose is a synthetic disaccharide. Taken orally, it is unaffected by small intestinal disaccharidases, is not absorbed and thus acts as an osmotic laxative. Tolerance may develop. Lactulose is also used in the treatment of hepatic encephalopathy (see Chapter 33).

Osmotic laxatives are frequently used to clear the colon for diagnostic procedures or surgery. Enemas containing phosphate or citrate effectively evacuate the distal colon and can be useful for treating obstinate constipation in elderly or debilitated patients. Oral preparations containing magnesium sulphate and citric acid (Citramag) or polyethylene glycol (Klean Prep, Movicol) are used in preparation for colonoscopy; they are made up with water to create an isotonic solution, and some patients find the large volumes difficult to tolerate.

FAECAL SOFTENERS (EMOLLIENTS)

The softening properties of these agents are useful in the management of anal fissure (see below) and haemorrhoids.

Docusate sodium (dioctyl sodium sulphosuccinate) softens faeces by lowering the surface tension of fluids in the bowel. This allows more water to remain in the faeces. It appears also to have bowel stimulant properties but these are relatively weak. Docusate sodium acts in 1–2 days. Poloxamers, e.g. poloxalkol (poloxamer 188), act similarly and are used in combination with other agents.

STIMULANT LAXATIVES

These drugs increase intestinal motility by various mechanisms; they may cause abdominal cramps, should be used only with caution in pregnancy, and never where intestinal obstruction is suspected.

Bisacodyl stimulates sensory endings in the colon by direct action from the lumen. It is effective orally in 6–10 h and, as a suppository, acts in 1 h. In geriatric

patients, bisacodyl suppositories reduce the need for regular enemas. There are no important unwanted effects.

Sodium picosulfate is similar and is also used to evacuate the bowel for investigative procedures and surgery.

Glycerol has a mild stimulant effect on the rectum when administered as a suppository.

The anthraquinone group of laxatives includes senna, danthron, cascara, rhubarb[5] and aloes. In the small intestine soluble anthraquinone derivates are liberated and absorbed. These are excreted into the colon and act there, along with those that have escaped absorption, probably after being chemically changed by bacterial action.

Senna, available as a biologically standardised preparation, is widely used to relieve constipation and to empty the bowel for investigative procedures and surgery. It acts in 8–12 h.

Danthron is available as a standardised preparation in combination with the faecal softeners poloxamer 188 (co-danthramer) and docusate sodium (as co-danthrusate). It acts in 6–12 h. Evidence from rodent studies indicates a possible carcinogenic risk, and long-term exposure to danthron should be avoided. It can be useful for treating constipation in terminally ill patients.

Drastic purgatives (castor oil, cascara, jalap,[6] colocynth, phenolphthalein and podophyllum) are obsolete.

SUPPOSITORIES AND ENEMAS

Suppositories (bisacodyl, glycerin) may be used to obtain a bowel action in about 1 h. Enemas produce defaecation by softening faeces and distending

---

[5]In the late 18th century Britain made approaches to trade with China that were met with indifference; it seems that the mandarins held the belief that the British feared death from constipation if deprived of rhubarb (*Rheum palmatum*), one of China's exports.

[6]In the 19th century 'young men proceeding to Africa' were advised to take pills named Livingstone's Rousers, consisting of rhubarb, jalap, calomel and quinine (British Medical Journal 1964; 2:1583).

---

[4]Epsom, a town near London, known for its now defunct mineral spring water, and for horse racing.

the bowel. They are used in preparation for surgery, radiological examination and endoscopy. Preparations with sodium phosphate, which is poorly absorbed and so retains water in the gut, are generally used. Arachis oil is included in enemas to soften impacted faeces.

MISUSE OF LAXATIVES

Dependence (abuse) may arise following laxative use during an illness or in pregnancy, or the individual may have the mistaken notion that a daily bowel motion is essential for health, or that the bowels are only incompletely opened by nature, and so indulge in regular purgation. This effectively prevents the easy return of normal habits because the more powerful stimulant purges empty the whole colon, whereas normal defaecation empties only the descending colon. Cessation of use after a few weeks is thus inevitably followed by a few days' constipation whilst sufficient material collects to restore the normal state; the delay may convince the patient of the continued need for purgatives. Laxative dependence, which may be solely *emotional* at first, may be followed by *physical dependence*, so that the bowels will not open without a purgative. Prolonged abuse can damage gut nerves and lead to an atonic colon.

Excessive use of stimulant purgatives[7] may, especially in the old, lead to severe water and electrolyte depletion, even to hypokalaemic paralysis, malabsorption and protein-losing enteropathy. Purgatives should not be given to patients with undiagnosed abdominal pain, inflammatory bowel disease or obstruction. Nor should they be used to empty the rectum of hardened faeces, for they will fail and cause pain. Initial treatment should be with enemas, but digital removal, generally ordered by a senior and performed by a junior doctor, may occasionally be required. A bulking agent or a faecal softener will help to prevent recurrence.

---

[7]The Roman Emperor Nero (AD 37–68) murdered his severely constipated aunt by ordering the doctors to give her 'a laxative of fatal strength'. He 'seized her property before she was quite dead and tore up the will so that nothing could escape him' (Suetonius (trans.) R Graves).

DIARRHOEA

Diarrhoea ranges from a mild and socially inconvenient illness to a major cause of death and malnutrition among children in less developed countries; acute diarrhoea from gastroenteritis causes 4 to 5 million deaths throughout the world annually. Drugs have a place in its management but the first priority of therapy is to preserve fluid and electrolyte balance.

SOME PHYSIOLOGY

In the normal adult, 7–8 L of water and electrolytes are secreted daily into the gastrointestinal tract. This, together with dietary fluid, is absorbed by epithelial cells in the small and large bowel. Water follows the osmotic gradients that result from shifts of electrolytes across the intestinal epithelium, and sodium and chloride transport mechanisms are central to the causation and management of diarrhoea, especially that caused by bacteria and viruses. The energy for the process is provided by the activity of Na^+/K^+-ATPase.

Absorption of sodium into the epithelium is effected by:

■ *Sodium–glucose-coupled entry.* Glucose stimulates the absorption of sodium and the resulting water flow also sweeps additional sodium and chloride along with it (solvent drag). This important mechanism remains active in diarrhoea of various aetiologies, and improvement of sodium and water absorption by glucose (and amino acids) is the basis of oral rehydration regimens (see below). Absorption of sodium and water in the colon is stimulated by short-chain fatty acids (see below, cereal-based oral rehydration therapy).

■ *Sodium–ion-coupled entry.* Na^+ and Cl^- enter the epithelial cell, either as a pair or, as seems more likely, there is a double exchange: Na^+ (extracellular) with H^+ (intracellular) and Cl^- (extracellular) with $2OH^-$ or $2HCO_3^-$ (intracellular). Oral rehydration solutions (see below) contain sodium, chloride and bicarbonate.

Secretion is the opposite process to absorption. In response to various stimuli, crypt cells actively transport chloride into the gut lumen, and sodium and water follow. This *stimulus–secretion coupling* is modulated by cyclic AMP and GMP, calcium, prostaglandins and leukotrienes.

Diarrhoea results from an imbalance between secretion and reabsorption of fluid and electrolytes; it has numerous causes, including infections with enteric organisms (which may stimulate secretion or damage absorption), inflammatory bowel disease and nutrient malabsorption due to disease. It also commonly occurs as a manifestation of disordered gut motility in the absence of demonstrable disease (see below). Rarely, it is due to secretory tumours of the alimentary tract, e.g. carcinoid tumour or vipoma (a tumour that secretes VIP, vasoactive intestinal peptide).

Motility patterns in the bowel. An important factor in diarrhoea may be loss of the normal segmenting contractions that delay passage of contents, so that an occasional peristaltic wave has a greater propulsive effect. Segmental contractions of the smooth muscle in the bowel mix the intestinal contents. Patients with diarrhoea commonly have less spontaneous segmenting activity in the sigmoid colon than do people with normal bowel habit, and patients with constipation have more. Antimotility drugs (see below) reduce diarrhoea by increasing segmentation and inhibiting peristalsis.

FLUID AND ELECTROLYTE TREATMENT

Oral rehydration therapy (ORT) with glucose–electrolyte solution is sufficient to treat the vast majority of episodes of watery diarrhoea from acute gastroenteritis. As a simple, effective, cheap and readily administered therapy for a potentially fatal condition, ORT must rank as a major advance in therapy. It is effective because glucose-coupled sodium transport continues during diarrhoea and so enhances replacement of water and electrolyte losses in the stool.

Oral rehydration salts (ORSs). The World Health Organization/UNICEF-recommended formulation is:

Sodium chloride	3.5 g/L
Potassium chloride	1.5 g/L
Sodium citrate	2.9 g/L
Anhydrous glucose	20.0 g/L.

This provides sodium 90 mmol/L, potassium 20 mmol/L, chloride 80 mmol/L, citrate 10 mmol/L, glucose 111 mmol/L (total osmolarity 311 mmol/L).[8]

Several other formulations exist, some with less sodium (see national formularies).[9]

Rehydration therapy with commercial soft drinks alone will fail because their sodium content is too low (usually less than 4 mmol/L). The glucose may be replaced by another substrate, such as glycine or rice powder. Indeed cereal-based ORSs, relying on starch (to produce glucose) from many sources (rice, wheat, corn, potato), have the advantage of controlling diarrhoea much more effectively than the glucose-based preparations. This may be because undigested starch is fermented in the colon to short-chain fatty acids, which stimulate colonic sodium and water absorption. Thus, almost every household in the world can find the essential components of an effective oral rehydration mixture: water, cereals and salt.

Most cases can be treated adequately by assiduous attention to oral intake, but fluid and electrolyte depletion is especially dangerous in children and intravenous fluid replacement in hospital may be needed. Antimotility drugs are inappropriate for severe diarrhoea in young children; any marginal effect they may have is liable to be counterbalanced by hazardous adverse effects (see below).

ANTIDIARRHOEAL DRUGS

There are two types of drug which are often used in combination.

Antimotility drugs

Codeine, *diphenoxylate* and *loperamide* all activate opiate receptors on the smooth muscle of the bowel to reduce peristalsis and increase segmentation

---

[8]Solutions with lower sodium content and thus reduced total osmolarity (250 mmol/L) are associated with less need for unscheduled intravenous fluid infusion, lower stool volume and less vomiting, and may now be preferred (Hahn S, Kim Y-J, Garner P 2001 Reduced osmolarity oral rehydration solution for treating dehydration due to diarrhoea in children: systematic review. British Medical Journal 323:81–85).
[9]The higher sodium content of the WHO/UNICEF formulation is based on sodium concentrations in diarrhoeal stools, but low-sodium, high-glucose formulations may be preferred for infants, whose faecal losses of sodium are less.

contractions. The actions of all three drugs are antagonised by naloxone. *Warning*: antimotility drugs should not be used for acute diarrhoea in children, especially babies, because they can cause respiratory depression. These drugs are also dangerous in patients with active inflammatory bowel disease, for they may cause paralytic ileus.

Drugs that directly increase the viscosity of gut contents

Kaolin and chalk are adsorbent powders. Their therapeutic efficacy is marginal as is shown by the fact that they are often combined with an opioid. Bulk forming agents such as ispaghula, methylcellulose and sterculia (see above) are useful for diarrhoea in diverticular disease, and for reducing the fluidity of faeces in patients with ileostomy and colostomy.

TRAVELLERS' DIARRHOEA

So familiar is diarrhoea to travellers that it has acquired regional popular names: the Aztec Two-step, Montezuma's Revenge, Delhi Belly, Rangoon Runs, Tokyo Trots, Gyppy Tummy, Hong-Kong Dog, Estomac Anglais and Casablanca Crud – all indicate some of the areas deemed dangerous by visitors. The Mexican name 'turista' indicates the principal sufferers.

Most cases are infective, and up to half of the diarrhoea that afflicts visitors to tropical and subtropical countries is associated with enterotoxigenic strains of *Escherichia coli*; other bacteria including *Shigella* and *Salmonella* spp., viruses including the Norwalk family, and parasites (particularly *Giardia lamblia*) have also been implicated. Recognition that transmission is almost invariably by ingestion of contaminated food and water points to the most effective way of reducing the risk.

Acute watery diarrhoea in adults can usually be controlled by oral rehydration solutions and one of the antimotility drugs, although in mild cases the abdominal bloating produced by the latter may be less acceptable than the loose stools. Although diarrhoea usually lasts only 2–3 days, this may still be socially inconvenient, and if symptomatic remedies fail an aminoquinolone, e.g. ciprofloxacin 500 mg b.d., will be effective. The use of antimicrobials for travellers' diarrhoea continues to evoke controversy but most sufferers will appreciate the relief that even one or two tablets can bring.

Prophylactic antimicrobial therapy has been shown to reduce the incidence of attacks of diarrhoea but its routine use carries the risk of hindering the diagnosis of serious infection. A wider issue is the possible development and spread of antibiotic-resistant organisms. Thus any benefits to the *individual* must be weighed against the risk to the *community* in the future. In most instances prophylactic antimicrobials should not be used but ciprofloxacin (500 mg once daily) may be justified for individuals who must remain well while travelling for short periods to high-risk areas.

SPECIFIC INFECTIVE DIARRHOEAS

Chemotherapy is available for certain specific organisms, e.g. amoebiasis, giardiasis, typhoid fever (see Index).

DRUG-INDUCED DIARRHOEA

Antimicrobials are the commonest drugs that cause diarrhoea, probably due to alteration of bowel flora. The diarrhoea may range from a mild inconvenience to a life-threatening antibiotic-associated (pseudomembranous) colitis, due to colonisation of the bowel with *Clostridium difficile*. The condition particularly affects elderly patients. Clindamycin and third-generation cephalosporins are especially prone to cause this complication, whereas it is uncommon with the quinolone and aminoglycoside groups. Treatment is with vancomycin or metronidazole.

Magnesium-containing antacids may also produce diarrhoea, as may non-steroidal anti-inflammatory drugs (NSAIDs) and lithium.

SECRETORY DIARRHOEAS

Octreotide, a synthetic peptide that shares amino acid homology with somatostatin (see p. 586), inhibits the release of peptides that mediate certain alimentary secretions, and may be used to relieve diarrhoea due to carcinoid tumours and vipomas.

INFLAMMATORY BOWEL DISEASE

The pathogenesis of inflammatory bowel disease is still poorly understood. Immune mechanisms are probably involved, and potential antigens include intestinal bacteria and intestinal epithelium. Abnormalities in inflammatory mediators have also been described; it has been suggested that an imbalance between pro-inflammatory and anti-inflammatory cytokines may determine susceptibility, although the abnormalities observed could simply be secondary to the disease process.

The main drugs used in the treatment of ulcerative colitis and Crohn's disease are the aminosalicylates and corticosteroids. Their mode of action is obscure. Other immunosuppressives also have a role and recent studies into the mechanisms of inflammation are leading to the introduction of novel therapies to inhibit the inflammatory process.

In acute exacerbations of inflammatory bowel disease a gastrointestinal infection should always be excluded by stool microscopy and culture, and testing for *Clostridium difficile* toxin. Measures to correct anaemia, fluid and electrolyte abnormalities, and to improve the general nutritional state, are also important. Antidiarrhoeals should be used only with extreme caution in active colitis and are contraindicated if the disease is severe. They can lead to toxic dilatation of the colon, with perforation.

ULCERATIVE COLITIS

Aminosalicylates

Aminosalicylates maintain remission in patients with ulcerative colitis (relapses are reduced by a factor of three), and may also be used for treatment of an acute attack (in addition to corticosteroid).

Sulfasalazine (salicylazosulfapyridine, Salazopyrin) consists of two compounds, sulfapyridine and 5-aminosalicylic acid, joined by an azo bond. Sulfasalazine is poorly absorbed from the small intestine, and colonic bacteria split the azo bond to release the component parts. The therapeutically active moiety is 5-aminosalicylic acid (5-ASA). Sulfapyridine is well absorbed, is acetylated in the liver and excreted in the urine; it has no therapeutic action in colitis but contributes to a mechanism for delivering 5-ASA to the colon.

Sulfasalazine is also used as a disease-modifying agent in rheumatoid arthritis (see p. 269), the condition for which it was originally introduced in the 1930s. It is available as a tablet, retention enema or suppository.

Adverse effects are due largely to the sulphonamide moiety and include headache, malaise, anorexia, nausea and vomiting; these are dose related and commoner in slow acetylators (of the sulphonamide). Allergic reactions include rash, fever and lymphadenitis; rarely leucopenia and agranulocytosis occur. Males may become infertile due to oligospermia and reduced sperm motility; this reverses if sulfasalazine is replaced with mesalazine. Body secretions may have an orange discoloration, which can stain soft contact lenses.

Mesalazine. Patients intolerant of sulfasalazine usually tolerate mesalazine, which is 5-ASA. Mesalazine is absorbed rapidly and completely in the upper jejunum, and is presented in various formulations that delay its release. Asacol tablets are coated in a resin, which dissolves only at pH 7 or higher, favouring its release in the ileum and colon. In contrast Pentasa has a slow-release but pH-independent coating so that 5-ASA is liberated throughout the gastrointestinal tract. 5-ASA that enters the blood is rapidly cleared by acetylation in the liver and renal excretion. In addition to oral formulations, mesalazine is available as an enema.

The profile of adverse effects includes nausea, watery diarrhoea (which can lead to diagnostic confusion in patients with inflammatory bowel disease), pancreatitis and interstitial nephritis. Renal function should be monitored regularly in patients taking 5-ASA, particularly with preparations that are extensively released in the small intestine.

Two other 5-ASA preparations effectively delay release of the active moiety until the preparation reaches the colon: olsalazine is two molecules of 5-ASA acid linked by an azo bond, whereas balsalazide comprises one molecule of 5-ASA acid linked by an azo bond to an inert carrier. 5-ASA is liberated after cleavage of the azo bonds by colonic bacteria.

Corticosteroid

Enemas and suppositories. When ulcerative colitis is restricted to the left hemicolon, exacerbations that do not respond to an aminosalicylate alone can often be controlled by steroid enemas. Properly administered, these will reach the splenic flexure, and for this to occur the patient should be instructed to lie down for at least 30 min after insertion of the enema. The foam-based preparations appear to coat the colonic mucosa more efficiently than the aqueous formulations.

In patients with disease limited to the distal few centimetres of the rectum, corticosteroid enemas may be ineffective because they will be delivered proximal to the inflamed segment. In this situation corticosteroid suppositories are often helpful. Patients with distal colitis are prone to faecal loading proximal to the inflamed segment and this can lead to overflow diarrhoea and worsening of inflammation. Faecal loading can be detected on straight abdominal radiography and is treated with laxatives; this is safe provided the inflammatory process is restricted to the distal colon. On no account should antidiarrhoeals be used as these will exacerbate the problem. Adequate quantities of dietary fibre and fluid should be encouraged, and stool bulking agents can also be helpful in protecting against faecal loading.

Systemic corticosteroid. *Moderately severe attacks* of ulcerative colitis should be treated with systemic corticosteroid, and oral preparations usually suffice. It is important to start with a dose that will bring the inflammatory process under control, e.g. prednisolone 60 mg/day by mouth. A response should start within 10–14 days, and if it does not the patient should be admitted to hospital for more intensive treatment including intravenous corticosteroid. Once remission has been attained the dose can be tailed down over a period of 6–8 weeks. This gradual decrease is important (in contrast, for example, to treating asthma where rapidly tailing regimens are appropriate).

Severe attacks of ulcerative colitis should be treated in hospital with intravenous corticosteroid. The main danger is toxic dilatation of the colon and perforation, which can occur insidiously. Regular measurements of abdominal girth and straight radiography of the abdomen are useful in monitoring response, which should be seen within 72 h. If there is no improvement a trial of ciclosporin (see below) may induce response. Treatment otherwise is by emergency colectomy.

Ciclosporin may induce remission in some patients with severe ulcerative colitis unresponsive to corticosteroid. The drug is given in a dose of 2–4 mg/kg i.v. until remission is attained. Renal function should be monitored closely as ciclosporin is nephrotoxic (see p. 197). For maintenance therapy azathioprine (see below) is often substituted. Ciclosporin use only delays surgery for many patients; after 1 year 50% will have relapsed and undergone colectomy.

Smoking aggravates Crohn's disease but (perversely) improves ulcerative colitis. Nicotine patches may provide benefit in ulcerative colitis but the effect is not sufficiently great to justify their routine use in management.

Maintenance of remission

Corticosteroids can be reduced slowly (see above) and maintenance therapy with an aminosalicylate started. If the disease is corticosteroid dependent, azathioprine or another immunosuppressive agent may be used (see below). Surgery is indicated if medical therapy fails to control the disease or is associated with unacceptable adverse effects.

CROHN'S DISEASE

Any part of the gastrointestinal tract may be involved, from mouth to anus, and treatment depends on the site of disease.

Management of colonic Crohn's disease is very similar to that of ulcerative colitis, with aminosalicylate and corticosteroid. These drugs are of less value in maintaining remission in Crohn's disease than in ulcerative colitis, although they do help to reduce recurrence of disease at sites of surgical anastomoses. Topical enema preparations are less useful because of the patchy distribution of inflammation and rectal sparing. In contrast to ulcerative colitis, about 50% of patients with Crohn's colitis will respond to *metronidazole* given for up to 3 months. The drug is also helpful in controlling perianal and small bowel disease, and it decreases the incidence of anastomotic recurrence after surgery. Adverse effects including alcohol intolerance, and peripheral neuropathy from such prolonged therapy often limit its use. Other antimicrobials, particularly *ciprofloxacin*, may also be effective.

Crohn's disease of the *small bowel* classically affects the ileocaecal region. Patients with small bowel involvement are frequently malnourished and specialist dietetic input is essential; enteral or parenteral nutrition may be required. Osteoporosis is common, particularly if corticosteroid consumption has been high.

Sulfasalazine, olsalazine and balsalazide are ineffective in small bowel Crohn's disease because these drugs are designed to liberate 5-ASA in the colon. Mesalazine preparations release 5-ASA higher in the gut and control mild to moderate exacerbations of ileocaecal disease in approximately 50% of patients, although high doses are needed (Asacol 2.4 g in divided doses, Pentasa 2 g b.d.).

In *more severe disease*, corticosteroid is needed to induce remission (prednisolone 60 mg/day by mouth until remission is induced, thereafter tailing the dose by 5 mg/day/week). Approximately 75% of patients respond. Budesonide, a potent topically active corticosteroid, is an alternative that can be administered either orally or as an enema. The oral preparation is presented as a delayed-release formulation which delivers drug to the terminal ileum and ascending colon. Extensive first-pass metabolism in the liver limits its systemic availability and potential for adverse effects. Budesonide is also useful as maintenance therapy of the 30% of patients with Crohn's disease whose condition is steroid dependent.

Maintenance of remission may require addition of azathioprine or another immunosuppressive drug (see below). Tobacco smoking definitely contributes to relapse and should be strongly discouraged.

Crohn's disease may be complicated by intestinal strictures, fistulae and intra-abdominal abscesses. Surgery is often necessary but strictures may be amenable to endoscopic balloon dilatation and abscesses can be drained under radiographic control.

Dietary therapy

There is evidence that liquid diets based on amino acids (elemental diets) or oligopeptides for 4–6 weeks are as effective as corticosteroids in controlling Crohn's disease, although relapse is common when the treatment stops. Elemental preparations are not particularly palatable and they often have to be administered through a nasogastric tube, which is unpopular with patients. They are worth trying in steroid-resistant cases and are particularly favoured by paediatricians, who prefer to avoid adrenal steroid because of its adverse effects on growth.

Antibodies to tumour necrosis factor (TNF)

TNFα causes activation of immune cells and release of inflammatory mediators. Evidence indicates that the inhibitors of TNF, *infliximab* and *etanercept* (see p. 267), give benefit in Crohn's disease. A single dose of anti-TNFα will induce remission in approximately one-third of patients with Crohn's disease resistant to conventional therapies, with improvement in a further third. A further dose after 8 weeks appears to produce longer-lasting remissions, and long-term maintenance therapy is currently being investigated. This treatment is also useful in treating Crohn's fistulae. Adverse reactions include headache, nausea and malaise; repeat infusions after prolonged drug-free intervals (1–2 years) may lead to hypersensitivity reactions. The efficacy of these drugs, and their potential for adverse effects in the long term (including development of malignancy), remain to be established but there is evidence that they lead to increased susceptibility to infection, particularly tuberculosis. There is no good evidence that anti-TNFα antibodies are effective for ulcerative colitis.

Immunosuppressant drugs

Azathioprine is effective as a *steroid-sparing* agent in maintenance therapy of Crohn's disease. A dose of up to 2 mg/kg may allow corticosteroid to be withdrawn altogether. Azathioprine is also used for this purpose in ulcerative colitis although evidence for its efficacy here is less persuasive. As the onset of action of azathioprine is delayed for about 8 weeks, it is not an appropriate drug for inducing remission, and reducing the corticosteroid dose in the first few weeks of azathioprine treatment may cause relapse.

As azathioprine can cause bone marrow suppression, the blood count should be monitored weekly for the first 2 months of therapy and every 2 months thereafter for as long as the drug is taken. Intolerance to azathioprine is shown by malaise, abdominal discomfort and sometimes fever. Pancreatitis occurs in up to 5%. These effects are usually due to the imidazole side-chain of the molecule, and *mercaptopurine* (which is azathioprine without the side-chain) may be better tolerated. The dose is 1–1.5 mg/kg daily.

Methotrexate can be helpful in controlling relapses of Crohn's disease unresponsive to corticosteroid or azathioprine. It has also been used with benefit in ulcerative colitis. Its short- and long-term uses are limited by a wide profile of adverse effects including bone marrow suppression and pulmonary and hepatic fibrosis (see p. 263).

Ciclosporin. There is no good evidence that ciclosporin is effective in Crohn's disease.

OTHER CONDITIONS

MICROSCOPIC COLITIS

This condition presents with diarrhoea; the colonic mucosa is macroscopically normal but histologically shows either lymphocytic infiltration of the mucosa (lymphocytic colitis) or subendothelial fibrosis (collagenous colitis). Treatment with aminosalicylate induces remission in about 50% and corticosteroid may also be needed.

Bile salt malabsorption

Failure of the terminal ileum to reabsorb bile salts may result from Crohn's disease or ileal resection, and occurs in many patients with microscopic colitis. The action of these salts in the colon causes diarrhoea. *Colestyramine* benefits the condition by binding with bile salts; the dose is titrated against symptoms, starting with 8 g b.d. Colestyramine can also bind to many drugs given by mouth and reduce their bio-availability (see p. 89).

IRRITABLE BOWEL SYNDROME (IBS)

This condition affects 20% of the population and is the commonest reason for referral to a gastroenterologist. It is manifested by a variety of gastrointestinal symptoms including disordered bowel habit (constipation, diarrhoea, or both), abdominal pain and bloating. Upper gastrointestinal symptoms manifest as non-ulcer dyspepsia (see Chapter 31). All of these symptoms occur in the absence of demonstrable pathology in the gastrointestinal tract, although patients with IBS often have abnormalities of gut motility. Another feature of the condition is visceral hypersensitivity; patients with IBS have lower thresholds for pain from colonic distension induced by inflating balloons placed in the bowel. A proportion of patients develop their IBS symptoms after an episode of gastroenteritis and, in many, emotional stress is an important precipitating factor. Associated psychopathology, with anxiety and sometimes depression, are common.

The mainstay of treatment, after investigation when appropriate, is to reassure the patient of the entirely benign nature of the disorder and the good prognosis. Those with predominant *constipation* should be encouraged to increase the fluid and fibre content of their diet. Unprocessed bran can lead to troublesome bloating and wind, and a bulking agent such as ispaghula husk is often better tolerated.

Diarrhoea can be treated with an antimotility drug such as loperamide, the dose being adjusted to symptoms. Codeine phosphate is effective although it may cause sedation.

Antispasmodics (see below) are given for *abdominal pain*, although there is little objective evidence for their therapeutic efficacy. The generation of evidence is complicated by the variable nature of IBS symptoms, the patients who suffer from them, and the high rate of placebo response in this condition. There are two main classes of antispasmodic, the antimuscarinic drugs and drugs that are direct smooth muscle relaxants.

Antimuscarinic drugs

These drugs block cholinergic transmission at parasympathetic postganglionic nerve endings and cause smooth muscle to relax. The synthetic antimuscarinics *dicyclomine* and *propantheline* are probably the most useful in IBS, but therapeutic efficacy is often limited by other anticholinergic effects. The drugs are contraindicated in patients with glaucoma and prostatism, and should be avoided in patients with gastro-oesophageal reflux.

Direct smooth muscle relaxants

Mebeverine is a reserpine derivative that has a direct effect on colonic muscle activity, especially, it appears, on colonic hypermotility. As it does not possess antimuscarinic activity, it does not exhibit the troublesome effects of that group of drugs.

Alverine and peppermint oil also have direct smooth muscle relaxing activity.

A trial of low dose *amitryptiline* (10–25 mg by mouth at night) is worthwhile in patients who do not respond to antispasmodics, and associated depression will be helped by conventional doses of this or other antidepressants. Relaxation therapy, hypnotherapy and cognitive behaviour therapy have a place in selected cases.

DIVERTICULAR DISEASE

Diverticular disease affects 5–10% of Western people over the age of 45 years; the incidence rises to 80% in those over 80 years. Colonic dysmotility with increased intracolonic pressure, and diets high in refined carbohydrate and low in fibre, are important pathogenic factors. Some patients experience abdominal pain from dysmotility, whereas others remain asymptomatic. Infection of diverticula occurs in a minority, giving potential for rupture or abscess formation.

Symptomatic diverticular disease often responds to an increase in dietary fibre and addition of a stool bulking agent. Antispasmodic drugs are helpful in controlling the pain of colon spasm but antimotility drugs encourage stasis of bowel contents, increase intracolonic pressure, and should be avoided. Diverticulitis requires treatment with broad-spectrum antimicrobials for 7–10 days (e.g. ciprofloxacin and metronidazole, or ampicillin, gentamicin and metronidazole).

ANAL FISSURE

Anal fissures are often intensely painful due to sphincter spasm. Anaesthetic ointments and stool softening agents have been widely used, with surgery (lateral internal sphincterotomy) for severely affected cases, but this procedure can cause incontinence from loss of sphincter control. An alternative is topical application of nitrate, which heals two-thirds of fissures. Preparations should be diluted to 0.2% as such use may be complicated by headache; tolerance can develop. Intrasphincteric injection of botulinum toxin has also been shown to be effective.

GUIDE TO FURTHER READING

Al-Abri S S, Beeching N J, Nye F J 2005 Traveller's diarrhoea. Lancet Infectious Diseases 5:349–360

Baumgart D C, Carding S R 2007 Inflammatory bowel disease: cause and immunobiology. Lancet 369:1627–1640

Baumgart D C, Sandborn W J 2007 Inflammatory bowel disease: clinical aspects and established and evolving therapies. Lancet 369:1641–1657

Cominelli F 2004 Cytokine-based therapies for Crohn's disease – new paradigms. New England Journal of Medicine 351:2045–2048

Lembo A, Camilleri M 2003 Chronic constipation. New England Journal of Medicine 349:1360–1368

Madoff R D 1998 Pharmacologic therapy for anal fissure. New England Journal of Medicine 338:257–259

Mertz H R 2003 Irritable bowel syndrome. New England Journal of Medicine 349:2136–2146

Midgley R, Kerr D 1999 Colorectal cancer. Lancet 353: 391–399

Nielsen O H, Vainer B, Schaffalitzky de Muckadell O B 2004 Microscopic colitis – a missed diagnosis? Lancet 364:2055–2057

Quartero A O, Meineche-Schmidt V, Muris J, Rubin G, de Wit N 2005 Bulking agents, antispasmodic and antidepressant medication for the treatment of irritable bowel syndrome. The Cochrane Database of Systematic Reviews (2)CD003460

Ransford R A J, Langman M J S 2002 Sulphasalazine and mesalazine; serious adverse reactions reevaluated on the basis of suspected adverse reaction reports to the Committee on Safety of Medicines. Gut 51(4):536–539

Shanahan F 2002 Crohn's disease. Lancet 359:62–69

Stollman N, Raskin J B 2004 Diverticular disease of the colon. Lancet 363:631–639

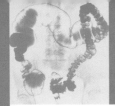

33

Liver, biliary tract, pancreas

SYNOPSIS

The liver is the most important organ in which drugs are structurally altered. Some of the resulting metabolites may be biologically inactive, some active and some toxic (see Chapter 7). The liver is exposed to drugs in higher concentrations than are most organs because most are administered orally and are absorbed from the gastrointestinal tract. Thus the whole dose must pass through the liver to reach the systemic circulation. Because of this the liver is a vulnerable target for injury from chemicals and drugs, and disordered hepatic function is an important cause of abnormal drug handling and response.

- Drugs and the liver
  - pharmacodynamic and pharmacokinetic changes
  - prescribing in liver disease
  - drug-induced liver injury
  - aspects of therapy
- Bile salts and gallstones
- Pancreas and drugs

EFFECTS OF LIVER DISEASE

PHARMACODYNAMIC CHANGES IN LIVER DISEASE

Patients with severe liver disease characteristically show abnormal end-organ response to drugs. For example:

- The sensitivity of the central nervous system (CNS) to opioids, sedatives and antiepilepsy drugs is increased.
- The effect of oral anticoagulants is increased because synthesis of coagulation factors is impaired.
- Fluid and electrolyte balance are altered. Sodium retention may be more readily induced by non-steroidal anti-inflammatory drugs (NSAIDs) or corticosteroids; ascites and oedema become more resistant to diuretics.

PHARMACOKINETIC CHANGES IN LIVER DISEASE

The liver has a large metabolic reserve, and it is only when disease becomes decompensated that important changes in drug handling occur. *Parenchymal* liver disease, e.g. chronic viral or alcoholic liver disease, has more impact on hepatic drug-metabolising enzyme activity than primarily *cholestatic* conditions, e.g. primary biliary cirrhosis, although clearance of drugs eliminated mainly by biliary excretion will be impaired in the latter.

Hepatocellular injury (toxic, infectious) leads to decreased activity of drug-metabolising enzymes, reflected in diminished plasma clearance of drugs that are metabolised. There is much variation between patients, and often overlap with healthy subjects.

HEPATIC BLOOD FLOW AND METABOLISM

Complex changes in blood flow occur with liver disease. Resistance to hepatic portal blood flow rises in cirrhosis, and portasystemic and intrahepatic shunts reduce drug delivery to hepatocytes. The pattern of change caused by disease relates to the manner in which the healthy liver treats a drug; there are two general classes:

- *Drugs that are rapidly metabolised and highly extracted in a single pass through the liver.* Clearance of such compounds is normally limited by *hepatic blood flow*, but in severe liver disease less drug is extracted from the blood as it passes through the liver owing to poor liver cell function, and portasystemic shunts allow a proportion of blood to bypass the liver altogether. Therefore the predominant change in the kinetics of drugs that are given orally is *increased systemic availability*. Accordingly the initial and maintenance doses of such drugs should be smaller than usual. When liver function is severely impaired the $t_{1/2}$ of drugs in this class may also be lengthened.

■ *Drugs that are slowly metabolised and are poorly extracted in a single pass through the liver*. The rate-limiting factor for elimination of this type of drug is *metabolic capacity*, and the major change caused by liver disease is *prolongation of $t_{1/2}$*. Consequently the interval between doses of such drugs may need to be lengthened, and the time to reach steady-state concentration in the plasma ($5 × t_{1/2}$) is increased.

PLASMA PROTEIN BINDING OF DRUG

Binding of drugs to albumin is reduced when plasma concentrations of the latter are low due to defective synthesis. Additionally, endogenous substances produced in liver disease may displace drugs from plasma protein binding sites. These changes provide scope to enhance the biological activity of drugs, but assume importance only for those that are extensively (>90%) protein bound.

OTHER CONSIDERATIONS

Patients with severe decompensated liver disease usually have associated renal impairment, with obvious consequences for drugs eliminated predominantly by the kidney. Where facilities exist, dosing should be guided by plasma concentration monitoring, e.g. gentamicin.

PRESCRIBING FOR PATIENTS WITH LIVER DISEASE

If liver disease is stable and well compensated, prescribing of most drugs is safe. Particular care should attend evidence of:

■ Impaired hepatic synthetic function (hypoalbuminaemia, impaired blood coagulation).
■ Current or recent hepatic encephalopathy.
■ Fluid retention and/or renal impairment.
■ Drugs with:
   – high hepatic extraction
   – high plasma protein binding
   – low therapeutic ratio
   – CNS depressant effect.

When a drug undergoes significant hepatic metabolism, a reasonable approach is to reduce the dose to 25–50% of normal and monitor the response carefully. The following are comments on specific examples.

CNS depressants. Sedatives, antidepressants and antiepilepsy drugs should be avoided or used with extreme caution in patients with advanced liver disease, particularly those with current or recent hepatic encephalopathy. Enhanced sensitivity of the CNS to such drugs is well documented and adds to the pharmacokinetic changes. Treatment of alcohol withdrawal in patients with established liver disease using clomethiazole is hazardous, especially when given intravenously. The temptation to give initial large doses to control agitation must be avoided because this drug, which normally has a high hepatic extraction, can readily accumulate to toxic concentrations. Chlordiazepoxide is preferred.

Analgesics. Opiates can precipitate hepatic encephalopathy in patients with decompensated liver disease. If required to control postoperative pain, doses should be reduced to 25–50% of normal. Constant intravenous infusions should be avoided if the patient is not to be overdosed insidiously. Codeine can precipitate hepatic encephalopathy by its constipating effect alone. Aspirin and other NSAIDs may exacerbate impaired renal function and fluid retention by inhibiting prostaglandin synthesis, and may also precipitate gastrointestinal bleeding.

Cardiovascular drugs. Propranolol (to prevent variceal bleeding) and diuretics (to treat ascites); see below.

Gastrointestinal system. Antacids that contain large quantities of sodium can precipitate fluid retention to cause ascites. Aluminium- and calcium-based preparations cause constipation and may thereby precipitate hepatic encephalopathy, as can antimotility drugs.

Hormone preparations. Use of contraceptives should be monitored carefully in patients with cholestatic liver disease, because jaundice may be exacerbated; continued use of oral contraceptives during an attack of acute hepatitis can have the same effect. Low-oestrogen preparations carry less risk of this complication.

DRUG-INDUCED LIVER DAMAGE

The spectrum of hepatic abnormalities caused by drugs is broad. Drugs tend to injure specific components of the hepatocyte, e.g. the cell membrane, canalicular apparatus, cytochrome P450 enzymes in the endoplasmic reticulum, mitochondria, and thus encompass the whole range of liver lesions from other causes. In general terms, drug injury results either from idiosyncrasy (not dose related) or as a result of increased or cumulative dose. Examples of drugs that cause such damage, with their sites and types of injury appear in Tables 33.1 and 33.2.

Additionally, certain drugs may *interfere with bilirubin metabolism and excretion* without causing morphological hepatic injury. Jaundice is induced selectively with minimal or no disturbance of other liver function test results; recovery ordinarily occurs on stopping the drug. Examples are:

- C-17α-substituted steroids impair bilirubin excretion into the hepatic canaliculi; the block is biochemical not mechanical. These include synthetic anabolic steroids and oestrogens used in oral contraceptives; jaundice due to the latter is rare with the low-dose formulations now preferred.
- Rifampicin impairs hepatic uptake and excretion of bilirubin; plasma unconjugated and conjugated bilirubin levels may be raised during the first 2–3 weeks of dosing.
- Fusidic acid interferes with hepatic bilirubin excretion to cause conjugated hyperbilirubinaemia, particularly in patients with sepsis.

DIAGNOSIS AND MANAGEMENT OF DRUG-INDUCED LIVER INJURY

- Always bear the possibility in mind. Take a careful *drug history,* including over-the-counter and complementary and alternative medicine remedies.
- In patients with *hepatitis* a viral aetiology should be excluded.
- *Cholestatic lesions,* which may resolve only slowly on drug withdrawal, have to be differentiated from other causes of obstructive jaundice, both intrahepatic and extrahepatic.

Table 33.1 Idiosyncratic drug reactions and the cell components that are affected

Type of reaction	Effect on cells	Examples of drugs
Hepatocellular	Direct effect or production by enzyme–drug combination leads to cell and membrane dysfunction	isoniazid, trazodone, diclofenac, nefazodone, venlafaxine, lovastatin
Immune mediated	Cytotoxic lymphocyte response directed at hepatocyte membranes altered by drug metabolite ± additional autoimmune component	nitrofurantoin, methyldopa, lovastatin, minocycline, halothane
Cholestasis	Injury to canalicular membrane and transporters	chlorpromazine, oestrogen, erythromycin and its derivatives
Granulomatous	Macrophages, lymphocytes infiltrate hepatic lobule	diltiazem, sulfa drugs, quinidine
Microvesicular fat	Altered mitochondrial respiration, β-oxidation leads to lactic acidosis and triglyceride accumulation	didanosine, tetracyclines, acetylsalicylic acid, valproic acid
Steatohepatitis (fatty liver)	Multifactorial	amiodarone, tamoxifen
Autoimmune	Cytotoxic lymphocyte response directed at hepatocytes membrane components	nitrofurantoin, methyldopa, lovastatin, minocycline
Fibrosis	Activation of stellate cells	methotrexate, excess vitamin A
Vascular collapse	Causes ischaemic or hypoxic injury	nicotinic acid, cocaine, methylenedioxymethylamfetamine (MDMA)
Oncogenesis	Encourages tumour formation	Oral contraceptives, androgens
Mixed	Cytoplasmic and canalicular injury, direct damage to bile ducts	amoxicillin–clavulanic acid, carbamazepine, herbs, ciclosporin, methimazole, troglitazone

Table 33.2   Effects of increased or cumulative doses of drugs[a]

Drug	Dose effect
amiodarone	Cumulative dose: steatohepatitis (fatty liver)
cocaine, phencyclidine	Increased dose: hepatocyte necrosis
cyclophosphamide	Increased dose: hepatocyte necrosis (worse with raised aminotransferase concentrations)
ciclosporin	Increased dose: cholestatic injury
paracetamol	Increased dose: hepatocytes necrosis, apoptosis
methotrexate	Increased or cumulative dose: hepatocyte necrosis, fibrogenesis
niacin	Increased dose: ischaemic necrosis
Oral contraceptives	Cumulative dose: associated with hepatic adenomas

[a]Although many of these reactions may be considered idiosyncratic, the individual or total dose has a role with these agents.
The authors are grateful for permission to reproduce and adapt the material in this table from Lee W M 2003 Drug-induced hepatotoxicity.
New England Journal of Medicine 349:474–485.

- *Underlying liver disease* can cause diagnostic confusion, e.g. the alcoholic patient receiving antituberculosis drugs. It is wise to perform liver function tests before starting treatment with any drug that has documented hepatotoxic potential.
- Liver biopsy is of only limited use in diagnosis, although certain features, e.g. eosinophil infiltration, may provide a pointer to drug-induced liver disease.
- Diagnostic challenge is extremely dangerous for hepatitic reactions because it may precipitate fulminant hepatic failure; the procedure is safer for cholestatic reactions.
- Monitoring liver function in the early weeks of therapy is useful in detecting an impending reaction to some drugs, e.g. isoniazid. Minor abnormalities (serum transaminase levels less than twice normal) are often self-limiting, and progress can be monitored. Increases greater than three-fold should be an indication for drug withdrawal, even if the patient is asymptomatic.

ASPECTS OF THERAPY

COMPLICATIONS OF CIRRHOSIS

Variceal bleeding

Varices are dilated anastomoses between the portal and systemic venous systems that form in an attempt to decompress the portal venous system when the pressure within undergoes a sustained increase. Those in the lower oesophagus or gastric body are prone to rupture because they are thin walled and lie just below the mucosa.

Portal pressure is a function of *resistance* in the portal venous system and the *flow* of blood through it. In cirrhosis, portal venous resistance is increased, and inflow of blood is increased by splanchnic vasodilatation and increased cardiac output. Variceal bleeding is increasingly likely as the pressure gradient between the portal and systemic venous systems rises beyond 12 mmHg.

Up to 50% of patients with portal hypertension bleed from oesophageal or gastric varices and half die from the complications of their first bleed. Hypovolaemia must be corrected with plasma expanders and blood transfusion. Sepsis is common; the incidence rises from 20% at 48 h to over 60% at 7 days, and antimicrobial prophylaxis should be given with ciprofloxacin (1 g/day). Some 70% will stop bleeding spontaneously but over half rebleed within 10 days.

Acute variceal bleeding

Management involves measures directed at the varices and also to reduce portal pressure by pharmacological methods and blood shunting procedures.

Direct treatment of varices by endoscopy is preferred. *Band ligation*, in which the varices are strangulated by application of small elastic bands, has fewer complications than *sclerotherapy*, which involves injecting sclerosant into and around the varices but may lead to oesophagitis, stricture or embolisation of sclerosant. Either technique can control bleeding in about 90% of patients, and rebleeding is reduced if this direct treatment is combined with reduction of portal pressure (see below).

Direct pressure on varices can be applied by inserting an inflatable triple-lumen (Sengstaken) tube that abuts the gastro-oesophageal junction and controls bleeding in 90%; rebleeding is common when the tube is withdrawn and its use may be accompanied by aspiration, oesophageal ulceration or perforation.

Reduction of portal pressure. *Vasopressin* (antidiuretic hormone, see p. 480), in addition to its action on the renal collecting ducts (through V_2 receptors), constricts smooth muscle (V_1 receptors) in the cardiovascular system (hence its name), and particularly in splanchnic blood vessels, so reducing blood flow in the portal venous system. Unfortunately, coronary vasoconstriction can also occur, and treatment has to be withdrawn from 20% of patients because of myocardial ischaemia. Glyceryl trinitrate (transdermally, sublingually or intravenously) reduces the cardiac risk and, advantageously, further reduces portal venous resistance and pressure.

Vasopressin is rapidly cleared from the circulation and must be given by continuous intravenous infusion. The synthetic analogue, *terlipressin* (triglycyl-lysine-vasopressin), is now preferred. This pro-drug (or hormogen) is converted in vivo to the vasoactive *lysine vasopressin*, which has biological activity for 3–4 h, and is effective by bolus injections 4-hourly; it is usually given for 48–72 h. It is a useful adjunct to endoscopic therapy and reduces rebleeding.

Somatostatin and its synthetic analogue *octreotide* reduce portal pressure by decreasing splanchnic blood flow. Octreotide has the advantage of a longer duration of action so that it can be given as a bolus injection rather than the constant intravenous infusion needed for administration of somatostatin. It can be used as an alternative to terlipressin, having similar efficacy and indications for use.

Patients who continue to bleed despite the above measures require surgery (ligation or transection of varices) or placement of a stent (tube) between intrahepatic branches of the portal and (systemic) hepatic veins under radiological control. The latter is now the technique of choice for the 10–15% of patients with acute bleeding resistant to conventional treatment, and also for long-term management of patients who are difficult to help by other methods (see below).

Prevention of variceal bleeding

Endoscopic therapy as above, preferably by band ligation, and repeated at weekly intervals until all varices are obliterated, is currently the treatment of choice; it reduces the incidence of rebleeding by 50–60%.

Pharmacological therapy. Non-selective β-blockers, e.g. propranolol or nadolol, reduce cardiac output (β_1-receptor antagonism) and induce splanchnic vasoconstriction (β_2-receptor antagonism allowing unopposed (α-adrenergic vasoconstriction). Recurrent bleeding is reduced by about 40%. As propranolol is extensively extracted in a single pass through the liver, its systemic availability may be unpredictable in patients with cirrhosis and portal hypertension due to variations in hepatic blood flow and portal/systemic shunts. Ideally, the dose of propranolol (given twice daily) should be adjusted by measuring the portal/systemic venous pressure gradient; if this is not feasible, the resting pulse rate is monitored, aiming at a 25% reduction. Decreased cardiac output can exacerbate impaired renal function and fluid retention. Nadolol, having a longer duration of action, is given only once daily.

ASCITES

About 50% of patients with cirrhosis develop ascites within 10 years of diagnosis and 50% of these will die within 2 years. The process by which ascites forms in cirrhosis is not fully understood but appears to involve the accumulation of vasodilator substances, activation of the renin–angiotensin–aldosterone system (causing renal *retention* of sodium and water), and the production of antidiuretic hormone (causing *hyponatraemia* due to dilution, not deficiency, of plasma sodium) (Fig. 33.1). Hypoalbuminaemia and portal hypertension favour transudation of fluid into the abdominal cavity to form ascites.

Management of ascites

The aim is to induce *natriuresis* with consequent loss of water. Fluid restriction is unnecessary unless the plasma sodium falls below 120 mmol/L. The initial management must include a diagnostic tap of the ascitic fluid as spontaneous bacterial peritonitis complicates up to 25% of patients on presentation.

A combination of bedrest (which lowers plasma renin activity) and dietary sodium restriction is effective in about 10% of patients but *diuretic therapy* is usually needed. The most useful drug is *spironolactone*, although its maximum effect can take up to 2 weeks to develop as it is metabolised to products with long duration of action, e.g. canrenone $t_{1/2}$ 10–35 h. A loop diuretic, e.g. *furosemide*, is therefore given in combination, as this also helps to counteract hyperkalaemia induced by spironolactone.

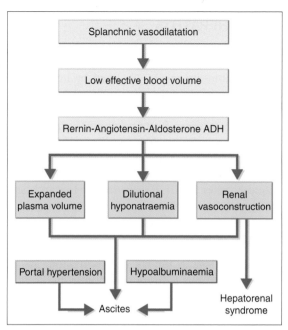

Fig. 33.1 Haemodynamic abnormalities in decompensated cirrhosis.

A dose ratio of spironolactone 100 mg and furosemide 40 mg o.d. works well, and can be increased every 3–4 days to a maximum of spironolactone 400 mg + furosemide 160 mg.

Body-weight and urinary sodium excretion should be monitored. Patients who have oedema as well as ascites exhibit rapid weight loss. When ascites alone is present, weight loss should not exceed 0.5 kg/day, which is the maximum rate with which fluid can move from the peritoneal cavity into the circulation. Creating a negative fluid balance runs the risk of hypovolaemia, electrolyte disturbance, renal impairment and, eventually, hepatic encephalopathy. Patients should lose weight if their urinary sodium excretion exceeds that provided by the diet; those who do not respond despite high urinary sodium outputs are almost certainly receiving additional sodium in their diet or medications, e.g. antacids. Should spironolactone cause painful gynaecomastia, amiloride is a useful substitute (10–40 mg/day) with a more rapid onset of action.

Abdominal paracentesis is useful particularly when ascites is tense; rapid drainage of 5 L leads to prompt relief of discomfort and improves circulatory dynamics. Provided renal function is not compromised, extensive paracentesis is safe and can be used as an adjunct to diuretic therapy to shorten hospital stay. When more than 5 L are drained it is customary to infuse colloid or albumin (6–8 g/L fluid removed) to prevent hypovolaemia.

Hepatorenal syndrome

This form of renal failure occurs in about 10% of patients with advanced cirrhosis and ascites, and is due to intense renal vasoconstriction (see Fig. 33.1). The outcome is poor, but up to two-thirds of patients will respond to vasoconstrictor agents, particularly terlipressin, over a 14-day interval. The drug is thought to improve renal perfusion by reducing the functional hypovolaemia caused by splanchnic vasodilatation. The optimal dose regime remains to be established. Concomitant administration of albumin appears to improve response. Dopamine is ineffective.

HEPATIC ENCEPHALOPATHY

Infection, gastrointestinal bleeding or injudicious use of sedatives and diuretics can precipitate hepatic encephalopathy in cirrhotic patients. The pathophysiology is complex but *ammonia* appears to hold a central role. Derived mainly from the action of colonic urease-containing bacteria, ammonia is normally extracted from the portal blood by the liver, but when there is portal/systemic shunting and impaired hepatic metabolism, it reaches high concentration in the blood and affects the brain adversely. Therapeutic measures that limit production of ammonia have therefore been developed.

Lactulose acts as an osmotic laxative to expedite clearance of potentially toxic substances from the gastrointestinal tract. In addition, colonic bacteria metabolise it to lactic and acetic acids, which inhibit the growth of ammonia-producing organisms and, by lowering pH, reduce non-ionic diffusion of ammonia (a basic substance) from the colon into the bloodstream. The correct dose is that which produces two to four soft acidic stools daily (usually 30–60 mL daily). Exceeding this dose can dehydrate the patient. As lactulose is intended for long-term use, there is no rational basis for giving it to patients after paracetamol overdose, as prophylaxis against hepatic encephalopathy.

Reduction of dietary protein reduces ammonia production and has long been used to prevent hepatic encephalopathy. Any potential benefit against encephalopathy must be tempered by the knowledge that most patients with severe liver disease are malnourished. Protein from vegetable sources is often better tolerated than animal-derived protein, at least in part due to its higher fibre content which accelerates transit through the gut.

Neomycin and *metronidazole* both inhibit urease-producing bacteria and are useful, but their long-term use is limited by toxicity.

IMMUNE-MEDIATED LIVER DISEASE

AUTOIMMUNE ACTIVE CHRONIC HEPATITIS

This chronic inflammatory disease of the liver is characteristically associated with circulating auto-antibodies and high serum immunoglobulin concentrations. Untreated, it progresses to cirrhosis, but the condition responds well to immunosuppressive drugs. Some 80% will benefit from *prednisolone*, which should be continued in the long term as most patients relapse if the drug is withdrawn. *Azathioprine* (1 mg/kg daily) is effective as a steroid-sparing agent, and usually permits reducing of prednisolone to 5–10 mg/day. Increasing azathioprine to 2 mg/kg allows further reduction in prednisolone dose, but haematological toxicity may result and the blood count must be monitored every 2 months.

PRIMARY BILIARY CIRRHOSIS (PBC)

This chronic cholestatic liver disease affects 1 in 4000 people in the UK. Pruritus is a common early symptom and can be helped by *colestyramine*, although its mechanism of action is obscure. Chronic cholestasis leads to malabsorption of fat-soluble vitamins, particularly vitamin D, deficiency of which must be corrected to avoid osteomalacia.

The aetiology of PBC is unknown but high titres of antimitochondrial antibody in the majority suggest involvement of immune mechanisms. There is no effective treatment. Adverse effects outweigh benefits from prednisolone, but budesonide is currently under assessment as it is highly extracted by the liver and thus poorly available to the systemic circulation. Ursodeoxycholic acid 10–15 mg/kg daily improves biochemical liver function test results, but appears not to lengthen survival or prevent complications.

VIRAL HEPATITIS

HEPATITIS A

Passive immunity can be obtained by intramuscular injection of globulin containing antibody to the virus (*normal immunoglobulin*, prepared from pooled plasma from known immune donors); this confers temporary protection for travellers visiting areas where the virus is endemic. Active immunisation with *hepatitis A vaccine* is now preferable; protective antibody takes about 2 weeks to develop and lasts for up to 10 years.

HEPATITIS B

Chronic carriage in the UK occurs in about 5% of those infected but is more common in the immunocompromised and in other high-risk groups including male homosexuals and intravenous drug abusers. In parts of Asia and Africa, chronic carriage occurs in up to 50% of the population. Worldwide there are about 300 million chronic carriers of hepatitis B virus and it is the most important cause of *primary hepatocellular carcinoma*.

Interferon-α (see p. 539) given for 4–6 months gives long-term clearance of hepatitis B virus from the plasma in 25–40% of patients. The effect is characteristically preceded by increased levels of serum transaminases, reflecting immune-mediated destruction of virus-infected hepatocytes. If liver function is impaired prior to therapy, use of interferon-α should be monitored carefully because it may precipitate hepatic failure.

Lamivudine, a nucleoside analogue, inhibits replication of hepatitis B virus DNA and reduces hepatic inflammation. The serum of about 17% of patients converts from positive to negative for antibodies to hepatitis B after 1 year of therapy. Long-term treatment is probably necessary and the drug is well tolerated.

Hepatitis B immunisation

Hepatitis B vaccine (inactivated B virus surface antigen adsorbed on aluminium hydroxide adjuvant) provides active immunity against hepatitis B infection, and in countries of low endemicity it is given to individuals at high risk, including health-care professionals. Immunity is conferred for at least 5 years and can be supplemented by booster inoculations given when the antibody concentration in plasma declines.

Hepatitis B immunoglobulin (pooled plasma selected for high titres of antibodies to the virus) provides passive immunity for post-exposure prophylaxis, e.g. after accidental needlestick injury.

In countries with a high prevalence of hepatitis B the virus is transmitted vertically (from mother to baby). Passive immunoprophylaxis with immune globulin given to the baby at birth, followed by vaccination, is effective at preventing chronic carriage. Mass vaccination should lead to a reduction in the incidence of primary hepatocellular carcinoma, but cannot yet be implemented in third world countries for want of funding.

HEPATITIS D

This virus replicates only in the presence of hepatitis B. Interferon-α is less effective than in other forms of viral hepatitis, giving sustained responses in about 15% of patients. There is no other useful therapy.

HEPATITIS C

Most individuals infected with the hepatitis C virus become long-term carriers. Chronic infection with hepatitis C virus affects an estimated 170 million individuals worldwide. Up to one-third of these will progress to cirrhosis with its attendant complications including hepatocellular carcinoma, over a period of 30–40 years. In the Western world, hepatitis C infection arises mainly from intravenous drug abuse.

Treatment with *interferon-α* leads to suppression of circulating hepatitis C viral RNA and improvement in hepatic inflammation in about 40%, but at least half relapse on cessation of treatment. Combination of interferon-α with *ribavirin* greatly enhances the response, achieving sustained remission in up to 70%; age, duration of infection and viral genotype are among the factors that determine the response. Interferon-α is cleared rapidly, mainly by the kidney ($t_{1/2}$ 4 h), and must be given by subcutaneous injection three times per week. Increasing the molecular weight of the drug by conjugation with polyethylene glycol (pegylation) prolongs the $t_{1/2}$ to 40 h, allowing single weekly injections. Pegylation also appears to enhance the efficacy of interferon-α, possibly by increasing exposure time to the virus.

Treatment should last for 6–12 months but should cease after 3 months if any viral RNA persists because this reliably predicts treatment failure.

Depression, agitation, headache and malaise may limit treatment. Its use is currently restricted to patients with severe necroinflammatory changes on liver biopsy (who are thought to be most at risk of progressing to cirrhosis).

GALLSTONES

Ursodeoxycholic acid can be used to dissolve cholesterol gallstones; it supplements the bile acid pool and thus improves the solubility of cholesterol in bile. Its use is limited to patients with a functioning gallbladder who have small stones that are not calcified. The dose is 8–12 mg/kg daily p.o.; treatment takes up to 2 years and recurrence is common.

PANCREAS

DIGESTIVE ENZYMES

In pancreatic *exocrine insufficiency* the aim of therapy is to prevent weight loss and diarrhoea, and in children to maintain adequate growth. The problem of getting sufficient enzyme to the duodenum concurrently with food is not as simple as it might appear. Gastric emptying varies with the composition of meals, e.g. high fat, calories or protein cause delay, and the pancreatic enzymes taken by mouth are destroyed by gastric acid. On the other hand, only one-tenth of the normal pancreatic output is sufficient to prevent steatorrhoea. Acid suppression by proton pump inhibitors improves the efficacy of pancreatic enzyme supplements.

Preparations are of animal origin and variable potency. *Pancreatin*, as Cotazym and Nutrizym, appears to be satisfactory. A reasonable course is to start the patient on the recommended dose of a reliable formulation and to vary this according to the individual's needs, and the size and composition of meals. Enteric-coated formulations (pancreatin granules, tablets) are available. High-potency pancreatic enzymes should not be used in patients with cystic fibrosis as they may cause ileocaecal and large bowel strictures.

ACUTE PANCREATITIS

Many drugs have been tested for specific effect, and none has shown convincing benefit. The main requirements of therapy are:

- To provide adequate *analgesia*. Opioids are generally satisfactory; their potential disadvantage of contracting the sphincter of Oddi (and retarding the flow of pancreatic secretion) appears to be outweighed by their analgesic efficacy; buprenorphine is often preferred.
- To correct *hypovolaemia* due to the exudation of large amounts of fluid around the inflamed pancreas. Plasma may be required, or blood if the haematocrit falls; in addition large volumes of electrolyte solution may be needed to maintain urine flow.
- To achieve biliary drainage (by endoscopic retrograde cannulation of the pancreas) early in the illness if gallstones are suspected.
- The value of additional interventions, including nutritional support and antibiotic prophylaxis, is as yet unproven.

DRUGS AND THE PANCREAS

Adverse effects are most commonly manifest as *acute pancreatitis*. The strongest association is with *alcohol* abuse. High plasma calcium concentration, including that caused by hypervitaminosis D, and parenteral nutrition also increase the risk. Corticosteroids, didanosine, azathoipurine, diuretics (including thiazides and furosemide), sodium valproate, mesalazine and paracetamol (in overdose) have also been causally related.

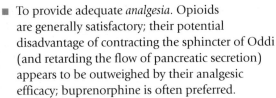

GUIDE TO FURTHER READING

Adams D H, Haydon G (eds) 2006 Liver disease. Clinical Medicine 6:19–46

Craig A S, Schaffner W 2004 Prevention of hepatitis A with the hepatitis A vaccine. New England Journal of Medicine 350:476–481

Ganem D, Prince A M 2004 Hepatitis virus B infection – natural history and clinical consequences. New England Journal of Medicine 350:1118–1129

Ginès P, Guevara M, Arroyo V, Rodés J 2003 Hepatorenal syndrome. Lancet 362:1819–1827

Ginès P, Cárdenas A, Arroyo V, Rodés J 2004 Management of cirrhosis and ascites. New England Journal of Medicine 350:1646–1654

Johnson C D 2005 UK guidelines for the management of acute pancreatitis. Gut 54:(Suppl iii):1–9

Kaplan M M, Gershwin M E 2005 Primary biliary cirrhosis. New England Journal of Mecicine 353:1261–1273

Kingsnorth A, O'Reilly D 2006 Acute pancreatitis. British Medical Journal 332:1072–1076

Krawitt E L 2006 Autoimmune hepatitis. New England Journal of Medicine 354:54–66

Lee W M 2003 Drug-induced hepatotoxicity. New England Journal of Medicine 349:474–485

Lok A S-F 2005 The maze of treatments for hepatitis B. New England Journal of Medicine 352:2743–2746

Navarro V J, Senior J R 2006 Drug-related hepatotoxicity. New England Journal of Medicine 354:731–739

Portincasa P, Moschetta A, Palasciano G 2006 Cholesterol gallstone disease. Lancet 368:230–239

Poynard T, Yuen M, Ratzin V, Lai C 2003 Viral hepatitis C. Lancet 362:2095–2100

Sharara A I, Rockey D C 2001 Gastroesophageal variceal hemorrhage. New England Journal of Medicine 345:669–681

Shawcross D, Jalan R 2005 Dispelling myths in the treatment of hepatic encephalopathy. Lancet 365:431–433

Wands J R 2004 Prevention of hepatocellular carcinoma. New England Journal of Medicine 351:1567–1570

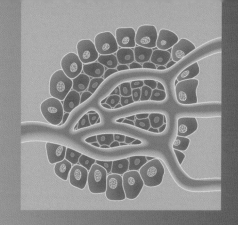

Section 8

ENDOCRINE SYSTEM, METABOLIC CONDITIONS

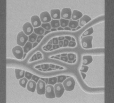

34

Adrenal corticosteroids, antagonists, corticotropin

SYNOPSIS

- Adrenocortical steroids and their synthetic analogues
  - mechanisms of action
  - actions: mineralocorticoid, glucocorticoid
  - individual adrenal steroids
  - pharmacokinetics
  - dosage schedules
  - choice of adrenal steroid
  - adverse effects of systemic pharmacotherapy
  - adrenal steroids and pregnancy
  - precautions during chronic therapy: treatment of intercurrent illness
  - dosage and routes of administration
  - indications for use
  - uses: replacement therapy, pharmacotherapy
  - withdrawal of pharmacotherapy
- Inhibition of synthesis of adrenal steroids
- Competitive antagonism
- Adrenocorticotrophic hormone (ACTH) (corticotropin)

In 1855, Dr Thomas Addison, assisted in his observations by three colleagues, published his famous monograph 'On the constitutional effects of disease on the suprarenal capsules' (Addison's disease). It was not until the late 1920s that the vital importance of the adrenal cortex was appreciated and the distinction made between the hormones secreted by the cortex and medulla.

By 1936, numerous steroids were being crystallised from cortical extracts, but the quantities were insufficient to provide supplies for clinical trial.

In 1948, cortisone was made from bile acids in quantity sufficient for clinical trial, and the dramatic demonstration of its power to induce remission of rheumatoid arthritis was published the following year. In 1950, it was realised that cortisone was biologically inert and that the active natural hormone is hydrocortisone (cortisol). Since then many steroids have been synthesised, covering the wide range of efficacy and potency required by the many indications for systemic and local use. Steroids derive from natural substances, chiefly plant sterols. The ideal steroid drug, providing all the desirable and none of the undesirable effects of cortisol, remains elusive. Research showing the multiple molecular actions of steroids within the target cell has explained the difficulty of achieving the ideal, but may help to bring this closer.

About the same time as cortisone was introduced, adrenocorticotrophin (ACTH) became available for clinical use. Its use is now largely for diagnostic tests of the pituitary–adrenal axis.

ADRENAL STEROIDS AND THEIR SYNTHETIC ANALOGUES

The adrenal is a composite endocrine gland, and each zone of the cortex synthesises a different predominant steroid; a mnemonic is offered in Figure 34.1.

The principal hormone is the glucocorticoid *hydrocortisone* (cortisol) secreted from the largest zone, the fasciculata; the mineralocorticoid, *aldosterone*, is secreted by the glomerulosa, and a number of *androgens* and *oestrogens* are secreted by the zona reticularis. The hypothalamic–pituitary system, through corticotropin releasing factor (CRF) and ACTH, controls hydrocortisone and, to a lesser extent, aldosterone secretion; synthesis and secretion of this hormone is regulated mainly by the renin–angiotensin system, and by variation in plasma K^+ levels.

When the adrenal cortex fails (Addison's disease) adrenocortical steroids are available for replacement therapy, but their chief use in medicine is for their anti-inflammatory and immunosuppressive effects (pharmacotherapy). These are obtained only

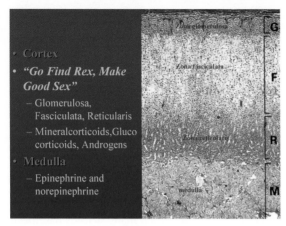

- **Cortex**
- **"Go Find Rex, Make Good Sex"**
  - Glomerulosa, Fasciculata, Reticularis
  - Mineralcorticoids, Gluco corticoids, Androgens
- **Medulla**
  - Epinephrine and norepinephrine

Fig. 34.1 The zones of the adrenal gland and the hormones they secrete.

when the drugs are given in doses far above those needed for physiological replacement. Various metabolic effects, which are of the greatest importance to the normal functioning of the body, then become adverse effects. Much successful effort has gone into separating glucocorticoid from mineralocorticoid effects[1] and some steroids, e.g. dexamethasone, have virtually no mineralocorticoid activity. But it has not yet proved possible to separate the glucocorticoid effects from one another, so that if a steroid is used for its anti-inflammatory action the risks, e.g. of osteoporosis, diabetes, remain.

In the account that follows, the effects of hydrocortisone will be described and then other steroids in so far as they differ. In the context of this chapter, 'adrenal steroid' means a substance with hydrocortisone-like activity. Androgens are described in Chapter 37.

MECHANISM OF ACTION

Glucocorticoids stimulate the cell through both a classical cytosolic receptor that, on binding with agonist, translocates to the nucleus, and an unidentified membrane-bound receptor (Fig. 34.2). The classical receptor is responsible for so-called genomic effects through either activation or repression of DNA transcription. Up-regulation of gene transcription occurs when the receptor dimerises on specific DNA glucocorticoid response elements

(GREs) with consequent recruitment of co-activator proteins. Many of the undesired effects of glucocorticoid occur through this pathway.

Repression of DNA transcription occurs at slightly lower cortisol concentrations than required for transactivation. Through protein–protein interaction, the glucocorticoid–receptor complex inactivates pro-inflammatory transcription factors such as nuclear factor (NF)-κB and activator protein 1 (AP-1), preventing their stimulation of inflammatory mediators: prostaglandins, leukotrienes, cytokines and platelet activating factor. These mediators would normally contribute to increased vascular permeability and subsequent changes including oedema, leucocyte migration, fibrin deposition.[2]

There is a distinction between *replacement therapy* (physiological effects) and the higher doses of *pharmacotherapy*.

On inorganic metabolism. Hydrocortisone is required for excretion of a water load. This action is unrelated to the apparently opposite, mineralocorticoid, action of hydrocortisone that occurs at supra-physiological concentrations.

On organic metabolism

- *Carbohydrate metabolism.* Gluconeogenesis is increased and peripheral glucose utilisation may be decreased (due to insulin antagonism) so that hyperglycaemia and sometimes glycosuria result. Latent diabetes becomes overt.
- *Protein metabolism.* Anabolism (conversion of amino acids to protein) decreases but catabolism continues unabated or even faster, so that there is a negative nitrogen balance with muscle wasting. Osteoporosis (reduction of bone protein matrix) occurs, growth slows in children, the skin atrophies and this, with increased capillary fragility, causes bruising and striae. Healing of peptic ulcers or of wounds is delayed, as is fibrosis.

---

[1]The introduction of a double bond transforms hydrocortisone to prednisolone, a big biological change; see Table 34.1 for relative potencies 1.0 : 1.0 to 4 : 0.8.

[2]Potency (the weight of drug in relation to its effect) rather than efficacy (strength of response); see page 79. If a large enough dose of a glucocorticoid, e.g. prednisolone, were administered, the Na⁺ retention would be almost as great as that caused by a mineralocorticoid. This is why, in practice, different (more selective, and potent) glucocorticoids, not higher doses of prednisolone, need to be used when maximal stimulation of glucocorticoid receptors is desired, e.g. in the treatment of acute transplant rejections.

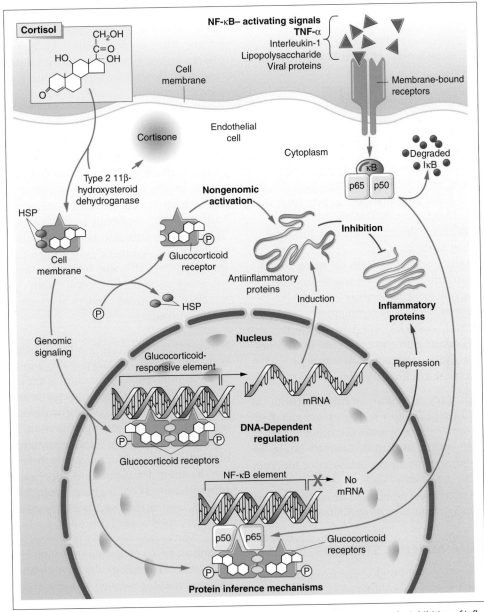

Fig. 34.2 Three general mechanisms of action of glucocorticoids and the glucocorticoid receptor in the inhibition of inflammation: non-genomic activation, DNA-dependent regulation, and protein interference mechanisms (e.g. NF-κB elements). Black arrows denote activation, the red line inhibition, the red dashed arrow repression, and the red X lack of product (i.e. no mRNA). HSP, heat-shock protein; mRNA, messenger RNA; NF, nuclear factor; P, phosphate; TNF, tumour necrosis factor. (Adapted from Rhen T, Cidlowski J A 2005 Antiinflammatory action of glucocorticoids – new mechanisms for old drugs. New England Journal of Medicine 353(16):1711–1723.)

- *Fat deposition.* This is increased on shoulders, face and abdomen.
- *Inflammatory response* is depressed, regardless of its cause so that, as well as being of great benefit in 'useless' or excessive inflammation, corticosteroids can be a source of danger in infections by limiting useful protective inflammation. Neutrophil and macrophage function are depressed, including the release of chemical mediators and the effects of these on capillaries.
- *Allergic responses* are suppressed. The antigen–antibody interaction is unaffected, but its

injurious inflammatory consequences do not follow.

- *Antibody production* is lessened by heavy doses.
- *Lymphoid tissue* is reduced (including leukaemic lymphocytes).
- *Renal excretion* of urate is increased.
- *Blood eosinophils* reduce in number.
- *Euphoria or psychotic* states may occur, perhaps due to central nervous system (CNS) electrolyte changes.
- *Anti-vitamin D action*, see calciferol (p. 663).
- *Reduction of hypercalcaemia*, chiefly where this is due to excessive absorption of calcium from the gut (sarcoidosis, vitamin D intoxication).
- *Urinary calcium excretion* is increased and renal stones may form.
- *Growth reduces* where new cells are being added (growth in children), but not where they are replacing cells as in adult tissues.
- *Suppression of hypothalamic–pituitary–adrenocortical feedback system* (with delayed recovery) occurs with chronic use, so that abrupt withdrawal leaves the patient in a state of adrenocortical insufficiency.

The average daily secretion of hydrocortisone is normally 10 mg (5.7 mg/m²)[3]. The exogenous daily dose that completely suppresses the cortex is hydrocortisone 40–80 mg, or prednisolone 10–20 mg, or its equivalent of other agents. Recovery of function is quick after a few days' use, but when used over months, recovery takes months. A steroid-suppressed adrenal gland continues to secrete aldosterone.

INDIVIDUAL ADRENAL STEROIDS

The relative potencies[2] for glucocorticoid and mineralocorticoid (sodium-retaining) effects (Table 34.1) are central to the choice of agent in relation to clinical indication.

---

[3]But this can be associated with an unphysiologically low plasma concentration of hydrocortisone in the late afternoon (with loss of well-being). Such patients may be best managed on three equal doses per day. Air travellers on long flights across longitude east to west (>12 h, i.e. longer day): take an extra dose near the end of the flight. For west to east flights (>8 h, i.e. shorter day): the normal evening dose may be taken sooner and the usual dose taken on the 'new' morning. Night-workers may adjust their dosage to their work pattern (Drug and Therapeutics Bulletin 1990; 28:71).

All drugs in Table 34.1 except aldosterone are active when swallowed, being protected from hepatic first-pass metabolism by high binding to plasma proteins. Some details of preparations and equivalent doses appear in the table. Injectable and topical forms are available (creams, suppositories, eye-drops).

The selectivity of hydrocortisone for the glucocorticoid receptor is due not to a different binding affinity of hydrocortisone to the two receptors but to the protection of the mineralocorticoid receptor by locally high concentrations of the enzyme 11β-hydroxysteroid dehydrogenase, which converts cortisol (hydrocortisone) to the inactive cortisone. This enzyme saturates at concentrations of cortisol (and some synthetic glucocorticoids) just above the physiological range, which explains the onset of mineralocorticoid action with pathological secretion of cortisol, and pharmacological use of glucocorticoids.

Hydrocortisone (cortisol) is the principal naturally occurring steroid; it is taken orally; a soluble salt can be given intravenously for rapid effect in emergency (whether due to deficiency, allergy or inflammatory disease). A suspension (Hydrocortisone Acetate Inj.) is available for intra-articular injection.

Parenteral preparation for systemic effect: the soluble Hydrocortisone Sodium Succinate Inj. gives quick (1–2 h) effect; for continuous effect about 6-hourly administration is appropriate. Prednisolone Acetate Inj. i.m. is an alternative, once or twice a week.

Tablet strengths, see Table 34.1.

Prednisolone is predominantly anti-inflammatory (glucorticoid), biologically active, and has little sodium-retaining activity; it is the standard choice for anti-inflammatory pharmacotherapy, orally or intramuscularly.

Methylprednisolone is similar to prednisone; it is used intravenously for megadose pulse therapy (see below).

Fluorinated corticosteroids (triamcinolone, fludrocortisone)

Triamcinolone has virtually no sodium-retaining (mineralocorticoid) effect but has the disadvantage that muscle wasting may occasionally be severe, and anorexia and mental depression more common at high dose.

Table 34.1 Relative potencies of adrenal steroids

Compound (tablet strength, mg)	Approximate relative potency		Equivalent[a] dosage (for anti-inflammatory effect, mg)[b]
	Anti-inflammatory (glucocorticoid) effect	Sodium-retaining (mineralocorticoid) effect	
cortisone (25)	0.8	1.0	25
hydrocortisone (20)	1.0	1.0	20
prednisolone (5)	4	0.8	5
methylprednisolone (4)	5	Minimal	4
triamcinolone (4)	5	None	4
dexamethasone (0.5)	30	Minimal	0.75
betamethasone (0.5)	30	Negligible	0.75
fludrocortisone (0.1)	15	150	Irrelevant
aldosterone (none)	none	500[c]	Irrelevant

[a]Note that these equivalents are in approximate inverse accord with the tablet strengths.
[b]The doses in the final column are in the lower range of those that may cause suppression of the hypothalamic–pituitary–adrenocortical axis when given daily continuously. Much higher doses, e.g. prednisolone 40 mg, can be given on alternate days or daily for up to 5 days without causing clinically significant suppression.
[c]Injected.

Fludrocortisone has a strong sodium-retaining effect. It can replace aldosterone where the adrenal cortex is destroyed (Addison's disease). Fludrocortisone is also the drug of choice in most patients with autonomic neuropathy, in whom volume expansion is easier to achieve than a sustained increase in vasoconstrictor tone. Much higher doses of fludrocortisone (0.5–1.0 mg) are required when the cause of hypotension is a salt-losing syndrome of renal origin, e.g. after an episode of interstitial nephritis.

Dexamethasone and betamethasone are similar, powerful, predominantly anti-inflammatory steroids. They are longer-acting than prednisolone and are used for therapeutic adrenocortical suppression.

Aldosterone ($t_{1/2}$ 20 min), the principal natural salt-retaining hormone, has been used intramuscularly for acute adrenal insufficiency. After oral administration, it is rapidly inactivated in the first pass through the liver.

Spironolactone (see p. 586) is a competitive aldosterone antagonist which also blocks the mineralocorticoid effect of other steroids; it is used in the treatment of primary hyperaldosteronism, as a diuretic in resistant hypertension, and when severe oedema is due to secondary hyperaldosteronism, e.g. cirrhosis, congestive cardiac failure. Long-term treatment increases survival in cardiac failure, possibly through blocking the fibrotic effect of aldosterone upon the heart.

Beclomethasone, budesonide, fluticasone, mometasone and ciclesonide are potent soluble steroids suitable for use by inhalation for asthma (see p. 501) and intranasally for hay fever. Patients swallow about 90% of an inhalation dose, which is then largely inactivated by hepatic first-pass. The drugs are listed in order of development; some newer agents possess properties (first-pass metabolism, high protein binding and lipophilicity) that may increase pulmonary residence time and reduce systemic effects. The main protection against these effects is simply that absorption through mouth, lungs and gut is low relative to the amounts used in systemic administration. The risk of suppression of the hypothalamic–pituitary–adrenal (HPA) axis is minimal.

PHARMACOKINETICS OF CORTICOSTEROIDS

Absorption of the synthetic steroids given orally is rapid. The plasma $t_{1/2}$ of most is 1–3 h but the maximum biological effect occurs after 2–8 h. Administration is usually two or three times a day. They are metabolised principally in the liver (some undergoing hepatic first-pass metabolism, see above) and some pass unchanged into the urine. Hepatic and renal disease prolongs and enzyme induction shortens $t_{1/2}$ to an extent that can be clinically important.

Topical application (skin, lung, joints) allows absorption, which can be enough to cause systemic effects.

In the blood, adrenal steroids are carried both free (and biologically active, 5%) and bound (95% in the case of hydrocortisone) to cortisol binding globulin (CBG, a globulin with high affinity, but low binding capacity) and, when the latter saturates, to albumin (80% in the case of hydrocortisone).

Because CBG is saturated at peak diurnal levels of cortisol, the free cortisol concentration ranges from approximately 1 nanomol/L at the diurnal trough to approximately 100 nanomol/L at the diurnal peak. CBG concentrations increase in the presence of oestrogens, e.g. pregnancy, oral contraceptives.

In patients with very low serum albumin, the steroid dose should be lowered to allow for reduced binding capacity. In liver disease, low albumin concentration may be accompanied by slow metabolism ($t_{1/2}$ of prednisolone may be doubled).

DOSAGE SCHEDULES

Various dosing schedules address the issue of limiting HPA suppression by allowing the plasma steroid concentration to fall between doses to provide time for pituitary recovery, e.g. prednisolone 40 mg on alternate days. None has been successful in both completely avoiding suppression and controlling symptoms. The following are examples:

- Where a *single daily dose* is practicable, give it in the early morning (to coincide with the natural activation of the HPA axis).
- *Alternate-day schedules* are worth using, especially where immunosuppression is the objective (organ transplants) rather than anti-inflammatory effect (rheumatoid arthritis).
- *Short courses* (a few days) may be practicable for some conditions without significant suppression, e.g. acute asthma of moderate severity.
- Another variant is to give *enormous doses* (grams, not mg), orally or intravenously, e.g. methylprednisolone 1.0 g i.v. on three consecutive days, at intervals of weeks or months (megadose pulses). The technique applies particularly in collagen diseases.

> **Choice of adrenal steroid: summary**
> - *For oral replacement therapy* in adrenocortical insufficiency, use *hydrocortisone* as the glucocorticoid. In primary adrenal failure (Addison's disease), use *fludrocortisone* as the mineralocorticoid to replace aldosterone.
> - *For anti-inflammatory and antiallergic (immunosuppressive) effect,* use *prednisolone* or *dexamethasone*. For inhalation, more potent adrenal steroids are required, e.g. *beclometasone* or *budesonide*.
> - *For hypothalamic–pituitary–adrenocortical suppression,* e.g. in adrenal hyperplasia, *prednisolone* or *dexamethasone*.

ADVERSE EFFECTS OF SYSTEMIC ADRENAL STEROID PHARMACOTHERAPY

These consist largely of over-production of the physiological or pharmacological actions listed under actions of hydrocortisone. Some occur only with systemic use and for this reason local therapy, e.g. inhalation, intra-articular injection, is preferred where practicable.

Unwanted effects generally follow prolonged administration and virtually do not occur with one or two doses, although some occur with a few days' use, e.g. spread of infection. The undesired effects recounted below should never be experienced in *replacement* therapy, but are sometimes unavoidable with steroid *pharmacotherapy*. Obviously, the nature of unwanted effects depends on the choice of steroid. Fludrocortisone (mineralocorticoid) in ordinary doses does not cause osteoporosis, and prednisolone (glucocorticoid) does not normally cause oedema.

In general, serious unwanted effects are unlikely if the daily dose is below the equivalent of hydrocortisone 50 mg or prednisolone 10 mg. The principal adverse effects of chronic corticosteroid administration are:

Endocrine. To greater or lesser degree features of Cushing's syndrome result in moon face, central obesity, oedema, hypertension, striae, bruising, acne, hirsutism. Major skin damage can result from minor injury. *Diabetes mellitus* may appear. *HPA suppression* is dependent on the corticosteroid used, its dose, duration and the time of administration. A regular single prednisolone dose of less than 20 mg in the morning may cause suppression, whereas 5 mg given late in the evening is likely to attenuate the essential early morning activation of the HPA axis (circadian rhythm). Substantial suppression of the HPA axis can occur within 1 week (but see below: Withdrawal of steroid therapy).

Musculoskeletal. *Proximal myopathy* and *tendon rupture* may occur. *Osteoporosis* develops insidiously leading to fractures of vertebrae, ribs, femora and feet. Pain and restriction of movement may occur months in advance of radiographic changes. A biphosphonate, with or without vitamin D, is useful for prevention and treatment. *Growth* in children is impaired. *Avascular necrosis* of bone (femoral heads) is a serious complication (at higher doses); it appears to be due to restriction of blood flow through bone capillaries.

Immune. *Suppression of the inflammatory response to infection and immunosuppression* causes some patients to present with atypical symptoms and signs, and to deteriorate quickly. The incidence of infection increases with high-dose therapy, and any infection can be more severe when it occurs. *Candidiasis* may appear, particularly in the alimentary tract. Previously dormant *tuberculosis* may become active insidiously. Intra-articular injections demand strict asepsis. *Live vaccines* become dangerous. Developing chickenpox may result in a severe form of the disease, and patients who have not had chickenpox should receive varicella-zoster immune globulin within 3 days of exposure. Similarly, avoid exposure to measles.

Gastrointestinal. Patients taking steroid regularly, especially in combination with a non-steroidal anti-inflammatory drug (NSAID), have an excess incidence of *peptic ulcer* and *haemorrhage* of about 1–2%. Prophylactic treatment with a proton pump inhibitor or histamine H_2-receptor blocker is appropriate when ulcer is particularly likely, e.g. in rheumatoid arthritis, or patients with a history of peptic ulcer disease. There is increased incidence of pancreatitis.

Central nervous system. *Depression* and *psychosis* can occur during the first few days of high-dose administration, especially in those with a history of mental disorder. Other effects include *euphoria, insomnia,* and *aggravation of schizophrenia* and *epilepsy.* Long-term treatment may result in *raised intracranial pressure* with papilloedema, especially in children.

Ophthalmic effects may include *posterior subcapsular lens cataract* (risk when dose exceeds prednisolone 10 mg/day or equivalent for more than a year), *glaucoma* (with prolonged use of eye drops), and *corneal* or *scleral thinning.*

Other effects include menstrual disorders, delayed tissue healing (including myocardial rupture after myocardial infarction), thromboembolism and, paradoxically, hypersensitivity reactions including anaphylaxis.

ADRENAL STEROIDS AND PREGNANCY

Adrenal steroids are teratogenic in animals. Although a relationship between steroid pharmacotherapy and cleft palate and other fetal abnormalities has been suspected in humans, there is no doubt that many women taking a steroid throughout have both conceived and borne normal babies. Adrenal insufficiency due to hypothalamic–pituitary suppression in the newborn occurs only with high doses to the mother.

Dosage during pregnancy should be kept as low as practicable and fluorinated steroids are best avoided as they are more teratogenic in animals (dexamethasone and betamethasone, triamcinolone and various topical steroids, e.g. fluocinolone). Hypoadrenal women who become pregnant may require an increase in hydrocortisone replacement therapy by about 10 mg/day to compensate for the increased binding by plasma proteins that occurs in pregnancy. Manage labour as for major surgery (below).

PRECAUTIONS DURING CHRONIC ADRENAL STEROID THERAPY

The most important precaution during replacement and pharmacotherapy is regular review for adverse effects including fluid retention (weight gain), hypertension, glycosuria, hypokalaemia (potassium supplements may be necessary) and back pain (osteoporosis), and for the serious hazard of patient non-compliance.

Mild withdrawal symptoms (iatrogenic cortical insufficiency) include conjunctivitis, rhinitis, weight loss, arthralgia and itchy skin nodules.

Patients must always:

- carry a steroid card giving details of therapy
- be impressed with the importance of compliance
- know what to do if they develop an intercurrent illness or other severe stress, i.e. double their next dose and consult their doctor. If a patient omits a dose, a replacement dose should be taken as soon as possible to maintain the same total daily intake, because every patient should be taking the minimum dose necessary to control the disease
- have access to parenteral hydrocortisone (their own supply for i.m. injection, if urgent medical referral is not always possible).

Treatment of intercurrent illness

The normal adrenal cortex responds to severe stress by secreting more than 300 mg cortisol daily. Intercurrent illness is stress and treatment is urgent, particularly of *infections*; a reasonable course is to double the dose of corticosteroid during the illness and gradually reduce it as the patient improves. Effective chemotherapy of bacterial infections is especially important.

Viral infections contracted during steroid therapy can be overwhelming because the immune response of the body may be largely suppressed. This is particularly relevant to therapeutically immunosuppressed patients exposed to varicella/herpes zoster virus, when fulminant illness may ensue. They may need passive protection with varicella-zoster immunoglobulin, VZIG, as soon as practicable. Continuous use of prednisolone 20 mg/day (or the equivalent) is immunosuppressive. But a corticosteroid may sometimes be useful therapy after the disease has begun (thyroiditis, encephalitis) and there has been time for the immune response to occur. Corticosteroid then acts by suppressing unwanted effects of immune responses and excessive inflammatory reaction.

Vomiting warrants parenteral steroid.

Surgery requires that patients receive hydrocortisone 100 mg i.m. or i.v. (or hydrocortisone 20 mg orally) with premedication. If there are any signs of cardiovascular collapse during the operation, infuse hydrocortisone (100 mg) i.v. at once. If surgery is uncomplicated, hydrocortisone 50 mg i.v. or orally every 6 h for 24–72 h is adequate for most patients on replacement therapy. Then reduce the dose by half every 24 h until the normal dose is reached.

Minor operations, e.g. dental extraction, may be covered by hydrocortisone 20 mg orally 2–4 h before operation, and the same dose afterwards.

In all of these situations, an intravenous infusion should be available for immediate use in case the recommendations above are insufficient. These precautions are particularly relevant for patients who have received substantial corticosteroid treatment within the previous year, because their HPA system, though sufficient for ordinary life, may fail to respond adequately to severe stress. If steroid therapy has been very prolonged, and in patients undergoing adrenalectomy for Cushing's syndrome (because the remaining adrenal gland is atrophic), the precautions apply for as long as 2 years afterwards, or until there is evidence of recovery of normal adrenal function.

DOSAGE AND ROUTES OF ADMINISTRATION

No single schedule suits every case, but examples appear below.

Systemic commencing doses:

- For a *serious disease* such as systemic lupus, dermatomyositis: prednisolone up to 0.75–2.0 mg/kg daily, orally in divided doses.
- If the condition is *life threatening*, give prednisolone up to 60 mg, or its equivalent of another steroid. The dose is then increased if necessary until the disease is controlled or adverse effects occur; prednisolone 2–3 mg/kg daily may be needed. Cyclophosphamide or azathioprine (see p. 264) are valuable adjuncts which may enhance the initial control of the disease and have a sparing effect on the maintenance dose of prednisolone.
- More usually now, megadose pulses (methylprednisolone 1.0 g i.v. daily for 3 days) are used, followed by oral maintenance with prednisolone and/or a steroid-sparing agent (above).
- For *less dangerous* disease, e.g. rheumatoid arthritis, give prednisolone 7.5–10.0 mg daily, adjusted later according to the response.
- In particular cases, including replacement of adrenal insufficiency, the dosage appears in the account of the disease.

■ For *continuous therapy,* give the minimum amount to produce the desired effect. Imperfect control may have to be accepted by the patient if full control, e.g. of rheumatoid arthritis, though obtainable, involves doses that will lead to toxicity, e.g. osteoporosis, if continued for years. The decision to embark on such therapy is a serious matter for the patient.

Topical applications (creams, intranasal, inhalations, enemas) are used in attempts, often successful, to obtain local effect, whilst avoiding systemic effects; suspensions of solutions are also injected into joints, soft tissues and subconjunctivally. All can, in heavy dose, be absorbed sufficiently to suppress the hypothalamus and cause other unwanted effects. Individual preparations appear in the text where appropriate.

The relatively high selectivity of inhaled beclometasone in asthma is due to a combination of route of administration, high potency and rapid conversion to inactive metabolites by the liver of any drug that is absorbed (see asthma, skin); yet hypothalamic–pituitary suppression and systemic toxicity occasionally occur.

Contraindications to adrenal steroids for suppressing inflammation are all relative, depending on the anticipated advantage. Where the patient has, e.g. diabetes, a history of mental disorder or peptic ulcer, epilepsy, tuberculosis, hypertension or heart failure, the reasons for use must be compelling. The presence of any infection demands that effective chemotherapy be begun before the corticosteroid, but there are exceptions (some viral infections, see above). Topical corticosteroid applied to an inflamed eye (with the very best of intention) can be disastrous if the inflammation is due to herpes virus.

Adrenal steroids containing fluorine (see above) intensify diabetes more than do others and are to be avoided in that disease.

Long-term use of adrenal steroids in children - presents essentially the same problems as in adults except that growth retards approximately in proportion to the dose. This is unlikely to be important unless therapy exceeds 6 months; there is a growth spurt after withdrawal. Intermittent dosage schedules (alternate day) may reduce the risk (rarely, corticotropin may be preferred, see p. 593).

Some problems loom larger in children than in adults. Common childhood viral infections may be more severe, and if a non-immune child taking an adrenal steroid is exposed to virus infection it is wise to try to prevent the disease with the appropriate specific immunoglobulin.

Live virus vaccination is unsafe in immunosuppressed subjects, e.g. systemic prednisolone, more than 2 mg/kg/day for more than 1 week in the preceding 3 months, as it may cause the disease, but active immunisation with killed vaccines or toxoids will give normal response unless the dose of steroid is high, when the response may be suppressed.

Raised intracranial pressure may occur more readily in children than in adults.

Indications for use of adrenal steroids
- Replacement of hormone deficiency.
- Inflammation suppression.
- Immunosuppression.
- Suppression of excess hormone secretion.

USES OF ADRENOCORTICAL STEROIDS

REPLACEMENT THERAPY

Acute adrenocortical insufficiency (Addisonian crisis)

This is an emergency; hydrocortisone sodium succinate 100 mg is given i.v. immediately it is *suspected,* or the patient may die.

■ An intravenous infusion of sodium chloride solution (0.9%) is set up immediately and a second 100 mg hydrocortisone is added to the first litre, which may be given over 2 h (several litres of fluid may be needed in the first 24 h).

■ The patient should then receive hydrocortisone 50 mg i.v. or i.m. 6-hourly for 24–72 h; thereafter a total of 30–40 mg/day orally in two or three divided doses usually suffices.

Treatment to restore electrolyte balance will depend on the circumstances. Seek and treat the cause of the crisis; it is often an infection. When the dose of hydrocortisone falls below 40 mg/day, supplementary mineralocorticoid (fludrocortisone) may be needed (see below).

The hyperkalaemia of Addison's disease will respond to the above regimen and must not be treated with insulin because the risk of hypoglycaemia is high.

Chronic primary adrenocortical insufficiency (Addison's disease)

Hydrocortisone is given orally (15–25 mg total daily) in two to three divided doses, according to the algorithm in Figure 34.3. The aim is to mimic the natural diurnal rhythm of secretion.[3] All patients also require mineralocorticoid replacement, and fludrocortisone, 50–100 micrograms orally once a day, suffices.

The dose of the hormones is determined in the individual by following general clinical progress and particularly by observing: weight, blood pressure, appearance of oedema, serum sodium and potassium concentrations, and haematocrit. If any complicating disease arises, e.g. infection, a need for surgery or other stress, the hydrocortisone dose is immediately doubled (as above). Where available, plasma renin assay is useful for titration of fludrocortisone dose. A suppressed value indicates overdosage, and vice versa.

If there is vomiting, the parenteral replacement hormone must be given without delay. There are no contraindications to replacement therapy. The risk lies in withholding rather than in giving it.

Chronic secondary adrenocortical insufficiency

This occurs in hypopituitarism. The need for hydrocortisone may be less than in primary insufficiency, especially when ACTH deficiency is partial. Some patients with borderline adrenocortical insufficiency may require steroid supplementation only during periods of stress, such as infection or surgery. Mineralocorticoid replacement is seldom required, for the pituitary has little control over aldosterone production. Other pituitary replacement is given as appropriate (see p. 637).

Iatrogenic adrenocortical insufficiency: abrupt withdrawal

(See also below: Withdrawal of corticosteroid pharmacotherapy) This occurs in patients who have recently received prolonged pharmacotherapy with a corticosteroid that inhibits hypothalamic production of the corticotropin releasing hormone and so results in secondary adrenal failure. Treat by reinstituting the original therapy or manage as for acute adrenal insufficiency, as appropriate. To avoid an acute crisis on discontinuing therapy, the corticosteroid must be withdrawn gradually to allow the hypothalamus, the pituitary and the adrenal to regain normal function. Treat patients taking corticosteroids who have an infection or surgical operation (major stress) as for primary insufficiency.

Sudden withdrawal of large doses of steroid hormone used to suppress inflammation or allergy may lead not only to an adrenal insufficiency crisis but also to relapse of the disease that is suppressed, not cured. Such relapse can be extremely severe, and sometimes life threatening.

PHARMACOTHERAPY

Suppression of adrenocortical function

In *congenital adrenal hyperplasia*, excess adrenal androgen secretion is suppressed by prednisolone or dexamethasone, which inhibit pituitary corticotropin production.

Use in inflammation and for immunosuppression

Drugs with primarily glucocorticoid effects, e.g. prednisolone, are chosen, so that the mineralocorticoid effects that are inevitable with hydrocortisone do not limit the dose.

It remains essential to use only the minimum dose that will achieve the desired effect. Sometimes therapeutic effects are partly sacrificed to avoid adverse effects, as it has not so far proved possible to separate all the glucocorticoid effects from one another; for example, it is not known whether it is possible to eliminate catabolic effects and yet retain anti-inflammatory action. In some conditions, e.g. nephrotic syndrome, the clinician cannot specify exactly what action they want the drug developer to provide.

Further specific uses

The decision to give a corticosteroid commonly depends on knowledge of the likelihood and amount of benefit (bearing in mind that very prolonged high dose inevitably brings serious complications), on the severity of the disease and on whether the patient has failed to respond usefully to other treatment.

Adrenal steroids are used in nearly all cases of:

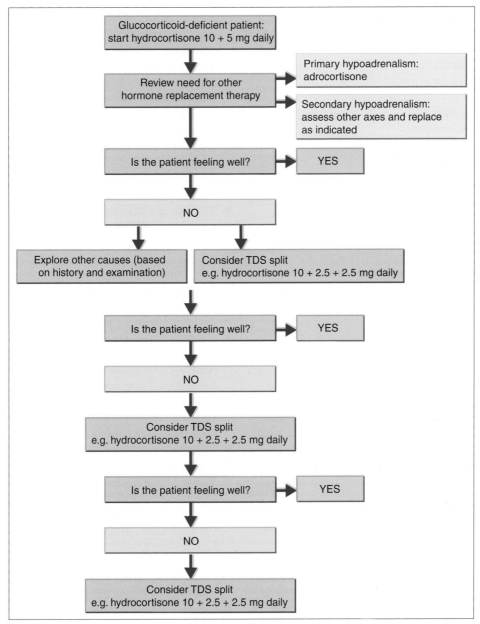

Fig. 34.3   Algorithm for treatment of the glucocorticoid-deficient patient. Patients should be reassessed at 6–8-week intervals while their treatment is optimised. (Adapted from Crown A, Lightman S 2005 Why is the management of glucocorticoid deficiency still controversial: a review of the literature? Clinical Endocrinology 63:483–492.)

- Exfoliative dermatitis and pemphigus, if severe.
- *Connective tissue diseases*, if severe, e.g. lupus erythematosus (systemic), polyarteritis nodosa, polymyalgia rheumatica and cranial giant cell arteritis (urgent therapy to save sight), dermatomyositis.
- *Severe asthma* (see p. 507).
- *Acute lymphatic leukaemia* (see p. 593).
- *Acquired haemolytic anaemia.*

- *Severe allergic reactions* of all kinds, e.g. serum sickness, angio-oedema, trichiniasis. Alone, they will not control acute manifestations of anaphylactic shock as they do not act quickly enough.
- *Organ transplant rejection.*
- *Acute spinal cord injury*: early, brief, and high dose (to reduce the oedema/inflammation).
- *Autoimmune active chronic hepatitis*: a corticosteroid improves well-being, liver

function and histological findings; prednisolone will benefit some 80% and should be continued in the long term, as most patients relapse if the drug is withdrawn.

Adrenal steroids are used in some cases of:

- *Rheumatic fever.*
- *Rheumatoid arthritis.*
- *Ankylosing spondylitis.*
- *Ulcerative colitis and proctitis.*
- *Regional enteritis* (Crohn's disease).
- *Hay fever* (allergic rhinitis); also some bronchitics with marked airways obstruction.
- *Sarcoidosis.* If there is hypercalcaemia or threat to a major organ, e.g. eye, adrenal steroid administration is urgent. Pulmonary fibrosis may be delayed and CNS manifestations may improve.
- *Acute mountain/altitude sickness*, to reduce cerebral oedema.
- *Prevention of adverse reaction* to radiocontrast media in patients who have had a previous severe reaction.
- *Blood diseases due to circulating antibodies*, e.g. thrombocytopenic purpura (there may also be a decrease in capillary fragility with lessening of purpura even though thrombocytes remain few); agranulocytosis.
- *Eye diseases.* Allergic diseases and non-granulomatous inflammation of the uveal tract. Bacterial and viral infections may be made worse and use of corticosteroids to suppress inflammation of infection is generally undesirable, is best left to ophthalmologists and must be accompanied by effective chemotherapy; this is of the greatest importance in *herpes virus infection.* Corneal integrity should be checked before use (by instilling a drop of fluorescein). Prolonged use of corticosteroid eye-drops causes glaucoma in 1 in 20 of the population (a genetic trait). Application is generally as hydrocortisone, prednisolone or fluorometholone drops, or subconjunctival injection.
- *Nephrotic syndrome.* Patients with minimal change disease respond well to daily or alternate-day therapy. With a total dose of prednisolone 60 mg/day, 90% of those who will lose their proteinuria will have done so within 4–6 weeks, and the dose is tapered off over 3–4 months. Longer courses only induce

adverse effects. Relapses are common (50%) and it is then necessary to find a minimum dose of adrenal steroid that will keep the patient well. If a corticosteroid is for any reason undesirable, cyclophosphamide or chlorambucil may be substituted. Membranous nephropathy may respond to high-dose corticosteroid with or without chlorambucil.

- *A variety of skin diseases*, such as eczema. Severe cases may involve occlusive dressings if a systemic effect is undesirable, though absorption can be substantial (see Chapter 16).
- *Aphthous ulcers.* Hydrocortisone 2.5 mg oromucosal tablets are allowed to dissolve next to an ulcer; beclometasone dipropionate inhaler 50–100 micrograms may be sprayed on the oral mucosa, or betamethasone soluble tablet 500 micrograms dissolved in water may be used (without swallowing) as a mouthwash.
- *Acute gout* resistant to other drugs (see p. 271).
- *Hypercalcaemia of sarcoidosis and of vitamin D intoxication* responds to prednisolone 30 mg daily (or its equivalent of other adrenal steroid) for 10 days. Hypercalcaemia of myeloma and some other malignancies responds more variably. Hyperparathyroid hypercalcaemia *does not respond* (see p. 665).
- *Raised intracranial pressure* due to cerebral oedema, e.g. in cerebral tumour or encephalitis. This is probably an anti-inflammatory effect, which reduces vascular permeability and acts in 12–24 h. Give dexamethasone 10 mg i.m. or i.v. (or equivalent) initially and then 4 mg 6-hourly by the appropriate route, reducing the dose after 2–4 days and withdrawing over 5–7 days. Much higher doses may be used in palliation of inoperable cerebral tumour.
- *Preterm labour*: (to mother) to enhance fetal lung maturation.
- *Aspiration of gastric acid* (Mendelsohn's syndrome).
- *Myasthenia gravis*: see page 397.
- *Cancer*, see Chapter 30.

Use in diagnosis: *dexamethasone suppression test.* Dexamethasone acts on the hypothalamus (like hydrocortisone) to reduce output of corticotropin releasing hormone (CRH), but it does not interfere with measurement of corticosteroids in blood or urine. Normal suppression of cortisol production after administering dexamethasone indicates that the HPA axis is intact. Failure of suppression implies pathological hypersecretion of ACTH by the pituitary or of cortisol by the adrenal or ectopic ACTH. Dexamethasone is used because its action is prolonged (24 h). There are several ways of carrying out the test.

WITHDRAWAL OF PHARMACOTHERAPY

The longer the duration of therapy the slower must be the withdrawal.

If use is less than 1 week, e.g. for acute asthma, although some hypothalamic suppression will have occurred, withdrawal can be safely accomplished in a few steps.

After use for 2 weeks, for rapid withdrawal, a 50% reduction in dose each day is reasonable.

If the duration of treatment is longer, dose reduction is accompanied by the dual risk of resurgence of the disease and iatrogenic hypoadrenalism; withdrawal should then proceed very slowly, e.g. 2.5–5 mg prednisolone or equivalent at intervals of 3–7 days.

An alternative scheme is to halve the dose weekly until it is 25 mg/day of prednisolone or equivalent, then to make reductions of about 1 mg/day every third to seventh day. Paediatric tablets (1 mg) can be useful during withdrawal.

These schemes may yet be too rapid (with the occurrence of fatigue, 'dish-rag' syndrome or relapse of disease). The rate of reduction may then need to be as slow as prednisolone 1 mg/day (or equivalent) per month, particularly as the dose approaches the level of physiological requirement (equivalent of prednisolone 5–7.5 mg daily).

The long tetracosactide test (see below) or plasma corticotropin concentration is useful to assess recovery of *adrenal* responsiveness. A positive result does not necessarily indicate full recovery of the patient's ability to respond to stressful situations; the latter is best shown by an adequate response to insulin-induced hypoglycaemia (which additionally tests *hypothalamic–pituitary* capacity to respond).

Corticotropin should not be used to hasten recovery of the atrophied cortex because its effects further suppress the hypothalamic–pituitary axis, on recovery of which the patient's future depends. Complete recovery of normal HPA function sufficient to cope with severe intercurrent illnesses or surgery is generally complete in 2 months but may take as long as 2 years.

There are many reports of collapse, even coma, occurring within a few hours of omission of adrenal steroid therapy, e.g. due to patients' ignorance of the risk to which their physicians are exposing them, or failure to carry their tablets with them. Patients must be instructed on the hazards of omitting therapy and, during intercurrent disease, intramuscular preparations should be freely used. For anaesthesia and surgery in adrenocortical insufficiency, see p. 601.

INHIBITION OF SYNTHESIS OF ADRENAL AND OTHER STEROID HORMONES

These agents have use in diagnosis of adrenal disease and in controlling excessive production of corticosteroids, e.g. by corticotropin-producing tumours of the pituitary (Cushing's syndrome) or by adrenocortical adenoma or carcinoma where the cause cannot be removed. Use of these drugs calls for special care as they can precipitate acute adrenal insufficiency. Some members inhibit other steroid synthesis.

Metyrapone inhibits the enzyme, steroid 11β-hydroxylase, which converts 11-deoxy precursors into hydrocortisone, corticosterone and aldosterone. It affects synthesis of aldosterone less than that of glucocorticoids.

Trilostane blocks the synthetic path earlier (3β-hydroxysteroid dehydrogenase) and thus inhibits aldosterone synthesis as well.

Formestane is a specific inhibitor of the aromatase that converts androgens to oestrogens. A depot injection of 250 mg i.m. is given twice a month to treat some patients with carcinoma of the breast who have relapsed on tamoxifen.

Aminoglutethimide blocks at an even earlier stage, preventing the conversion of cholesterol to pregnenolone. It therefore stops synthesis of all steroids, hydrocortisone, aldosterone and sex hormones (including the conversion of androgens to oestrogens); it has a use in breast cancer.

Ketoconazole is an effective antifungal agent by virtue of its capacity to block sterol/steroid synthesis (ergosterol in the case of fungi). In humans it inhibits adrenal steroid synthesis in gonads and adrenal cortex, and has been used in Cushing's syndrome and prostatic cancer.

Anastrozole is an adrenal aromatase inhibitor that finds use as *adjuvant* treatment of oestrogen receptor-positive early breast cancer in postmenopausal women. It is used as *sole* therapy, following

2–3 years of tamoxifen, in advanced breast cancer in postmenopausal women that is oestrogen receptor positive or responsive to tamoxifen. *Letrozole* and *exemestane* are similar.

COMPETITIVE ANTAGONISM OF ADRENAL STEROIDS

Spironolactone antagonises the sodium-retaining effect of aldosterone and other mineralocorticoids. It is used to treat primary and secondary hyperaldosteronism (see p. 597).

ADRENOCORTICOTROPHIC HORMONE (ACTH) (CORTICOTROPIN)

Natural corticotropin is a 39-amino-acid polypeptide secreted by the anterior pituitary gland; it is obtained from animal pituitaries.

The physiological activity resides in the first 24 amino acids (which are common to many species) and most immunological activity lies in the remaining 15 amino acids.

The pituitary output of corticotropin responds rapidly to physiological requirements by the familiar negative-feedback homeostatic mechanism. As the $t_{1/2}$ of corticotropin is 10 min and the adrenal cortex responds within 2 min, it is plain that corticosteroid output can adjust rapidly.

Synthetic corticotropins have the advantage of shorter amino acid chains (they lack amino acids 25–39) which are less likely to cause serious allergy, although this does occur. Additionally, they are devoid of animal proteins, which are potent allergens.

Tetracosactide (tetracosactin) consists of the biologically active first 24 amino acids of natural corticotropin (from humans or animals) and so it has similar properties, e.g. $t_{1/2}$ 10 min.

ACTIONS

Corticotropin stimulates the synthesis of corticosteroids (of which the most important is hydrocortisone) and to a lesser extent of androgens, by the cells of the adrenal cortex. It has only a minor (transient) effect on aldosterone production, which proceeds *independently*; in the absence of corticotropin the cells of the inner cortex atrophy.

The release of natural corticotropin by the pituitary gland is controlled by the hypothalamus through *corticotropin releasing hormone* (CRH, or corticoliberin), production of which is influenced by environmental stresses as well as by the level of circulating hydrocortisone. High plasma concentration of any adrenal steroid with glucocorticoid effect prevents release of CRH and so of corticotropin, lack of which in turn results in adrenocortical hypofunction. This is why catastrophe may accompany abrupt withdrawal of long-term adrenal steroid therapy with adrenal atrophy.

The effects of corticotropin are those of the steroids (hydrocortisone, androgens) liberated by its action on the adrenal cortex. Prolonged heavy dosage causes the clinical picture of Cushing's syndrome.

Uses. Corticotropin is used principally in diagnosis and rarely in treatment. It is inactive if taken orally and has to be injected like other peptide hormones.

Diagnostic use is to test the capacity of the adrenal cortex to produce cortisol. With the *short test*, the plasma cortisol (hydrocortisone) concentration is measured before and 30 min and 60 min after an intramuscular injection of tetracosactide (Synacthen); a normal response is a rise in plasma hydrocortisone concentration of more than 200 nanomol/L. In cases of uncertainty, the *longer* variants of the test require intramuscular injection of a depot (sustained-release) formulation, e.g. 1 mg daily for 3 days at 09:00 hours, with a short tetracosactide test performed on day 3.

Therapeutic use is seldom appropriate, as the peptide hormone must be injected. Selective glucocorticoid (without mineralocorticoid) action is not possible, and clinical results are irregular. Corticotropin cannot be relied on to restore adrenal cortisol output when a steroid is being withdrawn after prolonged therapy, as it does not restore function in the suppressed hypothalamic–pituitary part of the HPA axis.

PREPARATIONS

- *Tetracosactide Injection* is supplied as an ampoule for injection i.v., i.m. or s.c.
- *Tetracosactide Zinc Injection* (Synacthen Depot) i.m. in which the hormone is adsorbed on to zinc phosphate from which it is slowly released. This is the form used in the long tetracosactide test.

Summary
- Physiological concentrations of cortisol are essential for supporting the circulation and glucose production. Physiological concentrations of aldosterone are essential to prevent excessive sodium loss.
- For systemic pharmacological uses, prednisolone or other synthetic adrenocorticosteroids are used because they are more selective glucocorticoids, i.e. have less sodium-retaining activity.
- For local administration (skin, lung), more potent, fluorinated steroids may be required.
- Glucocorticoids inhibit the transcriptional activation of many of the inflammatory cytokines, giving them a versatile role in the treatment of many types of inflammation.
- Fludrocortisone is a valuable treatment for many sodium-losing states, and for most causes of autonomic neuropathy.
- Corticotropin is used to test the capacity of the adrenal gland to produce cortisol.

GUIDE TO FURTHER READING

Arlt W 2006 Junior doctors' working hours and the circadian rhythm of hormones. Clinical Medicine 6:127–129

Buttgereit F, Burmester G-R, Lipworth B J 2005 Optimised glucocorticoid therapy: the sharpening of an old spear. Lancet 365:801–803

Cooper M S, Stewart P M 2003 Corticosteroid insufficiency in acutely ill patients. New England Journal of Medicine 348:727–734

Hench P S et al 1949 The effect of a hormone of the adrenal cortex (17-hydroxy-11-dehydrocorticosterone: Compound E) and of pituitary adrenocorticotropic hormone on rheumatoid arthritis. Proceedings of the Staff Meetings of the Mayo Clinic 24:181, 277 (acute rheumatism)

The classic studies of the first clinical use of an adrenocortical steroid in inflammatory disease. See also page 298 for an account by E C Kendall of the biochemical and pharmaceutical background to the clinical studies. Kendall writes of his collaboration with Hench, 'he can now say "17-hydroxy-11-dehydrocorticosterone" and in turn I can say "the arthritis of lupus erythematosus". In sophisticated circles, however, I prefer to say, "the arthritis of L.E."'.

Hilditch K 2000 My Addison's disease. British Medical Journal 321:645 (a patient's account of the disease)

Hochhaus G 2004 New developments in corticosteroids. Proceedings of the American Thoracic Society 1:269–274

Lipworth B J 2000 Therapeutic implications of non-genomic glucocorticoid activity. Lancet 356:87–88

Løvås K, Husebye E 2005 Addison's disease. Lancet 365:2058–2061

Newell-Price J, Bertagna X, Grossman A B, Nieman L K 2006 Cushing's syndrome. Lancet 367:1605–1617

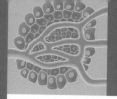

35

Diabetes mellitus, insulin, oral antidiabetes agents, obesity

SYNOPSIS

Diabetes mellitus affects 1–2% of many national populations. Its successful management requires close collaboration between the patient and the doctor.

- Diabetes mellitus and insulin
- Insulins in current use (including choice, formulations, adverse effects, hypoglycaemia, insulin resistance)
- Oral antidiabetes drugs
- Treatment of diabetes mellitus
- Diabetic ketoacidosis
- Surgery in diabetic patients
- Obesity and overweight

DIABETES MELLITUS AND INSULIN

HISTORY

Diabetes was known to ancient Greek medicine with the description of 'a melting of the flesh and limbs into urine … the patients never stop making water but the flow is incessant … their mouth becomes parched and their body dry'.[1]

Insulin (as pancreatic islet cell extract) was first administered to a 14-year-old insulin-deficient patient on 11 January 1922 in Toronto, Canada. An adult sufferer from diabetes who developed the disease in 1920 and who, because of insulin, lived until 1968, has told how:

Many doctors, after they have developed a disease, take up the speciality in it … But that was not so with me. I was studying for surgery when diabetes took me up. The great book of Joslin said that by starving you might live four years with luck. [He went to Italy and, whilst his health was declining there, he received a letter from a biochemist friend which said] there was something called 'insulin' appearing with a good name in Canada, what about going there and getting it. I said 'No thank you; I've tried too many quackeries for diabetes; I'll wait and see'. Then I got peripheral neuritis … So when [the friend] cabled me and said, 'I've got insulin – it works – come back quick', I responded, arrived at King's College Hospital, London, and went to the laboratory as soon as it opened … It was all experimental for [neither of us] knew a thing about it … So we decided to have 20 units a nice round figure. I had a nice breakfast. I had bacon and eggs and toast made on the Bunsen. I hadn't eaten bread for months and months … by 3 o'clock in the afternoon my urine was quite sugar free. That hadn't happened for many months. So we gave a cheer for Banting and Best.[2]

But at 4 pm I had a terrible shaky feeling and a terrible sweat and hunger pain. That was my first experience of hypoglycaemia. We remembered that Banting and Best had described an overdose of insulin in dogs. So I had some sugar and a biscuit and soon got quite well, thank you.[3]

Diabetes mellitus is classified broadly as:
- **Type 1** (formerly, insulin dependent diabetes mellitus, IDDM) which typically occurs in younger people who cannot secrete insulin.
- **Type 2** (formerly, non-insulin dependent diabetes mellitus, NIDDM), which typically occurs in older, often obese, people who retain capacity to secrete insulin but who are resistant to its action. These terms and abbreviations are used in this chapter.

[1]The Extant Works of Aretaeus, trans. Francis Adams (London 1856) p. 338 (quoted by Ackerknecht E H 1982 A short history of medicine. Johns Hopkins, Baltimore, pp. 71–72).

[2]F G Banting and C H Best of Toronto, Canada (see also Journal of Laboratory and Clinical Medicine 1922; 7:251).
[3]Abbreviated from Lawrence R D 1961 King's College Hospital Gazette 40:220. Transcript from a recorded after dinner talk to students' Historical Society.

SOURCES OF INSULIN

Insulin is synthesised and stored (bound to zinc) in granules in the β-islet cells of the pancreas. Daily secretion amounts to 30–40 units, which is about 25% of total pancreatic insulin content. The principal factor that evokes insulin secretion is a high blood glucose concentration. In healthy subjects, glucose elicits a robust first-phase secretion and then a more prolonged second-phase release into the portal circulation.

Insulin is a polypeptide with two peptide chains (A chain, 21 amino acids; B chain, 30) linked by two disulphide bridges. The basic structure having metabolic activity is common to all mammalian species but there are minor species differences:

- *Bovine* insulin differs from human insulin by three amino acids.
- *Porcine* insulin differs from human by only one amino acid.
- *Human* insulin is made either by enzyme modification of porcine insulin, or by using recombinant DNA to synthesise the pro-insulin precursor molecule for insulin. This is done by artificially introducing the DNA into either *Escherichia coli* or yeast.[4]
- *Insulin analogues* have small numbers of modifications to the α and/or β chains, which result in more rapid onset and offset of action (rapidly acting analogues), or slower offset (long-acting analogues) than naturally occurring insulin.

INSULIN RECEPTORS

Insulin binds to the β subunit of its receptor. The β subunit is a tyrosine kinase that is activated by insulin binding and is autophosphorylated. Tyrosine kinase also phosphorylates other substrates so that a signalling cascade is initiated and biological response ensues. Insulin receptors are present on the surface of the target cells (mostly liver, muscle, fat). Receptors vary in number inversely with the insulin concentration to which they are exposed, i.e. with high insulin concentration the number of receptors declines (*down-regulation*) and responsiveness to insulin also declines (insulin resistance); with low insulin concentration the number of receptors increases (*up-regulation*) and responsiveness to insulin increases. Patients with Type 2 diabetes have insulin resistance.

Hyperinsulinaemia predates the onset of Type 2 diabetes and the resistance is secondary to down-regulation of insulin receptors as well as post-receptor, intracellular events. Obesity is a major factor in the development of insulin resistance. Patients may recover insulin responsiveness as a result of dieting so that the insulin secretion decreases, cellular receptors increase and insulin sensitivity is restored.

ACTIONS OF INSULIN

The effects of stimulation of the insulin receptors include activation of glucokinase and glucose phosphatase. Insulin also increases glucose transport as well as its utilisation, especially by muscle and adipose tissue. Its effects include:

- *Reduction in blood glucose* due to increased glucose uptake in the peripheral tissues (which convert it into glycogen or fat), and reduction of hepatic output of glucose (diminished breakdown of glycogen and diminished gluconeogenesis). When the blood glucose concentration falls below the renal threshold (10 mmol/L or 180 mg/100 mL) glycosuria ceases, as does the osmotic diuresis of water and electrolytes. Polyuria with dehydration and excessive thirst are thus alleviated. As the blood glucose concentration falls, appetite is stimulated.
- *Other metabolic effects.* In addition to enabling glucose to pass across cell membranes, the transit of amino acids and potassium into the cell is enhanced. Insulin regulates carbohydrate utilisation and energy production. It enhances protein synthesis. It inhibits breakdown of fats (lipolysis). An insulin-deficient diabetic (Type 1) becomes dehydrated due to osmotic diuresis, and is ketotic because fats break down faster than the ketoacid metabolites can be metabolised.

USES

- Diabetes mellitus is the main indication.
- Insulin promotes the passage of potassium simultaneously with glucose into cells, and this

---

[4]The three forms of human insulin have the same amino acid sequence, but are separately designated as insulin emp (Enzyme Modified Porcine), prb (Pro-insulin Recombinant in Bacteria) and pyr (Precursor insulin Yeast Recombinant). Although one of the incentives for introducing human insulin was avoidance of insulin antibody production, the allergies to older insulins were caused largely by impurities in the preparations, and are avoided equally well by using the highly purified, monocomponent porcine and bovine insulins.

effect is utilised to correct hyperkalaemia (see p. 485).

- Insulin-induced hypoglycaemia can also be used as a test of anterior pituitary function (growth hormone and corticotropin are released).

PHARMACOKINETICS

Insulin, naturally secreted by the pancreas, enters the portal vein and passes straight to the liver, where half of it is taken up. The rest enters and is distributed in the systemic circulation so that its concentration (in fasting subjects) is only about 15% of that entering the liver.

When insulin is injected subcutaneously it enters the systemic circulation and both liver and other peripheral organs receive the same concentration.

In conventional use, insulin is injected (s.c., i.m. or i.v.) as it is digested when swallowed. It is absorbed into the blood and inactivated in the liver and kidney; about 10% appears in the urine. The $t_{1/2}$ is 5 min.

Insulin may be delivered by needles and syringes, insulin pens (supplied preloaded or with replaceable cartridges), and (within hospital) by external infusion. Some specialist centres employ implantable pumps.

DIFFERENCES BETWEEN HUMAN AND ANIMAL INSULINS

Human insulin is absorbed from subcutaneous tissue slightly more rapidly than animal insulins and has a slightly shorter duration of action.

Human insulin is less immunogenic than bovine, but not porcine, insulin. Rarely patients taking human insulin appear to experience more frequent or severe hypoglycaemic attacks, or to have lessened awareness of hypoglycaemia. Animal insulins are now used too little to permit or warrant a definite resolution of a possible species difference in tolerability. It is reasonable for the occasional patient to try switching from human to porcine insulin, or to remain on porcine insulin if well controlled.

PREPARATIONS OF INSULIN(see Table 35.1)

There are three major factors:

- Strength (concentration).
- Source (human, porcine, bovine).
- Formulation

– *short-acting* solution of insulin for use s.c., i.m., i.v., inhaled
– *intermediate and longer-acting* (sustained release) preparations in which the insulin has been modified physically by combination with protamine or zinc to give an amorphous or crystalline suspension; this is given subcutaneously and slowly dissociates to release insulin in its soluble form (given intramuscularly, which is not advised, the time course of release would be different).

Dosage is measured in *international units* standardised by chemical assay.

Diabetes mellitus may be managed from a choice of four types of insulin (animal or human) preparations, whose different time-courses of action are illustrated in Fig. 35.1.

1. *Short duration* of action (and rapid onset): Soluble Insulin (also called neutral or regular insulin). The most recent addition to this class of insulin, Insulin Lispro, is a modified human insulin in which the reversal of two amino acids (lysine and proline) has resulted in a very rapid onset of action (within 15 min of injection). Insulin Aspart is similar.
2. *Intermediate duration* of action (and slower onset): Isophane (NPH) Insulin, a suspension with protamine; Insulin Zinc Suspensions, amorphous or a mixture of amorphous and crystalline.
3. *Longer duration* of action: Insulin Zinc Suspension, crystalline, or Protamine Zinc Insulin (insulin in suspension with both zinc and protamine). The new additions to this group are the analogues Insulin Glargine and Insulin Detemir (Fig. 35.2).
4. *A mixture* of soluble and isophane insulins, officially called *biphasic* insulins, or of short-acting analogue insulins with isophane insulin.

NOTES FOR PRESCRIBING INSULIN

Allergy to purified or analogue insulins is very rare.

Antibodies to insulin can occur, but are no longer of clinical significance.

Compatibility. Soluble insulin may be mixed in the syringe with insulin zinc suspensions (amorphous,

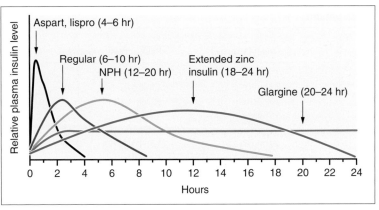

Fig. 35.1 Approximate pharmacokinetic profiles of human insulin and insulin analogues. The relative duration of action of the various forms of insulin is shown. The duration will vary widely both between and within persons. (Redrawn from Hirsch I B 2005 Insulin analogues. New England Journal of Medicine 352:174–183.)

crystalline) and with isophane and mixed (biphasic) insulin, and used at once. Long-acting analogue insulins, and protamine insulin suspensions, *should not be mixed* in a syringe with short-acting insulins.

Intravenous insulin. Only Soluble (neutral) Insulin Inj. should be used.

The standard strength of insulin preparations is 100 units/mL. Solutions of 40 and 80 units remain available in some countries, and health-care providers should be aware of this. Biological standardisation of insulin has been replaced by physicochemical methods (high-performance liquid chromatography, HPLC).

Inhaled insulin. One aerosol is available. Bio-availability is only 15%. In conjunction with an injected basal insulin, inhaled insulin maintains a level of glycaemic control comparable to that of patients taking multiple daily injections. The key benefit is likely to be improved patient satisfaction. Long-term safety remains to be determined.

CHOICE OF INSULIN PREPARATION

There are two types of regimen for patients requiring insulin:

1. *Intensive/flexible therapy.* This uses pens (or pumps) to administer multiple injections of short-acting insulin during the day to mimic prandial secretion of insulin by the pancreas, and a single night-time dose of long-acting insulin.

2. *Conventional therapy.* This involves two injections a day of biphasic insulin. Soluble insulin or one of the rapid-acting analogues is given subcutaneously three times a day. Soluble insulin is given 30 min before meals whilst the analogues have the advantage of being given immediately before, during or after the meal. Risk of hypoglycaemic reaction is lower with the analogues.

NPH insulin or one of the long-acting analogues is given at night. This mimics basal pancreatic insulin release. The long-acting analogues do this more effectively over 24 h than NPH insulin, and avoid risk of nocturnal hypoglycaemia (see Fig. 35.1). NPH and long-acting analogues may occasionally be given twice daily.

Biphasic insulins are a mixture of variable proportions of soluble insulin with NPH insulin, or of short-acting analogue with protamine insulin. The available mixtures are listed in Table 35.1. The most commonly used is 30:70 (soluble:NPH).

All of the above are normally administered subcutaneously. Soluble insulin may also be administered by intravenous infusion. This is the preferred method of delivery in diabetic ketoacidosis, in other critically ill patients, and in perioperative management of diabetes.

Use of a slow-infusion pump is recommended: 50 units soluble insulin is dissolved in 50 mL isotonic saline (i.e. insulin concentration 1 unit/mL). Insulin loss is minimised and control of dose is more

Table 35.1 Insulin preparations

Preparation	Onset (approx.)	Peak activity (approx.)	Duration of action (approx.)
Neutral Insulin Injection			
Actrapid	<30 min	1.5–3.5 h	7–8 h
Apidra (Insulin Glulisine)	10–20 min	55 min	1.5–4 h
Humalog (Insulin Lispro[a])	15 min	1.5 h	2–5 h
Humulin S	30 min to 1 h	1–6 h	6–12 h
Hypurin Bovine Neutral	30 min to 1 h	1.5–4.5 h	6–8 h
Hypurin Porcine Neutral	30 min to 1 h	1.5–4.5 h	6–8 h
Insuman Rapid	<30 min	1–4 h	7–9 h
NovoRapid (Insulin Aspart)	10–20 min	1–3 h	3–5 h
Pork Actrapid	<30 min	1.5–3 h	3–8 h
Velosulin	<30 min	1.5–3.5 h	7–8 h
Biphasic Insulin Injection[b]			
Humalog Mix25	15 min	2 h	22 h
Humalog Mix50	15 min	2 h	22 h
Humulin M3	30 min to 1 h	1–12 h	22 h
Hypurin Porcine 30/70	<2 h	4–12	24 h
Insuman Comb 15	30 min to 1 h	2–4 h	11–20 h
Insuman Comb 25	30 min to 1 h	2–4 h	12–19 h
Insuman Comb 50	<30 min	1.5–4 h	12–16 h
Mixtard 10	<30 min	2–8 h	24 h
Mixtard 20	<30 min	2–8 h	24 h
Mixtard 30	<30 min	2–8 h	24 h
Mixtard 40	<30 min	2–8 h	24 h
Mixtard 50	<30 min	2–8 h	24 h
NovoMix 30	<10–20 min	1–4 h	24 h
Pork Mixtard 30	30 min	4–8 h	24 h
Isophane Insulin Injection			
Humulin I	30 min to 1 h	1–8 h	22 h
Hypurin Bovine Isophane	<2 h	6–12 h	18–24 h
Hypurin Porcine Isophane	<2 h	6–12 h	18–24 h
Insulatard	<1.5 h	4–12 h	24 h
Insuman Basal	<1 h	3–4 h	11–20 h
Pork Insulatard	1.5 h	4–12 h	24 h
Hypurin Bovine Lente	2 h	8–12 h	30 h
Hypurin Bovine PZI	4–6 h	10–20 h	24–36 h
Lantus (Insulin Glargine)	2.5 h	–	24 h
Levemir (Insulin Detemir)	2.5 h	–	24 h
Exubera	10–20 min	2 h	6 h

Reproduced with permission from the Monthly Index of Medical Specialities. The chart is subject to change as companies develop their products. Source from emims: http://www.healthcarerepublic.com/mims/Tables/28933/insulin-preparations/

[a]Insulin Lispro, human insulin analogue.

[b]Speed of onset is proportional to amount of soluble insulin.

accurate than when more dilute solutions are used. For intravenous doses see diabetic ketoacidosis, below.

DOSE

The total daily output of endogenous insulin from pancreatic islet cells is 30–40 units (determined by the needs of completely pancreatectomised patients), and most insulin-deficient diabetics need 30–50 units insulin per day (0.5–0.8 units/kg).

Initial treatment for a Type 1 patient who does not present with ketoacidosis will usually be outside hospital with one of the regimens described above. A guide to initial daily dose requirement is:

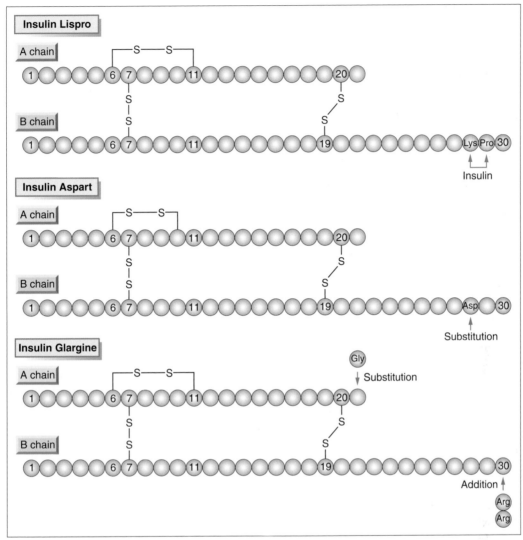

Fig. 35.2 Amino acid alterations in Insulin Lispro, Insulin Aspart and Insulin Glargine. (Redrawn from Hirsch I B 2005 Insulin analogues. New England Journal of Medicine 352:174–183.)

- 0.3 units/kg (16–20 units daily)
- increasing to 0.5 units/kg.

If using biphasic insulin, *two-thirds* of the daily dose may be given in the morning and *one-third* in the evening. If using the multiple injection regimen, a suggested initial dose is 10–15 units of long-acting insulin at night and 4–8 units of short-acting insulin with meals.

The dose is adjusted according to the blood glucose. Daily (total) dose increments should be 4 units at 3–4-day intervals.

Physical activity increases carbohydrate utilisation and insulin sensitivity, so that hypoglycaemia is likely if a well stabilised patient changes suddenly from an inactive existence to a vigorous life. If this is likely to happen the carbohydrate in the diet may be increased and/or the dose of insulin reduced by up to one-third and then readjusted according to need.

ADVERSE EFFECTS OF INSULIN

Adverse effects of insulin are mainly those of overdose. Because the brain relies on glucose as its source of energy, an adequate blood glucose concentration is just as essential as an adequate supply of oxygen, and *hypoglycaemia* may lead to coma, convulsions and even death (in 4% of diabetics aged less than 50 years).

Diagnosis of hypoglycaemia should generally be confirmed before administration of intravenous glucose to comatose diabetics. Glucose can cause a brisk and potentially hazardous rise in serum potassium levels, in contrast to effects in non-diabetics in whom glucose causes a fall in serum potassium concentration.

Hypoglycaemia may manifest itself as disturbed sleep (nightmares) and morning headache. For details of treatment see below.

Lipodystrophy (atrophy or hypertrophy) at the injection sites is rare with modern, purified insulins and patient education to rotate the site of injection. If lipodystrophy is present, the site should be avoided because of erratic absorption of insulin.

Generalised allergic reactions are very rare.

TREATMENT OF A HYPOGLYCAEMIC ATTACK

Prevention depends largely upon patient education, but it is an unavoidable aspect of intensive glycaemic control. Patients should not miss meals, must know the early symptoms of an attack, and always carry glucose with them.

Treatment is to give sugar, either by mouth if the patient can still swallow or glucose (dextrose) i.v. (20–50 mL 50% solution, i.e. 10–25 g). This concentration is irritant, especially if extravasation occurs; the veins of diabetics are precious, so compress the vein immediately after completion of injection. Administration of 50–100 mL 20% glucose, if available, is less thrombotic. The response is usually dramatic.

The patient should be given a snack containing slowly absorbable carbohydrate to avoid relapse.

After prolonged hypoglycaemia, cerebral oedema may occur. If the patient does not respond to i.v. glucose within 30 min, i.v. dexamethasone should be given.

After large overdoses of insulin or sulphonylurea, 20% glucose should be given by continuous i.v. infusion. Very severe attacks sometimes damage the central nervous system (CNS) permanently. (See also use of glucagon, below.)

After recovery from a severe attack and elucidation of the cause, the patient's treatment regimen should be carefully reviewed with appropriate educational input.

Hypoglycaemia due to other causes, e.g. alcohol, changes in diet or exercise activity, is treated similarly.

INSULIN RESISTANCE AND HORMONES THAT INCREASE BLOOD GLUCOSE

Insulin resistance may be due to a decline in number and/or affinity of receptors (see above) or to defects in postreceptor mechanisms.

A diabetic patient requiring more than 200 units/day is rare and regarded as insulin resistant (occasional patients have needed as much as 5000 units/day). Insulin resistance has become much less frequent since the advent of purified insulins. If the requirement is acquired and genuine, it is due to antibodies binding insulin or its receptor. This can occur in patients with systemic lupus erythematosus or lymphoma. Insulin resistance also occurs in a small number of genetic syndromes, e.g. due to mutations in *PPARγ*.[5] Severe cases of insulin resistance may be suspected from presence of the skin condition acanthosis nigricans.

Glucagon ($t_{1/2}$ 4 min) is a polypeptide hormone (29 amino acids) from the β-islet cells of the pancreas. It is released in response to hypoglycaemia and is a physiological regulator of insulin effect, acting by causing the release of liver glycogen as glucose. Glucagon is used as a stopgap treatment for insulin-induced hypoglycaemia. But in about 45 min from onset of coma the hepatic glycogen will be exhausted and glucagon will be useless. Its chief advantage is that, as it can be given s.c. or i.m. (1.0 mg), glucagon can be used in a severe hypoglycaemic attack by somebody, e.g. a member of the patient's family, who is unable to give an i.v. injection of glucose.

Glucagon has a positive cardiac inotropic effect by stimulating adenylyl cyclase. In acute overdose of β-adrenoceptor blockers, cardiogenic shock unresponsive to atropine is probably best treated with glucagon 2–10 mg i.v. in glucose 5% followed by infusion of 50 micrograms/kg/h (see p. 432).

---

[5] The importance of PPARγ (peroxisome proliferator-activated receptor γ) in insulin sensitivity was confirmed by the finding, in Cambridge, of two families presenting with severe insulin resistance in whom rare mutations of the *PPARγ* gene caused loss of PPARγ activity (Barroso I, Gurnell M, Crowley V E et al 1989 Dominant negative mutations in human PPARgamma associated with severe insulin resistance, diabetes mellitus and hypertension. Nature 402:880–883).

Adrenaline (epinephrine) raises the blood sugar concentration by mobilising liver and muscle glycogen (a β_2-adrenoceptor effect), and suppressing secretion of insulin (an α-adrenoceptor effect). Hyperglycaemia may occur in patients with phaeochromocytoma, and is usually reversed by α-adrenoceptor blockade (see p. 404).

Adrenal steroids, either endogenous or exogenous, antagonise the actions of insulin, although this effect is only slight with the primarily mineralocorticoid group; the glucocorticoid hormones increase gluconeogenesis and reduce glucose uptake and utilisation by the tissues. Patients with Cushing's syndrome thus develop diabetes very readily and may be resistant to insulin. Patients with Addison's disease, hypothyroidism and hypopituitarism are abnormally sensitive to insulin action.

Oral contraceptives can impair carbohydrate tolerance.

Growth hormone antagonises the actions of insulin in the tissues. Acromegalic patients may develop insulin-resistant diabetes.

Thyroid hormone increases the requirements for insulin.

ORAL ANTIDIABETES DRUGS

Oral antidiabetes drugs are of three kinds: *sulphonamide* derivatives (sulphonylureas), *guanidine* derivatives (biguanides) and *thiazolidinediones*. The discovery of sulphonylureas was serendipitous. In 1930 it was noted that sulphonamides could cause hypoglycaemia, and in 1942 severe hypoglycaemia was found in patients with typhoid fever during a therapeutic trial of sulphonamide. Sulphonylureas were introduced into clinical practice in 1954.

MODE OF ACTION

Sulphonylureas block the ATP-sensitive potassium channels on the β-islet cell plasma membrane. This results in the release of stored insulin in response to glucose. Sulphonylureas do not stimulate insulin synthesis. They appear to enhance insulin action on liver, muscle and adipose tissue by increasing insulin receptor number and by enhancing the complex post-receptor enzyme reactions mediated by insulin. The principal result is decreased hepatic glucose

output and increased glucose uptake in muscle. Sulphonylureas are ineffective in totally insulin-deficient patients, and successful therapy probably requires about 30% of normal β-cell function to be present. Their main *adverse effects* are hypoglycaemia and weight gain.

Secondary failure (after months or years) occurs due to declining β-cell function and to insulin resistance.

Biguanides have been avaialble since 1957. *Metformin* is now the only biguanide in use, and is a major agent in the management of Type 2 diabetes. Its cellular mode of action is uncertain but the most important effect is reduction of hepatic glucose production. Recent studies have identified the intracellular target of metformin in the liver as the enzyme adenosine monophosphate-activated protein kinase (AMPK). This is a conserved regulator of the cellular response to low energy, and is activated when intracellular ATP concentrations decrease and AMP concentrations increase. Such increases normally occur in response to reduced nutrient supply, or increased energy demands, e.g. exercise. In effect, therefore, metformin fools the liver into 'thinking' that the body is starved, or exercising, and that hepatic gluconeogenesis needs to be switched off.[6] Metformin may have other minor actions, including enhancement of peripheral insulin sensitivity increasing glucose uptake in peripheral tissues. The drug is ineffective in the absence of insulin.

Metformin can be used in combination with either insulin or other oral hypoglycaemic agents.

Thiazolidinediones. *Pioglitazone* and *rosiglitazone* reduce peripheral insulin resistance, leading to a reduction of blood glucose concentration. These drugs stimulate the nuclear hormone receptor, peroxisome proliferator-activated receptor (PPARγ), which causes differentiation of adipocytes. They are generally less effective in controlling diabetes than either metformin or sulphonylureas. In the UK, the National Institute for Health and Clinical Excellence (NICE) advises that the use of a thiazolidinedione is

---

[6]The discovery of the AMPK response, and of other players in the pathway, has enabled experiments to be performed in which the hepatic response to metformin is selectively knocked out. In the mouse, at least, these experiments show that actions of metformin at other sites are of little importance.

recommended only as a replacement for metformin or sulphonylurea in:

- patients who are unable to tolerate metformin and sulphonylurea in combination therapy, or
- patients in whom either metformin or a sulphonylurea is contraindicated.

Thiazolidinediones can cause 3–4 kg of weight gain in the first year of use, with peripheral oedema in 3–4% of patients. The hope that this class, by increasing insulin sensitivity, may have beneficial influence on cardiovascular outcome has not been supported. In the PROACTIVE study of 5238 patients with diabetes and macrovascular disease, pioglitazone achieved only a non-significant trend to reduction, compared with placebo, in the primary endpoint[7]. In the CHICAGO study, however, pioglitazone was more effective than a sulphonylurea in preventing carotid atherosclerosis in 462 patients with diabetes.[8] In the DREAM study of 5269 patients with impaired glucose tolerance, rosiglitazone slowed onset of diabetes, but by no more than could be explained by the fall in blood glucose.[9]

Other drugs

Meglitinides (Table 35.2) are short-acting insulin secretagogues that act like the sulphonylureas.

Incretin analogues and mimetics

Exenatide is a functional analogue of glucagon-like peptide-1 (GLP-1), a naturally occurring peptide that enhances insulin secretion in response to raised plasma glucose concentrations. It is indicated as adjunctive therapy to improve glycaemic control in patients with Type 2 diabetes mellitus who are taking metformin, a sulphonylurea, or a combination of both, but have not achieved adequate glycaemic control. A bonus may be slight reduction in weight, but the cost may be a small incidence of nausea and vomiting. The recommended dose is 5–10 micrograms twice daily, administered subcutaneously within the 60 min interval prior to the morning and evening meal.

Dipeptidyl peptidase-4 (DPP-4) inhibitors improve glucose control by inhibiting breakdown of GLP-1. Vildagliptin and sitagliptin are used at 100 mg daily.

INDIVIDUAL DRUGS

Absorption from the alimentary tract is satisfactory for all the oral agents. It is advisable to take drugs about 30 min before a meal. These three groups of drugs are effective only in the presence of insulin. If a patient fails to respond to one drug, response to another as single treatment is unlikely. Proceeding to a combination of drugs from different classes may then be effective, provided the patient is not insulin deficient.

Sulphonylureas (see also Table 35.2)

Several are available. Choice is determined by the duration of action as well as the patient's age and

[7]This was a composite of all-cause mortality, non-fatal myocardial infarction, stroke, acute coronary syndrome, endovascular or surgical intervention in the coronary or leg arteries, and amputation above the ankle (Dormandy J A, Charbonnel B, Eckland D J et al 2005 Secondary prevention of macrovascular events in patients with Type 2 diabetes in the PROACTIVE Study (PROspective pioglitAzone Clinical Trial In macroVascular Events): a randomised controlled trial. Lancet 366:1279–1289).

[8]CHICAGO, Carotid intima-media tHICkness in Atherosclerosis using pioGlitazOne (Mazzone T, Meyer P M, Feinstein S B et al 2006 Effect of pioglitazone compared with glimepiride on carotid intima–media thickness in type 2 diabetes: a randomized trial. Journal of the American Medical Association 296(21):2572–2581).

[9]DREAM, Diabetes REduction Assessment with ramipril and rosiglitazone Medication (Gerstein H C, Yusuf S, Bosch J et al 2006 Effect of rosiglitazone on the frequency of diabetes in patients with impaired glucose tolerance or impaired fasting glucose: a randomised controlled trial. Lancet 368:1096–1105).

Table 35.2 Principal oral antidiabetes drugs

Drug	Total daily dose (mg)	Dosing schedule (doses/day)	Duration of action (h)
Sulphonylureas			
glibeclamide	2.5–20	1–2	12–24
gliclazide	40–320	1–2	12–24
glipizide	2.5–40	1–2	12–24
glimepiride	1–6	1	16–24
Biguanide			
metformin	500–3000	2–3	8–12
Thiazolidinedione			
rosiglitazone	2–8	1–2	12–24
pioglitazone	15–30	1	16–24
Meglitinide			
repaglinide	0.5–16	3	3–4
nateglinide	60–180	3	2–3
α-glucosidase inhibitor			
acarbose	50–300	3	3–4

Other sulphonylureas include tolbutamide, gliquidone, glibornuride, tolazamide.

renal function, and unwanted effects. The long-acting sulphonylureas, e.g. *glibenclamide*, are associated with a greater risk of hypoglycaemia; for this reason they should be avoided in the elderly for whom the shorter-acting alternatives, such as *gliclazide* or *tolbutamide*, are preferred. Chlorpropamide is both long-acting and has more unwanted effects (see below); it is no longer recommended. In patients with impaired renal function, gliclazide, glipizide and tolbutamide are preferred as they are not excreted by the kidney. Generally, it is prudent to start at the lowest recommended dose in order to minimise risk of hypoglycaemia.

Sulphonamides, as expected, potentiate sulphonylureas by direct action and by displacement from plasma proteins.

Gliclazide is a commonly used second-generation agent. If the dose exceeds 80 mg, the drug should be taken twice daily before meals, or once daily if prescribed as a modified-release preparation.

Glimepiride is designed to be used once daily and provokes less hypoglycaemia than glibenclamide.

Repaglinide is a very short-acting oral hypoglycaemic agent ($t_{1/2}$ 1 h) whose action, like that of the sulphonylureas, is mediated through blockade of ATP-dependent potassium channels. It affects only postprandial insulin profiles, and should in theory reduce risk of hypoglycaemia.

Biguanides (see also Table 35.2)

Metformin ($t_{1/2}$ 5 h) is taken with or after meals. It has a mild anorexic effect which helps to reduce weight in the obese. Its chief use is in the obese patient with Type 2 diabetes either alone or in combination with a sulphonylurea.

Minor adverse reactions are common, including nausea, diarrhoea and a metallic taste in the mouth. These symptoms are usually transient or subside after reduction of dose. Heavy prolonged use can cause vitamin B_{12} deficiency due to malabsorption. With a biguanide, ketonuria may occur in the presence of normal blood sugar levels. This is not generally severe and responds to reduction of dose.

More serious, but rare, is *lactic acidosis*, which occurs in 0.03 cases per 1000 patient-years. When this condition does occur, it is usually against the background of renal impairment, liver failure, or cardiogenic or septic shock. Metformin is therefore contraindicated in these conditions, including relatively mild renal impairment (plasma creatinine >125 micromoles/L in women, >135 micromoles/L in men).

Metformin should also be withdrawn temporarily before general anaesthesia and administration of iodine-containing contrast media, which might precipitate renal impairment. During pregnancy, metformin should be substituted by insulin. Lactic acidosis is treated with large (i.v.) doses of isotonic sodium bicarbonate.

Thiazolidinediones (see also Table 35.2)

Pioglitazone is indicated once daily in patients not controlled by metformin alone. It is contraindicated by cardiac or hepatic failure. Weight gain and oedema are the main adverse effects.

Rosiglitazone is similar and is administered once or twice daily.

PRECAUTIONS WITH ORAL AGENTS

Hypoglycaemia is the most common adverse effect with sulphonylureas, but is less common than with insulin therapy. It can be severe and prolonged (for days), and may be fatal in 10% of cases, especially in the elderly and patients with heart failure. Erroneous alternative diagnoses such as stroke may be made.

Renal and hepatic disease. A biguanide should not be used in patients with either condition as the risk of lactic acidosis is too great. Sulphonylureas are potentiated in these diseases and a drug with a short $t_{1/2}$ (i.e. not glibenclamide) should be used in low dose.

Age adds to the hazard of oral agents.

Other adverse effects are rare but include skin rashes, gastrointestinal upset, minor derangement of haematological and hepatic indices.

Other oral agents

Acarbose is an α-glucosidase inhibitor that reduces the digestion of complex carbohydrates and slows their absorption from the gut; in high doses it may cause actual malabsorption. Acarbose reduces glycaemia after meals and may improve overall glycaemic control. The usual dose is 50–300 mg/day. *Adverse effects* are mainly flatulence and diarrhoea, which lead to a high discontinuation rate. The drug may be combined with a sulphonylurea.

Dietary fibre and diabetes. The addition of gel-forming (soluble) but unabsorbable fibre (guar gum, a hydrocolloidal polysaccharide of galactose and mannose from seeds of the 'cluster bean') to the diet of diabetics reduces carbohydrate absorption and flattens the postprandial blood glucose curve. Reduced need for insulin and oral agents has been reported, but adequate amounts (taken with lots of water) are unpleasant (flatulence) and patient compliance is therefore poor.

TREATMENT OF DIABETES MELLITUS

Doctor, nurse and patient are faced with a lifetime of collaboration. Compliance is not a one-sided process, and the patients need all the consideration and support they can get. They should learn about their disease and its management, including home monitoring of blood glucose, and about the need for appropriate diet, exercise and avoidance of smoking.

All Type 1 patients need immediate insulin therapy. Initial therapy in Type 2 patients should be by dietary means alone, for 2–3 months, but most patients will need oral antidiabetes drugs in addtion.

The *aims of treatment* are:

- to alleviate symptomatic hyperglycaemia and improve quality of life, while avoiding hypoglycaemia
- to avoid ketosis and infections
- to keep:
  - the fasting blood glucose at <6 mmol/L
  - the 1-h postprandial concentration at <9 mmol/L
  - the glycosylated haemoglobin (HbA1c) as close to normal (<6.2%) as possible.

In addition to optimal glycaemic control, other cardiovascular risk factors should be corrected:

- optimal blood pressure control <130/80 mmHg
- low-density lipoprotein (LDL) cholesterol <2.5 mmol/L[10]
- triglycerides <2.0 mmol/L
- by this regimen to avoid or delay long-term microvascular and macrovascular complications, and reduce mortality.

Each patient must be assessed individually; only an outline of the general principles involved can be given here.

Diet. Patients should be allowed to follow their own preferences as far as is practicable. They should receive dietary advice on a high complex carbohydrate diet (approx. 65% of total calories) with low fat (<30% of calories) and an emphasis on reduction in saturated fat in favour of mono- and poly-unsaturates. Calories should be restricted and patients encouraged to achieve an ideal body-weight. Diet should contain about 40 g fibre per day, with plenty of fresh fruit and vegetables.

The way in which carbohydrate is distributed through the day should correspond with the type of drug treatment, and especially the type of insulin in Type 1 patients.

Type 1 patients are initially underweight, whereas the reverse is true of Type 2. Although carbohydrate intake needs to be controlled in both types, overall energy intake is restricted initially only in the obese Type 2 patients. Other general factors that influence the diet, in both Types 1 and 2, are the:

- high incidence of ischaemic heart disease in diabetics, requiring restriction of saturated fat intake
- need to reduce protein intake in patients with established nephropathy.

Weight. Older overweight diabetics (70% of Type 2) have a relative deficiency of insulin but seldom develop ketosis. In these patients, a hypocaloric (weight-reducing) diet is vital, as weight loss dramatically improves glycaemic control and, indeed, glycosuria may cease when their weight is reduced. It is also likely that effective dieting helps to prevent macrovascular disease through improved control of blood lipids and blood pressure. Exercise is similarly beneficial. *Biguanide* treatment in particular helps weight reduction. Weight loss is associated with an increased number of insulin receptors, and so an increase in responsiveness to insulin. The use of anorectic agents is discussed below.

Young patients with Type 1 diabetes are often underweight and need insulin to restore normal

---

[10]European and American advice differs on treatment of hyperlipidaemia, reflecting the lack of evidence on thresholds and targets for treatment. The UK advice is to give a statin to all patients with diabetes aged more than 40 years, and to higher-risk patients younger than this. The LDL target recommended in the text is taken from the American Diabetes Association recommendation to achieve a LDL concentration of 100 mg/dL.

weight. Calorie restriction is not required initially in these patients. The blood of these young diabetics contains negligible insulin and they readily become ketotic.

SELECTION OF THERAPY FOR DIABETES

Patients are treated with:

- Diet alone
- Diet plus oral agent(s)
- Diet plus insulin
- Diet plus oral agent (metformin) plus insulin
- For ketoacidosis: soluble insulin, urgently.

Diabetic patients under 30 years: almost all need insulin; the exception is the rare single-gene disorder of maturity-onset diabetes of the young (MODY), which is usually due to mutations in the glucokinase gene.

Diabetic patients over 30 years: approximately one-third need insulin, one-third oral agents and one-third diet alone.

Type 1 diabetes: human insulin is used for new patients (for regimen see below).

Type 2 diabetes: careful trial is the only sure way of deciding who can be maintained on oral therapy rather than insulin. About 30% of patients will be adequately managed without oral therapy. When diet alone has failed to control Type 2 diabetes, it is necessary to add an oral agent; the choice should fall first on:

- *metformin* for the *obese* patient: the usual regimen is metformin 500 mg once or twice daily after meals, increasing at 2–4-week intervals to a maximum of 3 g/day.
- a *sulphonylurea* for the *non-obese*: an example regimen would be gliclazide 80 mg/day orally (or 40 mg in the small or aged) before the main meal of the day. The dose is adjusted, according to response, at 2–4-week intervals by increments of 40–80 mg, to a maximum of 320 mg/day. If control is incomplete, metformin may be added.

Insulin treatment in type 2 diabetes. When oral therapy fails, insulin treatment should be used alone or in combination with metformin. There is little advantage from adding insulin to a sulphonylurea. If a patient is taking metformin in combination with a sulphonylurea and/or a thiazolidinedione, the latter drugs should be discontinued when progressing to insulin. Definitive evidence that institution of insulin will reduce complications is lacking; however, there is an improvement in quality of life, with few patients requesting to stop insulin once they have started, and the improved glycaemic control can be assumed also to improve outcome. Initial treatment with a single injection of an intermediate-acting insulin (see Fig. 35.1) at night, or twice daily, may control hyperglycaemia. Fluctuations in blood glucose levels may be controlled with twice-daily mixed insulin or by multiple injections.

Re-evaluation of the requirement for drugs can be made after the patient has been controlled and stable for 3–6 months, but complete withdrawal of oral agents is unusual.

Monitoring of patients taking oral agents should be as close as those on insulin. The prognosis of poorly controlled Type 2 diabetes is serious.

Prevention of complications in Type 2 diabetics: the UK Prospective Diabetes Study (UKPDS).[11,12] This landmark study of Type 2 diabetes confirmed that good glycaemic control and aggressive blood pressure reduction independently improve outcome. For every 1% reduction in haemoglobin A1c (HbA1c) there was a 21% reduction in diabetes-related deaths and a 37% reduction in microvascular disease. The study disproved concerns about long-term safety of sulphonylureas, but suggested that metformin might be the preferred first-line pharmacological therapy in obese patients. Of highest importance was the finding that effective blood pressure control – regardless of the type of antihypertensive drug – was more influential than glycaemic control in preventing macrovascular complications. Reduction of blood pressure in 758 patients to a mean of 144/82 mmHg achieved a 32% reduction in deaths related to diabetes and a 37% reduction in microvascular endpoints,

[11]UK Prospective Diabetes Study (UKPDS) Group 1998 Effect of intensive blood-glucose control with metformin on complications in overweight patients with Type 2 diabetes (UKPDS 34). Lancet 352:854–865.

[12]UK Prospective Diabetes Study (UKPDS) Group 1998 Tight blood pressure control and risk of macrovascular and microvascular complications in Type 2 diabetes. British Medical Journal 317:703–713.

compared with findings in 390 patients treated to a blood pressure of 154/87 mmHg.

Type 1 treatment. The range of insulin formulations available allows flexible adjustment of the regimen to the patient's way of life. No single regimen suits all patients but one of the following regimens can suit most patients (see also Table 35.2):

- Three doses of prandial insulin (soluble given before main meals, analogue with meals) plus an intermediate-acting or long-acting insulin at bedtime.
- A biphasic or intermediate-acting insulin two or three times a day before meals.
- A single morning dose of a biphasic or intermediate-acting insulin before breakfast may suffice for some patients.

Injection technique has pharmacokinetic consequences according to whether the insulin is delivered into the subcutaneous tissue or (inadvertently) into muscle and patients should standardise their technique. The introduction of a range of needles of appropriate length and pen-shaped injectors has enabled patients to inject perpendicularly to the skin without risk of intramuscular injection. The absorption of insulin is as much as 50% more rapid from shallow intramuscular injection. Clearly factors such as heat or exercise that alter skin or muscle blood flow can markedly alter the rate of insulin absorption.

Inadvertent intramuscular injection of an overnight dose of an extended-duration insulin can lead to hypoglycaemia and inadequate early morning control of blood glucose. Sites of injection should be rotated to minimise the now rare local complications (lipodystrophy). Absorption is faster from arm and abdomen than it is from thigh and buttock.

Complications of diabetes. A well controlled diabetic is less liable to ketosis and infections. It is now certain that good control of glycaemia mitigates the serious microvascular complications of retinopathy, nephropathy, neuropathy and cataract. Too tight control of glycaemia can increase the frequency of attacks of hypoglycaemia. The question of whether good glycaemic control reduces the risk of cardiovascular complications has now been resolved by the EDIC extension of the DCCT. This showed that a 1.7% difference in HbA1c was associated, over 17 years, with a 57% reduction in the risk of

non-fatal myocardial infarction, stroke or death from cardiovascular disease ($P = 0.02$).[13]

SOME FACTORS AFFECTING CONTROL OF DIABETES

Intercurrent illnesses cause fluctuations in the patient's metabolic needs. If these are severe, e.g. myocardial infarction, it is prudent to substitute insulin for oral agents. Infections increase insulin need (20–50%), which may drop briskly on recovery. In patients with poor glycaemic control, it is preferable to use an insulin infusion and sliding scale, as described below for diabetic ketosis.

Surgery, see below.

Menstruation and oral contraception: insulin needs may rise slightly.

Use of glucocorticoids: insulin needs are increased.

In pregnancy close control of diabetes is of the first importance to avoid fetal loss at all stages, and in the first trimester to reduce fetal malformations. Insulin requirements increase steadily after the third month. Ideally, women of childbearing age should be advised to conceive during a period of stable, euglycaemic control.

During labour soluble insulin should be given by continuous i.v. infusion at about 1–2 units/h with i.v. infusion of 5% glucose 1.0 L in 8 h. Substantially less, e.g. 25%, insulin is likely to be needed immediately after delivery, when timing and dose of insulin injections should be carefully reconsidered lest hypoglycaemia occur. Insulin need remains lower during the first 6 weeks of lactation.

Blood glucose estimations are necessary during pregnancy, for glycosuria is not then a reliable guide. The renal threshold for glucose (also of lactose) falls, so that glycosuria and lactosuria may occur in the presence of a normal blood glucose.

Maternal hyperglycaemia leads to fetal hyperglycaemia with consequent fetal islet cell hyperplasia, high birth-weight babies and postnatal hypoglycaemia.

---

[13] The Diabetes Control and Complications Trial/ Epidemiology of Diabetes Interventions and Complications (DCCT/EDIC) Study Research Group 2005 Intensive diabetes treatment and cardiovascular disease in patients with Type 1 diabetes. New England Journal of Medicine 353:2643–2653.

Premature labour: use of β_2-adrenoceptor agonists and of dexamethasone (to prevent respiratory distress syndrome in the prematurely newborn) causes hyperglycaemia and increased insulin (and potassium) need.

Current practice for women on *oral hypoglycaemic* agents who are planning, or starting, a pregnancy is to change to insulin and continue on it throughout pregnancy. There is no definitive evidence that oral drugs are associated with fetal malformations.

INTERACTIONS WITH NON-DIABETES DRUGS

The subject is ill documented, but whenever a diabetic under treatment takes other drugs it is prudent to be on the watch for disturbance of control.

β-adrenoceptor blocking drugs impair the sympathetically mediated (β_2 receptor) release of glucose from the liver in response to hypoglycaemia and also reduce the adrenergically mediated symptoms of hypoglycaemia (except sweating). Insulin hypoglycaemia is thus both more prolonged and less noticeable. A diabetic needing a β-adrenoceptor blocker should be given a β_1-selective member, e.g. *bisoprolol*.

Thiazide diuretics at a higher dose than those now generally used in hypertension can precipitate diabetes.

Hepatic enzyme inducers may enhance the metabolism of sulphonylureas that are metabolised in the liver (tolbutamide). Cimetidine, an *inhibitor* of drug-metabolising enzymes, increases metformin plasma concentration and effect.

Monoamine oxidase inhibitors potentiate oral agents and perhaps also insulin. They can also reduce appetite and so upset control.

Interaction may occur with *alcohol* (hypoglycaemia with any antidiabetes drug).

Salicylates and *fibrates* can increase insulin sensitivity.

The action of *sulphonylureas* is intensified by heavy sulphonamide dosage, and some sulphonamides increase free tolbutamide concentrations, probably by competing for plasma protein binding sites. These examples suffice to show that the possibility of interactions of practical clinical importance is a real one.

DRUG-INDUCED DIABETES

Diazoxide (see p. 424) is chemically similar to thiazide diuretics, but stimulates the ATP-dependent K+ channel that is blocked by the sulphonylureas. Therefore its chronic use as an antihypertensive agent is precluded by the development of diabetes. Indeed its use in therapeutics should now be confined to the rare indication of treating hypoglycaemia due to islet-cell tumour (insulinoma). Adrenocortical steroids are also diabetogenic.

DIABETIC KETOACIDOSIS

The condition is discussed in detail in medical texts and only the more pharmacological aspects will be considered here.

The patients are always severely dehydrated and fluid replacement is the first priority. In severe ketoacidosis the patient urgently needs insulin to stop ketogenesis. The objective is to supply, as continuously as possible, a moderate amount of insulin.

Soluble insulin should be given by continuous i.v. infusion of a 1-unit/mL solution of insulin in isotonic sodium chloride. If a pump is not available, the insulin should be added in a concentration of 1 unit/mL to 50–100 mL sodium chloride in a burette. The infusion rate is determined by a sliding scale, as illustrated in Table 35.3. The rate is adjusted hourly using the same scale. Stringent precautions against septicaemia are necessary in these patients. Continuous i.m. (not s.c.) infusion can also be equally effective, provided the patient is not in shock and there is not an important degree of peripheral vascular disease.

Intermittent doses i.v. or i.m. may be used when circumstances demand. If the i.m. route is used, a priming dose of 10 units should be given at the outset and then 6–10 units hourly.

Table 35.3 Sliding scale of insulin doses according to blood glucose concentrations in diabetic ketoacidosis (see text)	
Blood glucose (mmol/L)	**Infusion rate (mL/h = units/h for 50-mL syringe containing 50 units insulin)**
≥22.0	10.0 (and check pump and connections)
19–21.9	8.0
16–18.9	6.0
12–15.9	4.0
8–11.9	2.0 (and change from saline to glucose infusion if blood glucose <10 mmol/L)
4–7.9	1.0
<3.9	0.5 (and increase glucose infusion)

Progress. When the patient can eat and drink, s.c. insulin is restarted. The rate of fall of blood glucose per hour is proportional to the rate of infusion of insulin over the range of 1–10 units/h. A reasonable rate of fall during treatment is 4–5.5 mmol/L (75–100 mg/100 mL) per hour.

Intravenous fluid and electrolytes. Patients are often more deficient in water than in saline and, although initial replacement is by isotonic (0.9%) sodium chloride solution, occurrence of hypernatraemia is an indication for half isotonic (0.45%) solution. A patient with diabetic ketoacidosis may have a fluid deficit of above 5 L and may be given:

- 1 L in the first hour, followed by
- 2 L in 4 h, then
- 4 L in the next 24 h, watching for signs of fluid overload.

Note that fluid replacement causes a fall in blood glucose concentration by dilution.

Glucose should be given only when its concentration in blood falls below the renal threshold, in practice starting when the blood glucose level falls to 10 mmol/L. If glucose is used at concentrations above the renal threshold it merely increases the diabetic osmotic diuresis, causing further dehydration and potassium and magnesium loss (but see Hypoglycaemia, above). When the blood glucose concentration falls to 10 mmol/L, the fluid replacement should be changed from saline to 5% glucose, at the same rate as detailed above.

Potassium. Even if plasma potassium concentration is normal or high, patients have a substantial total body deficit, and the plasma level will fall briskly with i.v. saline (dilution) and insulin, which draws potassium into cells within minutes. Potassium chloride should be added to the second and subsequent litres of fluid according to plasma potassium (provided the patient is passing urine):

- <3.5 mmol/L: add 40 mmol/L of fluid
- 3.5–5.0 mmol/L: add 20 mmol/L of fluid
- >5.0 mmol/L: none.

Bicarbonate (isotonic) should be used only if plasma pH is <7.0 and peripheral circulation is good; insulin corrects acidosis.

Success in treatment of diabetic ketoacidosis and its complications (hypokalaemia, aspiration of stomach contents, infection, shock, thromboembolism, cerebral oedema) depends on close, constant, informed supervision.

Mild diabetic ketosis. If the patient is fully conscious and there has been no nausea or vomiting for at least 12 h, intravenous therapy is unnecessary. It is reasonable to give small doses of insulin s.c. 4–6-hourly and fluids by mouth.

Hyperosmolar diabetic coma occurs chiefly in non-insulin-dependent diabetics who fail to compensate for their continuing osmotic glucose diuresis. It is characterised by severe dehydration, a very high blood sugar level (>33 mmol/L), and lack of ketosis and acidosis. Treatment is with isotonic (0.9%) saline, at half the rate recommended for ketoacidotic coma, and with less potassium than in severe ketoacidosis. Insulin requirements are less than in ketoacidosis, where the acidosis causes resistance to the actions of insulin, and should generally be half those shown in Table 35.3. Patients are more liable to thrombosis and prophylactic heparin is used.

SURGERY IN DIABETIC PATIENTS

PRINCIPLES OF MANAGEMENT:

- Surgery constitutes a major stress.
- Insulin needs increase with surgery.
- Avoid ketosis.
- Avoid hypoglycaemia.

High blood glucose concentration matters little over short periods, except in the critically ill. The programme for control should be agreed between anaesthetist and physician whenever diabetic patients must undergo general anaesthesia or modify their diets. There are many different techniques that can give satisfactory results.

TYPE 1 DIABETES

Elective major surgery

- Admit to hospital the day before surgery.
- Arrange surgery for the morning.
- Evening before surgery: give patient's usual insulin.

- Day of operation: omit morning s.c. dose; set up i.v. infusion: glucose 5% + KCl 20 mmol/L, infuse at 100 mL/h; insulin should be infused by pump at an approximate rate of 2 units/h and adjusted according to a sliding scale.
- Modify regimen during and after surgery according to monitoring; insulin doses should be adjusted according to similar scale as that in Table 35.3.
- Stop i.v. infusion 1 h after first post-surgical s.c. insulin.
- Insulin requirements may be high, 10–15 units/h, in cases of serious infection, corticosteroid use, obesity, liver disease.

Minor surgery

For example, simple dental extractions (for multiple extractions or when there is infection the patient should be admitted to hospital). A suitable postoperative diet of appropriate calorie and carbohydrate content must be arranged. Plan the operation for between 12 noon and 5 pm (17:00 hours). Omit the usual dose of long-acting insulin on the morning of the operation and substitute soluble insulin, one-quarter of the usual total daily dose, before a light breakfast 6 h before the operation. Arrange a light evening meal after the operation and soluble insulin, 10–20 units s.c., according to the blood glucose level. Return to the normal routine the next day.

Emergency surgery

When a surgical emergency is complicated by diabetic ketosis, an attempt should be made to control the ketosis before surgery. Management during the operation will be similar to that for major surgery except that more insulin will be needed.

In other cases small doses of soluble insulin are given 2–4-hourly (where pumps are not available), keeping the blood glucose concentration between 5 and 8 mmol/L.

TYPE 2 DIABETES

Elective and emergency surgery, and minor surgery if Type 2 is poorly controlled: use the same regimen as for Type 1.

Minor surgery: if diabetes is well controlled, omit the oral hypoglycaemic agent on the morning of surgery.

More than minor surgery: monitor blood glucose carefully, and use soluble insulin s.c. or by infusion if blood glucose concentration rises. If vomiting is likely, use insulin.

MISCELLANEOUS

Most patients with both Type 1 and Type 2 succumb to either the macrovascular or microvascular complications – especially ischaemic heart disease and diabetic nephropathy, respectively. Indeed diabetes is the major indication for dialysis and transplantation. As discussed in other chapters, the treatment of hypertension and hyperlipidaemia is particularly important in patients with diabetes. Patients with diabetic nephropathy should receive either an angiotensin converting enzyme (ACE) inhibitor or an angiotensin receptor antagonist, with the evidence for the latter's superiority in reducing progression to renal failure in comparison with other antihypertensive agents being particularly strong.[14] Addition of an ACE inhibitor to other drugs may also improve overall outcome in patients with diabetes.[15]

Most impressively, the Heart Protection Study showed that addition of simvastatin 40 mg daily to the treatment of 4000 patients with diabetes reduced all cardiovascular complications by 30%.

---

[14]Three trials compared an angiotensin blocker with other blood pressure lowering drugs and found a 20% reduction in the proportion of patients in whom proteinuria worsened or serum creatinine concentration doubled during follow-up: (1) Parving H H, Lehnert H, Brochner-Mortensen J et al 2001 The effect of irbesartan on the development of diabetic nephropathy in patients with Type 2 diabetes. New England Journal of Medicine 345:870–878; (2) Brenner B M, Cooper M E, de Zeeuw D et al 2001 Effects of losartan on renal and cardiovascular outcomes in patients with Type 2 diabetes and nephropathy. New England Journal of Medicine 345:861–869; (3) Lewis E J, Hunsicker L G, Clarke W R et al 2001 Renoprotective effect of the angiotensin-receptor antagonist irbesartan in patients with nephropathy due to Type 2 diabetes. New England Journal of Medicine 345:851–860.

[15]The HOPE study included patients with diabetes as one of its high-risk group of cardiovascular patients, in whom ramipril reduced further coronary heart disease endpoints by about 30%. Yusuf S, Sleight P, Pogue J et al 2000 Effects of an angiotensin converting enzyme inhibitor, ramipril, on cardiovascular events in high-risk patients. The Heart Outcomes Prevention Evaluation Study Investigators. New England Journal of Medicine 342:145–153.

SECTION 8

Summary

- Diabetes mellitus is important in global terms because of its chronicity, and high incidence and frequency of major complications. It is of two kinds: Type 1 (previously, insulin-dependent diabetes mellitus) and Type 2 (previously, non-insulin-dependent diabetes).
- Type 1 diabetes is commoner among young, thin patients with diabetes. Insulin may also be required when glycaemic control is not achieved by oral drugs in Type 2 patients.
- Insulin is given subcutaneously to stable patients, usually as a biphasic mixture of soluble, short-acting human insulin, and a longer-acting suspension of insulin with protamine or zinc.
- In the treatment of diabetic ketoacidosis, in the perioperative patient, and at other times of changing insulin requirement, insulin is best given by intravenous infusion of the soluble form.
- Diet plays a major role in the treatment of Type 2 diabetes with obesity.
- If a drug is required, a sulphonylurea is used as a first-line agent only for the non-obese, and metformin (a biguanide) for the obese. A thiazolidinedione is used as second-line treatment in patients intolerant of, or uncontrolled by, metformin or sulphonylurea.
- Aggressive treatment of Type 1, and probably Type 2, diabetes successfully reduces microvascular complications. Close attention to associated risk factors, especially hyperlipidaemia and hypertension, is important in reducing risk of macrovascular disease.

OBESITY AND APPETITE CONTROL

Overweight and obesity are the commonest nutritional disorders in developed countries. Between 1991 and 1998 the incidence of obesity rose from 12.0% to 17.9% in the USA. Obesity predisposes to several chronic diseases including hypertension, hyperlipidaemia, diabetes mellitus, cardiovascular disease and osteoarthritis, and aspects of these are discussed in the relevant sections of this book.

The body mass index[16] (BMI) correlates highly with the amount of body fat; individuals whose BMI lies between 25 and 30 kg/m^2 are considered *overweight* and those in whom it exceeds 30 kg/m^2 are defined as *obese*. Management of the condition involves a variety of approaches from nutritional advice to lifestyle alteration, drugs and, in extreme instances, gastric surgery. An evidence-based algorithm coordinates these.[17] The present account concentrates on pharmacological interventions.

Drugs for obesity act either on the gastrointestinal tract, lowering nutrient absorption, or centrally, reducing food intake by decreasing appetite or increasing satiety (appetite suppressants).

ORLISTAT

Orlistat is a pentanoic acid ester that binds to and inhibits gastric and pancreatic lipases; the resulting inhibition of their activity prevents the absorption of about 30% of dietary fat compared with a normal 5% loss. Weight loss is due to calorie loss but drug-related adverse effects also contribute by diminishing food intake. The drug is not absorbed from the alimentary tract.

Clinical trials have shown that patients who adhered to a low-calorie diet and took orlistat lost on average 9–10 kg after 1 year (compared with 6 kg in those taking placebo); in the following year those who remained on orlistat regained 1.5–3.0 kg (4–6 kg with placebo). Orlistat has found a place in the management of obesity in the UK but, not surprisingly, this is subject to stringent guidance from NICE, namely that it be initiated only in individuals:

- aged 18–75 years
- with a BMI of 28 kg/m^2 or more who also have cardiovascular risk factors, or 30 kg/m^2 or more without such co-morbidity, and
- who have lost at least 2.5 kg body-weight by dieting and increasing physical activity in the previous month.

The dose is 120 mg, taken immediately before, during or 1 h after each main meal, up to three times daily. If a meal is missed, or contains no fat, the dose of orlistat should be omitted.

Treatment should be accompanied by counselling advice and proceed beyond 3 months only in those who have lost more than 5% of their initial weight, beyond 6 months in those who have lost more than 10%, should not normally exceed 1 year, and never more than 2 years.

---

[16]The weight in kilograms divided by the square of the height in metres (kg/m^2).

[17]http://www.nhlbi.nih.gov/guidelines/obesity/practgde.htm

Adverse effects include flatulence and liquid, oily stools, leading to faecal urgency, abdominal and rectal pain. Symptoms may be reduced by adhering to a reduced-fat diet. Low plasma concentrations of the fat-soluble vitamins A, D and E have been found. Orlistat is *contraindicated* where there is chronic intestinal malabsorption or cholestasis.

SIBUTRAMINE

Sibutramine was originally developed as an antidepressant; it inhibits the reuptake of noradrenaline (norepinephrine) and serotonin at nerve endings, increasing the concentration of these neurotransmitters at postsynaptic receptors in the brain that affect food intake. It is also thought to stimulate energy expenditure.

The drug is rapidly absorbed from the gastrointestinal tract and extensively metabolised in the liver by cytochrome P450 3A4. These metabolites have a $t_{\frac{1}{2}}$ of 14–16 h and are responsible for its effects.

When taken with dietary advice, sibutramine can be expected to cause a loss of 5–7% of initial bodyweight but this tends to be regained once the drug is stopped.

Sibutramine should be prescribed only for individuals with a BMI of 27 kg/m^2 or more who have other cardiovascular risk factors, or 30 kg/m^2 or more in their absence. It should be discontinued if weight loss after 3 months is less than 5% of initial weight, if weight stabilises at less than 5% of initial weight thereafter, or if users regain more than 3 kg after previous weight loss. It should not be given for more than 1 year.

The dose is 10–15 mg/day by mouth.

Adverse effects include constipation, dry mouth and insomnia, which occur in more than 10% of users. Less commonly, nausea, tachycardia, palpitations, raised blood pressure, anxiety, sweating and altered taste may occur. Blood pressure should be monitored closely throughout use of sibutramine (twice weekly in the first 3 months). *Contraindications* include severe hypertension, peripheral occlusive arterial or coronary heart disease, cardiac arrhythmia, prostatic hypertrophy, and severe hepatic or renal impairment. Sibutramine should not be used to treat obesity of endocrine origin or those with a history of major eating disorder or psychiatric disease. Concomitant use with tricyclic antidepressants should be avoided (CNS toxicity).

RIMONABANT

The *endocannabinoid* system plays an important role in the control of appetite and food (see p. 112). Rimonabant is a recently developed selective cannabinoid (CB$_1$) receptor blocker. At a dose of 20 mg daily, it reduced weight by 5% more than placebo in 60% of participants who completed the RIO-Europe study.[18] Weight loss was associated with a waist circumference reduction, improvement in dyslipidaemia and fasting blood glucose. *Adverse effects* are depression, anxiety and nausea. It should not be used for women of childbearing age or in patients with depression.

The noradrenergic drugs fenfluramine, dexfenfluramine and phenteramine were formerly prescribed as appetite suppressants but were withdrawn when their use was found to be associated with cardiac valve disease and pulmonary hypertension.

The adipocyte-derived hormone leptin (Greek: *leptos*, thin) has a limited role in therapeutics for rare patients with genetic defects in the leptin or leptin receptor genes. Leptin acts on the hypothalamus to reduce appetite. Most obese patients have raised plasma leptin concentrations, to which they have become relatively resistant.

GUIDE TO FURTHER READING

Chan J L, Mantzoros C S 2005 Role of leptin in energy-deprivation states: normal human physiology and clinical implications for hypothalamic amenorrhoea and anorexia nervosa. Lancet 366:74–85

Daneman D 2006 Type 1 diabetes. Lancet 367:847–858

Dornhorst A 2001 Insulinotropic meglitinide analogues. Lancet 358:1709–1716

Drucker D J, Nauck M A 2006 The incretin system: glucagon-like peptide-1 receptor agonists and dipeptidyl peptidase-4 inhibitors in type 2 diabetes. Lancet 368:1696–1705

Eckel R H, Grundy S M, Zimmet P Z 2005 The metabolic syndrome. Lancet 365:1415–1428

Guber C 2005 Personal account: Type 2 diabetes. Lancet 365:1347

Haslam D W, James W P T 2005 Obesity. Lancet 366: 1197–1209

[18]Despres J-P, Golay A, Sjostrom L 2005 The Rimonabant in Obesity-Lipids Study G. Effects of rimonabant on metabolic risk factors in overweight patients with dyslipidemia. New England Journal of Medicine 353:2121–2134.

Hirsch I B 2005 Insulin analogues. New England Journal of Medicine 352:174–183

Marshall S M, Flyvbjerg A 2006 Prevention and early detection of vascular complications of diabetes. British Medical Journal 333:475–480

McMahon G T, Arky R A 2007 Inhaled insulin for diabetes mellitus. New England Journal of Medicine 356:497–502

Montori V M, Isley W L, Guyatt G H 2007 Waking up from the DREAM of preventing diabetes with drugs. British Medical Journal 334:882–884

Nutrition Committee of the Royal College of Physicians 2004 Anti-obesity drugs. Guidance on appropriate prescribing and management. Annals of Clinical Biochemistry 41(1):85

Padwal R S, Majumdar S R 2007 Drug treatments for obesity: orlistat, sibutramine, and rimonabant. Lancet 369:71–77

Stevens A B, Roberts M, McKane R et al 1989 Motor vehicle driving amongst diabetics taking insulin and non-diabetics. British Medical Journal 299:591–595

Stumvoll M, Goldstein B J, van Haeften T W et al 2005 Type 2 diabetes: principles of pathogenesis and treatment. Lancet 365:1333–1346

The Diabetes Control and Complications Trial/Epidemiology of Diabetes Interventions and Complications (DCCT/EDIC) Study Research Group 2005 Intensive diabetes treatment and cardiovascular disease in patients with Type 1 diabetes. New England Journal of Medicine 353:2643–2653

Wright J R 2002 From ugly fish to conquer death: J J R Macleod's fish insulin research, 1922–24. Lancet 359:1238–1242

Yki-Järvinen H 2004 Thiazolidinediones. New England Journal of Medicine 351:1106–1118

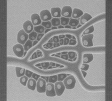

36

Thyroid hormones, antithyroid drugs

SYNOPSIS

- Thyroid hormones (thyroxine/levothyroxine T_4, liothyronine T_3)
- Use of thyroid hormone: treatment of hypothyroidism
- Antithyroid drugs and hyperthyroidism: thionamides, drugs that block sympathetic autonomic activity, iodide and radio-iodine ^{131}I, preparation of patients for surgery, thyroid storm (crisis), exophthalmos
- Drugs that cause unwanted hypothyroidism
- Calcitonin (see Chapter 38)

THYROID HORMONES

L-Thyroxine (T_4 or tetra-iodo-L-thyronine) and lio-thyronine (T_3 or tri-iodo-L-thyronine) are the natural hormones of the thyroid gland. T_4 is a less active precursor of T_3, which is the major mediator of physiological effect. In this chapter, T_4 for therapeutic use is referred to as *levothyroxine* (the rINN; see p. 69).

For convenience, the term 'thyroid hormone' is used to comprise T_4 plus T_3. Both forms are available for oral use as therapy.

Calcitonin. See page 665.

PHYSIOLOGY AND PHARMACOKINETICS

Thyroid hormone synthesis requires oxidation of dietary iodine, followed by iodination of tyrosine to mono- and di-iodotyrosine; coupling of iodotyrosines leads to formation of the *active molecules, tetra-iodothyronine*, (T_4 or L-thyroxine) and *tri-iodothyronine* (T_3 or L-thyronine).

These active thyroid hormones are stored in the gland within the molecule of thyroglobulin, a major component of the intrafollicular colloid. They are released into the circulation following reuptake of the colloid by the apical cells and proteolysis. The main circulating thyroid hormone is T_4. About 80% of the released T_4 is de-iodinated in the peripheral tissues to the biologically active T_3 (30–35%) and biologically inactive 'reverse' T_3 (45–50%); thus most circulating T_3 is derived from T_4. Further de-iodination, largely in the liver, leads to loss of activity.

In the blood both T_4 and T_3 are extensively (99.9%) bound to plasma proteins (thyroxine binding globulin [TBG] and thyroxine-binding prealbumin [TBPA]). The concentration of TBG is raised by oestrogens (physiological, e.g. pregnancy, and pharmacological, e.g. oral contraceptives) and prolonged use of neuroleptics. The concentration of TBG is lowered by adrenocortical and androgen (including anabolic steroid) therapy and by urinary protein loss in the nephrotic syndrome. Phenytoin and salicylates compete with thyroid hormone for TBG binding sites. Effects such as these would interfere with the assessment of the clinical significance of measurements of total thyroid hormone concentration but the availability of free thyroid hormone assay largely avoids such complicating factors. Normal values are: free T_4 9–25 picomol/L, free T_3 3–9 picomol/L.

T_4 and T_3 are well absorbed from the gut, except in myxoedema coma when parenteral therapy is required.

T_4 (levothyroxine). A single dose reaches its maximum effect in about 10 days (its binding to plasma proteins is strong as well as extensive) and passes off in 2–3 weeks ($t_{1/2}$ 7 days in euthyroid, 14 days in hypothyroid and 3 days in hyperthyroid subjects).

T_3 (liothyronine) is about five times as biologically potent as T_4; a single dose reaches its maximum effect in about 24 h (its binding to plasma proteins is weak) and passes off in 1 week ($t_{1/2}$ 2 days in euthyroid subjects).

PHARMACODYNAMICS

Thyroid hormone passes into the cells of target organs. T_4 is de-iodinated to T_3, which combines with specific nuclear receptors and induces characteristic metabolic changes:

- *Protein synthesis* during growth.
- *Increased metabolic rate* with raised oxygen consumption.
- *Increased sensitivity to catecholamines* with proliferation of β-adrenoceptors (particularly important in the cardiovascular system).

LEVOTHYROXINE FOR HYPOTHYROIDISM

The main indication for levothyroxine is treatment of deficiency (cretinism, adult hypothyroidism) from any cause. The adult requirement of hormone is remarkably constant, and dosage does not usually have to be altered once the optimum has been found. Patients should be monitored annually. Monitoring needs to be more frequent in children, who may need more as they grow. Similarly, pregnant women should be monitored monthly, and require a 50–100% increase in their normal dose of levothyroxine.

Early treatment of neonatal hypothyroidism (cretinism) (1 in 5000 births) is important if permanent mental defect is to be avoided. It must be lifelong.

Hypothyroidism due to panhypopituitarism requires replacement with glucocorticoids as well as with thyroid hormone. Use of levothyroxine alone can cause acute adrenal insufficiency.

Small doses of levothyroxine in normal subjects merely depress pituitary thyroid-stimulating hormone (TSH) production and consequently reduce the output of thyroid hormone by an equivalent amount.

Levothyroxine is used in some countries for the treatment of non-toxic nodular goitre, on the assumption that nodular thyroid tissue growth is dependent on TSH. The treatment is not curative. Levothyroxine should not be used to treat obesity (see Obesity, p. 624).

Treatment of hypothyroidism

Levothyroxine tabs contain pure L-thyroxine sodium and should be used.

The initial oral dose in young patients without cardiac disease is 50–100 micrograms/day. In the old and patients with heart disease or hypertension, this level should be achieved gradually (to minimise cardiovascular risk due to a too sudden increase in metabolic demand), starting with 12.5–25 micrograms daily for the first 2–4 weeks, and then increasing by 12.5 micrograms monthly until normal TSH levels are achieved.

The usual replacement dose at steady state is 75–150 micrograms in women, and 100–200 micrograms in men, as a single daily dose. This is usually sufficient to reduce plasma TSH to normal (0.3–3.5 mU/L), which is the best indicator of adequate treatment. Patients who appear to need more are probably not taking their tablets consistently. The maximum effect of a dose is reached after about 10 days and passes off over about 2–3 weeks. Absorption is more complete and less variable if levothyroxine is taken well apart from food.

Tablets containing physiological mixtures of levothyroxine and liothyronine are not sufficiently evaluated to recommend in preference to levothyroxine alone.

Hypothyroid patients tend to be intolerant of drugs in general owing to slow metabolism.

Liothyronine tabs. Liothyronine is the most rapidly effective thyroid hormone, a single dose giving maximum effect within 24 h and passing off over 24–48 h. It is not routine treatment for hypothyroidism because its rapid onset of effect can induce heart failure. Its main uses are myxoedema coma and psychosis, both rare conditions. A specialised use is during the withdrawal of levothyroxine replacement (to permit diagnostic radio-iodine scanning) in patients with thyroid carcinoma.

Myxoedema coma follows prolonged total hormone deficiency and constitutes an emergency. Liothyronine 5–20 micrograms is given intravenously every 12 h. Intravenous therapy is mandatory because drug absorption is impaired. Intravenous hydrocortisone is also needed, as prolonged hypothyroidism may be associated with adrenocortical insufficiency.

Subclinical hypothyroidism. This term has become an acceptable misnomer for a biochemical diagnosis in patients with normal free T_4 but raised TSH levels. The recommended indications for treatment in these patients are any one of the following: symptoms of hypothyrodism, TSH ≥10 mU/L, presence of a goitre, detectable thyroid antibodies, hypercholesterolaemia, pregnancy, or ovulatory dysfunction with infertility.

Adverse effects of thyroid hormone parallel the increase in metabolic rate. The symptoms and signs are those of hyperthyroidism. Symptoms of myocardial ischaemia, atrial fibrillation or heart failure are liable to be provoked by too vigorous therapy or in patients having serious ischaemic heart disease who may even be unable to tolerate optimal therapy. Should they occur, discontinue levothyroxine for at least a week, and recommence at lower dose. Only slight overdose may precipitate atrial fibrillation in patients aged over 60 years.

In pregnancy a hypothyroid patient should be assessed carefully and monitored monthly; optimal replacement is essential in the first trimester when the athyroid fetus is dependent on maternal supply. A 50–100% increase in dose of levothyroxine may be required. Breast-feeding is not contraindicated.

ANTITHYROID DRUGS AND HYPERTHYROIDISM

Drugs used for the treatment of hyperthyroidism include:

- *Thionamides*, which block the synthesis of thyroid hormone.
- *Iodine*: *radio-iodine*, which destroys the cells that make thyroid hormone; *iodide*, an excess of which reduces the production of thyroid hormone temporarily by an unknown mechanism (it is also necessary for the formation of hormone, and both excess and deficiency can cause goitre).

THIONAMIDES (THIOUREA DERIVATIVES) CARBIMAZOLE, METHIMAZOLE, PROPYLTHIOURACIL

Mode of action (Fig. 36.1)

The major action of thionamides is to reduce the formation of thyroid hormone by inhibiting oxidation and organification (incorporation into organic

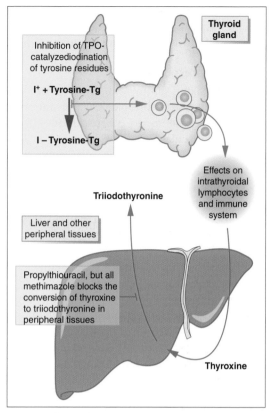

Fig. 36.1 Effects of antithyroid drugs. The multiple effects of antithyroid drugs include inhibition of thyroid hormone synthesis and a reduction in both intrathyroid immune dysregulation and (in the case of propylthiouracil) the peripheral conversion of thyroxine to tri-iodothyronine. Tyrosine-Tg, tyrosine residues in thyroglobulin; 1+, the iodinating intermediate; TPO, thyroid peroxidase. (Adapted from Cooper D S 2005 Antithyroid drugs. New England Journal of Medicine 352:905–917.)

form) of iodine (iodotyrosines). Maximum effect is delayed until existing hormone stores are exhausted (weeks, see below). With high dose, reduced hormone synthesis leads to hypothyroidism.

Carbimazole and methimazole (the chief metabolite of carbimazole) ($t_{1/2}$ 6 h) and propylthiouracil ($t_{1/2}$ 2 h) are commonly used, but the $t_{1/2}$ matters little because the drugs accumulate in the thyroid and act there for 30–40 h; thus a single daily dose suffices.

Propylthiouracil (PTU) differs from other members of the group in that it also inhibits peripheral conversion of T_4 to T_3, but only at the high doses used in treatment of thyroid storm (see p. 633). PTU differs from the other thionamides in its apparent radio-protective effect when used prior to radio-iodine.

Immunosuppression

In patients taking antithyroid drugs, serum concentrations of antithyrotropin receptor antibodies decrease with time, as do other immunologically important molecules, including intracellular adhesion molecule 1, and soluble interleukin-2 and interleukin-6 receptors. There is an increased number of circulating suppressor T cells and a decreased number of helper T cells. Antithyroid drugs may also induce apoptosis of intrathyroidal lymphocytes.

Doses

- *Carbimazole* 40 mg total/day is given orally (or *methimazole* 30 mg) until the patient is euthyroid (usually 4–6 weeks). Then either titrate (*titration regimen*) by decrements initially of 10 mg every 4–6 weeks to a maintenance dose of 5–10 mg/day; or continue (*block–replace regimen*) 40 mg once daily, and add levothyroxine 75–125 micrograms/day, with monitoring of free T_4 and TSH.
- *Propylthiouracil* 300–600 mg total/day is given orally until the patient is euthyroid: maintenance 50–100 mg total/day. Much higher doses (up to 2.4 g/day) with frequent administration are used for thyroid storm.

Use

It is probable that no patient is wholly refractory to these drugs. Failure to respond is likely to be due to the patient not taking the tablets or to wrong diagnosis. The drugs are used in hyperthyroidism as

- principal therapy
- adjuvant to radio-iodine, before and after administration, to control the disease until the radiation achieves its effect[1]
- to prepare patients for surgery.

Clinical improvement is noticeable in 2–4 weeks, and the patient should be euthyroid in 4–6 weeks.

---

[1]Use of a thionamide during the week before and after radio-iodine therapy may impair the response to radiation (Velkeniers B, Cytryn R, Vanhaelst L, Jonckheer M H 1988 Treatment of hyperthyroidism with radioiodine: adjunctive therapy with antithyroid drugs reconsidered. Lancet i: 1127–1129) (see Mode of action of thionamides, above).

The best guides to therapy are the patient's symptoms (decreased nervousness and palpitations), increased strength and weight gain, and pulse rate.

Symptoms and signs are, of course, less valuable as guides if the patient is also taking a β-adrenoceptor blocker, and reliance then rests on biochemical tests.

With optimal treatment the gland decreases in size, but over-treatment leading to low hormone concentrations in the blood activates the pituitary feedback system, inducing TSH secretion and goitre.

Adverse reactions

The thionamide drugs are all liable to cause adverse effects. *Minor* reactions include rash, urticaria, arthralgia, fever, anorexia, nausea, abnormalities of taste and smell. *Major* effects include agranulocytosis, thrombocytopenia, acute hepatic necrosis, cholestatic hepatitis, lupus-like syndrome, vasculitis.

Blood disorders (<3 per 10 000 patient-years) are most common in the first 2 months of treatment. Routine leucocyte counts to detect blood dyscrasia before symptoms develop are unlikely to protect, as agranulocytosis may be so acute that blood counts give no warning. Patients must be advised to stop the drug and have a leucocyte count performed if symptoms of a sore throat, fever, bruising or mouth ulcers develop. Any suggestion of anaemia should be investigated.

Cross-allergy between the drugs sometimes occurs, but is not to be assumed for agranulocytosis. Treatment of agranulocytosis consists of drug withdrawal, admission to hospital, and administration of broad-spectrum antibimicrobials plus granulocyte colony-stimulating factor.

Pregnancy. If a pregnant woman has hyperthyroidism (2 per 1000 pregnancies), she should be treated with the smallest possible amount of these drugs because they cross the placenta; over-treatment causes fetal goitre. Surgery in the second trimester may be preferred to continued drug therapy.

Propylthiouracil is the treatment of choice during breast-feeding, because little passes into breast milk.

CONTROL OF ANTITHYROID DRUG THERAPY

The aim of drug therapy is to control the hyperthyroidism until a natural remission takes place. The recommended duration of therapy is 12–18 months. Longer treatment is usual for young patients with large, vascular goitres, because of the higher risk of recurrence. Most patients enter remission, but some will relapse – usually during the first 3 months after withdrawal from treatment. Approximately 30–40% of patients remain euthyroid 10 years later. If hyperthyroidism recurs, there is little chance of a second course of thionamide achieving long-term remission. In such patients, indefinite low-dose antithyroid treatment is an alternative option to radio-iodine or surgery.

The use of levothyroxine concurrently with an antithyroid drug ('block and replace regimen') facilitates maintenance of a euthyroid state and reduces the frequency of clinic visits. There is a higher risk of the dose-related adverse effects of carbimazole, and no compensatory reduction in the incidence of relapse. Therefore, the 'titration' (see above) regimen is regarded as first-line treatment.

β-Adrenergic blockade. There is increased tissue sensitivity to catecholamines in hyperthyroidism with a rise in either the number of β-adrenoceptors or the second-messenger response (i.e. intracellular cyclic AMP synthesis) to their stimulation. Therefore, some of the unpleasant symptoms are adrenergic.

Quick relief can be obtained with a β-adrenoceptor blocking drug (judge the dose by heart rate), although these do not block all the metabolic effects of the hormone, e.g. on the myocardium, and the basal metabolic rate is unchanged. For this reason, β-blockade is not used as sole therapy except in mild thyrotoxicosis in preparation for radio-iodine treatment, and in these patients it should be continued until the radio-iodine has taken effect. β-Blockers do not alter the course of the disease, or affect biochemical tests of thyroid function. Any effect on thyroid hormonal action on peripheral tissues is clinically unimportant. Although atenolol is widely used, it is preferable to choose a drug that is *non-selective* for $β_1$ and $β_2$ receptors and *lacks partial agonist effect* (e.g. propranolol 20–80 mg 6–8-hourly, or timolol 5 mg once daily). The usual contraindications to β-blockade (see p. 427) apply, especially asthma.

IODINE (IODIDE AND RADIOACTIVE IODINE)

Iodide is well absorbed from the intestine, distributed like chloride in the body, and rapidly excreted by the kidney. It is selectively taken up and concentrated (about ×25) by the thyroid gland, more in hyperthyroidism and less in hypothyroidism. A deficiency of iodide reduces the amount of thyroid hormone produced; this stimulates the pituitary to secrete TSH. The result is hyperplasia and increased vascularity of the gland, with eventual goitre formation.[2]

Effects

The effects of iodide are complex and related to the dose and thyroid status of the subject.

In hyperthyroid subjects, a moderate excess of iodide may enhance hormone production by providing 'fuel' for hormone synthesis. But a substantial excess inhibits hormone release and promotes storage of hormone and involution of the gland, making it firmer and less vascular so that surgery is easier. The effect is transient and its mechanism uncertain.

In euthyroid subjects with normal glands an excess of iodide from any source can cause goitre (with or without hyperthyroidism), e.g. use of iodide-containing cough medicines, iodine-containing radiocontrast media, amiodarone, seaweed eaters.

A euthyroid subject with an autonomous adenoma (hot nodule) becomes hyperthyroid if given iodide.

Uses

Iodide (large dose) is used for thyroid storm (crisis) and in preparation for thyroidectomy because it rapidly benefits the patient by reducing hormone release and renders surgery easier and safer (above).

Potassium iodide in doses of 60 mg orally 8-hourly (longer intervals allow some escape from the iodide effect) produces some effect in 1–2 days, maximal after 10–14 days, after which the benefit declines as the thyroid adapts. A similar dose used for 3 days covers administration of some [131]I- or ^{123}I-containing preparations, for instance meta-iodobenzylguanidine (^{123}I-MIBG) (see p. 434).

Iodine therapy maximises iodide stores in the thyroid, which delays response to thionamides. Prophylactic iodide (1 part in 100 000) may be added to the salt, water or bread where goitre is endemic.

---

[2]Apparently from the beginning of time: Michaelangelo's image of the Separation of Light from Darkness on the ceiling of the Sistine Chapel in the Vatican depicts the Creator with a multinodular goitre (Bondeson L, Bondeson A-G 2003 Michaelangelo's divine goitre. Journal of the Royal Society of Medicine 96:609–611).

In economically deprived communities, a method of prophylaxis is to inject iodised oil intramuscularly every 3–5 years; given early to women, this prevents endemic cretinism but occasional hyperthyroidism occurs (see autonomous adenoma, above).

As an antiseptic for use on the skin, povidone–iodine (a complex of iodine with a sustained-release carrier, povidone or polyvinyl–pyrrolidone) can be applied repeatedly and used as a surgical scrub.

Bronchial secretions. Iodide is concentrated in bronchial and salivary secretions. It acts as an expectorant (see Cough, p. 495).

Organic compounds containing iodine are used as contrast media in radio-imaging. It is essential to ask patients specifically whether they are allergic to iodine before such contrast media are used. Severe anaphylaxis, even deaths, occur every year in busy imaging departments; iodine-containing contrast media are being superseded by so-called non-ionic preparations.[3]

Adverse reactions

Patients vary enormously in their tolerance of iodine; some are intolerant or allergic to it both orally and when it is applied to the skin.

Symptoms of iodism include: a metallic taste, excessive salivation with painful salivary glands, running eyes and nose, sore mouth and throat, a productive cough, diarrhoea, and various rashes that may mimic chickenpox. A saline diuresis enhances elimination.

Goitre can occur (see above) with prolonged use of iodide-containing expectorant by bronchitics and asthmatics. Such therapy should therefore be intermittent, if it is used at all.

Topical application of iodine-containing antiseptics to neonates has caused hypothyroidism. Iodide intake above that in a normal diet will depress thyroid uptake of administered radio-iodine, because the two forms will compete.

In the case of diet, medication, and water-soluble radio-diagnostic agents, interference with thyroid function will cease 2–4 weeks after stopping the source, but with agents used for cholecystography it may last for 6 months or more (because of tissue binding).

RADIO-IODINE (^{131}I)

^{131}I is treated by the body just like the ordinary non-radioactive isotope, so that when swallowed it is concentrated in the thyroid gland. It emits mainly β radiation (90%), which penetrates only 0.5 mm of tissue and thus allows therapeutic effects on the thyroid without damage to the surrounding structures, particularly the parathyroids. It also emits some γ rays, which are more penetrating and are detectable with a radiation counter.[4] ^{131}I has a physical (radioactive) $t_{1/2}$ of 8 days.

^{131}I is the preferred initial treatment for hyperthyroidism caused by Graves' disease in North America. It is contraindicated in children and pregnant or breast-feeding women, and can induce or worsen ophthalmopathy. It is used in combination with surgery in thyroid carcinoma.

In hyperthyroidism, the beneficial effects of a single dose may be felt in 1 month, and patients should be reviewed at 6 weeks to monitor for onset of hypothyroidism. The maximal effect of radio-iodine may take 3 months to achieve. β-Adrenoceptor blockade and, in severe cases, an antithyroid drug (but see footnote 1) will be needed to render the patient comfortable whilst waiting; this is more likely when radio-iodine is used for patients with relapsing thyrotoxicosis. Very rarely radiation thyroiditis causes excessive release of hormone and thyroid storm. Repeated doses may be needed.

Adverse effects of radio-iodine are as for iodism, above. In the event of inadvertent overdose, large doses of sodium or potassium iodide should be given to compete with the radio-iodine for thyroid uptake and to hasten excretion by increasing iodide turnover (increased fluid intake and a diuretic are adjuvants).

---

[3]The newer preparations approximately triple the cost of diagnostic investigations requiring contrast media. With a fatality rate of about 1 per 50 000 in patients receiving the older agents, hospitals are faced with an interesting cost–benefit equation.

[4]And emissions can be sufficient to activate airport radiation alarms. One victim was detained, strip-searched and interrogated, but released on producing his radionucleotide card (Gangopadhyay K K, Sundram F, De P 2006 Triggering radiation alarms after radioiodine treatment. British Medical Journal 333:293–294).

Radio-iodine offers the advantages that treatment is simple and carries no immediate mortality, but it is slow in acting and the dose that will render the patient euthyroid is difficult to judge. In the first year after treatment, 20% of patients will become hypothyroid. Thereafter, 5% of patients become hypothyroid annually, perhaps because the capacity of thyroid cells to divide is permanently abolished so that cell renewal ceases. There is therefore an obligation to monitor patients indefinitely after radio-iodine treatment, for most are likely to need treatment for hypothyroidism eventually. Realistically, because follow-up over years may fail and, because the onset of hypothyroidism is insidious and not easily recognised, some physicians prefer deliberately to render patients hypothyroid with the first dose and to educate them on the use of replacement therapy, which is safe and effective.

Risks

Experience had eliminated the fear that radio-iodine causes carcinoma of the thyroid, and led to its use in patients of all ages. The Chernobyl disaster subsequently revived concern about exposure of children and it would be wise again to restrict radio-iodine treatment to adults. Pregnant women should not be treated with radio-iodine (^{131}I) because it crosses the placenta.

There is a theoretical risk of teratogenic effect and women are advised to avoid pregnancy for an arbitrary 12 months after treatment.

Treatment of thyroid carcinoma requires larger doses of radio-iodine than are used for hyperthyroidism, and there is an increased incidence of late leukaemia in these patients. The management of thyroid carcinoma is highly specialised, and extends beyond the scope of this textbook.

RADIO-ISOTOPE TESTS

Radio-iodine uptake can be used to test thyroid function, although it has now been superseded by technetium-99m. Scanning the gland may be useful to identify solitary nodules and in the differential diagnosis of Graves' disease from the less common thyroiditides, e.g. de Quervain's thyroiditis. In thyroiditis, excessive thyroid hormone release caused by follicular cell damage can cause clinical and biochemical features of hyperthyroidism, but radionuclide uptake is reduced.

Choice of treatment of hyperthyroidism

- Antithyroid drugs
- Radio-iodine
- Surgery

Antithyroid drugs are generally preferred provided the goitre is small and diffuse. They may be used in pregnancy.

Radio-iodine is an alternative first-line treatment for adult patients, but not in pregnancy. It may be preferred to antithyroid drugs in patients with large or multinodular goitres, and in patients with a single hyperfunctioning adenoma ('hot nodule'). Preparation with antithyroid drugs is recommended in severe thyrotoxicosis.

Surgery is generally a second choice for thyrotoxicosis. It may be indicated if the thyroid contains a nodule of uncertain nature, or in patients with large, multinodular goitres causing tracheal compression.

PREPARATION FOR SURGERY

Routine reparation of hyperthyroid patients for surgery can be achieved satisfactorily by making them euthyroid with one of the above drugs plus a β-adrenoceptor blocker for comfort (see below) and safety,[5] and adding iodide for 7–10 days before operation (not sooner) to reduce the surgically inconvenient vascularity of the gland.

In an emergency, the patient is prepared with a β-adrenoceptor blocker (e.g. propranolol 6-hourly, with dose titration to eliminate tachycardia) for 4 days, continued through the operation and for 7–10 days afterwards. Iodide is also given (see p. 631). The important differences with this second technique are that the gland is smaller and less friable but the patient's tissues are still hyperthyroid and, to avoid a hyperthyroid crisis or storm, it is essential that the adrenoceptor blocker continue as above without the omission of even a single 6-hourly dose of propranolol.

THYROID STORM

Thyroid crisis, or storm, is a life-threatening emergency owing to the liberation of large amounts of

---

[5]No patient should be operated on with a resting pulse of 90 beats/min or above, and no dose of β-adrenoceptor blocker, including the important postoperative dose, should be omitted (Toft A D, Irvine W J, Sinclair I et al 1978 Thyroid function after surgical treatment of thyrotoxicosis. A report of 100 cases treated with propranolol before operation. New England Journal of Medicine 298:643–647).

hormone into the circulation. Surgical storm is rare with modern methods of preparing hyperthyroid patients for surgery. Medical thyroid storm may occur in patients who are untreated or incompletely treated. It may be precipitated by infection, trauma, surgical emergencies or operations, radiation thyroiditis, toxaemia of pregnancy or parturition.

Treatment is urgently required to save life. Propranolol should be given immediately, 60–80 mg orally every 6 h or i.v. slowly, initially 0.5–1 mg over 10 min with continuous cardiac rhythm monitoring; the i.v. dose may be repeated every few hours until the oral dose takes effect. Large doses of an antithyroid agent, preferably propylthiouracil 300–400 mg 4-hourly are required, down a nasogastric tube or per rectum. Thereafter, iodide is used to inhibit further hormone release from the gland (potassium iodide 600 mg to 1.0 g orally in the first 24 h) (see above). Lithium carbonate may be used in cases of iodide allergy. Large doses of adrenocorticoid, e.g. dexamethasone 2 mg 6-hourly, are given to inhibit both release of thyroid hormone from the gland and peripheral conversion of T_4 to T_3. Hyperthermia may be treated by cooling and aspirin; heart failure in the ordinary way; fluid deficit by a combination of normal saline and 5% dextrose.

EXOPHTHALMOS OF HYPERTHYROIDISM

The cause may involve an immunoglobulin that attacks the external ocular muscles and retrobulbar tissue. Antithyroid drugs do not help directly. Nevertheless, it is important that any thyroid dysfunction is treated meticulously, and the TSH concentration held within the normal range. Mild to moderate cases regress spontaneously. Artificial tears (hypromellose) are useful when natural tears and blinking are inadequate to maintain corneal lubrication. In severe cases, high doses of systemic prednisolone, alone or in combination with another immunosuppressive (azathioprine), may help. A course of low-dose orbital radiation achieves rapid regression of ophthalmopathy, and may avoid the need for prolonged immunosuppressive treatment. In severe cases, surgery may be required to remove optic nerve compression.

TREATMENT OF SUBCLINICAL HYPERTHYROIDISM

Like subclinical hypothyroidism, this term is an acceptable misnomer for the common biochemical diagnosis of a normal serum T_4 and T_3 but suppressed TSH concentrations. Some 5% of patients per annum progress to frank hyperthyroidism, and there is an increased risk of atrial fibrillation, stroke and osteoporosis in the elderly. The treatment of endogenous subclinical hyperthyroidism should be considered when the TSH level is less than 0.1 mU/L, especially in patients aged over 60 years, those with an increased risk for heart disease, osteopenia or osteoporosis, or with clinical symptoms suggestive of hyperthyroidism. Other patients should be monitored 6-monthly; eventually 50% become euthyroid.[6]

DRUGS THAT CAUSE HYPOTHYROIDISM

In addition to drugs used for their antithyroid effects, the following substances can cause hypothyroidism: lithium (for mania, bipolar disorder, recurrent depression), amiodarone (see below), β–interferon (hepatitis and multiple sclerosis), iodide (see above), resorcinol (leg ulcers). Effects may be reversible on withdrawal.

Amiodarone bears a significant structural resemblance to thyroxine. Each molecule of amiodarone contains two iodine atoms, constituting 37.5% of its mass. Hence, a patient taking a 200-mg/day dose ingests 75 mg organic iodine each day. Subsequent de-iodination through drug metabolism results in the daily release of approximately 6 mg free iodine into the circulation, which is 20 to 40 times higher than usual daily iodine intake of 0.15–0.30 mg. Amiodarone has a very long $t_{1/2}$ (54 days) on chronic dosing, mainly due to its storage in adipose tissue. Hence, the excess iodine clears slowly over months and the toxic effects of amiodarone can persist or can even occur well after its discontinuation.

Some 90% of patients receiving amiodarone remain euthyroid. Despite the exposure of the thyroid gland to an extraordinary load of iodine, important adjustments are made in thyroidal iodine handling and hormone metabolism; these are shown in Figure 36.2, and the consequences for thyroid function tests summarised in the Table 36.1.

[6]Consensus statement: Surks M I, Ortiz E, Daniels G H et al 2004 Subclinical thyroid disease: scientific review and guidelines for diagnosis and management. Journal of the American Medical Association 291:228–238.

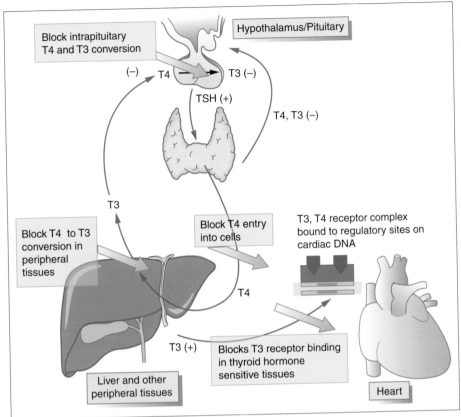

Fig. 36.2 Mechanisms by which amiodarone affects thyroid hormone metabolism. TSH, thyroid stimulating hormone. (Adapted from Basaria S, Cooper D S 2005 Amiodarone and the thyroid. American Journal of Medicine 118:706–714.)

Table 36.1 Effects of amiodarone on thyroid function tests in euthyroid subjects

Thyroid hormone	Acute effects (≤3 months)	Chronic effects (≥3 months)
Total and free T$_4$	↑50%	Remains ↑20–40% of baseline
T$_3$	↓15–20%, remains in low–normal range	Remains ↓20%, remains in low–normal range
Reverse T$_3$	↑>200%	Remains↑>150%
TSH	↑20–50%, transient, generally remains <20 mU/L	Normal

Amiodarone-induced *hypothyroidism* is more prevalent in iodine-sufficient areas of the world, whereas *thyrotoxicosis* is more prevalent in iodine-deficient regions. Amiodarone-induced hypothyroidism typically occurs between 6 and 12 months of treatment with amiodarone. The main risk factor is underlying Hashimoto's disease. In other patients, hypothyroidism resolves within 2–4 months of discontinuing amiodarone.

Thyrotoxicosis induced by amiodarone is of two types. Type 1 develops in individuals with underlying thyroid disease and is due to increased synthesis and release of thyroid hormone. Type 2 is a destructive thyroiditis in individuals with no underlying thyroid disease, and the hyperthyroidism is due to release of preformed thyroid hormone from damaged thyroid follicular epithelium. The two types are partially distinguished by measurement of interleukin-6 (normal or low in Type 1, raised in Type 2). In Type 1, amiodarone treatment should be discontinued, if possible. Large doses of thionamides are required, because high intrathyroidal iodine stores antagonise their inhibitory effect on thyroidal iodine utilisation. In patients who fail to respond after 2–3 months of treatment, potassium perchlorate 200–1000 mg daily can be a useful adjunct. Radio-iodine is rarely used because uptake is blocked by the high concentration of circulating iodine. In Type 2, prednisolone 40–60 mg leads to rapid improvement in thyroid function in most patients, often within 1 week, and amiodarone discontinuation may not be necessary. Iopanoic acid (an oral cholecystographic agent) has also been used to reduce T_4 to T_3 conversion, but is generally inferior to prednisolone. In resistant cases, other therapies have been recommended, including lithium, plasmapheresis and ultimately thyroidectomy in patients with severe thyrotoxicosis, whose amiodarone cannot be discontinued.

MISCELLANEOUS

Treatment of thyroiditis (Hashimoto's thyroiditis, subacute thyroiditis of de Quervain). Where hyperthyroidism is a feature, treatment is by a β-adrenoceptor blocking drug. Antithyroid drugs should not be used. Where there is permanent hypothyroidism, the treatment is thyroid hormone replacement.

Calcitonin. See Chapter 38.

Summary

- Autoimmune disease of the thyroid can cause over- or under-production of thyroid hormone.
- Hypothyroidism is readily treated with levothyroxine 50–200 micrograms daily by mouth, continued indefinitely.
- The treatment of hyperthyroidism due to Graves' disease is either 12–18 months' treatment with carbimazole or propylthiouracil, or a (usually) single dose of [131]I.
- The natural history of Graves' disease is of alternating remission and relapse. Progression to hypothyroidism can occur, especially after ^{131}I treatment. All patients require long-term follow-up.
- Severe forms of thyroid eye disease require adrenal steroid and immunosuppressants, or low-dose radiotherapy. Urgent surgical decompression can be required for optic nerve compression.

GUIDE TO FURTHER READING

Basaria S, Cooper D S 2005 Amiodarone and the thyroid. American Journal of Medicine 118:706–714

Biondi B, Palmieri E A, Klain M et al 2005 Subclinical hyperthyroidism: clinical features and treatment options. European Journal of Endocrinology 152(1):1–9

Cawood T, Moriarty P, O'Shea D 2004 Recent developments in thyroid eye disease. British Medical Journal 329: 385–390

Chan G W, Mandel S J 2007 Therapy insight: management of Graves' disease during pregnancy. Nature Clinical Practice Endocrinology and Metabolism 3:470–478

Cooper D S 2003 Hyperthyroidism. Lancet 362:459–468

Cooper D S 2005 Antithyroid drugs. New England Journal of Medicine 352:905–917

Dayan C M 2001 Interpretation of thyroid function tests. Lancet 357:619–624

Pearce E N, Farwell A P, Bravermen L E et al 2003 Thyroiditis. New England Journal of Medicine 348:2646–2655

Roberts C G P, Ladenson P W 2004 Hypothyroidism. Lancet 363:793–803

Vanderpump M P, Ahlquist J A, Franklyn J A, Clayton R N 1996 Consensus statement for good practice and audit measures in the management of hypothyroidism and hyperthyroidism. The Research Unit of the Royal College of Physicians of London, the Endocrinology and Diabetes Committee of the Royal College of Physicians of London, and the Society for Endocrinology. British Medical Journal 313:539–544

Van Nostrand D, Wartofsky L 2007 Radioiodine in the treatment of thyroid cancer. Endocrinology and Metabolism Clinics of North America 36:807–822

37

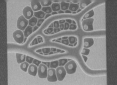

Hypothalamic, pituitary and sex hormones

SYNOPSIS

- Hypothalamic and pituitary hormones (anterior and posterior)
- Sex hormones and antagonists
  - androgens
  - antiandrogens
  - anabolic steroids
  - oestrogens
  - antioestrogens
  - progesterone and progestogens
  - antiprogestogens
  - danazol
- Fertility regulation
  - infertility
  - contraception by drugs and hormones
  - development of new contraceptives
- Menstrual disorders
- Myometrium
  - ergot and derivatives
  - oxytocin
  - uterine relaxants
  - prostaglandins
  - hormones, analogues and antagonists

Once the structure of natural hormones, local or systemic (including hormone-releasing hormones), is defined it becomes possible to synthesise not only the hormones themselves but also analogues and antagonists. Thus, increasingly, substances become available differing in selectivity and duration of action, and active by various routes of administration.

These hormones, analogues (agonists) and antagonists can be used:

- to analyse the functional integrity of endocrine control systems
- as replacement in hormone deficiency states
- to modify malfunction of endocrine systems
- to alter normal function where this is inconvenient, e.g. contraception.

The scope of the specialist endocrinologist continues to increase in amount and in complexity and only an outline is appropriate here.

HYPOTHALAMIC AND ANTERIOR PITUITARY HORMONES

The hypothalamus releases a number of locally active hormones that stimulate or inhibit pituitary hormone release (Fig. 37.1).

Some agents have restricted commercial availability. The $t_{1/2}$ of the polypeptide and glycoprotein hormones listed below is 5–30 min; they are digested if swallowed.

Corticotropin releasing hormone (CRH) is a hypothalamic polypeptide that has diagnostic use. It increases secretion of adrenocorticotrophin (ACTH) in Cushing's disease secondary to pituitary ACTH-secreting adenoma. It has no therapeutic use.

Adrenocorticotrophic hormone (ACTH). Corticotropin, see page 593.

Thyrotrophin releasing hormone (TRH) is a tripeptide amide formed in the hypothalamus and controlled by free plasma T_4 and T_3 concentration. It has been synthesised and can be used in diagnosis to test the capacity of the pituitary to release thyroid stimulating hormone (TSH), to determine whether hypothyroidism is due to primary thyroid gland failure or secondary to pituitary hypothalamic lesion, and in the differential diagnosis of borderline or subclinical thyrotoxicosis. TRH is also a potent prolactin releasing factor.

Thyroid stimulating hormone (TSH) thyrotrophin, a glycoprotein of the anterior pituitary, controls the synthesis and release of thyroid hormone from

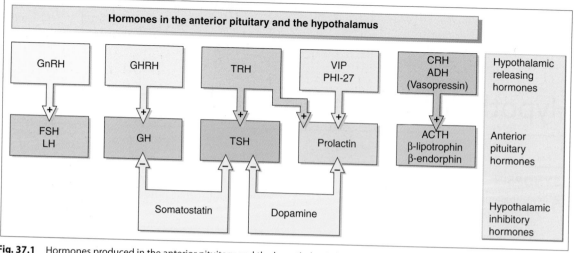

Fig. 37.1   Hormones produced in the anterior pituitary and the hypothalamic hormones that regulate their secretion. ACTH, adrenocorticotrophic hormone; ADH, antidiuretic hormone; CRH, corticotropin releasing hormone; FSH, follicle stimulating hormone; GH, growth hormone; GHRH, growth hormone releasing hormone; GnRH, gonadotrophin releasing hormone; TRH, thyrotrophin releasing hormone; TSH, thyroid stimulating hormone; VIP, vasoactive intestinal peptide.

the gland, and also the uptake of iodide. There is a negative feedback of thyroid hormones on both the hypothalamic secretion of TRH and pituitary secretion of TSH.

Antithyroid drugs, by reducing thyroid hormone production, cause increased formation of TSH which causes thyroid enlargement during excessive antithyroid drug therapy.

Growth hormone releasing hormone (GHRH) stimulates the release of growth hormone. It has been used to treat a variety of growth hormone-deficient states secondary to hypothalamic disease, idiopathic growth hormone deficiency and pituitary stalk severance.

Somatostatin is a 14 amino acid hypothalamic peptide. It inhibits growth hormone secretion.

Sermorelin is an analogue of the hypothalamic growth hormone releasing hormone (somatorelin); it is used in a diagnostic test for growth hormone secretion from the pituitary.

Growth hormone release inhibiting hormone, somatostatin, occurs in other parts of the brain as well as in the hypothalamus, and also in some peripheral tissues, e.g. pancreas, stomach. In addition to the action implied by its name, it inhibits secretion of thyrotrophin, insulin, gastrin and serotonin.

Octreotide is a synthetic analogue of somatostatin having a longer action ($t_{1/2}$ 1.5 h). It is administered subcutaneously two or three times daily; a depot formulation is available for deep intramuscular injection once a month. *Lanreotide* is much longer acting than octreotide, and is administered intramuscularly twice a month. Uses of the somatostatin analogues include acromegaly, carcinoid (serotonin-secreting) tumours and other rare tumours of the alimentary tract. An unlicensed use of octeotride is the termination of variceal bleeding (see p. 585). Radiolabelled somatostatin is used to localise, and in higher doses to treat, metastases from neuroendocrine tumours which often bear somatostatin receptors.

Growth hormone, somatrophin (Genotropin, Humatrope) is a biosynthetic form (191 amino acids) of growth hormone prepared by recombinant DNA technology, as is somatrem. Naturally occurring human growth hormone was extracted from cadaver pituitaries and its supply was therefore limited. In 1985 the use of natural growth hormone was terminated because of the risk of transmitting Creutzfeldt–Jacob disease, the fatal prion infection. Growth hormone acts on many organs to produce a peptide insulin-like growth factor IGF-1 (somatomedin), which causes muscle, bone and other tissues to increase growth, i.e. protein synthesis, and the size and number of cells.

Growth hormone is approved for treatment of children with short stature due not just to growth hormone deficiency, but also to Turner's syndrome, renal failure, small size for gestational age, Prader–Willi syndrome and, most recently, idiopathic short stature. Treatment is continued until closure of the epiphyses. Subsequent treatment into adulthood needs re-evaluation. Growth hormone therapy should be confined to specialist clinics.

The use of growth hormone in adults varies among different countries. In the UK, treatment is limited to growth hormone-deficient patients with severely impaired quality of life. Treatment improves exercise performance, increases lean body mass and overall quality of life. A low starting dose of 0.27 mg s.c. daily is used, and adjusted at 4–6-week intervals according to clinical response and IGF-1 levels. It is recommended by the National Institute for Health and Clinical Excellence (NICE) that treatment be discontinued in patients when quality of life improves by fewer than seven points on the Adult Growth Hormone Deficiency Assessment scale.

Adverse effects include increases in weight, blood pressure, and blood glucose and lipid levels. These should be monitored together with plasma haemoglobin A1c (HbA1c).

In *acromegaly*, excess growth hormone causes diabetes, hypertension and arthritis. The former two lead to a two-fold excess in cardiovascular mortality. Surgery is the treatment of choice. Growth hormone secretion is reduced by octreotide, lanreotide and other somatostatin analogues, and to a lesser degree by bromocriptine and cabergoline (see Index). If surgery fails (nadir growth hormone during oral glucose tolerance test >1 microgram/L) somatostatin analogues should be used. These bind to somatostatin receptors 2 and 5 to inhibit growth hormone production. About 60% of patients respond to somatostatin analogues.

Pegvisomant is a growth receptor antagonist. It binds to the receptor and prevents activation and production of IGF-1. As a result growth hormone increases with pegvisomant treatment, which is a specialist indication for the treatment of acromegaly in patients with inadequate response to pituitary surgery or radiation, and to somatostatin analogues.

Gonadotrophin releasing hormone (GnRH), gonadorelin, releases luteinising hormone (LH) and follicle stimulating hormone (FSH). It has a use in the assessment of pituitary function. In hypogonadotrophic hypogonadal men GnRH may be used to induce spermatogenesis and fertility. Pulsatile subcutaneous GnRH administration via a catheter attached to a mini-pump evokes secretion of gonadotrophins (LH and FSH) and is used to treat infertility. But continuous use evokes tachyphylaxis owing to down-regulation of its receptors, i.e. gonadotrophin release and therefore gonadal secretions are reduced.

Longer-acting analogues, e.g. *buserelin*, *goserelin*, *nafarelin*, *deslorelin* and *leuprorelin*, are used to suppress androgen secretion in prostatic carcinoma. Other uses may include endometriosis, precocious puberty and contraception.

Cetrorelix and *ganirelix* are luteinising hormone releasing hormone antagonists, which inhibit the release of gonadotrophins. They are used in the treatment of infertility by assisted reproductive techniques

All of these drugs need to be administered by a parenteral route. Their use should generally be in the hands of a specialist endocrinologist, oncologist or gynaecologist.

Follicle stimulating hormone (FSH) stimulates development of ova and of spermatozoa. It is prepared from the urine of postmenopausal women; *menotrophin* also contains a small amount of LH, and *urofollitrophin* is FSH alone. They are used in female and male hypothalamic hypophyseal infertility as an alternative to GnRH treatment. Pulsatile GnRH is more likely to result in development and ovulation of a single follicle than FSH. Recombinant FSH subunits (follitrophin α or β) are available for in vitro fertilization.

Chorionic gonadotrophin (human chorionic gonadotrophin, HCG) is secreted by the placenta and is obtained from the urine of pregnant women. Its predominant action is that of luteinising hormone (LH), which induces progesterone production by the corpus luteum in women, and in the male it is involved in spermatogenesis and gonadal testosterone production. It is also used to trigger ovulation in induction protocols, for corpus luteum support. In males, HCG is used in diagnostic tests of ambiguous genitalia; if HCG fails to induce testicular descent in prepubertal males, there is time for surgery to achieve a fully functioning testis. In older boys, HCG may be used to induce puberty where this is delayed.

Prolactin is secreted by the lactotroph cells of the anterior pituitary gland. Its control is by tonic hypothalamic inhibition through dopamine, which in turn acts on D_2 receptors of the lactotrophs. Its main physiological function is stimulation of lactation. Supra-physiological levels of prolactin inhibit gonadotrophin releasing hormone and gonadotrophin release as well as gonadal steroidogenesis.

Hyperprolactinaemia may be caused by drugs with antidopaminergic actions: antiemetics, major tranquillisers, second-generation neuroleptics, monoamine oxidase (MAO) inhibitors, tricyclic antidepressants and, to a lesser extent, oestrogens.

Hyperprolactinaemia may occur in primary hypothyroidism, in pituitary stalk disconnection or prolactin-secreting adenomas. Medical treatment is with *bromocriptine* started at 0.625 mg by mouth nightly, and titrated weekly to a maximum of 20 mg in divided doses. *Cabergoline* may be preferred as a more specific dopamine agonist than bromocriptine, which is taken once weekly, titrated from 500 micrograms to 2 mg. Higher doses of up to 6 mg weekly are necessary only in the treatment of macroprolactinomas. Other dopamine agonists are quinagolide 25–150 micrograms at bedtime.

In pregnancy, the dopamine agonists are discontinued in microadenomas, where the risk of enlargement is small. Treatment should continue for macroadenomas because the risk of enlargement is much higher, 15–30%. Both bromocriptine and cabergoline are safe to use, although cabergoline is not licensed in pregnancy.

Trasphenoidal surgery in a specialist unit is an alternative to medical therapy in patients who do not tolerate, or are resistant to, dopamine agonists.

HYPOPITUITARISM

In hypopituitarism there is a partial or complete deficiency of hormones secreted by the anterior and posterior lobe of the pituitary, although the latter is less common. Patients suffering from severe hypopituitarism may present in coma, in which case treatment is as for severe acute adrenal insufficiency. Maintenance therapy is required, using hydrocortisone, thyroxine, estradiol and progesterone (in women) and testosterone (in men), growth hormone and desmopressin, where indicated.

POSTERIOR PITUITARY HORMONES AND ANALOGUES

Vasopressin: antidiuretic hormone (ADH)

Vasopressin is a nonapeptide ($t_{1/2}$ 20 min) with two separate G-protein-coupled target receptors responsible for its two roles. The V_1 receptor on vascular smooth muscle cells is coupled to calcium-ion entry and is not usually stimulated by physiological concentrations of the hormone. The V_2 receptor is coupled to adenylyl cyclase, and regulates opening of the water channel, aquaporin, in cells of the renal collecting duct.

Secretion of the antidiuretic hormone is stimulated by any increase in the osmotic pressure of the blood supplying the hypothalamus and by a variety of drugs, notably nicotine. Secretion is inhibited by a fall in blood osmotic pressure and by alcohol.

In large non-physiological doses (*pharmacotherapy*) vasopressin causes contraction of all smooth muscle, raising the blood pressure and causing intestinal colic. The smooth muscle stimulant effect provides an example of tachyphylaxis (frequently repeated doses give progressively less effect). It is not only inefficient when used to raise the blood pressure, but is also dangerous, as it causes constriction of the coronary arteries and sudden death has occurred following its use.

For replacement therapy of pituitary diabetes insipidus the longer acting analogue desmopressin is used.

Desmopressin

Desmopressin (des-amino-D-arginine vasopressin, DDAVP) has two major advantages: the vasoconstrictor effect has been reduced to near insignificance and the duration of action with nasal instillation, spray or subcutaneous injection, is 8–20 h ($t_{1/2}$ 75 min) so that, using it once to twice daily, patients are not inconvenienced by polyuria and nocturia.

Desmopressin is available as oral or sublingual tablets, nasal spray and injection. The adult dose for intranasal administration is 10–20 micrograms daily. The dose for children is about half that for adults. The bio-availability of intranasal DDAVP is 10%. It is also the only peptide for which an oral formulation is currently available, albeit with a bio-availability of only 1%. Tablets of DDAVP are prescribed initially at 200–600 micrograms daily in three divided doses. The main complication of

DDAVP is hyponatraemia, which can be prevented by allowing the patient to develop some polyuria for a short period during each week. The dose requirement for DDAVP may decrease during intercurrent illness. It is therefore important to review the need for DDAVP daily in critically ill patients.

Nephrogenic diabetes insipidus, as is to be expected, does not respond to antidiuretic hormone.

In *bleeding oesophageal varices*, use is made of the vasoconstrictor effect of vasopressin (as terlipressin, a vasopressin pro-drug); see page 480.

In *haemophilia*, desmopressin can enhance blood concentration of factor VIII.

Felypressin is used as a vasoconstrictor with local anaesthetics.

Enuresis: see page 324.

DIABETES INSIPIDUS: VASOPRESSIN DEFICIENCY

Diabetes insipidus (DI) is characterised by persistent production of excess dilute urine (>40 mL/kg every 24 h in adults and >100 mL/kg every 24 h in children). DI is classified as cranial or nephrogenic. *Cranial* causes of DI are genetic, developmental or idiopathic. Acquired causes are head injury, surgery to the hypothalamic–pituitary region, tumours, inflammatory conditions such as granulomatous and infectious disease, vascular causes and external radiotherapy. *Nephrogenic* DI has a larger number of causes including drugs (lithium, demeclocycline) and several diseases affecting the renal medulla. The DNA sequencing of the receptor and aquaporins has also allowed identification of mutations in these that cause congenital DI.

Desmopressin replacement therapy is the first choice. Thiazide diuretics (and chlortalidone) also have paradoxical antidiuretic effect in diabetes insipidus. That this is not due to sodium depletion is suggested by the fact that the non-diuretic thiazide, diazoxide (see Index), also has this effect. It is probable that changes in the proximal renal tubule result in increased reabsorption and in the delivery of less sodium and water to the distal tubule, but the mechanism remains incompletely elucidated. Some cases of the nephrogenic form, which is not helped by antidiuretic hormone, may be benefited by a thiazide.

Chlorpropamide up to 300 mg/day (but not other sulphonylureas) and carbamazepine 200 mg o.d. or b.d. are effective in partial pituitary diabetes insipidus, because they act on the kidney, potentiating the effect of vasopressin on the renal tubule. Hypoglycaemia may be difficult to prevent with chlorpropamide, and neither of these drugs is the first choice for this disease.

SYNDROME OF INAPPROPRIATE ANTIDIURETIC HORMONE SECRETION (SIADH)

A variety of tumours, e.g. oat-cell lung cancer, can make vasopressin, and they are not, of course, subject to normal homeostatic mechanisms. SIADH also occurs in some central nervous system (CNS) and respiratory disorders (infection). Dilutional hyponatraemia follows, i.e. low plasma sodium with an inappropriately low plasma osmolality and high urine osmolality. When plasma sodium approaches 120 mmol/L, treatment should be with fluid restriction (e.g. 500 mL/day). Treatment is primarily of the underlying disorder accompanied by fluid restriction. Chemotherapy to the causative tumour or infection is likely to be the most effective treatment. *Demeclocycline*, which inhibits the renal action of vasopressin, is useful. Initially 0.9–1.2 g is given daily in divided doses, reduced to 600–900 mg daily for maintenance.

EMERGENCY TREATMENT OF HYPONATRAEMIA

Whereas most patients with a serum sodium concentration exceeding 125 mmol/L are asymptomatic, those with lower values may have symptoms, especially if the disorder has developed rapidly. These may be mild (headache, nausea) or severe (vomiting, disorientation). Complications are catastrophic: seizures, coma, permanent brain damage, respiratory arrest, brainstem herniation and death. Optimal treatment requires balancing the risks of hypotonicity against those of therapy, the most feared being central pontine myelinolysis. Infusion of isotonic or hypertonic saline is therefore reserved for extreme emergencies, associated with stupor, and undertaken with great caution.

The rate of correction must not exceed 0.5 mmol/L/h until the plasma sodium is 120–125 mmol/L. Over-correction (to plasma sodium >130 mmol/L) is unnecessary and potentially harmful. The predicted increase in plasma sodium per litre of infusate can be estimated from the formula:

$$(\text{infusate sodium concentration} - \text{plasma sodium concentration}) \div \text{total body water(litres)}$$

Body water is a fraction of body-weight in kilograms, being 0.6 in children and non-elderly men, 0.5 in elderly men and non-elderly women, and 0.45 in elderly women.

Oxytocin. See page 657.

SEX (GONADAL) HORMONES AND ANTAGONISTS: STEROID HORMONES

Steroid hormone receptors (for gonadal steroids and adrenocortical steroids) are complex proteins inside the target cell. The steroid penetrates, binds to the receptor and translocates into the cell nucleus, which is the principal site of action and where RNA synthesis occurs. Compounds that occupy the receptor without causing translocation into the nucleus or the replenishment of receptors act as antagonists, e.g. spironolactone to aldosterone, cyproterone to androgens, clomiphene to oestrogens.

Selectivity. Many synthetic analogues, although classed as, e.g. androgen, anabolic steroid, progestogen, are non-selective and bind to several types of receptor as agonist, partial agonist, antagonist. The result is that their effects are complex, as will be seen in the following account.

Pharmacokinetics. Steroid sex hormones are well absorbed through the skin (factory workers need protective clothing) and the gut. Most are subject to extensive hepatic metabolic inactivation (some so much that oral administration is ineffective or requires very large doses, if a useful amount is to pass through the liver and reach the systemic circulation).

There is some enterohepatic recirculation, especially of oestrogen, and this may be interrupted by severe diarrhoea, with loss of efficacy. Some non-steroidal analogues are metabolised more slowly. Sustained-release (depot) preparations are used. The hormones are carried in the blood extensively bound to sex hormone binding globulin. In general the plasma $t_{1/2}$ relates to the duration of cellular action, which is implied in the recommended dosage schedules.

ANDROGENS

Testosterone is the predominant natural androgen secreted by the Leydig cells of the testis; in a normal adult male testosterone production amounts to 4–9 mg/24 h. It circulates highly bound to a hepatic glycoprotein called sex hormone binding globulin (65%) and loosely bound to albumin (33%). Only 1–2% of circulating testosterone is unbound and freely available to tissues. It is converted by hydroxylation to the active dihydrotestosterone (DHT). Testosterone is necessary for normal spermatogenesis, for the development of the male secondary sex characteristics, sexual potency and for the growth, at puberty, of the genital tract.

Protein anabolism is increased by androgens, i.e. androgens increase the proportion of protein laid down as tissue, especially muscle and (combined with training, increase strength). Growth of bone is promoted, but the rate of closure of the epiphyses is also hastened, causing short stature in cases of precocious puberty or of androgen overdose in the course of treating hypogonadal children.

INDICATIONS FOR ANDROGEN THERAPY

Indications for testosterone treatment are primary testicular failure such as a result of bilateral anorchia, Klinefelter's (XXY) karyotype, surgery, chemotherapy and radiotherapy, or secondary testicular failure as a result of hypothalamic–pituitary disease.

Other conditions that require testosterone treatment are delayed puberty in boys aged 16 years or older, angioneurotic oedema and adrenal insufficiency in females.

Possible uses currently under investigation are hormonal male contraception, elderly men with low testosterone levels, female androgen insufficiency syndrome and wasting disease associated with cancer and HIV.

Testosterone replacement improves libido and overall sexual performance in hypogonadal men. Its effect on erectile response to sexual arousal is less clear.

PREPARATIONS AND CHOICE OF ANDROGENS

Testosterone given orally is subject to extensive hepatic first-pass metabolism and it is therefore usually given by other routes. Androgens are available for oral, buccal, transdermal or depot administration.

Oral preparations

Testosterone undecanoate is highly lipophilic. When given orally it is absorbed through the intestinal lymphatics, thereby bypassing otherwise extensive hepatic first-pass metabolism. Yet bio-availability is poor and variable. The $t_{1/2}$ is short and the dose is 40–120 mg t.d.s.

Mesterolone is a DHT derivative. It cannot be biotransformed into estradiol and therefore is an unsatisfactory preparation with only partial androgen effect.

Parenteral preparations

Sustanon is a mixed testosterone ester preparation normally given 2–4-weekly by deep i.m. injection; the usual dose is 250 mg (range 100–250). Other preparations, *testosterone enanthate* and *testosterone epionate*, are given at 1–2-week intervals. These preparations are widely used and have a good safety profile. Their main disadvantage is fluctuation of plasma testosterone concentrations, causing swings of mood and well-being. But *testosterone undecanoate* (1000 mg in 4 mL castor oil given by a depot i.m. injection) achieves stable physiological concentrations lasting for 3 months.

Transdermal preparations

Patches are available for scrotal and non-scrotal sites; they provide stable pharmacokinetics and are an alternative to painful injections. Absorption is superior at the scrotum because of its high skin vascularity. High concentrations of DHT are achieved because 5α-reductase is present in scrotal skin.

Non-scrotal patches are applied to the skin of the upper arms, back, abdomen and thighs.

Local skin reactions occur in 10% of cases and they are secondary to absorption enhancers. Application of corticosteroid ointment improves tolerability. Patches must be changed every 24 h.

Trandermal gels are hydroalcoholic gels for delivering testosterone transdermally. They are applied daily on the skin of the arms and torso. Showering must be avoided for 6 h, as well as intimate skin contact with others as transfer of testosterone may occur.

Buccal preparations

These are available in a sustained-release form. A tablet is placed in the small depression above the incisor tooth twice daily. Testosterone is absorbed and delivered into the superior vena cava, thereby bypassing hepatic first-pass metabolism. Steady-state testosterone and DHT concentrations are achieved in 24 h.

Testosterone implants

Pellets of crystallised testosterone are implanted subcutaneously under local anaesthesia by a small incision in the anterior abdominal wall, using a trocar and cannula. Three implanted pellets (total 600 mg) give hormone replacement for about 6 months. There is an approximately 10% risk of extrusion of the pellets; infection and haemorrhage are uncommon.

FEMALE ANDROGEN INSUFFICIENCY

Women with adrenal or pituitary insufficiency, premature ovarian failure or surgical menopause have reduced androgen production. This state may be associated with reduced libido, low mood and ill health.

Dehydroepiandrosterone benefits women with adrenal insufficiency but there is inadequate evidence for androgen supplement in other disease states.

See also: anabolic steroids, danazol (p. 648).

ADVERSE EFFECTS

Increased libido may lead to undesirable sexual activity, and virilisation is undesired by most women. Androgens have a weak salt and water retaining activity, which is not often clinically important. Liver injury (cholestatic) can occur, particularly with 17α-alkyl derivatives (ethylestrenol, danazol, oxymetholone); it is reversible but these agents should be avoided in hepatic disease. As androgens are contraindicated in carcinoma of the prostate, monitoring during treatment includes regular measurement of prostate specific antigen (PSA). Haemoglobin should also be monitored to avoid polycythaemia.

Effects on blood lipids are complex and variable, and the balance may be to disadvantage.

In patients with malignant disease of bone, androgen administration may be followed by hypercalcaemia. The less virilising androgens are used to promote anabolism and are discussed below.

ANTIANDROGENS (ANDROGEN ANTAGONISTS)

Oestrogens and progestogens are *physiological* antagonists to androgens. But compounds that compete selectively for androgen *receptors* have been made.

Cyproterone

Cyproterone is a derivative of progesterone; its combination of structural similarities and differences results in the following:

- Competition with testosterone for receptors in target peripheral organs (but not causing feminisation as do oestrogens); it reduces spermatogenesis even to the level of azoospermia (reversing over about 4 months after the drug is discontinued); abnormal sperm occurs during treatment.
- Competition with testosterone in the CNS, reducing sexual drive and thoughts, and causing impotence.
- Some agonist progestogenic activity on hypothalamic receptors, inhibiting gonadotrophin secretion, which also inhibits testicular androgen production.

Uses. Cyproterone is used for reducing male hypersexuality, and in prostatic cancer and severe female hirsutism. A formulation of cyproterone plus ethinylestradiol (Dianette) is offered for this latter purpose as well as for severe acne in women; this preparation acts as an oral contraceptive but does not have a UK licence, and should not be used primarily for this purpose.

Flutamide and bicalutamide are non-steroidal antiandrogens available for use in conjunction with the gonadorelins (e.g. goserelin) in the treatment of prostatic carcinoma.

Finasteride and *dutasteride* (see p. 492), which inhibit conversion of testosterone to dihydrotestosterone, have localised antiandrogen activity in tissues where dihydrotestosterone is the principal androgen; they are therefore useful drugs in the treatment of benign prostatic hypertrophy.

Spironolactone (see p. 597) also has antiandrogen activity and may help hirsutism in women (as an incidental benefit to its diuretic effect). Androgen secretion may be diminished by continued use of a gonadorelin (LHRH) analogue (see p. 639).

Ketoconazole (antifungal) interferes with androgen and corticosteroid synthesis and may be used in prostatic carcinoma and Cushing's syndrome.

ANABOLIC STEROIDS

(See also above.)

Androgens are effective protein anabolic agents, but their clinical use for this purpose is limited by the amount of virilisation that women will tolerate. Attempts made to separate anabolic from androgenic action have been only partially successful and *all anabolic steroids also have androgenic effects.*

They benefit some patients with *aplastic anaemia.*

Nandrolone 50 mg is given by deep intramuscular injection every 3 weeks. *Oxymetholone* tablets (available on named-patient basis from Cambridge) may be used in aplastic anaemia at a dose of 1–5 mg/kg daily for 3–6 months.

Hereditary angio-oedema (lack of inhibition of the complement C_1 esterase) may be prevented by *danazol.*

Anabolic steroids can prevent the calcium and nitrogen loss in the urine that occurs in patients bedridden for a long time, and have been used in the treatment of some severe fractures. The use of anabolic steroids in conditions of general wasting despite nutritional support may be justifiable in extreme debilitating disease, such as severe ulcerative colitis, and after major surgery. In the later stages of malignant disease they may make the patient feel and look less wretched.

Anabolic steroids do not usefully counter the unwanted catabolic effects of the adrenocortical hormones.

None of these agents is free from virilising properties in high doses; acne and greasy skin may be the early manifestation of virilisation (see also, Adverse effects of androgens, p. 634, and Drugs and sport, p. 147).

Oestrogens have only a modest anabolic effect.

Administration of anabolic steroids should generally be intermittent in courses of 3–12 weeks with similar steroid-free intervals, to reduce the occurrence of unwanted effects, especially liver injury.

OESTROGENS

Estrone and *estradiol* are both natural oestrogens. Oestrogens are responsible for the development of normal secondary sex characteristics in women, uterine growth, thickening of vaginal mucosa and the ductal breast system.

PHARMACOKINETICS

See page 80.

PREPARATIONS OF OESTROGENS

The dose varies according to whether replacement of physiological deficiencies is being carried out (replacement therapy) or whether pharmacotherapy is being used.

- *Ethinylestradiol* ($t_{1/2}$ 13 h) is a synthetic agent of first choice for *pharmacological* uses (mainly contraceptive, female hypogonadism and menstrual disorders); it is effective by mouth, dose 20–50 micrograms/day.
- *Estradiol* and *estriol* are orally active mixed natural oestrogens, dose 1–2 mg/day.
- *Conjugated oestrogens* (Premarin) are orally active mixed natural oestrogens containing 50–65% estrone obtained from the urine of pregnant mares, dose 0.625–1.25 mg.
- *Estropipate* (piperazine estrone sulphate) is an orally active synthetic conjugate.
- *Diethylstilbestrol* (stilboestrol) is the first synthetic oestrogen; it is rarely used in prostatic cancer, and occasionally in postmenopausal women with breast cancer.

CHOICE OF OESTROGEN

Ethinylestradiol, or its methylated derivative *mestranol* (synthetic), is a satisfactory first choice for pharmacotherapy. The weaker endogenous oestrogens, estradiol, estriol and estrone (natural), or the conjugated equine oestrogens (CEE) are preferable for physiological replacement. It remains uncertain whether all oestrogens have exactly similar hormonal and non-hormonal effects, including adverse effects.

Selective oestrogen receptor modulators (SERMS) combine oestrogenic and antioestrogenic properties (raloxifene and tibolone). *Raloxifene* has antioestrogenic effects on breast and endometrium, but oestrogenic effects on bone and is used for prevention and treatment of osteoporosis. It reduces risk of invasive breast cancer but increases risk of stroke and thromboembolism. It has no effect on vasomotor symptoms. *Tibolone* is licensed for short-term treatment of osteoporosis.

OESTROGEN FORMULATIONS AND ROUTES OF ADMINISTRATION

Oral. This is an easy and effective route but is subject to the first-pass effect through the liver, and higher doses are needed in comparison to other formulations.

Transdermal formulations are in the form of patches and gels. This route may eliminate the risk of thrombosis associated with oral oestrogen.

Subcutaneous implants. Crystalline pellets inserted into the anterior wall or buttock release hormone over several months. Used in women who undergo oophorectomy and hysterectomy, they are usually repeated at 6 months and tachyphylaxis may be a problem.

Vaginal (ring, cream, tablet or pessary). Low-dose oestrogen therapy is delivered for treatment of urogenital symptoms. If used for long periods, i.e. more than 2 years, progesterone should be added to avoid endometrial hyperplasia.

Others. A nasal spray is available. It delivers 300 micrograms of estradiol daily.

INDICATIONS FOR OESTROGEN THERAPY

Replacement therapy in hypo-oestrogenaemia

This term refers to decreased oestrogen production due to ovarian disease, or to hypothalamic–pituitary disease (hypogonadotrophic hypogonadism). Treatment is by *cyclic oestrogen* (estradiol 1–2 mg, conjugated oestrogens 0.625/1.25 mg daily or ethinylestradiol 20–30 micrograms continuously) plus a progestogen, *medroxyprogesterone* 2.5–10 mg daily for the last 10–14 days of oestrogen treatment. An alternative treatment is the oral contraceptive (see p. 650).

Postmenopausal hormone replacement therapy (HRT)

HRT refers to the use of oestrogen treatment in order to reverse or prevent problems due to the loss of ovarian hormone secretion after the menopause, whether physiological or induced. The tissues sensitive to oestrogen include brain, bone, skin, cardiovascular and genitourinary. The goal of HRT is to reduce the vasomotor symptoms of oestrogen loss – hot flushes, sleeplessness and vaginal dryness – without causing disorders that may be more common with oestrogen treatment such as breast and endometrial cancer.

All types of HRT (oestrogen with or without progestogen) are effective at reducing the hot flushes experienced by more than 50% of postmenopausal women. The benefit is most during the first year of treatment when 75% of women report a reduced likelihood. By year 3 of treatment the reduction in frequency decreases by 65% in comparison to placebo. The other major value of HRT is the relief of vaginal dryness. Vaginal administration is the most effective route for treatment of dyspareunia and related symptoms. Urinary incontinence does not respond to HRT.

The clinical evidence base for prescribing HRT has changed since the publication of trials showing excess risks of breast cancer and stroke that outweigh small benefits in reduction of fractures and risk of colonic cancer. HRT should not be used in the treatment of osteoporosis or for prevention of coronary heart disease.

Preparations used for HRT. There are three types of regimen:

1. Women *without* a uterus take continuous *oestrogen* alone.
2. Women *with* a uterus require *oestrogen combined with progestogen* to prevent endometrial proliferation and risk of endometrial cancer.
   a. In the commonest, *'sequential'*, regimen women take oestrogen without a break and add a progestogen from day 12–14 to day 28 of each cycle (different preparations vary in the exact length of progestogen prescribing). The first course is started on the first day of menstruation (if present), and 28-day cycles of treatment follow thereafter without interval.
   b. In the *'continuous'* regimen (appropriate only for women who have been amenorrhoeic for more than 1 year) fixed-dose combinations of oestrogen and progestogen are taken without a break. Continuous combination HRT regimens will eventually induce amenorrhoea in most women, thereby eliminating one of the major deterrents to HRT use, withdrawal bleeding.

Calendar packs are available. The oral preparations, Prempak C and Femoston, use, respectively, conjugated oestrogen and estradiol as their oestrogen. Oral progestogens include *dihydrogesterone, medroxyprogesterone, norgestrel* and *norethisterone*. Individual progestogens can be given orally in combination with an oestrogen, as subcutaneous depot injection or by transdermal patch. Some patches provide both hormones but obviously lack the facility for doses to

be separately titrated to provide the minimum necessary to prevent both flushing and (if undesired) withdrawal bleeding.

An alternative to oestrogen therapy is *tibolone* 2.5 mg, which is a synthetic oral steroid with weak oestrogenic, progestogenic and androgenic properties. Its main adverse effect is vaginal bleeding, which needs investigation if persistent. Vasomotor menopausal symptoms may occasionally be helped by low doses of clonidine (Dixarit).

Contraception. HRT in routine use does not provide contraception and any potentially fertile woman who requires HRT should take appropriate precautions. A woman is considered potentially fertile for 2 years after her last menstrual period if she is under 50 years of age, and for 1 year if she is aged over 50 years. A woman who is under 50 years and free of all risk factors for venous and arterial disease can use a low-oestrogen combined oral contraceptive pill to provide both relief of menopausal symptoms and contraception; it is recommended that the oral contraceptive be stopped at 50 years of age as there are more suitable alternatives.

Adverse effects of HRT. The commonest reasons for withdrawal are *irregular or withdrawal bleeding* and *breast pain*. Concerns about musculoskeletal symptoms and weight gain have not been substantiated in the long-term trials. Transdermal patches were associated with skin reactions but as the alcohol content has been reduced in the newer formulations the incidence has been reduced.

The more serious complications are venous thromboembolism and cancer of the endometrium or breast. These risks are small in absolute terms, particularly so for the risks of cancer during the first 5 years of treatment.

For *venous thromboembolism*, the excess risk is 4 per 1000 woman-years, which may be considered clinically insignificant except in women with predisposing factors, e.g. previous personal or family history of thromboembolism, or recent surgery.

The risk of *carcinoma of the endometrium* is increased two-fold during 5 years, rising to sevenfold with longer treatment. Because endometrial cancer is uncommon, the absolute risk is about one-tenth that of thromboembolic disease; the risk subsides over 5–10 years after stopping treatment.

Carcinoma of the breast can occur with any type of HRT. Some 45 in every 1000 women aged 50 years will have breast cancer over the next 20 years, rising by only 2, 6 and 12 cases, respectively, for women who take HRT for 5, 10 or 15 years. A family history of breast cancer does not increase the risks from HRT.

The risk of *gallstones* may be increased up to two-fold. HRT does not increase risk of ovarian cancer.

Blood lipids: the effect of oestrogens is on balance favourable, but the addition of a progestogen (unless gestodene or desogestrel) reverses the balance.

Contraindications to oestrogen therapy include recent arterial or venous thromboembolic disease, and history of oestrogen-dependent neoplasm, e.g. breast cancer. Hypertension, liver disease or gallstones, migraine, diabetes, uterine fibroids or endometriosis may all be made worse by oestrogen. These are very variable, and are not absolute contraindications.

PHARMACOTHERAPY

Contraception. See page 654.

Menstrual disorders. See page 656.

Vaginitis. Senile vaginitis usually responds to daily use of an oestrogen pessary or cream (which can also be used in small girls with vaginitis). Absorption can occur sufficiently to cause systemic effects in both the subject and her male sexual partner.

Androgen-dependent carcinoma. Diethylstilbestrol (stilboestrol) is rarely used to treat prostate cancer because of its adverse effects. It is occasionally used in postmenopausal women with breast cancer. Toxicity is common.

Osteoporosis. See SERMS above (p. 667).

Epistaxis: as a last resort in recurrent cases, e.g. telangiectasia.

Atrophic rhinitis may benefit, as also may *acne*.

ANTI-OESTROGENS

Selective antagonists of the oestrogen receptor are used either to induce gonadotrophin release in anovulatory infertility or to block stimulation of oestrogen receptor-positive carcinomas of the breast.

Clomifene is structurally related to diethylstilbestrol; it is a weak oestrogen agonist having less activity than natural oestrogens, so that its occupation of receptors results in antagonism, i.e. it is a partial agonist. Clomifene blocks hypothalamic oestrogen receptors so that the negative feedback of natural oestrogens is prevented and the pituitary responds by increased secretion of gonadotrophins, which may induce ovulation.

Clomifene is administered during the early follicular phase of the menstrual cycle (50 mg daily on days 2–6) and is successful in inducing ovulation in about 85% of women. Multiple ovulation with multiple pregnancy may occur and this is its principal adverse effect, which can be limited by using ultrasonography. There have been reports of an increased incidence of ovarian carcinoma following multiple exposure, and the number of consecutive cycles for which clomiphene may be used to stimulate ovulation should be limited to 12.

Cyclofenil acts similarly to clomiphene.

Tamoxifen is a non-steroidal competitive oestrogen antagonist on target organs. Although available for anovulatory infertility (20 mg daily on days 2, 3, 4 and 5 of the cycle), its main use now is in the treatment of *oestrogen-dependent breast cancer* (see p. 550). Treatment with tamoxifen delays the growth of metastases and increases survival; if tolerated it should be continued for 5 years.

Tamoxifen is also the hormonal treatment of choice in women with oestrogen receptor-positive *metastatic* breast cancer. Approximately 60% of such patients respond to initial hormonal manipulation, whereas less than 10% of oestrogen receptor-negative tumours respond.

Severe adverse effects are unusual with tamoxifen but patients with bony metastases may experience an exacerbation of pain, sometimes associated with hypercalcaemia; this reaction commonly precedes tumour response. Amenorrhoea commonly develops in premenopausal women. Patients should be told of the small risk of endometrial cancer and encouraged to report relevant symptoms early. They can be reassured that the benefits of treatment far outweigh the risks.

PROGESTERONE AND PROGESTOGENS

Progesterone ($t_{1/2}$ 5 min) is produced by the corpus luteum and converts the uterine epithelium from the proliferative to the secretory phase. It is thus necessary for successful implantation of the ovum and is essential throughout pregnancy, in the last two-thirds of which it is secreted in large amounts by the placenta. It acts particularly on tissues that are sensitised by oestrogens. Some synthetic progestogens are less selective, having varying oestrogenic and androgenic activity, and these may inhibit ovulation, though not very reliably. Progestogens are of two principal kinds:

- *Progesterone and its derivatives*: dydrogesterone, hydroxyprogesterone, medroxyprogesterone ($t_{\frac{1}{2}}$ 28 h).
- *Testosterone derivatives*: norethisterone and its pro-drug ethynodiol ($t_{\frac{1}{2}}$ 10 h), levonorgestrel, desogestrel, gestodene, gestronol, norgestimate.

Drospirenone is a derivative of the synthetic aldosterone antagonist, spironolactone (see p. 597). It therefore has antimineralocorticoid activity, reducing salt retention and blood pressure. It also exhibits partial antiandrogenic activity, about 30% of that of cyproterone acetate. It is available as a combination with ethinylestradiol for use as a contraceptive.

Most progestogens can virilise directly or by metabolites (except progesterone and dydrogesterone), and fetal virilisation to the point of sexual ambiguity has occurred with vigorous use during pregnancy (see also Contraception, p. 654).

Megestrol is used only in cancer; it causes tumours in the breasts of beagle dogs.

USES

The clinical uses of progestational agents are ill defined, apart from *contraception*, the *menopause* and *postmenopausal hormone replacement* therapy (see above).

Other possible uses include: menstrual disorders, e.g. menorrhagia, endometriosis, dysmenorrhoea and premenstrual syndrome (doubtful efficacy), breast and endometrial cancer.

PREPARATIONS

Available progestogens (some used only in combined formulations) include:

- *Oral*: norethisterone, dydrogesterone, gestodene, desogestrel, levonorgestrel, megestrol, medroxyprogesterone.
- *Suppositories* or *pessaries*: progesterone.
- *Injectable*: progesterone, hydroxyprogesterone, medroxyprogesterone.

Adverse effects of prolonged use include virilisation (see above), raised blood pressure and an adverse trend in blood lipids. Gestodene, desogestrel and norgestimate may have less affinity for androgen receptors and therefore fewer unfavourable effects on blood lipids; however, the first two of these may have a higher risk of thrombosis.

ANTIPROGESTOGENS

Menstruation (in its luteal phase) is dependent on progesterone, and uterine bleeding follows antagonism of progesterone. Pregnancy is dependent on progesterone (for implantation, endometrial stimulation, suppression of uterine contractions and placenta formation), and abortion follows progesterone antagonism in early pregnancy.

Mifepristone is a pure competitive antagonist at progesterone and glucocorticoid receptors. Clinical trials of oral use in hospital outpatients have shown it to be safe and effective in terminating pregnancy. Efficacy is enhanced if its use is followed by vaginal administration of a prostaglandin (gemeprost) to produce uterine contractions (the success rate is raised from 85% to more than 95%).

Adverse effects of the combined treatment include nausea and vomiting, dizziness, asthenia, abdominal pain; uterine bleeding may be heavy. Mifepristone also offers the opportunity for mid-trimester terminations. These are likely to become more frequent with rise in the number of inherited syndromes amenable to antenatal diagnosis at this stage.

Guidelines may vary in detail and the following are general regimens:

- For gestation of up to 1 week where the fetus is deemed viable, mifepristone 600 mg by mouth followed 36–48 h later by gemeprost 1 mg by vagina.
- For mid-trimester medical abortion (13–24 weeks), mifepristone 600 mg by mouth followed 36–48 h later by gemeprost 1 mg every 3 h by vagina to a maximum of 5 mg.

Other progesterone derivatives

Danazol (Danol) is a derivative of the progestogen, ethisterone. It has partial agonist androgen activity and is described as an 'impeded' androgen; it has little progestogen activity. It is a relatively selective inhibitor of pituitary gonadotrophin secretion (LH, FSH) affecting the surge in the mid-menstrual cycle more than basal secretion. This reduces ovarian function, which leads to atrophic changes in endometrium, both uterine and elsewhere (ectopic), i.e. endometriosis. In males it reduces spermatogenesis. Unwanted androgenic effects occur in women (acne, hirsutism and, rarely, enlargement of the clitoris).

It is used chiefly for: endometriosis, fibrocystic mastitis, gynaecomastia, precocious puberty, menorrhagia and hereditary angio-oedema (see p. 656).

Gestrinone is similar.

FERTILITY REGULATION

INFERTILITY

The treatment of infertility in either sex is a highly specialised business, requiring a detailed understanding of reproductive physiology and analysis of the cause.

Depending on the cause, the following agents, already described, are used:

For women, ovulation induction:

- Hypothalamic hormone: gonadorelin (p. 639).
- Anterior pituitary hormones: follicle stimulating hormone (p. 639); chorionic gonadotrophin (p. 639).
- Anti-oestrogens: clomifene, etc. (p. 647).
- Bromocriptine for hyperprolactinaemia (p. 382).

For men, induction of spermatogenesis: the same agents as for ovulation are used.

POLYCYSTIC OVARY SYNDROME (PCOS)

The diagnosis requires at least two of the following features:

- Polycystic ovaries.
- Oligo-ovulation or anovulation.
- Clinical and/or biochemical evidence of androgen excess.

Management of PCOS includes:

- *Treatment of infertility.* Induction of ovulation can be accomplished in 75–80% of women with PCOS by the use of anti-oestrogens, typically clomifene citrate. More recent data indicate that metformin (see below) may improve ovulation rates in women with PCOS when given alone or in combination with clomifene.
- *Menstrual regulation* in those who do not desire pregnancy. A low-dose combined oral contraceptive (containing ethinylestradiol, 20–35 micrograms) may be the most convenient form of treatment, although cyclical progestogen is a reasonable alternative. Norgestimate and desogestrel are the preferred progestins, having virtually no androgenic properties.
- *Treatment of associated symptoms of hyperandrogenism.* Management of hirsutism usually involves cosmetic treatment to remove unwanted hair and, in more severe cases, antiandrogen therapy. The most commonly used antiandrogen is cyproterone acetate. This also has progestogenic activity and can be combined with ethinylestradiol to provide cycle control in addition to management of hyperandrogenic symptoms. Drospirenone (see above) is ideal in PCOS because of its antiandrogen and antimineralocorticoid properties. Spironolactone can be used at high doses, 100–200 mg. Flutamide is a potent non-steroidal antiandrogen that is effective in the treatment of hirsutism. Concern about inducing hepatocellular dysfunction has limited its use.
- Prevention of the possible long-term consequences of the metabolic disturbance characteristic of anovulatory women with PCOS.

Calorie restriction in obese women with PCOS improves insulin sensitivity and glucose tolerance, and leads to resumption of spontaneous ovulatory cycles and normal fertility in many cases. Metformin may be a safe and effective means of improving metabolic profile and reproductive function in both lean and obese women with PCOS.

CONTRACEPTION BY DRUGS AND HORMONES

The requirements of a successful hormonal contraceptive are stringent, for it will be used by millions of healthy people who wish to separate sexual relations from physical reproduction. The following represent the ideal:

- It must be extremely *safe* as well as highly effective.
- Its action must be *quick* in onset and quickly and completely reversible, even after years of continuous use.
- It must not affect *libido*.

The fact that alternative methods are less reliable implies that their use will lead to more unwanted pregnancies with their attendant inconvenience, morbidity and mortality, and this must be taken into account in deciding what risks of hormonal contraception are acceptable.

POSSIBLE MODES AND SITES OF ACTION

1. *Direct inhibition of spermatogenesis*: this presents many problems including the lag in onset of effect due to storage of mature spermatozoa until they are ejaculated or die from old age.
2. *Indirect inhibition of spermatogenesis* by suppression of hypothalamic–pituitary activity, which controls it, e.g. by progestogen–androgen combinations; see gonadorelin.
3. *Immunological techniques* (vaccines) to induce antibodies to pituitary gonadotrophins, sperm, or other components of the reproductive process in either sex; these are being developed.
4. *Inhibition of ovulation* presents a different and easier biological problem. There is no need to suppress continuous formation of the gametes, as in the male, but only to prevent their release from the ovary approximately 13 times a year. Either the pituitary gonadotrophin may be inhibited or the ovary may be made unresponsive to it.
5. *Prevention of fertilisation*: the female genital tract may be made inhospitable to spermatozoa, e.g. by altering cervical mucus or fallopian tube function.
6. *Antizygotic drugs*: compounds effective in the rat have been developed.
7. *Inhibition of implantation*: implantation does not occur unless the endometrium is in the right state, and this depends on a delicate balance between oestrogen and progesterone. This balance can readily be disturbed.
8. *Use of spermicides in the vagina* (in combination with barrier methods). This is strictly chemical

rather than hormonal contraception, as also are intrauterine devices that contain copper, which is gametocidal.

Hormonal contraception in women comprises:

- Oestrogen and progestogen (combined and phased administration).
- Progestogen alone.

COMBINED CONTRACEPTIVES (THE 'PILL')

Combined oestrogen–progestogen oral contraceptives (COCP) have been used extensively since 1956. The principal mechanism is inhibition of ovulation (4, above) through suppression of LH surge by hypothalamus and pituitary. In addition the endometrium is altered, so that implantation is less likely (7, above) and cervical mucus becomes more viscous and impedes the passage of the spermatozoa (5, above).

The combination is conveniently started on the first day of the cycle (first day of menstruation) and continued for 21 days (this is immediately effective, inhibiting the first ovulation). It is followed by a period of 7 days when no pill is taken, and during which bleeding usually occurs. Thereafter, regardless of bleeding, a new 21-day course is begun, and so on, i.e. active tablets are taken daily for 3 weeks out of 4. For easy compliance, some combined pills are packaged so that the woman takes one tablet every day without interruption (21 active then 7 dummy).

In some instances, the course is not started on the first day of menstruation but on the second to the fifth day (to give a full month between the menses at the outset). An alternative method of contraception should then be used until the seventh pill has been taken, as the first ovulation may not have been suppressed in women who have short menstrual cycles.

The pill should be taken at about the same time (to within 12 h) every day to establish a routine. The monthly bleeds that occur 1–2 days after the cessation of active hormone administration are hormone withdrawal bleeds not natural menstruation. They are not an essential feature of oral contraception, but women are accustomed to monthly bleeds and they provide monthly reassurance of the absence of pregnancy.

Numerous field trials have shown that progestogen–oestrogen combinations, if taken precisely as directed, are the most reliable reversible contraceptive known. (The only close competitors are depot progestogens and progestogen-releasing intrauterine devices.)

Important aspects

Subsequent fertility. After stopping the pill, fertility that is normal for the age the woman has now reached is restored, although conception may be delayed for a few months longer in younger, and for as much as a year in older, users than if other methods had been used.

Effect on an existing pregnancy. Although progestogens can masculinise the female fetus, the doses for contraception are so low that risk of harming an undiagnosed pregnancy is extremely small, probably less than 1 in 1000 (the background incidence of birth defects is 1–2%).

Carcinomas of the breast and cervix are slightly increased in incidence;[1] the incidence of hepatoma (very rare) is increased. The risk to life seems to be less than that of moderate smoking (10 cigarettes/day). The risk of carcinoma of the ovary and endometrium is substantially reduced. The overall incidence of cancer is unaltered.

The effect on menstruation (it is not true menstruation, see above) is generally to regularise it, and often to diminish blood loss, but amenorrhoea can occur. In some women 'breakthrough' intermenstrual bleeding occurs, especially at the outset, but this seldom persists for more than a few cycles. Premenstrual tension and dysmenorrhoea are much reduced.

Libido is greatly subject to psychosocial influences, and removal of fear of pregnancy may permit enthusiasm for the first time. It is likely that direct pharmacological effect (reduction) is rare. There is evidence that the normal increase in female-initiated sexual activity at time of ovulation is suppressed.

---

[1] A meta-analysis of 54 studies concluded that use of the COCP was associated with a relative risk of 1.24, which disappears over 10 years after stopping the COCP. A higher relative risk in women who started taking the COCP at a young age is explained by the lower background rate and there is little added effect from long-term COCP ingestion. (Collaborative Group on Hormonal Factors in Breast Cancer. *Lancet* 1996; **347**:1713–27).

Cardiovascular complications. The incidence of *venous thromboembolism* is increased in pill users. It is lowest in the 20–35-microgram pill and rises progressively with the 50- and 100-microgram preparations; it is not known whether there is any difference between doses of 20 and 35 micrograms. The small increase in hypertension, cerebrovascular events and acute myocardial infarction is confined principally to smokers.

Increased arterial disease also appears to be associated with the type of progestogen in the combined pill. The 'third-generation' pills (see below) appear to carry a higher risk of venous thrombosis, but may have a lower risk of arterial thrombosis because their lower androgen activity leads to slightly higher high-density lipoprotein (HDL) levels than older pills. The progestogen-only pill does not significantly affect coagulation.

Major surgery (in patients taking oestrogen–progestogen contraceptives and postmenopausal hormone replacement therapy). Because of the added risk of venous thromboembolism (surgery causes a fall in antithrombin levels), oral contraceptives should be withdrawn, if practicable, 4 weeks before all lower limb operations or any major elective surgery (and started again at the first menstruation to occur more than 2 weeks after surgery). But increase in clotting factors may persist for many weeks and there is also the risk of pregnancy to be considered. An alternative for emergencies is to use low molecular weight heparin (although this may not reverse all the oestrogenic effects on coagulation) and other means (mechanical stimulation of venous return) to prevent postoperative thrombosis.

Hepatic function may be impaired as may drug-metabolising capacity ($t_{1/2}$ of antipyrine, a general indicator of the drug-metabolising capacity, may increase by 30%). Gallbladder disease is more common, and highly vascular hepatocellular adenomas occur (rare).

Cervical ectropion (erosion) incidence is doubled (it is a harmless condition).

Crohn's disease is more frequent.

Decreased glucose tolerance occurs, perhaps owing to a peripheral effect reducing the action of insulin.

Plasma lipoproteins may be adversely affected; least where the progestogen is desogestrel or low-dose norethisterone.

Plasma proteins. Oestrogens cause an increase in proteins, particularly the globulins that bind hydrocortisone, thyroxine and iron. As a result, the total plasma concentration of the bound substances is increased, although the concentration of free and active substance remains normal. This can be misleading in diagnostic tests, e.g. of thyroid function. This effect on plasma proteins passes off about 6 weeks after cessation of the oestrogen.

Other adverse effects

Often more prominent at the outset and largely due to oestrogen, these include: nausea and, rarely, vomiting; breast discomfort, fluid retention, headache (including increase in migraine), lethargy, abdominal discomfort, vaginal discharge or dryness. Depression may occur but most depression in pill users is not due to the contraceptive.

The above account gives rise to guidelines for use:

Absolute contraindications include:

- A personal history of thromboembolic venous, arterial or cardiac disease, or severe or multiple risk factors for these.
- Transient cerebral ischaemic attacks without headache.
- Infective hepatitis, until 3 months after liver function test results have become normal, and other liver disease including disturbances of hepatic excretion, e.g. cholestatic jaundice, Dubin–Johnson and Rotor syndromes.
- Migraine, if there is a typical aura, focal features, or if it is severe and lasts for more than 72 h despite treatment, or is treated with an ergot derivative (use with caution is acceptable if there is no aura, focal features, or if it is controlled with a 5HT$_1$ receptor agonist).
- Carcinoma of the breast or genital tract, past or present.
- Other conditions including: systemic lupus erythematosus, porphyria, following evacuation of a hydatidiform mole (until urine and plasma gonadotrophin concentrations are normal), undiagnosed vaginal bleeding.

Relative contraindications or uses with caution, include:

- Family history of venous thromboembolism, arterial disease or a known prothrombotic condition, e.g. factor V Leiden (pretreatment coagulation investigation is advised).
- Diabetes mellitus, which may be precipitated or become more difficult to control (avoid if there are diabetic complications).
- Hypertension (avoid if blood pressure exceeds 160/100 mmHg).
- Smoking more than 40 cigarettes per day (15 cigarettes/day enhances the risks of circulatory disease three-fold, and constitutes an absolute contraindication for women over 35 years).
- Age over 35 years (avoid if older than 50 years).
- Obesity (avoid if body mass index exceeds 39 kg/m^2).
- Long-term immobility, e.g. due to leg plaster, confinement to bed.
- Breast-feeding (until weaning or for 6 months after birth).

Duration of use does not enhance risks of itself. The increase in risk with increased duration of use is due to increasing age. The approaching menopause presents an obvious problem. Because cyclical bleeding will continue to occur under the influence of the drugs even after the natural menopause, the only way of deciding whether contraception can be permanently abandoned is by abandoning it (and using another technique) for 3 months annually to see whether natural menstruation is resumed, or by stopping the combined pill for 1 month and measuring luteinising hormone (LH)/follicle stimulating hormone (FSH) concentration in the blood, which indicates the state of pituitary function.

Benefits additional to contraception

The oestrogen–progestogen pill is associated with a reduced risk of functional ovarian cysts and cancer, of endometrial cancer and of benign breast disease; there is a reduced risk of uterine fibroids and they bleed less; menses are regular and blood loss is not excessive; menses are accompanied by less premenstrual tension and dysmenorrhoea. When oestrogen is combined with the antiandrogen cyproterone acetate as the progestogenic agent 'Dianette', the combined pill is useful treatment for acne in young women.

Conclusions

Serious adverse effects of the combined pill are rare and 'several times a rare event is still a rare event'.

Precise figures on risk with current low-dose formulations are not available. The major studies, involving, e.g. 23 000 women, used higher-dose formulations and cannot be repeatedly replicated (cost, logistics) to keep up with developments.

Overall mortality amongst users (having low risk factors) is either unaffected or only slightly increased.

Formulations of oestrogen–progestogen combination

Oestrogen: ethinylestradiol or mestranol.

Progestogen:

- Second generation: norethisterone, levonorgestrel.
- Third generation: desogestrel, gestodene, norgestimate.

Combined oral contraceptives are defined as second or third generation by the progestogen component (first-generation progestogens are obsolete). Those containing a fixed amount of oestrogen and progestogen in each active tablet are termed 'monophasic'. Other pills employ variable ratios between oestrogen and progestogen, in two (biphasic) or three (triphasic) periods within the menstrual cycle. The dose of progestogen is low at the beginning and higher at the end, the oestrogen remaining either constant or rising slightly in mid cycle. The objective is to achieve effective contraception with minimal distortion of natural hormonal rhythms.

The advantages claimed for these techniques are diminished adverse metabolic changes, e.g. blood lipids, and a particularly reliable monthly bleeding pattern without loss of contraceptive efficacy. Preparations include BiNovum, TriNovum, Logynon.

It is now appreciated that the earlier preparations had much more oestrogen than was necessary for efficacy. It seems probable that 20 micrograms is about the limit below which serious loss of efficacy can be expected. Indeed, in patients whose hepatic enzymes are likely to be induced, e.g. those taking antiepileptic or some antirheumatic drugs, it is advisable to use a preparation containing 50 micrograms oestrogen or more to avoid loss of efficacy due to increased oestrogen metabolism (elimination of breakthrough bleeding is a guide to adequacy of dose).

Choice of oestrogen–progestogen combination

There is a wide choice of formulations, with the dose of *ethinylestradiol* varying from 20–35 micrograms. In general, users should be prescribed the lowest total hormone dose that suits them (good cycle control and minimal side-effects) and should make a start with the first preparation given above, recognising that compliance is particularly important with the 20-microgram dose.

Common problems

Missed pill. The following refers to the combined pill (see later for the progestogen-only pill):

- If an omitted dose is remembered within 12 h, it should be taken at once and the next dose at the usual time, and all should be well.
- If more than 12 h have elapsed, the above procedure should be followed but an additional barrier method of contraception should be used for 7 days (or abstinence). Although the protective effect of cervical mucus returns within 48 h, this 7-day period is needed to ensure effective suppression of an ovulation that may have been initiated by the missed pill.

Intercurrent gut upset. If vomiting occurs more than 3 h after a pill, behave as for a missed pill (above). The hormones are rapidly absorbed and only severe diarrhoea would interfere significantly with efficacy. But if there is doubt, it would be prudent to use a barrier method during and for 7 days after the episode.

Changing of preparation. If a woman is unhappy on one preparation she may be changed to another containing a different dose of oestrogen and/or progestogen. The new preparation should start the day after she has finished a cycle on the previous preparation. If this is done no extra risk of pregnancy occurs.

Breakthrough bleeding (bleeding on days of active pill taking) can mean that a higher dose of oestrogen or progestogen is required. Note that missed or late pills, drug interaction (see below) or sexually transmitted infection, e.g. due to chlamydia, can also cause breakthrough bleeding.

PROGESTOGEN-ONLY CONTRACEPTION

Progestogen-only pills (POPs) are indicated where oestrogen is contraindicated (see above, p. 644) and in lactating women. Progestogens render cervical mucus less easily penetrable by sperm and induce a premature secretory change in the endometrium so that implantation does not occur. Older POPs became unreliable if not taken at the same time of day, because their effect on cervical mucus wears off after 3 h and their additional action to inhibit ovulation occurs in only 40% of cycles. There is also liability to breakthrough bleeding.

A newer POP containing 75 micrograms *desogestrel* inhibits ovulation in 97–99% of cycles, resulting in an efficacy similar to that of the COCP. A further advantage of the newer POP is that no extra contraceptive cover is required if the exact time of dose is missed, provided the delay is no more than 12 h. Ectopic pregnancy may be more frequent due to a fertilised ovum being held up in a functionally depressed fallopian tube.

Medroxyprogesterone acetate and its metabolites are excreted in breast milk, so women who breast-feed should wait until 6 weeks postpartum before starting Depo-Provera, when the infant's enzyme system should be more mature. *Norethisterone enantate* 200 mg (Noristerat) is shorter-acting than Depo-Provera, 8 weeks, and is used to provide contraception after administration of the rubella vaccine, and until a partner's vasectomy has taken effect. It can also be used in the longer-term but only on a 'named patient' basis.

Subdermal implantations that release hormone for several years are in use; they can be removed surgically if adverse effects develop or pregnancy is desired. For example, a flexible rod containing *etonorgestrel* (Implanton) inserted into the lower surface of the upper arm provides contraception for 3 years (2 years for overweight women because they have lower blood concentrations). The rod must be removed when its effective period has elapsed.

Two depot injections of *intramuscular progestogen* are available, equal in efficacy to the combined pill. Medroxyprogesterone (Depo-Provera) ($t_{1/2}$ 28 h) is a sustained-release (aqueous suspension) deep i.m. injection given 3-monthly. When injected between day 1 and day 5 of the menstrual cycle, contraception starts immediately. If given after day 5, a barrier contraceptive is needed for 7 days.

POSTCOITAL ('MORNING AFTER PILL') AND EMERGENCY CONTRACEPTION

This is not a new concept: post-ejaculation douching has been advocated from ancient to modern times, using substances ranging from ground cabbage blossoms to Coca-Cola.

The overall risk of pregnancy following a single act of unprotected intercourse on any day in the menstrual cycle is 2–4%. The risk from a single act is highest (20–30%) in the days before and just after ovulation. Pregnancy may be prevented before implantation by disrupting the normal hormonal arrangements; the mode of action is probably by delaying or preventing ovulation or by preventing implantation of the fertilised ovum.

Progestogen-only treatment is preferred. *Levonorgestrel* 1500 micrograms is taken within 72 h of unprotected sexual intercourse. It can be taken more than once in a cycle, if required, and there is no upper limit to how many times it can be taken in a year. Contraindications to hormonal emergency contraception include current or suspected pregnancy, multiple episodes of unprotected sexual intercourse more than 72 h earlier, and sensitivity to the components of the progestogen-only preparation. Some women complain of nausea and vomiting, which responds best to domperidone.

DRUG INTERACTION WITH STEROID CONTRACEPTIVES

Particularly now that the lowest effective doses are in use there is little latitude between success and failure if absorption, distribution and metabolism are distrubed. Any additional drug-taking must be looked at critically lest it reduces efficacy.

Enzyme induction. The rifamycins, rifampicin and rifabutin, are potent inducers of hepatic drug-metabolising enyzmes. The classic example of failure with the combined pill is breakthrough bleeding and pregnancy in young women being treated with rifampicin for tuberculosis, or meningitis including eradication of the carrier state. The enhanced metabolism of the steroids results in contraceptive failure.

Antiepileptics (phenytoin and carbamazepine but not sodium valproate) create a similar risk. Indeed, all drugs that induce metabolising enzymes (see

p. 589), whether prescribed or self-administered (alcohol, tobacco smoking), constitute a risk to contraceptive efficacy and prescribing should be specifically reviewed for the effect.

Broad-spectrum antimicrobials, e.g. ampicillin, doxycillin, can reduce the efficacy of combined oral contraceptives by diminishing the bacterial flora that metabolise ethinylestradiol in the large bowel and make it available for recycling. Additional contraceptive measures should be taken during a short course of antimicrobial, and for 7 days thereafter. When the course is long, i.e. more than 3 weeks, the bacteria have time to recover by developing resistance, and additional precautions are unnecessary after the first 14 days.

HYPOTHALAMIC/PITUITARY HORMONE APPROACH TO CONTRACEPTION

(See gonadorelin.)

OTHER METHODS OF CONTRACEPTION

Copper intrauterine devices are widely used and highly effective (>99% at 1 year) for 5 years, and some for 10 years. They are especially useful in the over-40s, in whom oral contraceptives may become progressively contraindicated and for whom one IUD will last into the menopause. The IUD prevents implantation of the fertilised ovum, and has an additional antifertilisation effect enhanced by the toxic effect of copper ions on the gametes.

The intrauterine levonorgestrel system Mirena is used as a contraceptive, as a medical treatment for idiopathic menorrhagia and as the progestogen component of hormone replacement therapy. It is popular because of reduced dysmenorrhoea and lighter menses. Mirena contains 52 mg levonorgestrel surrounded by a Silastic capsule, and releases 20 micrograms/day over 5 years, after which the device should be changed.

Vaginal preparations, used to immobilise or kill (spermicide) spermatozoa, are used to add safety to various mechanical contraceptives. They are very unreliable and should be used alone only in an emergency. Substances used include nonoxinols (surfactants that alter the permeability of the sperm liporotein membrane) as pessary, gel or foam.

Oil-based lubricants cause failure of rubber condoms and contraceptive diaphragms; many 'lubricants', e.g. hand or baby creams, wash off readily, but are nevertheless oil-based. Barrier contraceptive devices made of polyurethane, e.g. the female condom (Femidom), are not so affected.

RISKS OF CONTRACEPTION IN RELATION TO BENEFIT

Despite the small risk of thromboembolism, the death rate from taking oral contraceptives is less than that from playing cricket, and much less than that from swimming or driving a car.

MALE CONTRACEPTION (SYSTEMIC)

Suppression of spermatogenesis may be achieved by interfering with:

- Extragonadal endocrine control, i.e. the hypothalamic–pituitary–gonadal axis.
- Direct action on gonadal spermatogenesis.
- Vaccines to produce antibodies to sperm.

Approaches include testosterone or combinations of androgen with danazol, or progestogens, or gonadotrophin releasing hormone (GnRH) antagonists.

In practice, the condom and vasectomy are the only commonly used forms of male contraception.

Summary
- Many of the pituitary hormones and their hypothalamic releasing factors are used in diagnosis or therapy.
- The main therapeutic use of pituitary hormones is of growth hormone (anterior pituitary) and those from the posterior pituitary: oxytocin and vasopressin.
- Vasopressin (antidiuretic hormone) is used both for its vasoconstrictor effect (in the treatment of oesophageal varices) and for its antidiuretic action.
- The main hypothalamus–pituitary target organ axis for therapeutic intervention is that controlling reproductive hormones, especially in women.
- Suppression of oestrogen and/or androgen production is used in the treatment of tumours stimulated by these: breast and prostate.
- Therapy in women is used to suppress ovulation (contraceptives), to stimulate ovulation (fertility treatment) or to mimic ovarian endocrine function (postmenopausal hormone replacement therapy, HRT).

MENSTRUAL DISORDERS

Amenorrhoea, primary or secondary, requires specialist endocrinological diagnosis. Where the cause is failure of hormone production, cyclical replacement therapy is indicated.

Menorrhagia can be associated with both ovulatory and anovulatory ovarian cycles. It is important to distinguish the menstrual consequences of each cycle. *Ovulatory* ovarian cycles give rise to *regular* menstrual cycles, whereas *anovulatory* cycles result in *irregular* menstruation or, extremely, amenorrhoea. This distinction is critical in management.

Both ovulatory and anovulatory cycles can give rise to excessive menstrual loss in the absence of any other abnormality, so-called dysfunctional uterine bleeding. Endocrine disorders do not cause excessive menstrual loss, with the exception of the endocrine consequences of anovulation. Equally, haemostatic disorders are rare causes of menorrhagia. One consequence of excessive menstrual loss is iron deficiency anaemia. In the Western world menorrhagia is the commonest cause of iron deficiency anaemia.

Medical treatment of menorrhagia is either *non-hormonal* or *hormonal* therapy. As there is no hormonal defect, the use of hormonal therapy does not correct an underlying disorder but merely imposes an external control of the cycle. For many women, cycle control is as important an issue as the degree of menorrhagia.

The two main first-line treatments for menorrhagia associated with ovulatory cycles are non-hormonal, namely *tranexamic acid* (an antifibrinolytic) and a non-steroidal anti-inflammatory drug (NSAID), e.g. *mefenamic acid* 500 mg when the blood loss becomes heavy, followed by 250 mg t.d.s. for 3 days. The effectiveness of these treatments has been shown in randomised trials and reported in systematic reviews of treatment. Tranexamic acid reduces menstrual loss by about a half and NSAIDs reduced it by about a third. Both have the advantage of being taken only during menstruation itself and are particularly useful in women who either do not require contraception or do not wish to use a hormonal therapy. They are also of value in treating excessive menstrual blood loss associated with the use of non-hormonal intrauterine contraceptive devices.

Hormonal therapy should be regarded as a third-choice treatment only in women not requiring contraception as a parallel objective. Progestogens are effective only when given for 21 days in each cycle. Combined oral contraceptives are useful for anovulatory bleeding as they impose a cycle. The levonorgestrel releasing intrauterine system (Mirena) is advocated as an alternative to surgery.

The timing of menstruation. Sometimes there are pressing reasons to prevent menstruation at the normal time but obviously this cannot be done at the last moment.

Menstruation can be *postponed* by giving oral *norethisterone* 5 mg t.d.s., starting 3 days before the expected onset; bleeding occurs 2–3 days after withdrawal. Users of the combined oral contraceptive pill (having a 7-day break) can simply continue with active pills where they would normally stop for 7 days.

Although there is no evidence that harm follows such manoeuvres, it is obviously imprudent to practise them frequently.

Note. These uses of progestogen should not be undertaken if there is any possibility of pregnancy.

Endometriosis. Medical treatments for endometriosis have focused on the hormonal alteration of the menstrual cycle in an attempt to produce a pseudo-pregnancy, pseudo-menopause or chronic anovulation. Each of these situations is believed to cause a suboptimal milieu for the growth and maintenance of endometrium and, by extension, of implants of endometriosis. *Danazol* 600–800 mg/day causes anovulation by attenuating the mid-cycle surge of luteinising hormone secretion, inhibiting multiple enzymes in the steroidogenic pathway, and increasing plasma free testosterone concentrations.

Medroxyprogesterone causes the decidualisation of endometrial tissue, with eventual atrophy.

Adverse effects occur at low (20–30 mg/day) or high (100 mg/day) dose, and include abnormal uterine bleeding, nausea, breast tenderness, fluid retention and depression. These resolve after the discontinuation of the drug.

Gestrinone 5–10 mg/week is an antiprogestational steroid that causes a decline in the concentrations of oestrogen and progesterone receptors, and a 50% decline in plasma estradiol concentrations. Androgenic adverse effects, such as a deepening of the voice, hirsutism and clitoral hypertrophy, are potentially irreversible. A combination of an *oestrogen and a progestogen* induces a hormonal pseudo-pregnancy. The oral contraceptive is used either continuously or cyclically (21 active pills followed by 7 days of placebo). Both regimens are effective; the amenorrhea of continuous administration is advantageous for women with dysmenorrhea.

Gonadotrophin-releasing hormone (GnRH) agonists diminish the secretion of follicle stimulating hormone and luteinising hormone, resulting in hypogonadotrophic hypogonadism, endometrial atrophy and amenorrhoea. The GnRH agonist can be given intranasally, subcutaneously or intramuscularly, with a frequency of administration ranging from twice daily to every 3 months. The unwanted effects are the menopausal-type symptoms of hypo-oestrogenism (such as transient vaginal bleeding, hot flushes, vaginal dryness) and can be prevented by concurrent administration of HRT in postmenopausal doses.

Although most treatments for endometriosis are directed at the hormones themselves, the symptoms can be also treated directly. NSAIDs such as diclofenac, ibuprofen and mefenamic acid are often given to relieve the pain associated with endometriosis. These drugs are frequently the first-line treatment in women with pelvic pain whose cause has not yet been proved to be endometriosis.

Dysmenorrhoea is due to uterine contractions resulting from excess prostaglandins in the uterus during ovulatory cycles. It can be treated by suppressing ovulation (using the combined pill or norethisterone), or by using inhibitors of prostaglandin synthesis, e.g. aspirin, indometacin, naproxen. The analgesic prostaglandin synthase inhibitor (NSAID) may need to be given for several days before menstruation, or only at the time of the pain.

Premenstrual tension syndrome may be due to an imbalance of natural oestrogen and progesterone secretion, but knowledge of the syndrome remains imprecise. Psychosocial factors can be important. Placebo effects are strong. Drugs are not necessarily the preferred treatment. There is evidence for and against the following:

- Restriction of salt and fluid plus a thiazide diuretic in the second half of the menstrual cycle where symptoms suggest fluid retention.
- Pyridoxine (vitamin B_6, a coenzyme): try 100 mg/day orally (not more) for 3 months

and abandon if there is no benefit. It may help depression and irritability in particular.
- Oestrogen–progestogen oral contraceptive combination.
- High-dose transdermal oestrogen patch.
- Bromocriptine, especially where there is breast pain.
- Prostaglandin synthase inhibition, e.g. mefenamic acid.
- Fluoxetine.

Cyclical breast pain or mastalgia, when severe, may respond to continuous use of gamolenic acid (Efamast) by mouth; it is an essential unsaturated fatty acid for cell membranes (patients have low concentrations); it may act by reducing cellular uptake of prolactin and ovarian hormones. Danazol and bromocriptine also help.

MYOMETRIUM

Oxytocics, i.e. drugs that hasten childbirth, and prostaglandins induce uterine contractions. They are used to induce abortion, to induce or augment labour, and to minimise blood loss from the placental site.

OXYTOCICS

Oxytocin is a peptide hormone of the posterior pituitary gland. It stimulates the contractions of the pregnant uterus, which becomes much more sensitive to it at term. Patients with posterior pituitary disease (diabetes insipidus) can, however, go into labour normally.

Oxytocin is released reflexly from the pituitary following suckling (also by manual stimulation of the nipple) and produces an almost immediate contraction of the myoepithelium of the breast; it can be used to enhance milk ejection (nasal spray). The only other clinically important effect is on the blood pressure, which may fall if an overdose is given.

Synthetic oxytocin (Syntocinon) is pure and is not contaminated with vasopressin as is the natural product, which is obsolete.

Oxytocin is used intravenously in the induction of labour and sometimes for uterine inertia, haemorrhage or during abortion. It produces, almost immediately, rhythmic contractions with relaxation between, i.e. it mimics normal uterine activity.

The decision to use oxytocin requires special skill. It has a $t_{1/2}$ of 6 min and is given by intravenous infusion using a pump (see below); it must be closely supervised; the dose is adjusted by results; overdose can cause uterine tetany and even rupture. The utmost care is required.

Oxytocin is structurally close to vasopressin and it is no surprise that it also has antidiuretic activity (see p. 480). Serious water intoxication can occur with prolonged intravenous infusions, especially where accompanied by large volumes of fluid. The association of oxytocin with neonatal jaundice appears to be due to increased erythrocyte fragility causing haemolysis.

Oxytocin has been supplanted by the ergot alkaloid, *ergometrine*, as prime treatment of postpartum haemorrhage.

Ergometrine is used to contract the uterus. It is an α-adrenoceptor and dopamine receptor agonist and acts almost immediately when injected intravenously. The uterus is stimulated at all times, but is much more sensitive in late pregnancy (see also ergotamine, p. 310).

Ergometrine and oxytocin differ in their actions on the uterus. In moderate doses, oxytocin produces slow generalised contractions with full relaxation in between; ergometrine produces faster contractions superimposed on a tonic contraction. High doses of both substances produce sustained tonic contraction. It will be seen, therefore, that *oxytocin* is more suited to *induction of labour* and *ergometrine* to the prevention and treatment of *postpartum haemorrhage*, the incidence of which is reduced by its routine prophylactic use (generally intramuscularly).

There are advantages in a mixture of oxytocin and ergometrine (Syntometrine).

PROSTAGLANDINS

(For a general account of the prostaglandins see Chapter 15.)

Prostaglandins that soften the uterine cervix (by an action on collagen) and have a powerful oxytocic effect include:

Dinoprost (prostaglandin $F_2\alpha$; $PGF_2\alpha$) (Prostin F2 alpha) and *dinoprostone* (prostaglandin E_2; PGE_2) (Prostin E2). They are used to induce labour and to terminate pregnancy, including missed or partial abortion and in the treatment of hydatidiform mole; they are given by intra- or extra-amniotic injection, by vaginal tablet, or intracervical gel, by intravenous infusion or by mouth. Their safe and effective use (including choice of route) requires special skill.

Adverse effects include vomiting, diarrhoea, headache, pyrexia and local tissue reaction.

Gemeprost (prostaglandin E_1 analogue) (Cervagem) is used intravaginally to soften the cervix before operative procedures in the first trimester of pregnancy and for abortion, alone and in combination with an antiprogestogen (mifepristone, see p. 648).

Carboprost (prostaglandin F_2 analogue) is used for postpartum haemorrhage (resistant to ergometrine and oxytocin) for its oxytocin action. It is highly effective. *Adverse effects* include hypertension, asthma and pulmonary oedema.

INDUCTION OF ABORTION

Gemeprost, administered vaginally as pressaries, is the preferred prostaglandin for the medical induction of late therapeutic abortion. Gemeprost ripens and softens the cervix before surgical abortion, particularly in primigravida. *Misoprostol* by mouth or by vaginal administration, or gemeprost, may be given to induce medical abortion (an unlicensed indication in the UK). Pretreatment with *mifepristone* (see p. 648) can facilitate the process, by sensitising the uterus to the prostaglandin so that abortion occurs in a shorter time and with a lower dose of prostaglandin.

INDUCTION AND AUGMENTATION OF LABOUR

Oxytocin is administered by slow intravenous infusion as below, usually in conjunction with amniotomy, and *dinoprostone* by vaginal tablets, pressaries and vaginal gels. *Misoprostol* may be used orally or vaginally to induce labour (an unlicensed indication in the UK).

The UK National Institute for Health and Clinical Excellence has recommended that:

■ Dinoprostone is preferable to oxytocin for induction of labour in women with intact membranes, regardless of parity or cervical favourability.
■ Dinoprostone and oxytocin are equally effective for the induction of labour in women with ruptured membranes, regardless of parity or cervical favourability.

- Intravaginal dinoprostone preparations are preferable to intracervical preparations.
- Oxytocin should not be started for 6 h following administration of vaginal prostaglandins.
- When used to induce labour, the recommended dose of oxytocin by intravenous infusion is initially 0.001–0.002 units/min, increased at intervals of at least 30 min until a maximum of three to four contractions occurs every 10 min (0.012 units/min is often adequate); the maximum recommended rate is 0.032 units/min (licensed max. 0.02 units/min).

PREVENTION AND TREATMENT OF UTERINE HAEMORRHAGE

Bleeding due to incomplete abortion can be controlled with *ergometrine* and *oxytocin* (Syntometrine) given intramuscularly. Their combination is more effective in early pregnancy than either drug alone.

For the routine management of the third stage of labour *ergometrine* 500 micrograms with oxytocin 5 units (Syntometrine 1 mL) is given by i.m. injection on delivery of the anterior shoulder or, at the latest, immediately after the baby is delivered. In pre-eclampsia, *oxytocin* may be given alone by i.m. injection. These regimens are also used for the treatment of postpartum haemorrhage. The same drugs may be given i.v. for excessive uterine bleeding caused by uterine atony. *Carboprost* is an alternative for haemorrhage unresponsive to ergometrine and oxytocin.

UTERINE RELAXANTS

β_2-Adrenoceptor agonists relax the uterus and are given by i.v. infusion by obstetricians to inhibit premature labour, e.g. *isoxsuprine, terbutaline, ritodrine, salbutamol*. Their use is complicated by the expected cardiovascular effects, including tachycardia, hypotension. Less easy to explain, but more devastating on occasion to the patient, is severe left ventricular failure. The combination of fluid overload (due to the vehicle) and increased oxygen demand by the heart are possible factors; the risk is higher in multiple pregnancy, pre-existing cardiac disease or maternal infection. It is important to administer the β_2 agonist with minimum fluid volume using a syringe pump with 5% dextrose (not saline) as diluent, and to monitor the patient closely for signs of fluid overload.

The dose of *ritodrine* for i.v. administration is: initially 50 micrograms/min, increased gradually according to response by 50 micrograms/min every 10 min until contractions stop or maternal heart rate reaches 140 beats per min; continue for 12–48 h after contractions cease (usual rate 150–350 micrograms/min).

GUIDE TO FURTHER READING

Barrett-Connor E L, Mosca L, Collins P et al 2006 Effects of raloxifene on cardiovascular events and breast cancer in postmenopausal women. New England Journal of Medicine 355(2):125–137

Brandes J L 2006 The influence of estrogen on migraine: a systematic review. Journal of the American Medical Association 295(15):1824–1830

Coombs N J, Taylor R, Wilcken N, Boyages J 2005 Hormone replacement therapy and breast cancer: estimate of risk. British Medical Journal 331:347–349

Dattani M, Preece M 2004 Growth hormone deficiency and related disorders: insights into causation, diagnosis, and treatment. Lancet 363:1977–1987

Ehrmann D A 2005 Polycystic ovary syndrome. New England Journal of Medicine 352(12):1223–1236

Federman D D 2006 The biology of human sex differences. New England Journal of Medicine 354:1507–1514

Giudice L C, Kao L C 2004 Endometriosis. Lancet 364:1789–1799 (Note also the 'Personal account: coping with endometriosis' by C Y Wang on p. 1800)

Hickey M, Davis S R, Sturdee D W et al 2005 Treatment of menopausal symptoms: what shall we do now? Lancet 366:409–421

Lee M M 2006 Idiopathic short stature. New England Journal of Medicine 354(24):2576–2582

Liu P Y, Swerdloff R S, Christenson P D, Handelsman D J, Wang C 2006 Rate, extent, and modifiers of spermatogenic recovery after hormonal male contraception: an integrated analysis. Lancet 367:1412–1420

Melmed S 2006 Medical progress: acromegaly. New England Journal of Medicine 355:2558–2573

Nelson H D, Vesco K K, Haney E et al 2006 Nonhormonal therapies for menopausal hot flashes: systematic review and meta-analysis. Journal of the American Medical Association 295(17):2057–2071

Peterson H B, Curtis K M 2005 Long-acting methods of contraception. New England Journal of Medicine 353(20):2169–2175

Proctor M, Farquhar C 2006 Diagnosis and management of dysmenorrhoea. British Medical Journal 332:1134–1138

Schlechte J A 2007 Long-term management of prolactinomas. Journal of Clinical Endocrinology and Metabolism 92:2861–2865

Westhoff C 2003 Emergency contraception. New England Journal of Medicine 349:1830–1835

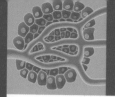

38

Vitamins, calcium, bone

SYNOPSIS

In general, the *pharmacological* aspects of vitamins appear here. The *nutritional* aspects, physiological function, sources, daily requirements and deficiency syndromes (primary and secondary) are to be found in any textbook of medicine.

- Vitamin A: retinol
- Vitamin B: complex
- Vitamin C: ascorbic acid
- Vitamin D, calcium, parathyroid hormone, calcitonin, bisphosphonates, bone
- Treatment of calcium and bone disorders
- Vitamin E: tocopherol

Vitamins[1] are substances that are essential for normal metabolism but are supplied chiefly in the diet.

Humans cannot synthesise vitamins in the body except some vitamin D in the skin and nicotinamide from tryptophan. Lack of a particular vitamin may lead to a specific deficiency syndrome. This may be *primary* (inadequate diet) or *secondary*, due to failure of absorption (intestinal abnormality or chronic diarrhoea) or to increased metabolic need (growth, pregnancy, lactation, hyperthyroidism).

Vitamin deficiencies are commonly multiple, and complex clinical pictures occur. There are numerous single and multivitamin preparations to provide prophylaxis and therapy.

There has recently been great interest in the suggestion that subclinical vitamin deficiencies may be a cause of chronic disease and liability to infection. The idea prompted a number of clinical trials that examined the potential benefit of vitamin supplementation in the prevention of cancer,

cardiovascular disease and other common diseases. There is little robust evidence to support this claim and, for most consumers, 'over the counter' vitamin preparations are probably little more than placebo value. Fortunately, most of the vitamins are comparatively non-toxic, but prolonged administration of *vitamins A and D* can have serious ill-effects.

Vitamins fall into two groups:

- *water-soluble vitamins*: the B group and vitamin C
- *fat-soluble vitamins*: A, D, E and K.

VITAMIN A: RETINOL

Vitamin A is a generic term embracing substances having the biological actions of retinol and related substances (called *retinoids*). The principal functions of retinol are to:

- sustain normal epithelia
- form retinal photochemicals
- enhance immune functions
- protect against infections and probably some cancers.

Deficiency of retinol leads to blindness, squamous metaplasia, hyperkeratosis and impairment of the immune system.

Therapeutic uses

Retinol and derivatives provide therapeutic benefit in a number of clinical areas.

Psoriasis

Tazorotene, a retinoid, is an effective topical agent in the treatment of chronic stable plaque psoriasis. Skin irritation is common, making it unsuitable for the treatment of inflammatory forms of psoriasis. *Acitretin* is a retinoic acid derivative ($t_{1/2}$ 48h) that is used orally for psoriasis (see p. 283, as well as other disorders of keratinisation).

---

[1]The term was coined by Casimir Funk in 1912 from the Latin *vita* meaning life and the (mistaken) belief that the organic compounds involved were amines. See: Hardy A 2004 Historical keywords. Vitamin. Lancet 364:323.

Acne

Tretinoin is retinoic acid and is used in acne by topical application (see p. 288). *Isotretinoin* is a retinoic acid isomer ($t_{1/2}$ 20 h) given orally for acne (see p. 287). It is also effective for preventing second tumours in patients following treatment for primary squamous cell carcinoma of the head and neck.

Acute promyelocytic leukaemia

Tretinoin can be used to induce remission in acute pro-myelocytic leukaemia in conjunction with chemotherapy. Initially, it proved remarkably successful, but the high doses given caused the fatal 'retinoic acid syndrome' (respiratory distress, fever and hypotension) and the duration of treatment is now shorter.

Vitamin A deficiency

Retinol is used to prevent and treat deficiency ($t_{1/2}$ 7–14 d).

Adverse effects

Acute toxicity occurs in adults with a single dose of more than 600 000 IU/day. Symptoms include headache, nausea, vomiting and drowsiness. Travellers have become ill by eating the livers of Arctic carnivores:

> Eskimos never eat polar-bear liver, knowing it to be toxic, and husky dogs, with instinctive wisdom, also avoid it. Those who pooh-pooh the Eskimos' fears of the husky dogs' instincts and are tempted to enjoy a man's portion of polar-bear liver – appetites get sharp near the North Pole – will consume anything up to 10 000 000 IU of vitamin A (normal daily requirement is 5000 IU). This is too much of a good thing, and the diner will probably soon find himself drowsy then overcome by headache and vomiting, and finally losing the outer layer of his skin.[2]

Chronic toxicity occur with prolonged high intake (in children 25 000–50 000 IU/day, 10 times the Recommended Daily Allowance, RDA).

A diagnostic sign is the presence of painful tender swellings on long bones. Anorexia, skin lesions, hair loss, hepatosplenomegaly, papilloedema, bleeding and general malaise also occur. Vitamin A accumu-lates in liver and fat, and effects take weeks to wear off. Most cases of vitamin A poisoning have been due to mothers administering large amounts of fish-liver oils to their children in the belief that it was good for them. Chronic overdose also causes an increased liability of biological membranes and of the outer layer of the skin to peel.

Teratogenicity. Vitamin A and its derivatives are tera-togenic at pharmacological doses (for precautions, see use in acne and psoriasis, p. 284). Supplements should not exceed 8000 IU (2400 micrograms) per day.

VITAMIN B COMPLEX

A number of widely differing substances are now, for convenience, classed the 'vitamin B complex'. Those used for pharmacotherapy include the following:

Thiamine (B_1) is used orally for nutritional purposes, but is given intravenously in serious emergencies, e.g. Wernicke–Korsakoff syndrome. Give the injection over 10 min (or intramuscularly); it can cause anaphylactic shock.

Cobalamins (B_{12}): see Chapter 29.

Folic acid: see Chapter 29.

Pyridoxine (B_6) is a co-enzyme in the metabolic transformation of many amino acids, including decarboxylation and transamination. Normal adult requirements are about 2 mg/day. As *pharmacotherapy*, pyridoxine is given to treat certain pyridoxine-dependent inborn errors of metabolism, e.g. homocystinuria, hereditary sideroblastic anaemia and primary hyperoxaluria. Deficiency may be induced by drugs such as isoniazid, hydralazine and penicillamine; pyridoxine 10 mg/day prevents the development of peripheral neuritis without interfering with therapeutic action.

Pyridoxine, in doses sometimes exceeding 100 mg/day, has found use for a variety of conditions including premenstrual tension, vomiting in pregnancy and radiation sickness. Concerns that prolonged exposure to such doses may be harmful, e.g. causing sensory neuropathy, are not resolved.

Niacin (nicotinic acid, B_7) is converted to nicotinamide, and subsequently to nicotinamide adenine

---

[2]Editorial 1962 British Medical Journal i:855.

dinucleotide (NAD) and nicotinamide adenine dinucleotide phosphate (NADP), the co-factors that are essential for the oxidation–reduction reactions that comprise tissue respiration. *Nicotinamide* is used for nutritional purposes. *Nicotinic acid* provides *pharmacotherapy* for some hyperlipidaemias (see p. 469), but in doses well in excess of those required for vitamin effect and causing adverse effects that include peripheral vasodilatation, unpleasant flushing, itching and fainting.

VITAMIN C: ASCORBIC ACID

Deficiency of ascorbic acid leads to *scurvy*,[3] which is characterised by petechial haemorrhages, haematomas, bleeding gums (if teeth are present) and anaemia. It has a memorable place in the history of therapeutic measurement. Scurvy had been a scourge for thousands of years, particularly amongst sailors on long voyages. In 1753, Dr James Lind performed a simple controlled therapeutic trial on 12 sailors with advanced scurvy. They were all on the same basic diet and were living in the same quarters on board ship at sea. He divided them into pairs and dosed each pair separately on cider, sulphuric acid, sea water, vinegar, a concoction of garlic, mustard, balsam and myrrh, and two oranges and a lemon. The pair receiving the oranges and lemon recovered and were back on duty within a week; of the others, only the pair taking cider was slightly improved. The efficacy of oranges and lemons in the prevention and cure of scurvy was repeatedly confirmed. Eventually the British Navy provided a regular daily allowance of lemon juice, unfortunately later replaced by the cheaper lime[4] juice which contained insufficient ascorbic acid to prevent scurvy completely.[5]

Function

Ascorbic acid is required for the synthesis of collagen. It is also a powerful *reducing agent* (antioxidant) and plays a part in intracellular oxidation–reduction systems, and in mopping up oxidants (free radicals) produced endogenously or in the environment, e.g. cigarette smoke (see Vitamin E).

Indications

- The prevention and cure of scurvy.
- Urinary acidification (rarely appropriate).
- Methaemoglobinaemia, for its properties as reducing agent (see below).

Adverse effects

High doses may cause sleep disturbances, headaches and gut upsets. Ascorbic acid is eliminated partly in the urine unchanged and partly metabolised to oxalate. Doses above 4g/day (taken over long periods in the hope of preventing coryza) increase urinary oxalate concentration sufficiently to form oxalate stones. Intravenous ascorbic acid may precipitate a haemolytic attack in subjects with glucose-6-phosphate dehydrogenase deficiency.

Methaemoglobinaemia

A reducing substance is needed to convert the methaemoglobin (ferric iron) back to oxyhaemoglobin (ferrous iron) whenever enough has formed seriously to impair the oxygen-carrying capacity of the blood. Ascorbic acid is non-toxic (it acts by direct reduction) but is less effective than *methylene blue* (methylthioninium chloride). Both can be given orally, intravenously or intramuscularly. Excessive doses of methylene blue can cause methaemoglobinaemia (by stimulating NADPH-dependent enzymes).

Methaemoglobinaemia may be induced by oxidising drugs: sulphonamides, nitrites, nitrates (may also occur in drinking water), primaquine, -caine local anaesthetics, dapsone, nitrofurantoin, nitroprusside, vitamin K analogues, chlorates, aniline and nitrobenzene. In the rare instance of there being urgency, methylene blue 1 mg/kg slowly i.v. benefits within 30 min. (Ascorbic acid competes directly with the chemical cause but is inadequate in severe cases, which are the only ones that need treatment.)

In the *congenital form*, oral methylene blue with or without ascorbic acid gives benefit in days to weeks.

Methylene blue turns the urine blue and high concentrations can irritate the urinary tract, so that fluid intake should be high when large doses are used.

---

[3]Only humans (and other primates), guinea-pigs, the Indian fruit bat and the red-vented bulbul (a bird) get scurvy; other animals are able to synthesise ascorbic acid for themselves.
[4]Hence the term 'limey' for British sailors; generally used pejoratively, but obsolete except in Australia.
[5]For a more detailed account see: Tröhler U 2005 Lind and scurvy: 1747 to 1795. Journal of the Royal Society of Medicine 98(11):519–522.

VITAMIN D, CALCIUM, PARATHYROID HORMONE, CALCITONIN, BISPHOSPHONATES, BONE

The agents are closely interrelated and are discussed together.

VITAMIN D

Vitamin D comprises a number of structurally related sterol compounds having similar biological properties (but different potencies) in that they prevent or cure the vitamin D deficiency diseases, rickets and osteomalacia. The important forms (Fig. 38.1) are:

- D_2 or *ergocalciferol* (calciferol) made by ultraviolet irradiation of ergosterol in plants. This is not the naturally occurring form.
- D_3 or *colecalciferol* made by ultraviolet irradiation of 7-dehydrocholesterol; this is the form that occurs in natural foods and is formed in the skin.

Vitamins D_2 and D_3 undergo two successive hydroxylations: first in the liver to form 25-hydroxyvitamin D and second in the proximal tubules of the kidney (under the control of parathyroid hormone, PTH) to form $1\alpha,25$-dihydroxyvitamin D_3, the most *physiologically active* form of vitamin D, i.e. *calcitriol*.

There exist also a variety of synthetic vitamin D analogues, developed to treat vitamin D deficiency and hypoparathyroidism. The newer vitamin D derivative 1α-hydroxycolecalciferol (*alfacalcidol*) requires only hepatic hydroxylation to become calcitriol. The usual adult maintenance dose, 0.25–1 micrograms/day, indicates its extraordinary potency.

There are four other 1α-hydroxylated vitamin D analogues: *paricalcitol, doxercalciferol, falecalcitriol* and *22-oxacalcitriol*. All are effective in renal failure as they bypass the defective renal hydroxylation stage. In addition, a structural variant of vitamins D_2 and D_3, dihydrotachysterol (ATIO, Tachyrol), is also biologically activated by hepatic 25-hydroxylation.

Pharmacokinetics

Alfacalcidol and *dihydrotachysterol* have a fast onset and short duration of clinical effect (days) which renders them suitable for rapid adjustment of plasma calcium, e.g. in hypoparathyroidism. Such factors are not relevant to the slower adjustment of plasma calcium (weeks) with vitamins D_2 and D_3 in the ordinary management of vitamin D deficiency.

Actions are complex. Vitamin D promotes the active transport of calcium and phosphate in the gut (increased absorption) and renal tubule (reduced excretion), and thus controls, with PTH, the plasma calcium concentration and the mineralisation of bone (see Fig. 38.1). After a dose of D_2 or D_3 there is a lag of about 21 h before the intestinal effect begins; this is probably due to the time needed for its metabolic conversion to the more active forms. With the biologically more active *calcitriol*, the lag is only 2 h.

A large single dose of vitamin D has biological effects for as long as 6 months (because of metabolism and storage). Thus, the agent is cumulative and overdose by a mother anxious that her child shall have strong bones can cause serious toxicity.

Pharmacotherapy

Indications for vitamin D are the prevention and cure of rickets of all kinds and osteomalacia, the symptomatic treatment of some cases of hypoparathyroidism; psoriasis and secondary hyperparathyroidism in renal failure. In general, use of vitamin D as pharmacotherapy requires monitoring of plasma calcium.

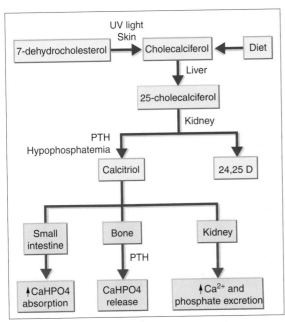

Fig. 38.1 Metabolism of vitamin D. 24, 25-D, ???; PTH, parathyroid hormone.

Vitamin D deficiency

Vitamin D deficiency can be treated with a variety of vitamin D analogues. Selecting the appropriate preparation requires a knowledge of the underlying aetiology.

Primary vitamin D deficiency is not uncommon in Asians consuming unleavened bread and in the elderly living alone; it can be prevented by taking an oral supplement of *ergocalciferol* 20 micrograms (800 units) daily.

Vitamin D deficiency resulting from *intestinal malabsorption or chronic liver disease* usually requires vitamin D in pharmacological doses, e.g. *ergocalciferol* tablets up to 1 mg (40 000 units) daily. The maximum antirachitic effect of vitamin D occurs after 1–2 months, and the plasma calcium concentration reflects the dosage given days or weeks before. Frequent changes of dose are therefore not required.

Vitamin D deficiency in *chronic renal failure* results from reduced synthesis of *calcitriol*. The final rate-limited renal 1α-hydroxylation is inadequate, and the less biologically active precursors lack adequate efficacy. Failure of 1α,25-dihydroxy-vitamin D_3 to occupy receptors on the parathyroid glands leads to increased release of PTH. The aim of treatment is to suppress this (secondary) hyperparathyroidism, normalise plasma Ca^{2+} levels and prevent renal osteodystrophy.[6] *Calcitriol* and vitamin D analogues (e.g. *alfacalcidol*, above) inhibit PTH gene transcription by the vitamin D receptor and increase the serum concentration of Ca^{2+}, which acts on the parathyroid Ca^{2+} receptor further to inhibit PTH secretion. Calcitriol (or a 1α analogue) is instituted in end-stage renal failure once plasma PTH concentrations reach 300 picograms/mL, i.e. to achieve the aim of preventing hyperparathyroidism, rather than treating established osteodystrophy. Note that vitamin D analogues, by increasing intestinal phosphate absorption, can worsen hyperphosphataemia.

Osteoporosis

Calcitriol is licensed for the management of postmenopausal osteoporosis (see below).

Hypoparathyroidism

The hypocalcaemia of hypoparathyroidism may require ergocalciferol in doses of up to 2.5 mg (100 000 units) daily to achieve normocalcaemia, but the dose is difficult to titrate and hypercalcaemia from overdose may take weeks to resolve. *Alfacalcidol* and *calcitriol* are therefore preferred as their rapid onset and offset of action makes for easier control of plasma calcium levels. Supplementary calcium by mouth may be needed.

Psoriasis

Calcipotriol and tacalcitol are vitamin D analogues available as creams or ointments for the treatment of psoriasis (see p. 284).

Symptoms of overdose are due mainly to an excessive increase in plasma calcium concentration. General effects include: malaise, drowsiness, nausea, abdominal pain, thirst, constipation and loss of appetite. Other long-term effects include ectopic calcification almost anywhere in the body, renal damage and an increased calcium output in the urine; renal calculi may form. It is dangerous to exceed 10 000 units daily of vitamin D in an adult for more than about 12 weeks.

Vitamin D toxicity may arise from well meaning, but needless, administration by parents. Dietary supplements should not exceed 400 units a day.

Patients with *sarcoidosis* have increased sensitivity to vitamin D including to physiological amounts synthesised in skin in response to sunlight. Overproduction of calcitriol by macrophages may be activated by interferon and is reversed by corticosteroid, which is also used in the treatment of severe hypervitaminosis D (see below).

Epileptic patients taking enzyme-inducing drugs long term can develop osteomalacia (adults) or rickets (children). This may arise from the accelerated metabolism, increasing vitamin D breakdown and causing deficiency, or from inhibition of one of the hydroxylations that increase biological activity.

TREATMENT OF CALCIUM AND BONE DISORDERS

HYPOCALCAEMIA

In *acute hypocalcaemia* requiring systemic therapy, give *calcium gluconate injection* as a 10% solution,

---

[6]This term covers the various forms of bone disease that may accompany chronic renal failure, i.e. hyperparathyroid bone disease, osteomalacia, osteoporosis and osteosclerosis.

10–20 mL at a rate of about 2 mL/min, followed by a continuous intravenous infusion containing 40 mL (9 mmol) in 1 L saline over 4–8 h, with monitoring of plasma calcium. Avoid infusing with solutions containing bicarbonate or phosphate, which cause calcium to precipitate. Intramuscular injection is contraindicated as it is painful and causes tissue necrosis. Calcium glubionate (Calcium Sandoz) can be given by deep intramuscular injection in adults.

For *chronic use*, e.g. hypoparathyroidism, dietary calcium is increased by oral *calcium gluconate* (an effervescent tablet is available) or *lactate*. When this is insufficient, use calfacalcidol or calcitriol. Alternatively, *aluminium hydroxide* binds phosphate in the gut causing hypophosphataemia, which stimulates renal formation of the most active vitamin D metabolite and usefully enhances calcium absorption.

Adverse effects of intravenous calcium may be very dangerous. An early sign is a tingling feeling in the mouth and of warmth spreading over the body. Serious effects are those on the heart, which mimic and synergise with digitalis, and it is advisable to avoid intravenous calcium administration in any patient taking a digitalis glycoside (except in severe symptomatic hypocalcaemia). The effect of calcium on the heart is antagonised by potassium, and similarly the toxic effects of hyperkalaemia in acute renal failure may be to an extent counteracted by calcium.

HYPERCALCAEMIA

Treatment of severe acute hypercalcaemia causing symptoms is needed whether or not the cause can be removed; generally a plasma concentration of 3.0 mmol/L (12 mg/100 mL) needs urgent treatment if there is also clinical evidence of toxicity (individual tolerance varies greatly).

Temporary measures

After taking account of the patient's cardiac and renal function, the following measures may be employed selectively:

- *Physiological saline solution* is important, firstly to correct sodium and water deficit, and secondly to promote sodium-linked calcium diuresis in the proximal renal tubule. Initially, 500 mL 0.9% saline should be given i.v. every 4–6 h for

2–3 days and continued at a rate of 2 L/day until the plasma Ca^{2+} level falls below 3.0 mmol/L and the oral intake is adequate. The regimen requires careful attention to fluid and electrolyte balance, particularly in patients with renal insufficiency secondary to hypercalcaemia or heart failure who are unable to excrete excess sodium. The use of furosemide to enhance renal Ca^{2+} excretion has been largely abandoned owing to the exacerbation of electrolyte disturbances and the increased availability of newer agents.

- *Bisphosphonates* are the agents of choice in severe hypercalcaemia. *Pamidronate*[7] is infused according to the schedule in Table 38.1; it is active in a wide variety of hypercalcaemic disorders. A fall in the serum calcium concentration begins within the first day, reaches a nadir in 5–6 days and lasts for 20–30 days. *Etidronate* may be given i.v. in hypercalcaemia of malignant disease. It acts in 1–2 days and a dose lasts for 3–4 weeks; it may also provide benefit for neoplastic metastatic disease in bone. The long infusion period renders it a less attractive choice. *Clodronate* (oral or i.v.) and *zoledonic* acid (i.v.) are alternatives. Zoledonic acid has the advantage of being more potent and can be administered over a shorter time (15 min versus 2 h). It is a convenient regimen for patients with hypercalcaemia of malignancy.
- *Calcitonin.* When the hypercalcaemia is at least partly due to mobilisation from bone, calcitonin can be used to inhibit bone resorption, and may enhance urinary excretion

Table 38.1 Treatment of hypercalcaemia with disodium pamidronate

Calcium (mmol/L)	Pamidronate (mg)
<3.0	15–30
3.0–3.5	30–60
3.5–4.0	60–90
>4.0	90

Infuse slowly, e.g. 30 mg in 250 mL 0.9% saline over 1 h. Expect a response in 3–5 days.

---

[7] Formerly called aminohydroxypropylidenediphosphonate disodium, APD.

of calcium. The effect develops in a few hours but responsiveness is lost over a few days owing to tachyphylaxis. Calcitonin is not as effective as the bisphosphonates in reducing hypercalcaemia.

- An *adrenocortical steroid*, e.g. prednisolone 20–40 mg/day orally, is effective in particular situations; it reduces the hypercalcaemia of vitamin D intoxication (which is due to excessive intestinal absorption of calcium) and of sarcoidosis (principally by its disease-modifying effect). Corticosteroid may be effective in the hypercalcaemia of malignancy where the disease itself is responsive, e.g. myeloma of lymphoma. Patients with hyperparathyroidism do not respond.
- *Phosphate* i.v. is quickly effective but lowers calcium by precipitating calcium phosphate in bone and soft tissues and inhibiting osteoclastic activity; it should be used only when other methods have failed.
- *Dialysis* is quick and effective and is likely to be needed in severe cases or in those with renal failure.

The above measures are only temporary, giving time to tackle the cause.

Longer-term treatment

Sodium cellulose phosphate (Calcisorb) is an oral ion exchange substance with a particular affinity for calcium which is bound in the gut, and the complex eliminated in the faeces. It is effective for patients who over-absorb dietary calcium and develop hypercalciuria and renal stones.

Inorganic phosphate, e.g. sodium acid phosphate (Phosphate Sandoz), taken orally also binds calcium in the gut. It is of particular use for hypercalcaemia resulting from increased intestinal absorption of calcium, e.g. vitamin D intoxication, or increased calcitriol production (as seen with chronic granulomatous disease).

HYPERCALCIURIA

In renal stone formers, in addition to general measures (low calcium diet, high fluid intake), urinary calcium may be diminished by a *thiazide* diuretic (with or without citrate to bind calcium) and oral *phosphate* (see above). See also Nephrolithiasis, page 490.

PARATHYROID HORMONE

Parathyroid hormone (PTH) acts chiefly on the kidney, increasing renal tubular reabsorption of calcium and excretion of phosphate; it increases calcium absorption from the gut, indirectly, by stimulating the renal synthesis of $1\alpha,25$-vitamin D (see above and Fig. 38.1). PTH increases the rate of bone remodelling (mineral and collagen) and osteocyte activity with, at *high* doses, an overall balance in favour of resorption (*osteoclast activity*) with a rise in plasma calcium concentration (and fall in phosphate); but, at *low* doses, the balance favours bone formation (*osteoblast activity*).

CALCITONIN

Calcitonin is a peptide hormone produced by the C cells of the thyroid gland (in mammals). It acts on bone (inhibiting osteoclasts) to reduce the rate of bone turnover, and on the kidney to reduce reabsorption of calcium and phosphate. It is obtained from natural sources (pork, salmon, eel) or synthesised. The $t_{1/2}$ varies according to source; the human $t_{1/2}$ is 10 min. Antibodies develop particularly to pork calcitonin and neutralise its effect; synthetic salmon calcitonin (salcatonin) is therefore preferred for prolonged use; loss of effect may also be due to down-regulation of receptors.

Calcitonin is used (subcutaneously, intramuscularly or intranasally) for Paget's disease of bone (relief of pain, and compression of nerves, e.g. auditory cranial), metastatic bone cancer pain, postmenopausal osteoporosis, and occasionally to control hypercalcaemia (rapid effect).

Adverse effects include allergy, nausea, flushing and tingling of the face and hands.

BISPHOSPHONATES

Bisphosphonates are synthetic, non-hydrolysable analogues of pyrophosphate (which inhibits bone mineralisation) in which the central oxygen atom of the -P-O-P- structure is replaced with a carbon atom to give the -P-C-P- group. The class includes *alendronate, clodronate, etidronate, ibandronate, pamidronate, risedronate, tiludronate* and *zoledronate*.

Actions. These compounds are effective calcium chelators that rapidly target exposed bone mineral surfaces, are imbibed by bone-resorbing osteoclasts, inhibit their function and cause osteoclast apoptosis. An additional action may be to stimulate bone formation by osteoblasts, but the therapeutic utility of bisphosphonates rests on their capacity to inhibit bone resorption.

Bisphosphonate binding to hydroxyapatite crystals can, in high doses, *inhibit* bone mineralisation (potentially causing osteomalacia), an effect that is unrelated to their anti-resorptive efficacy. This disadvantageous effect, prominent with earlier bisphosphonates, is less with newer members. Thus, etidronate is administered cyclically to prevent demineralisation, whereas alendronate does not appear to exert this effect at anti-resorptive doses and can be used continuously.

Pharmacokinetics. Bisphosphonates are poorly absorbed after ingestion. Absorption is further impaired by food, drinks, and drugs containing calcium, magnesium, iron or aluminium salts. A proportion of bisphosphonate that is absorbed is rapidly incorporated into bone; the remaining fraction is excreted unchanged by the kidneys. Once incorporated into the skeleton, bisphosphonates are released only when the bone is resorbed during turnover. They may be given orally or intravenously.

Uses. Four bisphosphonates (*alendronate, etidronate, risedronate, ibandronate*) are currently licensed in the UK for the treatment of osteoporosis (*zoledronate* is also effective). Alendronate can be taken weekly (70 mg) instead of daily (10 mg). *Pamidronate, clodronate* and *zoledronate* are used in Paget's disease of bone and in hypercalcaemia due to cancer. Bisphosphonates may also provide benefit for neoplastic disease that has spread to bone; evidence indicates that *clodronate* by mouth and *pamidronate* i.v. are effective in the secondary prevention of bone metastases due to multiple myeloma and breast cancer.

Adverse effects include gastrointestinal disturbances, and oesophageal irritation is a particular problem with alendronate. This drug should be taken at least 30 min before food, with the patient remaining erect during this period. Disturbances of calcium and mineral metabolism (e.g. vitamin D deficiency, PTH dysfunction) should be corrected before starting a bisphosphonate. Increased bone pain (as well as relief) and fractures (high dose, prolonged use only) can occur due to bone demineralisation.

OSTEOPOROSIS

Osteoporosis is a disease characterised by increased skeletal fragility, low bone mineral density (less than 2.5 standard deviations below the mean for young people; Fig. 38.2) and deterioration of bone microarchitecture. It occurs most commonly in postmenopausal women and patients taking long-term corticosteroid. Exclude underlying causes such as hyperthyroidism, hyperparathyroidism and hypogonadism (in both sexes) before treatment is initiated.

Postmenopausal osteoporosis is due to gonadal deficiency; it can be *prevented*. In the UK, one in four women in their sixties and one in two in their seventies experience an osteoporotic fracture. Prevention with combined oestrogen–progestogen therapy was widespread until data from the UK Women's Health Initiative showed an increased risk of breast cancer, stroke and venous thromboembolic disease (see p. 521).

Now, patients at risk of osteoporosis are advised to increase daily exercise, stop smoking and optimise diet to ensure sufficient calories and an adequate intake of calcium and vitamin D. The recommended daily calcium intake of 1500 mg can be achieved with calcium supplementation. Vitamin D supplementation with ergocalciferol (10 micrograms/400 IU) can be given to ensure a daily intake of 800 IU.

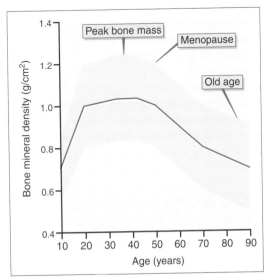

Fig. 38.2 Bone mineral density of the lumbar spine in women. The shaded area represents two standard deviations above and below the mean for bone mineral density.

Pharmacotherapy

Bisphosphonates are the first-line treatment for postmenopausal osteoporosis. Alendronate and risendronate are effective both at preventing post-menopausal osteoporosis and at reducing fracture incidence. They are administered either once daily or once weekly. Ibandronate is effective as a once-monthly preparation, or intravenously every 3 months for those unable to tolerate oral bisphosphonates.

Selective oestrogen receptor modulator. Raloxifene is effective for both the prevention and treatment of osteoporosis; it reduces the incidence of vertebral but not of non-vertebral fractures. It is probably less effective than bisphosphonates but no direct comparisons have been made. Raloxifene reduces the risk of breast cancer (see p. 550) but there is a three-fold increase in the risk of venous thromboembolic disease.

Parathyroid hormone. PTH increases bone resorption but the synthetic PTH, teriparatide, administered intermittently (20 micrograms/day s.c.), *stimulates* bone formation and reduces the risk of fracture. It is indicated for severe postmenopausal osteoporosis or where bisphosphonates have proved to be ineffective.[8]

Oestrogen–progestogen therapy, although now out of favour (see above), may yet be indicated in a small proportion of postmenopausal women with documented osteoporosis or osteopenia, or those at increased risk of osteoporosis, who do not have a personal or family history of breast cancer or other contraindications and are unable to tolerate alternative anti-resorptive agents.

Calcitonin. The mode of administration (s.c., i.m. or nasally) and possible tachyphylaxis make calcitonin a less suitable choice for treatment of osteoporosis. Additionally, the increase in bone mineral density and reduction in fracture risk is small compared with alternative agents.

Strontium ranelate may stimulate bone formation and reduce resorption, but the mechanism is unclear and evidence for either mechanism is also uncertain. The drug reduces the risk of spine and non-spine fracture, and carries a small risk of thromboembolism. It is reserved for patients intolerant of bisphosphonates.

Fracture is the only important outcome of osteoporosis and the evidence to support the efficacy of various interventions appears in Table 38.2.

Corticosteroid-induced osteoporosis. Most bone loss occurs during the first 6–12 months of use. Patients taking the equivalent of prednisolone 7.5 mg or more each day for more than 3 months should be considered for prophylactic treatment, and is mandatory in those aged over 65 years. All patients should receive vitamin D and calcium supplements. Bisphosphonates are first line for both the prophylaxis and treatment;

Table 38.2 Anti-fracture efficacy of interventions in postmenopausal osteoporotic women: grades of recommendation

	Spine	Non-vertebral	Hip
Alendronate	A	A	A
Calcitonin	A	B	A
Calcitriol	A	A	ND
Calcium	A	B	B
Calcium plus vitamin D	ND	A	A
Cyclical etidronate	A	B	B
Hip protectors	–	–	A
HRT	A	A	B
Physical exercise	ND	B	B
Raloxifene	A	ND	ND
Risedronate	A	A	A
Tibolone	ND	ND	ND
Vitamin D	ND	B	B

Grade A: meta-analysis of randomised controlled trials, or from at least one randomised controlled trial, or from at least one well designed controlled study without randomisation.
Grade B: from at least one other type of well designed, quasi-experimental study, or from well designed, non-experimental studies (e.g. comparative studies, correlation studies, case–control studies).
Grade C: from expert committee reports/opinions and/or clinical experience of authorities.
ND: not demonstrated.
Data from the Royal College of Physicians and the Bone and Tooth Society.

[8]In a pivitol 19-month trial, teripatide increased bone mineral density in the spine and femoral neck, and rates of new vertebral fractures and non-vertebral fractures were 5% and 6.3% compared with 14.3% and 9.7% respectively for placebo (Neer R M, Arnaud C D, Zanchetta J R et al 2001 Effect of parathyroid hormone (1–34) on fractures and bone mineral density in postmenopausal women with osteoporosis. New England Journal of Medicine 344(19):1431–1441).

calcitonin may be considered where bisphosphonates are contraindicated or not tolerated.

RENAL BONE DISEASE

Typically patients with chronic renal failure have hyperphosphataemia, hypocalcaemia, low calcitriol levels and secondary hyperparathyroidism. Treatment is aimed at replacing vitamin D to suppress PTH, and normalisation of serum calcium and phosphate levels.

Phosphate binders are used in the management of hyperphosphataemia. These include *calcium carbonate, calcium acetate* and less frequently *aluminium hydroxide*. Aluminium toxicity (manifested as osteomalacia, microcytic anaemia and encephalopathy) limits its safety in chronic use. Newer, non calcium-based phosphate agents e.g. *sevelamer* and *lanthanum carbonate* should be used in patients who are hypercalcaemic.

Vitamin D replacement is the cornerstone of treatment for secondary hyperparathyroidism (see p. 000). In addition, calcimimetics are increasingly used where vitamin D is not sufficient.

Cinacalcet is a calcium analogue that competes with Ca^{2+} for binding to the Ca^{2+} receptor in the parathyroids. It is indicated for patients on renal dialysis with secondary hyperparathyroidism, or for severe hypercalcaemia associated with parathyroid carcinoma.

OSTEOMALACIA

Osteomalacia is due to *primary* or *secondary* vitamin D deficiency. In secondary cases, e.g. malabsorption or renal disease, high doses of vitamin D are sometimes needed.

PAGET'S DISEASE OF BONE

This disease is characterised by bone turnover (resorption and formation) being increased as much as 50 times normal; the result is large, vascular, deformed and painful bones that fracture.

Bisphosphonates (etidronate, pamidronate, tiludronate) are effective because they inhibit crystal formation, growth and dissolution, such as must occur in bone mineralisation and demineralisation. Their response is dose related and remission after a course may last for up to 2 years.

Calcitonin (which also inhibits bone resorption) has been largely superseded by the bisphosphonates but retains usefulness because it reduces bone blood flow before surgery.

VITAMIN E: TOCOPHEROL

The functions of vitamin E may be to take up (scavenge) the free radicals generated by normal metabolic processes and by substances in the environment, e.g. hydrocarbons. This prevents free radicals from attacking polyunsaturated fats in cell membranes with resultant cellular injury.

A deficiency syndrome is recognised, including peripheral neuropathy with spinocerebellar degeneration, and a haemolytic anaemia in premature infants.

α-Tocopheryl acetate (Ephynal) pharmacotherapy may benefit the neuromuscular complications of congenital cholestasis and abetalipoproteinaemia.

VITAMIN K

See page 514.

GUIDE TO FURTHER READING

Bischoff-Ferrari H A, Dawson-Hughes B, Willett W C et al 2004 Effect of vitamin D on falls: a meta-analysis. Journal of the American Medical Association 291(16): 1999–2006

El-Kadiki A, Sutton A J 2005 Role of multivitamins and mineral supplements in preventing infections in elderly people: systematic review and meta–analysis of randomised controlled trials. British Medical Journal 330:871–876

Farford B, Prescutti R J, Moraghan T J 2007 Nonsurgical management of primary hyperparathyroidism. Mayo Clinic Proceedings 82:351–355

Holick M F 2007 Vitamin D deficiency. New England Journal of Medicine 357:266–281

Lambrinoudaki I, Christodoulakos G, Botsis D 2006 Biphosphonates. Annals of the New York Academy of Science 1092:403–407

Lucock M 2004 Is folic acid the ultimate functional food component for disease prevention? British Medical Journal 328:211–214

Rosen C J 2005 Postmenopausal osteoporosis. New England Journal of Medicine 353(6):595–603

Sambrook P, Cooper C 2006 Osteoporosis. Lancet 367: 2010–2018

Seeman E, Delmas P D 2006 Bone quality – the material and structural basis of bone strength and fragility. New England Journal of Medicine 354:2250–2261

Simon L S 2007 Osteoporosis. Rheumatic Disease Clinics of North America 33:149–176

Steddon S J, Cunningham J 2005 Calcimimetics and calcilytics – fooling the calcium receptor. Lancet 365: 2237–2239

Venning G 2005 Recent developments in vitamin D deficiency and muscle weakness among elderly people. British Medical Journal 330:524–526

Wharton B, Bishop N 2003 Rickets. Lancet 362: 1389–1400

Whyte M P 2006 Paget's disease of bone. New England Journal of Medicine 355:593–600

Willett W C, Stampfer M J 2001 What vitamins should I be taking, doctor? New England Journal of Medicine 345:1819–1824

Index

A

Abacavir, 229
Abbreviations
  prescription, 29, 30
  weights and measures, 31
Abciximab, 438, 526
Abdominal paracentesis, 587
Abelcet, 235
Abortion
  adverse effects of drugs, 126
  induction of, 658
Abscesses, 224
Absence seizures, 377
Absolute risk, 56–7
Absorption, 88–93
  bioavailability, 89–91
  in disease, 111
  in the elderly, 109
  enteral administration advantages and
    disadvantages, 91
  enterohepatic circulation, 89
  gastrointestinal tract, 88–9
  parenteral administration advantages and
    disadvantages, 91–3
  in pregnancy, 110
  reduction of time of, 102–3
  systemic availability, 89–91
  through the skin See Topical application
    of medication
  zero-order, 85
Abuse, drug, 142–72
  dependence, 143, 144–7, 148
    designer drugs, 147
    escalation, 147
    mortality, 146–7
    physical (physiological), 145
    prescribing for, 146
    psychological, 145
    route of administration and effective,
      145–6
    sites and mechanisms of action, 145
    treatment of, 146
  drives to, 143–4
  drugs as adjuvants to crime, 172
  ethanol See Ethanol (alcohol)
  individual rewards, 144
  pattern of use, 144
  principal forms, 143–4
  psychodysleptics/hallucinogens, 162–7
  psychostimulants, 167–71
  social aspects, 142–4
  and sport, 147–8
  terminology, 143–4
  tobacco See Smoking
  types of, 148
  volatile substance abuse, 138, 171–2
Acamprosate, 154
Acarbose, 616, 617
Accelerated phase hypertension, 442–3
Acceptable risk, 10
ACD scheme, antihypertensives, 441–2
ACE inhibitors See Angiotensin converting
  enzyme (ACE) inhibitors
Acenocoumarol, 520
Acetaldehyde, 149
Acetaminophen See Paracetamol
Acetazolamide, 487

Acetic acids, 258
Acetylation, 107
Acetylcholine, 367, 393
  antagonists of, 321
  cholinergic drugs, 391–2
  drugs that oppose, 399–402
  gastric acid secretion, 561
  parkinsonism, 380
Acetylcholinesterase, 78, 367
Acetylcysteine, 132
Acetylsalicylic acid See Aspirin
Aciclovir, 225–7, 284
Acid-fast bacilli, antibiotic choice, 186
Acid groups ionisation, 82
Acidification of urine, 134, 488
Acipimox, 476
Acitretin, 287, 660
Acne, 283, 287–8
  hormone replacement therapy, 647
  vitamin A, 661
Acquired immunodeficiency syndrome
  (AIDS), 228, 284
Acrivastine, 500
Acromegaly, 639
Actinic keratoses, 285
Actinomycetes, antibiotic choice, 186
Actinomycosis, 224
Action, drug
  prolongation of, 102
  See also specific drug
Action potentials, 294, 449
Activated charcoal, 99, 130–1, 133,
  139, 259
Activated partial thromboplastin time
  (APTT), 521
Active substances, 96
Activity, altering biological, 96
Acute coronary syndromes, 437
Acute lymphatic leukaemia (ALL), 603
Acute myeloblastic leukaemia (AML),
  539
Acute promyelocytic leukaemia, 661
Acute stress disorder, 355
Adalimumab, 267
Adapalene, 288
Adaptive immune response, 250, 252–3
Addiction, drug, 143
  See also Abuse, drug
Addisonian anaemia, 534–5
Addisonian crisis, 601–2
Addison's disease, 593, 602
Adefovir, 229
Adenosine
  for cardiac arrhythmia, 451, 456
  plasma half-life of, 87
Adenosine diphosphate (ADP), 525
Adenosine monophosphate-activated
  protein kinase (AMPK), 615
Adenylyl cyclase, 76
Adhesion molecules, 251
Adjustment disorder, 355
Adjuvants, 306–8
  cancer therapy, 541
  definition of, 296
Administration route
  drug abuse, effect, 145–6
  See also specific route
Adrenal cortex, 593

Adrenaline
  discovery of, 403
  effect on blood glucose, 615
  nomenclature, 69
  as a procoagulant, 516
  for shock, 412–13
  uses of, 408–9
Adrenal steroids See Corticosteroids
Adrenergic mechanisms, 403
Adrenergic nerve terminals, 403
Adrenergic neurone blocking drugs, 434
Adrenoceptor agonists, 403, 406
  See also α-Adrenoceptor agonists;
    β-Adrenoceptor agonists
Adrenoceptor antagonists/blockers, 90,
  426–34
  See also α-Adrenoceptor antagonists/
    blockers; β-Adrenoceptor
    antagonists/blockers
Adrenoceptors
  consequences of activation, 405–6
  selectivity for, 406–8. See also
    β-Adrenoceptors
Adrenocortical function suppression, 602
Adrenocortical insufficiency
  acute, 601–2
  chronic, 602
  iatrogenic, 602
Adrenocortical steroids See Corticosteroids
Adrenocorticotrophic hormone (ACTH),
  147–8, 593, 605, 606
Adsorbents, oral, 130–1
Advanced life support, 462
Adverse drug reactions, 115–28
  affecting the skin, 282–4
  allergy See Allergy
  attribution and degrees of conviction,
    116–17
  background, 115
  cannabis, 166
  definitions, 115–16
  drug-induced illness, 117–18
  drugs and skilled tasks, 119, 165, 369
  effects of prolonged administration,
    125–6
  hallucinogens, 166–7
  medical record linkage, 59
  pharmacoepidemiology, 117–19
  pharmacovigilance, 117–19
  population statistics, 59
  practicalities of detecting rare, 117
  predisposition to, 119
  prescription event monitoring, 59
  on reproduction, 126–8
  sources of, 119–21
  voluntary reporting of, 58–9
  See also specific drug
Advertising, 28
Aerosols
  for asthma, 505
  inhaled, 92
African sleeping sickness, 246
Afterload, 462, 464–5
Age
  effect on adverse drug reaction, 120, 617
  effect on drug action, 108–10
Agonists, 76
  see also specific agonist

Agranulocytosis, 123
AIDS (Acquired immunodeficiency syndrome), 228, 284
Airway
  increased resistance due to smoking, 159
  maintenance, poisoning, 135
Akathisia, 345
Albendazole, 247
Albumin
  binding, 95, 583
  low levels of, 95, 111
Alcohol See Ethanol (alcohol)
Alcohol dehydrogenase, 78, 149
Aldehyde, 137
Aldehyde dehydrogenase, 149
Aldesleukin, 268
Aldosterone, 420, 593, 597
  potency, 597
Alfacalcidol, 663, 664
Alfentanil, 302
Alginic acid, 562
Alimentary tract See Gastrointestinal tract
Alkaline groups ionisation, 82
Alkalinisation of urine, 134, 488
Alkaloids with cholinergic effects, 393–4
Alkylating agents, 266–7, 544, 546
Allergic vasculitis, 283
Allergy, drug, 121–5
  anaphylactic shock, 122–3
  angioedema, 122
  aplastic anaemia, 124
  aspirin, 261
  blood disorders, 123
  cholestatic jaundice, 124
  collagen diseases, 124
  corticosteroids, 280
  cross-allergy, 122
  cytotoxic drug-induced, 546
  desensitisation, 124–5
  diagnosis of, 124
  fever, 124
  granulocytopenia, 123
  haemolysis, 124
  hepatitis, 124
  lymphoid system diseases, 122
  nephropathy, 124
  non-urticarial rashes, 122
  penicillin, 189–90
  prevention of, 125
  principle clinical manifestations and treatment, 122–4
  pseudo-allergic reactions, 125
  pulmonary reactions, 123
  serum sickness syndrome, 123
  thrombocytopenia, 123
  type III reactions, 121–2
  type II reactions, 121
  type I reactions, 121
  type IV reactions, 122
  urticarial rashes, 122
Allergy, general, 499–501
  asthma See Asthma
  corticosteroids, 603
  drug management of, 501
  effect of corticosteroids on, 595–6
Allodynia, 296
Allopathy, 6
Allopurinol, 264, 272
  nephrolithiasis, 491
All-trans-retinoic acid (ATRA), 551–2
Allylamine, 238
Alopecia, 283
  androgenic, 285
  cytotoxic drug-induced, 545

Alopecia areata, 285
α_1-Acid glycoprotein, 95
α-Adrenoceptor agonists, 406
α_1-Adrenoceptor agonists
  effects, 405
  selectivity for, 406
α_2-Adrenoceptor agonists, 435
  selectivity for, 406
α-Adrenoceptor antagonists/blockers, 404
  for arrhythmias, 453–4
  for benign prostatic hyperplasia (BPH), 492
  combined with β_1-adrenoceptor blocker, 434
  in hypertension, 426–7
α_1-Adrenoceptor antagonists/blockers, 426–7, 436
α_2-Adrenoceptor antagonists/blockers, 426–7
α_2-Antiplasmin, 523
α-Glucosidase inhibitor, 616, 617
α-Methylnoradrenaline, 435
α-Tocopherol acetate, 476, 669
Alprostadil, 253, 425, 493
Alteplase, 437, 523
Alternative medicine, 13–17
  regulation, 67
Altitude sickness, 487, 604
Aluminium hydroxide, 562, 665
Alzheimer's disease, drugs for, 367–8
Amantadine, 231, 384, 385
AmBisome, 235
Amblyopia, tobacco, 535
Amenorrhoea, 656
Amfetamines, 168, 410
Amide compounds, 324, 325–6
Amikacin, 198
Amiloride, 79, 480, 481, 483
Amino acids, 579
Aminoglutethimide, 550, 605
Aminoglycosides, 188, 196–8
D-Aminolaevulinic acid (ALA) synthase, 120
Aminophylline, 170, 497, 504
4-Aminoquinolone, 240
8-Aminoquinolone, 240
Aminosalicylates, 577
5-Aminosalicylic acid (5-ASA), 577
Amiodarone, 451, 454
  cumulative dose effects, 585
  hypothyroidism, 634–6
Amisulpride, 346
Amitriptyline, 335, 337, 427, 580
Amlodipine, 420
Ammonia, 587
Amnesia, 93, 314–15
Amoebiasis, 246–7
Amotivational syndrome, 166
Amoxicillin, 192, 489
  plasma half-life of, 87
Amphetamines, 365–6
Amphocil, 235
Amphotericin, 235–6
Ampicillin, 192
Anabolic steroids, 644
  abuse of, 147–8
Anabolism, 594
Anaemia, 531–2
  acquired haemolytic, 603
  aplastic, 124, 540
  of chronic renal failure, 537
  pernicious, 534–5
  sickle cell, 538–9
Anaerobic microorganisms, pneumonia due to, 212
Anaerobic vaginosis, 218

Anaesthesia, 312–29
  and antihypertensives, 444
  in the diseased, 328–9
  dissociative, 314
  drugs that affect, 327–8
  general, 312–20
    dissociative, 314, 319
    history/development, 312
    inhalation anaesthetics, 315–18
    intravenous, 318–20
    during labour, 327
    mode of action of anaesthetics, 315
    oxygen in, 317–18
    pharmacokinetics, 315–16, 318–20
    pharmacology of anaesthetics, 315
    phases of, 313–14
    special techniques, 314–15
    vomiting after, 570
  local, 323–6
    adverse reactions, 325
    desired properties, 323
    individual, 325–6
    mode of action, 323
    for neuropathic pain, 307
    other effects, 324
    pharmacokinetics, 323–4
    prolongation of action by vasoconstrictors, 324
    topical, 277
    uses, 324–5
  obstetric, 326–7
  in particular patient groups, 328–9
  in patients already taking medication, 327–8
Anagrelide, 539
Anakinra, 268
Analeptics, 497–8
Anal fissure, 580–1
Analgesia
  after surgery, 313
  for bone pain, 308
  mechanism of, 296–7
  obstetric, 326–7
  in opioid addicts, 305–6
  in palliative care, 308–9
  before surgery, 313
Analgesics, 293–311
  and anticoagulants, 519
  chronic daily headache associated with, 310
  definition of, 296
  in liver disease, 583
  non-opioid, 296–7
  NSAIDs, 255
  opioid See Opioids
  presystemic elimination, 90
  topical, 277
Anaphylactic shock, 122–3, 499
  adrenaline in, 408
Anaphylactoid reactions, 125, 323, 499
Anaphylaxis, 121, 283
  neuromuscular block, 323
Anastrozole, 605–6
Androgen-dependent carcinoma, 647
Androgenic alopecia, 285
Androgen(s), 550, 593, 642–3
  adverse effects, 643
  antagonists, 643–4
Angel dust See Phencyclidine
Angina pectoris
  β-adrenoceptor blockers, 430
  drugs used in, 416–36
  drug treatment of, 436–7
  how drugs act, 415
  prophylaxis, 436–7
  unstable, 438

Angiogenesis, 553
Angio-oedema, 122, 284, 288–9
  ACE inhibitor induced, 422
  hereditary, 524, 644
Angiotensin (AT) II receptor blockers
    (ARBs), 420–3
  adverse effects, 423
  cautions, 422
  for heart failure, 464–5
  interactions, 423
    with NSAIDs, 257
  sexual function and, 444
  uses of, 421–2
Angiotensin converting enzyme (ACE)
    inhibitors, 420–3
  adverse effects, 422
  cautions, 422
  for heart failure, 464–5
  interactions, 423
    with azathioprine, 264
    with NSAIDs, 257
  for myocardial infarction, 438
  pregnancy hypertension, 443–4
  sexual function and, 444
  uses of, 421–2
Animal insulins, 609, 610
Animals (Scientific Procedures) Act 1986,
    38
Animal studies, 36–8
  animal models of human disease, 35
  ethics and legislation, 37–8
  transgenic animals, 35
Anion-exchange resins See Bile
    acid-binding resins
Ankylosing spondylitis, 271
  corticosteroids for, 604
Anogenital infections, 217
Anopheles mosquitoes, 239–40
Anorexia, 308
Anovulatory ovarian cycles, 656
Antacids, 562–3
  in GORD, 567
  in liver disease, 583
Antagonism, 112–13
Antagonists, 76–7
  see also specific antagonist
Anthelminthic drugs, 176, 247–9
Anthracyclines, 544, 547
Anthraquinone laxatives, 573
Antiandrogens, 643–4
Antianginal drugs, 416–36, 436–7
Antiarrhythmics, 448–62
  and anticoagulants, 519
  in breast milk, 100
  class I, 450
  class IA, 450–2
  class IB, 452
  class IC, 452–3
  class II, 450, 453–4
  class III, 450, 454
  class IV, 450, 454–5
  classification of, 449–50
  objectives of treatment, 448
  proarrhythmic drug effects, 457
Anti-asthma drugs in breast milk, 100
Antibacterial drugs, 176, 188–206
  cell wall synthesis inhibition, 188,
    189–96
  classification, 188–9
  nucleic acid synthesis inhibition, 188–9,
    203–6
  protein synthesis inhibition, 188,
    196–203
  See also specific class; specific drug
Antibiotic cycling, 183
Antibodies, 596

Anticancer drugs
  in breast milk, 100. See also
    Chemotherapy, cytotoxic
Anticholinesterase drugs, 322, 394–6
  and anaesthesia, 327
  poisoning, 395–6
Anticoagulants, 517–22
  action of, 108
  and alcohol, 157
  under development, 522
  effect on other drug action, 108
  interaction with NSAIDs, 258
  reversal of anticoagulation, 518
  surgery in patients receiving, 519–20
  uses of, 519
  withdrawal of, 518
Anticonvulsant embryopathy, 375
Anticonvulsants See Antiepileptics
Antidepressants, 331–41
  adverse effects, 336–8
  and anaesthesia, 328
  and anticoagulants, 519
  for anxiety disorders, 354, 357
  augmentation, 336
  in breast milk, 100
  changing and stopping, 335–6
  classification of, 331
  electroconvulsive therapy, 341
  indications for, 370
  for insomnia, 364
  interactions, 338–40
    pharmacodynamic, 338–9
    pharmacokinetic, 339
  in liver disease, 583
  mechanism of action, 331–3
  mode of use, 335
  for neuropathic pain, 306–7
  pharmacokinetics, 333–4
  selection of, 335
  St John's wort, 340–1
  therapeutic efficacy, 335
  tricyclic See Tricyclic antidepressants
    See also Monoamine
      oxidase inhibitors (MAOIs);
      Novel compounds; Selective
      serotonin-reuptake inhibitors (SSRIs)
Antidiabetes drugs, 615–18
  interactions, 621
Antidiarrhoeal drugs, 575–6
Antidiuretic hormone (ADH), 480, 586,
    640, 641
Antidotes, 131, 132
Antiemesis drugs, 568–9
Antiepileptics, 372–80, 377
  and alcohol, 157
  and anaesthesia, 327
  and anticoagulants, 519
  in breast milk, 100
  dosage and administration, 373
  and folic acid, 537
  interaction with NSAIDs, 258
  in liver disease, 583
  mode of action, 372
  monitoring blood concentrations of, 373–4
  for neuropathic pain, 307
  and oral contraceptives, 375, 654–5
  pharmacology of, 376–80
  teratogenicity of, 375
  withdrawal, 373, 374
Antifibrinolytics, 524
Antifols, 244
Antifungal drugs, 176, 233–8
  classification of, 235
Antihelminthic drugs, 176, 247–9
Antihistamines See H₁-receptor antagonists
    (antihistamines)

Antihypertensive drugs, 416–36, 439–44
  ACD scheme, 441–2
  aim of treatment, 439
  and anaesthesia, 327
  interactions, 444
    with NSAIDs, 258
  principles of therapy, 440
  sexual function and, 444–5
  threshold and targets for treatment, 439–40
Anti-IL-1 agents, 268
Anti-inflammatory drugs, 250–73
  for asthma, 506
  in breast milk, 100
Antilymphocyte immunoglobulin (ALG),
    540, 557
Antimalarials, 238–46
  history of, 175
  photosensitivity, 281
  and pregnancy, 243
Antimetabolites, 240, 262–3, 544, 546–7
Antimicrobials
  for acne, 288
  and anaesthesia, 327
  in animal feeds, 121
  and anticoagulants, 519
  in breast milk, 100
  chemoprophylaxis, 178, 180–1
  choice of, 178–80
  classification of, 176–7
  combinations, 180
  diarrhoea induced by, 576
  drugs of choice, 184–6
  masking of infections, 184
  minor, 206
  neuromuscular transmission
      disorders, 398
  and oral contraceptives, 655
  polypeptide antibiotics, 206
  principles of chemotherapy, 177–8
  problems with, 181–4
  resistance to, 179, 180, 181–3, 202–3
  selection of, 178
  sites of action, 177
  superinfection, 183–4
  use of, 178–81
  See also specific class; specific drug
Antimotility drugs, 575–6
Antimuscarinics, 399–402
  for abnormal micturition, 491
  bronchodilators, 504
  chronic obstructive pulmonary disease
      (COPD), 508
  for irritable bowel syndrome, 580
  for parkinsonism, 384, 385
  peptic ulcer, 564
  before surgery, 313
  uses of, 400, 401
  for vomiting, 568
Antimuscarinic syndromes, 135, 347
Antinicotinic drugs, 399
Antinuclear antibodies, 268
Antioestrogens, 647
Antiplatelet drugs, 525–8
  angina pectoris, 436
  interaction with NSAIDs, 258
  for myocardial infarction, 437–8
  NSAIDs as, 255–6
  uses of, 527
Antiprogestogens, 648–9
Antiprotozoal drugs, 176, 238–47
Antipruritics, 277–8
Antipseudomonal penicillins, 189, 192–3
Antipsychotics, 341–8
  action of, 106–7
  adverse effects, 345–8
  in breast milk, 100

673

Antipsychotics (*Continued*)
classical versus atypical, 348
classification of, 341–2
drug-induced parkinsonism, 385–6
efficacy, 343
indications for, 342, 370
for insomnia, 364–5
long-acting depot injections, 344
mechanism of action, 342
mode of use, 344–5
pharmacokinetics, 343
rapid tranquillisation, 345
Antipyretics, NSAIDs as, 255
Antiretroviral therapy, 227–31
Anti-riot agents, 139–40
Antispasmodics, 580
Antistaphylococcal penicillins, 191
Antithrombin, 520
Antithymocyte globulin (ATG), equine, 540
Antithyroid drugs, 629–34, 638
control of therapy, 630–1
Anti-TNFα agents, 267
Antituberculous drugs, 219–20, 221–3
Antitussives, 495–6
Antiviral drugs, 176, 225–33
interaction with NSAIDs, 258
Antizygotic drugs, 650
Anxiety disorders, 330, 336, 342, 351–7
classification of, 351–7
general comments about treating, 356–7
properties of drugs for, 357
Anxiolytics, 313
and anticoagulants, 519
in breast milk, 100
Aortic dissection, 430
Aortic stenosis, 422
Aphthous ulcers, 604
Aplastic anaemia, 124, 540
Apnoea, 498
Apomorphine, 383, 385, 493
Apoptosis, 543
Appetite control, 624–5
Aprotinin, 524
Aqueous channels, 83
Arabinosides, 547
Area under the plasma concentration-time curve (AUC), 89
Arecoline, 394
Argatroban, 522
Aripiprazole, 346
Aromatase inhibitors, 544
for breast cancer, 550
Aromatic retinoids, 284
Arrhythmia, 448–62
choice of treatment, 457–8
drugs for *See* Antiarrhythmics
physiology and pathophysiology, 448–9
poisoning, 135
Arsenic, 131
Arsenic trioxide, 553–4
Artemether, 240, 245
Artemisinin, 245
Arterial occlusion, 524
Artesunate, 240, 245
Arthritis
corticosteroids for, 604
psoriatic, 271
rheumatoid, 269–70
septic, 218–19
Arylaminoalcohols, 240
Ascites, 484, 586–7
Ascorbic acid, 531, 536, 662
Asparaginase, 547
Aspergillosis, 234

Aspirin, 260–1
adverse effects of, 256–7
antiplatelet action of, 255–6, 525–6, 527
ionisation, 82
for myocardial infarction, 438
Asthenia, 6
Asthma, 501–8
acute severe, 507–8
approaches to treatment, 502–4
chest infections, 507
constant and intermittent, 505–6
corticosteroids in, 603
drug allergy, 123
drug treatment, 505–8
drug variations in, 111
inhalation drug therapy, 505
pathophysiology, 502
types of, 502
Astringents, 278
Atenolol, 433, 489
plasma half-life of, 87
Atheroma, 416
Atom oxetine, 368
Atonic seizures, 377
Atopic dermatitis, 289
Atorvastatin, 474
Atovaquone, 246
ATRA (all-*trans*-retinoic acid), 551–2
Atracurium, 321
Atrial ectopic beats, 458
Atrial fibrillation, 455, 458–9
Atrial flutter, 456, 459
Atrial tachycardia, 458, 459
Atrioventricular (AV) node, 448–9
Atrophic rhinitis, 647
Atropine
acetylcholine opposition, 399–400
β-adrenoceptor blocker overdose, 432
in poisoning, 132, 396
vagus nerve activity, 457
Atropinic effects of toxic plants, 139
Attention deficit hyperactivity disorder (ADHD), 368–9
Audit, 42
Auranofin, 266
Autoimmune active chronic hepatitis, 588
Automaticity, heart, 448
Autonomic ganglion blocking drugs, 435
Autonomic nervous system
cholinergic drugs, 392
effects of antiarrhythmics, 456–7
Autonomy, 28
Aversion therapy, 140–1
Azathioprine, 264, 272, 284
for autoimmune active chronic hepatitis, 588
in Crohn's disease, 579
Azithromycin, 200
Azoles, 188–9, 205–6, 236–8
Aztreonam, 192

B
Bacille Calmette-Guérin (BCG), 545
Bacilli, antibiotic choice, 185–6
Baclofen, 322–3
Bacteria
knowledge of, 179
resistance of, 179, 180, 181–3
response to antimicrobials, 177
Bacterial infections chemotherapy, 208–24
skin, 289
See also specific infection
Bacterial vaginosis, 218
Bactericidal drugs, 176
Bacteriostatic drugs, 176

Bacteriuria, asymptomatic, 216
Bacteroides spp, 181
Band ligation of varices, 585
Barbiturates, 364
in alcohol abuse, 157
for epilepsy, 379
Baroreceptor reflexes, 441
Barrier preparations, 276–7
Bartter's syndrome, 256
B cells, 252–3
BCG (bacille Calmette-Guérin), 545
Beclomethasone, 279, 597
Bendroflumethiazide, 79, 482
Beneficence, 43
Benign malaria, 241–2
Benign prostatic hyperplasia (BPH), 491–2, 551
Benoxaprofen, 62
Benzatropine, 132
Benzhexol, 401
Benznidazole, 246
Benzodiazepines, 77
antagonist, 363
for anxiety disorders, 354, 357
as co-analgesics, 306
indications for, 370
for sleep disorders, 361–3
Benzyl benzoate, 282
Benzylpenicillin, 189, 190–1
adverse effects, 191
plasma half-life of, 87
preparations and dosage, 191
uses, 190–1
β-Adrenoceptor agonists, 405
selectivity for, 406
β$_1$-Adrenoceptor agonists, 406
β$_2$-Adrenoceptor agonists, 406
in asthma, 503
chronic obstructive pulmonary disease (COPD), 508
inhaled, 506
as a uterine relaxant, 659
β-Adrenoceptor antagonists/blockers, 404, 427–34
abuse of, 148
action of, 427–8, 436
adverse reactions, 431–2
and anaesthesia, 327
in breast milk, 100
classification of, 430
effects, 428
for heart failure, 465
hyperthyroidism, 631
interactions, 433
with antidiabetes drugs, 621
interference with self-regulating systems, 104
for myocardial infarction, 437–8
notes on individual, 433–4
overdose, 432–3
peripheral vascular disease, 426
pharmacokinetics, 429–30
in pregnancy, 433
pregnancy hypertension, 443
properties, 429
selectivity, 428–9
uses of, 430–1
for variceal bleeding, 586
withdrawal, 428, 432
β$_1$-Adrenoceptor antagonists/blockers, 434
β-Adrenoceptors, 76
β-Carbolines, 77
β-Endorphin, 298
β-Lactamase inhibitors, 188
β-Lactams, 188, 189–93
Betamethasone, 597
Bethanechol, 393

Bevacizumab, 553
Bias in trials, 51–2
Bicalutamide, 644
Bicarbonate in diabetic ketoacidosis, 622
Biguanides, 615, 616, 617
Bile acid-binding resins, 471, 475
Bile salts, 89
  malabsorption, 580
Biliary cirrhosis, primary (PBC), 588
Biliary excretion, 99
Bilirubin, 584
Binding
  receptor, 77
  tissue, 95
Bioassay, 80
Bioavailability, 89–91
Bioequivalence, 45–6, 51
Biological activity, altering, 96
Biological agents as weapons, 139
Biological assay, 80
Biological standardisation, 80
Biological variations in drug effects, 105–8
Biotechnology, 35
  animal studies, 37
Biphasic insulin, 611–12
Bipolar affective disorder, 348–9
Birth defects See Teratogenicity
Bisacodyl, 573
Bismuth chelate, 564
Bisoprolol, 433
Bisphosphonates, 270, 666–7
  for bone pain, 308
  for hypercalcaemia, 665
  for osteoporosis, 668
  for Paget's disease of bone, 669
Bites, infected, 223–4
Bivalirudin, 522
Black cohosh, 15
Black triangle, inverted, 65
Bladder, urinary
  cholinoceptors, 392
  decreased activity, 491
  unstable, 491
Blastomycosis, 234
Blinding in trials, 51–2
Blockers See Antagonists; specific blocker
Blood
  disorders, 123
  doping, 148
  flow, reduced, 431
  infections, 208–9
  lipoproteins, 152
  volume increase, 440
Blood-brain barrier, 83
Blood dyscrasias
  ACE inhibitor-induced, 422
  antipsychotic-induced, 347
Blood lipids
  effect of xanthines on, 171
  hormone replacement therapy, 647
Blood pressure, 415
  control in diabetic patients, 619–20
  control in phaeochromocytoma, 446–7
  emergency reduction of, 442–3
  See also Antihypertensive drugs;
    Hypertension; Hypotension
Blood vessels
  cholinoceptors, 393
  effect of histamine on, 499
Body mass index (BMI), 624
Body weight See Weight (body)
Bone(s)
  adjuvant used for pain in, 308
  disorders, 667–9
  infections of, 218–19
  marrow suppression, 543–5

Bortezomib, 554
Bosentan, 445
Bovine insulin, 609, 610
Bowel
  infection, 214–16
  irrigation, 131
  lumen amoebiasis, 246
  motility patterns, 575
Bowen's disease, 285
Bradycardia, 446, 460
  sinus, 458
Bradykinin, 421
Brain
  capillary endothelial cells, 97
  drug passage, 83
Brain-derived neurotrophic factor (BDNF),
  333
Bran, 572
Breast cancer, 550
  effect of combined contraceptives,
    651
  hormone replacement therapy, 646–7
  tamoxifen, 647
Breast feeding
  drug elimination from, 100
  See also Lactation
Breast pain, 657
Breathing disorders, sleep-related, 365
Brinzolamide, 487
British Approved Name (BAN), 69
British National Formulary (BNF), 29
Broad-spectrum penicillins, 189, 191–2
Bromocriptine, 382, 657
  hyperprolactinaemia, 640
Bronchi
  cholinoceptors, 392
  dilatation of narrowed, 503–4
  reduction of inflammation of, 503
Bronchial decongestants, 410–11
Bronchial infection, 210–12
Bronchitis, 210
Bronchoconstriction, 431
Bronchodilators, 503–4
Bronchogenic carcinoma, 160
Brown, John, 6
Buccal administration/absorption, 89, 91
Budesonide, 579, 597
Bulimia nervosa, 336
Bullous pemphigoid, 283
Bumetanide, 481
Bupivacaine, 325–6
Buprenorphine, 302–3
Bupropion, 162, 333
Burns, infected, 223, 289
Buspirone, 357
Busulfan, 539
Butorphanol, 303

C

Cabergoline, 382
  hyperprolactinaemia, 640
Caffeine, 169–71
Calamine lotion, 278
Calcareous stones, 490–1
Calciferol, 663
Calcineurin antagonists, 262, 265
Calcipotriol, 287
Calcitonin, 665–6, 666
  for osteoporosis, 668
Calcitriol, 663, 664
Calcium
  and cardiac cells, 454–5
  homeostasis, 486
  See also Hypercalcaemia; Hypercalciuria;
    Hypocalcaemia

Calcium channel blockers, 418–20, 454–5
  action of, 436
  adverse effects, 419
  arrhythmias, 450
  indications, 419
  interactions, 419
  pharmacokinetics, 419
  pregnancy hypertension, 443
  sexual function and, 444
  vascular smooth muscle cells, 418–19
Calcium glubionate, 665
Calcium gluconate, 132, 137, 665
Calcium-phase resin, 487
Campylobacter jejuni, 215
Cancer, 541–51
  chemoprevention of, 555
  chemotherapy
    See Chemotherapy, cytotoxic
  colon, NSAIDs in, 256
  corticosteroids for, 604
  cures: unproven remedies, 555–6
  development of anticancer
    therapy, 552
  effect on drug action, 107
  hormonal influence on, 550–1
  immunotherapy in, 551–2
  lung, 160
  pain related to, 295
  systemic therapy, 541–2
  targeted biological cancer therapies, 552–5
  treatments and outcomes, 541–2
  See also specific cancer
Candida infections, 183, 234
  skin, 289–90
Cannabinoid receptor blocker, 625
Cannabinoids, 295
Cannabis, 164–6
  adverse effects, 166
  pharmacodynamics, 164–5
  pharmacokinetics, 164
  uses, 165–6
Capreomycin, 223
Capsaicin, 307
Capsule, definition of, 89
Captopril, 423, 489
Carbachol, 393
Carbamazepine, 307, 351, 376
Carbapenems, 188, 189, 195
Carbaryl, 395
Carbidopa, 78
Carbimazole, 629
Carbocisteine, 496
Carbohydrate
  intolerance, 486
  metabolism, 594
Carbonic acid (H$_2$CO$_3$), 486
Carbonic anhydrase inhibitors, 486–7
Carbon monoxide
  poisoning, 136
  in smoking, 159
Carboprost, 253, 658, 659
Carboxypenicillins, 192–3
Carcinogenicity, 116, 126
  animal studies, 37
  cytotoxic drugs, 546
  immunosuppression, 557–8
Carcinoma, bronchogenic, 160
Cardiac arrest, 459
Cardiac arrhythmia See Arrhythmia
Cardiac cycle, 449–50
Cardiac glycosides, 455–7
Cardiac output (CO), 462
Cardiovascular system
  abrupt drug withdrawal, 104
  anaesthesia in patients with diseases
    of, 328

Cardiovascular system (*Continued*)
  effects of antipsychotics on, 347
  effects of atropine on, 400
  effects of β-adrenoceptor blockers, 427–8
  effects of combined contraceptives on, 651
  effects of nicotine on, 160
  effects of NSAIDs on, 257
  effects of opioids on, 299
  effects of propofol on, 318
  effects of thiopental on, 319
  effects of toxic plants on, 139
  effects of xanthines on, 169–70
  sexual intercourse and the, 445
Car driving, 119
  and alcohol, 152–4
  and epilepsy, 374
  psychotropic drugs, 369
Carminatives, 568
Carotid sinus massage, 457
Carrier-mediated transport, 83–4, 97
  drug interactions, 113
Case-control studies, 58, 59
Case reports, 59
Caspofungin, 238
Cataplexy, 365
Catecholamines, 76, 408–9
  blockers, 450, 453–4
  in phaeochromocytoma, 446
  pharmacokinetics, 407
  synthetic non-, 407
Catechol-*O*-methyltransferase (COMT), 384
Cation-exchange resins, 487
CD20, 554
Ceftriaxone, 193–5
Cell(s)
  cardiac, 449, 454–5
  effect of chronic pharmacology on, 105
  membrane *See* Membranes, cell (humans), drug passage across
  wall
    antimicrobial action on, 177
    synthesis inhibition, 188, 189–96
Central nervous system
  abrupt drug withdrawal, 104
  bleeding into the, 518
  cholinoceptors, 393
  effects of atropine on, 400
  effects of corticosteroids on, 599
  effects of opioids on, 298–9
  effects of prolonged drug administration, 125
  effects of propofol on, 318
  effects of thiopental on, 319
  hypertensives acting on, 435–6
Cephalosporins, 188, 193–5
  adverse effects, 193–5
  classification and uses, 193
  mode of action, 193
  pharmacokinetics, 193
Cephamycins, 188
Cerebrospinal fluid (CSF), drug passage, 83
Cervical carcinoma, 651
Cervical ectropion, 651
C₁-esterase inhibitor, 288
Cestodes, 247
Cetirizine, 500
Cetrorelix, 639
Cetuximab, 553
CFCs (chlorofluorocarbons), 505
Chagas' disease, 246
Chalk, 576
Chancroid, 218
Charcoal, activated, 99, 130–1, 133, 139, 259

Cheese reaction, monoamine oxidase inhibitors, 383
Chelating agents, 131–3
Chemical interaction, 76
Chemoimmunotherapy, 553
Chemokines, 251
Chemoprevention of cancer, 555
Chemoprophylaxis, 178, 180–1
  of malaria, 242–3
  meningitis, 214
  streptococcal throat infection, 209–10
  tuberculosis, 220
  urinary tract infections, 217
Chemoresistant cancers, 542
Chemotaxis inhibitors, 261–2
Chemotherapy, cytotoxic
  adverse effects of, 543–6
  classes of drugs for, 543, 544–5, 546–7
  in clinical practice, 547–50
  drug interactions, 550
  drug resistance, 549
  drug use and tumour cell kinetics, 547–8
  immunosuppression, 556
  improving efficacy of, 549
  rationale for, 542
  staff hazards, 549
Chemotherapy of infections, 175–87
  bacterial *See* Bacterial infections chemotherapy
  drug choice, 184–6
  drug classification, 176–7
  history, 176
  malaria, 240–2
  principles of, 177–8
  See also Antimicrobials
Chest infections in asthma, 507
Chickenpox, 226
Children
  anaesthesia in, 329
  drug response in, 108–9
  epilepsy in, 375
  long-term corticosteroids use, 601
  psychiatric illness in, 369
Chlamydiae
  antibiotic choice, 186
  conjunctivitis, 219
  endocarditis, 213
Chloral hydrate, 364
Chloramphenicol, 201
Chlordiazepoxide, 154
Chlormethiazole, 364
Chloroguanide *See* Proguanil
Chloroquine, 240, 243
Chlorphenamine, 501
Chlorpromazine, 341, 346, 427
Chlorpropamide, 641
Chlortalidone, 482
Cholera, 215
Cholestatic jaundice, 124
Cholesterol, 469
Choline esters, 393
Cholinergic crisis, 398
Cholinergic drugs, 391–8
  antagonism of atropine, 400
  classification, 391
  pharmacology, 392–6
  sites of action, 391–2
  uses of, 391
Cholinergic syndromes, 135
Cholinergic transmission, 367
Cholinoceptors, 392
Cholinomimetics *See* Cholinergic drugs
CHOP regimen, 548
Chorea, 386
Chorionic gonadotrophin, 639
  in sportsmen, 147–8

Chronic obstructive pulmonary disease (COPD), 508–9
  asthma associated with, 502
  long-term oxygen therapy, 509
Chronic pharmacology, 103–5
Chylomicrons, 469
CIBIS–2 trial, 466–7
Ciclesonide, 597
Ciclosporin, 284, 287, 556–7
  in Crohn's disease, 579
  increased dose effects, 585
  interaction with NSAIDs, 258
  in ulcerative colitis, 578
Cidofovir, 232
Cimetidine, 563
  interactions with antidiabetes drugs, 621
Cinacalcet, 664
Ciprofloxacin, 205
Circadian rhythm disorders/disruption, 359–61, 367
Cirrhosis
  complications of, 585–6
  primary biliary, 588
Cisatracurium, 321
Cisplatin, 552
Clarithromycin, 200
  resistance, 566
Classification of drugs, 69
Claudication, intermittent, 425
Clavulanic acid, 192
Clearance, drug, 100
Clindamycin, 201
Clinical equivalence trials, 51
Clobetasol, 279
Clodronate, 665
Clofazimine, 223
Clomethiazole, 154, 157
Clomifene, 647
Clonazepam, 379
Clonidine, 307, 369, 414, 435
Clopidogrel, 438, 526
Clostridium spp., 181
  colitis, 183
Clotrimazole, 236
Clotting *See* Coagulation
Cloxacillin, 191
Clozapine, 341–2, 344, 346, 347–8
CN (chloroacetophenone) gas, 140
Coagulant factors, 514
  concentrates, 515–16
  See also specific factor
Coagulation, 513–22, 525
  See also Anticoagulants
Co-amoxiclav, 192
Co-analgesics, 306–8
  definition of, 296
Cobalamins, 534–5
  deficiency, 536
Co-beneldopa, 382
Cocaine, 167–8, 323, 326
  increased dose effects, 585
Co-careldopa, 382
Cocci, antibiotic choice, 184
Coccidioidomycosis, 234
Codeine, 298, 301
Cohort studies, 57–8, 59
Colchicine, 261–2, 284
Colecalciferol, 663
Colesevelam, 475
Colestipol, 475
Colestyramine, 475, 580
  for primary biliary cirrhosis, 588
Coliforms, 181
Colistin, 206

Colitis
  antibiotic-associated, 183
  microscopic, 579–80
  ulcerative, 577–8, 604
Collagen diseases, 124
Collecting duct, 480
Colloidions, 276
Colloids, 413
Colon cancer, NSAIDs in, 256
Colony-stimulating factors, 538
Combinations, drug
  antimicrobials, 180
  fixed-dose, 103
Combinatorial chemistry, 34–5
Combined oestrogen-progestogen oral
    contraceptives (COCP), 650–3, 657
Combivir, 230
Comfrey, 15
Compensation, 44
Competitive antagonism, 77, 321–2
Complementary and alternative medicine
    (CAM), 13–17
  regulation, 67
Compliance, 22–5
  doctor, 25
  patient, 22–5
Compound A, 317
Compound Benzoic Acid Ointment, 233
Concentration, drug
  change in with change/cessation of
    dosing, 86–7
  decrease in after intravenous bolus
    injection, 85–6
  increase with constant dosing, 86
  measurement interpretation, 88
  steady state, 85–7
  time course of, 85–8
Confidence intervals, 48–9
Congenital adrenal hyperplasia, 602
Congestive cardiac failure, 483
Conjugated oestrogens, 645
Conjugation, 97
Conjunctivitis, chlamydial, 219
Connective tissue disease, 603
Consent, 20–1
  research ethics, 42–3
Constipation, 572–4
  due to opioids, 299
  in dying patients, 308
  in irritable bowel syndrome (IBS), 580
Consumer rights, 28
Containers, medicine, 30
Continuous long-term domiciliary oxygen
    therapy, 498
Contraception
  drug interactions with, 654–5
  by drugs and hormones, 649–55 (See also
    Oral contraceptives)
  hormone replacement therapy, 646
  male, 655
  oral See Oral contraceptives
  possible modes and sites of action, 650
  postcoital/emergency, 654
  progestogen-only, 654
  risks in relation to benefits, 655
Contractility, 462
Control, 4
Convoluted tubules, 478, 480
Convulsions
  poisoning, 135
  from poisonous plants, 139
  See also Antiepileptics; Epilepsy
Copper intrauterine devices, 655
Cornea
  deposits of chloroquine, 243
  opacities, antipsychotics, 347

Coronary artery thrombolysis, 523–4
Coronary heart disease (CHD), 161
Corticosteroids, 253–4, 593–607
  action of, 251
  adverse effects of systemic
    pharmacotherapy, 598–9
  and anaesthesia, 327
  for cancer, 551
  choice of, 598
  as co-analgesics, 306
  competitive antagonism of, 606
  contraindications, 601
  Crohn's disease, 579
  dosage schedules, 598, 600–1
  effect on blood glucose, 615
  fluorinated, 596–7
  for hypercalcaemia, 666
  inhibition of lymphocyte activation,
    262–3
  inhibition of synthesis of, 605–6
  interference with cytokine expression or
    signalling, 267–8
  long-term use in children, 601
  for multiple sclerosis, 386–7
  osteoporosis induced by, 668–9
  pharmacokinetics of, 597–8
  precautions during therapy, 599–600
  and pregnancy, 599
  replacement therapy, 601–2
  routes of administration, 600–1
  systemic, 578
  topical, 277, 278–80, 287
  and tuberculosis, 220
  for ulcerative colitis, 577–8
  uses of, 601–5
  withdrawal, 600, 602, 605
  See also Glucocorticoids;
    Mineralocorticoids
Corticotrophin, 147–8, 593, 605, 606
Corticotrophin releasing hormone (CRH),
    605, 606, 637
Corticotropin releasing factor (CRF), 593
Cortisol See Hydrocortisone
Cortisol binding globulin (CBG), 598
Cortisone, 593
  potency, 597
Cost-benefit analysis, 27
Cost-containment in prescribing, 19–20
Cost-effectiveness analysis, 27
Cost-minimisation analysis, 27
Costs, 27
Cost-utility analysis, 27
Co-trimoxazole, 203
  interaction with methotrexate, 264
Cough, 495–7
  ACE inhibitor induced, 422
  due to opioids, 299
  mixtures, 497
  See also Antitussives
Coumarins, 515, 517
  action of, 108
Counterfeit drugs, 67
Counterirritants, 277
Coxib, 256–7, 297
Coxiella spp., 213
CR (dibenzoxazepine), 140
Creams, 275
Creatinine clearance, 490
Crime, drugs as adjuvants to, 172
Critical care units, sedation in, 329
Crohn's disease, 578–9
  corticosteroids for, 604
  effect of combined contraceptives, 651
Cromolyn sodium, 261
Cross-allergy, 122
  penicillin, 190

Cross-over designs, 52
Cross-sectional surveys, 59
Cryptococcosis, 234
Crystalloid solutions, 413
CS (chlorobenzylidene malononitrile) gas,
    139–40
Cullen, William, 6
Cults, 14–15
Culture-negative endocarditis, 213
Curare, 320
Cure, drugs that, 8
Cushing's syndrome, 606
Cutaneous drug reactions, 282–4
Cutaneous irritation from toxic
    plants, 139
Cyanide, 424
  poisoning, 136
Cyclic AMP, 76
Cyclic AMP response element binding
    (CREB) protein, 333
Cyclin-dependent kinase inhibitors, 553
Cyclin-dependent kinases, 553
Cyclins, 553
Cyclofenil, 647
Cyclo-oxygenase (COX), 566
  in analgesia, 296–7
  aspirin and, 78, 525–6
  eicosanoids synthesis, 251
  NSAIDs mode of action, 254–5
Cyclophosphamide, 262, 266–7
  increased dose effects, 585
Cycloserine, 223
Cyproterone, 644
Cytochrome 3A4 enzyme, 334
Cytochrome 2D6 enzyme, 333–4, 453
Cytochrome P450 enzymes, 96–7,
    106, 230
  antidepressants, 333–4
  induction, 16
  inhibition, 16
  porphyrias, 120
Cytokines, 538
  drugs that interfere with expression of, 262
  interference with expression or signalling
    of, 267–8
  recombinant, 268
Cytomegalovirus (CMV), 232
  drugs of choice for, 226
Cytoplasmic membrane, antimicrobial
    action on, 177
Cytosolic receptors, 76
Cytotoxic chemotherapy See Chemotherapy,
    cytotoxic
Cytotoxics
  immunosuppression, 556
  interaction with NSAIDs, 258
  vomiting induced by, 570
  See also Chemotherapy, cytotoxic

D

Danaparinoid sodium, 522
Danazol, 644, 648–9, 656
Dandruff, 286
Danthron, 573
Dantrolene, 323, 328
Dapsone
  acetylation, 107
  for leprosy, 223
  for malaria, 240
  pyrimethamine with, 245
  safety monitoring, 284
Daptomycin, 196
Darbepoietin, 538
Daunorubicin, 547
Death rattle, 309

Decarboxylase inhibitors, 381
Decongestants, mucosal, 410–11
Decontamination of the gut, selective, 215–16
Deep vein thrombosis (DVT), 524
    International Normalised Ratio (INR), 518
Deferiprone, 534
Dehydroemetine, 246
Delavirdine, 230
Delirium, 309
Demeclocycline, 641
Dementia, drugs for, 367–8
Dental procedures prophylaxis, 213
Dependence, drug
    amfetamines, 168
    opioids, 305
    xanthines, 170
    See also Abuse, drug; specific drug
Depolarising neuromuscular blocker, 321
Depot preparations
    antipsychotics, 343
    for prolongation of drug action, 102
    sex hormones, 642
Depression, 330–70, 342, 349
    effect on drug action, 107
    See also Antidepressants
Dermal pharmacokinetics, 274–82
Dermatitis, 283
    atopic, 289
    corticosteroids in, 603
Dermatitis herpetiformis, 285
Dermatophyte infections, 233
Desensitisation to drug allergy, 124–5
Desferrioxamine, 132, 533
Desflurane, 316, 317
Designer drugs, 147
Desmopressin (DDAVP), 516, 640–1
    replacement therapy, 641
Desogestrel, 654
Detrusor, 491
Development, drug
    animal studies, 36–8
    orphan drugs and diseases, 39
    phases of, 45
    preclinical, 32–6
    prediction, 39
Development, human, toxic effects on, 37
Dexamethasone, 597
    potency, 597
    suppression test, 604–5
Dexamfetamine, 365, 368, 410
Dextran 70, 413
Dextrans, 527
    with iron, 532
Dextromethorphan, 496
Dextropropoxyphene, 519
Diabetes insipidus, 641
    nephrogenic, diuretics in, 483
Diabetes mellitus, 608–23
    complications of, 620
    and dietary fibre, 618
    drug-induced, 621
    drugs for, 615–18
    factors affecting control of, 620–1
    history, 608
    interactions with non-diabetes drugs, 621
    selection of therapy, 619–20
    surgery in patients with, 622–3
    treatment of, 618–21
    type 1, 608
        surgery in patients with, 622–3
        treatment for, 612–13, 619, 620
    type 2, 608
        surgery in patients with, 623
        treatment for, 619
Diabetic ketoacidosis, 621–2

Diabetic nephropathy, 421–2
Diagnostic tests for infections, 179
Dialysis, 134, 666
3,4-Diaminopyridine (3,4-DAP), 398
Diamorphine, 300–1
Diarrhoea, 574–6
    cytotoxic drug-induced, 545
    drug-induced, 576
    fluid and electrolyte treatment, 575
    in irritable bowel syndrome (IBS), 580
    physiology, 574–5
    secretory, 576
    specific infective, 576
    travellers, 576
Diazepam, 396
    plasma half-life of, 87
Diazoxide, 424, 621
Di Bella therapy, 556
Dichlorphenamide, 487
Dicobalt edetate, 132, 133, 136
Dicyclomine, 401
Didanosine, 228–9
Diet
    and Crohn's disease, 579
    in diabetic patients, 618
    fibre in, 572
        and diabetes, 618
    hyperlipidaemias, 471, 473
    potassium intake, 484
    sodium intake, 484
Diethylcarbamazine, 247
Diethylstilbestrol, 645
Diffusion
    facilitated, 84
    hypoxia, 315–16
    passive, 81–2
Digestive enzymes, 589
Digitalis, 455
Digoxin, 451, 489
    for arrhythmias, 455–6
    for heart failure, 465
    interaction with amiodarone, 454
Digoxin-specific antibody fragments (FAB), 132
Dihydrocodeine, 301
Dihydrofolate reductase, 263
Dihydrofolic acid (DHF) synthase, 203
Dihydro-orotate dehydrogenase, 264
Dihydrotachysterol, 663
Diloxanide furoate, 246
Diltiazem, 420
Dimercaprol, 131–3, 132, 137
2,3-dimercaptosuccinic acid (DMSA), 137
Dimeticone, 562–3
Dinitro-compounds, 138
Dinoprost, 658
Dinoprostone, 253, 658–9
Diphenhydramine, 501
Diphtheria, 210
Diphyllobothrum latum, 535
Dipyridamole, 526
Diquat, 138
Direct current (DC) electric shock, 457–8
Directly observed therapy (DOT), 23–4
Disabling agents, 139–40
Discontinuation syndrome, 26, 145
Discovery, drug, 34–6
Disease
    anaesthesia and, 328–9
    animal models of, 35
    drug response in, 111
    effect of chronic pharmacology on, 105
    effect on binding, 95
    enzyme induction and, 98
    orphan, 39
    physician-induced, 12–13

Disease-modifying antirheumatic drugs (DMARDs), 262, 265–6
Disopyramide, 451, 452
Disseminated intravascular coagulation (DIC), 513
Dissociative anaesthesia, 314, 319
Distal convoluted tubule, 480, 488–9
Distigmine, 395
Distribution, drug, 93–5
    alcohol, 149
    in disease, 111
    in the elderly, 109
    interactions during, 113
    plasma protein and tissue binding, 94–5
    in pregnancy, 110–11
    volume, 93–4
    in the young, 108
Disulfiram, 154–5
Diuresis, 133–4
Diuretic effect of alcohol, 151
Diuretics, 478–86
    abuse of, 486
    adverse effects characteristic of, 484–6
    and anaesthesia, 328
    for ascites, 586
    classification, 480–1
    definition of, 478
    for heart failure, 464
    high-efficacy See Loop diuretics
    in hypertension, 416, 442
    indications for, 483–6
    interactions, 486
        with NSAIDs, 258
    low-efficacy, 480–1, 482–3
    methylxanthines, 486
    moderate-efficacy See Thiazides
    osmotic, 478, 486
    potassium-sparing See Potassium-sparing diuretics
    sites and modes of action, 478–80
Diverticular disease, 580–1
DNA
    alteration of, 126
    genetic medicines, 35
Dobutamine, 409
    plasma half-life of, 87
    for shock, 412
Docusate sodium, 573
Domperidone, 569
Donepezil, 367
Dopa decarboxylase, 78
    inhibitors, 381–2
Dopamine, 78, 403
    action of, 409
    agonists, 382–3
    inhibition of metabolism, 383
    parkinsonism, 380
    release, 384
Dopamine D_2 receptors, 342
    antagonists, 568
Dopaminergic drugs, 381–4
Dopexamine, 409
Dornase, 496–7
Dorsal horn neurones, 295
Dorzolamide, 487
Dose-response relationships, 79
Dose-response trials, 50–1
Doses/dosing, 100–3
    calculation by body-weight and surface area, 102
    change in plasma concentration with cessation of, 86–7
    drug development, 32, 46
    increase in plasma concentration with constant, 86
    missed, clinical importance of, 26

schedules, 101–3
underdosing, 25–6
in the young, 109 See also Poisoning and
overdose
Dosulepin, 87
Dothiepin, 337
Double-blind trials, 52
Down-regulation, 104
Doxapram, 497
Doxazosin, 427
Doxorubicin, 547
Doxycycline, 199, 239, 240
D-Penicillamine, 266
Drastic purgatives, 573
DRESS, 282
Drinks containing xanthine, 170–1
Driving, car See Car driving
Drospirenone, 648
Drug discontinuation syndromes, 104
Drug-drug interactions, 112
Drug-food interactions, 112
Drug-herb interactions, 112
Drug history, 18–19
Drug holidays, 105
Drug-induced illness, 117–18
Drug-induced injury, 12–13
Drug(s)
abuse See Abuse, drug
adverse reactions See Adverse drug reactions
and breast feeding See Breast feeding;
Lactation
classification, 69
consumption, 18–22
counterfeit, 67
criticisms of modern, 11
definition of, 4
dependence on/misuse, 30
development See Development, drug
discovery, 34–6
essential, 21–2
evaluation See Animal studies; Humans,
drug evaluation in
good/beneficial, 7, 8–10
and haemostasis, 513–28
harmful, 7 (See also Risk(s))
interactions. See Interaction, drug
licensed. See Licence
modification of structure, 78
new
introducing to humans, 45–8
regulatory review of applications for,
63–5
nomenclature, 69–72
non-proprietary names, 70–1
proprietary names, 71–2
orphan, 39
photosensitivity, 280–1
public view of, 10–11
quality of, 36
and skilled tasks, 119, 165, 369
and the skin See Skin
therapeutic monitoring, 87–8
treating patients with, 7–8
unlicensed, 66
unwanted, 30
use of, 4, 8
Drug Safety Research Unit, 65
Drug-specific rashes, 283–4
Drug targeting, 78
Dry mouth, 308
Dry powder inhalers, 505
Dual-reuptake inhibitors, 306
Duloxetine, 338
Dutasteride, 644
Dyaesthesia, 296
Dynorphin, 298

Dyskinesia, 385
tardive, 345–7
Dysmenorrhoea, 657
Dyspepsia, non-ulcer, 568
Dyspnoea, 309, 463
Dystonias, 345
drug-induced, 386

E

Ear infection, 209
Echinocandins, 238
Econazole, 236
Economics, 18–22, 26–7
Ecstasy, 163–4
Eczema See Dermatitis
Edrophonium, 395, 397
Efalizumab, 265
Efavirenz, 230
Effect, (drug)
therapeutic, 46
time course of concentration and, 85–8
Effectors, 250, 251
Efficacy, 79–80
drug development, 47
of drugs, 7
homeopathic remedies, 16
missed doses, 26
pharmacological, 79
therapeutic, 79
Efflux transporters, 97
Eflornithine, 247
Ehrlich, Paul, 32, 80
Ehrlichia spp., 186
Eicosanoids, 251, 253
Elderly
anaesthesia in the, 329
drug response in, 109–10
prescribing rules, 110
Electroconversion, 457–8
Electroconvulsive therapy (ECT), 341
Electrolytes
in diabetic ketoacidosis, 622
treatment of diarrhoea, 575
Elemental diets, 579
Elimination, 98–100
in disease, 111
in the elderly, 109–10
in pregnancy, 111
presystemic, 90–1
in the young, 109
Emboli, 519
Embryo, drugs affecting, 126–7
See also Teratogenicity; specific drug
Emesis See Vomiting
Emollients, 276, 573
Empyema, 212
Emtricitabine, 229
Emulsifying ointment, 276
Enalapril, 78, 423
Enantiomorphs, 78–9
Encephalitis, herpes, 226
Encephalopathy, hepatic, 587–8
Endocannabinoids, 165, 625
Endocarditis, 212–13
dose regimens, 212–13
principles for treatment, 212
prophylaxis, 213
Endocrine system
abrupt drug withdrawal, 104
β-adrenoceptor blockers, 431
chronic pharmacology, 103
effect of corticosteroids on, 598–9
Endocrine therapy, 550–1
Endometrial carcinoma, 646
Endometriosis, 656–7

Enemas, 573–4, 577–8
Energy, alcohol as a source of, 151
Enflurane, 316, 317
Enfuvirtide, 230
Enkephalin, 298
Enolic acids, 258
Enoximone, 465
Entacapone, 384
Enteral administration, 91
Enterococci, 213
Enterocytes, 97
Enterohepatic circulation, 89
Entonox, 315, 327
Entry inhibitor, 230–1
Environment
effect on adverse drug reactions, 121
effect on drug action, 108–12
poisons from the, 130
Enzyme(s), 78
induction, 97–8, 339
phenytoin, 378
inhibition, 76, 98, 99
and antihypertensives, 444
effect of antidepressants on, 339
phenytoin, 378
Eosinophilic bronchitis, 495
Eosinophils, 596
Ephedrine, 410
Epidermal growth factor receptors (EGFs),
553, 554
Epidural administration of opioids, 300
Epidural local anaesthesia, 325, 327
Epilepsy, 372–80, 487
in children, 375
classification of, 372
driving regulations and, 374
drugs of choice for, 377
and oral contraceptives, 375
pregnancy and, 374–5
principles of management, 372–6
Epinephrine See Adrenaline
Epistaxis, 647
Epithelial Na channel, 480
Eplerenone, 483
Epoetin, 537–8
Epoprostenol, 253, 526
Epoxides, 97
Eptifibatide, 526–7
Epzicom, 230
Equine antithymocyte globulin (ATG), 540
Equivalence trials, 47–8, 51
Erectile dysfunction, 128, 492–4
Ergocalciferol, 663, 664
Ergometrine, 658, 659
Ergosterol, 236, 238
Ergotamine, 310–11
Ermorelin, 638
Errors in trials, 49–50, 54
Ertapenem, 195
Erysipelas, 209
Erythema multiforme, 283
Erythema nodosum, 283
Erythrocyte cycle of malaria, 240
Erythromycin, 199–200
Erythropoietin, 148, 537–8
Escherichia coli, 181
intestinal infection, 215
meningitis, 214
Esmolol, 451
Essential drugs, 21–2
Essential tremor, 386
Ester compounds, 324, 326
Estradiol, 644, 645
Estriol, 645
Estrone, 644
Estropipate, 645

Etanercept, 267–8
Ethacrynic acid, 481
Ethambutol, 222
Ethanol (alcohol), 78, 480
    abuse of, 148–57
        alcohol dependence syndrome, 154–6
        car driving and, 152–4
        chronic consumption, 152
        effects of, 151–2
        and other drugs, 157
        pharmacodynamics, 150–1
        pharmacokinetics, 149–50
        pregnancy/fetus/lactation, 156–7
        safe limits for chronic consumption,
            155–6
        treatment of dependence, 154–5
        withdrawal, 154
    acute poisoning, 152
    as an antidote, 132, 137
    and antihypertensives, 444
    kinetics, 84–5
    miscellaneous uses of, 157
    poisoning, 136
Etherified starch, 413
Ethics
    animal studies, 37–8
    of research in humans, 42–3
Ethinylestradiol, 645
Ethionamide, 223
Ethosuximide, 380
    plasma half-life of, 87
Ethylene glycol poisoning, 137
Etidronate, 665
Etomidate, 319
Etonorgestrel, 654
EU Clinical Trial Directive
    2001/20/EC, 63
European Medicines Agency
    (EMA), 63
Evidence, strength of, 59
Exanthematic reactions, 283
Excretion of drugs
    biliary, 99
    delayed for prolongation of drug
        action, 102
Execution, drugs used for judicial,
    140–1
Exenatide, 616
Exercise
    asthma induced by, 502
    incapacity for vigorous, 431
Exfoliative dermatitis, 603
Exfoliative erythroderma, 283
Exocrine glands, 392
    effect of atropine on, 399
Exophthalmos of hyperthyroidism, 634
Expectorants, 497
Experimental studies, 117
Experimental therapeutics, 41–5
Explanatory trials, 47
Exponential processes See First-order
    processes
Extradural anaesthesia, 325
Extrapyramidal symptoms, antipsychotics,
    345, 347
Eye(s)
    cholinoceptors, 392
    corneal deposits of chloroquine, 243
    disease, corticosteroids for, 604
    effects of antipsychotics on, 347
    effects of atropine on, 399
    effects of corticosteroids on, 599
    effects of prolonged drug administration,
        125
    infections, 219
Ezetimibe, 471, 475

F

Facilitated diffusion, 84
Factor II, 518
Factor VII, 513, 518
Factor VIII, 515, 516
Factor IX, 513, 516, 518
Factor X, 513, 518
Factor Xa, 520
Factorial designs, 52–3
Faeces
    bulking agents, 572
    elimination, 99
    softeners, 573
Falciparum malaria, 241
Famciclovir, 227
Familial combined hyperlipidaemia
    (FCHL), 470
Familial hypercholesterolaemia, 470
Familial hypertriglyceridaemia (FHTG), 470
Familial hypoalphalipoproteinaemia
    (FHA), 470
Famotidine, 563
Fat deposition, 595
Fatigue, 463
Febrile convulsions, 375
Feedback systems, 103
FEIBA, 516
Felypressin, 324, 641
Females
    adverse drug reactions in, 120
    androgen insufficiency, 643
    hirsutism, 285
    infertility, 649
    and smoking, 161
Fenamic acid, 258
Fenoprofen, 79
Fentanyl, 302
Fenticonazole, 236
Ferritin, 529, 530
Ferroportin, 529–30
Ferrous fumarate, 531–2
Ferrous gluconate, 531–2
Ferrous succinate, 531–2
Ferrous sulphate, 531–2
Fertilisation prevention, 650
Fertility
    after taking combined contraceptives, 651
    regulation, 649–55
    See also Contraception; Reproduction,
        toxic effects on
Fetal alcohol syndrome, 156–7
Fetus, drugs affecting, 126–7
    alcohol, 156–7
    smoking/nicotine, 161
Fever
    in chemotherapy patients, 545
    drug allergy, 124
Fibrates, 471, 474–5
    interactions with antidiabetes drugs, 621
Fibre, dietary, 572
    and diabetes, 618
Fibric acid derivatives See Fibrates
Fibrin, 520, 522–3, 525
Fibrin glue, 516–17
Fibrinogen, 516–17, 525
Fibrinolysis, 522–4
    drugs that prevent, 524
    drugs that promote, 523–4
Filtration, 83
Finasteride, 492, 644
First-order processes, 84
First pass elimination, 90–1
Fixed dose, 100
    combination products, 46, 103
Fixed eruptions, 283

Fixed sample size trials, 54
Flavoxate, 401, 491
Flecainide, 451, 452–3
Flucloxacillin, 191
Fluconazole, 236–7
Flucytosine, 238
Fludrocortisone, 597
    potency, 597
Fluid treatment
    of diabetic ketoacidosis, 622
    of diarrhoea, 575
Flukes, 248
Flumazenil, 132, 363
Flunitrazepam, 172
Fluoroquinolones See Quinolones
5-Fluorouracil (5FU), 546–7
Fluoxetine, 336, 657
Flutamide, 545, 644
Fluticasone, 597
Fluvastatin, 474
Folic acid/folate, 263, 535–7
    antagonists, 287
    contraindications, 537
    deficiency, 532–3, 536
    functions, 536
    indications, 536–7
    occurrence and requirements, 536
    preparations and dosage, 537
Folinic acid, 132, 536
    rescue, 546
Follicle stimulating hormone (FSH), 639
Fomivirsen, 232
Fondaparinux, 520
Food
    drug-food interactions, 112
    effect on drugs, 111–12
    and monoamine oxidase inhibitors
        (MAOIs), 339–40
Food and Drug Administration (FDA), 63
Formaldehyde, 137
Formestane, 605
Formic acid, 78
Formularies, 21–2
Foscarnet, 232
Fosphenytoin, 378
Foxglove, 15
Framycetin, 198
Fraudulent medicines, 67
Fresh frozen plasma (FFP), 515–16
Friedlander's pneumonia, 211
Fuller's earth, 131
Fungal infections, 233–8
    drugs of choice for, 234
    endocarditis, 213
    skin, 289–90
    superficial, 233–4
    systemic, 234–5
Fungating tumours, 309
Furosemide, 79, 480, 481, 486
    for ascites, 587
Fusariosis, 234
Fusidic acid, 584

G

$GABA_A$-benzodiazepine receptor complex,
    361, 364
Gabapentin, 295, 307, 380
Galactorrhoea, 347
Galantamine, 367
Gallstones, 589, 647
γ-Aminobutyric acid (GABA), 77, 295
γ-Hydroxybutyrate (GHB), 157
Gamolenic acid, 657
Ganciclovir, 232
Ganirelix, 639

Gases, anaesthesia, 315–16
Gas gangrene, 223
Gastric acid
  aspiration, 604
  drug destruction by, 90
  inhibition and neutralisation of, 561–2
  secretion, 561
  suppression in GORD, 567
Gastric lavage, 130
Gastric mucosa
  alcohol-related injury, 151
  enhancing resistance of, 564–6
  mechanism of toxicity, 566
Gastrin, 561
Gastrointestinal tract
  candidiasis, 234
  drugs and breast feeding, 100
  drugs for and anticoagulants, 519
  effects of corticosteroids on, 599
  effects of histamine on, 499
  effects of NSAIDs, 256–7
  effects of opioids on, 299
  effects of toxic plants, 139
  flora, 113, 215
  interactions in the, 113
  motility, 113
  poisons from the, 130–1
  symptoms in dying patients, 308
Gastro-oesophageal reflux disease (GORD),
    567
Gelatin products, 413
Gels, 276
Gemeprost, 253, 658
General anaesthesia See Anaesthesia, general
Generalised anxiety disorder, 352–3, 355–6
Generalised convulsive status epilepticus,
    375–6
Generic substitution, 19
Gene therapy, 35
Genetic medicines, 35
Genetic polymorphism, 106
Genital herpes, 226
Genital tract infections, 217–18
Genital warts, 226
Genotoxicity, 36–7
Gentamicin, 197, 489
Germ cells, 546
Germ theory, 6
Gestation prolongation, NSAIDs, 256
Gestrinone, 649, 656
Giant cell arteritis (GCA), 272–3
Giardiasis, 246
Ginseng, 15, 171
Glibeclamide, 616
Gliclazide, 616, 617
Glimepiride, 617
Glomerular damage, 488
Glomerular filtration, 99
Glucagon, 132, 614
  β-adrenoceptor blocker overdose, 432
Glucagon-like peptide-1 (GLP-1), 616
Glucocorticoids, 594
  for asthma, 503
  and diabetes, 620
  inhaled, 506
Glucose
  actions of insulin, 609
  decreased tolerance due to combined
    contraceptives, 651
  in diabetic ketoacidosis, 622
  hormones that increased blood, 614–15
  sodium absorption, 574
  tolerance, effect of alcohol on, 151
Glucose-6-phosphate dehydrogenase
    (G6PD) deficiency, 107, 244
Glue sniffing, 138, 171–2

Glutamate, 294–5
Glutathione, 97, 259
Glycerol, 573
Glyceryl trinitrate, 417–18, 586
Glycoprotein Ib, 525
Glycoprotein IIb/IIIa receptor, 438, 525
  antagonists, 526–7
Glycopyrronium, 401
Goitre, 632
Gold, 266
Gold, Harry, 4
Gonadorelin, 639
Gonadotrophin releasing hormone (GnRH),
    639, 657
Gonorrhoea, 217
Good Laboratory Practice (GLP), 36
Goserelin, 545
Gout, 271–2
  corticosteroids for, 604
G-protein-coupled receptor systems, 76
Gramicidin, 206
Gram-negative organisms, antibiotic choice,
    184–6
Gram-positive organisms, antibiotic choice,
    184–5
Grand mal seizures, 377
Granulocyte colony-stimulating factors
    (G-CSF), 538
Granulocytopenia, 123
Granuloma inguinale, 218
Greeks in history, 6
Grey baby syndrome, 201
Griseofulvin, 238
Growth hormone, 639
  effect on blood glucose, 615
  in sportsmen, 147–8
Growth hormone releasing hormone
    (GHRH), 638
Guidelines, 21–2
Gut cholinoceptors, 392

H

Haem, 120
Haemochromatosis, 533
Haemodialysis, 134
Haemofiltration, 134
Haemoglobin, 529
Haemolysis, 124, 125
Haemoperfusion, 134
Haemophilia, 516, 641
Haemophilus influenzae meningitis, 214
Haemopoietic growth factors, 537–8
Haemosiderin, 529, 530
Haemostasis, drugs and, 513–28
Hahnemann, Samuel, 16
Hair invasion, dermatophyte, 290
Hair loss, 283, 285, 545
Hallucinogens, 162–7
  cannabis See Cannabis
  experiences with, 162–3
  lysergide (LSD), 163–4
  management of adverse reactions to,
    166–7
  toxic plants, 139
Halofantrine, 240, 243–4
Halogenated anaesthetics, 316–17
Haloperidol, 346
Halothane, 316, 317
Harassing agents, 139–40
Hard drugs, 143
Harvey, William, 6
Hashimoto's thyroiditis, 636
Hashish See Cannabis
Hay fever, 501
  corticosteroids for, 604

Headache
  analgesic-associated chronic daily, 310
  migraine See Migraine headache
Heart
  block, 459
  cholinoceptors, 392
  disease, heparin in, 522
  failure, 456
  rate, intrinsic, 427–8
  tissue types, 448–9
  See also Cardiac
Heartburn, 567
Heart failure, 462–8
  ACE inhibitors in, 421, 422
  β-adrenoceptor blockers, 430–1, 431
  chronic, 465–7
  classification of drugs, 464–5
  congestive, 483
  definition of chronic, 462–3
  drug management of, 465–7
  natural history of chronic, 463
  objectives of treatment, 464
  physiology and pathophysiology, 462
  Starling curve and, 463
  surgery for, 467
Helicobacter pylori, 565–6
Helminthic infections, 247–9
Heparin, 83, 520–2
  action of, 108, 520
  adverse effects, 521
  monitoring, 521
  pharmacokinetics, 521
  reversal, 521
  surgery in patients receiving, 519–20
  use of, 521–2
Heparin-induced thrombocytopenia (HIT),
    521
Heparinoids, 522
Hepatitis, 588–9
  alcohol-induced, 152
  autoimmune active chronic, 588
  corticosteroids for, 604
  drug allergy, 124
  drugs of choice for, 226
Hepatocellular injury, 582
Hepatolenticular degeneration, 386
Hepatorenal syndrome, 587
Hepatotoxic effects of toxic plants, 139
Hepcidin, 529–30
Herbal medicine
  drug-herb interactions, 112
  for insomnia, 365
  regulation, 67
Herbal teas, 15
Herbicide poisoning, 138
Her2/neu (erbB2) cell surface receptor,
    552–3, 554
Heroin See Diamorphine
Herpes keratitis, 219, 226
Herpes simplex virus, 225–7
Herxheimer reaction, 218
Hexamethonium, 435
Hiccough, 309
High-altitude sickness, 487
High concentration oxygen therapy, 498
High-density lipoprotein (HDL), 469, 470–1
Highly active antiretroviral therapy
    (HAART), 227
Hippocratic corpus, 6
Hirsutism, female, 285
Hirudin, 522
Histamine, 251, 499–501
  gastric acid secretion, 561
  for pruritus, 277
Histoplasmosis, 234
Historical controls, 53

History of clinical pharmacology, 6
HIV *See* Human immunodeficiency virus (HIV)
Homatropine, 401
Homeostasis, 103
Homoeopathy, 16–17
 regulation, 67
Hormone antagonists, 519
Hormone replacement therapy (HRT), 645–7
 adverse effects of, 646–7
 contraception, 646
 contraindications, 647
 preparations used for, 646
Hormones
 for acne, 288
 in breast milk, 100
 as cytotoxic drugs, 544–5
 influence on cancer, 550–1
 in liver disease, 583
 long-term use of, 126
 that increase blood glucose, 614–15
Horse chestnut, 15
Host influences on drug action, 108–12
H_1-receptor antagonists (antihistamines), 499–502
 actions, 500
 adverse effects, 500, 501
 for insomnia, 364
 urticaria, 288
H_2-receptor antagonists, 499–500
 in GORD, 567
 peptic ulcer, 562, 563
$5HT_3$-receptor antagonists, 568
Human chorionic gonadotrophin (HCG), 639
Human Genome Project, 32
Human immunodeficiency virus (HIV), 227–31
 drugs of choice for, 226
 entry inhibitor, 230–1
 general comments, 227–8
 non-nucleoside reverse transcriptase inhibitors, 230
 nucleoside reverse transcriptase inhibitors, 228–9
 protease inhibitors, 229–30
Human insulin, 609, 610
Human leucocyte antigen (HLA) molecules, 252
Humans, drug evaluation in, 41–60
 evidence strength, 59
 experimental therapeutics, 41–5
 meta-analysis, 54–5
 need for statistics, 48–50
 pharmacoepidemiology, 57–9
 rational introduction of a new drug to humans, 45–8
 results, implementation, 55–7
 types of therapeutic trials, 50–4
Humours, 6
Hyaluronidase, 103
Hydralazine, 424
 for heart failure, 464
Hydrocarbons, poisoning, 138
Hydrocortisone, 279, 593, 596
 action of, 594
 potency, 597
Hydrocyanic acid, 136
Hydrofluoroalkanes (HFAs), 505
Hydrogen ions, 82, 480
Hydrogen peroxide, 236
Hydrolysis, 97
Hydromorphone, 301
Hydrophilic drugs, 274
Hydroxycarbamide, 539
Hydroxychloroquine, 266

Hydroxycobalamin, 136, 535
Hydroxymethylglutaryl coenzyme A (HMGCoA) reductase, 474
5-Hydroxytryptamine (5HT), 336
Hyoscine, 401
Hyoscine butylbromide, 401
Hyperaldosteronism, 484
Hyperalgesia, 296
Hyperbaric oxygen, 136
Hypercalcaemia, 665–6
 corticosteroids for, 604
 diuretics in, 483
Hypercalciuria, 666
 diuretics in, 483
Hyperglycaemia, maternal, 620
Hyperhidrosis, 285
Hyperinsulinaemia, 609
Hyperkalaemia, 485, 487
Hyperlipidaemias, 469–76
 drugs used in treatment of, 474–6
 management, 471–3
 pathophysiology, 469
 secondary, 471
 sites of drug action, 471
Hyperosmolar diabetic coma, 622
Hyperplasminaemic bleeding state, 524
Hyperprolactinaemia, 640
Hypersomnia, 359, 365–6
Hypertension
 accelerated phase, 442–3
 ACE inhibitors in, 421
 alcohol-induced, 152
 β-adrenoceptor blockers, 430, 431
 diuretics in, 483
 drugs used in, 416–36
 drug treatment of, 439–44
 emergency treatment, 442–3
 hepatic portal, 430
 how drugs act, 415
 monitoring, 442
 and monoamine oxidase inhibitors (MAOIs), 339
 pregnancy, 443–4
 pulmonary, 445
 severe, 442
 treating, 441–2
Hyperthermia, 135
Hyperthyroidism, 629–34
 β-adrenoceptor blockers, 431
 exophthalmos of, 634
 subclinical, 634
Hypertrichosis, 283, 424
Hyperuricaemia, 485
 alcohol-induced, 151
Hypnogram, 357, 358
Hypoalbuminaemia, 95, 111
Hypocalcaemia, 665
Hypoglycaemia, 613–14
 alcohol-induced, 151
 β-adrenoceptor blockers, 431
 drug-induced, 617
 treatment of attack, 614
Hypoglycaemic drugs, 258
 See also Antidiabetes drugs
Hypokalaemia, 484, 535
Hypomania, 349
Hyponatraemia, 198, 485
 ACE inhibitor induced, 422
 emergency treatment of, 641–2
Hypo-oestrogenaemia, 645
Hypoparathyroidism, 664
Hypoperfusion, 411
Hypopituitarism, 640
Hypoproteinaemia, 490
Hyposensitisation, 501

Hypotension, 412
 β-adrenoceptor blockers, 431
 chronic orthostatic, 413–14
 due to opioids, 299
 poisoning, 135
 postural, 434
Hypothalamic hormones, 637–40
Hypothalamic-pituitary-adrenal axis, 333
Hypothalamic-pituitary system, 593
Hypothalamic-pituitary-thyroid axis, 333
Hypothesis of no difference, 48
Hypothyroidism, 628–9
 drugs that cause, 634–6
 subclinical, 628–9
 treatment of, 628–9
Hypovolaemia, 485
 in acute pancreatitis, 590
Hypoxia, 315–16

I

Iatrogenic disease, 12–13
Ichthammol, 282
Idiosyncrasy, 116, 124
Idoxuridine, 227
Imatinib, 553
Imidazoles, 233, 236
Imidazolines, 426
Imipenem, 195
Imiquimod, 233
Immobility from poisoning, 135
Immune inflammation, abrupt drug withdrawal, 104
Immune-mediated liver disease, 588
Immune system
 drugs that modulate the host, 233
 effect of corticosteroids on, 599
Immunisation
 for hepatitis B, 588–9
 during immunosuppressive therapy, 558
 in patients taking corticosteroids, 601
Immunocompromised patients, antituberculous therapy in, 220–1
Immunoglobulin E (IgE), 121
Immunoglobulin G (IgG), 553
Immunological memory, 250
Immunomodulator drugs, 262–8
Immunopharmacology, 35
Immunosuppression, 126, 556–8
 active immunisation during, 558
 antithyroid drugs, 630
 corticosteroids, 602
 in Crohn's disease, 579
 hazards of life, 557–8
 myasthenia gravis, 397
Immunotherapy, 545, 551–2
Impetigo, 285
Impotence, 128, 492–4
Inactive substances, 96
Incapacitating agents, 139–40
Indanediones, 515
Indapamide, 482
Individual variations in drug effects, 105–8
 opioids, 300
Indometacin, 256
Indoramin, 427
Infants
 drug response in, 108–9
 premature, 536
 See also Children
Infection(s)
 bacterial *See* Bacterial infections chemotherapy
 blood, 208–9
 bones, 218–19

chemotherapy of *See* Antimicrobials;
Chemotherapy of infections
ears, 209
eye, 219
fungal *See* Fungal infections
genital tract, 217–18
helminthic, 247–9
intestinal, 214–16
joints, 218–19
lung, 210–12
masking of, 184
mycobacterial, 219–24
opportunistic, 183–4, 228
paranasal sinuses, 209
protozoal, 238–47
skin, 289–90
throat, 209–10
urinary tract, 216–17
viral *See* Viral infections/viruses
See also specific infection
Infectious mononucleosis, 122
Infertility, 649
See also Reproduction, toxic effects on
Inflammation, 250–3
acute, 251
chronic, 251–2
corticosteroids, 278, 602
drugs for *See* Anti-inflammatory drugs
effect of corticosteroids on, 595
pharmacological manipulation of
inflammatory mediators, 253–68
Inflammatory bowel disease, 576–9
Infliximab, 267
Influenza, 231–2
drugs of choice for, 226
pneumonia following, 211
Inhalation therapy
advantages and disadvantages, 92
anaesthetics, 315–18
for asthma, 505
Inherited influences on drug effects, 105–8,
120–1
Initial dose, 101
Injectable preparations, 102
See also Depot preparations
Innate immune response, 250, 252
Inorganic phosphate, 666
Inorganic salts, 573
Inosine monophosphate dehydrogenase,
264
Inosine pranobex, 233
Inositol, 349
Inositol nicotinate, 425
Insecticides, 121
Insect repellents, 282
Insomnia, 309, 359–65
drugs for, 361–5
precipitating factors for, 360
Insulin, 608–23
actions of, 609
adverse effects of, 613–14
allergy, 610
analogues, 609
biphasic, 611–12
choice of preparation, 611–12
in diabetic ketoacidosis, 621–2
differences between human and animal,
610
dose, 612–13
history, 608
inhaled, 611
intravenous, 611
NPH, 611
pharmacokinetics, 610
preparations of, 610
prescribing, 610–11

receptors, 609
resistance, 614–15
sources of, 609
uses, 609–10
Insulin-dependent diabetes mellitus
(IDDM) *See* Diabetes mellitus, type 1
Interaction, drug, 112–14
with amfetamines, 168
clinical importance of, 112
drug-drug, 112
drug-food, 112
drug-herb, 112
effect of chronic pharmacology on, 105
enzyme induction and, 98
with herbal medicine, 16
with nicotine, 161
pharmacological basis of, 112–14
studies, 46
tetracycline, 199
See also specific drug
Inter-ethnic variation in tolerance, 152
Interferon-α (INFα), 539, 545
for hepatitis B, 588
for hepatitis C, 589
Interferons, 233, 387
for cancer, 551
Interim analyses, 54
Interleukin (IL), 268
for cancer, 551
Interleukin 2 (IL2), 545
Intermittent claudication, 425
International Conferences on
Harmonisation (ICH), 63
International Covenant on Civil and
Political Rights, 42
International normalised ratio (INR),
259, 515
for thrombotic disorders, 519
Interrogation, drugs used for, 140–1
Intertrigo, 285
Intestine *See* Bowel
Intolerance, 116
of alcohol, 152
of NSAIDs, 257
Intracranial pressure, raised
anaesthesia and, 329
corticosteroids for, 604
Intramuscular injection
advantages and disadvantages, 92
antimicrobials, 179
in the young, 108
Intraocular pressure reduction, 487
Intrathecal administration
local anaesthesia, 325
of opioids, 300
Intrauterine devices, 655
Intravascular volume restoration, 413
Intravenous injection
advantages and disadvantages, 91–2
anaesthetics, 318–20, 325
antimicrobials, 179
decrease in plasma concentration after,
85–6
opioids, 300
Intrinsic heart rate, 427–8
Intrinsic sympathomimetic activity (ISA), 77
Inverse agonists, 77
Iodide, 629, 631–2
Iodine, 629, 631–3
Iodoquinol, 247
Ion channels, ligand-gated, 76
Ionic movements, cardiac cells, 449
Ionisation
drugs capable of, 81
drugs incapable of, 81–2
Ipratropium, 401

Iron, 529–34
interactions, 531
kinetics, 529–31
therapy, 531–4
chronic overload, 533–4
oral, 531–2
overdose/poisoning, 533
parenteral, 532–3
Irreversible inhibition, 78
Irritable bowel syndrome (IBS), 580
Ischaemic stroke, 524
Isoconazole, 236
Isoenzymes, 96
Isoflurane, 316–17
Isoniazid, 221
Isoprenaline, 132, 409
Isoprotenerol, 457
Isosorbide dinitrate, 418
Isosorbide mononitrate, 418
Isotretinoin, 288, 661
Ispaghula husk, 572
Itching *See* Pruritus
Itraconazole, 233, 237
Ivermectin, 247

J

Japanese Pharmaceutical Affairs Bureau, 63
Jarisch-Herxheimer reaction, 218
Jaundice, antipsychotic-induced, 347
Joint(s)
disease management, 268–73
infection of, 218–19
Judicial execution, drugs used for, 140–1
Justice, 43

K

Kaletra, 230
Kaolin, 576
Keratin, 238
Keratitis, herpes, 219, 226
Keratolytics, 281
for acne, 288
Ketamine, 164, 308, 319–20
Ketoacidosis, diabetic, 621–2
Ketoconazole, 236, 605
as an antiandrogen, 644
Ketosis, diabetic, 622
Ketotifen, 503
Khat, 171
Kidney(s), 478–80
adverse effects of NSAIDs, 257
clearance, 100
disease
anaesthesia in patients with, 328
dose adjustment for patients with, 490
drug-induced, 488–9, 617
prescribing in, 489–90
drugs and, 488–90
effects of prolonged drug administration,
125
effects of xanthines on, 170
elimination, 99
failure, chronic, effect on binding, 95
oedema, 484
stones, 490–1
tubular cells, 97
tubular diffusion, 99
tubular transport, 99
Klebsiella pneumoniae, 211

L

Labetalol, 427, 434
Labial herpes, 226

Labour
   augmentation of, 658–9
   corticosteroids for preterm, 604
   and diabetes, 620
   drugs given during, 127
Lactation
   alcohol and, 157
   antiepileptics, 374–5
   antiretroviral therapy, 228
   xanthines and, 171
Lactic acidosis, 617
Lactulose, 573
   in hepatic encephalopathy, 587
Laetrile, 555–6
Lambert-Eaton syndrome, 398
Lamifiban, 526
Lamivudine, 229
   for hepatitis B, 588
Lamotrigine, 379–80
Lanosterol 14-α-demethylase, 236
Lanreotide, 638
Larva migrans, 285
Lavoisier, Antoine, 6
Law of Mass Action, 84
Laxatives
   misuse of, 574
   osmotic, 572–3
   stimulant, 573
L-dopa See Levodopa
Lead poisoning, 137
Leaky epithelia, 81
Leflunomide, 264
Left ventricle
   failure, acute, 467
   outflow tract obstruction, 422
Legal hazards, 21
Legionnaires' disease, 212
Legislation in animal studies, 37–8
Leishmaniasis, 246
Lens opacities, antipsychotics, 347
Leprosy, 223
Leptin, 625
Leptospirosis, 224
Leucocytes, 121, 251
Leukaemia
   acute lymphatic, 603
   acute myelodysplastic, 539
   acute promyelocytic, 661
Leukocytes, 268
Leukotriene receptor antagonists, 504
Leuprolelin, 545
Levamisole, 247
Levetiracetam, 380
Levobupivacaine, 326
Levodopa, 78, 381–2, 385
Levofloxacin, 205
Levome promazine, 306
Levonorgestrel, 654, 655
Levothyroxine (T$_4$), 627–9
   for hypothyroidism, 628–9
Liability, no-fault, 12–13
Libido, effect of combined contraceptives on, 651
Lice, 286
Licence
   accelerated, 66
   application, 46
   granting of, 63
   post-licensing responsibilities, 64–5
   regulation, 61–2
   unlicensed indications, 66
   variations to, 65
Lichenoid eruption, 283
Lichen planus, 285
Lichen simplex, 285
Lidocaine, 325, 326, 451, 452
Ligand-gated ion channels, 76

Lily of the valley, 15
Linctus, 495
   definition of, 89
Linezolid, 202–3
Liothyronine (T$_3$), 627–9
Lipid-lowering drugs, 471–6
   and anticoagulants, 519
Lipid(s)
   disorders, 469–71
   solubility, 81–2
      reducing, 95
Lipid-soluble substances, 81
   β-adrenoceptor blockers, 429
   blood-brain barrier, 83
   gastrointestinal tract absorption, 89
   placenta, 83
Lipodystrophy, 614
Lipolysis, 609
Lipo-oxygenase, 251
Lipophilic drugs, 274
Lipoprotein, 152, 469, 652
   binding, 95
   plasma, 432
Lipoprotein lipase (LPL), 469
   efficiency, 470
Liquid formulations, topical, 275
Liquorice, 15
Liquorice derivatives, 565
Lisinopril, 423
Listeria monocytogenes meningitis, 214
Lisuride, 382–3
Lithium
   interaction with NSAIDs, 258
   neuromuscular transmission disorders, 398
Lithium carbonate, 336, 349–50
   indications for, 370
Liver
   ascites, 484
   blood flow, 582–3
   cells, 97
   clearance, 100
   cycle of malaria, 239–40
   drug absorption, 89
   effects of alcohol abuse on, 149–50
   effects of combined contraceptives on, 651
   effects of prolonged drug administration on, 125
   encephalopathy, 587–8
   metabolism, 582–3
      in pregnancy, 111
   portal hypertension, 430
Liver disease
   anaesthesia in patients with, 328
   cholestatic, 582
   chronic, effect on binding, 95
   drug-induced, 584–5, 617
   hepatic blood flow and metabolism, 582–3
   immune-mediated, 588
   parenchymal, 582
   pharmacodynamic changes in, 582
   pharmacokinetic changes in, 582
   plasma protein binding of drug, 583
   prescribing for patients with, 583
Loading dose, 101
Local anaesthesia See Anaesthesia, local
Long QT syndromes, 460
Long-term domiciliary oxygen therapy, 498
   chronic obstructive pulmonary disease
      (COPD), 509
Long term drug therapy See Chronic
      pharmacology
Loop diuretics, 480, 481
   for ascites, 586
   interactions, 486
   potassium depletion, 484
Loop of Henle, 478–80

Lopinavir, 230
Loratadine, 500
Losartan, 423
Lotions, 275
Low concentration oxygen therapy, 498
Low-density lipoprotein (LDL), 469, 470–1
Lower urinary tract infection, 216
Low molecular weight heparin (LMWH), 520
LSD (lysergide), 163–4
Lubricants, oil-based, 655
Lumefantrine, 240, 245–6
Lungs
   abscess, 212
   cancer, 160
   chronic disease of, 161
   drug elimination, 99–100
   effects of prolonged drug administration,
      125
   infection, 210–12
Lupus erythematosus, 283, 285
Luteinising hormone (LH), 639
Lyme disease, 224
Lymphocytes, 432
   inhibition of activation, 262–5
Lymphoid system diseases, 122
Lymphoid tissue, 596
Lymphoreticular system suppression, 543–5
Lysergide (LSD), 163–4
Lysine vasopressin, 586

M

MacKenzie skin blanching test, 278
Macrolides, 188, 199–201, 223
Macromolecules, 413
Macrophages, 251
Maculopapular reactions, 283
Magnesium deficiency, 485–6
Magnesium hydroxide, 562, 573
Magnesium oxide, 562
Magnesium sulphate, 131, 573
Main-stream smoke, 158
Maintenance dose, 101–2
Malabsorption syndromes, 535, 536
Malaria, 238–46
   chemoprophylaxis of, 242–3
   chemotherapy of acute, 240–2
   drug-resistant, 240
   life cycle of malaria parasite, 239–40
   sites of drug action, 239–40
Males
   contraception, 655
   infertility, 649
   reproductive function, drug effect on, 128
Malignant hyperthermia, 328
Malignant malaria, 241
Malnutrition, alcohol-induced, 152
Malpractice See Negligence
Mania, 342, 348–9
Mannitol, 486
Marijuana See Cannabis
Marketing Authorisation Holders (MAHs), 61
Masking creams, 277
Mastalgia, 657
Mast cells, 251
   stabilisers, 261–2
Maternal hyperglycaemia, 620
Maximum tolerated dose, 101
MDMA, 163–4
MDR1 transporter, 99
   drug interactions, 113
Mebendazole, 247
Mebeverine, 580
Mecillinam, 189, 192
Mecysteine, 496
Medical record linkage, adverse reactions, 59

Medicines Monitoring Unit (MEMO), 65
Medroxyprogesterone, 656
Medroxyprogesterone acetate, 545, 654
Mefloquine, 240, 244
Meglitinides, 616
Meglumine antimonate, 247
Melarsoprol, 247
Melatonin for insomnia, 365
Memantine, 368
Membranes, cell (humans), drug passage
    across, 81–4
Membrane stabilising activity, 450
Men See Males
Menadiol, 515
Menadione, 514
Meningeal tuberculosis, 220
Meningitis, 213–14
Meningococcal meningitis, 214
Menorrhagia, 656
Menotrophin, 639
Mensa, 267
Menstrual disorders, 656–7
Menstruation, 648
    and diabetes, 620
    effect of combined contraceptives on, 651
    timing of, 656
Mental disorders in dying patients, 309
Mental performance, effect of xanthines
    on, 169
Mepacrine, 247
Meperidine, 303, 327
Meptazinol, 303
Mercaptopurine, 264
MERIT-HF trial, 466–7
Meropenem, 195
Merozoites, 239, 240
Mesalamine, 265
Mesalazine, 577
Mescaline, 163
Mesterolone, 643
Meta-analysis, 54–5, 59
Metabolism, 95–8
    alcohol, 149–50
    altering biological activity, 96
    in disease, 111
    effects of antidepressants on, 339
    effects of chronic pharmacology on, 105
    effects of corticosteroids on, 594–5
    effects of histamine on, 499
    effects of nicotine on, 160
    in the elderly, 109
    interactions during, 113
    phase I, 96–7
    phase II, 97
    in pregnancy, 111
    process of, 96–7
    slowing for prolongation of drug action, 102
    in the young, 108–9
Meta-iodobenzylguanidine (MIBG), 434, 447
Metformin, 615, 616, 617, 619
Methadone, 299, 301–2
Methaemoglobinaemia, 662
Methanol, 78
    poisoning, 137
Methimazole, 629
Methionine, 132, 259
Methohexitone, 319
Methotrexate, 263–4, 546
    in Crohn's disease, 579
    increased dose effects, 585
    psoriasis, 287
    safety monitoring, 284
    staff hazards, 549
Methotrimeprazine, 306
Methylamfetamine, 168
Methylcellulose, 572

Methyldopa, 435–6
Methylene blue, 662
Methylenedioxymethamfetamine, 163–4
Methylphenidate, 366, 368
Methylprednisolone, 386–7, 596
    potency, 597
Methylxanthines See Xanthines
Meticillin, 191
Meticillin-resistant Staphylococcus aureus
    (MRSA), 181
Metirosine, 434–5, 447
Metoclopramide, 568–9
Metolazone, 482
Metriphonate, 247
Metronidazole, 205–6
    Crohn's disease, 578
    in hepatic encephalopathy, 588
    resistance, 566
Metyrapone, 605
Mexiletine, 451, 452
Miconazole, 236
Microscopic colitis, 579–80
Micturition, pharmacological aspects of, 491
Midazolam, 87
Midodrine, 414
Mifepristone, 648, 658
Migraine headache, 309–11
    management of, 310–11
    preventative treatment for, 311
Milrinone, 465
Mineralocorticoids, 594
Minimal risk, 9–10
Minimum tolerated dose, 101
Minocycline, 199, 240
Minoxidil, 423–4
Miosis, opioid-induced, 299
Mirena, 655
Mirtazapine, 338
Misoprostol, 253, 564–5, 658
Missed doses, clinical importance of, 26
Mistletoe, 15
Mitotic spindle inhibitors, 544
Mivacurium, 321
Mixture, definition of, 89
Moclobemide, 340
Modafinil, 365
Model List of Essential Medicines, 22
Modified-release (m/r) formulations, 89
Molecular medicine, 32
Molecular modelling, 34
Molluscum contagiosum, 226
Mometasone, 597
Monoamine hypothesis, 331–2
Monoamine oxidase inhibitors (MAOIs), 331
    adverse effects, 338
    and alcohol, 157
    interactions, 339–40
        with antidiabetes drugs, 621
        with levodopa, 382
    mechanism of action, 332
    overdose, 340
Monoamine oxidase (MAO) enzymes, 383
Monobactams, 188, 189, 192
Monoclonal antibodies, 553
Mononucleosis, infectious, 122
Montelukast, 253, 504
Mood stabilisers, 348–51
Moraxella catarrhalis, 211
Morbilliform rashes, 283
Morning after pill, 654
Morphine, 300
    tolerance, 80
Morphine-6 glucuronide (M6G), 300
Mortality in drug abuse, 146–7
Mosquitoes, anopheles, 239–40
Motility patterns, bowel, 575

Motion sickness, 569–70
Motor neurone disease, 387
Mountain sickness, 487
    corticosteroids for, 604
Mouth, dry, 308
Mouth ulcers, cytotoxic drug induced, 545
Moxifloxacin, 205
MRSA See Meticillin-resistant Staphylococcus
    aureus (MRSA)
Mucolytics, 496–7
    chronic obstructive pulmonary disease
    (COPD), 509
Mucormycosis, 234
Mucosal decongestants, 410–11
Mucus hypersecretion, 161
Müller procedure, 457
Multicentre trials, 53
Multiple drug resistance (MDR), 549
Multiple sclerosis (MS), 386–7
Mupirocin, 206
Muscarine, 392, 394
Muscarinic effects of plants, 139
Muscarinic syndromes, 135
Muscle diseases and anaesthesia, 328–9
Muscle relaxants, 320–3
    for irritable bowel syndrome, 580
Muscle spasm, involuntary, 386
Musculoskeletal system, effect of
    corticosteroids on, 599
Mutagenicity, 116
Mutagenic substances, 36
Myasthenia gravis, 396–8
    corticosteroids for, 604
    drug variations in, 111
Myasthenic crisis, 398
Mycobacterial infections, 219–24
Mycophenolate, 557
Mycophenolate mofetil, 264
Mycophenolic acid, 264
Mycoplasma spp., antibiotic choice, 186
Mycoses See Fungal infections
Myelosuppression, 543–5
Myocardial infarction
    ACE inhibitors in, 422
    β-adrenoceptor blockers, 430
    drug treatment of, 437–9
    drug variations in, 111
    secondary prevention, 438–9
Myocardium stimulation, 465
Myoclonic seizures, 377
Myometrium, 657–9
Myotonia, 386
Myotonic seizures, 377
Myxoedema, 628

N

Nabilone, 569
N-acetylcysteine (NAC), 259–60
N-acetyl-p-benzoquinoneimine (NABQ1),
    259
Naftidrofuryl, 425
Nail invasion, dermatophyte, 290
Nalbuphine, 303
Nalidixic acid, 204, 205
Naloxone, 132, 304
Naltrexone, 304
Names of drugs See Nomenclature
Nandrolone, 644
Nappy rash, 285
Narcolepsy, 365
Narrow-spectrum penicillins, 189,
    190–1
Nasal decongestants, 410–11
National Health Service (NHS),
    economics, 27

National Institute for Health and Clinical Excellence (NICE), economics, 27
Natriuresis, 586
Natural products, drug discovery, 35–6
Nausea
    cytotoxic drug-induced, 543
    due to opioids, 299
    in dying patients, 308
    postoperative, 314
    See also Vomiting
Nebivolol, 433
Nebulisers, 505
Nedocromil, 261
    for asthma, 503
Nefopam, 297
Negative reactors, 18
Negligence, 12–13, 21, 25
Negligible risk, 10
Neisseria meningitidis, 214
Nematodes, 247
Neoadjuvant cancer therapy, 541
Neomycin, 198
    in hepatic encephalopathy, 588
Neonates
    congenital heart defects, 253, 256
    drug response in, 108–9
    grey baby syndrome, 201
    iodine-containing antiseptics, 632
    menadiol, 515
    meningitis in, 214
    septicaemia, 208
Neoplastic disease *See* Cancer
Neostigmine, 395, 396–7
    as an antidote, 132
    antagonism, 322
Nephrogenic diabetes insipidus, 483
Nephrolithiasis, 490–1
Nephron, 479
Nephropathy, 124
Nephrotic syndrome, 604
Nephrotoxicity, aminoglycosides, 197
Nerve block, 324–5
Netilmicin, 198
Neural tube defect prevention, 536
Neuraminidase inhibitors, 231–2
Neurodermatitis, 285
Neuroleptic malignant syndrome, 348
Neuroleptics, 306
Neuromuscular blockade, 320–3
    aminoglycosides, 197
Neuromuscular junction, 392–3
Neuromuscular transmission disorders, 396–8
    drug-induced, 398
Neuropathic pain, 295, 306–8
Neuropsychiatric events due to mefloquine, 244
Neutropenia, 422
Neutrophils, 251
Nevirapine, 230
New York Heart Association (NYHA) classification of heart failure, 463
Niacin, 471, 476, 661–2
    increased dose effects, 585
Niclosamide, 247
Nicorandil, 424–5, 436
Nicotinamide, 662
Nicotinamide adenine dinucleotide (NAD), 661–2
Nicotinamide adenine dinucleotide phosphate (NADP), 662
Nicotine, 393–4
    pharmacology, 159–60, 392
    replacement, 162
    tobacco composition, 158
    See also Smoking

Nicotinic acid *See* Niacin
Nicotinic effects of toxic plants, 139
Niemann-Pick C1-like 1 (NCPC1L1) transporter, 475
Nifedipine, 419–20
Nifurtimox, 247
Night cramps, 425
Nightmares, 366
Night terrors, 366
Nimodipine, 420
Nitrates, 416–17
    action of, 436
    for heart failure, 464
    tolerance, 80
Nitric oxide, 416, 492
Nitrodilators, 416
Nitrofurantoin, 217
Nitrous oxide, 316
    and oxygen, 327
Nizatidine, 563
N-methyl-D-aspartate (NMDA) receptors, 295
Nociception, 294–5
N-of-1 trial, 53
Nomenclature, 69–72
    non-proprietary names, 69–70, 70–1
    proprietary names, 69–70, 71–2
Non-acidic NSAIDs, 258
Non-coronary thrombolysis, 524
Non-emulsifying ointment, 276
Non-gonococcal urethritis, 217
Non-inferiority, 51
Non-insulin-dependent diabetes mellitus (NIDDM) *See* Diabetes mellitus, type 2
Non-maleficence, 43
Non-nucleoside reverse transcriptase inhibitors, 230
Non-respiratory tuberculosis, 220
Non-starch polysaccharides (NSPs), 572
Non-ST elevation myocardial infarction (non-STEMI), 437
Non-steroidal anti-inflammatory drugs (NSAIDs), 251, 254–61
    adverse effects of, 256–7
    as analgesics, 296–7
    and anticoagulants, 519
    classes of, 258
    interactions, 257–8
        with azathioprine, 264
        with β-adrenoceptor blockers, 433
    for menorrhagia, 656
    mode of action, 254–5
    pharmacokinetics, 255
    and the stomach, 566–7
    topical, 261, 277
    uses, 255–6
Noradrenaline, 69, 403
    deficiency, 331–2
    depletion of, 434
    effects of, 409
    for shock, 412
Norepinephrine *See* Noradrenaline
Norethisterone, 656
Norethisterone enantate, 654
Norfloxacin, 205
Novel compounds, 331
    adverse effects, 338
NPH insulin, 611
Nuclear receptors, 76
Nucleic acid, 35
    inhibition of synthesis, 188–9, 203–6
    metabolism, 177
    See also DNA; RNA
Nucleoside analogues, 544
Nucleoside reverse transcriptase inhibitors, 228–9
Null hypothesis, 48

Number needed to treat, 56
Nystatin, 236

O
Obesity, 624–5
Observational studies, 57–8, 59, 117
Observed minus expected values, 55
Obsessive-compulsive disorder, 352–3, 356
Obstetric analgesia and anaesthesia, 326–7
Obstructive lung disease, 161
Octreotide, 576, 586, 638
Oculomucocutaneous syndrome, 432
Odds ratio, 55
Oedema, 483, 484
Oestrogen-progestogen oral contraceptives (COCP), 650–3, 657
    See also Oral contraceptives
Oestrogen(s), 644–5
    for abnormal micturition, 491
    for acne, 288
    as an antiandrogen, 643–4
    in cancer, 550
    choice of, 645
    formulations, 645
    indications for, 645–7
    in menstrual disorders, 656–7
    for osteoporosis, 668
    pharmacotherapy, 647
    preparations of, 645
    route of administration, 645
    secretion, 593
Ofloxacin, 205
Oil-in-water creams, 275
Ointments, 276
Olanzapine, 346
Oligopeptides, 579
Omega–3 marine triglycerides, 476
Omeprazole, 563–4
Ondansetron, 569
Onychomycosis, 286
Open trials, 52
Opioids, 295, 297–306
    with actions on other systems, 303–4
    addiction, 304–5
    adverse effects of, 298
    agonist-antagonist mixed, 303
    agonist(s), 300–3
        partial, 302–3
    antagonist(s), 304
    choice of, 304
    classification of, 298, 304
    for coughs, 496
    dependence, 304–5
    interaction with monoamine oxidase inhibitors, 340
    in liver disease, 583
    mechanism of action, 298
    oral analgesic equivalents, 305
    pain in addicts of, 146
    pharmacokinetics, 299–300
    pharmacology of individual, 300–4
    poisoning, 136
    receptors, 298
    regional anaesthesia, 325
    relative potency of, 305
    systemic effects of, 298–300
    tolerance, 80, 304–5
    vomiting induced by, 570
Opportunistic infections, 183–4, 228
    cytotoxic drug-induced, 545
Opportunity cost, 27
Oral adsorbents, 130–1
Oral contraceptives, 650–5
    adverse effects, 652
    and anaesthesia, 328

combined contraceptive, 650–3
common problems, 653
and diabetes, 620
effect on blood glucose, 615
and epilepsy, 375
increased dose effects, 585
Oral rehydration salts (ORSs), 575
Oral rehydration therapy (ORT), 575
Oral route of administration
antimicrobials, 179
opioids, 300
See also Buccal administration/absorption;
Inhalation therapy; Sublingual
administration; Swallowing
medication
Order of reaction, 84–5
Organophosphate, 395, 396
Organophosphorus pesticides, 138
Organ transplant rejection, 604
Orlistat, 476, 624–5
Orphan drugs/diseases, 39
Orthostatic hypotension, chronic, 413–14
Oseltamivir, 231–2
Osmosis, 76
Osmotic diuretics, 478, 481, 486
Osmotic laxatives, 572–3
Osteoarthritis, 268–9
Osteomalacia, 669
Osteomyelitis, 218
Osteoporosis, 664, 667–8
antipsychotic-induced, 347
and heparin, 521
Osteoprotection, 269–70
OTC See Over-the-counter (OTC)
medicines
Otitis media, 209
Ototoxicity, aminoglycosides, 197
Over-compliance, 24
Overdose See Poisoning and overdose
Over-the-counter (OTC) medicines, 28
Overton-Meyer hypothesis, 315
Overweight, 624–5
Ovulation inhibition, 650
Ovulatory ovarian cycles, 656
Oxacillin, 191
Oxcarbazepine, 376
Oxidation, 96–7
Oxpentifylline, 425
Oxybutynin, 401, 491
Oxycodone, 301
Oxygen, 498
in acute severe asthma, 507
in anaesthesia, 317–18
as an antidote, 132
Oxytocics, 657–8
Oxytocin, 657–8, 659

P

P450 enzymes See Cytochrome P450 enzymes
Pacemaker cells, 455
Paget's disease of bone, 669
Pain, 293–311
acute, 295
bone, 308
cancer-related, 295
chronic, 295
classification of clinical, 295
definition of, 293–4
evaluation of, 295–6
neuropathic, 295, 306–8
nociception, 294–5
in opioid addicts, 146
relief of, 305–6
relief See Analgesia
Palivizumab, 232–3

Palliative care, 308–9
cancer, 542
Pamidronate, 308, 665
p-aminobenzoic acid (PABA), 203
Pancreas, 589–90
drugs and the, 590
Pancreatin, 589
Pancreatitis, acute, 589–90
Pancuronium, 322
Panic disorder, 351–4
Papaveretum, 302
Papaverine, 425, 493
Papillomavirus, 226
Para-amino phenol, 258
Paracelsus, 32
Paracentesis, abdominal, 587
Paracetamol, 258–60
adverse effects, 259
as an analgesic, 297
dose, 259
increased dose effects, 585
mode of action, 258–9
overdose, 259–60
pharmacokinetics, 259
plasma half-life of, 87
Paracoccidioidomycosis, 234
Paraesthesia, 296
Parallel group designs, 52
Paranasal sinuses infection, 209
Paraquat, 138
Parasitic infections
skin, 290
See also specific parasite
Parasomnias, 359, 366
Parasympathetic nervous system, 392
Parasympathomimetics, 491
Parathyroid hormone (PTH), 666, 668
Parenteral administration
advantages and disadvantages of, 91–3
antimicrobials, 179
Parkinsonism/Parkinson's disease, 345,
380–6
drug-induced, 385–6
drugs for, 381–4
objectives of therapy, 381
on-off phenomenon, 104, 380, 385
pathophysiology, 380–1
treatment of, 384–6
Paromomycin, 247
Paroxysmal supraventricular tachycardia, 458
Partial agonists, 77
Passive diffusion, 81–2
Pastes, 276
Patch skin testing, 124
Patents ductus arteriosus, 256
Patient-controlled analgesia (PCA), 300
Patient information leaflets (PILs), 21, 24,
46, 64
Patient preference trials, 51
Patient selection, 33
Pediculosis, 286
Pegfilgrastim, 538
Pegvisomant, 639
Pelvic inflammatory disease, 217
Pemphigoid, 286
Pemphigus, 283, 286
corticosteroids in, 603
Penciclovir, 227
Penicillamine, 132, 133
neuromuscular transmission disorders,
398
Penicillin G See Benzylpenicillin
Penicillin(s), 188, 189–93
adverse effects, 189–90
airborne, 121
antipseudomonal, 189, 192–3

antistaphylococcal, 191
broad-spectrum, 189, 191–2
carbapenems, 188, 189
discovery of, 175–6
mecillinam, 189, 192
in milk, 121
mode of action, 189
monobactam, 188, 189, 192
narrow-spectrum, 189
pharmacokinetics, 189
Penicillin V See Phenoxymethylpenicillin
Pentaerythritol tetranitrate, 418
Pentamidine, 247
Pentazocine, 303
Peptic ulcer, 561–2
effect on drug action, 107
NSAID-induced
prevention of, 567
treatment of, 566
Percentages, 31
Performance
drug effect on, 119
enhancement of, 147–8
mental See Mental performance
Pergolide, 382
Periodic limb movements of sleep (PLMS),
366
Periodic paralysis, 487
Peripheral arterial occlusion, 522
Peripheral blood flow, 431
Peripheral sensitisation, 296
Peripheral sympathetic nerve terminal,
434–5
Peripheral vascular disease, 425–6
Peritoneal dialysis, 134
Peritonitis, 216
Pernicious anaemia, 534–5
Personal injury claims, 12–13
Pessary, definition of, 89
Pesticide poisoning, 138
Pethidine, 303, 327
Petit mal seizures, 377
P-glycoprotein (Pgp), 549
pH
drugs that ionise according to, 82
urine, 133–4, 488
Phaeochromocytoma, 435, 445–7
β-adrenoceptor blockers, 431
Pharmacodynamics, 4, 75–80
alcohol abuse, 150–1
animal studies, 36
cannabis, 164–5
in disease, 111
drug interaction, 112
in the elderly, 110
nicotine, 159–60
qualitative aspects, 75–9
quantitative aspects, 79–80
in the young, 109
Pharmacoeconomics See Economics
Pharmacoepidemiology, 57–9, 117–19
Pharmacogenetics, 33, 105–8
Pharmacogenomics, 32, 46
Pharmacokinetics, 4, 45–6, 80–114
alcohol abuse, 149–50
amfetamines, 168
animal studies, 36
antimicrobials, 178
cannabis, 164
in disease, 111
drug interaction, 112
nicotine, 159
skin, 274–82
xanthines, 169
See also specific drug
Pharmacological efficacy, 79

Pharmacological testing, 39
Pharmacology history, 3
Pharmacopoeia, 62
Pharmacovigilance, 58–9, 117–19
Pharyngeal gonorrhoea, 217
Pharyngitis, 209–10
Phase 1/2/3/4 studies, 45, 47–8, 57–8, 65
Phenanthrene methanol, 240
Phencyclidine, 164
    increased dose effects, 585
Phenoxybenzamine, 132, 427, 446
Phenoxy herbicides, 138
Phenoxymethylpenicillin, 191
Phentolamine, 132, 427, 446
Phenylephrine, 410
Phenylpropanolamine, 410
Phenytoin, 85
    for epilepsy, 378
    neuromuscular transmission disorders, 398
    for neuropathic pain, 307
Phobia, simple, 352–3, 356
Phocomelia, 62
Pholcodine, 496
Phosphate, 666
Phosphodiesterase (PDE) inhibitors, 417
    in asthma, 503
Phosphodiesterase type 5 (PDE5), 493
Phosphodiesterase type 6 (PDE6), 493
Phospholipase A_2, 251
Phospholipids, 525
Photoallergy, 281
Photosensitivity, 280–1, 283
    drug, 280–1
Phototoxicity, 281
pH partition hypothesis, 82
Physical (physiological) drug dependence, 145
Physician-induced disease, 12–13
Physiological antagonism, 77–8
Physostigmine, 394
Phytomenadione, 132, 515
Pigmentation, 283
Pilocarpine, 394
Pindolol, 414
Pioglitazone, 615, 617
Piperacillin, 193
Piperazine, 247
Piperine, 16
Piretanide, 481
Piroxicam, 87
Pituitary hormones
    anterior, 637–40
    posterior, 640–2
Pityriasis rosea, 286
Pityriasis versicolor, 289–90
Pivmecillinam, 192
Pizotifen, 311
Placebo controlled trials, 43–4
Placebo medicines, 17–18
Placebo-reactors, 18
Placenta, drug passage through, 83
Plants
    alkaloids, 547
    poisoning, 138–9
Plasma
    analysis for poisoning, 130
    half-life ($t_{1/2}$), 85–7
        biological effect, 87
    protein, 94–5
Plasmin, 522
Plasminogen activator inhibitors, 523
Plasminogen activators, 522–3, 523–4
Plasmodium spp., 240, 241
Platelet-activating factor (PAF), 251, 253
Platelet function, 525–8

Platinum drugs, 544, 547
Plural infection, 210–12
Pneumococcal meningitis, 214
Pneumocystosis, 235
Pneumonia, 210–12
    community acquired, 210
    due to anaerobic microorganisms, 211
    hospital acquired, 210
    in immunocompromised patients, 210–11
    legionnaires' disease, 211
    in people with chronic lung disease, 210
Poisoning and overdose, 129–41
    acceleration of elimination of poison, 133–4
    amfetamines, 168
    anticholinesterase drugs, 395–6
    antidotes, 131, 132
    aspirin, 261
    atropine, 400
    β-adrenoceptor blockers, 432
    biological agents and weapons, 139
    by biological substances, 138–9
    characteristic toxic syndromes, 135–6
    chelating agents, 131–3
    cocaine, 167–8
    digoxin, 456
    drugs used for torture, interrogation and judicial execution, 140–1
    general measures, 134–5
    by herbicides and pesticides, 138
    identification of poison(s), 129–30
    incapacitating agents, 139–40
    initial assessment and resuscitation, 134–5
    iron, 533
    mood stabilisers, 350
    by (non-drug) chemicals, 136–8
    paracetamol, 259–60
    prevention or further absorption, 130–1
    principles of health treatment, 129
    psychiatric and social assessment, 135
    self-poisoning, 129
    supportive treatment, 135
    sympathomimetics, 408
    theophylline, 504
    tricyclic antidepressants, 337
    xanthines, 169, 170–1
Polycystic ovary syndrome (PCOS), 649
Polycythaemia vera, 539–40
Polyene antibiotics, 235–6
Polyethylene glycol-electrolyte solution, 131
Polymerase chain reaction (PCR), 179
    drug discovery, 35
Polymorphisms, 97
    genetic, 106
    transporter, 108
Polymyxin B, 206
Polypeptide antibiotics, 206
POM *See* Prescription-only medicines (POM)
POM-OTC/POM-P switch, 28
Population statistics of adverse reactions, 59
Porcine insulin, 609, 610
Porphyrias, 120–1
Portal hypertension, 585
    β-adrenoceptor blockers, 430
Posaconazole, 237–8
Positron emission tomography (PET), 35
Postcoital contraception, 654
Postmenopausal hormone replacement therapy (HRT) *See* Hormone replacement therapy (HRT)
Postoperative nausea and vomiting (PONV), 314
Post-traumatic stress disorder, 352–3, 355
Postural hypotension, 434

Potassium
    depletion, diuretics, 484
    in diabetic ketoacidosis, 622
    in hypertension, 442
    sympathomimetics and plasma, 408
Potassium channel blockade, 454
Potassium citrate, 491
Potassium ferric hexacyanoferrate, 132
Potassium iodide, 631–2
Potassium ions, 480
Potassium-sparing diuretics, 480, 485
Potency, 79–80
Potentiation, 113, 180
Powders, inhaled, 92
Power curves, 49
Practolol, 62
Pragmatic trials, 47
Pralidoxime, 132, 396
Pramipexole, 383
Praziquantel, 247
Prazosin, 426–7
Pre-consent randomisation, 51
Prediction, 39
Prednisolone, 596
    acute severe asthma, 507
    for autoimmune active chronic hepatitis, 588
    oral, 506
    potency, 597
Pre-emptive suppressive therapy, 180–1
Pre-excitation syndrome, 459
Pregabalin, 307
Pregnancy, 648
    ACE inhibitors in, 422
    adverse effects in, 126–8
    and alcohol, 156–7
    antimalarial drugs and, 243
    antiretroviral therapy, 228
    benzodiazepines in, 363
    and β-adrenoceptor blockers, 433
    corticosteroids and, 599
    diabetes in, 620–1
    drug response in, 110–11
    effect of combined contraceptives on, 651
    and epilepsy, 374–5
    folate deficiency in, 532–3
    folic acid in, 536
    hypertension in, 443–4
    iron in, 531
    smoking in, 161
    tetracycline in, 198–9
    thionamides in, 630
    thyroid hormones in, 629
    tuberculosis treatment during, 220
    use of ketamine in, 320
    vomiting in, 570
    warfarin in, 518
Preload, 462, 464–5
Premature infants, folic acid in, 536
Premenstrual tension syndrome, 657
Pre-randomisation, 51
Prescription, 18–22, 29–30
    for drug dependence, 146
    inappropriate, 19
    non-presentation, 22
    public view of, 10–11
    repeat, 20
    rules for the elderly, 110
    underprescribing, 20
Prescription event monitoring (PEM), 57–8, 65
    of adverse reactions, 59
Prescription-only medicines (POM), 28
Pressurised aerosols, 505
Presynaptic inhibition, 294

Presystemic elimination, 90–1
Prevention, drugs for See Prophylaxis
Prilocaine, 325
Primaquine, 239, 240, 244
Primary biliary cirrhosis (PBC), 588
Priming dose, 101
Proarrhythmic drug effects, 457
Probenecid, 113
Procaine penicillin, 191
Procoagulant drugs, 514–17
Proctitis, 604
Product Licence of Right (PLR), 67
Progesterone, 550, 647–8
Progestogen-only contraception, 654
Progestogen(s), 647–8
    as an antiandrogen, 643–4
    in menstrual disorders, 656–7
    for osteoporosis, 668
Proguanil, 239, 240, 244–345
Pro-kinetic drugs, 567
Prolactin, 347, 640
Prolonged administration effects, 125–6
Promethazine, 501
Propafenone, 451, 453
Propantheline, 401, 491
Prophylaxis, 8
    angina, 436–7
    See also Chemoprophylaxis
Propionic acids, 258
Propiverine, 401
Propofol, 318
Proportions, 31
Propranolol, 132, 433, 451
    in liver disease, 583
Propylthiouracil (PTU), 629–30
Prostacyclin (PGI$_2$), 256, 525–6
Prostaglandins, 253, 255, 256, 658
    and antihypertensives, 444
Prostaglandin synthase inhibition, 657
Prostanoids, 296–7
Prostatic cancer, 551
Prostatitis, 216
Protamine, 132, 521
Protease inhibitors, 229–30, 554–5
Protein C, 517
Protein kinase receptors, 76
Protein S, 517
Protein(s)
    effect of oestrogen on, 652
    as medicines, 35
    metabolism, 594
    plasma, 94–5
    reduction of dietary, 587–8
    synthesis, 177
        inhibition, 188, 196–202
Proteins induced in vitamin K absence
        (PIVKAs), 515, 517
Prothionamide, 223
Prothrombin See Factor II
Proton pump inhibitors (PPIs), 561–2
    action of, 107
    in GORD, 567
    peptic ulcer, 563–4
Protozoal infections, 238–47
Proximal convoluted tubule, 478, 488–9
Pruritus, 277–8, 283
    in dying patients, 309
    in primary biliary cirrhosis, 588
Pruritus ani, 278
Prussian blue, 132
Prussic acid, 136
Pseudallescheriasis, 234
Pseudo-allergic reactions, 125
Pseudocholinesterase, 394
    deficiency
        anaesthesia and, 329

effect on drug action, 107
    plasma, 322
Pseudomonads, 183
Psilocybin, 163
Psoralens, 281
    See also PUVA
Psoriasis, 283, 284–7, 660, 664
Psoriatic arthritis, 271
Psychiatric disorders, 330–70
    classification of, 330–1
Psychodysleptics See Hallucinogens
Psychological drug dependence, 145
Psychosis, 106–7
Psychostimulants, 167–71
Psychotherapy, 330–1
Psychotic disorders, 330
Psychotropic drugs, 330–70
    and anaesthesia, 328
    diagnostic issues, 330
    and skilled tasks, 369
    See also specific class
Pteroylglutamic acid See Folic
        acid/folate
Pulmonary elimination, 99–100
Pulmonary emboli, 519
Pulmonary hypertension, 445
Pulmonary surfactant, 498
Pulmonary tuberculosis, 219–23
    principles of therapy, 219–20
Pure antagonists, 77
Purgatives, drastic, 573
Purine antagonists, 547
Purpura, 283
Pustular rash, 283
PUVA, 287
P value, 48–9, 54
Pyelonephritis, acute, 216
Pyoderma gangrenosum, 286
Pyrantel, 247
Pyrazinamide, 222
Pyridostigmine, 395
Pyridoxine, 657, 661
Pyrimethamine, 240, 245
    with dapsone, 245
    with sulfadoxine, 245
Pyrimidine antagonists, 546–7

Q
Quality, drug, 36
Quality-adjusted life-year (QALY), 27
Quality of life, 27
Quetiapine, 346
Quinacrine, 247
Quinapril, 423
Quinidine, 245, 450–2
Quinine, 239, 240, 245
Quinolones, 188, 204–5, 223
    interaction with NSAIDs, 257
Quinupristin-dalfopristin, 202

R
Rabbit antilymphocyte globulin (ALG), 540
Radioimmunotherapy, 553
Radio-iodine, 629, 632–3
Radio-isotope tests, 633
Radiophosphorus, 539–40
Raised intracranial pressure See Intracranial
        pressure, raised
RALES trial, 467
Raloxifene, 645, 668
Ramipril, 423
Randomisation in trials, 51
Randomised controlled trials (RCTs), 50, 59
    ethics, 43–4

Ranitidine, 563
Rapamycin, 553
Rapid eye movement (REM) sleep, 358
Rashes, drug allergy, 122, 282–4
Rationing, 26
Raynaud's phenomenon, 425, 426
Rebound phenomenon, 104
Reboxetine, 337
Receptors, 76–8
    binding, 77
    regulation of, 104
Reclassifications of drugs, 65
Recombinant activated protein C (APC)
        drotrecogin α, 412
Recombinant cytokines, 268
Recombinant factor VIIa, 516
Recombinant tissue plasminogen activator
        (rtPA), 437
Recommended International Non-
        proprietary Names (rINNs), 69
Recreational use of drugs See Abuse, drug
Rectal administration
    advantages and disadvantages of, 91
    in the young, 108
Reflectant sunscreens, 280
Refractoriness
    lengthening of, 450–2, 454
    minimal effect on, 452–3
    shortening of, 452
Regional anaesthesia, 324–5
Regret avoidance, 67
Regulations
    animal studies, 36
    introduction of new drugs to humans,
        45–6
    of medicines, official, 61–8
        basis for, 61–3
        complementary and alternative
            medicine (CAM), 67
        counterfeit drugs, 67
        current systems, 62–3
        discussion, 65–8
        the future, 68
        historical background, 62
        requirements, 63–5
Regulatory review, 63–4
Relative risk, 56–7
    hypertension, 439–40
Relenza See Zanamivir
REM behaviour disorder, 366
Remifentanil, 299, 302
Remnant removal disease (RRD), 470
Renal artery stenosis, 422
Renin, 420, 440
Renin-angiotensin-aldosterone system, 586
Renin-angiotensin system, 593
Repaglinide, 616, 617
Reproduction, toxic effects on, 126–8
    animal studies, 37
    cytotoxic drugs, 546
    of nicotine/smoking, 161
Research
    ethics, in humans, 42–3
    injury to subjects, 44
    involving human subjects, 42–5
    payment of subjects, 44–5
    See also Animal studies
Reserpine, 434
Resistance, drug
    antimicrobials, 179, 180, 181–3, 202–3
    cytotoxic drugs, 549
    tuberculosis, 220
Respiratory distress syndrome (RDS), 498
Respiratory failure, 498
Respiratory syncytial virus (RSV), 226,
        232–3

Respiratory system, 495–509
  anaesthesia in patients with diseases of, 328
  drug variations affecting, 111
  effects of opioids on, 298
  effects of propofol on, 318
  effects of thiopental on, 319
  effects of xanthines on, 169
  stimulants, 497–8
  symptoms in dying patients, 309
Restless legs syndrome (RLS), 366–7, 386
Resurgence, disease, 104
Resuscitation of poisoned patients, 134–5
Reteplase, 523
Retinal pigmentation, antipsychotics, 347
Retinoic acid See Vitamin A
Retinoids, 660
  aromatic, 284
Retinol See Vitamin A
Reverse transcriptase inhibitors, 341
  in HIV, 227
  See also Non-nucleoside reverse
    transcriptase inhibitors; Nucleoside
    reverse transcriptase inhibitors
Reversible inhibition, 78
Reye's syndrome, 261
Rhabdomyolysis, 135
Rheumatic fever, 604
Rheumatoid arthritis, 269–70
  corticosteroids for, 604
Rheumatoid disease, 262
Rhinitis, atrophic, 647
Riamet, 245–6
Ribavirin, 232
  for hepatitis C, 589
Rickets, 663, 664
Rickettsia spp., antibiotic choice, 186
Rifabutin, 222
Rifampicin, 221–2, 223, 584
Rifaximin, 222
Rimonabant, 625
Ringworm, 233
Risk(s)
  absolute, 56–7
  categories of, 9
  elements of, 9–10
  grades of, 10
  reduction of, 9
  relative, 56–7
  research subjects, 44
  of taking drugs, 7, 8–10
  unavoidable, 8–9
Risperidone, 346
Ritodrine, 659
Ritonavir, 230
Rituximab, 268, 545, 552
Rivastigmine, 367
RNA, genetic medicines, 35
Rocuronium, 321
Rodenticides, 138
Ropinirole, 383
Ropivacaine, 326
Rosacea, 286
Rosiglitazone, 615, 616, 617
Rosuvastatin, 474
Routes of administration See specific route
Rubefacients, 277

S

Safety
  animal studies, 38
  drug development, 46
  of drugs, 7
  monitoring, 284
  in self-medication, 28
  surveillance methods, 48

Salbutamol, 410
  acute severe asthma, 507
Salicylates, 621
Salicylic acid, 258
  ionisation, 82
Salicylism, 260
Saline solution, 665
Salmeterol, 410
Salmonella, 215
Sarcoidosis, 664
  corticosteroids for, 604
Sassafras, 15
Saturation kinetics See Zero-order
    processes
Scabies, 286
Scarlet fever, 209
Schistosomiasis, 248
Schizonts, 239, 240
Schizophrenia, 342
  symptoms of, 343
Scleroderma-like rashes, 283
Sclerosing agents, 517
Sclerotherapy, 585
Scurvy, 662
Seborrhoeic dermatitis, 286
Secondary effects, 116
Sedation
  anaesthesia, 314–15
  for coughs, 496
  in critical care units, 329
  effects of opioids, 298
  in psychotic illness, 347
Sedatives
  and anticoagulants, 519
  in breast milk, 100
  in liver disease, 583
  poisoning, 136
Seizures
  antipsychotic-induced, 347
  types of, 377
Selective decontamination of the gut,
    215–16
Selective delivery, 78
Selective distribution, 94
Selective 5-HT₁ agonists, 310–11
Selective oestrogen receptor modulators
    (SERMs), 645
  for osteoporosis, 668
Selective serotonin-reuptake inhibitors
    (SSRIs), 16, 62, 331
  adverse effects, 337–8
  interactions, 338–9
  mechanism of action, 332
  for neuropathic pain, 306
Selectivity, 32, 78–9
Selegiline, 368, 383–4
Self-medication, 28
Self-poisoning, 129
Self-regulating systems, interference with,
    103–4
Sengstaken tube, 585–6
Senna, 573
Septicaemia, 208–9
Septic arthritis, 218–19
Septic shock, 412
Sequential designs, 54
Serendipity, 36
Serotonin deficiency, 331–2
Serotonin syndrome, 338, 348
Serpin, 517
Serum sickness, 123, 283
Sesquiterpenes, 240
Sevoflurane, 316, 317
Sex, effect on adverse drug reaction, 120
Sex hormones, 642
  and anticoagulants, 519

Sexual dysfunction
  antipsychotic-induced, 347
  See also Erectile dysfunction
Sexual forms of malaria, 240
Sexual function
  alcohol effects on, 151
  and cardiovascular drugs, 444–5
  and the cardiovascular system, 445
  effect of β-adrenoceptor blockers on, 432
Shigella, 215
Shingles, 226
Shock, 411–13
  anaphylactic See Anaphylactic shock
  choice of drug in, 412
  definition of, 411
  monitoring drug use in, 412–13
  in poisoning, 134
  septic, 412
  treatment, 411
  types of, 411–12
Sibutramine, 333, 625
Sickle cell disease, 329, 538–9
Side-effects definition, 115
  See also Adverse drug reactions
Siderosis, transfusion, 533
Side-stream smoke, 158
Signal transduction, 33
  inhibitors, 553
Significance tests, 48–9
Sildenafil, 444, 493
Silicone sprays, 277
Silver sulfadiazine, 203
Simvastatin, 474
Sinoatrial (SA) node, 448–9
Sinus bradycardia, 458
Sinusitis, 209
Sirolimus, 262, 265
Skeletal muscle, effects of xanthines
    on, 169
Skilled tasks and drugs, 119
  cannabinoids, 165
  psychotropic drugs, 369
Skin
  allergy testing, 124
  cutaneous drug reactions, 282–4
  disease, corticosteroids for, 604
  disinfection and cleansing of the, 290
  disorders, 284–90
  drugs and the, 274–90
  effects of antipsychotics on, 347
  effects of histamine on, 499
  effects of toxic plants, 139
  infections, 289–90
  pharmacokinetics, 274–82
  See also Topical application of medication
Skin prick tests, 124
Sleep
  disorders, 357–67
Sleep
  disorders
    normal sleep, 357–8
    types of, 359
  effects of xanthines on, 169
  hygiene programme, 359
  scheduling disorders, 367
Sleep-related breathing disorders, 365
Sleep-walking, 366
Small intestine, absorption, 88–9
Smoking, 157–62
  anaesthesia and, 328
  coughs, 495
  and Crohn's disease, 579
  effects of, 159–60
    chronic, 160–1
  nicotine pharmacology, 159–60
  starting and stopping use, 161–2

tobacco composition, 158
tobacco dependence, 158–9
and ulcerative colitis, 578
and women, 161
Smooth muscle
  effects of atropine on, 399
  effects of histamine on, 499
  effects of xanthines on, 170
Social anxiety disorder, 352–3, 354
Social aspects of drug abuse, 142–4
Social habits, effect on adverse drug
    reactions, 121
Sodium
  absorption, 574
  in antacids, 562
  dietary, 484
Sodium aurothiomalate, 266
Sodium bicarbonate, 134, 137, 562
Sodium calciumedetate, 132, 133, 137
Sodium cellulose phosphate, 491, 666
Sodium channel blockers, 450–3
Sodium cromoglicate, 503
Sodium fusidate, 201–2
Sodium ions, 480
Sodium nitrite, 136
Sodium nitroprusside, 424, 446
Sodium-phase resin, 487
Sodium picosulphate, 573
Sodium stibogluconate, 247
Sodium thiosulphate, 136
Sodium valproate, 307, 351, 378–9
Soft drugs, 143
Solid preparations, topical, 276
Solubility
  lipid, 81–2
  water, 81–2
Solvent abuse, 138, 171–2
Somatostatin, 586, 638
Somatotrophin, 638–9
Somatrem, 638
Sotalol, 451
Spasticity, 386
Special risk groups, prescribing for, 105
Specificity of antimicrobials, 178
Spectinomycin, 198
Spermatogenesis, 128
  inhibition, 650
Spermicides, 650
Spina bifida prevention, 536
Spinal anaesthesia, 325, 327
Spinal cord injury, 604
Spindle poisons, 547
Spirochaetes, antibiotic choice, 186
Spironolactone, 597
  aldosterone antagonism, 606
  as an antiandrogen, 644
  for ascites, 586–7
  as a diuretic, 480, 481, 482–3
  in heart failure, 465
Splenectomy patients, septicaemia risk,
    208–9
Spondyloarthritis, 271
Sporotrichosis, 234
Sporozoites, 239
Sport, drugs and, 147–8
Stagnant loop syndrome, 535
Standardisation, biological, 80
Staphylococci
  endocarditis, 213
  methicillin-resistant, 181
  penicillins, 191
  septicaemia, 208
Starling curve, 463
Statins, 471, 474
Statistical significance test, 48–9
Statistics, need for, 48–50

Status asthmaticus, 507–8
Status epilepticus, 375–6
Stavudine, 229
Steam inhalation, 496
ST elevation myocardial infarction (STEMI),
    437
Stereoselectivity, 78–9
Steroid hormone receptors, 642
Steroids
  adrenal See Corticosteroids
  anabolic See Anabolic steroids
  sex See Sex hormones
Stevens-Johnson syndrome, 283
Sthenia, 6
Stimulant laxatives, 573
Stimulants, abuse of, 148
St John's wort, 16, 340–1
Stomach
  absorption, 89
  acid See Gastric acid
  and NSAIDs, 566–7
Stones, renal, 490–1
Stools See Faeces
Streptococci
  in colorectal surgery, 181
  meningitis, 214
  throat infection, 209–10
  viridans group, 212
Streptokinase, 437, 523
Streptomycin, 196, 198
Stress disorder, acute, 355
Strontium ranelate, 668
Structural modification of drugs, 78
  for prolongation of drug action, 102
Subarachnoid block, 325
Subclinical hyperthyroidism, 634
Subclinical hypothyroidism, 628–9
Subcutaneous injection
  advantages and disadvantages, 92
  opioids, 300
  in the young, 108
Sublingual administration, 91
Substance abuse See Abuse, drug
Substance P, 295
Substitution, generic and therapeutic, 19
Succimer, 137
Succinimides, 380
Succinylcholine See Suxamethonium
Sucralfate, 564
Sucrose with iron, 532
Sulconazole, 236
Sulfadiazine, 203
Sulfadoxine, 240, 245
Sulfapyridine, 265, 577
Sulfasalazine
  adverse effects, 107
  as a disease-modifying antirheumatic drug
      (DMARD), 265–6
  interaction with azathioprine, 264
  nucleic acid synthesis inhibition, 203–4
  for ulcerative colitis, 577
Sulfinpyrazone, 272
Sulphonamides
  as an antidiabetes drug, 615
  interactions
    with antidiabetes drugs, 621
    with methotrexate, 264
  nucleic acid synthesis inhibition, 188,
      203–4
Sulphonamide-trimethoprim combination,
    203
Sulphonylureas, 615, 616–17, 619
Sulpiride, 346
Sumatriptan, 310
Summation, 113
Sunburn, 280–1

Sunscreens, 280–1
Superinfection, 183–4
Superiority, 51
Superstatins, 474
Suppositories
  advantages and disadvantages, 91
  for constipation, 573–4
  definition of, 89
  ulcerative colitis, 577–8
Suppression, drugs for, 8
Suramin, 247
Surface area, dose calculation by, 102
Surgery
  chemoprophylaxis in, 181
  in diabetic patients, 622–3
  effect of combined contraceptives, 651
  for hyperthyroidism, 633
  in patients receiving anticoagulants,
      519–20
  for patients taking corticosteroids, 600
Surrogate effect, 46–7
Surveillance systems, 58–9
Sustained-release preparations, 102
Sustanon, 643
Suxamethonium, 321, 322
  resistance to, 107
Swallowing medication, 91
Sympathetic nervous system, 392
  effects of antiarrhythmics, 457
Sympathomimetics
  adverse effects, 407–8
  and antihypertensives, 444
  classification of, 403–8
  effects of, 406–7
  history, 404–5
  interactions of, 404
  mode of action, 403–6
  overdose, 408
  and plasma potassium, 408
Sympathomimetic syndromes, 136
Syndrome of inappropriate secretion of
    antidiuretic hormone (SIADH), 483,
    641
Synergism, 113
Synergy, 180
Synthetic oxytocin, 657
Syphilis, 218
Syrup, definition of, 89
Systematic reviews, 55, 59
Systemic availability, 89–91
Systemic lupus erythematous, 272

T
Tablet, definition of, 89
Tacalcitol, 287
Tachyarrhythmias, 430
Tachycardia, 446, 461
  atrial with variable AV block, 459
  paroxysmal supraventricular, 458
  ventricular, 459
Tachyphylaxis, 76, 80, 404
  to LSD, 163
Tacrolimus, 556, 557
  interaction with NSAIDs, 258
Tamiflu, 231–2
Tamoxifen, 544, 550, 647
  action of, 107
  in sportsmen, 147–8
Tamsulosin, 492
Tapeworms, 247
Tardive dyskinesia, 345–7
Target difference, 50
Targeted biological cancer therapies, 552–5
Tar in tobacco, 158
Tars, 281–2

Taxanes, 544
Taxoids, 547
Tazorotene, 660
T cells, 252–3
Teeth discoloration, tetracycline, 198–9
Teicoplanin, 195–6
Telithromycin, 200–1
Temperature regulation, 347
Tenamfetamine, 163–4
Tenecteplase, 523
Tenofovir, 229
Teratogenicity, 116, 126–7, 127–8
    of antiepileptics, 375
    of corticosteroids, 599
    See also specific drug
Terbinafine, 233, 238
Terfenadine, 288, 500
Terlipressin, 586
Terminology, drug abuse, 143–4
Testosterone, 642–3
Testosterone undecanoate, 643
Tetanus, 387
Tetracosactride, 606
Tetracosactride Injection, 606
Tetracosactride test, 605, 606
Tetracosactride Zinc Injection, 606
Tetracyclines, 188, 198–9
    for malaria, 240
Tetrahydrocannabinol (THC), 164
Tetrahydrofolic acid (THF), 203, 536, 546
Thalidomide, 62, 223, 268, 551
Theobromine, 169–71
Theophylline, 169–71
    in asthma, 503–4
    chronic obstructive pulmonary disease
        (COPD), 509
Therapeutic drug monitoring, 87–8
Therapeutic effect, 46
Therapeutic efficacy, 79
Therapeutic evaluation, 4, 47–8
Therapeutic index, 79–80
Therapeutic investigations, 46–8
Therapeutics
    evolution of, 4–7
    experimental, 41–5
Therapeutic situation, 4–11
Therapeutic substitution, 19
Therapeutic trials See Trials
Thiacetazone, 223
Thiamine, 661
Thiazides, 480, 481–2, 486
    diuretics related to the, 482
    for hypertension, 416
    interactions with antidiabetes drugs, 621
    nephrolithiasis, 490
Thiazolidinediones, 615–16, 616, 617
Thiocyanate, 424
Thiomethylpurine transferase (TMPT),
    264
Thionamides, 629–30
    adverse reactions, 630
    mode of action, 629–30
    in pregnancy, 630
    use, 630
Thiopental, 318–19
Thioridazine, 346
Throat infection, 209–10
Thrombin, 514, 516–17, 517
Thrombin-activatable fibrinolysis inhibitor
    (TAFI), 523
Thrombocytopenia, 123, 524
    heparin-induced (HIT), 521
Thromboembolism, venous, 521–2
Thrombolysis, 437–8, 522–4, 523–4
Thrombolytic drugs, 523–4
Thrombopoietin (TPO), 538

Thrombosis, 519
    with heparin-induced thrombocytopenia,
        521
Thromboxane, 256, 525
Thromboxane A_2, 525–6
Thymectomy, 397
Thymidine kinase, 225
Thymoxamine, 427
Thyroglobulin, 627
Thyroid hormones, 627–9
    effect on blood glucose, 615
    for hypothyroidism, 628–9
    pharmacodynamics, 628
    pharmacokinetics, 627
    physiology, 627
    in pregnancy, 629
Thyroiditis, 633, 636
Thyroid-stimulating hormone (TSH), 628,
    637–8
Thyroid storm, 633–4
Thyrotoxicosis, 635
Thyrotrophin, 637–8
Thyrotrophin releasing hormone (TRH),
    637
Thyroxine See Levothyroxine (T_4)
Thyroxine binding globulin (TBG), 627
Tiabendazole, 249
Tibolone, 645
Ticarcillin, 193
Ticlopodine, 526
Tigecycline, 199
Tight epithelia, 81
Tinea, 233, 234, 286
Tinidazole, 206
Tioconazole, 233, 236
Tiotropium, 401
Tirofiban, 526
Tissue binding, 95
Tissue factor pathway inhibitor (TFPI),
    514
Tissue factor (TF), 513–14
Tissue-invading amoebiasis, 246
Tissue plasminogen activator (tPA), 522–3
Tobacco
    amblyopia, 535
    composition, 158
    dependence, 158–9
    See also Smoking
Tobramycin, 197
Tocopherol, 476, 669
Tolbutamide, 87
Tolerance, 80, 145
    of alcohol, 151
    cannabis, 166
    enzyme induction and, 98
    local, animal studies, 37
    nicotine, 160
    opioids, 305
    xanthines, 170
    See also Intolerance; Tachyphylaxis
Tonic-clonic seizures, 377, 487
Tonics, 18
Topical application of medication
    advantages and disadvantages, 92–3
    analgesics, 277
    antimicrobials, 179
    molecular size, 274
    NSAIDs, 261
    vehicles for, 275–6
    in the young, 108
Topiramate, 380
Topoisomerase I inhibitors, 544, 547
Torasemide, 481
Torture, drugs used for, 140–1
Total body clearance, 100
TOXBASE, 129

Toxic epidermal necrolysis (TENS), 283
Toxicity
    chronic organ, 125–6
    definition, 116
    enzyme induction and, 98
    mechanism of gastric mucosal, 566
        See also Adverse drug reactions; specific
            drug
Toxicology
    animal studies, 36
    testing, 39
    See also Adverse drug reactions
Toxic shock syndrome, 208
Toxic syndromes, 135–6, 208
Toxoplasmosis, 246
Traditional medicine, 13–17, 36
    regulation, 67
Tramadol, 303–4
Tranexamic acid, 524, 656
Tranquilisation, rapid, 345
Transdermal delivery systems, 274–5
    See also Topical application of
        medication
Transferrin, 529
Transfusion siderosis, 533
Transgenic animals, 35
Transient hypercoagulable state, 517
Translational science, 33
Transport
    carrier-mediated, 83–4, 97, 113
    inhibition of, 76
Transporters, 97
    polymorphisms, 108
Trastuzumab, 545, 552
Traveller's diarrhoea, 576
Trazodone, 338
Tremor, essential, 386
Treponema pallidum, 218
Tretinoin, 288, 661
Trials
    authorisation for in the UK, 63
    complementary and alternative
        medicine, 15
    design of, 51–3
    errors in, 49–50
    meta-analysis, 54–5, 59
    results, 55–7
    sensitivity of, 54
    size of, 53–4
    therapeutic, 47–8
    types of therapeutic, 50–4
        See also Placebo medicines; specific
            type of trial
Triamcinolone, 596–7
    potency, 597
Triamterene, 480, 481, 483
Triazoles, 236
Tribavirin, 232
Trichloroethanol, 364
Trichomoniasis, 246
Tricyclic antidepressants, 331
    for abnormal micturition, 491
    action of, 107
    for ADHD, 369
    adverse effects, 337
    with α_2-adrenoceptor agonists, 435
    interactions, 338–9
        with monoamine oxidase inhibitors,
            340
    mechanism of action, 332
    for neuropathic pain, 306
    overdose, 337
Trifluoperazine, 346
Triglycerides, 470
Tri-iodothyronine (T3), 336
Trilostane, 605

Trimetaphan, 435
Trimethoprim, 203, 204
  interaction with methotrexate, 264
Tripotassium dicitratobismuthate, 564
Triptans, 310–11
Trizivir, 230
Tropicamide, 401
Truvada, 230
Trypanosomiasis, 246
Tryptophan, 336
Tuberculosis
  of the genitourinary tract, 217
  pulmonary See Pulmonary tuberculosis
Tubocurarine, 322
Tubule, renal
  damage, 488–9
  distal convoluted, 480
  obstruction, 489
  proximal convoluted, 478
Tumour cell kinetics, 547–8
Tumour necrosis factor-α (TNFα), 251, 267
  antibodies to, 579
Type I error, 49–50, 54
Type II error, 50, 54
Typhoid fever, 215
Tyramine, 339
Tyrosine hydroxylase, 434–5
Tyrosine kinase inhibitors (TKIs), 553

U

Ubiquitin-proteasome pathway, 554
UK Prospective Diabetes Study (UKPDS),
  619–20
Ulcerative colitis, 577–8
  corticosteroids for, 604
Ultraviolet (UV) solar radiation, 280, 287
Umbrella branding, 72
Unacceptable risk, 10
Underdosing, 25–6
Underprescribing, 20
Unfractionated heparin (UFH), 520
Unithiol, 132, 133
Unstable angina, 438
Upper urinary tract infection, 216
Up-regulation, 104
Uptake transporters, 97
Urate nephropathy, 545–6
Urate retention, 485
Urea, 282
Ureidopenicillins, 193
Ureters, 392
Urethral sphincter dysfunction, 491
Urethritis, non-gonococcal, 217
Uric acid, 271–2
Urinary retention, 485
Urinary tract
  infection, 216–17
    septicaemia related to, 208
    symptoms in dying patients, 309
    tuberculosis, 217
Urine pH alteration, 133–4, 488
Urofollitrophin, 639
Urogenital tract, effects of opioids on,
  299
Urokinase plasminogen activator (uTA),
  522–3
Ursodeoxycholic acid
  for gallstones, 589
  for primary biliary cirrhosis, 588
Urticaria, 122, 284, 288–9
  ACE inhibitor induced, 422
Uterus
  contractions, 658
  prevention of haemorrhage, 659
  relaxants, 659

V

Vaginal candidiasis, 234
Vaginitis
  bacterial, 218
  hormone replacement therapy, 647
Vagus nerve stimulation, 457
Valaciclovir, 226
Valganciclovir, 232
Valproic acid, 307, 351, 378–9
Valsalva manoeuvre, 457
Vancomycin, 195
  chemoprophylaxis, 181
Variability, enzyme induction and, 98
Variable dose, 101
Variation in drug effects
  biological, 105–8
  individual, 105–8
  opioids, 300
Variceal bleeding, 585–6, 641
Varicella-zoster virus, 225–7
Vascular smooth muscle cells, 418–19
Vasculitis, allergic, 283
Vasculoendothelial growth factor (VEGF),
  553, 554
Vasoconstriction
  corticosteroids, 278
  prolongation of drug action, 102
Vasoconstrictors, 324
Vasodilators, 416–26
  in peripheral vascular disease, 425–6
Vasopressin, 480, 586, 640
  deficiency, 641
Vaughan-Williams classification of
  antiarrhythmics, 450
Vecuronium, 321
Venepuncture, 418
Venlafaxine, 335, 338
Venn diagram, 443
Venous leg ulcers, 286, 289
Venous thromboembolism, 521–2, 646
  effect of combined contraceptives, 651
Ventilation of poisoned patients, 135
Ventricular fibrillation, 459
Ventricular outflow obstruction, 430
Ventricular premature beats, 459
Ventricular tachycardia, 459
Verapamil, 420, 445, 451, 455
Verotoxic Escherichia coli (VTEC), 215
Vertigo, 570–1
Very-low-density lipoprotein (VLDL),
  469, 470–1
Vibrio cholerae, 215
Vigabatrin, 379
VIGOR trial, 256–7
Vinca alkaloids, 544
Vincent's infection, 210
Vincristine, 549
Viral infections/viruses, 225–33
  contracted during steroid therapy, 600
  drugs of choice for, 226
  skin, 290
  See also specific virus
Viral warts, 286
Viridans group streptococci, 212
Viscous fibres, 572
Vitamin A, 660–1
  for acne, 288
  deficiency, 661
  for psoriasis, 287
Vitamin B$_1$, 661
Vitamin B$_6$, 657, 661
Vitamin B$_7$ See Niacin
Vitamin B$_{12}$, 534–5
  deficiency, 536
Vitamin C, 531, 536, 662

Vitamin D, 588, 663–4
  deficiency, 663, 664
  overdose, 664
  in rheumatoid arthritis, 270
Vitamin E, 476, 669
Vitamin K, 514–15
Vitamins, 660–4
  See also specific vitamin
Volatile liquids, anaesthesia, 315–16
Volatile solvent abuse, 138, 171–2
Voltage-operated ion channels
  (VOCs), 418
Voluntary reporting of adverse reactions,
  58–9
Vomiting, 130, 568–71
  alcohol-induced, 151
  antiemesis drugs See Antiemesis drugs
  cytotoxic drug-induced, 543
  drug-induced, 570
  due to opioids, 299
  in dying patients, 308
  physiology, 568
  postoperative, 314
  treatment of various forms of, 569–71
Von Willebrand factor (vWF), 516
Von Willebrand's disease (VWD), 516
Voriconazole, 237

W

Warfarin, 78–9, 517–19
  adverse effects, 518
  dose, 518
  embryopathy, 518
  interactions, 518–19
  mode of action, 517
  pharmacokinetics, 517–18
  reversal of anticoagulation, 518
  surgery in patients receiving, 519–20
  uses, 518
  withdrawal, 518
Warnings, 20–1
Warts, viral, 286
Water
  inhalation, 496
  solubility, 81–2
Water-in-oil creams, 275
Water-soluble agents
  β-adrenoceptor blockers, 430
  ointments, 276
Weapons, biological agents as, 139
Weight (body)
  in diabetic patients, 618–19
  dose calculation by, 102
  gain, 347
  See also Obesity; Overweight
Weight in volume, 31
Weights and measures, 31
White blood cells, 251
Whitfield's ointment, 233
Whole-bowel irrigation, 131
Whooping cough, 210
Wilson's disease, 386
Wind-up, 295
Withdrawal, drug, 145, 146
  abrupt, 104
  alcohol, 154
  cannabis, 166
  corticosteroids, 600, 602, 605
  opioids, 305
  syndrome, 104
  See also specific drug
Wolff-Parkinson-White syndrome, 459
Women See Females
World Medical Association declaration of
  Helsinki, 42

693

Worms *See* Helminthic infections
Wound(s)
    delayed healing, 546
    infections, 223–4

X

Xanthine oxidase, 264, 272
Xanthines, 169–71, 486
    drinks containing, 170–1
Xipamide, 482

Y

Yellow Card system, 58–9, 62, 64

Z

Zafirlukast, 253, 504
Zalcitabine, 229
Zaleplon, 364
Zanamivir, 231
Zero-order processes, 84–5

Zidovudine, 228
Zinc oxide, 282
Zoledonic acid, 665
Zolpidem, 364
Zopiclone, 363–4
Zuclopenthixol, 346
Zymogens, 518